CURRENT
Diagnosis & Treatment
Geriatrics

a LANGE medical book

CURRENT
Diagnosis & Treatment
Geriatrics

Second Edition

Editors

Brie A. Williams, MD, MS
Associate Professor of Medicine
Associate Director, Program for the Aging Century
Division of Geriatrics
University of California, San Francisco
Medical Director, Geriatrics Clinic
San Francisco VA Medical Center
San Francisco, California

Anna Chang, MD
Associate Professor of Medicine
Associate Director, Program for the Aging Century
Division of Geriatrics
Department of Medicine
Director, Foundations of Patient Care
University of California, San Francisco
San Francisco, California

Cyrus Ahalt, MPP
Clinical Research Coordinator
Division of Geriatrics
University of California, San Francisco
San Francisco, California

Rebecca Conant, MD
UCSF Housecalls Physician
Medical Director, UCSF Home Health
Associate Clinical Professor of Medicine
Division of Geriatrics
University of California, San Francisco
San Francisco, California

Christine Ritchie, MD, MSPH
Professor of Medicine
Harris Fishbon Distinguished Professor
University of California, San Francisco
The Jewish Home of San Francisco
The San Francisco VA Medical Center
San Francisco, California

Helen Chen, MD
Chief Medical Officer
Hebrew SeniorLife Health Care Services
and Hebrew Rehabilitation Center
Boston, Massachusetts
Clinical Professor of Medicine
Division of Geriatrics
University of California, San Francisco
San Francisco, California

C. Seth Landefeld, MD
Spencer Chair of Medical Science
Leadership
Chair, Department of Internal Medicine
University of Alabama at Birmingham
Birmingham, Alabama

Michi Yukawa, MD, MPH
Medical Director of the Community
Living Center
San Francisco VA Medical Center
Associate Clinical Professor of Medicine
Division of Geriatrics
University of California, San Francisco
San Francisco, California

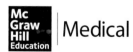

New York   Chicago   San Francisco   Athens   London   Madrid
Mexico City   Milan   New Delhi   Singapore   Sydney   Toronto

Current Diagnosis & Treatment: Geriatrics, Second Edition

2 3 4 5 6 7 8 9 0   DOC/DOC 19 18 17 16 15 14

ISBN 978-0-07-179208-0
MHID 0-07-179208-2
ISSN 1549-5736

Notice

Medicine is an ever-changing science. As new research and clinical experience broaden our knowledge, changes in treatment and drug therapy are required. The authors and the publisher of this work have checked with sources believed to be reliable in their efforts to provide information that is complete and generally in accord with the standards accepted at the time of publication. However, in view of the possibility of human error or changes in medical sciences, neither the authors nor the publisher nor any other party who has been involved in the preparation or publication of this work warrants that the information contained herein is in every respect accurate or complete, and they disclaim all responsibility for any errors or omissions or for the results obtained from use of the information contained in this work. Readers are encouraged to confirm the information contained herein with other sources. For example and in particular, readers are advised to check the product information sheet included in the package of each drug they plan to administer to be certain that the information contained in this work is accurate and that changes have not been made in the recommended dose or in the contraindications for administration. This recommendation is of particular importance in connection with new or infrequently used drugs.

This book was set in Minion by Thomson Digital.
The editors were Jim Shanahan and Harriet Lebowitz.
The production supervisor was Richard Ruzycka.
Project Management was provided by Ritu Joon, Thomson Digital.
RR Donnelley was printer and binder.

This book is printed on acid-free paper.

Contents

Section IV. Common Clinical Scenarios in Geriatrics

Section V. Broadening Clinical Practice

Authors

Gallane D. Abraham, MD
Assistant Professor
Department of Emergency Medicine
Icahn School of Medicine at Mount Sinai
New York, New York
*Providing Quality Care to Older Adults in the
Emergency Department*

Gunnar Akner, MD, PhD
Professor in Geriatric Medicine
Senior Physician Specialized in Geriatric Medicine
Internal Medicine and Clinical Nutrition
School of Health and Medical Sciences
Örebro University
Örebro, Sweden
International Perspectives in Geriatric Care (Sweden)

Cathy A. Alessi, MD
Professor of Medicine
Director, Geriatric Research, Education and
    Clinical Center (GRECC)
Chief, Division of Geriatrics
VA Greater Los Angeles Healthcare System
Department of Medicine
VA Greater Los Angeles Healthcare System
David Geffen School of Medicine at University of
    California, Los Angeles
Los Angeles, California
Sleep Disorders

Gretchen E. Alkema, PhD
Vice President, Policy and Communications
The SCAN Foundation
Long Beach, California
Public Policy Intersecting with an Aging Society

Theresa A. Allison, MD, PhD
Associate Professor of Medicine and Family
    & Community Medicine
Division of Geriatrics
University of California, San Francisco
San Francisco, California
Long-Term Care, Nursing Home, & Rehabilitation

Katherine Anderson, MD
Assistant Professor
Division of Geriatrics
Department of Internal Medicine
University of Utah
Salt Lake City, Utah
Treating Headaches in Older Adults

Sik Kim Ang, MB, BCh, BAO
Consultant in Geriatric and Palliative Medicine
Department of Internal Medicine
RIPAS Hospital
Bandar Seri Begawan, Brunei Darussalam
*Peripheral Arterial Disease & Venous Thromboembolism;
    Chronic Venous Insufficiency & Lymphedema*

Daniel Antoniello, MD
Assistant Professor of Neurology
Department of Neurology
Montefiore Hospital/Albert Einstein College of Medicine
Bronx, New York
Cerebrovascular Disease

Louise Aronson, MD, MFA
Associate Professor of Medicine
Division of Geriatrics
Department of Medicine
University of California, San Francisco
San Francisco, California
The Interprofessional Team

Kristen L. Barry, PhD
Research Professor
Department of Psychiatry
University of Michigan
Ann Arbor, Michigan
*Managing Misuse of Alcohol & Psychoactive
    Prescription Medications in Older Adults*

Lisa C. Barry, PhD, MPH
Assistant Professor
Department of Psychiatry
UCONN Center on Aging at the University
    of Connecticut Health Center
Farmington, Connecticut
*Understanding the Effects of Criminal Justice
    Involvement on Older Adults*

Rebecca J. Beyth, MD, MSc
Associate Professor of Medicine
Department of Medicine
North Florida/South Georgia GRECC,
    and the University of Florida
Gainesville, Florida
Considering Anticoagulation in Older Adults

Frederic C. Blow, PhD
Professor
Department of Psychiatry
University of Michigan
Ann Arbor, Michigan
*Managing Misuse of Alcohol & Psychoactive Prescription
    Medications in Older Adults*

Katrina Booth, MD
Assistant Professor
Division of Gerontology, Geriatrics, and Palliative Care
University of Alabama at Birmingham
Birmingham, Alabama
Chronic Kidney Disease

C. Barrett Bowling, MD, MSPH
Assistant Professor
Division of General Medicine & Geriatrics
Emory University
Birmingham, Alabama
Chronic Kidney Disease

Cynthia M. Boyd, MD, MPH
Associate Professor, Health Policy and Management
Geriatric Medicine and Gerontology
Department of Medicine
Johns Hopkins Center on Aging and Health
Baltimore, Maryland
Addressing Multimorbidity in Older Adults

Jennifer S. Brach, PhD, PT
Associate Professor
Department of Physical Therapy
University of Pittsburgh
Pittsburg, Pennsylvania
Determining the Appropriate Use of Exercise for Older Adults

Rebecca Brown, MD, MPH
Assistant Adjunct Professor of Medicine
Division of Geriatrics
University of California, San Francisco/San Francisco
    Veterans Affairs Medical Center
San Francisco, California
*Understanding the Effects of Homelessness and Housing
    Instability on Older Adults*

John G. Cagle, PhD, MSW
Assistant Professor
University of Maryland, Baltimore School of Social Work
Baltimore, Maryland
Geriatrics & Palliative Care

Kellie Hunter Campbell, MD, MA
Assistant Professor of Medicine
Geriatrics and Palliative Medicine
Department of Medicine
University of Chicago Medicine
Chicago, Illinois
Fluid & Electrolyte Abnormalities

Teresa L. Carman, MD
Director, Vascular Medicine
Assistant Professor of Medicine
Division of Cardiovascular Medicine
University Hospitals Case Medical Center
Case Western Reserve University School of Medicine
Cleveland, Ohio
*Peripheral Arterial Disease & Venous Thromboembolism;
    Chronic Venous Insufficiency & Lymphedema*

Tessa del Carmen, MD
Assistant Professor of Medicine
Division of Geriatrics and Gerontology
Weill Cornell Medicine College
New York, New York
Detecting, Assessing, & Responding to Elder Mistreatment

Anna Chang, MD
Associate Professor of Medicine
Associate Director, Program for the Aging Century
Division of Geriatrics
Department of Medicine
Director, Foundations of Patient Care
University of California, San Francisco
San Francisco, California
*Transforming the Care of Older Adults: Knowledge,
    Skills, & System Change*

Serena Chao, MD, MSc
Assistant Professor
Section of Geriatrics, Department of Medicine
Boston University School of Medicine
Boston, Massachusetts
Benign Prostatic Hyperplasia & Prostate Cancer

Gerald Charles, MD
Professor of Medicine, Emeritus
Department of Medicine
University of California, San Francisco
San Francisco, California
The Aging Traveler

Melvin Cheitlin, MD
Emeritus Professor of Medicine
Department of Medicine, Cardiology Division
San Francisco General Hospital
San Francisco, California
Coronary Disease

Helen Chen, MD
Chief Medical Officer
Hebrew SeniorLife Health Care Services
    and Hebrew Rehabilitation Center
Boston, Massachusetts
Clinical Professor of Medicine
Division of Geriatrics
University of California, San Francisco
San Francisco, California
The Social Context of Older Adults

Jane Chen, MD
Associate Professor of Medicine
Department of Internal Medicine
Cardiovascular Division
Washington University School of Medicine
St. Louis, Missouri
Heart Failure & Heart Rhythm Disorders

Bruce Allen Chernof, MD, FACP
President and CEO
The SCAN Foundation
Long Beach, California
Public Policy Intersecting with an Aging Society

Ryan Chippendale, MD
Assistant Professor
Section of Geriatrics, Department of Medicine
Boston University School of Medicine
Boston, Massachusetts
Benign Prostatic Hyperplasia & Prostate Cancer

Anna H. Chodos, MD, MPH
Research Fellow
Division of Geriatrics
Department of Medicine
University of California, San Francisco
San Francisco, California
Helping Older Adults with Low Health Literacy

Teena Chopra, MD, MPH
Assistant Professor
Division of Infectious Diseases
Wayne State University
Physician
Detroit Medical Center
Detroit, Michigan
Common Infections

Jessica L. Colburn, MD
Assistant Professor of Medicine
Division of Geriatric Medicine and Gerontology
Johns Hopkins University School of Medicine
Baltimore, Maryland
Home-Based Care

Jessamyn Conell-Price, MS
Medical Student
School of Medicine
The UCSF-UC Berkeley Joint Medical Program
San Francisco, California
Diabetes

Leo M. Cooney Jr, MD
Humana Foundation Professor of Geriatric Medicine
Department of Internal Medicine, Section of Geriatrics
Yale University School of Medicine
New Haven, Connecticut
Managing Back Pain in Older Adults

Kenneth E. Covinsky, MD, MPH
Professor of Medicine
Department of Medicine
University of California, San Francisco
San Francisco, California
Applying Evidence-Based Medicine to Older Patients

Sanket Dhruva, MD
Cardiology Fellow
Division of Cardiovascular Medicine
Department of Internal Medicine
University of California Davis Medical Center
Sacramento, California
Coronary Disease

Manuel Eskildsen, MD, MPH
Associate Professor of Medicine
Division of General Medicine and Geriatrics
Department of Medicine
Emory University School of Medicine
Atlanta, Georgia
Meeting the Unique Needs of LGBT Older Adults

Kathryn J. Eubank, MD
Associate Clinical Professor of Medicine
Medical Director
Division of Geriatrics
Department of Medicine
Acute Care for Elders (ACE) Unit
University of California, San Francisco
San Francisco VA Medical Center
San Francisco, California
Hospital Care

Emily Finlayson, MD, MS
Assistant Professor of Surgery
Department of Surgery
Institute of Health Policy Studies
University of California, San Francisco
San Francisco, California
Perioperative Care in Older Surgical Patients

Joseph H. Flaherty, MD
Department of Internal Medicine
Division of Geriatrics
Saint Louis University School of Medicine
St. Louis, Missouri
International Perspectives in Geriatric Care (China)

Lynn A. Flint, MD
Assistant Clinical Professor
Staff Physician
Division of Geriatrics
University of California, San Francisco
San Francisco VA Medical Center
San Francisco, California
Transitions and Continuity of Care

Sara J. Francois, PT, DPT, MS
Research Physical Therapist
Program in Physical Therapy
Washington University in St. Louis School of Medicine
St. Louis, Missouri
Determining the Appropriate Use of Exercise for Older Adults

Nicholas B. Galifianakis, MD, MPH
Assistant Professor of Neurology
San Francisco VA Parkinson's Disease Research, Education, & Clinical Center (PADRECC)
University of California, San Francisco
San Francisco, California
Parkinson Disease & Essential Tremor

Steven R. Gambert, MD
Professor of Medicine
Associate Chair for Clinical Program Development
Director of Medical Student Programs
Co-Director, Division of Gerontology and Geriatric Medicine
Director of Geriatric Medicine
Department of Medicine
University of Maryland School of Medicine
University of Maryland Medical Center and R. Adams Cowley Shock Trauma Center
Baltimore, Maryland
Thyroid, Parathyroid, & Adrenal Gland Disorders

Julie K. Gammack, MD
Associate Professor of Medicine
Program Director, Geriatric Medicine Fellowship Program
Division of Geriatrics
Saint Louis University School of Medicine
Saint Louis, Missouri
Urinary Incontinence

Dane J. Genther, MD
Resident
Department of Otolaryngology–Head and Neck Surgery
Johns Hopkins University School of Medicine
Baltimore, Maryland
Managing Hearing Impairment in Older Adults

Angela Gentili, MD
Professor of Internal Medicine
Director, Geriatrics Fellowship Program
Internal Medicine, Division of Geriatric Medicine
McGuire VAMC & Virginia Commonwealth University Health System
Richmond, Virginia
Sexual Health & Dysfunction

A. Ghazinouri, MD
Staff Physician
Geriatrics, Palliative and Extended Care
San Francisco VA Medical Center
San Francisco, California
Parkinson Disease & Essential Tremor

Michael Godschalk, MD
Professor of Internal Medicine
Director, Geriatric Health Care Center
Internal Medicine, Division of Geriatric Medicine
McGuire VAMC & Virginia Commonwealth University Health System
Richmond, Virginia
Sexual Health & Dysfunction

Dick Gregory, DDS, FASGD
Postdoctoral Scholar-Fellow
Multidisciplinary Fellowship in Dentistry, Medicine,
    and Mental/Behavioral Health
The Department of Preventive and Restorative Dental
    Sciences
University of California, San Francisco
San Francisco, California
Oral Diseases & Disorders

Corita R. Grudzen, MD, MSHS, FACEP
Associate Professor
Department of Emergency Medicine
Brookdale Department of Geriatrics and
    Palliative Medicine
Icahn School of Medicine at Mount Sinai
New York, New York
*Providing Quality Care to Older Adults in the
    Emergency Department*

Karen E. Hall, MD, PhD
Clinical Professor
Research Scientist
Division of Geriatric and Palliative Medicine
Department of Internal Medicine
Geriatric Research and Extended Care Center (GRECC)
Medical Director, Acute Care for Elders Unit (ACE)
University of Michigan
Ann Arbor VA Healthcare System
St. Joseph Mercy Health, Ann Arbor
Ann Arbor, Michigan
Gastrointestinal & Abdominal Complaints

Susan E. Hardy, MD, PhD
Associate Medical Director
Summit ElderCare
Worcester, Massachusetts
Consideration of Function & Functional Decline

G. Michael Harper, MD
Professor of Medicine
Division of Geriatrics
University of California, San Francisco
San Francisco VA Medical Center
San Francisco, California
Valvular Disease

Jennifer L. Hayashi, MD
Assistant Professor of Medicine
Director, Elder House Call Program
Johns Hopkins University School of Medicine
Johns Hopkins Bayview Medical Center
Baltimore, Maryland
Home-Based Care

Holly M. Holmes, MD
Associate Professor
Division of Internal Medicine
Department of General Internal Medicine
The University of Texas MD Anderson Cancer Center
Houston, Texas
Principles of Prescribing for Older Adults

Miwako Honda, MD
Director, General Medicine
Department of General Medicine
National Hospital Organization Tokyo Medical Center
Meguro, Tokyo, Japan
International Perspectives in Geriatric Care (Japan)

Tammy Ting Hshieh, MD
Associate Physician
Division of Aging
Brigham and Women's Hospital
Boston, Massachusetts
Delirium

Yong Gil Hwang, MD
Assistant Professor of Medicine
Division of Rheumatology and Clinical Immunology
University of Pittsburgh School of Medicine
Pittsburgh, Pennsylvania
Osteoarthritis

Susan Hyde, DDS, MPH, PhD, FACD
Associate Professor
The Department of Preventive and Restorative
    Dental Sciences
UCSF School of Dentistry
University of California, San Francisco
San Francisco, California
Oral Diseases & Disorders

Sharon K. Inouye, MD, MPH
Professor of Medicine
Milton & Shirley F. Levy Family Chair
Director, Aging Brain Center
Department of Medicine/Institute for Aging Research
Harvard Medical School
Beth Israel Deaconess Medical Center
Hebrew Senior Life
Boston, Massachusetts
Delirium

Jeremy M. Jacobs, MBBS
Senior Lecturer
Department of Geriatrics and Rehabilitation
Hadassah University Hospital Mt. Scopus, and Hebrew
    University Hadassah Medical School
Jerusalem, Israel
International Perspectives in Geriatric Care (Israel)

Diana V. Jao, MD
Staff Physician
Department of Primary Care: Ron Robinson Senior Care
San Mateo Medical Center
San Mateo, California
Sleep Disorders

Bree Johnston, MD, MPH
Director, Clinical Professor of Medicine
Palliative and Supportive Care
Division of Geriatrics
PeaceHealth St. Joseph Medical Center
University of California, San Francisco
Bellingham, Washington
San Francisco, California
Geriatric Assessment

Susan M. Joseph, MD
Assistant Professor of Medicine
Division of Cardiology, Heart Failure
    and Transplant Section
Department of Internal Medicine
Washington University School of Medicine
Saint Louis, Missouri
Heart Failure & Heart Rhythm Disorders

Deborah M. Kado, MD, MS
Associate Professor
Departments of Family & Preventive Medicine
    and Internal Medicine
University of California, San Diego
San Diego, California
Falls & Mobility Disorders

Ravi Kant, MD
Fellow
Division of Endocrinology
University of Maryland School of Medicine
Baltimore, Maryland
Thyroid, Parathyroid, & Adrenal Gland Disorders

Helen Kao, MD
Associate Professor of Medicine
Medical Director, Geriatrics Clinical Programs
Division of Geriatrics
Department of Medicine
University of California, San Francisco
San Francisco, California
Ambulatory Care & the Patient-Centered Medical Home

Keith S. Kaye, MD, MPH
Professor of Internal Medicine and Infectious Diseases
Division of Infectious Diseases
Detroit Medical Center
Wayne State University
Detroit, Michigan
Common Infections

Leslie Kernisan, MD, MPH
Clinical Instructor
Division of Geriatrics
Department of Medicine
University of California, San Francisco
San Francisco, California
Addressing Dyspnea in Older Adults

Margot Kushel, MD
Professor of Medicine
Division of General Internal Medicine
University of California, San Francisco/San Francisco
    General Hospital and Trauma Center
San Francisco, California
*Understanding the Effects of Homelessness and Housing
    Instability on Older Adults*

C. Kent Kwoh, MD
Professor of Medicine and Medical Imaging
Division of Rheumatology and University of Arizona
    Arthritis Center
University of Arizona College of Medicine
Tucson, Arizona
Osteoarthritis

Mark S. Lachs, MD, MPH
Co-Chief
Professor of Medicine
Director, Center for Aging Research and Clinical Care
Division of Geriatrics and Gerontology
Weill Cornell Medical College
Director, Geriatrics
New York-Presbyterian Health System
Detecting, Assessing, & Responding to Elder Mistreatment

C. Seth Landefeld, MD
Spencer Chair of Medical Science Leadership
Chair, Department of Internal Medicine
University of Alabama at Birmingham
Birmingham, Alabama
Hospital Care

Bonnie Lederman, DDS, BSDH
Postdoctoral Scholar-Fellow
Multidisciplinary Fellowship in Dentistry, Medicine,
    and Mental/Behavioral Health
The Department of Preventive and Restorative
    Dental Sciences
University of California, San Francisco
San Francisco, California
Oral Diseases & Disorders

Kewchang Lee, MD
Associate Clinical Professor
Department of Psychiatry
University of California, San Francisco
Site Director, Psychiatry Medical Student Education
Director, UCSF Psychosomatic Medicine Fellowship
    Program
San Francisco VA Medical Center
San Francisco, California
Depression & Other Mental Health Issues

Sei Lee, MD, MAS
Associate Professor of Medicine
Senior Scholar, VA National Quality Scholars Fellowship
    Program
Staff Physician
Division of Geriatrics
University of California, San Francisco
San Francisco VA Medical Center
San Francisco, California
Diabetes

Bruce Leff, MD
Professor of Medicine
Associate Director, Elder House Call Program
Johns Hopkins University School of Medicine
    and the Johns Hopkins University
    Bloomberg School of Public Health
Johns Hopkins Bayview Medical Center
Baltimore, Maryland
Home-Based Care

Frank R. Lin, MD, PhD
Assistant Professor
Core Faculty
Departments of Otolaryngology–Head and Neck Surgery,
    Geriatric Medicine, Mental Health, and Epidemiology
Johns Hopkins Center on Aging and Health
Johns Hopkins University School of Medicine
Bloomberg School of Public Health
Baltimore, Maryland
Managing Hearing Impairment in Older Adults

Milta O. Little, DO
Assistant Professor of Geriatric Medicine
Internal Medicine-Division of Gerontology and Geriatric
    Medicine
Saint Louis University School of Medicine
Saint Louis, Missouri
*Assessing Antiaging Therapies for Older Adults;
    Considering Complementary & Alternative Medicines
    for Older Adults*

Dandan Liu, MD
Volunteer Assistant Clinical Professor; Staff Physician
Division of Geriatrics
University of California, San Francisco; On Lok Lifeways
San Francisco, California
Prevention & Health Promotion

David Liu, MD, MS
Assistant Clinical Professor
Department of Psychiatry and Behavioral Sciences
University of California Davis
Sacramento, California
Depression & Other Mental Health Issues

Bernard Lo, MD
President
The Greenwall Foundation
New York, New York
Ethics & Informed Decision Making

Daniel S. Loo, MD
Associate Professor of Dermatology
Tufts University School of Medicine
Boston, Massachusetts
Common Skin Disorders

Una E. Makris, MD
Assistant Professor
Department of Internal Medicine
Division of Rheumatic Diseases
University of Texas Southwestern Medical Center
Dallas, Texas
Managing Back Pain in Older Adults

Rubina A. Malik, MD, MSc
Assistant Professor of Medicine
Department of Medicine
Division of Geriatrics
Albert Einstein College of Medicine/ Montefiore
　　Medical Center
Bronx, New York
Osteoporosis & Hip Fractures

Alayne Markland, DO, MSc
Associate Professor
Department of Medicine
Division of Gerontology, Geriatrics, and Palliative Care and
　　the Department of Veterans Affairs, Birmingham/Atlanta
　　Geriatrics Research, Education, and Clinical Center
Birmingham Veterans Affairs Medical Center and the
　　University of Alabama at Birmingham
Birmingham, Alabama
Constipation

Janet E. McElhaney, MD
HSN Volunteer Chair in Geriatric Research
Health Sciences North and Advanced Medical Research
　　Institute of Canada
Sudbury, Ontario, Canada
Common Cancers

Barbara Messinger-Rapport, MD, PhD
Associate Professor
Director
Center for Geriatric Medicine
Cleveland Clinic Lerner College of Medicine
　　of Case Western Reserve University
Cleveland Clinic
Cleveland, Ohio
Hypertension

Myron Miller, MD
Professor
Divisions of Endocrinology and of Geriatric Medicine
　　and Gerontology
Johns Hopkins University School of Medicine
Baltimore, Maryland
Thyroid, Parathyroid, & Adrenal Gland Disorders

Lona Mody, MD, MSc
Associate Professor
Geriatric Medicine
Department of Internal Medicine
University of Michigan
Ann Arbor, Michigan
Common Infections

Sandra Y. Moody, MD, BSN, AGSF
Associate Clinical Professor
Professor-in-Residence
Department of Medicine
Medicine/Graduate Medical Education
University of California, San Francisco
San Francisco Veterans Affairs Medical Center
Kameda Medical Center
San Francisco
Kamogawa City, Chiba, Japan
International Perspectives in Geriatric Care (Japan)

John E. Morley, MB, BCh
Dammert Professor of Gerontology
Director
Geriatric Research Education & Clinical Center
St. Louis University Medical School
St. Louis VA Medical Center
St. Louis, Missouri
Assessing Antiaging Therapies for Older Adults;
　　Considering Complementary & Alternative Medicines
　　for Older Adults

Joanne E. Mortimer, MD, FACP
Director, Womens Cancers Program
Vice Chair
Professor
Medical Oncology
Division of Medical Oncology & Experimental Therapeutics
City of Hope Comprehensive Cancer Center
Duarte, California
Common Cancers

Mary A. Norman, MD
Vice President and Regional Medical Director
Erickson Retirement Communities
Dallas, Texas
Depression & Other Mental Health Issues

Lawrence Oresanya, MD
Postdoctoral Fellow
Department of Surgery
Philip R. Lee Institute for Health Policy Studies
University of California, San Francisco
San Francisco, California
Perioperative Care in Older Surgical Patients

Miguel Paniagua, MD, FACP
Director, Internal Medicine Residency Program
Department of Internal Medicine
Saint Louis University School of Medicine
Saint Louis, Missouri
Addressing Chest Pain in Older Adults

Christina Paruthi, MD
Resident
Internal Medicine
Saint Louis University School of Medicine
Saint Louis, Missouri
Addressing Chest Pain in Older Adults

Carla M. Perissinotto, MD, MHS
Assistant Professor of Medicine
Division of Geriatrics
University of California, San Francisco
San Francisco, California
Atypical Presentations of Illness in Older Adults

Vyjeyanthi S. Periyakoil, MD
Clinical Associate Professor
Department of Medicine
Stanford University School of Medicine
Palo Alto, California
Managing Persistent Pain in Older Adults

Edgar Pierluissi, MD
Professor of Clinical Medicine
Medical Director
Department of Medicine, Divisions of Geriatrics and
    Hospital Medicine
Acute Care for Elders (ACE) Unit
University of California
San Francisco General Hospital
San Francisco, California
Hospital Care

Anita Rajasekhar, MD, MS
Assistant Professor of Medicine
Department of Medicine
University of Florida
Gainesville, Florida
Considering Anticoagulation in Older Adults

Scott Reeves, PhD
Professor
Department of Social & Behavioral Sciences
UCSF School of Nursing
University of California, San Francisco
San Francisco, California
The Interprofessional Team

David B. Reuben, MD
Chief Director
Archstone Professor of Medicine
Division of Geriatrics
Multicampus Program in Geriatric Medicine
    and Gerontology
University of California, Los Angeles
Los Angeles, California
Geriatric Assessment

Michael W. Rich, MD
Professor of Medicine
Division of Cardiology
Department of Internal Medicine
Washington University School of Medicine
Saint Louis, Missouri
*Heart Failure & Heart Rhythm Disorders;
    Valvular Disease*

James Riddell IV, MD
Associate Professor of Internal Medicine
Division of Infectious Disease
University of Michigan Health System
Ann Arbor, Michigan
Common Infections

Christine Ritchie, MD, MSPH
Professor of Medicine
Harris Fishbon Distinguished Professor
University of California, San Francisco
The Jewish Home of San Francisco
The San Francisco VA Medical Center
San Francisco, California
*Atypical Presentations of Illness in Older Adults; Addressing
    Multimorbidity in Older Adults*

Josette A. Rivera, MD
Associate Professor of Medicine
Division of Geriatrics
Department of Medicine
University of California, San Francisco
San Francisco, California
The Interprofessional Team; Diabetes

Brooke Salzman, MD
Assistant Professor
Division of Geriatric Medicine and Palliative Care
Jefferson University Hospitals
Philadelphia, Pennsylvania
Chronic Obstructive Pulmonary Disease

Natalie A. Sanders, DO, FACP
Assistant Professor of Medicine
Internal Medicine, Division of Geriatrics
University of Utah
Salt Lake City, Utah
Assessing Older Adults for Syncope Following a Fall

David Sengstock, MD, MS
Program Director
Geriatrics Fellowship and Clinical Assistant Professor
Internal Medicine
Oakwood Hospital and Medical Center
Wayne State University School of Medicine
Dearborn, Michigan
Addressing Polypharmacy & Improving Medication Adherence in Older Adults

Mark Simone, MD
Instructor of Medicine
Division of Geriatric Medicine
Mount Auburn Hospital, Harvard Medical School
Cambridge, Massachusetts
Meeting the Unique Needs of LGBT Older Adults

Bobby Singh, MD
Health Sciences Associate Clinical Professor
Department of Psychiatry
University of California, San Francisco
San Francisco, California
Depression & Other Mental Health Issues

Kaycee M. Sink, MD, MAS
Director of the Kulynych Memory Assessment Clinic
Associate Professor
Section on Gerontology and Geriatric Medicine
Sticht Center on Aging
Wake Forest School of Medicine
Winston-Salem, North Carolina
Cognitive Impairment & Dementia

Daniel Slater, MD, FAAFP
Associate Clinical Professor
Department of Family & Preventive Medicine
University of California, San Diego
San Diego, California
Falls & Mobility Disorders

Alexander K. Smith, MD, MS, MPH
Assistant Professor of Medicine
Division of Geriatrics
University of California, San Francisco
San Francisco, California
Goals of Care & Consideration of Prognosis; Ethics & Informed Decision Making

Danielle Snyderman, MD
Assistant Professor
Division of Geriatric Medicine and Palliative Care
Jefferson University Hospitals
Philadelphia, Pennsylvania
Chronic Obstructive Pulmonary Disease

Margarita M. Sotelo, MD
Assistant Professor of Medicine
Division of Geriatrics
University of California, San Francisco
Medical Director, Acute Care for Elders Clinic (ACE) Unit
San Francisco General Hospital
San Francisco, California
Valvular Disease

Michael A. Steinman, MD
Associate Professor of Medicine
Division of Geriatrics
University of California, San Francisco
San Francisco VA Medical Center
San Francisco, California
Principles of Prescribing for Older Adults

Caroline Stephens, PhD, MSN
Assistant Professor
UCSF School of Nursing
University of California, San Francisco
San Francisco, California
Evaluating Confusion in Older Adults

Jochanan Stessman, MD
Professor of Medicine/Geriatrics
The Jerusalem Institute of Aging Research
Hadassah University Hospital Mt. Scopus, and Hebrew
    University Hadassah Medical School
Jerusalem, Israel
International Perspectives in Geriatric Care (Israel)

Lisa Strano-Paul, MD
Associate Professor of Clinical Medicine
Co-Director, Ambulatory Care Clerkship
Core Faculty, Long Island Geriatric Education
    Center (LIGEC)
Division of General Medicine and Geriatrics
    Department of Internal Medicine
Stony Brook Medicine
Stony Brook, New York
Managing Joint Pain in Older Adults

Stephanie Studenski, MD, MPH
Professor Staff Physician
Division of Geriatrics
Department of Medicine
University of Pittsburgh School of Medicine, VA Pittsburgh
    GRECC
Pittsburgh, Pennsylvania
Determining the Appropriate Use of Exercise for Older Adults

Rebecca L. Sudore, MD
Associate Professor in Residence
Division of Geriatrics
University of California, San Francisco
San Francisco VA Medical Center
San Francisco, California
Helping Older Adults with Low Health Literacy

Mark A. Supiano, MD
Professor of Medicine
Marjorie Rosenblatt Goodman and Jack Goodman Family
    Professor of Geriatrics
Chief, Division of Geriatrics; University of Utah School of
    Medicine
Director, VA Salt Lake City Geriatric Research, Education
    and Clinical Center
Executive Director, University of Utah Center on Aging
Department of Internal Medicine, Division of Geriatrics
University of Utah
George E Whalen Veterans Affairs Health System
Salt Lake City, Utah
Assessing Older Adults for Syncope Following a Fall

Quratulain Syed, MD
Assistant Professor of Medicine
Center for Geriatric Medicine
Cleveland Clinic
Cleveland, Ohio
Hypertension

David R. Thomas, MD, FACP, AGSF, GSAF
Medical Director
Program for All-Inclusive Care of the Elderly (PACE)
Saint Louis, Missouri
Pressure Ulcers

Christine O. Urman, MD
Assistant Professor
Department of Dermatology
Tufts University School of Medicine
Boston, Massachusetts
Common Skin Disorders

Gary J. Vanasse, MD
Assistant Professor of Medicine
Hematology Division
Brigham and Women's Hospital
Harvard Medical School
Boston, Massachusetts
Anemia

Louise C. Walter, MD
Professor of Medicine
Chief, Division of Geriatrics
University of California, San Francisco
San Francisco VA Medical Center
San Francisco, California
Prevention & Health Promotion

Shuang Wang, MD
Department of Geriatrics
West China Hospital, Sichuan University
Chengdu, Sichuan, China
International Perspectives in Geriatric Care (China)

Meredith Whiteside, OD
Associate Clinical Professor
School of Optometry
University of California
Berkeley, California
Managing Vision Impairment in Older Adults

Eric W. Widera, MD
Associate Clinical Professor
Program Director, Geriatrics Fellowship Director
Division of Geriatrics
Hospice and Palliative Care
University of California, San Francisco
San Francisco VA Medical Center
San Francisco, California
*Goals of Care & Consideration of Prognosis; Geriatrics
& Palliative Care*

Brie A. Williams, MD, MS
Associate Professor of Medicine
Associate Director, Program for the Aging Century
Division of Geriatrics
University of California, San Francisco
Medical Director, Geriatrics Clinic
San Francisco VA Medical Center
San Francisco, California
*Transforming the Care of Older Adults: Knowledge, Skills,
& System Change; Understanding the Effects of Criminal
Justice Involvement on Older Adults*

Jana Wold, MD
Assistant Professor
Division of Geriatrics
Department of Internal Medicine
University of Utah
Salt Lake City, Utah
Treating Headaches in Older Adults

Mariko Koya Wong, MD
Assistant Professor
Section of Geriatrics
The University of Chicago
Chicago, Illinois
Fluid & Electrolyte Abnormalities

Kristine Yaffe, MD
Roy and Marie Scola Endowed Chair in Psychiatry
Associate Chair of Clinical and Translational Research
Professor
Department of Psychiatry, Neurology, and Epidemiology
    and Biostatistics
University of California, San Francisco
Chief, Geriatric Psychiatry
Director of the Memory Disorders Clinic
San Francisco VA Medical Center
San Francisco, California
Cognitive Impairment & Dementia

Michi Yukawa, MD, MPH
Medical Director of the Community Living Center
San Francisco VA Medical Center
Associate Clinical Professor of Medicine
Division of Geriatrics
University of California, San Francisco
San Francisco, California
Defining Adequate Nutrition for Older Adults

Jonathan Zimmerman, MD, MBA, FACP
Program Director, Internal Medicine Residency and
    Clinical Assistant Professor
Internal Medicine
Oakwood Hospital and Medical Center and Wayne State
    University School of Medicine
Dearborn, Michigan
*Addressing Polypharmacy & Improving Medication
    Adherence in Older Adults*

Preface

Current Diagnosis and Treatment: Geriatrics, 2nd Edition, is written for clinicians who provide care to older adults. In the context of our evolving health care system and a rapidly aging population, clinicians are continually adapting their practice to meet the needs of their older patients. *Current Diagnosis and Treatment: Geriatrics* provides a framework for using the functional and cognitive status, prognosis, and social context of patients to guide diagnosis and treatment of medical conditions. In this edition, authors apply the **principles of geriatric medicine**, in different **care settings** to address **common clinical scenarios** and **common geriatric conditions** encountered by clinicians in the care of older adults.

In the first section, **Principles of Geriatric Medicine**, the authors examine how the care of older adults differs from the more disease- or organ-focused care geared toward younger adults. The introductory chapter describes the theoretical framework of geriatric care. Each subsequent chapter provides an in-depth review of fundamental components of care, for example, the correlation between a person's physical function and their living environment, and the management of multiple chronic conditions and medications in older adults. This section concludes with a discussion of the intersection between geriatrics and palliative care and the application of ethics and informed decision-making principles in the care of older adults.

Care Settings, the second section, presents the different health care system settings in which clinicians provide care to older adults. Beginning with an overview of transitions in care between settings, the section focuses on the cornerstones of care for older adults in the ambulatory clinic setting, in the emergency department, in the hospital, in long-term care facilities, and in home care settings. Also included are special situations such as addressing the needs of older patients in the perioperative period or the needs of those with chronic health conditions who are planning to travel.

In the third section, **Common Geriatric Conditions**, authors discuss approaches to managing medical conditions in older adults, applying and integrating the current knowledge base to guide decision-making. Some of the clinical challenges included are evaluating delirium, dementia, and cognitive impairment, managing gastrointestinal and abdominal complaints, and responding to sleep disorders in the older adult.

The **Common Clinical Scenarios** section addresses some of the special considerations and unique needs encountered in clinical practice with older adults, such as treating vulnerable subpopulations of older adults (eg, those who are lesbian or gay, those with low literacy, or those who are homeless).

The final section is **Broadening Clinical Practice**, which guides clinicians in weighing evidence from new studies to optimize their ability to provide evidence-based care to older adults. The section ends with a broader look at how healthcare systems in the United States and internationally (Japan, Israel, China, and Sweden) are responding to population aging.

We thank our authors for their contributions to the second edition of *Current Diagnosis and Treatment: Geriatrics*, and we look forward to advancing the care of older adults.

Brie A. Williams, MD, MS, and Anna Chang, MD
Cyrus Ahalt, MPP
Helen Chen, MD
Rebecca Conant, MD
C. Seth Landefeld, MD
Christine Ritchie, MD, MSPH
Michi Yukawa, MD, MPH

Transforming the Care of Older Adults: Knowledge, Skills, & System Change

Anna Chang, MD
Brie A. Williams, MD, MS

Populations are aging worldwide. This demographic shift will dominate the social, political and public health landscape of the 21st century. The medical and social science literature is replete with commentaries and interventions designed to address the magnitude and consequences of this phenomenon. Many of these opinions and discoveries have led to improvements in medical and social care for older adults and their caregivers. Such advances have addressed diverse areas of care, including transitions in medical care, medication prescribing practices, fall reduction, pain and symptom control, and decreasing caregiver burden, to name just a few.

Yet, as clinicians who focus on enhancing the care of older adults, we note that a disconnect often remains between what happens in clinicians' offices and what patients and their caregivers need at home. Although the principles of geriatric medicine aim to bridge such gaps, many clinicians leave their training ill-equipped to incorporate the fundamental principles of geriatric medicine into their care of older adults.

GUIDING PRINCIPLES

Five principles guide the care of older adults:

A. The Impact of Decreased Physiologic Reserve

Older adults have lower physiologic reserve in each organ system when compared with younger adults, placing them at risk for more rapid decline when faced with acute or chronic illness. Some contributors to decreased physiologic reserve may include decreases in muscle mass and strength, bone density, exercise capacity, respiratory function, thirst and nutrition, or ability to mount effective immune responses. For these reasons, older adults are often more vulnerable, for example, to periods of bedrest and inactivity, external temperature fluctuations, illnesses that are otherwise self-limited

in younger adults, and complications from common infectious diseases. Although preventive measures, such as vaccinations, may be beneficial, decreased physiologic reserve may also impair older adults' ability to mount an effective immune response to vaccines. These processes can also delay or impair recovery from serious events or illnesses such as hip fractures or pneumonia. As a result of the interplay of multiple medical conditions in the context of decreased physiologic reserve, older adults are prone to developing complex geriatric syndromes, such as frequent falls.

B. The Importance of Functional and Cognitive Status

In older adults, cognitive and physical functional status are often more accurate predictors of health, morbidity, mortality, and health care utilization than are individual diseases. Cognitive status includes domains of executive function, memory, mental status, and clinical decision-making ability. Functional status includes the physical requirements necessary to maintain independence in one's own environment, often assessed using activities of daily living (ADLs) and instrumental activities of daily living (IADLs). Decreased cognitive abilities put older adults at risk (eg, for medication errors caused by an inability to follow instructions about complex medication regimens), can create significant stress on caregivers, and increase the possibility of elder abuse (eg, financial abuse). If cognitive disorders such as dementia are present, relying solely on patient history may result in inaccurate diagnosis and treatment. Functional status can also strongly affect health outcomes. Decreased functional status in the hospital setting, for example, increases the likelihood of nursing home placement and death after discharge. Thus, a comprehensive understanding of cognitive and functional status is critical to providing care to the older adult, planning for the older adult's future medical and social care needs, prognosticating, and providing caregiver support.

C. Using Goals of Care and Prognosis in Clinical Decision Making

Clinicians should begin the clinical evaluation of older adults by assessing their goals of care and decision-making capacity. This approach focuses the clinical encounter on targeting diagnostic and therapeutic plans based on the stated needs and goals of the patient and the patient's caregivers, and identifying the patient who needs the help of surrogate decision makers. Experts in geriatrics and palliative medicine have developed tools and approaches to explore patients' and their caregivers' goals of care as an important starting place in the clinical encounter. To further enhance individualized decision making, geriatrics applies a consideration of prognosis to assess benefits and harms of proposed evaluations and interventions. While the science of prognostication is still catching up to clinical need, prognostication models based on more than age alone can be used to determine more accurate estimates of life expectancy. Considering such estimates in the context of patients' goals of care represents an appropriate starting place for guiding decisions and treatment plans.

D. The Social Context of Care

Caring for the older adult is most effective when the broader context of the older adult's family, friends, and community is taken into account. The social network of an older person's life plays a significant role in identifying the individual's preferences, resources, and support infrastructure in times of need. While younger adults may thrive with relative independence in accessing resources, older adults may rely more on their social network to provide care during episodes of acute illness or exacerbations of chronic illness. In managing a complex therapeutic plan at home (eg, one that involves managing multiple medications, dressing changes), effective compliance with therapy may hinge on the availability of financial resources, the ability of the patient to remain mobile in the residence and in the community, and the helping hands of family or friends. In the setting of acute unexpected events, an older adult's survival may depend on having maintained routine contact with a social network. In addition, meeting the needs of the older adult is often contingent upon adequate care and support for caregivers who often suffer from caregiver burden, stress, and health effects of their own, particularly when caring for an older adult with advanced cognitive impairment. Thus, planning effective medical care of the older adult is inseparable from the thorough consideration of his or her social context.

E. The Impact of Multiple Conditions, Medications, and Settings of Care

Because of the complex interactions between physiologic reserve, functional and cognitive status, and social and/or caregiver support, older adults are particularly vulnerable when faced with multiple chronic conditions, many medications, and transitions across settings of care. When treating multiple conditions, the clinician caring for the older adult will be challenged by conflicting clinical care guidelines, as well as by the polypharmacy that often results when following several clinical guidelines simultaneously. As a result, the older adult often experiences new symptoms that represent adverse drug effects or interactions from multiple medications. During times of transition, for example, from hospital to home or from nursing home to emergency room, the older adult is particularly at risk for poor outcomes from incomplete medication reconciliation processes, inadequate hand-off communication, and additional potential harms, such as pressure ulcers from waiting an excessive amount of time on gurneys and falls related to hazards such as intravenous tubing. When caring for an older adult, multiple dimensions of care must be taken into account, guided by the patients' goals and prognosis.

As older adults age, interaction with the medical system becomes, on average, a bigger part of their lives. Unfortunately, suffering amongst older adults and their caregivers remains too common. Because of older adults' significant medical and social complexities, the typical medical encounter may be insufficient to identify or address the etiology of this suffering. In an increasingly global community, now is the time to learn from models of care that have been tried in different communities, populations, and countries. It is essential that clinicians are adept at applying and integrating the proven principles of geriatrics—accounting for decreases in physiologic reserve and cognitive and functional abilities, considering prognosis and goals of care, understanding the social context of the patient, and responding to the complex needs of patients with multiple conditions and medications across diverse care settings—to optimize the health of an aging society.

Creditor MC. Hazards of hospitalization of the elderly. *Ann Intern Med.* 1993;118:219-223.

Landefeld C, Winker MA, Chernof B. Clinical care in the aging century—announcing "Care of the Aging Patient: From Evidence to Action." *JAMA.* 2009;302(24):2703-2704.

Reuben DB. Medical care for the final years of life: "when you're 83, it's not going to be 20 years." *JAMA.* 2009;302(24):2686-2694.

Consideration of Function & Functional Decline

2

Susan E. Hardy, MD, PhD

GERIATRIC PRINCIPLES

Maintenance of function is a main goal of geriatric care and is an important element of successful aging. Like other geriatric syndromes, functional decline is multifactorial; medical, psychological, social, and environmental factors can all contribute to impaired functional status. The revised World Health Organization's International Classification of Functioning, Disability and Health (ICF) provides a framework for the evaluation of function and the prevention and treatment of functional decline that emphasizes the interrelation of contributing factors. The ICF classifies abnormalities in organ system structure or physiologic function as impairments. These impairments lead to difficulties with individual activities, and the limitations and barriers associated with those difficulties lead, in turn, to reduced participation in society. Environmental factors (eg, ramps and grab-bars) and personal factors (eg, education or social support) that do nothing to address underlying impairment can nonetheless influence the effect of impairments on activities and social participation. For example, a woman with severe benign essential tremor (impairment) may have difficulty eating (activity) and therefore not go out to lunch with friends (participation). Interventions to improve function in older adults can address not only the underlying impairments, but also the relevant personal and environmental factors.

Clinicians often think of function in terms of specific important activities, such as the basic and instrumental activities of daily living (ADLs, Box 2–1). Basic ADLs refer to capacities required for personal care, including walking, dressing, bathing, using the toilet, transferring from the bed to a chair, grooming, and eating. Instrumental ADLs, such as shopping, housework, transportation, using the telephone, managing finances, and managing medications, are necessary for living independently in the community. Awareness of functional deficits that often precede ADL problems can help clinicians anticipate potential ADL difficulties. In particular, problems with mobility, such as walking a quarter mile or climbing stairs, and upper-extremity limitations, such as difficulty lifting an object over one's head or grasping small objects, often precede difficulty in ADLs and put older adults at risk for further functional decline. Early detection of mobility difficulty, upper-extremity limitations, or declines in performance measures, such as gait speed, may allow for interventions to prevent progression to ADL disability.

Functional deficits in older adults are not the simple product of their medical diagnoses, but rather a key element in quality of life and the main determinant of the ability to live independently in the community. Given that many diseases and impairments of older adults cannot be cured or eliminated, prevention and treatment of functional decline must involve not only medical treatment of disease, but also environmental alterations to circumvent refractory impairments, psychological interventions to alleviate the fears and frustrations associated with physical impairment, and the marshalling of resources to provide the support necessary to keep older adults safely in the community.

EPIDEMIOLOGY OF FUNCTIONAL LIMITATIONS

More than half of older adults report difficulty with mobility, IADLs, or ADLs. In 2010, 32% of adults older than age 65 years in the United States, representing almost 13 million people, had difficulty with basic ADLs. Functional limitations increase with age and are more common in women than men (Figure 2–1). Although functional decline with age is often incorrectly assumed to be inevitable and steadily progressive, more recent research has shown that many adults maintain their independence in old age and that the majority of older adults who develop disability later regain their independence, at least temporarily. Approximately 6% to 10% of community-dwelling older adults independent in their basic ADLs will report a decline in ADL dependence 1 year later. Among those with ADL dependence at baseline, approximately 20%

Box 2-1. Activities of Daily Living (ADL) and Instrumental Activities of Daily Living (IADL) Sample Form

Activity	Independent	Needs Help	Example of Needing Help
Dressing			Needs help with any item of clothing
Bathing			Needs help getting in or out of tub
Toileting			Needs help transferring or cleaning
Transferring			Needs help moving from bed to chair
Grooming			Needs help with daily hygiene
Eating			Needs help getting food to mouth
Shopping			Needs to be accompanied
Housework			Does not perform any housekeeping
Transportation			Requires assistance for travel
Using the Telephone			Does not use the telephone
Managing Finances			Can't handle money day-to-day
Managing Medications			Requires medications are prepared

decline. The immobility, poor nutrition and hydration, and delirium that frequently accompany hospital care put older adults at high risk for deconditioning and functional decline. Restricted activity, such as staying in bed or cutting back on usual activities, is also associated with development of disability. Falls, even without injury, can be associated with subsequent fear of falling, leading to activity restriction and disability.

Functional status is consistently one of the strongest predictors of morbidity and mortality among older adults. Functional limitations are associated with low quality of life, institutionalization, and mortality, as well as increased health care utilization and costs. Compared to older adults with no ADL disability, those with ADL disability are 5 times more likely to be institutionalized and 3 times more likely to be deceased 2 years later. The yearly cost in 1991 dollars of caring for disabled older persons in the community ranged from $6340 for the least disabled to $17,017 for the most disabled. Similar results are found for mobility disability. Compared to older adults without difficulty walking one-quarter mile (and after adjusting for multiple other risk factors), those who could walk one-quarter mile only with difficulty were 1.6 times more likely to die and almost 3 times as likely to develop new basic or instrumental ADL disability. Total annual health care costs were $2773 higher in older adults with difficulty walking one-quarter mile than in those without difficulty. The morbidity and cost associated with disability combined with the anticipated growth in the number of older adults over the next several decades make prevention of functional decline a major public health and policy issue.

ASSESSMENT OF FUNCTIONAL STATUS

Functional status can be assessed by self-report or proxy report, by physical performance tests, or by direct observation of task performance. These different methods provide complementary information. A simple clinical screen for functional difficulties should include self-report of difficulty or requiring help with basic and instrumental ADLs as well as observation of the older adult's transfers and ambulation. In older adults with evidence of cognitive impairment, it is important to confirm self-reported ability to perform ADLs with a caregiver or other appropriate informant. Proxy informants tend to overestimate functional deficits, but their accuracy improves as their amount of contact with the patient increases.

Simple physical performance measures have been shown to be feasible in primary care settings, where they have provided important prognostic information. Gait speed, which can be easily measured with a stopwatch and 4-meter distance markings on the floor, is highly correlated with subsequent functional decline and mortality. Clinical cutpoints for gait speed make it easily interpretable: faster than 1.0 m/s suggests intact mobility and between 0.6 and 1.0 m/s indicates high risk; most older adults with a gait

will report independence 1 year later. However, many older adults will also have experienced transient episodes of disability during that year. In 1 cohort of community-dwelling independent adults older than 70 years, 11% reported ADL disability at 1 year. However, 24% of the cohort had experienced an episode of disability during the year and 14% had experienced at least 2 consecutive months of disability. Most disability episodes are transient. Among older adults who develop new ADL disability, 81% regain independence. Even among those who experience 3 consecutive months of disability, 60% regain independence. However, even brief episodes of disability are associated with increased risk of recurrent disability and death.

Acute illnesses, particularly those requiring hospitalization, are the most common events that precipitate functional

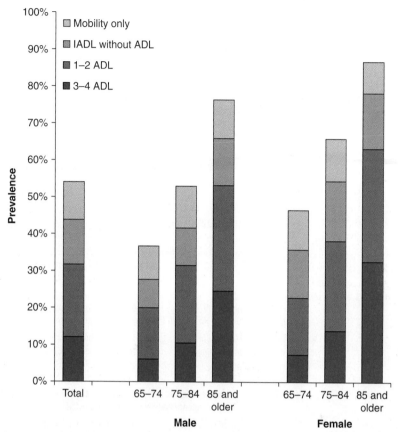

▲ **Figure 2–1.** Prevalence of functional limitations by age group and gender. ADL limitations refer to difficulty performing (or inability to perform for a health reason) 1 or more of the following tasks: bathing, dressing, eating, getting in/out of chairs, walking, using the toilet. IADL limitations refer to difficulty performing (or inability to perform for a health reason) 1 or more of the following tasks: using the telephone, light housework, heavy housework, meal preparation, shopping, managing money. Mobility limitations refers to difficulty walking (or inability to walk) one-quarter mile.

speed less than 0.6 m/s already have ADL difficulties. A change over time of 0.1 m/s is clinically significant. Gait speed and other standardized assessments of functional status can be particularly helpful in monitoring function over time. Different rehabilitation settings use specific tools to assess functional status and changes in function. Table 2–1 presents some of the most commonly used functional assessment tools.

Reported difficulties in ADLs or observed problems with gait and transfers should trigger a more detailed evaluation to identify potentially modifiable contributors to functional decline. Evaluation of these high-risk older adults should include cardiopulmonary status, strength, balance, functional range of motion, cognition, mood, pain, and nutritional status. Physical and occupational therapists can provide a more detailed assessment of function and mobility.

RISK FACTORS FOR FUNCTIONAL DECLINE

In addition to demographic factors such as age and gender, many biopsychosocial factors are associated with functional decline. Limitations in physical performance are a strong risk factor for subsequent disability in mobility as well as basic and instrumental ADLs. Compared to older adults with a usual gait speed of 1 m/s or greater, those with a gait speed less than 1 m/s are twice as likely to become unable to walk one-half mile or climb stairs, and 3 times as likely to develop new ADL dependence. Prior transient episodes of disability are also associated with recurrence. Compared to older adults with no disability in the prior 18 months, older adults who had experienced an episode of ADL dependence were twice as likely to experience a subsequent episode of disability. Older adults with greater comorbidity, more medications,

Table 2-1. Commonly used functional assessment tools.

Tool	Description	Reference
Barthel Index	Self- or proxy-reported assessment of basic ADLs and mobility. Scores range from 0–20 with lower scores representing lower function. When used over time, a change of 2 or more points is meaningful.	Collin 1988
Katz Index of ADL	Evaluation of independence in basic ADLs. Classifies patients by degree of independence. Has been used to assess need for assistance and to measure change over time.	Katz 1970
Lawton IADL Index	Assesses ability to perform 8 IADLs: telephone use, shopping, meal preparation, housekeeping, laundry, transportation, medication management, and managing finances. Useful for care planning and assessing needs for community-dwelling older adults.	Lawton 1971
Palliative Performance Scale	Assesses the physical and functional status of patients receiving palliative care on a scale from 0 (death) to 100 (normal). Used to evaluate disease progression, prognosis, care needs, and timing of hospice referral.	Anderson 1996
Karnofsky Performance Scale	Assesses the degree of functional impairment in patients with chronic or advanced illness on a scale from 0 (death) to 100 (normal). Used in oncology and palliative care.	Schag 1984
Global Assessment of Functioning Scale	Assessment of psychological, social and occupational functioning across a spectrum of mental health states, scored from 0 to 100 with higher scores representing better function. Included in the DSM IV as the axis V assessment.	American Psychiatric Association 2000
FIM (formerly the Functional Independence Measure)	Mandatory assessment for inpatient rehabilitation facilities. The FIM score is composed of 18 items assessing self-care, sphincter control, transfers, locomotion, communication, and social cognition, with the score on each item ranging from 1 (total assistance) to 7 (complete independence).	Dodds 1993
Minimum Data Set (MDS)–Activities of Daily Living (ADL)	The MDS-ADL is required for all residents of CMS-certified nursing homes. It assesses basic ADL self-performance and level of support provided.	MDS 3.0 RAI Manual
Outcome and Assessment Information Set (OASIS) Functional Assessment	The OASIS functional measure is part of the comprehensive assessment required for all CMS-certified home care agencies. It assesses basic and instrumental ADLs.	OASIS-C Manual
Timed Up-and-Go Test	A simple physical performance measure assessing transfers and ambulation.	Podsiadlo 1991
Short Physical Performance Battery	A physical performance test that includes gait speed, chair stands, and balance. Scored from 0 to 12, with higher scores representing better function.	Guralnik 1994

CMS, Centers for Medicare and Medicaid Services.

more depressive symptoms, low physical activity, obesity or low weight, malnutrition, dehydration, lower social interactions, hearing deficits, and visual deficits are all more likely to experience functional decline. Current smoking and excessive alcohol consumption also are associated with increased risk of functional decline. In addition to protein-calorie malnutrition, low intake of folate and vitamins D, E, and C is associated with functional decline in some studies. Polypharmacy generally, as well as specific medications, including anticholinergic drugs and benzodiazepines, are associated with functional decline. Among comorbid conditions, arthritis, chronic cardiopulmonary disease, neurologic diseases, and chronic pain place patients at a greater risk.

Hospitalization is a main precipitant of functional decline; more than one-third of older adults hospitalized for an acute medical condition experience decline in their ability to perform basic ADLs. Risk factors for functional decline

during hospitalization include older age, prehospitalization functional limitations, use of an assistive device, depressive symptoms, and cognitive deficits. Pressure ulcers, bedrest, and delirium during a hospitalization are also associated with functional decline. The Hospital Admission Risk Profile categorizes newly admitted older adults as high, intermediate, or low risk for functional decline based on age, cognitive function, and preadmission IADL function. This instrument can be used to target preventive interventions to those patients most likely to benefit.

PREVENTION OF FUNCTIONAL DECLINE

▶ Community-Dwelling Older Adults

Increased physical activity is the best intervention to prevent functional decline or improve functional status in older adults. Progressive resistance training, aerobic exercise, and balance training have all been shown to prevent functional decline in older adults. The National Institute on Aging has produced a handbook for older adults that provides information about the health benefits of exercise, as well as information to help start and maintain a safe program of physical activity. Older adults without acute cardiac symptoms generally do not need additional testing before beginning an exercise program. Although standard group exercise can be beneficial in higher-functioning older adults, most successful interventions in frail older adults have involved individualized exercise programs developed by a physical therapist or other trained professional.

Comprehensive geriatric assessment and home visit interventions that include multidimensional assessment of risk factors and follow-up visits also have been shown to prevent functional decline. Management of cardiovascular risk factors may prevent functional decline among relatively healthy older adults. Although no good evidence shows that nutritional interventions prevent functional decline in community-dwelling older adults, addressing nutritional deficiencies may have a beneficial effect on function.

▶ Hospitalized Older Adults

Many interventions have been developed to prevent functional decline in hospitalized older adults. Key features of successful interventions include assessment of risk factors; nursing protocols to improve self-care, continence, nutrition, mobility, sleep, skin care, and cognition; daily multidisciplinary team rounds; careful attention to hydration and nutritional status; minimization of catheterization, potentially inappropriate medications, and mobility restrictors (lines, tubes, and restraints); environmental enhancements (handrails, uncluttered hallways, large clocks and calendars, elevated toilet seats); and encouraging getting out of bed and walking. Acute Care for the Elderly units and Geriatric Evaluation and Management programs, which incorporate many of these features, have reduced hospitalization-associated functional decline in some studies. The Hospital Elder Life Program, designed to prevent delirium, has also been effective at preventing functional decline.

REHABILITATION: THE TREATMENT OF FUNCTIONAL DECLINE

Like other geriatric syndromes, functional decline is usually multifactorial, and rehabilitative care must address multiple medical, psychological, and social factors. Settings for rehabilitative care vary depending upon the circumstances and the patient's needs. Older adults with functional difficulties in the outpatient setting can receive an office-based comprehensive geriatric evaluation and can be referred to home-based or outpatient physical and occupational therapy. Upon discharge, hospitalized older adults can receive rehabilitative services in an inpatient rehabilitation facility, in a skilled nursing facility, through home health, or as outpatients. Regardless of setting, the multidisciplinary nature and the key components of rehabilitation are similar.

Treatment of functional decline requires attention to the full range of factors that affect function. A comprehensive assessment must identify potential diseases, symptoms, and impairments, as well as the personal or environmental factors that contribute to an individual's functional decline. The treatment plan is then tailored to the individual's specific deficits. For example, a patient whose participation in therapy is limited by symptomatic heart failure may benefit from more intense medical management. However, a patient with heart failure whose ambulation is limited by severe orthostatic hypotension may need less-intensive heart failure management in order to preserve standing blood pressure.

Each member of the interdisciplinary team has an important role in rehabilitation. In addition to treatment of uncontrolled acute or chronic medical conditions, medical assessment of the rehabilitation patient needs to include factors that may impede functional recovery, such as orthostatic hypotension, poor pain control, delirium, and depressive symptoms. A pharmacist can provide valuable assistance in review of the medications regimen to identify potentially inappropriate medications or medications contributing to delirium, fatigue, or mobility difficulty. Physical and occupational therapists evaluate and treat deficits in balance, strength, range of motion, and endurance. They also use modalities such as heat, cold, electrical stimulation, and ultrasound to treat pain and as adjuncts to therapeutic exercise. Therapists also determine the most appropriate assistive device for an individual and provide training in the proper use of assistive devices. Occupational therapists focus on functional tasks and can provide adaptive equipment and recommend environmental changes to promote safety and independence. Nutritionists can assist in assessment of nutritional status, and provide dietary recommendations. Speech therapists also help ensure adequate nutrition by assessing the mechanics of eating; in addition, they can provide cognitive therapy for patients with cognitive deficits. The interdisciplinary team must also include the patient and caregivers, who will be responsible for maintaining functional gains once rehabilitation is complete.

American Psychiatric Association. *Diagnostic and Statistical Manual of Mental Disorders*, 5th Edition. Washington DC: American Psychiatric Association; 2013.

Anderson F, Downing GM, Hill J. Palliative performance scale (PPS): a new tool. *J Palliat Care*. 1996;12(1):5-11.

Center for Medicare and Medicaid Services. *Long-Term Care Facility Resident Assessment Instrument User's Manual: MDS 3.0*. April 2012. U.S. Department of Health and Human Services. Available at https://www.cms.gov/Medicare/Quality-Initiatives-

Patient-Assessment-Instruments/NursingHomeQualityInits/MDS30RAIManual.html

Centers for Medicare and Medicaid Services. *Outcome and Assessment Information Set: OASIS-C Guidance Manual.* December 2011. U.S. Department of Health and Human Services. Available at http://www.cms.gov/Medicare/Quality-Initiatives-Patient-Assessment-Instruments/HomeHealthQualityInits/HHQIOASISUserManual.html

Collin C, Wade DT, Davies S, Horne V. The Barthel ADL Index: a reliability study. *Int Disabil Stud.* 1988;10(2):61-63.

Dodds TA, Martin DP, Stolov WC, Deyo RA. A validation of the functional independence measurement and its performance among rehabilitation inpatients. *Arch Phys Med Rehabil.* 1993;74:531-536.

Gill TM, Hardy SE, Williams CS. Underestimation of disability among community-living older persons. *J Am Geriatr Soc.* 2002;50:1492-1497.

Guralnik JM, Ferrucci L, Pieper CF, et al. Lower extremity function and subsequent disability: consistency across studies, predictive models, and value of gait speed alone compared with the short physical performance battery. *J Gerontol A Biol Sci Med Sci.* 2000;55(4):M221-M231.

Guralnik JM, Simonsick EM, Ferrucci L, et al. A short physical performance battery assessing lower extremity function: association with self-reported disability and prediction of mortality and nursing home admission. *J Gerontol.* 1994;49(2):M85-M94.

Hardy SE, Gill TM. Recovery from disability among community-dwelling older persons. *JAMA.* 2004;291:1596-1602.

Katz S, Downs TD, Cash HR, Grotz RC. Progress in development of the index of ADL. *Gerontologist.* 1970;10(1):20-30.

Kleinpell RM, Fletcher K, Jennings BM. Reducing functional decline in hospitalized elderly. In: *Patient Safety and Quality: An Evidence-Based Handbook for Nurses.* AHRQ Publication No. 08-0043. Rockville, MD: Agency for Healthcare Research and Quality; 2008. Available at http://www.ahrq.gov/qual/nurseshdbk

Lawton MP. The functional assessment of elderly people. *J Am Geriatr Soc.* 1971;19(6):465-481.

Liu CJ, Latham NK. Progressive resistance strength training for improving physical function in older adults. *Cochrane Database Syst Rev.* 2009;3:CD002759.

Peron EP, Gray SL, Hanlon JT. Medication use and functional status decline in older adults: a narrative review. *Am J Geriatr Pharmacother.* 2011; 9:378-391.

Podsiadlo D, Richardson S. The timed "Up and Go" test: a test of basic functional mobility for frail elderly persons. *J Am Geriatr Soc.* 1991;39:142-148.

Rodgers AB, Pocinki KM. *Exercise & Physical Activity: Your Everyday Guide from the National Institute on Aging.* NIH Publication no. 09-4258. Gaithersburg, MD: National Institute on Aging; 2009.

Sager MA, Rudberg MA, Jalaluddin M, et al. Hospital admission risk profile (HARP): identifying older patients at risk for functional decline following acute medical illness and hospitalization. *J Am Geriatr Soc.* 1996;44:251-257.

Schag CC, Heinrich RL, Ganz PA. Karnofsky performance status revisited: reliability, validity, and guidelines. *J Clin Oncol.* 1984;2:187-193.

Stuck AE, Egger M, Hammer A, Minder CE, Beck JC. Home visits to prevent nursing home admission and functional decline in elderly people: systematic review and meta-regression analysis. *JAMA.* 2002;287:1022-1028.

Stuck AE, Walthert JM, Nikolaus T, Bula CJ, Hohmann C, Beck JC. Risk factors for functional status decline in community-living elderly people: a systematic literature review. *Soc Sci Med.* 1999;48:445-469.

USEFUL WEBSITES

Go4Life: An exercise and physical activity campaign from the National Institute on Aging which offers exercises, motivational tips, and free resources to help older adults get ready, start exercising, and keep going. The Go4Life campaign includes an evidence-based exercise guide in both English and Spanish, an exercise video, and many other resources. http://go4life.nia.nih.gov/

Hartford Institute for Geriatric Nursing. Assessment Tools: Try This. A series of articles describing assessment tools for use in older adults, many with videos demonstrating their use. http://hartfordign.org/practice/try_this

The Hospital Elder Life Program (HELP): http://www.hospitalelderlifeprogram.org/public/public-main.php

Iowa Geriatric Education Center. Geriatric Assessment Tools: An online library of standardized tools, including several tools for assessment of functional status and physical performance. http://www.healthcare.uiowa.edu/igec/tools

Goals of Care & Consideration of Prognosis

3

Eric W. Widera, MD

Alexander K. Smith, MD, MS, MPH

GOALS OF CARE DISCUSSIONS

Goals of care discussions provide a broad framework for decision making, helping align patients' underlying values and hopes with the realistic and achievable options for care given the current medical circumstances. This is no easy task, however, as patients and their family members may simultaneously express multiple goals for their health care, which may include maintenance of independence, prevention of illness, prolongation of life, relief of suffering, and maximization of time with family and friends. The relative importance placed on each goal may change over time as new information is shared with the patient or family, such as new diagnosis or a worsening prognosis. These goals should serve as a guide from which patients and their physicians can develop specific plans for treatment when dealing with acute or chronic illness.

A PRACTICAL GUIDE TO GOALS OF CARE DISCUSSIONS

Goals of care can provide a guide for various decisions, including immediate decisions regarding life-sustaining treatments, decisions regarding preferences for preventive therapies such as cancer screening, and for the completion of advance directives. There is no one right way of having these discussions; however, the following outlines 7 practical steps for having a discussion (see Table 3–1 for words to use, and Table 3–2 for words to avoid).

1. *Prepare:* Clinicians should establish an appropriate setting, one that is quiet with enough space for all participants to sit down. The clinician should identify appropriate participants, including extended family, other consultants, or team members, such as social work or chaplaincy. A facilitator should be identified in advance if more than one clinician or team member will be present. Also, ensure adequate time is set aside for the meeting and that interpreters are used if needed.

2. *Create structure:* At the start of the meeting, all participants should introduce themselves. The purpose of the meeting should be made explicit. Clinicians should also ask about patient and family preferences for information sharing and decision making.

3. *Explore understanding of medical situation and underlying values:* Effective decision making depends on both health care providers and patients having an understanding of the patient's illness and prognosis. Clinicians should determine what the patient and family members understand about the patient's illness and its expected natural course. Information should be given in small, easy-to-understand statements with frequent checks to assess for comprehension. This is also a time to explore what outcomes patients and families are hoping for and which ones they would want to avoid, as well as what is most important in their lives and what they would like most to accomplish.

4. *Define overarching goals:* Based on what was learned about the patient's and family's hopes and expectations, providers can explore or suggest overarching goals. This should also be a time to address hopes and goals that may be unreasonable or unrealistic given the current health state or future prognosis.

5. *Assist in making a decision based on the patient's beliefs and values:* Discuss how goals can be achieved by discussing treatment options consistent with the patient's goals of care. This should include the potential benefits, harms, and burdens associated with various therapies, and the likelihood that the proposed intervention will accomplish the goals that have been specified.

6. *Plan for follow-up:* Goals and preferences may change over time, so these discussions should be considered part of an ongoing process.

7. *Document goals and decisions:* This may include documentation in the chart, in advance directives, or if preferences for potentially life-prolonging therapies are clear, in state authorized portable orders such as the physician orders for life-sustaining treatments (POLST).

Table 3–1. Words that may be useful when discussing goals.

1	Prepare	"At our next visit, I would like to talk about your health and the ways we can go forward with your care. Is there someone who you think should be at this meeting?"
2	Create structure	"Some patients feel it is important to know all the details of their illness, prognosis, and treatment options; others don't and want others to make decisions for them. How do you feel?"
3	Explore understanding and values	"Tell me how things are going for you?" "What do you understand about your current health?" "Given what we know about your health and prognosis, what things are most important to you? What are your hopes? Fears?" "When you think about getting very sick, what worries you the most?"
4	Define overarching goals	"It seems to me that what is most important to you is that you remain comfortable and that we get you back to your home. Is that correct?"
5	Assist in making a decision	Considering how important being pain free and remaining at home appears to be for you, I recommend that we...."
6	Plan for follow-up	"It sounds like you could use some more time to think about these issues and discuss them with your family. Can we talk more tomorrow afternoon?" "I am sure you will have lots of questions later. Here is how to reach me."
7	Document goals and decisions	"Considering your wishes, I think it would be important to document this in orders by using a physician order for life-sustaining treatment (POLST) form, which can help ensure that your preferences for end-of-life care are followed."

IMPORTANCE OF SURROGATE DECISION MAKERS

One out of 4 older adults may require surrogates to make or help make medical treatment decisions before death. Physicians have a responsibility to help these surrogates make decisions consistent with the preferences, values, and goals for care of the patient. However, because of the often uncertain and unanticipated nature of medical illness, even if specific preferences have been laid out in advance directives, these directives may not address the decision at hand and may still require interpretation by the surrogate. Complicating matters further, older adults may desire that future decisions be made on wishes and interests of family members, not just their own stated preferences for care.

Involving surrogates in advance care planning discussions with the patient prior to incapacitation may help increase the chances that the wishes of a patient are known to the surrogate and may help lessen the burden of surrogate decision making. These discussions should focus on preparing surrogates for future decisions, including appointing a health care proxy to serve as a surrogate in the event of incapacity, clarifying and articulating patients values and preferences, and addressing how much leeway surrogates have in decision-making.

Table 3–2. Words to avoid when discussing goals.

Words to Avoid	Rationale
"There is nothing more we can do"	There is always something more that can be done, including symptomatic relief and psychosocial support to patients and family members.
"We plan to withdraw care"	Care is never withdrawn. We always continue to care.
"Heroic measures"	Too vague of a term. Who would not want to be a hero?
"Your diagnosis is terminal"	Sounds cold (like the terminator), as if the patient is cut off from all options.
"Would you like us to do everything possible?"	Everything possible is too vague, and everything possible may include contradictory treatments. Hospice care and ICU level care may both be possible, for example.

PROGNOSTICATION

Prognostication can be divided into 2 parts. The first is the estimation of the patient's prognosis by the clinician. The second is communicating the prognosis to the patient and/or family. Prognostication involves more than predictions of survival or mortality. Older adults care about their prognosis for remaining independent, functional, and free from dementia. However, life and death predictions are often implied when individuals ask about "prognosis." Clinicians should ask patients to clarify the outcome they are concerned about.

Why Prognosis in Older Adults Is Important

Prognostication is a key component in clinical decision making. Prognostication provides patients and families with information to determine realistic, achievable goals of care. It targets interventions to those likely to live long enough to realize the beneficial outcomes. It establishes patients' eligibility for care programs such as hospice or advance illness management programs. It also impacts decisions outside of the health care setting, including how individuals decide to spend time and their money.

A key part of decision making based on goals of care is the need for explicit consideration of the likely outcomes of possible medical interventions. Simply asking a patient's preferences for an intervention such as cardiopulmonary resuscitation (CPR) is rather meaningless unless there is consideration of likelihood that the intervention will produce a desirable outcome consistent with the individual's goals. Furthermore, if outcomes are not explicitly discussed, patients may hold on to erroneous ideas about the likelihood of particular outcomes. However, if misconceptions are corrected and outcomes are clearly discussed, patients may change their preferences for certain interventions to those more consistent with the underlying values.

There are 3 important concepts to remember when considering prognosis in the older adult. The first is that estimating prognosis in older adults is made more complicated in that they are more likely to have more than one chronic progressive illness that impacts life expectancy. In these individuals, it would be inadequate to focus on only 1 problem when estimating prognosis, as it would not take account of the interaction of their medical problems. The second is that most prognostic algorithms in younger patients are based on specific diseases; in the oldest old, however, functional limitations are greater predictors of mortality than chronic conditions. Most disease-specific prognostic algorithms do not adequately account for functional status. The third is that clinical decision making must take into account the likelihood that a patient will live long enough to survive to benefit from a proposed intervention. For example, preventative therapies, such as cancer screening, blood pressure management, and glycemic control, have all been shown to be effective in healthier, highly functional cohorts of older adults. As the benefits of these treatments all require many years to accrue, frail older adults may not realize the benefit in the time they have left to live. They are though exposed to the harms of the intervention, which often occur much earlier than the delayed benefits.

Estimating Prognosis

The most common type of prognostication is simply using clinician judgment and experience. Prognostication based on clinician judgment is correlated with actual survival, however, it is subject to various shortcomings that limit prognostic accuracy. Clinicians are more likely to be optimistic and tend to overestimate patient survival by a factor of between 3 and 5. Clinical predictions also tend to be more accurate for short-term prognosis than long-term prognosis. The length of doctor–patient relationships also appears to increase the physician's odds of making an erroneous prognostic prediction. Accuracy of clinician predictions may be improved by integrating clinical predictions with some other form of estimating prognosis such as life tables or prognostic indices.

Life tables estimate remaining life by comparing to national averages for individuals of similar age, sex, and race. These estimates give information on median life expectancy, although the heterogeneity in health states and prognosis among older adults of the same age significantly decreases its value. Using clinical characteristics such as comorbidities and functional status to estimate whether a patient will live shorter or longer than the median life expectancy may help individualize prognostic estimates in the clinical setting.

Prognostic indices are a useful adjunctive in prognostication. Clinicians should select indices that predict mortality over a time frame equal to that time to benefit for the intervention. Clinicians should also select indices that have been tested in settings that resemble the patient's clinical situation, that have reasonable accuracy in predicting risk, and that use readily available data as its variables. A helpful repository of published geriatric prognostic indices can be found at www.ePrognosis.org. Prognostic indices are intended to supplement rather than replace the clinical judgment of clinicians based upon their assessment of the patient's condition. When using any of these methods to estimate prognosis, it is important to know that it is not a one-time event. Rather, it is a process that involves periodic reassessment.

Non–Disease-Specific Prognosis

Many older adults do not die from a single disease; instead, they die from the interacting effects of multiple chronic conditions, functional impairment, and cognitive decline. Several non–disease-specific prognostic indices have been created in recognition of this fact. These indices were the subject of a systematic review. Here we list some of the highest-quality indices, commenting on their practical application in clinical settings.

- *Schonberg 5- and 9-year index for community-dwelling older adults:* This index was developed from a nationally representative survey of older adults. Included risk measures are generally aspects of clinical care that most geriatric providers would have access to, including history of diabetes, cancer, independence in instrumental activities of daily living (IADLs), and mobility. The only exception is self-rated health. The 9-year time frame may be particularly useful for making long-term screening decisions.

- *Lee 4-year index for community-dwelling older adults:* Similar to the Schonberg index, this index was also developed from a national representative survey of older adults. Included risk measures are clinically accessible.

- *Walter 1-year index for hospitalized older adults:* This index was developed from the Acute Care for Elders dataset from 2 hospitals in Cleveland, OH. All risk measures would be easy to locate in the patient's medical record, including admission creatinine and albumin, and activities of daily living (ADL) disability at the time of discharge. For decisions about hospice eligibility at hospital discharge, the risk of death at 6-months crosses the 50% threshold in the highest-risk group.

- *Porock 6-month index for nursing home residents:* All risk measures are derived from the minimum dataset, and should be readily accessible to the clinician.

PROGNOSIS RELATED TO SPECIFIC DISEASES

▶ Advanced Dementia

The long clinical course of advanced dementia makes estimating an accurate short-term prognosis difficult. Individuals with advanced disease may survive for long periods of time with severe functional and cognitive impairments. They are also at risk of sudden, life-threatening complications of advanced dementia, such as pneumonias and urinary tract infections. These complications can serve as a marker of a very poor short-term survival. In one prospective study of advanced dementia residing in a nursing home, the 6-month mortality rates after the development of pneumonia, a febrile episode, or eating problems, were 47%, 45%, and 39%, respectively. Short-term survival rates are similar for individuals with advanced dementia who are admitted to the hospital with either pneumonia or a hip fracture, with 6-month mortality rates exceeding 50%.

Several validated indices have been developed to predict survival in advanced dementia; however, their ability to predict the risk of death within 6 months is poor. An example of a mortality index that can be used in nursing home residents with advanced dementia is the Advanced Dementia Prognostic Tool (ADEPT). The ADEPT can help identify nursing home residents with advanced dementia who are at high risk of death within 6 months, although only marginally better than current hospice eligibility guidelines.

▶ Congestive Heart Failure

The majority of deaths from advanced heart failure are preceded by a period of worsening symptoms, functional decline, and repeated hospitalizations as a result of progressive pump failure. Despite significant advances in the treatment of heart failure, the prognosis in patients who have been hospitalized

for heart failure remains poor, with a 1-year mortality rates ranging from 20% to 47% after discharge. The prognosis only worsens for those with multiple hospitalizations. In one prospective study, the median survival after the first, second, third, and fourth hospitalization was 2.4, 1.4, 1.0, and 0.6 years, respectively. Advanced age also worsens prognosis as the median survival decreases to 1 year for 85-year olds after 1 hospitalization and approximately 6 months after 2 hospitalizations.

Other indicators of a poor prognosis in heart failure include patient demographic factors, heart failure severity, comorbid diseases, physical examination findings, and laboratory values. Heart-failure-specific prognostic indices often combine many of these factors to help identify patients who are have a high short-term mortality. The Seattle Heart Failure Model is a well-validated index composed of 14 continuous and 10 categorical variables that provides accurate estimates on 1-, 2-, and 5-year mortality, as well as mean life expectancy both pre- and postintervention. An online calculator is available at http://depts.washington.edu/shfm/.

▶ Chronic Obstructive Pulmonary Disease

Severity of disease, comorbidities, and, to a lesser degree, acute exacerbations influence prognosis in chronic obstructive pulmonary disease (COPD). The most widely studied mortality index in COPD is the BODE index (Table 3–3). It includes 4 variables known to influence mortality in COPD: weight (body mass index [BMI]), airway obstruction (forced expiratory volume at 1 second [FEV_1]), dyspnea (Medical

Table 3–3. BODE index.

Variable	Points on BODE Index			
	0	1	2	3
FEV_1 (% predicted)	≥65	50-64	36-49	≤35
6-minute walk test (meters)	≥350	250-349	150-249	≤149
MMRC dyspnea scale	0-1	2	3	4
Body mass index	>21	≤21		

Higher BODE scores correlate with an increasing risk of death	
BODE Index Score	Approximate 4-Year Survival
0-2	80%
3-4	67%
4-6	57%
7-10	18%

Data from Celli BR, Cote CG, Marin JM, et al. The body-mass index, airflow obstruction, dyspnea, and exercise capacity index in chronic obstructive pulmonary disease. *N Engl J Med.* 2004;350:1005-1012.

Research Council dyspnea score), and exercise capacity (6-minute walk distance). The BODE index has been shown to be more accurate than mortality predications based solely on FEV_1. However, the BODE index is not useful in predicting short-term life expectancy (in weeks to months).

▶ Cancer

Prognosis for earlier stage cancer is primarily based on tumor type, disease burden, and aggressiveness suggested by clinical, imaging, laboratory, pathologic, and molecular characteristics. Tumor-specific factors tend to lose prognostic significance for patients with very advanced cancer. For these advanced cancers, patient-related factors, such as performance status and clinical symptoms, have increasing significance in regards to short-term mortality. Performance status has consistently been found to be a strong predictor of survival in cancer patients. Several different measures of performance status have been developed, including the Eastern Cooperative Oncology Group (ECOG) (Table 3–4) and the Karnofsky Performance Status Score (KPS) (Table 3–5). High performance status score does not necessarily predict long survival, although low or decreasing prognostic scores have been shown to be reliable in predicting a poor short-term prognosis. Symptoms that are associated with a poor short-term prognosis in advanced cancer include dyspnea, dysphagia, weight loss, xerostomia, anorexia, and cognitive impairment. The Palliative Prognostic Index (PPI) is an example of a tool that predicts short-term survival of advanced cancer patients in the palliative care setting by combining functional status with presence of symptoms of edema, delirium, dyspnea at rest, and oral intake.

Table 3–4. The Eastern Cooperative Oncology Group (ECOG) Performance Status.

Grade	Criteria
0	Fully active, able to carry on all predisease performance without restriction
1	Restricted in physically strenuous activity but ambulatory and able to carry out work of a light or sedentary nature (eg, light house work, office work)
2	Ambulatory and capable of all self-care but unable to carry out any work activities; up and about more than 50% of waking hours
3	Capable of only limited self-care, confined to bed or chair more than 50% of waking hours
4	Completely disabled; cannot carry on any self-care; totally confined to bed or chair
5	Dead

Table 3–5. The Karnofsky Performance Status.

Value	Level of Functional Capacity
100	Normal, no complaints, no evidence of disease
90	Able to carry on normal activity, minor signs or symptoms of disease
80	Normal activity with effort, some signs or symptoms of disease
70	Cares for self, unable to carry on normal activity or to do active work
60	Requires occasional assistance, but is able to care for most needs
50	Requires considerable assistance and frequent medical care
40	Disabled, requires special care and assistance
30	Severely disabled, hospitalization is indicated although death is not imminent
20	Hospitalization is necessary, very sick, active supportive treatment necessary
10	Moribund, fatal processes progressing rapidly
0	Dead

COMMUNICATING PROGNOSIS TO PATIENT OR SURROGATE

Communicating bad news, such as a poor prognosis, to a patient or a patient's family is one of the most difficult tasks in medicine. Most physicians are not trained in how to communicate about prognosis, most believe their training in prognostication is deficient, and the prognosis clinicians communicate to family tends to be overly optimistic. Yet, the majority of patients and families prefer to discuss prognosis with physicians, even in the face of uncertainty. The consequences of failing to communicate prognosis with patients and their surrogates are great. For instance, patients are more likely to receive aggressive end-of-life care and less likely to receive symptom-directed care when they have a poor understanding of their prognosis.

The SPIKES mnemonic is one way to help remember key steps in deliver bad news such as a poor prognosis (Table 3–6). Prognosis should be framed in the context of ones illness, and be framed in both the positive and negative (eg, "If there were 100 patients in your father's current condition, in 5 years roughly 80 would die and 20 would survive. I am basing this on his advanced heart failure and his worsening functional status."). Technical language should be avoided. For example, most individuals do not understand the term "median" survival when used by their physicians. Similarly, vague language such as "good" or "poor" chance of survival may also lead to misinterpretations. Combining both qualitative and numeric language may improve comprehension of prognostic statements.

Table 3-6. The SPIKES pneumonic for delivering bad news.

S	Setting up the interview
P	Patient's Perception (assessing what they understand of their illness and prognosis)
I	Obtain the patient's Invitation (ask about the readiness to discuss prognostic information)
K	Give Knowledge and information (give prognosis in the context of the patients illness)
E	Address the patient's Emotions with empathic response
S	Strategy and Summary (establish and summarize a clear care plan)

Exploring patient and surrogate understanding and personal beliefs about prognosis is imperative in these discussions, as there may exist poor concordance in what information the professional perceived was given and information the patient or surrogate understood from a conversation. In addition, few surrogates report basing their view of their loved one's prognosis solely on the physician's prognostic estimate. Rather, most attempt to balance the physicians judgment of prognosis with other factors, including (a) their own knowledge of the patient's intrinsic qualities and will to live; (b) their observations of the patient; (c) their belief in the power of their support and presence; and (d) optimism, intuition, and faith. Furthermore, even in the face of poor prognostic information, patients and surrogates remain optimistic and overestimate survival.

SUMMARY

Accurate prognostication allows for clinicians to provide patients and families with realistic options for care given current medical circumstances, and aids in determining which interventions offer little chance of benefit because of competing risks of morbidity and mortality. The use of structured approaches, such as SPIKES, is one way to ensure that this information is delivered in an effective and empathic manner. Prognostic information should be used along with consideration of other health priorities, such as maintaining independence, as part of shared decision making with older adults and their family members.

Abadir PM, Finucane TE, McNabney MK. When doctors and daughters disagree: twenty-two days and two blinks of an eye. *J Am Geriatr Soc.* 2011;59:2337-2340.

Baile WF, Buckman R, Lenzi R et al. SPIKES—a six-step protocol for delivering bad news: application to the patient with cancer. *Oncologist.* 2000;5:302-311.

Christakis NA, Iwashyna TJ. Attitude and self-reported practice regarding prognostication in a national sample of internists. *Arch Intern Med.* 1998;158:2389-2395.

Feudtner C. The breadth of hopes. *N Engl J Med.* 2009;361: 2306-2307.

Glare P, Virik K, Jones M, Hudson M, Eychmuller S, Simes J, Christakis N. A systematic review of physicians survival predictions in terminally ill cancer patients. *BMJ.* 2003;327(7408):195-198.

Knaus WA, Harrell FE Jr, Lynn J, et al. The SUPPORT Prognostic Model: Objective Estimates of Survival for Seriously Ill Hospitalized Adults. *Ann Intern Med.* 1995;122(3):191-203.

Lee SJ, Go AS, Lindquist K, Bertenthal D, Covinsky KE. Chronic conditions and mortality among the oldest old. *Am J Public Health.* 2008;98(7):1209-1214.

Mack JW, Weeks JC, Wright AA, Block SD, Prigerson HF. End-of-life discussions, goal attainment, and distress at the end of life: predictors and outcomes of receipt of care consistent with preferences. *J Clin Oncol.* 2010;28:1203-1208.

Mitchell SL, Miller SC, Teno JM, Kiely DK, Davis RB, Shaffer ML. Prediction of 6-month survival of nursing home residents with advanced dementia using ADEPT vs. hospice eligibility guidelines. *JAMA.* 2010;304(17):1929-1935.

Silveira MJ, Kim SY, Langa K. Advance directives and outcomes of surrogate decision making before death. *N Engl J Med.* 2010;362(13):1211-1218.

Setoguchi S, Stevenson LW, Schneeweiss S. Repeated hospitalizations predict mortality in the community population with heart failure. *Am Heart J.* 2007;154(2):260-266.

Yourman LC, Lee SJ, Schonberg MA, Widera EW, Smith AK. Prognostic indices for older adults: a systematic review. *JAMA.* 2012;307(2):182-192.

USEFUL WEBSITES

ePrognosis: www.eprognosis.org (a repository of geriatric prognostic indices)

Seattle Heart Failure Index: http://depts.washington.edu/shfm/

EPERC: http://www.eperc.mcw.edu/EPERC (accessible and clinically relevant monographs on palliative care topics)

The Social Context of Older Adults

4

Helen Chen, MD

"No man is an island, entire of itself."

John Donne, *Meditation XVII*

Care of the older adult must occur within the context of her community and social environment, of which health care is only a small part. Geriatric care is most effectively provided within the framework of an integrated care team that includes members well versed in care coordination who have expertise and knowledge regarding community resources available to assist older adults and their caregivers. This is particularly important for older adults facing functional decline and frailty. The Disablement Process delineated by Verbrugge and Jette demonstrates how intraindividual and extraindividual factors cumulatively interact with pathophysiologic changes to result in disability. Using this conceptual model, "society," broadly defined as the person's entire social and physical environment, and the individual, both present opportunities to intervene to delay or prevent functional loss. For example, a person with age-related eye changes may be able to mitigate functional loss through interventions involving her community, such as adequate refraction and correction or increased font size on written materials. The typical older adult may also face multiple concurrent pathophysiologic changes, such as decreased renal function, cardiovascular disease, and joint changes from arthritis. Thus, appropriate interventions for one condition may interact negatively with other interventions to increase the risk for functional loss and disablement. Because of the physiologic changes and complexities faced by many older adults, the Environmental Press model (Nahemow, Lawton, and Center) also applies. This model describes the interaction between a person's ability to function and her exposure to environmental demands. Many older adults may have a lower physiologic baseline than younger adults and may not have the "physiologic reserve" to manage new environmental or psychosocial demands (eg, the death of a caregiver) or medical insults from new or exacerbations of existing disease. When the demand exceeds the person's reserve, she may become unable to function in her community. In addition, older adults may be dependent on extraindividual supports, such as modifications to their housing and built environment, financial entitlements, and paid or casual (unpaid) caregiving. This chapter discusses the significance of the social environment and context as it affects the health and care of older adults, focusing on the following areas:

- Financial issues
- Food insecurity
- Housing and long-term care
- Caregiving

FINANCIAL ISSUES IN THE THIRD AGE

The Social Security Act was signed into law in 1935. The first monthly benefits began to be paid in 1940. Despite this benefit, more than a third of older Americans lived below the poverty line well into the 1960s. It was not until the 1970s, some 10 years after the enactment of Medicare, that this began to significantly improve, suggesting that medical issues and the lack of medical coverage were important factors in the impoverishment of older adults throughout most of the 20th century. Although adults older than age 65 years are currently the least likely age group to be officially defined as "poor," those who depend primarily on Social Security may find it difficult to pay for basic needs, such as housing, medical costs, and transportation. The UCLA Center for Health Policy Research has defined an "Elder Economic Security Index" for estimated baseline living costs that in some metropolitan areas in California is over twice the average Social Security benefit. For example, in San Francisco, the Elder Index in 2010 was $27,622 roughly $13,000 more than the average Social Security payment that year, increasing the likelihood that an older adult whose sole income in retirement was Social Security would have difficulty paying for basic needs.

FOOD INSECURITY AND OLDER ADULTS

Even though most older adults do not live in poverty, they may still have difficulty meeting their basic needs. The U.S. Department of Agriculture (USDA) defines food security as the ability for all persons in a household to have ready access to nutritionally adequate, safe foods through socially acceptable means (ie, not through means such as stealing or scavenging). By this definition, fewer than 10% of older adults experience food insecurity. However, organizations, such as the Meals on Wheels Association of America, report that up to 15% of older adults experienced some form of food insecurity in 2010. The risk of being food-insecure was higher in southern U.S. states, for Hispanic or African American older adults, those who live alone or in rural areas, and those in households with children. Population studies demonstrate that older adults who are food insecure are at higher risk for chronic disease and cognitive impairment.

The Supplemental Nutrition Assessment Program (SNAP), formerly the food stamp program, provides cash allowances for food purchases. Specific eligibility criteria vary from state to state, but are primarily linked to income and assets. "Elderly" (defined as older than age 60 years by the USDA) adults may qualify even if they exceed the income limits on the basis of disability, receive Supplemental Security Income (SSI), or they reside in federally subsidized housing for the elderly. Yet, even with expanded eligibility, older adults are less likely to participate in SNAP than the general population. According to the USDA, only 9% of SNAP participants were older than age 60 years, and only 35% of eligible older adults participate, compared with two-thirds of all eligible younger individuals. It is not clear why older adults have a lower participation in SNAP. Potential reasons include reluctance to accept the benefit or logistical challenges related to the application process (such as requiring in-person applications or applications being written at a high level of literacy).

Another option to address food insecurity in older adults may be congregate meal programs such as senior center lunches or home-delivered meals, for example, "Meals on Wheels," which is available in many communities. Although these programs are generally low cost or operate on a sliding scale, most do require some payment. Given the linkages between adequate nutrition and positive outcomes for chronic conditions such as diabetes and cardiovascular disease, health care professionals who care for older adults should routinely assess for issues related to food access or food preparation (see Chapter 6, "Geriatric Assessment").

MEDICARE

Signed into law in 1965, Medicare is a primary reason why most U.S. seniors no longer live in poverty. Traditional Medicare is a single-payer, federally managed form of health insurance coverage for older adults that covers hospital care and, with additional optional premiums, outpatient services and pharmaceuticals. Despite funding issues, Medicare remains a popular U.S. government entitlement. Although there have been several important additions (eg, hospice services in 1989; prescription drugs in 2006), Medicare continues to have notable coverage gaps. Beneficiaries are required to pay significant amounts in the form of deductibles and copayments. For lower-income beneficiaries, these out-of-pocket costs may represent a significant proportion of their monthly incomes (Figure 4–1). Some older adults, the "dual eligibles" may also qualify for Medicaid, a state and federally funded health insurance program that is limited to those with very low incomes. The coverage provisions and eligibility criteria for Medicaid vary from state to state.

In 2012, even those older adults whose incomes qualify them for Medicaid face copayments for their medications. It is important for prescribers to inquire about enrollment in low income subsidy plans for drug coverage. In addition, some patients may practice "economic nonadherence" and self-ration, dose adjust, or fail to obtain medications because of unaffordable copayments for medications or other financial considerations such as deductibles or insurance premiums. Although it is hoped that economic nonadherence has declined as a result of the availability of Medicare D in 2006, even a full subsidy, low-income beneficiary may be required to pay several dollars' copayment per prescription. Considering that recommended, guideline-driven care for type 2 diabetes alone may result in the prescription of 5 or more medications, those with multiple chronic conditions may find the cumulative associated costs for medications overly burdensome. Financial issues as a reason for nonadherence should be considered when patients do not respond in expected ways to appropriately prescribed medications.

HOUSING AND LONG-TERM CARE

Most U.S. older adults live in their own homes, with a relatively small percentage (4% according to the Administration on Aging in 2011) residing in long-term care facilities. An increasing proportion of older adults are redefining the concept of home. According to the National Center for Assisted Living, nearly 1 million adults in the United States today reside in assisted-living facilities. "Assisted living" is not a regulated term and its definition may vary regionally. Assisted-living services may be provided in a variety of venues—from a private home with several extra bedrooms to large facilities that may appear similar in concept to nursing homes. However, all assisted-living facilities differ from nursing homes or skilled nursing facilities in that they are not licensed to provide skilled nursing care (eg, wound care, rehabilitation, and medication titration) and may have regulatory restrictions limiting or prohibiting the admission of medically acute or functionally impaired residents. In some communities, older adults have creative arrangements, such as naturally occurring retirement communities (NORCs).

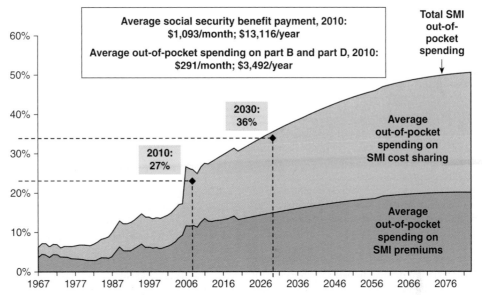

▲ **Figure 4–1.** Total Part B and Part D (SMI) Out-of-Pocket Spending as a Share of the Average Social Security Benefit, 1967–2084. (Reproduced with permission from The Henry J. Kaiser Family Foundation, "A Primer on Medicare Financing." January 2011. Available at: http://www.kff.org/health-reform/issue-brief/a-primer-on-medicare-financing/. Based on Kaiser Family Foundation analysis of data from 2010 Annual Report of the Boards of Trustees of the Federal Hospital Insurance and Federal Supplementary Medical Insurance Trust Funds, Figure III.C1.)

Residents in NORCs live in their own homes but contribute services or funds to obtain services such as housekeeping or transportation that enable them to remain safely in the community. The goal of these models is to avoid institutional long-term custodial care for as long as possible.

Although Medicare covers a limited number of days of skilled nursing facility care in association with a qualifying hospitalization, the majority of nursing home days are deemed "custodial" and are not covered by Medicare. Custodial care is defined as unskilled personal care provided for patients who need assistance with activities of daily living, such as bathing or eating. Many older adults are concerned about future needs for long-term care (LTC) and are looking for options to be able to remain independent at "home" as long as possible. If long-term, custodial care is needed, the costs are usually initially paid by individuals and families, and later by Medicaid as financial assets are "spent down" to meet eligibility levels. LTC insurance is available for purchase, although many older adults may find the premiums cost-prohibitive relative to the potential benefit. Most reputable plans pay a per-diem rate for LTC services provided either in the home or a facility. The per-diem rate may not cover the entire cost of the service, but may enable some individuals to remain at home or choose a higher-quality nursing facility. There have also been highly publicized cases of insurers refusing or being slow to pay LTC insurance benefits. Patients

or their families seeking to purchase LTC insurance should research the financial health and benefit payment record of insurance providers under consideration.

Alternatives to institutional LTC include adult day health centers or social adult day centers. The availability and funding for such programs varies across states. Depending on the program and its focus, these services may include physical therapy, meals, socialization, nursing/medical care, transportation, and supervision. Many of these programs are designed to allow families to safely manage older adults with cognitive impairments in a safe environment with social stimulation during the day when caregivers need to work outside the home. The Program for All-Inclusive Care for the Elderly (PACE) is an integrated social and health maintenance organization model that began with On-Lok in San Francisco in 1971. PACE became an established Medicare benefit in 1997, although state Medicaid programs may opt not to participate. As of 2012, there are 89 PACE organizations in 30 states, serving fewer than 12,000 beneficiaries. The program was designed primarily for dual-eligible participants (ie, those covered by both Medicare and Medicaid) who meet eligibility criteria for nursing home care. The goal of PACE is to prevent or delay nursing home placement with additional social, medical, and caregiving supports that enable participants to remain in their communities as long as possible. PACE organizations are paid a higher capitated rate compared with other Medicare Advantage/ Health Maintenance Organization (HMO) plans in exchange for assuming full risk for all needed care, including nursing home stays, whether intermittent or permanent. The cost, complexity, and regulatory requirements of the PACE model have limited its dissemination and impact.

CAREGIVING

Many older adults and their families are surprised to learn that Medicare, with very limited exceptions such as hospice, does not cover unskilled personal care such as bathing or feeding. Older adults may elect to pay out of pocket to receive care at home, but as care needs increase, these costs may increase to become comparable with nursing home care costs. Although Medicaid may provide limited coverage for personal care aides in some states, and the Veterans Health Affairs provides some coverage for eligible veterans, the burden of caregiving typically falls on family or other unpaid caregivers. AARP estimates that 43.5 million adults in the United States are caregivers for older adults. Most caregivers are female, with an average age of 50 years. Most of these unpaid caregivers who are providing care for a family member also work outside the home. Four in 10 caregivers felt that they did not have a choice regarding caregiving. Although most reported good health status, 32% reported a high caregiving burden. Increased age and poorer health status in caregivers were associated with a perception of high burden. Of those who also work outside the home, 64% needed scheduling accommodations to meet their caregiving responsibilities, often in the form of arriving late, leaving early, or taking time off.

Medical providers may not view the caregiver of their patients as the providers' principal health concern. However, most caregivers provide care because of the recipients' age, chronic medical conditions, or Alzheimer disease or other dementing illness, with the goal of allowing independent living at home. Many frail and dependent older adults are "one caregiver away" from a crisis that leads to placement in institutional care. In addition, caregiver stress and burden are risk factors for elder abuse and most health care professionals are mandated reporters (see Chapter 72, "Detecting, Assessing, & Responding to Elder Mistreatment"). Validated instruments, such as the Caregiver Strain Index (CSI) can be used to more objectively assess for stress and burden. The CSI is easy to administer and a score of >7 should prompt intervention to assist the caregiver. Caregivers report that they need information regarding respite care, self-care, and stress management, and options for extended or LTC, but do not always know where to find it. Some may turn to the Internet, but 30% will ask a doctor, nurse, or other health care professional. Organizations such as the Family Caregiver Alliance (www.caregiver.org) and the Alzheimer's Association (www.alz.org) have free educational resources and information regarding support groups and respite care

that may be useful to caregivers. While many primary care providers may view caregiver education and support as the responsibility of social services clinicians, only 2% of caregivers reported that they would seek advice from a social worker. This may either reflect a lack of knowledge of or access to social services in the health care systems known to these caregivers.

RECOMMENDATIONS FOR CLINICIANS

The social context and environment of their patients may be unknown to many health care professionals. Problems, such as financial stress or lack of adequate caregiving, may have a negative impact on health and functional status as much as or more than chronic diseases. Older adults who do not live in a health care facility spend <1% of their lives in contact with health care professionals and >99% of their time self-managing their chronic conditions and functional issues in their social environment. Physicians and other primary care providers are important sources of health-related information for older adults and may be asked to advise patients and families about their options or to refer to other services available in their own communities. Clinicians who wish to expand their effectiveness in caring for older adults should:

- Become familiar with the health impact of limitations in Medicare coverage
- Remain vigilant for evidence of elder abuse or mistreatment in caregiving situations
- Learn about available community resources, for example via the Area Agency on Aging (AAA), direct service providers or clearinghouses for information and referrals. The national roster of AAAs can be accessed at http://www.n4a.org/about-n4a/?fa=aaa-title-VI

Nahemow L, Lawton MP, Center PG. Toward an ecological theory of adaptation and aging. 1.3. *Environ Des Res.* 1973;4(1):24.

National Association for Caregiving and AARP. *Caregiving in the US, 2009.* Accessed November 2012. http://www.caregiving.org/data/Caregiving_in_the_US_2009_full_report.pdf

Sullivan MT. *Caregiver Strain Index.* New York, NY: The Hartford Institute for Geriatric Nursing. February 2002. Accessed November 2012. http://medschool.ucsf.edu/sfghres/fhc/pdf/Caregiver_strain.pdf

Supplemental Nutrition Assistance Program. Accessed November 2012. http://www.fns.usda.gov/snap/

UCLA Center for Health Policy Research. *Elder Economic Security™ Index for California Counties, 2011.* January 2012. Accessed November 2012. http://www.healthpolicy.ucla.edu/elder_index12jan.aspx

Verbrugge LM, Jette AM. The disablement process. *Soc Sci Med.* 1994; 38(1):1-14.

The Interprofessional Team

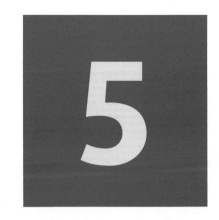

Josette A. Rivera, MD
Scott Reeves, PhD
Louise Aronson, MD, MFA

Nationally and worldwide, interprofessional teamwork is increasingly recognized as a means to address the challenges of the current health care system. Patients with complex problems and diverse needs require the expertise of different health professionals, ideally working together. A series of landmark Institute of Medicine reports recommended interprofessional teams and training of all health care workers in teamwork as a key mechanism to increase health care safety and quality. Additional factors driving the need for effective teamwork include patient expectations; a primary care workforce shortage; new models of team care that demonstrate efficiency, lower cost, and improved outcomes; and national policy changes that incentivize the creation of these models.

Older adults, with their high prevalence of chronic conditions, functional decline, geriatric syndromes, and terminal illness, are high utilizers of the health care system and its teams. The American Geriatrics Society has developed and supported 2 position statements that underscore the benefits of interprofessional team care for older adults, and endorses interprofessional team training for all professions. This chapter defines the multiple types of interprofessional work in health care, describes practice-based interprofessional geriatrics innovations, reviews the evidence for interprofessional collaboration in the care of older adults, provides resources for building interprofessional skills and teams, and discusses barriers and future steps to improve interprofessional teamwork in geriatrics.

Mion L, Odegard PS, Resnick B, et al. Interdisciplinary care for older adults with complex needs: American Geriatrics Society position statement. *J Am Geriatr Soc.* 2009;57(10):1917.

Partnership for Health in Aging Workgroup on Interdisciplinary Team Training. *Position Statement on Interdisciplinary Team Training in Geriatrics: an Essential Component of Quality Healthcare for Older Adults.* 2011. http://www.americangeriatrics.org/pha

Young HM, Siegel EO, McCormick WC, Fulmer T, Harootyan LK, Dorr DA. Interdisciplinary collaboration in geriatrics: Advancing health for older adults. *Nurs Outlook.* 2011;59:243-250.

KEY DEFINITIONS AND CONCEPTS

The teamwork literature consists of a wide array of terms, used interchangeably, to describe this phenomenon—from interdisciplinary, to multidisciplinary, to interprofessional. In addition to this terminologic uncertainty, different authors describing "interdisciplinary teamwork" often employ very differing conceptualizations related to team composition, function, and outcome. It is possible, however, to distinguish the different types of teamwork as follows: "interprofessional teamwork" involves different *health care professionals* who share a team identity, have clarity of roles, work in an interdependent and integrated fashion, and have a shared responsibility to solve problems and deliver services. This contrasts to "interdisciplinary teamwork," which is seen as a collaborative activity undertaken by individuals from different *disciplines*, such as psychology, anthropology, economics, medicine, political science, and computer science. This, in turn, contrasts with "multidisciplinary teamwork," which is regarded as an approach like interprofessional teamwork, but different in that the team members come from different academic disciplines (psychology, sociology, mathematics) rather than from different professions, such as medicine, nursing and social work. In health care, "multidisciplinary team" also refers to teams in which health professionals may share information regarding a patient, but do not formulate a treatment plan together. Although the term *interdisciplinary teamwork* has been prevalent for the past 30 years in U.S. medicine, including in geriatrics, scholars increasingly contend that applying this term in a health care setting is conceptually incorrect, as the notion of interprofessional teamwork more accurately describes the essence of health care teams (including geriatric teams) who work together to deliver services.

It is also important to distinguish interprofessional education, an increasingly common learning activity in health care, from interprofessional practice. "Interprofessional education" is an activity that occurs when members (or students/trainees) of 2 or more health care professions engage in learning with, from, and about each other to improve interprofessional teamwork and the delivery of care. Interprofessional practice centers on the provision of patient care and has a range of differing configurations. Interprofessional teamwork is a "tighter" more integrated type of work where members share a team identity and work in an integrated and interdependent manner to provide care to patients. Examples of interprofessional practice teams include geriatrics teams, intensive care teams and emergency room teams. This is a different arrangement to interprofessional collaboration which is a "looser" type of work, where membership is more fluid and shared membership less important. Examples of this type of work can be found in primary care and general medical settings.

Reeves S, Goldman J, Gilbert J, et al. A scoping review to improve conceptual clarity of interprofessional interventions. *J Interprof Care*. 2011;25:167-174.

Reeves S, Lewin S, Espin S, et al. *Interprofessional Teamwork for Health and Social Care*. London, UK: Blackwell-Wiley; 2010.

INTERPROFESSIONAL TEAM INNOVATIONS IN GERIATRICS

In the United States, the care of older adults has been a major impetus for innovations in interprofessional education and practice. Accordingly, there are many geriatric models of care where teamwork is fundamental (Table 5–1). These teams vary widely with respect to their goals, procedures, setting, number and type of professionals, and membership stability.

The earliest training initiatives, Interdisciplinary Team Training in Geriatrics, were developed by the Department of Veterans Affairs in the 1970s. This was followed by the creation of 2 programs administered by the Health Resources and Services Administration of the U.S. Department of Health and Human Services. Geriatric Education Centers, founded in the 1980s, support collaboration between health professions schools and health care clinics, facilities, and systems to provide training in geriatrics and team care that must be offered to 4 or more professions. Geriatric Academic Career Awards, which originated in the 1990s, support the career development of junior faculty to become academic geriatricians and to provide clinical geriatrics training to interprofessional teams.

The John A. Hartford Foundation has significantly supported the development of team training and models of care for older adults. In 1997, the Hartford Geriatric Interdisciplinary Team Training (GITT) initiative funded 8 institutions to develop innovative models of formal team training, resulting in a repository of teaching materials and a collectively produced curriculum and implementation guide described in more detail under "Resources" below. In 2000, Hartford funded the Geriatric Interdisciplinary Teams in Practice initiative that supported the design and testing of models of interprofessional team care of older adults with chronic illnesses. Four models that transformed team care in everyday practice and demonstrated positive impact on patient outcomes and cost have been widely adopted nationally: (a) the Care Transitions Intervention, developed at the University of Colorado Health Sciences Center; (b) the Care Management Plus model, developed by Intermountain Health Care and Oregon Health & Science University; (c) the Senior Health and Wellness Clinic model developed by PeaceHealth Oregon Region; and (d) the Virtual Integrated Practice model, developed at Rush University Medical Center.

Geriatrics also has led innovations in team-based models of care. The Program of All-Inclusive Care for the Elderly (PACE) is a capitated, joint Medicare-Medicaid program that provides comprehensive, team-based care for frail, nursing-home-eligible older adults living in the community. In the inpatient setting, the Acute Care for Elders (ACE) unit provides hospitalized older adults with an interprofessional team that aims to preserve function and to avoid unnecessary procedures and medications. As of 2011, there are 82 PACE programs in 29 states, and an estimated 100 ACE units nationally. Both the PACE and ACE models have been shown to improve patient outcomes while reducing costs.

Table 5–1. Examples of team care in geriatrics.

Disease specific	Heart Failure
	Diabetes
	Poststroke
Program specific	Hospice
	Geriatric assessment/consultative clinics
	Program of All Inclusive Care for the Elderly
	Geriatric Resources for Assessment and Care of Elders
Site specific	Home care
	Rehabilitation settings
	Adult day health centers
	Nursing homes
	Acute care for the elderly units

Ahmed NN, Pearce SE. Acute care for the elderly: a literature review. *Popul Health Manag*. 2010;13(4):219-225.

Coleman EA, Parry C, Chalmers S, Min SJ. The care transitions intervention: results of a randomized controlled trial. *Arch Intern Med*. 2006;166(17):1822-1828.

Hirth V, Baskins J, Dever-Bumba M. Program of all-inclusive care (PACE): past, present, and future. *J Am Med Dir Assoc*. 2009;10(3):155-160.

Stock R, Mahoney ER, Reese D, Cesario L. Developing a senior healthcare practice using the chronic care model: effect on physical function and health-related quality of life. *J Am Geriatr Soc*. 2008;56(7):1342-1348.

Wieland D, Kinosian B, Stallard E, Boland R. Does Medicaid pay more to a program of all-inclusive care for the elderly (PACE) than for fee-for-service long term care? *J Gerontol A Biol Sci Med Sci*. 2013;68(1):47-55.

EVIDENCE OF INTERPROFESSIONAL TEAMS IN THE CARE OF OLDER ADULTS

Substantial research shows benefits of geriatric interprofessional team care for specific diseases and geriatric syndromes, across models of care, and in settings from acute care and skilled nursing facilities to rehabilitation and outpatient clinics. Team-based models of care, such as PACE and the Geriatric Resources for Assessment and Care of Elders (GRACE), have demonstrated improved quality of care and reduced utilization of services. Team care has reduced morbidity and mortality after a stroke, and shown improvement in behavioral and psychological symptoms without a significant increase in medications among patients with Alzheimer disease. Team-based approaches reduce the prevalence of delirium and the incidence of falls and related injuries. Interprofessional teams have also been shown to improve medication adherence and reduce adverse drug reactions.

Overall, results are mixed regarding the ability of interprofessional teams to reduce health services utilization and costs. Boult et al offer possible explanations for the difficulty in demonstrating these reductions in older adults with multimorbidity, which include unavoidable exacerbations requiring acute care in multimorbid patients, and not knowing which patients benefit most from team care or what aspects of team care reduce utilization and costs. Moreover, quality team care may also increase utilization by high-risk patients. Finally, clinical trial duration may be too short to capture the cost savings "downstream" that could offset the initial and operating costs of a team-based model.

In addition to the evidence on teamwork, there exists a deep and intuitive logic for why effective teamwork is needed: patients frequently have conditions that have multiple causes and require multiple treatments from a range of health care professionals with different skills and expertise. As it is unusual for one profession to deliver a complete episode of care in isolation, good quality care depends upon professions working together in interprofessional teams. In general, when a team works "well" it does so because every member has a role. Every member not only knows and executes his or her own role with great skill and creativity, each member also knows the responsibilities and activities of every other role on the team, and understands the personal nuances that each individual brings to his or her role. As has been shown in military training and the aviation industry, when understanding of each person's role is achieved, interprofessional teamwork becomes an essential ingredient for reducing duplication of effort, improving coordination, enhancing safety, and delivering high-quality outcomes.

Boult C, Reider L, Leff B, et al. The effect of guided care teams on the use of health services. *Arch Intern Med.* 2011;171(5): 460-466.

Callahan CM, Boustani MA, Unverzagt FW, et al. Effectiveness of collaborative care for older adults with Alzheimer disease in primary care: a randomized controlled trial. *JAMA.* 2006;295(18):2148-2157.

Counsell SR, Callahan CM, Clark DO, et al. Geriatric care management for low-income seniors: A randomized controlled trial. *JAMA.* 2007;298(22):2623-2633.

Mion L, Odegard PS, Resnick B, et al. Interdisciplinary care for older adults with complex needs: American Geriatrics Society position statement. *J Am Geriatr Soc.* 2009;57(10):1917.

Partnership for Health in Aging Workgroup on Interdisciplinary Team Training. *Position Statement on Interdisciplinary Team Training in Geriatrics: an Essential Component of Quality Healthcare for Older Adults.* 2011. http://www.americangeriatrics.org/pha

RESOURCES AND TOOLS FOR TEAMWORK

Literature describing program development strategies and the educational goals of team training is emerging. In 2010, the Interprofessional Education Collaborative, which consists of 6 national health professions education associations, convened an expert panel to develop interprofessional competencies as a means of providing a framework to move interprofessional education forward. The competency domains identified were:

- Values/ethics for interprofessional practice,
- Roles/responsibilities for collaborative practice,
- Interprofessional communication, and
- Interprofessional teamwork and team-based care.

The competencies identify behaviors that reflect underlying attitudes, knowledge, and values essential for effective, patient-centered teamwork. The domains provide a guide for individual learning and practice improvement, curriculum and program development, and for setting accreditation and licensing standards for schools and professionals alike.

Salas et al detail principles for team training, which include using teamwork competencies to focus the training content, which should align with desired outcomes and local resources; concentrating on teamwork and excluding individual level tasks; providing hands-on practice in as authentic an environment as possible; providing detailed, timely feedback by team skills experts; evaluating knowledge, behaviors, and patient level outcomes; and sustaining teamwork through continued coaching, incentives, and performance evaluations.

The best way to improve an individual's teamwork skills is in interprofessional teams. Health care teams may improve their teamwork by focusing explicitly on underlying processes and by creating a culture of openness. An initial step is identification of team goals and objectives and what is needed to achieve them, clarification of roles and responsibilities, and specification of team procedures and ground rules. Salas et al provide practical guidelines and tips for improving teamwork based on their framework of communication, coordination, and cooperation. An overarching theme is the creation of an environment that encourages open discussion and input from all members. This includes ensuring time for members to jointly reflect upon their team performance and to give "process feedback" that is descriptive and specific. Team members should also reflect upon their own and other members' behaviors, while both eliciting and providing constructive feedback along with ideas for improvement.

Two well-developed team training programs offer practical guidelines and tools for teamwork available on the internet. The Hartford Foundation's GITT Program includes paper-based and video-based complex cases, exercises for discussion, and didactic material on team training in the care of older adults. Although designed for trainees, the content is relevant to practicing professionals. A companion implementation manual offers a synthesis of guidance, lessons learned, and tools from the 8 GITT sites on the implementation of a team training program. The GITT Interdisciplinary Team Training Pocket Card contains 8 principles of successful teamwork, a 7-step meeting process, a team dynamics checklist, tips on how to be an effective team member, and guidelines for dealing with conflict.

The TeamSTEPPS program, developed by the Department of Defense, is not geriatrics-specific but presents an evidence-based teamwork training system for health professionals. Like the GITT Program, it offers a curriculum and implementation guide accessible from the Internet, but the materials are more extensive and contain slide sets with speaker notes, handouts, videos, and assessment and evaluation tools. The training system provides detailed guidance on its 3-step process that includes a local needs assessment, planning and training, and sustainment. Practical communication tools and strategies are a prominent part of the curriculum. Unlike the GITT Program, TeamSTEPPS is an ongoing effort that offers webinars and in-person training sessions nationwide for master trainers.

Interprofessional Education Collaborative Expert Panel. *Core Competencies for Interprofessional Collaborative Practice: Report of an Expert Panel.* Washington, DC: Interprofessional Education Collaborative; 2011.

Salas E, Almeida SA, Salisbury M, et al. What are the critical success factors for team training in health care? *Jt Comm J Qual Patient Saf.* 2009;35(8):398-405.

Salas E, Wilson KA, Murphy CE, King H, Salisbury M. Communicating, coordinating, and cooperating when lives depend on it: tips for teamwork. *Jt Comm J Qual Patient Saf.* 2008;34(6):333-341.

The John A. Hartford Foundation, Inc. Geriatric Interdisciplinary Team Training Program. http://www.gittprogram.org

U.S. Department of Health and Human Services. *TeamSTEPPS: National Implementation.* http://teamstepps.ahrq.gov

BARRIERS TO THE ADVANCEMENT OF TEAMWORK

Despite the potential benefits of teamwork for patients and professionals alike, the underlying processes are fraught with challenges. Teamwork has received relatively little attention in both preprofessional and continuing education; consequently, despite the data on its benefits to patients, most practicing professionals have received minimal or no relevant training, and efforts to increase interprofessional teamwork often meet attitudinal, educational, and fiscal barriers. One challenge relates to the medical profession's history of unchallenged authority and attitudes toward teams. Physician attitudes towards teamwork in general are particularly problematic. Reasons may include medical training that rewards autonomy and individual efforts, lack of perceived value added by teamwork, and perceived losses of power, time, and money. With a paucity of role models and strong cultural influences, it is not surprising that medical trainees have rated lower agreement with respect to the benefits of teamwork compared with nursing and social work students.

Additional barriers to improving interprofessional teamwork are systems based. First, despite the ubiquity of health care teams, widespread formal education on teamwork has lagged in the United States. Consequently, because teams in practice do not use principles of teamwork, little informal team training occurs. Second, few incentives exist for implementing or improving interprofessional education and practice. There is currently no reimbursement for the implementation of innovative educational programs or for team services provided by practicing health professionals. In addition, few medical schools or medical practices recognize teamwork skills for the purposes of individual advancement or promotion. Third, logistical barriers are a prevalent problem that often centers on finding time for teaching or participating in teamwork. At the trainee level, hindrances include different academic calendars and training sites, while tension in the practice setting centers on balancing release time for team training with staffing needs of hospitals and clinics.

Leipzig, RM, Hyer K, Ek K, et al. Attitudes toward working on interdisciplinary health care teams: a comparison by discipline. *J Am Geriatr Soc.* 2002;50(6):1141-1148.

Young HM, Siegel EO, McCormick WC, Fulmer T, Harootyan LK, Dorr DA. Interdisciplinary collaboration in geriatrics: advancing health for older adults. *Nurs Outlook.* 2011;59(4):243-250.

FUTURE STEPS

Interprofessional education and practice must develop in tandem to transform the standard of health care in the United States. Widespread implementation of both will require culture change and investment of time and resources.

Differences in professional identities and cultures must be reconciled, with the recognition that everyone, from early learners to seasoned professionals, harbors biases, stereotypes, and inadequate knowledge of other professions. Program leaders need to address the practical problems of differences in roles, priorities, service needs, schedules, and licensure and accreditation requirements among health professionals and students. Research is needed to determine the most effective timing, teaching strategies, methods, settings, and assessment tools, as well as the impact of interprofessional education and practice on health service utilization and cost. Professional and faculty development courses should train a cadre of health professionals who effectively teach and role model teamwork skills. Accreditation, licensure, and regulation are powerful ways through which to advance interprofessional education and practice. The Patient Protection and Affordable Care Act of 2010, particularly its support of team-based care via the Patient Centered Medical Home model, has potential to disseminate interprofessional practice in response to public health needs.

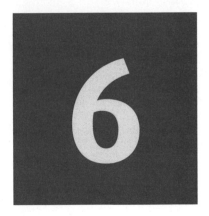

6

Geriatric Assessment

Bree Johnston, MD, MPH
David B. Reuben, MD

Geriatric assessment is a broad term that describes a clinical approach to older patients that goes beyond a traditional medical history and physical exam to include functional, social, and psychological domains that affect well-being and quality of life. Although geriatric assessment has been adapted to different settings, structures, and models of care, 4 key concepts inform the approach: the clinical site of care, prognosis, patient goals, and functional status.

TEAMS AND CLINICAL SITES OF CARE

Although geriatric assessment may be comprehensive and involve multiple team members (eg, social workers, nurses, physicians, rehabilitation therapists, pharmacists), it may also involve just a single clinician and be much more simple in approach. In general, teams that use an *interdisciplinary* or *interprofessional* approach (teams in which multiple disciplines meet together to develop a single comprehensive treatment plan for a patient) are most common in settings that serve primarily frail, complex patients, such as inpatient units, rehabilitation units, PACE (Program for All-Inclusive Care of the Elderly), and long-term care facilities. In outpatient settings, teams are less likely to be formalized, and if present, are more likely to be virtual, asynchronous and *multidisciplinary* (teams in which each discipline develops its own assessment and treatment plan) than interdisciplinary. (For more information, see Chapter 5, "The Interprofessional Team.")

Regardless of team composition, the setting and functional level of the patient population being served will determine what assessment tools are most appropriate. For example, long-term care settings are likely to focus on basic activities of daily living (eg, bathing), whereas outpatient teams are more likely to focus on higher levels of functioning, such as mobility and ability to prepare meals. In inpatient settings, the focus is on preventing deconditioning, providing medical support (eg, nutrition), and discharge planning, including assessing rehabilitation potential and best setting for discharge. Regardless of the team structure, site, and tools being used, many of the principles of assessment are the same.

PROGNOSIS

An older adult's prognosis can be critically important in determining which interventions are likely to beneficial or burdensome for that individual. In community-dwelling older persons, prognosis can be estimated initially by using life tables that consider the patient's age, gender, and general health. For example, <25% of men age 95 years will live 5 years, whereas nearly 75% of women age 70 years will live 10 years. However, persons with chronic diseases may have substantially shorter survival. When an older patient's clinical situation is dominated by a single disease process (eg, lung cancer metastatic to brain), prognosis can sometimes be estimated well with a disease-specific instrument. Even when disease-specific prognostic information is available, frequently the range of survival is wide. Moreover, prognosis generally worsens with age (especially age >90 years) and with the presence of serious age-related conditions, such as dementia, malnutrition, or impaired ability to walk. See Chapter 3, "Goals of Care & Consideration of Prognosis," for a more comprehensive approach to prognostication in the older patient.

When an older person's life expectancy is >10 years (ie, 50% of similar persons live longer than 10 years), the appropriateness of tests and treatments is generally the same as for younger persons. When life expectancy is <10 years (and especially when it is much less), choices of tests and treatments should be made on the basis of their ability to improve that particular patient's prognosis and quality of life in the context of that patient's life expectancy. The relative benefits and harms of tests and treatments often change as prognosis worsens.

Palliative care services should be considered for any patient with a life-limiting illness, particularly when the prognosis is less than 18 months. If the prognosis is 6 months or less, hospice should be considered, if consistent with the patient's goals of care.

PATIENT GOALS

Although patients vary in their values and preferences, many frail older adults prioritize maintaining their independence or relieving pain or other symptoms over prolonging survival. Values and preferences are determined by speaking directly with a patient or, when the patient cannot express preferences reliably, with the patient's surrogate. Even patients who cannot make complicated decisions can often express preferences, and should be involved in decision making as much as they are able. See Chapter 12, "Ethics & Informed Decision Making," for a more thorough discussion of patient decision making.

Values and preferences are often easiest to assess in the context of a specific medical decision. For example, the clinician might ask a patient considering chemotherapy for a new cancer, "Tell me about the risk and discomfort you are willing to go through to achieve an increased chance of living an extra 6 months." In assessing values and preferences, it is important to keep in mind that patients should be definitive sources of information about their preferences for outcomes and experiences; however, they usually do not have adequate information to express informed preferences for specific tests or treatments, and require guidance from a clinician who can explain how the tests or treatments might help achieve the patient's goals. Therefore, it is often more useful to ask about values ("What is the least acceptable quality of life for you?" or "If you were critically ill, would you like us to focus more on comfort and quality of life or prolonging life?") rather than interventions lacking a context ("Would you want pressors?"). Patients' preferences often change over time. For example, some patients find living with a disability more acceptable than they would have before experiencing it. Some patients change their values based on important events, such as their desire to live to see the graduation or birth of a grandchild.

Every older person should be encouraged to complete advance directives for both health care and finances, to designate a surrogate decision maker, and to discuss their values and preferences with their surrogate and with their health care clinicians. Many states honor a specific advance directive form that is signed by both patient and physician and serves as both an advance directive and order sheet that is portable across different sites of care. Examples of this form would include the POLST or MOLST (physician or medical orders for life-sustaining treatment).

FUNCTIONAL ASSESSMENT

Functional status can be viewed as a summary measure of the overall impact of health conditions in the context of a patient's physical and psychosocial environmental. Functional status information is important for planning, monitoring responses to therapy, and for determining prognosis. Functional impairment is common in older adults and has many potential causes, including age-related physiological and cognitive changes, disuse, disease, social factors, and the interplay between any of these. According to the 2007 Centers for Medicare and Medicaid Services, Medicare Current Beneficiary Survey, 29% of patients age 65 years and older had limitations in basic activities of daily living (ADLs: bathing, dressing, eating, transferring, continence, toileting) and 14% had limitations in instrumental ADLs (IADLs; transportation, shopping, cooking, using the telephone, managing money, taking medications, cleaning, laundry). IADLs are activities that are essential for independent living. Subtle or new declines in IADL function may be an early sign of dementia, or other disease, such as Parkinson disease. Loss of ADL or IADL function often signals a worsening disease process or the combined impact of multiple comorbidities. Level of ADL and IADL impairment can usually be determined by self- or proxy report, but should be corroborated when possible. When accurate functional information is essential for planning, direct observation by a physical or occupational therapist can be invaluable.

For highly functional independent elders, standard functional screening measures will not capture subtle functional impairments. One technique that may be useful for these elders is to identify and regularly query about a target activity, such as playing bridge, golf, or fishing that the patient enjoys and regularly participates in (advanced ADLs). Although many of these activities reflect patient preferences that may change over time, if the patient begins to drop the activity, it may indicate an early impairment, such as dementia, incontinence, or worsening vision or hearing loss.

Functional status should be assessed initially and periodically thereafter, particularly after hospitalization, severe illness, or after the loss of a spouse or caregiver. Unexpected changes in functional status should prompt a comprehensive evaluation. If no reversible cause of functional decline is found after a reasonable medical search, the clinician should focus on supportive services, and when necessary, placement in a different living setting. For more information about functional ability and assessment in older persons, refer to Chapter 2, "Consideration of Function & Functional Decline."

PREVENTIVE SERVICES

Preventive services include counseling on healthy behaviors, screening to detect asymptomatic disease, and vaccinations.

Specific preventive interventions for an individual patient should be based upon evidence-based guidelines, the patient's estimated life expectancy, and the patient's values and goals. The U.S. Preventive Services Task force has an interactive website with specific recommendations based on the patient's age, gender, tobacco use, and sexual activity (http://epss.ahrq.gov/PDA/about.jsp) (see Chapter 8, "Prevention & Health Promotion").

FALLS AND GAIT IMPAIRMENT

Falls are the leading cause of nonfatal injuries and unintentional injury and death in older persons. Every older person should be asked about falls at least annually. Because gait and balance impairments commonly coexist with falls, a gait assessment is important to perform in older people and is likely to be more sensitive for abnormalities (which are commonly multifactorial because of muscular weakness and arthritis, as well as specific neurologic impairments) than other components of the neurologic examination.

Components of the gait exam include observing if the patient can get up from a chair without using the hands (to test quadriceps strength), observing symmetry, stride length, step height, and width of stance. Balance can be tested by observing stability with eyes closed, with a sternal nudge, with a 360-degree turn, and ability to maintain side by side, tandem, and semitandem stance for 10 seconds. The "Timed Up and Go" tests a person's ability to get up from a chair, walk 3 meters, return, and sit down. Although a variety of cut-off scores are used for this test, inability to complete the task in fewer than 15 seconds is generally considered abnormal, and longer times are associated with a greater risk of functional impairments. Patients with an abnormal gait evaluation should be evaluated further for potentially reversible causes (see Chapter 25, "Falls & Mobility Disorders," and Chapter 59, "Assessing Older Adults for Syncope Following a Fall").

VISION IMPAIRMENT

The prevalence of cataract, age-related macular degeneration, glaucoma, and need for corrective lenses increases with advancing age. Given the commonness of eye problems in older people and the inability of most primary care physician's offices to perform high-quality, comprehensive eye examinations, periodic examinations by an optometrist or ophthalmologist are reasonable for older people, particularly those who have diabetes or are at high risk of glaucoma, such as African Americans.

Vision screening in the primary care setting, with a Snellen eye chart for far vision and a Jaeger card for near vision, is relatively easy to perform and may provide valuable on-the-spot information for the practitioner. A vision screening question such as, "Do you have difficulty driving, watching television, reading or doing any of your daily activities because of your eyesight, even while wearing glasses?," is helpful but may not be sensitive enough to replace a formal vision assessment (see Chapter 61, "Managing Vision Impairment in Older Adults").

HEARING IMPAIRMENT

More than 33% of individuals older than age 65 years and 50% of those older than age 85 years have some hearing loss. Hearing loss is correlated with social and emotional isolation, clinical depression, and limited activity.

The optimal screening method for hearing loss in older adults is undetermined. The whispered voice test is easy to perform but many patients will still require formal follow up testing; sensitivities and specificities range from 70% to 100%. Handheld audiometry with the Welch-Allyn AudioScope can increase the accuracy of screening if performed in a quiet environment. The U.S. Screening and Prevention Task Force recommends using screening questions about hearing loss in older adults. Structured questionnaires such as the Hearing Handicap Inventory for Elderly–Screening are most useful for assessing the degree to which hearing loss interferes with functioning (see Chapter 62, "Managing Hearing Impairment in Older Adults").

DEMENTIA

Dementia is common in older adults but is commonly missed by primary care practitioners. Early diagnosis of Alzheimer disease and related disorders is important in order to identify potentially treatable contributors (which are uncommon), and to involve the patient in advance care planning for health care and finances. As medications and treatments for Alzheimer disease become more effective, early screening will become more important. The 3-item recall, in combination with the clock draw (the mini-cog) is a brief screen that is sensitive for detecting dementia. Patients who fail the mini-cog should be followed up with a more in-depth mental status examination.

Patients who screen positive for possible dementia should also have further assessment of whether or not they have advance directives, have decision making capacity, and whether they have processes in place for protecting their finances (see Chapter 22, "Cognitive Impairment & Dementia" and Chapter 52, "Evaluating Confusion in Older Adults").

INCONTINENCE

Incontinence in older adults is common but often goes unmentioned. Women are twice as likely as older men to be incontinent; overall, approximately 6% to 14% of older women experience incontinence daily. Ask a simple question, such as, "Is inability to control your urine a problem for you?" or "Do you have to wear pads, diapers, or briefs because of urine leakage?" Positive answers should be followed up with a more complete assessment, as determined by the patient's goals (see Chapter 39, "Urinary Incontinence").

DEPRESSION

Depression is commonly missed in primary care. Although major depression is no more common in older adults than in younger populations, depressive symptoms are more common in older adults. In ill and hospitalized older patients, the prevalence of depression is ≥25%. The PHQ-2 is a sensitive screening tool for depression. Positive responses should be followed up with more extensive screen (eg, the PHQ-9), and, if positive, a comprehensive interview conducted (see Chapter 45, "Depression & Other Mental Health Issues").

NUTRITION

Nutritional problems among the elderly include obesity, undernutrition, and specific vitamin and nutrient deficiencies. Unintentional loss of >5% of body weight should trigger further evaluation, which should include consideration of oral health issues (eg, loss of dentures), medical issues (eg, dementia or malignancy), and social issues (eg, loss of transportation). Loss of 5% of body weight in 1 month or 10% of body weight over 6 months is associated with increased morbidity and mortality.

Increasingly, obesity is becoming a problem in the elderly and is associated with multiple morbid conditions, including diabetes, osteoarthritis, poor mobility, and obstructive sleep apnea. Obesity in the older adult is defined as a body mass index (BMI) of ≥30 kg/m^2 (see Chapter 68, "Defining Adequate Nutrition for Older Adults").

MEDICATION USE

The average older person takes 4–5 medications, and many older adults receive medications from more than 1 physician, which increases the risk for medication discrepancies and adverse drug events. Medications should be reviewed with the primary care practitioner, pharmacist, or nurse at every visit. Patients should be encouraged to bring all of their medications, including nonprescription drugs, (the "brown bag assessment") to every visit. Regular pharmacy reviews and commercially available medication management programs can help primary care providers monitor for potential inaccuracies and potential drug–drug interactions

(see Chapter 9, "Principles of Prescribing for Older Adults," and Chapter 53, "Addressing Polypharmacy & Improving Medication Adherence in Older Adults").

CAREGIVER SUPPORT

Providing primary care for a frail older adult requires that attention be paid to family caregivers as well as to the patient, because the health and well-being of the patient and caregivers are intricately linked. High levels of functional dependence place an enormous burden on a caregiver. Burnout, depression, and poor self-care are possible consequences of high caregiver loads. Asking the caregiver about stress, burnout, anger, and guilt is often instructive. For the stressed caregiver, a social worker can often identify helpful programs such as caregiver support groups, respite programs, adult day care, and hired home health aides.

FINANCIAL, ENVIRONMENTAL AND SOCIAL RESOURCES

Old age can be a time of reduced resources, both social and financial. The old are at particular risk of social isolation and poverty. Screening questions about social contacts and financial resources are often helpful in guiding providers in designing realistic treatment and social service planning. Every older person should be encouraged to engage in advance financial planning when they are being encouraged to complete medical advance directives.

Assessment of the patient's environment should include asking about their ability to access needed community resources (eg, banking, grocery, pharmacy) either themselves or via proxy, the safety of their home, and the appropriateness of their environment for their level of functional impairment. When the safety of the home is in question, a home safety assessment by a home health care agency is appropriate.

ABUSE

Because of the possibility of abuse, vulnerable elders should have the opportunity to be interviewed alone. Direct questioning about abuse and neglect is may be useful, particularly under circumstances of high caregiver load. Clues to the possibility of elder abuse include observation of behavioral changes in the presence of the caregiver, delays between injuries and seeking treatment, inconsistencies between an observed injury and an associated explanation, lack of appropriate clothing or hygiene, and unfilled prescriptions. A simple question—"Do you ever feel unsafe or threatened?"—is a reasonable initial screen (see Chapter 72, "Detecting, Assessing, & Responding to Elder Mistreatment").

GERIATRIC ASSESSMENT IN PRIMARY CARE

A number of strategies can help make the process of geriatric assessment more efficient for busy primary care practices, such as using previsit screening questionnaires, using nonphysician personnel to help perform standard geriatric assessments, and having standardized protocols for following up on positive results. Screening instruments such as the ones by Lachs et al and Moore et al (Figure 6–1) are useful in the primary care setting. A number of well-designed previsit questionnaires for elders are available (eg, www.geronet.ucla.edu/images/stories/docs/professionals/Geri_Pre-visit_Questionnaire.pdf). The Medicare Annual Wellness Visit also can facilitate the performance of many

Patient name _____

Source: Patient _____ Other_____   Date _____

History items	Abnormal	Action	Result and comments
"Have you had any falls in the last year?"	Yes	Gait assessment _____ Further exam, home eval & PT Osteoporosis and injury risk assess	
"Do you have trouble with stairs, lighting, bathroom, or other home hazards?"	Yes to any	Home eval &/or PT _____	
"Do you have a problem with urine leaks or accidents?"	Yes	Rule out reversible (DIAPPERS[a])_____ History (stress, urge), exam, PVR	
"Over the past two weeks, have often been bothered by feeling sad, depressed, or hopeless?" "During the two weeks, have you often been bothered by little interest or pleasure in doing things?"	Yes to either	Quantify with PHQ-2 _____ GDS or PHQ-9	
Do you ever feel unsafe where live? Does anyone threaten you or hurt you?	Yes	Explore further, social work, APS _____	
Is pain a problem for you?	Yes __No ___	Evaluate _____	

Do you have any problems with any of the following areas? Who assists? / do you use any devices? (For "Yes" answers, consider causes, social services and/or home eval/PT/OT)

Doing strenuous activities like fast walking/bicycling?	Yes __No ___	_____
Cooking	Yes __No ___	_____
Shopping	Yes __No ___	_____
Doing heavy housework like washing windows	Yes __No ___	_____
Doing laundry	Yes __No ___	_____
Getting to a place beyond walking distance by driving or taking a bus	Yes __No ___	_____
Managing finances	Yes __No ___	_____
Getting out of bed/transfer	Yes __No ___	_____
Dressing	Yes __No ___	_____
Toileting	Yes __No ___	_____
Eating	Yes __No ___	_____
Walking	Yes __No ___	_____
Bathing (sponge bath, tub, or shower)	Yes __No ___	_____

▲ **Figure 6–1.** Simple geriatric screen. (Reproduced with permission from C. Bree Johnston, MD, based on data from Moore AA, Siu AL. Screening for common problems in ambulatory elderly: clinical confirmation of a screening instrument. *Am J Med.* 1996;100(4):483-443, and Lachs MS, Feinstein AR, Cooney LM Jr, et al. A simple procedure for general screening for functional disability in elderly patients. *Ann Intern Med.* 1990;112(9):699-706.)

	Abnormal	Action	Comments
Review medications that patient brought in	Confusion about meds >5 meds Doesn't bring in	Consider simplification Medi-set or other aid Consider home visit	_____
Also ask about herbs, vitamins, supplements, and nonprescription meds			

Physical exam items
(The next few items will be performed by nursing staff in some settings)

	Abnormal	Action	Comments
Weight/BMI And ask "have you lost weight?" If so, how much?	BMI <21 Loss of 5% since last visit Or 10% over one year	Alert provider Or nutrition eval Consider medical, dental, social	_____
Do you have problems with your teeth or gums?	Yes	Dental referral	_____
Perform oral exam	Abnormal exam		
Jaeger Card or Snellen eye chart Test each eye (with glasses)	Can't read 20/40	Alert provider or refer	_____
Whisper short sentences @ 6–12 inches (Out of visual view) or audioscopy	Unable to hear Retest/refer/ Hearing handicap inventory	Cerumen check	_____
Name three objects/re-ask in 5 minutes Clock draw test (mini-cog)	Misses any or unable	MOCA, MMSE full cognitive evaluation	_____
"Rise from your chair (do not use arms to get up), walk 10 feet, turn, walk back to the chair and sit down (Timed up and go)	Observed problem or longer than 15 sec	Further gait & neuro exam; Home eval & PT	_____
"Touch the back of your head with your hands. Pick up the pencil"	Unable to do either	Further exam Consider OT	_____

(Remember to ask recall of the 3 items from mini-cog!)

Other areas of concern: Caregiver stress, alcohol, social isolation, advance directives and health care wishes.

[a]**D**elirium, **I**nfection, **A**trophic urethritis, **P**harmaceuticals, **P**sychological, **E**xcessive excretion, **R**estricted mobility, **S**tool impaction

▲ **Figure 6–1.** (*continued*)

of these assessment in a separate visit that does not need to address the patient's ongoing medical problems. New reimbursement models for team based medical homes may make performing geriatric assessment in primary care more practical for many practices than it is currently.

Boult C, Wieland GD. Comprehensive primary care for older patients with multiple chronic conditions: "nobody rushes you through." *JAMA*. 2010;304(17):1936-1943.

Reuben DB. Medical care for the final years of life "when you're 83, it's not going to be 20 years." *JAMA*. 2009;302:2686-2694.

USEFUL WEBSITES

Agency for Healthcare Research and Quality. *Search for Recommendations*. http://epss.ahrq.gov/ePSS/search.jsp

Centers for Disease Control and Prevention. http://www.cdc.gov/mmwr/PDF/wk/mm753-Immunization.pdf

Social Security Administration. *Life Expectancy Tables*. http://www.ssa.gov/OACT/STATS/table4c6.html

UCLA GeroNet. Healthcare office forms. http://geronet.ucla.edu/centers/acove/office_forms.htm

U.S. Preventive Services Task Force. Home page. http://www.uspreventiveservicestaskforce.org/

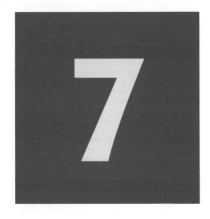

Atypical Presentations of Illness in Older Adults

Carla M. Perissinotto, MD, MHS

Christine Ritchie, MD, MSPH

Traditional education of health care clinicians hinges on typical presentations of common illnesses. Yet, what is often left out from medical training is the frequent occurrence of atypical presentations of illness in older adults. These presentations are termed "*atypical*" because they lack the usual signs and symptoms characterizing a particular condition or diagnosis. In older adults, "atypical" presentations are actually quite common. For example, a change in behavior or functional ability is often the *only* sign of a new, potentially serious illness. Failure to recognize atypical presentations may lead to worse outcomes, missed diagnoses, and missed opportunities for treatment of common conditions in older patients.

In medical education, teaching about atypical presentations of medical illness in the older patient offers a unique opportunity to introduce key geriatric principles to trainees at all levels of training. Furthermore, atypical medical presentations in the older adult are now an Accreditation for Graduate Medical Education (ACGME) Geriatrics competency, underscoring the importance of integrating this concept into medical education for all learners.

DEFINING ATYPICAL PRESENTATIONS

The definition of an atypical presentation of illness is: *when an older adult presents with a disease state that is missing some of the traditional core features of the illness usually seen in younger patients*. Atypical presentations usually include one of 3 features: (a) vague presentation of illness, (b) altered presentation of illness, or (c) nonpresentation of illness (ie, underreporting).

IDENTIFYING PATIENTS AT RISK

The prevalence of atypical presentation of illness in older adults increases with age. With the aging of the world's population,

atypical presentations of illness will represent an increasingly large proportion of illness presentations. The most common risk factors include:

- Increasing age (especially age 85 years or older)
- Multiple medical conditions ("multimorbidity")
- Multiple medications (or "polypharmacy")
- Cognitive or functional impairment

Understanding which patients may be more at risk of atypical disease presentation will guide clinicians to more astutely pick up subtle signs of illness. Rather than approaching a patient visit in the "traditional" way, the clinician may also need to expand beyond the "typical" evaluation of illness and incorporate questions or exam findings that correlate with an atypical presentation (Table 7–1). For example, recognition of an atypical presentation of illness requires a clinician to pay more attention to small changes in cognition compared to baseline. In the case of a patient with dementia, this can be difficult to determine as some older adults with dementia still experience minor daily variations in cognition. Gathering this baseline level of information requires patience, time, and having reliable caregivers and family member informants. Many times, in order to arrive at an accurate history of present illness, the clinician will have to undertake a systematic investigative approach.

▶ Common Signs and Symptoms of Atypical Disease Presentation in Older Adults

The first step to assessing an older person for atypical presentation of disease is to recognize the common warning signs and symptoms frequently present across a wide spectrum of illness in the older adult. In an older adult, a common warning sign of a looming infection or critical illness may be a

Table 7–1. Potential questions to uncover common symptoms characteristic of an "*atypical*" presentation of illness.

Symptom	Question
• Acute confusion (ie, delirium) • Anorexia (change in appetite) • Absence of fever • Absence of pain, or pain in alternate location • Generalized weakness • Fatigue • New urinary incontinence • New functional decline (ie, change in mobility)	• Is the patient usually quiet and nonconversant or is this a change? • Have you noticed the patient to be more "fidgety" or more hyperactive? • Has there been any weight loss? • Are there any new medications that were started when the symptoms started? • In the past, when patient has had an infection, what signs has the patient had? • I see the patient is in a wheelchair, can the patient walk, or is this a new change?

new decline in function (eg, new incontinence, new difficulty walking). Similarly, a change in behavior (eg, agitation or increased confusion) in either cognitively impaired or intact people may be the only indication to caregivers or family members (who are most in-tune to the individual's normal cognition and behavior) that "something is going on." Other indicators of a new, potentially serious illness include, but are not limited to, falls, anorexia, and generalized weakness.

▶ Unique Presentations of Commons Conditions in the Older Adult

Examples of atypical presentations exist across a variety of disease states, including infectious pulmonary, cardiovascular, and psychiatric diseases. In the care of an older adult, atypical presentations of illness are sometimes more common than a classic textbook presentation, such that a clinician must maintain a wide differential diagnosis, and be prepared to find coexisting new diagnoses before too rapidly arriving at a single explanation for the clinical findings. The principle of Occam's razor, in which there exists 1 unifying diagnosis to explain all of the patient's symptoms and findings, is a rarity in geriatric care. For example, a patient with community-acquired pneumonia and kidney failure may present without a fever and without the ability to describe key symptoms, such as nausea, cough, or pleuritic chest pain. Ultimately, atypical presentations occur because of a combination of factors that coexist in older adults: physiologic changes of aging, loss of physiologic reserve, and a combination of acute and multiple comorbidities and geriatric syndromes which all converge to confound the diagnosis and make the presentation of a new illness uncharacteristic. Some common examples are included in Table 7–2 and are described in greater detail below.

A. Dehydration

Dehydration is the most common fluid and electrolyte problem in older adults. This is a result of normal age-related physiologic changes, which include decreases in total-body water, alterations in thirst perception, and reduced renal function leading to decreased urine-concentrating ability. As in other atypical presentations, the signs and symptoms of dehydration in the older adult may be vague or even absent. For example, older adults will be more prone to dehydration with infection, tube feedings, and medication-related side effects. Additional risk factors for dehydration include delirium and mobility disorders, both of which can lead to decreased fluid intake. Vital signs may not be revealing; cardiac conduction disturbances or medications such as β blockers may mask the usual tachycardic response seen in volume depletion. Skin turgor in the older adult is unreliable, and intake–output charts are likely to be inaccurate in the setting of incontinence. Lastly, oral dryness may be misleading given the prevalence of mouth breathing or mouth dryness as a result of medications with anticholinergic properties. Consequently, the clinician must be aware of the vulnerability posed by older adult physiology and the possibility that dehydration may manifest itself only as constipation or slight orthostatic hypotension. In most cases, the clinician will need to rely on a combination of symptoms, signs, and possible laboratory abnormalities in order to accurately detect severe dehydration.

B. The Acute Abdomen

Acute abdominal pain in older adults is often underrecognized, with some studies indicating that as much as 40% of older patients are misdiagnosed. Some of the most common causes of abdominal pain in the older adult include cholecystitis, bowel obstruction, diverticular disease, complications of cancer, and medication side effects. In these medical conditions, rather than having localizing signs to specific abdominal quadrants, pain may be more diffuse, mild, or absent altogether. Patients may also lack a fever, and instead present with hypothermia. They may lack an elevated white count, and have reduced rebound secondary to decreased abdominal wall musculature. In cholecystitis, only 25% of adults actually present with biliary colic; consequently, a wide differential should be considered when older adults present with vague abdominal complaints. In addition to different and vague symptom presentation, the diagnosis of acute abdomen in the older adult may be difficult as a result of challenges in obtaining an accurate history, and confounding signs and symptoms because of presentation later in the illness course; multiple comorbid conditions; and illness-related complications. Because of delayed presentations and difficult diagnoses, the mortality rate and complications of the acute abdomen are much greater in older adults. As in other illnesses, some of the reasons for delayed presentation may be caused by social factors, such as lack of caregiver, lack

Table 7–2. Examples of atypical presentation of illness in older adults.

Altered Presentation of Illness in Elderly Persons	
Illness	**Atypical Presentation**
Infectious diseases	Absence of fever Sepsis without usual leukocytosis and fever Falls, decreased appetite or fluid intake Confusion Change in functional status
"Silent" acute abdomen	Absence of symptoms (silent presentation) Mild discomfort and constipation Some tachypnea and possibly vague respiratory symptoms
"Silent" malignancy	Back pain secondary to metastases from slow-growing breast masses Silent masses of the bowel
"Silent" myocardial infarction	Absence of chest pain Vague symptoms of fatigue, nausea and a decrease in functional status Classic presentation: shortness of breath is a more common complaint than chest pain
Nondyspneic pulmonary edema	May not subjectively experience the classic symptoms of paroxysmal nocturnal dyspnea or coughing Typical onset may be insidious with change in function, food or fluid intake, or confusion
Thyroid disease	Hyperthyroidism presenting as "apathetic thyrotoxicosis" (ie, fatigue and a slowing down) Hypothyroidism presenting with confusion and agitation
Depression	Lack of sadness Somatic complaints: appetite changes, vague gastrointestinal symptoms, constipation, and sleep disturbances Hyperactivity Sadness misinterpreted as normal consequence of aging Medical problems that mask depression
Medical illness that presents as depression	For example, hypothyroid and hyper disease that presents as diminished energy and apathy

Reproduced with permission from Ham R, Sloane D, Warshaw G. *Primary Care Geriatrics: A Case-Based Approach.* St. Louis, MO: Mosby; 2002:32-33.

of transportation, the fear of being hospitalized, and the risk of losing independence.

C. Infection

Although a new infection can present in the usual way with fever and leukocytosis in older adults, it is just as common for an older adult to present with vague symptoms, no fever, no elevation in white count, and no localizing signs. Older adults generally have a lower basal body temperatures due to reduced muscle and meal-induced thermogenesis; therefore a temperature >37.3°C may be more likely to be indicative of infection. Frequently, a change in functional status and mental status is the only sign of underlying infection. The urinary tract infection is one of the best examples of this phenomenon. Rather than present with dysuria and frequency, both older men and older women may instead present with confusion, incontinence, and anorexia. Similarly, pneumonia can present with the absence of cough, incomplete radiographic findings or shortness of breath and instead present with general malaise and confusion. Although leukocytosis is less common in older adults, even in the absence of an elevated white blood cell count, a left shift is usually observed and indicative of infection. Attending to these subtle cues are important as the consequences of missing atypical infection presentations could lead to sepsis, prolonged hospitalization, and even death.

D. Cardiovascular Disease

Classic symptoms of cardiovascular disease, specifically myocardial infarction, are hard to miss: crushing substernal chest pain, shortness of breath, and nausea. But in the older adult, myocardial infarction can present as mild pain or a complete absence of pain, and can occur in the absence of dyspnea. Instead, myocardial infarction in the very old often presents as new-onset fatigue, dizziness, or confusion. Similarly, although heart failure is increasingly prevalent in older-age groups, clinicians must be attuned to both the typical and atypical presentations of heart failure. Common symptoms in older patients can include fatigue and loss of appetite rather than breathlessness. In other illnesses, such as peripheral artery disease, comorbidities may obscure typical symptoms, such as claudication. For example, preexisting neuropathy can lead to a baseline alteration in pain perception and a relative lack of physical activity can make it easy for clinicians to miss this common and potentially dangerous diagnosis.

E. Depression

The prevalence of depression among patients older than age 65 years in medical outpatient clinics ranges from 7% to 36% and increases to 40% in those who are hospitalized. Because early treatment of depression may improve quality of life and functional status, the recognition of depression is important. The typical symptoms of depression such as malaise and depressed mood are well-captured in the PHQ-9. In older adults, other common more atypical symptoms may include anxiety symptoms, diminished self-care, irritability, weight loss, new cognitive impairment, and higher rates of somatic symptoms and insomnia. Depression in older adults is often overlooked or misdiagnosed because some of these "atypical" symptoms are erroneously labeled as a normal part of aging.

F. Cognitive Impairment

Cognitive impairment and dementia continue to be difficult diagnoses to make for many clinicians. As a result, patients may be incorrectly diagnosed with a primary psychiatric illness and/or miss the opportunity to engage in meaningful goal setting and advanced care planning while they are still able. The patterns of cognitive domains affected can help clinicians identify which type of dementia a patient may have. For example, in Alzheimer disease, memory and language are the domains primarily affected. However, it is less appreciated that cognitive changes outside of these 2 domains can also signify a neurodegenerative process. Changes in behavior, visuospatial function, or executive function, for example, although not as typical in early Alzheimer disease, can be a hallmark of early frontotemporal dementia. It is critical that clinicians elicit information about all cognitive domains, not just memory, so that non-Alzheimer neurodegenerative disorders are also diagnosed. (For more information, see Chapter 21, "Delirium," and Chapter 22, "Cognitive Impairment & Dementia.")

SUMMARY

Recognizing atypical presentations of illness in older adults is an underappreciated but essential component of high-quality geriatric care. Delay in the recognition of acute illness can lead to adverse health outcomes such as prolonged hospitalization, iatrogenesis, and increased risk of death. For example, failure to recognize pneumonia in an older adult who presents with isolated confusion can result in delay of antibiotics, prolonged hospital stay, and death. As the population ages, increasing numbers of adults with geriatric syndromes and multiple medical conditions will present to hospitals and primary care offices with serious illnesses in the absence of typical clinical features. Recognition of common serious illnesses in the setting of atypical presentations in older patients is becoming an increasingly essential skill in clinical diagnosis and treatment. Optimal treatment of older adults with an atypical presentation of disease fundamentally requires knowledge of the manners in which illness may present atypically in the older adult; recognition of the common signs and symptoms of acute disease presentation in the older adult; and familiarization with the common conditions presenting atypically in older adults. By becoming more familiar with these common, yet underrecognized, presentations, health care clinicians can optimize the care of older adults and more effectively train future health care clinicians to do the same.

Bayer AJ, Chadha JS, Farag RR, Pathy MS. Changing presentations of myocardial infarction with increasing old age. *J Am Geriatr Soc.* 1986;34(4):263-266.

Chang CC, Wang SS. Acute abdominal in the elderly. *Int J Gerontol.* 2007;1(2):77-82.

Cooper N, Mulley G. Introducing geriatric medicine. In: Cooper N, Forest K, Mulley G, eds. *ABC of Geriatric Medicine.* West Sussex, UK: Blackwell Publishing; 2009:1-3.

Crystal S, Sambamoorthi U, Walkup JT, Akincigil A. Diagnosis and treatment of depression in the elderly Medicare population: predictors, disparities and trends. *J Am Geriatr Soc.* 2003;51:1718-1728.

Dang C, Aguilera P, Dang A, Salem L. Acute abdominal pain: four classifications can guide assessment and management. *Geriatrics.* 2002;57(3):30-32, 35-36, 41-42.

Emmett KR. Nonspecific and atypical presentation of disease in the older patient. *Geriatrics.* 1998;53(2):50-52, 58-60.

Gavazzi G, Krause KH. Aging and infection. *Lancet Infect Dis.* 2002;2(11):659-666.

Ham R, Sloane D, Warshaw G. *Primary Care Geriatrics: A Case-Based Approach.* St Louis, MO: Mosby; 2002:32-33.

Khouzam HR. Depression in the elderly: when to suspect. *Consultant.* 2012 (March):225-240.

Kroenke K, Spitzer RL, Williams JB. The PHQ-9: validity of a brief depression severity measure. *J Gen Intern Med.* 2001;16(9): 606-613.

Lavizzo-Mourey R. Dehydration in the elderly: a short review. *J Natl Med Assoc.* 1987;79(10):1033-1038.

Lyon C, Park D. Diagnosis of acute abdominal pain in older patients. *Am Fam Physician.* 2006;74(9):1537-1544.

Musgrave T, Verghese A. Clinical features of pneumonia in the elderly. *Semin Respir Infect.* 1990;5(4):269-275.

Norman DC. Fever in the elderly. *Clin Infect Dis.* 2000;31(1):148-151.

Oudejans I, Mosterd A, Bloemen JA, et al. Clinical evaluation of geriatric outpatients with suspected heart failure: value of symptoms, signs and additional tests. *Eur J Heart Fail.* 2011;13(5):518-527.

Pathy MS. Clinical presentation of myocardial infarction in the elderly. *Br Heart J.* 1967;29(2):190-199.

Rich MW. Epidemiology, clinical features, and prognosis of acute myocardial infarction in the elderly. *Am J Geriatr Cardiol.* 2006;15(1):7-11.

Tseng Y, Hwang L, Chang W. Delayed diagnosis in an elderly patient with atypical presentation of peripheral artery occlusion disease. *Int J Gerontol.* 2011;5:59-61.

van Duin D. Diagnostic challenges and opportunities in older adults with infectious diseases. *Clin Infect Dis.* 2012;54(7):973-978.

Waterer GW, Kessler LA, Wunderink RG. Delayed administration of antibiotics and atypical presentation in community-acquired pneumonia. *Chest.* 2006;130(1):11-15.

Weinberg AD, Minaker KL. Dehydration. Evaluation and management in older adults. Council on Scientific Affairs, American Medical Association. *JAMA.* 1995;274(19):1552-1556.

Prevention & Health Promotion

Dandan Liu, MD
Louise C. Walter, MD

8

SCREENING ISSUES FOR THE GERIATRIC POPULATION

Even in the very elderly, preventive interventions can limit disease and disability. The heterogeneity of the older population in terms of medical conditions, life expectancy, and goals of treatment, however, requires a more thoughtful and individualized application of prevention guidelines rather than a one-size-fits-all approach based solely on age.

Since the 1980s, the U.S. Preventive Services Task Force (USPSTF) has provided evidence-based scientific reviews of preventive health services to guide primary care decision making. The fundamental standard applied by the task force is whether the intervention leads to improved health outcomes (eg, reduced disease-specific morbidity and mortality). In 1998, the Assessing Care of Vulnerable Elders project began developing quality indicators specific for vulnerable older persons (defined as age >65 years and life expectancy <2 years). This project concluded that high-quality evidence about benefits and harms is often limited for interventions in older adult populations. In addition, trials generally show the average effectiveness of an intervention, so it is always necessary to incorporate individual characteristics (eg, life expectancy, goals of care, function, and comorbidities) into screening decisions because such characteristics may change the likelihood that a person will receive benefit versus harm from a preventive intervention.

The framework for individualized decision making (Table 8–1) is anchored by considering an individual's life expectancy. Rather than using the average life expectancy for a given age, the person's health status should be incorporated into preventive decisions (Figure 8–1). Persons with several comorbid medical conditions or functional impairments likely have a life expectancy that is lower than average for their age, whereas those without any significant medical conditions or functional impairment likely will live longer than average (see Chapter 3, "Goals of Care & Consideration of Prognosis"). The risk of experiencing the adverse effects

of a condition and the potential benefit from early detection should be considered in the context of a person's estimated life expectancy. The last component of the framework is to assess how individuals view these potential harms and benefits, and integrate their values and preferences into screening decisions.

Table 8–2 summarizes conditions for which screening or other prevention interventions have been shown to result in net benefit for some older people based on USPSTF and geriatrics-focused guidelines. The table also provides general guidance for individualized recommendations by incorporating a person's function, health, life expectancy, and goals of care. Screening for some conditions is not recommended when potential harms of screening (and the procedures that emanate from screening) outweigh potential benefits based on an individual's characteristics.

American Geriatric Society. *AGS Guidelines & Recommendations.* http://www.americangeriatrics.org/health_care_professionals/clinical_practice/clinical_guidelines_recommendations/

Gnanadesigan N, Fung CH. Quality indicators for screening and prevention in vulnerable elders. *J Am Geriatr Soc.* 2007;55 Suppl 2:S417-S423.

Lee SJ, Walter LC. Quality indicators for older adults: preventing unintended harms. *JAMA.* 2011;306(13):1481-1482.

Walter LC, Covinsky KE: Cancer screening in elderly patients: a framework for individualized decision making. *JAMA.* 2001;285(21):2750-2756.

U.S. Preventive Services Task Force. Home page. http://www.uspreventiveservicestaskforce.org/

GERIATRIC SYNDROMES

Common geriatric conditions (called syndromes to reflect the multifactorial etiologies) include falls, poor nutrition, vision and hearing loss, and cognitive impairment. These conditions are often underrecognized despite causing

Table 8–1. Steps to individualize decision making for screening tests.

1. Estimate the individual's life expectancy.
2. Estimate the risk of dying from the condition.
3. Determine the potential benefit of screening.
4. Weigh the direct and indirect harms of screening.
5. Assess the patient's values and preferences.

Reproduced with permission from Walter LC, Covinsky KE. Cancer screening in elderly patients: a framework for individualized decision making. *JAMA*. 2001;285(21):2750-2756.

significant burdens to quality of life and function. Therefore, detection of these conditions is recommended to evaluate the etiology of functional limitations in frail elders. USPSTF and Assessing Care of Vulnerable Elders (ACOVE)-3 guidelines are discussed here; see Chapter 6, "Geriatric Assessment," for a more detailed discussion of geriatric syndromes.

▶ **Falls**

The USPSTF concludes that there is strong evidence that several types of primary care-relevant interventions (eg, comprehensive multifactorial assessment and management, exercise/physical therapy interventions, and vitamin D supplementation) reduce falls among older adults at high risk for falling. Components most commonly included in effective multifactorial trials, and thus recommended, are home safety modifications; balance, gait and strength training; and withdrawal or minimization of psychoactive and other medications. Harms of these interventions appear minimal. The most frequently recommended screening test for falls is the Get Up and Go Test, which takes less than 1 minute. Any unsafe movement during the test suggests an increased risk of falling and should prompt the provider to refer the patient to physical therapy for complete evaluation. The American Geriatric Society has also published guidelines on falls and recommends asking older people annually if they have fallen in the past year.

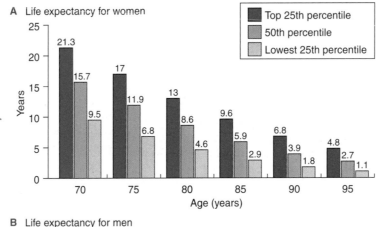

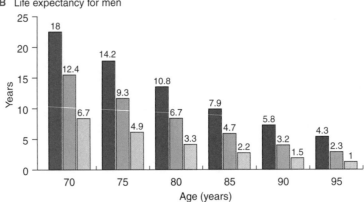

▲ **Figure 8–1.** Life expectancy quartiles by age. (Reproduced with permission from Walter LC, Covinsky KE: Cancer screening in elderly patients: a framework for individualized decision making. *JAMA*. 2001;285(21):2750-2756.)

Table 8–2. Individualized decision making.

Topics by System	Recommendations		Individualized Decision Making (Function, Health, Prognosis, Goals)		
	Please Refer to Text for More Information		High Independence Healthy Life Expectancy >10 Years Longevity	Limited function Multiple Comorbidities Life Expectancy 2–10 Years Preserving Function	Dependent End Stage Disease Life Expectancy <2 Years Comfort-Palliation
Geriatric syndromes[a]	Falls	Annually	Yes	Yes	Yes
	Depression	Annually	Yes	Yes	Yes
	Nutrition	Weigh at each visit	Maybe	Yes	Yes
	Hearing	Initially then unclear frequency	Maybe	Maybe	Maybe
	Vision	Initially then every 2 years	Maybe	Maybe	Maybe
	Incontinence	Initially then unclear frequency	Maybe	Maybe	Maybe
	Cognition	Patient preference specific	Maybe	Maybe	Maybe
	Elder abuse	No formal screening, but be vigilant for signs of mistreatment	Maybe	Maybe	Maybe
Health-related behaviors	Exercise	Annually	Yes	Yes	Yes
	Substance use	Annually	Yes	Yes	Yes
	Sexual Health	Annually	Yes	Yes	Yes
Immunizations	Influenza	Annually	Yes	Yes	Maybe
	Pneumococcal	Once after age 65 years[b]	Yes	Yes	Maybe
	Tetanus	Booster every 10 years	Yes	Yes	Maybe
	Herpes zoster	Once after age 50 years	Yes	Yes	Maybe
Endocrine	Osteoporosis	Initially women >65 years, men >70 years	Yes	Yes	Maybe
	Diabetes	Initially if hypertension or hyperlipidemia, then every 3 years	Yes	Maybe	No
Cardiovascular	Hypertension	Initially, then based on blood pressure	Yes	Yes	No
	Hyperlipidemia	Initially, then every 5 years	Yes	Yes	No
	Aortic aneurysm	Once in men age 65–75 years who ever smoked	Yes	Maybe	No
	Aspirin use (81 mg)	Initially (men age 55–79 years to prevent myocardial infarction women age 55–79 years to prevent cardiovascular accident) if outweighs risk of gastrointestinal bleeding	Yes	Maybe	No
Cancer screening	Colorectal	Fecal Immunochemical Test (FIT) annually or colonoscopy every 10 years	Yes	Maybe	No
	Breast	Mammogram every 2 years	Yes	Maybe	No
	Cervical	Stop at age 65	No[c]	No	No
	Prostate	Patient preference specific	Maybe	No	No

[a]Although evidence is limited, these conditions are underdiagnosed and may reveal etiology of impaired function and quality of life.
[b]If vaccinated before age 65 years, should receive 1 revaccination 5 years from last dose.
[c]If no previous screening or at high risk for cervical cancer (ie, immunosuppressed), discuss with patients their preference.

Michael YL, Whitlock EP, Lin JS, Fu R, O'Connor EA, Gold R; US Preventive Services Task Force. Primary care-relevant interventions to prevent falling in older adults: a systematic evidence review for the U.S. Preventive Services Task Force. *Ann Intern Med.* 2010;153(12):815-825.

Summary of the updated American Geriatrics Society/British Geriatrics Society clinical practice guideline for prevention of falls in older persons. *J Am Geriatr Soc.* 2011;59(1):148-157.

Depression

Depression is not a normal part of aging. It is associated with decreased quality of life, function, and higher mortality. The USPSTF recommendation is to screen if a system to support treatment of depression exists (eg, mental health treatment or care coordination). The Patient Health Questionnaire 2 (PHQ-2) is a screening tool that has been validated in adults age 65 years and older (sensitivity 100% and specificity 77%):

- Over the past month, have you often had little interest or pleasure in doing things?
- Over the past month, have you often been bothered by feeling down, depressed, or hopeless?

If the person answers yes to either of these questions, then a more detailed assessment (ie, PHQ-9) along with consideration of other medical explanations (ie, hypothyroidism, medication side effect, or substance use) is required.

Depression causes high morbidity, especially at the end of life, and a range of effective therapies exist. Treatments, including antidepressants and psychotherapy, are effective in older adults, and in contrast to young adults, antidepressants reduce suicidal behaviors. Supportive counseling and psychotherapy, when available, should be offered. When adding antidepressants, providers should consider pharmacokinetics in older adults and start with a lower dose, choose agents to minimize anticholinergic side effects, and weigh the time to benefit (usually 4–6 weeks) against a person's goals and prognosis.

O'Connor EA, Whitlock EP, Beil TL, Gaynes BN. Screening for depression in adult patients in primary care settings: a systematic evidence review. *Ann Intern Med.* 2009;151(11):793-803.

Unützer J. Clinical practice. Late-life depression. *N Engl J Med.* 2007;357(22):2269-2276.

Nutrition

For the general population, the USPSTF recommends dietary counseling to reduce fats and salt and to increase fruits, vegetables, and grain products containing fiber because these diets are associated with better health outcomes. Counseling can improve dietary behaviors, including reduction in dietary fat and salt and increases in fruit and vegetable intake. None of the studies, however, were designed to assess the adverse effects of dietary counseling, especially in chronically ill older

adults for whom protein-calorie malnutrition becomes an important concern. For older adults at risk for malnutrition or weight loss, restrictive diets should be avoided. ACOVE-3 recommends assessing weight at each visit for frail elders to identify undernourishment.

Suboptimal levels of vitamins may be risk factors for chronic disease such as cardiovascular disease, cancer, and osteoporosis. For most individuals, a single multivitamin should provide adequate levels. Because the recommended intake of vitamins B_{12} and D is closer to twice the recommended daily intake, it is reasonable to recommend multivitamin supplements with additional vitamin D and B_{12}.

Fairfield KM, Fletcher RH. Vitamins for chronic disease prevention in adults: scientific review. *JAMA.* 2002;287(23):3116-3126.

Lin JS, O'Connor E, Whitlock EP, et al. *Behavioral Counseling to Promote Physical Activity and a Healthful Diet to Prevent Cardiovascular Disease in Adults: Update of the Evidence for the U.S. Preventive Services Task Force.* Rockville, MD: Agency for Healthcare Research and Quality; 2010. (Evidence Syntheses, No. 79.)

Reuben DB. Quality indicators for the care of undernutrition in vulnerable elders. *J Am Geriatr Soc.* 2007;55 Suppl 2:S438-S442.

Vision

Up to 50% of older adults have undetected vision impairment. ACOVE-3 recommends a comprehensive eye exam (including acuity, dilation of pupil, intraocular pressure measurement, and retina) every 2 years. There is little evidence, however, that screening for vision loss improves functional outcomes or quality of life, and some treatments carry a small risk for serious complications, including acute vision loss. In most primary care clinics, routine screening is completed with the Snellen eye chart, which can identify impaired visual acuity (defined as best corrected vision worse than 20/50), but does not screen for macular degeneration, cataracts, or glaucoma. There is insufficient evidence for or against screening for these problems, given little evidence that early treatment improves vision-related function. Therefore, in clinical settings, screening for visual problems is a preference-sensitive decision.

Rowe S, MacLean CH. Quality indicators for the care of vision impairment in vulnerable elders. *J Am Geriatr Soc.* 2007;55 Suppl 2:S450-S456.

U.S. Preventive Services Task Force. Screening for impaired visual acuity in older adults: U.S. Preventive Services Task Force recommendation statement. *Ann Intern Med.* 2009;151(1):37-43.

Hearing

ACOVE-3 recommends screening for hearing loss in vulnerable adults during initial evaluation with no specific recommendation on repeat screening. The USPSTF evidence review did find good evidence screening detects hearing loss, but only 1 good-quality randomized trial showing benefit on quality of life with immediate hearing aids. Screening for hearing loss carries little risk, and hearing impairment is a prevalent problem in older persons. Examples of screening include a brief question ("Would you say you have any difficulty hearing?"), finger rub (failure to identify rub in ≥2 of 6 trials), or audiometric testing. If a patient wants to pursue amplification there are effective treatments (hearing aids); therefore, screening for hearing loss is a preference-sensitive decision.

Chou R, Dana T, Bougatsos C, Fleming C, Beil T. Screening adults aged 50 years or older for hearing loss: a systematic evidence review for the U.S. Preventive Services Task Force. *Ann Intern Med.* 2011;154(5):347-355.

Pacala JT, Yueh B. Hearing deficits in the older patients. *JAMA.* 2012;307:1185-1194.

Cognitive Impairment

The USPSTF gives no formal recommendation for routine screening of dementia. Although some screening tests have good sensitivity to detect cognitive impairment (eg, Minicog, Mini Mental State Examination [MMSE], and Montreal Cognitive Assessment [MOCA]), the limited efficacy of therapies (both pharmacologic and behavioral) and the potential distress of being labeled with dementia in face of limited treatment options have to be considered. ACOVE-3 recommends an initial cognitive assessment to allow for early implementation of nonpharmacologic interventions and earlier advanced planning, while also recognizing the lack of evidence. Given the risk of harm, the decision to screen an asymptomatic person should be preference-specific and may include discussion with a caregiver to determine if this is desired by the person. If memory has been raised as a concern by the person or caregiver, then the above tests can be performed as part of an initial diagnostic workup.

Brayne C, Fox C, Boustani M. Dementia screening in primary care: is it time? *JAMA.* 2007;298(20):2409-2411.

Feil DG, MacLean C, Sultzer D. Quality indicators for the care of dementia in vulnerable elders. *J Am Geriatr Soc.* 2007;55 Suppl 2: S293-S301.

Elder Abuse

Elder Abuse is not addressed by USPSTF, but it is estimated to have a prevalence of 2% to 10%, even with underreporting. The definition of abuse includes both intentional actions that cause or increase risk of harm and failure to satisfy an elder's needs or protect the elder from harm. Although there is no formal recommendation for screening, there is a need for health care providers to be vigilant to the signs and symptoms of abuse.

Lachs MS, Pillermer K. Elder abuse. *Lancet.* 2004;364(9441): 1263-1272.

National Center on Elder Abuse. http://www.ncea.aoa.gov

HEALTH-RELATED BEHAVIORS

Exercise

The benefits of as little as 30 minutes per day of walking on most days of the week to prevent coronary artery disease (CAD), hypertension, diabetes, obesity, and osteoporosis are well established. A Cochrane Review of progressive resistance strength training in older adults, including persons who were healthy, frail, or institutionalized, found it improved strength and performance (gait speed and transfer from chair). Resistance training and exercises such as tai chi, dance, and yoga also have been shown to improve balance. Although the USPSTF does not make a recommendation to counsel on exercise, the review does recognize that multicomponent interventions, including goal setting, written exercise prescriptions, and follow-up, may help increase physical activity. Exercise prescriptions include frequency, intensity, type, timing, and progression of exercise.

Howe TE, Rochester L, Neil F, Skelton DA, Ballinger C. Exercise for improving balance in older people. *Cochrane Database Syst Rev.* 2011;(11). Art. No.: CD004963. DOI: 10.1002/14651858. CD004963.pub3.

Liu CJ, Latham NK. Progressive resistance strength training for improving physical function in older adults. *Cochrane Database Syst Rev.* 2009;(3). Art. No.: CD002759. DOI: 10.1002/14651858. CD002759.pub2.

McDermott AY, Mernitz H. Exercise and older patients: prescribing guidelines. *Am Fam Physician.* 2006;74(3):437–444.

Substance Abuse

Tobacco, alcohol, and drug use have adverse impacts on health and are prevalent in older persons, as well as in younger persons. There is good evidence that even older smokers derive benefit from quitting tobacco, including decreased cardiovascular events. The USPSTF recommends asking all adults about tobacco use and providing tobacco cessation interventions if they screen positive. Issues specific to older adults include different pharmacokinetics with aging that may require gentle initiation of pharmacotherapy and inclusion of caregivers in counseling as they may be the source of tobacco.

Screening for alcohol use is also recommended by USPSTF, with a similar recommendation for behavioral counseling if the person screens positive for alcohol overuse. Although the prevalence of alcohol use decreases with age, an estimated 38% of people older than age 65 years drink alcohol, of whom 7.6% drink 5 or more servings a day. Unlike tobacco, there are safe amounts of alcohol consumption. Low-risk consumption is no more than 1 standard drink/day in people age 65 years and older, although in an individual with cognitive impairment, history of falls, liver disease, or a pattern of substance abuse, there may not be a safe amount. There is also controversy around the potential health benefits (reduction in heart disease, stroke, and possibly dementia) from moderate alcohol intake. Screening tests (such as CAGE [cutting, annoyance, guilt, eye-opener], Michigan Alcoholism Screening Test–Geriatric Version, and Alcohol Use Disorders Identification Test) have been validated in primary care settings, but primarily in younger populations. There also is growing interest in using a new single screening question: "In the past year, have you had any times when you had 4 or more drinks at 1 sitting?" (sensitivity 74.3%, specificity 95.6% among people age 65 years and older). The recommended follow-up to a positive screen is counseling and referral to therapy (treatment locator can be found at www.samhsa.gov).

Illicit substance use is a growing problem in the United States, although its prevalence remains lower in older adults than in younger adults (12.9% among ages 30–34 years vs. 1.1% among ages 65 years and older). The question, "How many times in the past year have you used an illegal drug or used a prescription medication for nonmedical reasons?," was highly sensitive and specific for detection of a drug use disorder in 1 study that included participants up to age 82 years.

AGS Clinical Practice Guidelines Position Paper. Alcohol use disorders in older adults. *Ann Longterm Care.* 2006;14(1):23-26. Available at: http://www.annalsoflongtermcare.com/article/5143

Kleykamp BA, Heishman SJ. The older smoker. *JAMA.* 2011;306(8):876-877.

McCance-Katz EF, Satterfield J. SBIRT: a key to integrate prevention and treatment of substance abuse in primary care. *Am J Addict.* 2012;21(2):176-177.

Smith PC, Schmidt SM, Allensworth-Davies D, Saitz R. A single question screening test for drug use in primary care. *Arch Intern Med.* 2010;170(13):1155-1160.

U.S. Preventive Services Task Force. Counseling and interventions to prevent tobacco use and tobacco-caused disease in adults and pregnant women: U.S. Preventive Services Task Force reaffirmation recommendation statement. *Ann Intern Med.* 2009;150(8):551-555.

Whitlock EP, Polen MR, Green CA, Orleans T, Klein J; U.S. Preventive Services Task Force. Behavioral counseling interventions in primary care to reduce risky/harmful alcohol use by adults: a summary of the evidence for the U.S. Preventive Services Task Force. *Ann Intern Med.* 2004;140(7):557-568.

▶ Sexual Health

The USPSTF recommends counseling to reduce sexually transmitted infections (STIs) in adults at increased sexual risk, meaning history of any STI in the past year or multiple sexual partners. STIs among older people are on the rise, including HIV, and assessing a person's sexual behaviors and attitudes is a way to better direct counseling. Assessing sexual health also may reveal psychosocial issues and medication side effects that may have otherwise been missed.

Ginsberg TB. Aging and sexuality. *Med Clin North Am.* 2006;90(5):1025-1036.

IMMUNIZATIONS

Several vaccinations are widely recommended because they result in net benefit for the majority of older adults. Although vaccination of older adults with moderate or severe acute illness should generally be deferred until the acute illness has improved or resolved, vaccination should not be delayed because of mild respiratory illnesses (with or without fever).

▶ Influenza Vaccine

The effectiveness of the influenza vaccination depends on the recipient's age and immunocompetence. Among community-dwelling adults older than age 60 years, the vaccine has been 56% effective in reducing influenza-related illness. Among older long-term care residents, vaccine effectiveness in preventing influenza may only be 30% to 40%; however, it may be 50% to 60% effective in preventing pneumonia and hospitalization, and 80% effective in preventing deaths. Seasonal trivalent inactivated influenza vaccine ("flu shot"), either standard-dose or high-dose formulation, is recommended annually for adults age 65 years and older starting in late summer or early fall—as soon as the vaccine is available. Live, attenuated influenza vaccine ("nasal spray") is not recommended for adults older than age 49 years. Flu shot side effects are typically minor and last less than 3 days. Because the vaccine comes from highly purified inactivated flu virus grown in eggs, influenza vaccination is contraindicated in persons with severe egg allergy.

▶ Pneumococcal Vaccine

The 23-valent pneumococcal vaccine represents 85% to 90% of the serotypes that cause invasive disease in the United States and has been shown to be 56% to 81% effective in preventing invasive disease. The Advisory Committee on Immunization Practices (ACIP) recommends pneumococcal immunization once for all adults age 65 years and older. A one-time pneumococcal revaccination is recommended for those age 65 years and older who received their initial vaccination before age 65. The vaccine has rarely been associated with major side effects, although up to half of vaccine recipients will have a mild local reaction that usually persists for less than 48 hours.

Tetanus/Diphtheria and Tetanus/ Diphtheria/Pertussis Vaccines

Cases of tetanus and diptheria in the United States are rare and mostly occur in unvaccinated people. Pertussis is an acute infectious cough illness that remains endemic in the United States. ACIP recommends a booster dose of tetanus-diphtheria toxoid (Td) vaccine every 10 years. For adults age 65 years and older who anticipate contact with an infant, a one-time booster of Tdap (tetanus, diphtheria, and acellular pertussis) vaccine should be given in place of the Td booster. Tdap vaccine can be administered regardless of the interval since the most recent Td vaccine. If an adult has never been vaccinated against tetanus, diptheria, or pertussis, then 3 doses are required (Tdap followed by Td ≥4 weeks later and another dose of Td 6–12 months later). Local reactions are common after these vaccines and a nodule may be palpable at the injection site for several weeks.

Herpes Zoster (Shingles) Vaccine

Zoster is a localized painful cutaneous eruption that is caused by reactivation of latent varicella zoster virus (VZV), often decades after initial varicella infection ("chicken pox"). Zoster vaccine is partially efficacious at preventing zoster, at reducing the severity and duration of pain, and at preventing postherpetic neuralgia. ACIP recommends a one-time herpes zoster (shingles) immunization for immunocompetent adults who are age 60 years and older. Shingles vaccine is a live, attenuated strain of VZV, the same strain used in varicella vaccines, but the shingles vaccine is much more potent. Persons with a history of zoster can be vaccinated. The few adults older than age 65 years who have received the varicella vaccine (began in the United States in 1995) do not need shingles vaccination. Injection site adverse effects may occur in up to half of vaccine recipients, although varicella-like rashes are rare. Shingles vaccination is contraindicated in persons with serious allergies to gelatin or neomycin.

Advisory Committee on Immunization Practices. Recommended adult immunization schedule: United States, 2012. *Ann Intern Med.* 2012;156(3):211-217.

ENDOCRINE DISORDERS

Diabetes Mellitus

The USPSTF recommends screening for diabetes mellitus in adults with hypertension or hyperlipidemia because treatment goals for those conditions might be altered with this additional diagnosis. Other organizations also recommend using HbA1c (glycosylated hemoglobin) ≥6.5% as a threshold for a diagnosis of diabetes, but this is controversial, especially among frail elders (eg, life expectancy <5 years and limited

function) for whom HbA1c treatment goal of <8% has been suggested to balance risks of hypoglycemia. Clinical trials to prevent microvascular complications of diabetes have shown that approximately 8 years of treatment are needed to benefit. For individuals whose life expectancy is less than that, benefits of lowering HbA1c are uncertain. Treatment carries the risk of hypoglycemia and burden of injection. For some persons, quality of life may outweigh any potential benefit of treating asymptomatic diabetes.

Brown AF, Mangione CM, Saliba D, Sarkisian CA; California Healthcare Foundation/American Geriatrics Society Panel on Improving Care for Elders with Diabetes. Guidelines for improving the care of the older person with diabetes mellitus. *J Am Geriatr Soc.* 2003;51(5 Suppl Guidelines):S265-S280.

Lee SJ, Boscardin WJ, Cenzer IS, Huang ES, Rice-Trumble K, Eng C. The risks and benefits of implementing glycemic control guidelines in frail elders with diabetes. *J Am Geriatr Soc.* 2011;59(4):666-672.

Thyroid Disorders

The USPSTF concludes there is insufficient data to recommend for or against screening for thyroid disorders in asymptomatic people. Many older adults, however, may have symptoms suggestive of hypothyroidism such as constipation, fatigue, depression, or weight gain. For adults with these symptoms, the preferred diagnostic test is a thyroid-stimulating hormone (TSH) level. In cases of normal free thyroxine (T_4) despite elevated TSH, subclinical hypothyroidism is suspected. A 2009 review found that for subclinical hypothyroidism, replacement therapy with levothyroxine neither improves survival nor quality life; treatment also does not decrease cardiovascular morbidity and has a small risk of harm (eg, unintended weight loss).

Villar HCCE, Saconato H, Valente O, Atallah ÁN. Thyroid hormone replacement for subclinical hypothyroidism. *Cochrane Database Syst Rev.* 2007;(3). Art. No.: CD003419. DOI: 10.1002/14651858. CD003419.pub2.

Osteoporosis

USPSTF recommends screening with a dual-energy x-ray absorptiometry (DXA) scan of hip and lumbar spine in women age 65 years and older, with at least a 2-year gap between repeat DXA scans. Although USPSTF makes no recommendations on testing in men, other organizations have recommended DXA in men based on individual risk assessment or age >70 years. Osteoporosis will affect as many as 1 in 2 women and 1 in 5 men. As women age, the number needed to treat to prevent 1 fracture over 5 years decreases to as low as 43 by ages 75–79. The FRAX score can further predict individual fracture risk. All guidelines emphasize that decisions to treat should be individualized because all current therapies, even calcium supplementation, although effective, do carry some potential risks.

American College of Physicians. *ACP Clinical Practice Guidelines.* http://www.acponline.org/clinical_information/guidelines/guidelines/

National Osteoporosis Foundation. *Clinician's Guide to Prevention and Treatment of Osteoporosis.* Washington, DC: National Osteoporosis Foundation; 2013. http://nof.org/files/nof/public/content/resource/913/files/580.pdf

Qaseem A, Snow V, Shekelle P, Hopkins R, Jr., Forciea MA, Owens DK. Clinical Efficacy Assessment Subcommittee of the American College of Physicians. Screening for osteoporosis in men: a clinical practice guideline from the American College of Physicians. *Ann Intern Med.* 2008 May;148(9):680-684.

U.S. Preventive Services Task Force. *Screening for Osteoporosis.* http://www.uspreventiveservicestaskforce.org/uspstf/uspsoste.htm

CARDIOVASCULAR DISEASE

CAD has remained the leading cause of death in the United States over the last 75 years. To date, using laboratory biomarkers and resting electrocardiograph as screening tests in asymptomatic people has not been shown to be beneficial. Rather, screening should focus on modifiable risk factors for cardiovascular disease, including hyperlipidemia, hypertension, tobacco use, diabetes, obesity, and physical inactivity.

Scott IA. Evaluating cardiovascular risk assessment for asymptomatic people. *BMJ.* 2009;338:a2844.

▶ Hyperlipidemia

The USPSTF recommends continued screening for hyperlipidemia in persons older than age 65 years with incorporation of some assessment of overall CAD risk (eg, Framingham or Adult Treatment Panel [ATP] III risk models). The Framingham equation, however, only includes ages up to 79 years, and it is unclear if risk should be extrapolated to older adults (eg, add additional points for each 5-year category thereafter).

In people with known CAD, excellent evidence supports screening and treating hyperlipidemia even up to age 80 years to reduce risk of myocardial infarction, stroke, and mortality. Systematic reviews of treating hyperlipidemia in elders with CAD have shown 25% to 30% reductions in 5-year coronary disease outcomes. Updated in 2004, the Third Report of the National Cholesterol Education Program (ATP III) recommends the low-density lipoprotein (LDL) cholesterol target should be <100 mg/dL for persons with CAD, and an expert-opinion-based recommendation suggests an LDL target <70 mg/dL for those at very high risk for vascular events (known CAD with comorbid diabetes, metabolic syndrome, or continued smoking). For very elderly individuals,

clinicians will need to carefully weigh life expectancy, goals of care, and potential side effects from therapies (eg, undernutrition from diet restrictions, myalgias from statins, and drug–drug interactions).

In people up to age 80 years without known CAD, there is 1 randomized control trial (Anglo-Scandinavian Cardiac Outcomes Trial [ASCOT]) that provided some evidence for hyperlipidemia screening and treatment (average LDL approximately 80 mg/dL postintervention). Specific treatment targets in older adults without CAD, however, are uncertain. Incorporation of a CAD risk score should guide application of ATP III guidelines. Although USPSTF recommends repeat screening every 5 years, guidelines recognize lipid levels are less likely to rise after age 65 years. In general, 3–5 years of treatment are required to derive benefit from lipid-lowering therapies, suggesting that for individuals with life expectancy less than 3–5 years, screening is likely to cause more harm than benefit.

Grundy SM, Cleeman JI, Merz CN, et al. Implications of recent clinical trials for the National Cholesterol Education Program Adult Treatment Panel III guidelines. *Circulation.* 2004 Jul 13;110(2):227-239.

Shah K, Rogers J, Britigan D, Levy C. Clinical inquiries. Should we identify and treat hyperlipidemia in the advanced elderly. *J Fam Pract.* 2006;55(4):356-357.

▶ Hypertension

The definition for hypertension among older adults remains unclear. Report 7 of the Joint National Commission on Detection, Evaluation and Treatment (JNC7) defines hypertension as >140/90 mm Hg regardless of age. Based on this definition, the USPSTF recommends screening for hypertension in all adults older than age 18 years, with no special recommendations for those older than age 65 years. Most guidelines recommend at least 2–3 different office measures taken on at least 2 different office visits to define hypertension. Frequency of screening is also guided by JNC7 guidelines, recommending intervals of 1–2 years depending on severity of hypertension.

The JNC7 guidelines, however, may be too stringent for older people without CAD. Sclerotic arteries can cause elevations in systolic blood pressure, causing "pseudohypertension," and at least 1 study among men age 85 years and older found a higher systolic blood pressure (SBP) (>180 mm Hg) was associated with greater survival compared to those who had a SBP <130 mm Hg. The landmark Hypertension in the Very Elderly Trial (HYVET) randomized controlled trial, however, demonstrated benefits of treating hypertension to prevent stroke, death, and CAD in generally healthy asymptomatic people age 60 years and older. This study treated to targets of SBP <150 mm Hg and diastolic blood pressure (DBP) <80 mm Hg. One stroke resulting in death or disease was prevented for every 50 people treated over 4.5 years. Death or disease from coronary heart disease was also reduced (number needed to treat = 100 over 4.5 years). Among the very old (age >80 years), the numbers were similar for stroke (absolute risk reduction of 1.8%, with number needed to treat of 56 over 2.2 years), with no decrease in coronary heart disease.

There is clear benefit in treating hypertension among those with CAD or equivalents regardless of age. The time of 3–5 years to these end points of decreased CAD and cardiovascular accident (CVA), coupled with potential side effects of treatment (fall, bradycardia, electrolyte abnormalities depending on the drug chosen) suggests that in those with limited life expectancy, risks may outweigh the benefit of screening and treatment. If treatment is considered, a higher target blood pressure should be considered.

Aronow WS, Fleg JL, Pepine CJ, et al: ACCF/AHA 2011 expert consensus document on hypertension in the elderly: a report of the American College of Cardiology Foundation Task Force on Clinical Expert Consensus Documents developed in collaboration with the American Academy of Neurology, American Geriatrics Society, American Society for Preventive Cardiology, American Society of Hypertension, American Society of Nephrology, Association of Black Cardiologists, and European Society of Hypertension. *J Am Soc Hypertens.* 2011;5(4):259-352.

Musini VM, Tejani AM, Bassett K, Wright JM. Pharmacotherapy for hypertension in the elderly. *Cochrane Database Syst Rev.* 2009;(4):CD000028.

Satish S, Freeman DH Jr, Ray L, Goodwin JS. The relationship between blood pressure and mortality in the oldest old. *J Am Geriatr Soc.* 2001;49(4):367-374.

▶ Abdominal Aortic Aneurysm

In men age 65–75 years with a history of tobacco use, the USPSTF recommends a one-time screening for abdominal aortic aneurysm by ultrasound to allow early detection and elective repair. An abdominal aortic aneurysm diameter of 5.5 cm or more is associated with increased risk of rupture and interventional management is generally recommended. Both endovascular and open repair carry risks for mortality and may require substantial recovery time. Therefore, in individuals with multiple comorbidities or limited life expectancy, the risk of screening and intervention may outweigh the benefits of early detection.

Fleming C, Whitlock EP, Beil TL, Lederle FA. Screening for abdominal aortic aneurysm: a best-evidence systematic review for the U.S. Preventive Services Task Force. *Ann Intern Med.* 2005;142(3):203-211.

Greenhalgh RM, Powell JT. Endovascular repair of abdominal aortic aneurysm. *N Engl J Med.* 2008;358(5):494-501.

▶ Aspirin

Aspirin for prophylaxis in persons without cardiovascular disease has been proposed to reduce the risk of several diseases: CVA, CAD, and colorectal cancer. The USPSTF weighed the reduced incidence of colorectal cancer against the increased risk of gastrointestinal bleed and hemorrhagic stroke from aspirin 325 mg and recommended against taking aspirin for colorectal cancer prevention.

Also, the benefits of aspirin in reducing the risk of CVA and CAD vary by sex: aspirin decreases CVA in women and decreases CAD in men. USPSTF recommends initiation of low-dose aspirin (75 mg/day was as effective as 325 mg/day in persons without cardiovascular disease) when the benefit (eg, Framingham calculators for CAD or CVA) outweighs the risk for gastrointestinal bleed. Concurrent use of nonsteroidal antiinflammatory drugs triples to quadruples the rate of gastrointestinal bleed from aspirin. Duration of aspirin therapy in trials has ranged from 3–10 years, and the USPSTF recommends reassessment of aspirin risks and benefits every 5 years. There is insufficient evidence to make recommendations for people >80 years old. Also, older individuals with less than a 5-year life expectancy or multiple comorbidities that place them at increased risk of gastrointestinal bleed are likely to experience net harm from initiating aspirin.

U.S. Preventive Services Task Force. Aspirin for the prevention of cardiovascular disease: U.S. Preventive Services Task Force recommendation statement. *Ann Intern Med.* 2009;150(6):396-404.

CANCER

▶ Breast Cancer

The USPSTF concludes that current evidence is insufficient to assess the balance of benefits and harms of screening mammography in women age 75 years and older because older women were not included in mammography trials. However, indirect evidence suggests mammography every 2 years is likely to result in net benefit for some older women in good health. For example, older women have a higher absolute risk of dying of breast cancer, mammography is more accurate in older women, and there is no evidence that the benefit of screening ceases at a specific age. Therefore, decisions to stop screening should be individualized based on whether a woman has comorbidities that limit her life expectancy to less than 5 years and her values and preferences regarding the potential benefits and harms of screening. Women with limited life expectancy are at risk for harms that happen around the time of screening while they have no chance for potential survival benefit, which only happens several years after the actual screening test. Harms of screening include false-positive results that may lead to a cascade of medical testing and psychological distress, as well as the overdetection and overtreatment of inconsequential disease that would never have come to clinical attention had the woman not been screened. Therefore, a screening mammography is likely to cause net harm in women with limited life expectancy and in those who place high importance on avoiding the harms of screening.

For all age groups, current evidence is insufficient to assess the additional benefits and harms of magnetic resonance imaging or clinical breast examination beyond mammography for breast cancer screening. In addition, teaching women to perform breast self-examination has been shown to cause net harm and is not recommended at any age. Of course, women should be encouraged to report breast changes or abnormalities they discover to their clinician.

Schonberg MA, Silliman RA, Marcantonio ER. Weighing the benefits and burdens of mammography screening among women age 80 years or older. *J Clin Oncol.* 2009;27(11):1774-1780.

U.S. Preventive Services Task Force. Screening for breast cancer: U.S. Preventive Services Task Force recommendation statement. *Ann Intern Med.* 2009;151(10):716-726.

Colorectal Cancer

The USPSTF recommends colorectal cancer screening in adults age 50 through 75 years; recommends individualized decision making for adults age 76 through 85 years; and recommends against screening adults older than age 85 years. These cutoffs are based on average life expectancy at each age and should be used as general guides rather than applied rigidly. For example, screening is not recommended for persons of any age who have a life expectancy less than 5 years, and screening may be appropriate for a very healthy 88-year-old person who has never been screened. Advancing age increases the absolute risk of dying of colorectal cancer.

There are multiple acceptable measures of colorectal cancer screening. These tests include high sensitivity gFOBT (guaiac-based fecal occult blood testing) or iFOBT (immunologic fecal occult blood test)/FIT (fecal immunochemical test) annually, or sigmoidoscopy every 5 years, or colonoscopy every 10 years. Older adults are more likely to have cancer in the right half of the colon, decreasing the sensitivity of sigmoidoscopy, which examines only the left half of the colon. Also, choice of screening test should consider availability and individual preferences. gFOBT requires dietary and medication restrictions 7 days prior to screening, whereas iFOBT/FIT eliminates the need for these restrictions. Bowel preparations are required prior to sigmoidoscopy and colonoscopy. The standard follow-up of any positive test is a diagnostic colonoscopy, such that people who would never accept or tolerate colonoscopy should not be screened. Risks of colonoscopy increase with age and comorbidity burden. It is estimated that perforation, hemorrhage, or cardiovascular/pulmonary events occur in 26 per 1000 colonoscopies for adults age 65 years and older and in approximately 35 per 1000 colonoscopies for adults age 85 and older.

For all ages there is insufficient evidence to weigh the potential benefits of computer tomographic colonography against the likely harms of the test. Barium enema is the least-sensitive screening test for colorectal cancer and is no longer recommended for screening.

Day LW, Kwon A, Inadomi JM, Walter LC, Somsouk M. Adverse events in older patients undergoing colonoscopy: a systematic review and meta-analysis. *Gastrointestinal Endoscopy* 2011;74(4): 885-896.

Pignone M, Rich M, Teutsch SM, Berg AO, Lohr KN. Screening for colorectal cancer in adults at average risk: a summary of the evidence for the U.S. Preventive Services Task Force. *Ann Intern Med.* 2002;137(2):132-141.

Cervical Cancer

The USPSTF recommends against screening for cervical cancer in women older than age 65 years who have had adequate prior screening and are not otherwise at high risk for cervical cancer (such as women with history of a high-grade precancerous lesion or cervical cancer, in utero exposure to diethylstilbestrol, or who are immunocompromised). Older women with adequate prior screening are at extremely low risk for developing cervical cancer, even if they have substantial life expectancy or a new sexual partner. Adequate prior screening is defined as 3 consecutive negative cytology results or 2 consecutive negative HPV (human papillomavirus) results within 10 years before cessation of screening, with the most recent test occuring within 5 years. Women older than age 65 years who have an inadequate screening history or those who have never been screened should receive screening with cytology (Papanicolaou smear) every 2 to 5 years, ending at age 70 to 75. Women at any age who have had a hysterectomy with removal of the cervix for a benign condition are not at risk for cervical cancer and should not be screened. Harms of cervical cancer screening include false-positive results. Mucosal atrophy, which is common after menopause, may predispose older women to false-positive cytology and lead to additional testing and invasive diagnostic procedures, such as colposcopy and cervical biopsy, as well as psychological distress. In addition, many precancerous cervical lesions (such as CIN2) will spontaneously regress such that screening may cause harm through the identification and treatment of inconsequential disease.

For all ages there is limited evidence on the benefits and harms of HPV testing alone as a screening strategy. HPV testing combined with cytology every 5 years may be a reasonable alternative in younger women who want to lengthen the screening interval.

Moyer VA; U.S. Preventive Services Task Force. Screening for cervical cancer: U.S. Preventive Services Task Force recommendation statement. *Ann Intern Med.* 2012;156(12):880-891.

Prostate Cancer

There is considerable controversy surrounding prostate-specific antigen (PSA) screening for men of all ages because of the lack of conclusive evidence that screening reduces mortality from prostate cancer. All guidelines, however, agree that screening men with a life expectancy less than 10 years is not recommended because they have little chance for any potential survival benefit. The USPSTF recommends against PSA screening in all men, whereas other organizations suggest screening might be warranted in men in good health who value the small or uncertain benefits of screening over the substantial known harms. Guidelines generally agree that among men with long life expectancy the decision to undergo PSA screening is a preference-sensitive decision that should be informed. Clinicians should inform men of the potential benefits, limits/gaps in current evidence, and known harms of screening. Harms include false-positive results that may lead to additional testing and prostate biopsies, as well as overdetection and overtreatment of clinically inconsequential prostate cancers that would never have progressed to cause illness in a man's lifetime. In addition, treatment of prostate cancer often results in serious adverse effects in older men (such as incontinence, impotence, radiation proctitis or hip fractures).

For all age groups digital rectal examination is not recommended for prostate cancer screening. Also, there is no evidence that the use of free PSA or PSA density, velocity, or doubling time improves health outcomes and some of these strategies may increase harm.

U.S. Preventive Services Task Force. *Screening for Prostate Cancer: U.S. Preventive Services Task Force Draft Recommendation Statement.* Available at: http://www.uspreventiveservicestaskforce.org/uspstf12/prostate/draftrecprostate.htm

▶ Other Cancers

The USPSTF recommends against routine screening for pancreatic or ovarian cancer for persons of all ages. There is no evidence that screening for pancreatic cancer (using abdominal palpation, ultrasonography, or serologic markers) or ovarian cancer (using CA-125 or transvaginal ultrasonography) is effective in reducing mortality, and there is potential for significant harm because of the limited accuracy of available screening tests, invasive nature of diagnostic tests, and the poor outcomes of treatment.

The USPSTF concludes that there is insufficient evidence to assess the balance of benefits and harms of screening for lung or skin cancer for persons of all ages. One randomized trial has shown low-dose computed tomography screening can reduce lung cancer mortality in current or former smokers age 55 to 74 years. However, the harms were substantial, including complications from invasive diagnostic procedures, such as bronchoscopy or lung biopsy, which may be greater in older adults. Therefore, lung cancer prevention efforts should still focus on encouraging older smokers to quit. Also, although there is no evidence to support total body skin examinations clinicians should remain alert for skin lesions with malignant features (eg, rapidly changing lesions and those with asymmetry, border irregularity, or color variability).

U.S. Preventive Services Task Force Guidelines. Available at http://uspreventiveservicestaskforce.org/uspstopics.htm#AZ

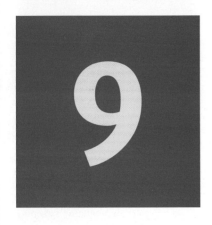

Principles of Prescribing for Older Adults

Michael A. Steinman, MD
Holly M. Holmes, MD

GERIATRIC PRINCIPLES

On the surface, prescribing for older adults is similar to prescribing for younger adults, requiring understanding of drug indications, dosing, potential adverse reactions, and drug–drug interactions. However, prescribing for older adults is complicated by a variety of factors. Physiologic changes as patients get older result in alterations in drug metabolism and susceptibility to adverse events. The presence of multiple chronic conditions and multiple medications leads to potentially complex drug–drug and drug–disease interactions, as well as the need to balance multiple competing recommendations. Changes in cognitive function, manual dexterity, and social supports complicate adherence to medications, and heterogeneous goals of care require special attention. Because clinical trials that inform many practice guidelines are often conducted in younger patients, there can be ambiguity about the extent to which these evidence-based recommendations apply to older adults. Thus, mastering prescribing for older patients requires expertise not only in technical elements of drug use, but also in synthesizing evidence and biomedical and psychosocial factors into a coordinated plan of care that meets each individual's unique needs. More details about polypharmacy can be found in Chapter 53, and more details about extrapolating the evidence from clinical research to older patients can be found in Chapter 74.

DRUG METABOLISM AND PHYSIOLOGIC EFFECTS IN OLDER ADULTS

► Pharmacokinetics

Pharmacokinetics refers to how the body handles a drug from the time it is ingested to the time it is excreted. This includes the processes of absorption, distribution, metabolism, and elimination. While each of these processes can vary with age, they are typically more influenced by genetic factors and by an individual's diseases, environment, and other medications. For most older patients, changes in renal function have the greatest impact on pharmacokinetics.

A. Absorption

Absorption of drugs is impacted by the size of the absorptive surface, gastric pH, splanchnic blood flow, and gastrointestinal (GI) tract motility. Most of these are relatively unaffected by age, but can be substantially affected by certain diseases and medications. Some medications, including vitamin B_{12}, calcium, and iron, have decreased absorption in older adults as a result of reduced activity of active transport mechanisms.

B. Distribution

Older patients have an increased fat-to-lean body mass ratio, decreased total-body water, and sometimes decreased serum albumin. Drugs that distribute in fat (eg, diazepam) may thus have a larger volume of distribution. Hydrophilic medications (eg, digoxin) will have a decreased volume of distribution, resulting in higher serum levels. Drugs that bind to serum proteins reach an equilibrium between bound (inactive) and free (active) drug. Use of 2 or more drugs that compete for protein binding (eg, thyroid hormone, digoxin, warfarin, phenytoin) can result in higher levels of free drug, requiring careful monitoring of drug levels and effects. In the case of testosterone, age-associated increases in sex-hormone binding globulin can result in normal serum levels of total testosterone, even while levels of serum free testosterone (the bioactive form) are reduced.

C. Metabolism

The cytochrome P450 system assists with drug metabolism through oxidation and reduction (known as Phase 1 metabolism). There may be an age-related decline in Phase 1 activity as a result of reductions in hepatic blood flow and liver size. Nonetheless, the cytochrome P450 system is typically far more impacted by genetic polymorphisms that result in some individuals being "fast" or "slow" metabolizers, and by the use of other drugs and foods that can inhibit or induce specific P450 enzymes, resulting in slowed or accelerated drug metabolism. (See the section "Adverse Drug Reactions" below for information on cytochrome P450-mediated drug–drug interactions.) Phase II hepatic metabolism, otherwise known as conjugation, follows phase I metabolism. It typically makes drugs biologically inactive and facilitates their excretion. It is not affected by age.

D. Excretion

Renal function often decreases with age, involving loss of both glomerular filtration rate and tubular function. Because muscle mass declines in older age, renal function can often be substantially impaired even in the presence of a normal serum creatinine. Thus, estimation of creatinine clearance (or the closely related glomerular filtration rate) is essential. Mathematically complex formulas such as the Chronic Kidney Disease Epidemiology Collaboration (CKD-EPI) and Modification of Diet in Renal Disease (MDRD) formulas tend to more accurately reflect renal function compared to the Cockroft-Gault equation (shown below). However, each is imperfect and should be interpreted as providing only a rough estimate of renal function. In situations of rapidly changing renal function, neither formula performs well. Nonetheless, it is far better to have (and use) an easy-to-obtain rough estimate of renal function than none at all.

$$\text{Creatinine clearance} = \frac{(140 - \text{age}) \times \text{weight (kg)}}{\text{Serum creatinine} \times 72}$$

(multiply by 0.85 for women to allow for 15% less muscle mass).

▶ Pharmacodynamics

Pharmacodynamics refers to how the drug affects the body; that is, the physiologic effects exerted by a drug's action on end-organ receptors. Pharmacodynamics has not been as carefully studied in older adults as pharmacokinetics. Older adults are more sensitive to medications that depress the central nervous system, which can result in delirium, confusion, and agitation. The frequent use of multiple medications in older adults often leads to the simultaneous use of 2 or more drugs that have mutually reinforcing physiologic effects, which can result in harm. Examples include bleeding with simultaneous use of anticoagulant drugs (eg, warfarin) and nonsteroidal antiinflammatory drugs (NSAIDs) or aspirin; and orthostatic hypotension with various blood pressure medications and α blockers.

GERIATRIC THERAPEUTICS

▶ Adverse Drug Reactions

A. Epidemiology and Risk Factors

Adverse drug reactions (ADRs) are substantially more common in older than in younger adults. Up to 35% of ambulatory older adults experience 1 or more ADRs annually, 5% to 10% of hospital admissions in older adults are ascribable to ADRs, and 5% or more of older hospitalized patients experience an ADR during their inpatient stay. Simply being old does not meaningfully increase ADR risk. Rather, it is the number of medications taken and the burden of disease (which often, but not always, increases as patients get older) that are the strongest risk factors for ADRs in the outpatient setting.

Several observational studies have failed to find a globally increased risk of ADRs in older adults with impaired functional status and geriatric syndromes. However, the risk of ADRs may increase with specific drugs that can interact with specific impairments. For example, central nervous system-acting drugs may have a particularly high risk of causing ADRs in patients with underlying cognitive impairment.

A note on terminology: "Adverse drug reactions" refers to the unwanted effects of drugs at normal dosage and use. "Adverse drug events" refers to a broader range of potential harms associated with the drug, including overdose, withdrawal reactions from abrupt discontinuation of a drug, and more.

B. Causes of Adverse Drug Reactions

ADRs are commonly classified into 2 predominant types. Type A ADRs result from expected yet unwanted or exaggerated physiologic effects of the drug. For example, β blockers may cause bradycardia that results in syncope. Type B ADRs, which are less common, result from idiosyncratic effects unrelated to the drug's usual physiologic targets; for example, anaphylaxis to penicillin.

In older adults, type A ADRs often arise from the interaction of a drug and underlying characteristics of the patient. Medications with a narrow therapeutic index and prolonged half-life cause the most trouble for the older patient. Patients with multiple medications, disease states, and/or subclinical physiologic changes associated with aging can be more susceptible to unwanted effects of a drug.

Drug–drug interactions can lead to ADRs by pharmacokinetic and pharmacodynamic mechanisms. In the former, Drug A inhibits the activity of a cytochrome P450 isoenzyme, resulting in delayed clearance of Drug B which is metabolized by that isoenzyme. This results in excessive tissue levels of Drug B, and resultant adverse effects. Common culprits that inhibit P450 activity include antimicrobials such as ciprofloxacin, fluconazole, and clarithromycin; some selective serotonin reuptake inhibitors; amiodarone; and verapamil and diltiazem. For example, diltiazem inhibits cytochrome

P450 isoenzyme 3A4 (CYP3A4). Atorvastatin and several other (but not all) statin medications are metabolized by CYP3A4. Thus, if a patient is taking both diltiazem and atorvastatin, atorvastatin will accumulate because the enzyme that metabolizes it has been rendered less active. Tissue levels of atorvastatin will rise, potentially to the level where they cause substantial toxicity (ie, increase the risk of rhabdomyolysis and liver injury).

Cytochrome P450 isoenzymes can also be induced ("sped up"). This induction results in rapid clearance and thus decreased effectiveness of drugs metabolized by the affected isozyme. Medications that are potent inducers of P450 enzymes include rifampin, barbiturates, carbamazepine, and phenytoin. In general, cytochrome P450-mediated interactions are most important when induction or inhibition is potent (eg, greater than 5-fold change in enzyme activity) and the substrate drug has a narrow therapeutic index (eg, warfarin, sulfonylureas). In contrast, drug interactions that involve weak induction or inhibition and a substrate drug with a wide safety margin are less likely to be clinically relevant.

Use of 2 or more drugs with mutually reinforcing physiologic effects can also result in harms. For example, third-degree heart block may occur in a patient prescribed digoxin and a β blocker, as both suppress conduction of atrial impulses through the atrioventricular node.

Drug–disease interactions occur when an underlying disease state makes a patient more susceptible to the unwanted physiologic effects of a drug. Not every potential interaction results in harm. For example, many patients with mild or moderate chronic obstructive pulmonary disease can tolerate β blockers without adverse effects, although some will develop worse pulmonary symptoms in this setting.

In addition to ADRs, an expanded range of adverse events can occur from misuse of drugs. This can include complications of excessive doses of a drug, failure to prevent or treat disease because of nonadherence to or insufficient dosing of a drug, or withdrawal reactions caused by abrupt discontinuation of a drug to which the body has physiologically adapted (ie, chronic opioids).

C. Preventing Adverse Drug Reactions and the Role of Monitoring

Fewer than one-quarter of ADRs in ambulatory older adults are a result of clinicians making clearly inappropriate prescribing decisions. In contrast, most ADRs result from drugs that were reasonable to prescribe, and represent the known but unwelcome potential adverse reactions of a given drug. Warfarin and insulin are the most common causes of ADRs severe enough to precipitate an emergency room visit. Nonetheless, these drugs have an important place in the therapeutic armamentarium for older adults. In fact, warfarin is often underprescribed, as for many patients the benefits of preventing a stroke or pulmonary embolism outweigh the risk of hemorrhage.

True prevention is difficult in this setting, as it can be difficult to precisely predict which patients will be helped or harmed by a drug. Yet, many ADRs can be detected and managed early, sparing the patient prolonged symptoms or a cascade of ever-worsening adverse effects (such as untreated orthostasis resulting in a fall with fracture). Monitoring older adults for emerging ADRs thus plays a critical role in reducing the burden of ADRs, yet is often not done well. One important impediment to monitoring is that both patients and physicians may falsely attribute a new symptom to an underlying disease state or "getting old," rather than recognizing it as an adverse drug reaction. This leads patients to underreport potential ADRs and to physicians not properly diagnosing a symptom as an ADR even when the patient reports it. The mantra "any symptom in an older adult is a medication side effect until proven otherwise" provides a useful reminder to always keep ADRs on the differential diagnosis when evaluating a new or worsened complaint.

> *Any symptom in an older adult is a medication side effect until proven otherwise.*

Dedicated nurse-led and pharmacist-led programs are effective strategies for ADR monitoring, best exemplified by anticoagulation clinics. Although little data are available to support simple in-office or bedside tools for ADR monitoring, expert opinion suggests that several strategies may be helpful. These include: (a) at the time a drug is prescribed, warning the patient of which adverse reactions to watch for; (b) at the next patient encounter, use a combination of open-ended questions and specific prompts to query for adverse reactions (eg, "Are you having any side effects or problems from Drug X?" followed by specific questions about dangerous and common adverse reactions); and (c) using a similar strategy to query for adverse reactions during annual medication review.

▶ Multiple Medication Use

A. Epidemiology and Potential Harms and Benefits of Using Multiple Medicines

Nearly 20% of adults age 65 years and older use 10 or more medications. This use of multiple medications is commonly referred to as "polypharmacy." This term carries a pejorative connotation, in part for good reason. Use of multiple medications substantially increases the risk of drug–drug interactions and of adverse drug events, can impose substantial cost burdens on patients, complicates adherence, and is associated with increased risk of using inappropriate medications. On the other hand, older patients often have multiple chronic conditions that can be substantially helped by medications. In many such patients, the use of multiple drugs is an appropriate therapeutic choice. Thus, while use of multiple medications is a risk factor for medication problems—and should prompt close attention to reducing unnecessary medications—the focus on reducing medications needs to be balanced with the harms to longevity and quality of life that arise from undertreated chronic conditions (see Chapter 53, "Addressing Polypharmacy & Improving Medication Adherence in Older Adults").

B. The Prescribing Cascade

One important contributor to multiple medication use is "the prescribing cascade," in which the adverse effects of one drug are treated with another drug, which itself causes adverse effects that are treated with a third drug, and so forth. This can result from misinterpreting a sign or symptom as the manifestation of an underlying disease process, rather than as an adverse drug effect. As noted above, remembering the mantra "any symptom in an older adult is a medication side effect until proven otherwise" can help guard against potential prescribing cascades. Except in unusual circumstances, it is typically better to withdraw or substitute the offending drug rather than treating its adverse effects with another drug.

▶ Overuse, Misuse, and Underuse of Medications

For many older adults, the question is not whether a patient is taking too many or too few medications, but whether the patient is taking the right medications given the patient's diseases, preferences, and ability to adhere. Deviations from an optimal regimen can be viewed as problems of overuse (use of a drug where no medication therapy is needed), misuse (use of a drug where a better alternative is available), and underuse (nonuse of a drug that would be beneficial).

A. Overuse and Misuse

Overuse and misuse of drugs are common. Approximately 20% to 30% of older ambulatory adults use at least 1 drug that consensus criteria recommend avoiding in older patients. Expert review of medication regimens in outpatient, inpatient, and nursing home settings has also identified large proportions of patients taking drugs that are not indicated, ineffective for the condition being treated, or otherwise problematic. It is common for drugs to be continued long after they are no longer necessary. For example, roughly half of patients who are started on a proton pump inhibitor for stress ulcer prophylaxis during a hospital stay are continued on these medications after discharge, for no discernible reason.

Several explicit criteria, commonly called "drugs-to-avoid lists," have been developed to identify medications and therapeutic situations that are potentially inappropriate for older adults. These tools have proved useful for quality improvement, including flagging instances of such prescribing for special scrutiny and review. Nonetheless, clinical judgment needs to be applied for individual patients, as there are situations in which use of many of these drugs is reasonable.

The *Beers criteria* of potentially inappropriate medications are shown in Table 9–1. The most frequently cited part of these criteria concern drugs that are potentially inappropriate in any setting. Commonly used medications on this "drugs-to-avoid" list include first-generation antihistamines (eg, diphenhydramine and hydroxyzine), tertiary-amine tricyclic antidepressants, use of benzodiazepines for insomnia, agitation, or delirium, long-acting sulfonylureas (eg, glyburide), and sliding-scale insulin.

The *STOPP* (Screening Tool of Older Person's Prescriptions) *criteria* define an extensive list of specific clinical situations in which drug use is potentially inappropriate (Table 9–2). Examples include use of loop diuretics for ankle edema in the absence of heart failure; selective serotonin reuptake inhibitors in patients with a history of hyponatremia; and use of NSAIDs in patients with heart failure or moderate-to-severe hypertension.

The *ACOVE* (Assessing Care of Vulnerable Elders) *criteria* for vulnerable older adults cover a wide range of topics, including a number of criteria related to medication use. ACOVE criteria address not only potentially inappropriate medications but also recommended care practices, including patient education about medications and regular medication review.

B. Underuse

Although use of inappropriate drugs is commonly discussed in older adults, equally important is the undertreatment of conditions that could be helped by drug therapy. Older adults are less likely to receive indicated medications than their younger counterparts, even after accounting for contraindications to these therapies. Excessive fear of causing adverse events, distraction by other clinical issues, a sense of futility, and subtle ageism likely contribute to this pattern. In addition, treatable conditions are often underdiagnosed in older patients, and symptoms such as pain, fatigue, depressed mood, or orthostasis may be incorrectly attributed to "getting old."

The *START* (Screening Tool to Alert doctors to Right Treatment) *criteria* are consensus criteria that identify potential underuse of beneficial medications in older adults (Table 9–3). As with other explicit criteria, these are intended as a guide but not as a substitute for clinical judgment for individual patients. Examples of drugs which the START criteria recommend should routinely be used include warfarin for chronic atrial fibrillation (in the absence of contraindications); regular inhaled β-agonist or anticholinergic therapy for patients with mild to moderate asthma or chronic obstructive pulmonary disease (COPD); and bisphosphonates in patients on chronic corticosteroid therapy.

The ACOVE criteria also identify instances of potential underuse for a variety of chronic illnesses. This includes not only omissions of specific medication but other

Table 9–1. Potentially inappropriate medications in older adults—Beers criteria (selected examples).[a]

Criterion	Rationale
First-generation antihistamines (eg, diphenhydramine, chlorpheniramine)	Highly anticholinergic; risk of confusion, dry mouth, constipation, and other anticholinergic effects
Antiarrhythmic drugs as first-line treatment of atrial fibrillation (acceptable as backup therapy)	Data suggest that rate control yields better balance of benefits and harms than rhythm control for most older adults. Amiodarone associated with multiple toxicities
Digoxin >0.125 mg/day	In heart failure, higher dosages associated with no additional benefit and may increase risk of toxicity; slow renal clearance may lead to risk of toxic effects
Tertiary tricyclic antidepressants (eg, amitriptyline)	Highly anticholinergic, sedating, and cause orthostatic hypotension
Antipsychotics for behavioral problems of dementia unless nonpharmacologic options have failed and patient is a threat to self or others	Increased risk of cerebrovascular accident (stroke) and mortality in persons with dementia
Benzodiazepines for treatment of insomnia, agitation, or delirium	Older adults have increased sensitivity to benzodiazepines and slower metabolism of long-acting agents. In general, all benzodiazepines increase risk of cognitive impairment, delirium, falls, fractures, and motor vehicle accidents in older adults
Chloral hydrate	Tolerance occurs within 10 days, and risks outweigh benefits in light of potential for overdose
Nonbenzodiazepine hypnotics (eg, zolpidem, eszopiclone) for chronic use (>90 days)	Adverse events similar to those of benzodiazepines in older adults (eg, delirium, falls, fractures); minimal improvement in sleep latency and duration
Male androgens unless indicated for moderate to severe hypogonadism	Potential for cardiac problems and contraindicated in men with prostate cancer
Long-acting sulfonylureas (eg, glyburide, chlorpropamide)	Risk of severe prolonged hypoglycemia
Meperidine	Not an effective oral analgesic in dosages commonly used; may cause neurotoxicity
Non–cyclooxygenase-selective NSAIDs; avoid chronic use unless other alternatives are not effective and patient can take gastroprotective therapy (eg, proton pump inhibitor)	Increases risk of GI bleeding and peptic ulcer disease in high-risk groups; use of proton pump inhibitor or misoprostol reduces, but does not eliminate, risk
Skeletal muscle relaxants	Poorly tolerated by older adults because of anticholinergic adverse effects, sedation, risk of fracture

[a]For the full list of Beers criteria, see American Geriatrics Society 2012 Beers Criteria Update Expert Panel. American Geriatrics Society updated Beers criteria for potentially inappropriate medication use in older adults. *J Am Geriatr Soc.* 2012;60(4):616-631.

recommended care processes, including annual medication review, educating patients about their medications, and monitoring for medication effectiveness and toxicity.

▶ High-Risk Medications

The following medications are often associated with adverse reactions and merit special caution in prescribing.

A. Warfarin and Other Anticoagulants

The benefits of warfarin for stroke prevention in atrial fibrillation and for the treatment of venous thromboembolism (VTE) outweigh the risk of hemorrhage for most patients, even for patients older than age 80 years and patients with a history of falls. Yet, warfarin is the most common medication implicated in emergency room visits and hospitalizations for

ADRs. Safe use requires close monitoring to keep patients in the target anticoagulation range and attention to the increased risk of hemorrhage when used with antiplatelet agents. Close to 700 known medications, supplements, and foods interact with warfarin, either by inhibiting cytochrome P450 enzyme activity, displacing plasma protein binding, affecting vitamin K metabolism, or potentiating bleeding risk through other antithrombotic mechanisms. Antibiotics, antiplatelet agents, and amiodarone are commonly implicated as the source of drug–drug interactions that result in bleeding. Patients receiving warfarin must be monitored closely to keep the international normalized ratio (INR) in target range, as well as for drug–drug interactions whenever a new medication is added.

Despite the risks of warfarin, newer anticoagulant medications have not yet displaced its use. Dabigatran is an oral direct thrombin inhibitor that is approved for stroke

Table 9–2. Potentially inappropriate medications in older adults—STOPP criteria (selected examples).[a]

Criterion	Rationale
Loop diuretic for dependent ankle edema only (ie, no clinical signs of heart failure)	No evidence of efficacy, compression stockings usually more appropriate
Use of diltiazem or verapamil with NYHA class III or IV heart failure	May worsen heart failure
Aspirin with no history of coronary, cerebral, or peripheral vascular symptoms or occlusive arterial event	Not indicated
Long-term (ie, >1 month) neuroleptics as long-term hypnotics	Risk of confusion, hypotension, extra-pyramidal side effects, falls
SSRIs with a history of clinically significant hyponatremia	SSRIs can precipitate hyponatremia
Diphenoxylate, loperamide, or codeine phosphate for treatment of diarrhea of unknown origin	Risk of delayed diagnosis; may exacerbate constipation with overflow diarrhea; may precipitate toxic megacolon in inflammatory bowel disease; may delay recovery in unrecognized gastroenteritis
Theophylline as monotherapy for COPD	Safer, more effective alternative; risk of adverse effects because of narrow therapeutic index
Bladder antimuscarinic drugs with dementia	Risk of increased confusion, agitation
Neuroleptic drugs in patient prone to fall	May cause gait dyspraxia, parkinsonism
Use of long-term powerful opiates (eg, morphine or fentanyl) as first-line therapy for mild-moderate pain	World Health Organization analgesic ladder not observed
Regular opiates for more than 2 weeks in those with chronic constipation without concurrent use of laxatives	Risk of severe constipation

COPD, chronic obstructive pulmonary disease; NYHA, New York Heart Association; SSRI, selective serotonin reuptake inhibitor.

[a]For the full list of STOPP criteria, see Gallagher P, O'Mahony D. STOPP (Screening Tool of Older Persons' potentially inappropriate Prescriptions): application to acutely ill elderly patients and comparison with Beers' criteria. *Age Ageing.* 2008;37(6):673-679.

prevention in nonvalvular atrial fibrillation and is used outside the United States for VTE prophylaxis after hip or knee replacement surgery. Dabigatran overdose cannot be reversed, and thus, the risk of severe, or even fatal, hemorrhage may make warfarin a more desirable choice. Reduced dosing is recommended in renal impairment. In Canada, doses are reduced for people age 80 years and older, although at this writing the labeling in the United States does not recommend any alteration in dose based on age.

B. Insulin

Older age is associated with increased risk of drug-induced hypoglycemia. Insulin is the second-most common cause

Table 9–3. START criteria: medications that should be used in older adults (barring extenuating circumstances).

- Warfarin in the presence of chronic atrial fibrillation[a]
- Aspirin or clopidogrel with a documented history of coronary, cerebral or peripheral vascular disease in patients in sinus rhythm[a]
- Angiotensin-converting enzyme (ACE) inhibitor in chronic heart failure[a]
- Regular inhaled β_2-agonist or anticholinergic agent for mild to moderate asthma or COPD
- L-DOPA (levodopa) in idiopathic Parkinson' disease with definite functional impairment and resultant disability
- Antidepressant in the presence of clearcut depressive symptoms, lasting at least 3 months
- Proton pump inhibitor in the presence of chronic severe gastroesophageal acid reflux or peptic stricture requiring dilatation
- Bisphosphonate in patients taking glucocorticoids for more than 1 month (ie, chronic corticosteroid therapy)
- Metformin with type 2 diabetes ± metabolic syndrome (in the absence of renal impairment)
- ACE inhibitor or angiotensin receptor blocker in diabetes with nephropathy

[a]Where therapy is not contraindicated.

For the full list of 22 criteria, see Barry PJ, Gallagher P, Ryan C, O'Mahony D. START (screening tool to alert doctors to the right treatment)—an evidence-based screening tool to detect prescribing omissions in elderly patients. *Age Ageing.* 2007;36(6):632-638.

of ADRs that lead to emergency room visits in older adults. Although insulin has a useful place in the treatment of diabetes, caution in prescribing is merited. Special attention should be paid to factors that may increase the risk and consequences of severe hypoglycemia. These risk factors include diminished renal function, use of medications that may interact with insulin's effects, and impaired cognitive function (which may interfere both with proper use and with the patient's ability to obtain help if hypoglycemia begins to occur). Long-acting basal insulins (eg, insulin glargine and insulin detemir) are less likely to cause hypoglycemia than neutral protamine Hagedorn (NPH) insulin. Sliding-scale insulin should be avoided, as it increases the risk of hypoglycemia without yielding improved glycemic control. (See also Chapter 42, "Diabetes.")

C. Long-acting Sulfonylureas

All sulfonylureas have the potential to cause hypoglycemia. In older adults, the risk of adverse events is particularly high with the long-acting sulfonylureas, including glyburide (also known as glibenclamide) and chlorpropamide. This excess risk is partly a consequence of accumulation of these drugs in patients with diminished drug clearance. If a sulfonylurea is used, a shorter-acting version, such as glipizide, is preferred.

D. Digoxin

Digoxin toxicity is common, often manifesting as neurologic abnormalities (including fatigue, confusion, or changes in color perception) and/or GI disturbances. Toxic effects including arrhythmias are accentuated in the presence of hypokalemia, which commonly occurs in patients who are also receiving loop diuretics. Impaired renal function and drug–drug interactions often result in elevated serum digoxin levels in older adults, although toxicity can occur even at serum digoxin levels within the normal range. Other agents are typically preferred for management of heart failure and atrial fibrillation with rapid ventricular response, although digoxin may be appropriate in select patients. If used, digoxin should be prescribed at doses ≤0.125 mg/day and patients carefully monitored for serum digoxin levels (aiming for the low-normal range), electrolytes (particularly hypokalemia), and for clinical signs of toxicity. New or worsening neurologic, GI, or cardiac signs or symptoms in a patient taking digoxin should be considered an adverse drug reaction until proven otherwise.

E. NSAIDs

NSAID-induced peptic ulcer disease and renal impairment occur more commonly in older adults than in younger adults. In addition, these drugs exacerbate hypertension, promote fluid retention in patients with heart failure, and antagonize the cardioprotective effects of aspirin through competitive inhibition of the cyclooxygenase (COX)-1 enzyme. The Beers

criteria and pain guidelines from the American Geriatrics Society discourage regular, chronic use of systemic NSAIDs in older adults, preferring acetaminophen, and in many cases opioids, for pain control. NSAIDs are contraindicated in patients with heart failure, renal dysfunction, and those at high risk of peptic ulcer-induced GI bleeding. Risk of this latter complication increases substantially in patients also taking warfarin, selective serotonin reuptake inhibitors (SSRIs), or systemic corticosteroids. If NSAIDs are used for longer than brief episodic use, the following considerations are advised: (a) use at the lowest dose and for the shortest duration possible; (b) coadminister proton pump inhibitors or misoprostol for gastroprotection; (c) maximize the time between taking cardioprotective aspirin and taking an NSAID (ie, take aspirin upon awakening, delay taking NSAIDs until at least 2 hours later); and (d) consider followup in 2–4 weeks after starting an NSAID to evaluate for renal dysfunction, fluid retention, and blood pressure elevation. NSAIDs with a balanced inhibition of COX-1 and COX-2 are preferred in patients who are at risk of cardiovascular disease. Consistent with this, some data suggest that naproxen has among the most favorable cardiovascular risk profiles. Topical NSAIDs, such as topical diclofenac gel, have relatively minimal systemic absorption and thus substantially lower risk of causing systemic toxicity.

F. Anticholinergics

Drugs that block the action of acetylcholine include sedatives, antihistamines, antidepressants, antipsychotics, bladder and GI antispasmodics, muscle relaxants, and antiemetics (see examples in Table 9–4). The cumulative burden of multiple anticholinergic drugs has been associated with an increased risk of falls, functional decline, and impaired cognition in older persons. If a medication with anticholinergic properties is considered necessary, substitution with a less anticholinergic medication in the same therapeutic category should be attempted when possible.

G. Opioids

Opioids are useful to treat moderate to severe pain in older persons, but opioids may be underused because of difficulty in diagnosing and assessing pain and concerns about safety and correct use of opioids. Safety concerns include an increased risk of delirium, GI side effects, and ventilatory depression. However, untreated pain can result in delirium, depression, decreased mobility, and impaired sleep. Changes in pharmacokinetics, as well as the increased pharmacodynamic effects of opioids, increase the risk of ADRs. Nonetheless, opioids can often be used safely when keeping these age-related changes in mind. In general, the dosing interval should be the same for an older person of any age, but it is typically appropriate to start with a low dose and titrate up the dose slowly, often termed 'start low and go slow.' Drug–drug interactions need to be kept in mind, as many opioids are

Table 9–4. Medications with anticholinergic properties.

Drug Type	Strong Anticholinergic Properties	Moderate Anticholinergic Properties
Anticonvulsants		Carbamazepine (Tegretol)
Antidepressants	Amitriptyline (Elavil) Desipramine (Norpramin) Doxepin (especially at doses >6 mg/day)	Paroxetine (Paxil)[a]
Antihistamines	Chlorpheniramine (Chlor-Trimeton) Diphenhydramine (Benadryl) Hydroxyzine (Atarax)	
Antipsychotics	Clozapine (Clozaril) Thioridazine (Mellaril)	Loxapine(Loxitane) Pimozide (Orap) Olanzapine (Zyprexa)[a] Quetiapine (Seroquel)[a]
Cardiovascular		Disopyramide (Norpace)
GI antispasmodics	Dicyclomine (Bentyl)	
H₂ antagonists		Cimetidine (Tagamet) Ranitidine (Zantac)
Muscle relaxants	Orphenadrine (Norflex)	Cyclobenzaprine (Flexeril)
Parkinson disease	Benztropine (Cogentin) Trihexyphenidyl (Artane)	
Urinary antispasmodics	Oxybutynin (Ditropan) Tolterodine (Detrol)	
Vertigo	Dimenhydrinate (Dramamine) Meclizine (Antivert) Scopolamine (TransDerm Scop)	

[a]Data from the Anticholinergic Drug Scale and Anticholinergic Cognitive Burden Scale (see the original scales for a complete list of medications with anticholinergic properties). These scales disagree on the degree of anticholinergic activity of olanzapine, paroxetine, and quetiapine.

substrates for P450 enzymes. Finally, tailoring treatment for renal or liver dysfunction may be necessary. For those with substantial renal impairment, morphine should be avoided, and hydromorphone, fentanyl, and methadone may be preferred alternatives. Methadone and codeine should not be used in severe liver impairment, and, in general, opioid dose should be reduced even further, with a longer dosing interval.

H. Antipsychotics in Dementia

The use of antipsychotics to treat behavioral and psychological symptoms of dementia is associated with increased likelihood of myocardial infarction, stroke, falls, fractures, VTE, and mortality. As a result, FDA warnings, practice guidelines, and initiatives from the Centers for Medicare and Medicaid Services have decreased their use. Older antipsychotics also have significant anticholinergic and extrapyramidal side effects. When possible, behavioral and psychological symptoms of dementia should be treated by nonpharmacologic means. When antipsychotics are deemed necessary for symptoms causing severe distress or harm, benefits and risks should be discussed with a patient's family or caregiver, the discussion should be clearly documented, and the antipsychotics should be used for a minimum duration of therapy with attempts to taper and discontinue the medication when possible.

PRESCRIBING FOR OLDER ADULTS

Explicit drugs-to-avoid criteria, attention to specific high-risk medications, and an understanding of technical elements of prescribing are important. Yet, these discrete skills address only a small proportion of potentially inappropriate prescribing in older adults. In most situations, close attention to several principles can be the most useful guide to optimizing prescribing decisions for older adults.

▶ Goals of Care

In younger and physically robust adults, there are typically standardized guidelines about the use of common drugs. These guidelines (both formal and informal) are based not only on the risks and benefits of drug therapy for an average patient, but also on the expectation that most people share similar values about what benefits and potential harms are most important to them. In contrast, older patients may have a different profile of benefits and risks than the "average" adult. Moreover, older adults hold widely varying views about what benefits they want their drugs to achieve and what harms are most important for them to avoid. For example, some older adults place great value on extending longevity and preventing future disease, whereas others are more interested in minimizing symptoms (both from their diseases and from drug side effects) and place a lower priority on life extension. Careful elicitation of a patient's goals of care—and keeping these goals of care in mind when prescribing—can help target therapy to achieve the goals most important to the patient and minimize the unwanted consequences most concerning to them.

▶ Time to Benefit

Medications used to prevent future health events (such as fracture, myocardial infarction, or renal failure) typically have a delayed time to benefit, with a meaningful reduction in risk not achieved until 1-2 or many years after the patient starts taking the drug. In contrast, adverse drug effects typically begin soon after a drug is started. Patients with limited life expectancy may thus spend the final period of their lives exposed to the harms of a drug, without living long enough to reap the benefits. (See tools for estimating life expectancy in Chapter 3, "Goals of Care & Consideration of Prognosis.") There are limited data on time to benefit for specific drugs in older adults, because most clinical trials of medications exclude older persons and those with multiple comorbid conditions. General estimates of time to benefit include:

- Glycemic control for patients with diabetes—at least 3 years for macrovascular complications (eg, myocardial infarction stroke) and 7 years for microvascular complications (eg, nephropathy, neuropathy)
- Bisphosphonates for osteoporosis—1.5 years to prevent fracture
- HMG-CoA reductase inhibitors ("statins") for patients with chronic cardiovascular disease—1 to 2 years to prevent cardiovascular events, and more than 3 years to prevent strokes

▶ Attention to Dose

Because older adults are more susceptible to adverse drug effects, it is often helpful to "start low and go slow," meaning to use a low starting dose and to advance the dose slowly. For many drugs, it is useful to start at half the regular adult starting dose. This can often be accomplished by splitting tablets using an inexpensive pill splitter. Of note, some patients with limited manual dexterity have difficulty splitting pills, and pills with sustained-release delivery mechanisms should not be split.

Careful attention should be placed on renal dysfunction and other characteristics that may result in increased serum levels, and dose escalation should stop at the lowest effective dose. Nevertheless, some older adults require the full dose of a drug, and many older patients are undertreated as a result of clinician reluctance to escalate the dose. This phenomenon is well-documented in the treatment of depression in older adults. Thus, continued dose escalation to the maximum dose is usually advisable if lower doses do not yield the desired effect and the patient is tolerating the drug.

▶ Monitoring

At the time a clinician prescribes a medication, she makes an educated guess that the probability of benefit exceeds the probability of harm, without definitively knowing which beneficial and harmful outcome(s) will occur. Monitoring for benefit and harm as determined by symptoms, signs, and laboratory tests can help determine to what extent a drug is actually helping or harming a patient, and thus plays a key role in individualizing care. Unfortunately, monitoring is often not consistently performed.

Few guidelines are available to guide the frequency of monitoring, either for laboratory values or for signs and symptoms. In the absence of specific evidence-based recommendations, a general approach can be helpful. Patients often underreport ADRs, and clinicians misinterpret these symptoms as markers of an underlying disease. Thus, once the decision is made to prescribe a drug patients should be educated and activated to understand and report medication-related problems (Figure 9–1). Then, at regular intervals the drug should be monitored for potential adverse effects and effectiveness, for patient adherence, and to assess whether the drug is still needed. Following subsequent modifications to the regimen (or not), the cycle repeats again. Although ongoing monitoring is important, in many cases adverse effects and effectiveness become apparent within the first several weeks of use, so particular attention should be paid to monitoring during this time. It is almost always useful to inquire about drug effectiveness, harms, and adherence in the first follow-up visit after a drug is started or changed.

▶ Adherence

Medications are not useful if patients don't take them. See "Adherence" below.

▶ Discontinuing Medications

Approximately 25% of patients suffer an adverse reaction upon withdrawing a medication, either because of return of the underlying disease or a physiologic withdrawal reaction (such as one might encounter with abrupt discontinuation of an opioid analgesic). To distinguish between drugs that can be stopped abruptly and those that need to be slowly tapered off, a rule of thumb is that if a drug generally requires a titration up from lower to higher doses, it should be titrated down instead of abruptly stopped. Examples of drugs that should not be discontinued abruptly are opioid analgesics, antidepressants, β blockers, and anticonvulsants such as gabapentin. In most cases, the rate of down-titration should match the rate at which one can safely up-titrate the drug. In contrast, drugs that can safely be started at maximum dose can typically be stopped abruptly without risking a physiologic withdrawal reaction. Examples include proton pump inhibitors and NSAIDs. In all cases, patients discontinuing a drug should be monitored for the return of signs or symptoms the drug was used to treat.

▶ Applying Clinical Trial Evidence and Evidence-Based Guidelines

Clinical trials that have established the efficacy of commonly used therapies have largely been conducted in relatively young and otherwise healthy populations. As a result, many have questioned the applicability of these findings to the care

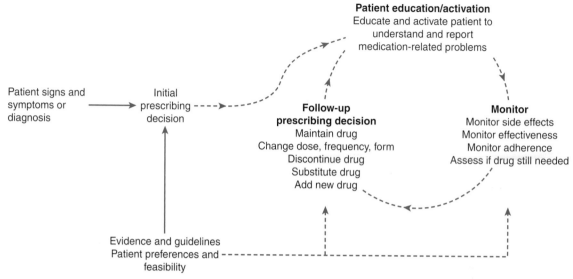

▲ **Figure 9–1.** Approach to monitoring for drug effectiveness, adverse events, and adherence. (Reproduced with permission from Steinman MA, Handler SM, Gurwitz JH, Schiff GD, Covinsky KE. Beyond the prescription: medication monitoring and adverse drug events in older adults. *J Am Geriatr Soc.* 2011;59:1513-1520.)

of clinically complex older adults. In addition, many clinical practice guidelines provide limited guidance about how their recommendations apply to adults who are frail or in the upper reaches of life span.

Despite this uncertainty, many of these therapies are likely beneficial for the majority of older adults. In some cases older adults may achieve greater benefits from drugs than the younger populations in which trials were conducted. Because older patients typically have a greater risk of developing the outcomes the drug is used to prevent, the relative reduction in risk associated with the drug translates to a greater absolute reduction in risk in older adults. Thus, while older adults can be more likely to suffer harms from drug therapy, in many cases they can have the most to gain. (See also Chapter 74 on extrapolating the evidence from clinical research to older patients).

Prescribing at the End of Life

Prescribing for patients with limited life expectancy typically requires a rebalancing of the benefits and harms of drug therapy. For many patients near the end of life, prevention of long-term outcomes through drugs used to prevent myocardial infarction, fracture, and other such outcomes is less relevant because of delayed time to benefit. Goals of care may shift to prioritizing quality of life and the minimization of medical interventions, and drugs to alleviate symptoms may continue to be highly valued. Difficulty swallowing can also complicate the delivery of oral therapies.

Several consensus recommendations have been published recommending drugs to be avoided in patients with limited life expectancy (typically less than 6 months to 1 year) and/or advanced dementia. Although there is no universal consensus, several groups recommend against routinely using bisphosphonates, cholesterol-lowering therapy, and warfarin. In contrast, bothersome symptoms are often underrecognized and undertreated in the patient in the terminal phase of life, and careful attention should be paid to pain control, constipation, and other symptoms. (See also Chapter 11, "Geriatrics & Palliative Care.")

ADHERENCE

Medication adherence refers to a patient actively participating in a therapeutic plan that has been agreed upon by a health care provider and the patient. Persistence refers to a patient taking a therapy for a necessary duration of time. Nonadherence and nonpersistence are prevalent problems, especially in the treatment of chronic, asymptomatic conditions like hypertension or hyperlipidemia. Nonadherence is associated with failure to achieve disease control, misdiagnoses, increased emergency room visits and hospitalizations, increased health care costs, and in some cases, higher mortality. Up to 40% of patients in the United States do not take their medications correctly, and failure to appreciate this could result in overprescription of additional medication. It is thus important to assess adherence regularly during clinical visits. Assessing adherence in a nonjudgmental fashion, such as asking how many doses are missed in a week, is a quick way to gauge adherence. Validated tools could also be used for regular monitoring, including the Morisky Medication Adherence Scale.

Major risk factors for nonadherence in chronic disease therapy include patients' beliefs that medications are not necessary or are harmful, side effects, cost and copay, and well as increased number of medications. Understanding the reason for nonadherence is essential for designing strategies to improve adherence. For example, if a patient is nonadherent because of high out-of-pocket costs for obtaining the drug, less-expensive drug alternatives or pharmaceutical assistance programs may be useful to consider. If a patient is nonadherent because the patient does not know what the drug is for, or believes that the drug is not providing benefit, educating the patient can be helpful. (Alternatively, if a patient taking a drug used to control symptoms believes the drug is not helping, this may be a sign to try another drug.) Drugs that require dosing 3 or 4 times per day can be difficult to take, and switching patients to a drug regimen that requires only once- or twice-daily dosing has proven to be one of the most successful strategies for improving adherence.

MANAGING COMPLEXITY

Optimizing prescribing for older adults is a complex process that requires balancing multiple considerations. While seemingly daunting, several strategies can be helpful to unpack this complexity and approach these issues in a systematic manner.

▶ Regular Medication Review

Experts recommend that regular medication review occur at least annually. Patients with multiple medication changes may benefit from more frequent review.

A. Brown Bag Review

A highly effective technique for medication review is the "brown bag review," in which the patient is instructed to put all of their medications (including over-the-counter, herbal, and other products) into a bag and bring it to clinic for inspection. In addition to reconciling the medications taken by a patient, this review provides a valuable opportunity to assess patient understanding and adherence. Multiple bottles of the same medicine, prescriptions whose label indicates that they were dispensed many months (or years) ago, and other visual clues can help identify potential problems. For each drug, asking "Do you know what this is for?"; "How do you take this?"; and "Do you sometimes not take it or miss a dose?" (and if yes, inquiring why) can provide valuable clues to improve adherence. Finally, asking the patient "Are you having any problems with this drug" and probing for common and dangerous adverse effects can help elicit previously underreported adverse drug effects.

B. Critically Reviewing the Medication List

Another important goal of medication review is to provide the clinician an opportunity to think critically and holistically about the medication regimen, rather than the piecemeal approach that often accompanies a typical visit in which the focus is on 1 or 2 specific diseases. This holistic review can include identifying drugs that are no longer needed (ie, overuse), drugs with inadequate or excessive doses or instances where an alternative drug is likely to be safer or more effective (ie, misuse), and omissions of potentially beneficial drugs (ie, underuse). The Medication Appropriateness Index provides a useful list of 10 questions to consider for each drug a patient is taking (Table 9–5).

A helpful strategy for reviewing the medication list is to group medicines by the patient's diseases or syndromes they are used to treat. This way of organizing medication information can highlight potential problems. If the patient is taking a drug with no corresponding disease on the patient's problem list, it may be unnecessary. For example, if a patient is taking a proton pump inhibitor and does not have a diagnosis of gastroesophageal reflux disease (GERD) or is not a chronic user of NSAIDs, the drug may be unnecessary. If a patient has a disease with no corresponding medication, this may represent underuse. For example, if an older male has bothersome lower urinary tract symptoms that persist despite lifestyle modifications, a trial of an α-blocker may be warranted. If a patient has poorly controlled disease for which the patient is taking multiple medications, this might indicate suboptimal doses, poor adherence, or a complicating factor. For instance, if an older patient has poorly controlled hypertension and is taking 4 antihypertensive medications, further investigation for nonadherence and potential secondary causes of hypertension may be useful. Finally, careful review of medications can identify other potential problems. For example, if

Table 9–5. Questions to consider during a medication review.

1. Is there an indication for the drug?
2. Is the medication effective for the condition?
3. Is the dosage correct?
4. Are the directions correct?
5. Are the directions practical?
6. Are there clinically significant drug-drug interactions?
7. Are there clinically significant drug-disease/condition interactions?
8. Is there unnecessary duplication with other drugs?
9. Is the duration of therapy acceptable?
10. Is this drug the least-expensive alternative compared with others of equal utility?

Adapted and reproduced with permission from the Medication Appropriateness Index in Hanlon JT, Schmader KE, Samsa GP, et al. A method for assessing drug therapy appropriateness. *J Clin Epidemiol.* 1992;45(10):1045-1051.

a patient is taking a medication with strong anticholinergic properties, it is worth inquiring about anticholinergic side effects and considering if there is another medicine that can provide the same benefit with less potential for harm.

Interdisciplinary Care

Careful attention to pharmaceutical care for older adults is time-consuming, and is best done using a team approach where feasible. Pharmacists can play an essential role, bringing both content expertise and dedicated time to assessing potential medication problems, reconciling medications, and evaluating and improving patient adherence. The emergence of patient-centered medical home models of care is increasingly integrating pharmacists into primary care clinics, providing opportunities to share workload and expertise. Several other opportunities are also available. Under Medicare Part D (the prescription drug benefit), health plans are required to offer medication therapy management services to high-risk older adults, including comprehensive medication review conducted in-person or by phone at least annually. The scope and impact of these programs is evolving and has yet to be clearly determined. Community pharmacists can work with prescribers and patients, and consultant pharmacists (expert consultants in geriatric pharmacotherapy) can be engaged to provide comprehensive medication review and reconciliation, monitor medications, improve adherence, identify prescription assistance programs to help lower drug costs, and more. In the inpatient setting, hospital pharmacists rounding with teams reduces ADRs, and pharmacists have been widely employed to assist with medication reconciliation at admission and discharge. Nurses can also be valuable partners, helping to reconcile medications, screen for adverse events, and monitor drug effectiveness (eg, through structured protocols for hypertension management, keeping track of overdue laboratory tests for drug monitoring, and so forth).

PRESCRIBING ACROSS THE CARE CONTINUUM

Although general principles of prescribing apply to different care settings, certain considerations merit special mention in the hospital and nursing home.

Prescribing in the Hospital

Hospitalized older adults are particularly prone to medication misadventures for a number of reasons. Errors in medication reconciliation and communication between providers commonly occur at various stages of transition, including admission, transfer between hospital units, and discharge. Ensuring that patients continue to receive the right medications as they move between providers and locations is critical. Hospital-based pharmacists have been shown to be helpful in improving outcomes related to medication reconciliation during these transitions and should be involved when possible. Medications started for transient reasons during hospital stays are often mistakenly continued at discharge, and may become a permanent fixture on the patient's medication regimen. Careful attention should be paid to discontinuing proton pump inhibitors that may have been started for stress ulcer prophylaxis (itself a questionable indication), analgesic medications for pain that is no longer present, and so forth.

Clinicians may be tempted to change medication regimens for chronic diseases during hospital stays. In many cases, this temptation should be resisted. Measures of chronic disease control measured during a hospital stay (ie elevated blood pressure and worse lipid profiles) may not be representative of the patient's usual status, and contextual factors, such as contraindications for a drug, may be known by the primary care provider but not by the inpatient team. Changing multiple medications also increases the risk of adverse drug events. Yet, if important quality gaps are identified, hospital stays can provide an opportune time to rectify these problems if done in consultation with the patient's primary care clinician.

Sedative/hypnotic drugs or anticholinergic agents such as diphenhydramine are often prescribed "as needed" to hospitalized older adults to aid sleep. These drugs increase the risk of falls and delirium and should be avoided if possible. Instead, environmental interventions such as limiting nighttime vital signs and reducing noise and light stimulation are preferable.

Prescribing in Nursing Homes

Patients in long-term care often have multiple medication conditions, physical frailty and/or cognitive impairment, and use an average of 7 to 8 medications. Prescribing for such patients is complex, and they are at high risk of adverse drug events.

Antipsychotic medications are prescribed to roughly one-quarter to one-third of nursing home residents in the United States, often to manage behavioral problems of dementia. Unfortunately, these drugs confer a substantially increased risk of death in older adults with dementia. Use should be avoided for behavioral management unless nondrug interventions have failed and the patient is a threat to himself or herself or others. Because psychotropic medications have long been prescribed at inappropriately high rates to nursing home patients, federal regulations require that each patient receiving these medicines has ongoing documentation of the reason for treatment, how medication effectiveness and adverse effects will be monitored, and plans for dose reduction or treatment continuation.

Federal regulations also require a pharmacist to conduct monthly medication review of patients in long-term care facilities. Unfortunately, such reviews have at times been found to be deficient, and should not be relied on to catch prescribing problems.

Bain KT, Holmes HM, Beers MH, Maio V, Handler SM, Pauker SG. Discontinuing medications: a novel approach for revising the prescribing stage of the medication-use process. *J Am Geriatr Soc.* 2008;56(10):1946-1952.

Boyd CM, Darer J, Boult C, Fried LP, Boult L, Wu AW. Clinical practice guidelines and quality of care for older patients with multiple comorbid diseases: implications for pay for performance. *JAMA.* 2005;294(6):716-724.

Gurwitz JH. Polypharmacy: a new paradigm for quality drug therapy in the elderly? *Arch Intern Med.* 2004;164(18): 1957-1959.

Holmes HM, Hayley DC, Alexander GC, Sachs GA. Reconsidering medication appropriateness for patients late in life. *Arch Intern Med.* 2006;166(6):605-609.

Mallet L, Spinewine A, Huang A. The challenge of managing drug interactions in elderly people. *Lancet.* 2007;370(9582):185-191.

Marcum ZA, Gellad WF. Medication adherence to multidrug regimens. *Clin Geriatr Med.* 2012;28(2):287-300.

Osterberg L, Blaschke T. Adherence to medication. *N Engl J Med.* 2005;353(5):487-497.

Schiff GD, Galanter WL. Promoting more conservative prescribing. *JAMA.* 2009;301(8):865-867.

Scott IA, Gray LC, Martin JH, Mitchell CA. Minimizing inappropriate medications in older populations: a 10-step conceptual framework. *Am J Med.* 2012;125(6):529-537.

Steinman MA, Handler SM, Gurwitz JH, Schiff GD, Covinsky KE. Beyond the prescription: medication monitoring and adverse drug events in older adults. *J Am Geriatr Soc.* 2011;59: 1513-1520.

Steinman MA, Hanlon JT. Managing medications in clinically complex elders: "There's got to be a happy medium." *JAMA.* 2010;304:1592-1601.

USEFUL WEBSITES

ACOVE-3 Criteria. *Introduction to Quality Indicators* (explicit criteria to identify potentially inappropriate medication use and to identify potential underuse of medications). http://www.rand.org/health/projects/acove/acove3.html

Age and Ageing. START criteria (in START [screening tool to alert doctors to the right treatment]—an evidence-based screening tool to detect prescribing omissions in elderly patients) (complete article; explicit criteria to identify potential underuse of medications) http://ageing.oxfordjournals.org/content/36/6/632.long

American Geriatrics Society. *AGS Beers Criteria 2012* (explicit criteria to identify potentially inappropriate medication use). http://www.americangeriatrics.org/health_care_professionals/clinical_practice/clinical_guidelines_recommendations/2012/

American Pharmacists Association. *What is Medication Therapy Management?* http://www.pharmacist.com/MTM

American Society of Consultant Pharmacists. *Medication Management.* http://www.ascp.com

Anticholinergic drug scale. http://www.ncbi.nlm.nih.gov/pubmed/18332297

DailyMed (information from package inserts). http://dailymed.nlm.nih.gov

GlobalRPh. Calculators including renal function online calculator. http://www.globalrph.com/multiple_crcl.htm

Indiana University Department of Medicine. *Cytochrome P450 Drug Interaction Table* (drug–drug interactions). http://medicine.iupui.edu/clinpharm/DDIs/

Indianapolis Discovery Network for Dementia. *Anticholinergic Cognitive Burden Scale.* http://www.indydiscoverynetwork.org/AnticholinergicCognitiveBurdenScale.html

Medline Plus. *Drugs, Supplements, and Herbal Information* (drug information for patients). http://www.nlm.nih.gov/medlineplus/druginformation.html

Morisky Medication Adherence Scale. http://www.acpinternist.org/archives/2009/02/adherence.pdf

National Council on Patient Information and Education (NCPIE). *Medication Use Safety Training (MUST) for Seniors.* http://www.mustforseniors.org

Proprietary drug–drug interaction programs, including www.epocrates.com (free), and www.lexicomp.com and www.micromedex.com (subscription only)

STOPP Criteria (explicit criteria to identify potentially inappropriate medication use). http://www.ncbi.nlm.nih.gov/pubmed/18218287

Addressing Multimorbidity in Older Adults

10

Cynthia M. Boyd, MD, MPH

Christine Ritchie, MD, MSPH

BACKGROUND AND DEFINITIONS

Multimorbidity is often defined as the presence of 2 or more chronic co-occurring conditions. Although this is the formal definition, most clinicians consider multimorbidity to be particularly vexing when it involves a broad array of conditions and is also accompanied by functional limitations, cognitive impairment or mental health concerns, as well as interactions between the conditions themselves and their treatments.

Among older adults, multimorbidity is the rule rather than the exception: almost half of those age 65–69 years old have 2 or more chronic conditions; this proportion increases to 75% among those age 85 years or older. Thanks to public health interventions, technology and overall population aging, the proportion of older adults with multimorbidity has grown significantly in the past decade. Among those age 65 years or older, the number of those with 2 or more conditions (from among 9 measured conditions) grew 22%. Clearly, multimorbidity will play a growing role in routine medical practice.

MULTIMORBIDITY AND HEALTH OUTCOMES

Multimorbidity is associated with a number of negative health outcomes, including accelerated declines in functional status, increased symptom burden, reduced quality of life, and mortality. Increasing numbers of chronic conditions place older adults at higher risk of hospitalization and nursing home placement. Accordingly, increased costs of care follow increased numbers of chronic conditions. In a study of more than 1 million Medicare beneficiaries, when 7 conditions were considered, average per-person cost of care increased from $211/year with no chronic conditions to $1870 with 2 or more conditions to $8159 for those with 5 conditions. Those with 7 or more conditions averaged more than $23,000 per year. As health care systems become increasingly accountable for care across care settings, development of effective approaches to support older adults with multimorbidity will likely become a growing priority.

CLINICIAN CHALLENGES IN THE CARE OF OLDER ADULTS WITH MULTIMORBIDITY

Clinicians caring for older adults with multimorbidity face a number of challenges in their management. This is true for both specialists and primary care clinicians, which may include physicians and allied health professionals. First, there is a disturbing lack of evidence for specific treatments among those with multiple chronic conditions as these individuals are commonly excluded from clinical trials. In a study examining a sample of randomized controlled trials (RCTs) published from 1995 to 2010 in the 5 highest-impact-factor general medical journals, individuals with multimorbidity were excluded in 63% of the 284 RCTs identified. In a separate examination of 11 Cochrane Reviews evaluating clinical trials of treatments for 4 chronic diseases (diabetes, heart failure, chronic obstructive pulmonary disease, and stroke), less than half described the prevalence among trial participants of any comorbidity co-occurring with the index condition. In addition to being excluded from many RCTs, multimorbidity is often not accounted for in clinical guidelines. If clinical practice guidelines for a particular condition acknowledge the presence of comorbid conditions, they often do not offer recommendations that take into account these other co-occurring conditions. This is particularly true if the condition is discordant (eg, the condition is pathophysiologically distinct from the condition of interest and therefore does not share treatments—in contrast to treatment concordant conditions that share treatments, such as diabetes and hypertension). For suggestions about how to apply clinical evidence from research to the older patient, see Chapter 74.

Second, older adults with multimorbidity frequently present special management challenges. Their medical and social complexity often leads to complicated treatment regimens that are difficult for patients to understand and challenging for clinicians to explain. Communication requirements are often intensified as a result of the need to coordinate with other clinicians and interact with patients and their family members. Goal setting and discussion of benefits and burdens of treatment also become more demanding when benefits of one treatment potentially contribute to burdens of another condition. All of these challenges are amplified in the setting of cognitive impairment. Time demands leave many clinicians feeling like they cannot go in-depth with these patients and contribute to frustration and a sense of incompetence.

Finally, financial compensation for patients with multimorbidity rarely corresponds to the time and effort required to appropriately care for these patients. Even with extended visit codes, the effort required to review long medication lists and medical records, communicate with other clinicians, and interact with family members generally exceeds reimbursement, particularly as many of these tasks fall outside the in-person visit itself.

GENERAL CONSIDERATIONS IN THE CARE OF MULTIMORBID OLDER ADULTS

Despite the challenges intrinsic to caring for someone with multimorbidity, provision of higher quality, more gratifying care can occur when a few guiding principles are taken into account. These guiding principles were initially developed by a national expert panel on multimorbidity of the American Geriatrics Society. The panel performed an extensive review of the literature and synthesized these findings into practical perspectives for clinicians. We discuss 3 steps that can support clinicians in their care of older adults with multimorbidity: ascertainment of prognosis, elicitation of patient preferences, and assessment and management of treatment complexity.

Because, in older adults with multimorbidity, tension exists between benefit from a particular intervention and possible harm from complications or interactions with other conditions, it is very important to ascertain as best as possible the older person's prognosis. Prognosis ideally should be considered not just for survival but also for function and quality of life (see Chapter 3, "Goals of Care & Consideration of Prognosis," for more details). Determination of prognosis can provide the appropriate context for elicitation of preferences for particular treatments. It offers the backdrop for decisions related to (a) disease prevention or treatment (eg, whether or not to start or stop a medication or insert or replace a device); (b) disease screening (eg, cancer); and (c) use of specific services (eg, whether or not to admit a patient to the hospital or enroll them into hospice).

Elicitation of patient preferences can help guide the management of older adults with multimorbidity. Patient preferences take many forms: preferences regarding the importance of any one condition over another, preferences regarding

states of being and how much burden is acceptable in order to achieve a particular state of being (also called an outcome; eg, survival, higher functional status, or better quality of life), and preferences regarding particular treatments in light of potential benefits and burdens associated with that treatment.

Involving patients and their caregivers (when appropriate) is particularly important when treatment decisions are preference-sensitive. Preference-sensitive decisions are those that (a) relate to therapies that might help one condition but lead to worse outcomes in another (antiinflammatory agents that might reduce pain but increase risk for gastrointestinal bleeding); (b) therapies that may be beneficial over the long term but are at risk for causing short-term harm (anticoagulants for stroke prevention); or (c) therapies that may include multiple medications with potential harmful interactions (such as heart failure medications and medications for chronic obstructive pulmonary disease). Table 10–1 offers some language for elicitation of preferences.

It is also important that patients and their caregivers understand as well as is possible the potential benefits and harms of a particular treatment. Unfortunately, the evidence base for risks and benefits for many treatments are not evaluated in the context of multimorbidity and must be extrapolated from single condition studies and observational studies. Regardless, it is incumbent on clinicians to communicate what is known in language that makes sense to patients. Table 10–2 provides some general suggestions for ways to communicate benefits and harms.

Treatment complexity is common in patients with multimorbidity. The Medication Regimen Complexity Index

Table 10–1. Language for eliciting patient preferences.

Question Purpose	Question
To understand patient's view of their quality of life	How would you consider your current quality of life?
To understand patient's view of their future	What sort of things have you been thinking about especially as you think about the future?
To learn patient's values	What kinds of things are important to you now? (*Or if surrogate:* If your loved one were able to tell us what she is thinking, what things would she think are important now?)
To learn patient's preferences	Some people want to live as long as possible no matter the risks, including being willing to accept hospitalizations and less independence. Other people are less willing to compromise their quality of life or independence and would defer [treatment] knowing this may limit their survival. Do you have an idea of what kind of person you might be?

Table 10–2. Strategies to communicate risks and benefits of treatments or diagnostic tests.

Do	Don't
Use numerical likelihoods	Use words like "rarely" and "frequently"
Provide the likelihood of an event both occurring and not occurring	Provide the likelihood in only 1 direction either in favor of benefit or harm
Provide absolute risks	Provide relative risks
Offer visual aids and assess understanding	Assume the patient understands

Table 10–3. Tools to identify treatment complexity.

Tool	Description
Medication Management Ability Assessment	Role-play task that simulates a prescribed medication regimen, similar in complexity to one to which an older person is likely to be exposed
Drug Regimen Unassisted Grading Scale	DRUGS- (1) *identification:* showing the appropriate medications, (2) *access:* opening the appropriate containers, (3) *dosage:* dispensing the correct number per dose, and (4) *timing:* demonstrating the appropriate timing of do
Hopkins Medication Schedule	Role play that includes the following: "Read the medication instructions below. Assume that you eat breakfast, lunch, and dinner at the following listed times. Please indicate at what times you should take each medication and how many you need to take. Also, indicate when your should drink water and eat any snacks."
Medication Management Instrument for Deficiencies in the Elderly	Twenty item assessment that covers three domains relevant to medication adherence (knowledge of medications, how to take medications, and procurement) and yields a total score of 13 or less.

(MRCI) captures some of the elements of complexity by capturing (a) the steps in the task, (b) the number of choices, (c) the duration of execution, (d) the process of administration, and (e) the patterns of intervening and potentially distracting tasks. It highlights the multiple dimensions of treatment patients have to contend with when managing their conditions. For clinicians who strictly follow individual clinical practice guidelines, regimens for patients can be both complex and also onerous and costly. Boyd et al described the implications of following individual practice guidelines for an older woman with the following conditions of *moderate severity:* chronic obstructive pulmonary disease (COPD), hypertension (HTN), diabetes mellitus (DM), osteoporosis, osteoarthritis. If clinical practice guidelines were followed, the patient would be taking 19 doses per day at 4 different time points. Assuming no prescription drug coverage, this regimen would cost $407 per month and $4877 per year. Complex treatment regimens increase risk for nonadherence, adverse reactions, reduced quality of life, financial burden, and caregiver stress.

Given the problems associated with complex treatment regimens, it is worthwhile to consider ways to reduce or mitigate treatment burden or complexity. A number of tools have been developed that can assist the provider in both identifying complex medication regimens that pose potential difficulties for patient self management along with strategies to reduce treatment complexity and optimize outcomes. Table 10–3 lists tools that can be used to assess treatment complexity and ability to manage it. Table 10–4 lists a few approaches that can be used by a patient's clinical team to address candidate medications to discontinue to decrease treatment complexity.

SUMMARY

Addressing multimorbidity in clinical practice is essential. Cumulatively adding treatments and interventions for individual conditions in persons with multimorbidity may be harmful for patients by increasing the risk for interactions between treatments and between treatments and other conditions, as well as by affecting adherence and quality of life. Thus, an individualized approach to care is necessary to make the complex decisions about which treatments and interventions are most likely to help an individual patient, and is based on the elicitation of patient preferences, assessment of prognosis for all outcomes, and minimization of treatment complexity and burden.

Table 10–4. Strategies to reduce treatment complexity and burden.

Tool	Description
Screening Tool to Alert to Right Treatment and Screening Tool of Older Persons' potentially inappropriate Prescriptions (START/STOPP)	Algorithm of medications that should be considered in certain conditions and medications that may be inappropriate to use in certain conditions
Good-Palliative Geriatric Practice (GP-GP) algorithm	Series of questions that can provide guidance of the ongoing utility or value of continuing a medication based on the patient's prognosis or the underlying evidence base

American Geriatrics Society Expert Panel on the Care of Older Adults with Multimorbidity. Guiding principles for the care of older adults with multimorbidity: an approach for clinicians. *J Am Geriatr Soc.* 2012;60(10):E1-E25.

Boult C, Wieland GD. Comprehensive primary care for older patients with multiple chronic conditions: "nobody rushes you through." *JAMA.* 2010;304(17):1936-1943.

Boyd CM, Darer J, Boult C, Fried LP, Boult L, Wu AW. Clinical practice guidelines and quality of care for older patients with multiple comorbid diseases: implications for pay for performance. *JAMA.* 2005;294(6):716-724.

Fried TR, Tinetti M, Agostini J, Iannone L, Towle V. Health outcome prioritization to elicit preferences of older persons with multiple health conditions. *Patient Educ Couns.* 2011;83(2):278-282.

Gallagher P, O'Mahony D. STOPP (Screening Tool of Older Persons' potentially inappropriate Prescriptions): application to acutely ill elderly patients and comparison with beers' criteria. *Age Ageing.* 2008;37(6):673-679.

Jadad AR, To MJ, Emara M, Jones J. Consideration of multiple chronic diseases in randomized controlled trials. *JAMA.* 2011;306(24):2670-2672.

Orwig D, Brandt N, Gruber-Baldini AL Medication management assessment for older adults in the community. Gerontologist. 2006;46(5):661-668.

The American Geriatrics Society 2012 Beers Criteria Update Expert Panel. American Geriatrics Society updated Beers criteria for potentially inappropriate medication use in older adults. *J Am Geriatr Soc.* 2012;60(4):616-631.

Wolff JL, Starfield B, Anderson G. Prevalence, expenditures, and complications of multiple chronic conditions in the elderly. *Arch Intern Med.* 2002;162(20):2269-2276.

Geriatrics & Palliative Care

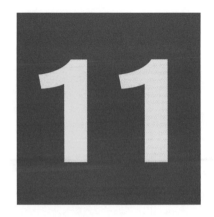

John G. Cagle, PhD, MSW
Eric W. Widera, MD

OVERVIEW OF PALLIATIVE CARE

Palliative care is a specialized form of interdisciplinary care for individuals with serious and life-threatening illnesses. An overarching goal of palliative care is to enhance quality of life for patients, which often involves high-quality pain and symptom management, clear communication about medical conditions, and matching a patient's goals of care with the appropriate treatments. This model of care is patient/family-centered, honoring patient/family values and preference through a shared decision-making process. It also recognizes and attempts to address the complex multidimensional needs of older adults and their families, including social, psychological/emotional, spiritual, and medical aspects (Figure 11–1).

Palliative care is a fast-growing form of care across settings that can generally be delivered concurrently with life-prolonging treatments and is not prognosis dependent. Hospice is a form of palliative care given to patients who meet certain conditions formalized under the Hospice Medicare Benefit. According to Medicare eligibility criteria, hospice care is only available to individuals who: (a) agree to forgo Medicare coverage of curative treatments for their terminal disease, and (b) have an estimated prognosis of 6 months or less to live if the illness progresses as expected. Hospice care is usually delivered in the patient's home or current place of residence, such as a nursing home or assisted-living community. Older adults with multiple chronic conditions are often not offered hospice even though it might be beneficial, because prognostication is more difficult in this population. Studies consistently demonstrate that both hospice and nonhospice palliative care can improve outcomes across diverse health care settings, including better pain management, lower rehospitalization, and greater family satisfaction.

PSYCHOLOGICAL, SPIRITUAL, AND SOCIAL ISSUES

Patients and families express a wide variety of psychological, spiritual, and social needs during the advent of serious illness. Preserving control and independence, accessing information (eg, regarding disease progression and expectations), managing anxiety and depression, dealing with financial burdens, and spiritual support are frequently cited concerns. Active collaboration with core members of the palliative care team, such as the social worker, chaplain, nurse, and nurse aide, is highly advised to help coordinate care, improve transitions between settings, and address the multidimensional needs of patients and their families. Supporting family members and informal caregivers is also a central focus of high-quality palliative care. Networks of family and friends often provide the bulk of hands-on assistance for sick and frail older adults, particularly those who are community dwelling. Thus, members of these informal care networks often require basic education about activities of daily living (ADLs) and instrumental activities of daily living (IADLs) assistance (eg, how to transfer the patient or administer medication), and knowledge of and access to community resources, such as emotional and spiritual support.

Illness, dying, and death are culturally defined phenomena and, thus, clinicians should be prepared to honor a range of diverse belief systems—which may, in some cases, conflict with conventional practice approaches. For example, discussing prognosis may be considered culturally taboo for some patients, or a shared decision-making process maybe preferred over a self-directed approach to care.

COMMUNICATION, DECISION MAKING, AND ADVANCE CARE PLANNING

Good communication is critical to ensuring high-quality palliative care. Shared decision making is a widely espoused process of communication between health care providers and family members that involves: (a) a review of the decisions that need to be made; (b) exchanging information about patient/family values, the patient's current health status, and the risks and benefits of available treatment options; (c) ensuring that all parties understand the information

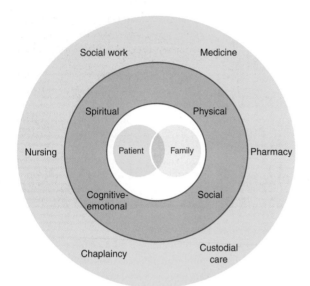

▲ Figure 11–1. The interdisciplinary model of care. This figure illustrates how core members of the palliative care team work together to meet the needs of the patient and family.

being provided; (d) a discussion of preferred roles in decision making; and (e) reaching an agreement about treatment that is congruent with patient/family values and preferences. All pertinent health care preferences and decisions should be documented in advance directives and honored by the attending health professionals. When initiating discussions about advance care planning, it may be helpful for physicians to begin by exploring the patient's priorities in terms of comfort, longevity, or functionality. Because goals and preferences can change over time, these discussions should be considered part of an ongoing dialogue; revising advance directives accordingly. In the course of caring for someone with a chronic progressive disease like Alzheimer' dementia, it is imperative that these discussions occur early on with both patients and their families, as a patient's capacity to make health care decisions may diminish over time.

Because palliative care patients are often coping with serious, complex, and life-threatening conditions, it is essential that clinicians prepare themselves to broach these difficult topics. Breaking bad news, such as a life-threatening illness or the lack of effective treatment options, can be very troubling for clinicians. When delivering bad news, the SPIKES (setup, perception, invitation, knowledge, empathize, summarize and strategize) model provides a framework when preparing for difficult conversations.

- *Setup*—Try to find a private space; prepare yourself for some of the difficult questions and emotions that may arise during the meeting.

- *Perception*—Begin by asking what the patient/family already know or what they think is going on.

- *Invitation*—Explore how much information the patient/family need and want.

- *Knowledge*—Give the facts of the situation in clear, easy to understand language; also discuss the unknown factors.

- *Empathize*—Acknowledge that this is difficult news to digest.

- *Summarize and Strategize*—Review what was discussed, including any decisions that were made, and talk about next steps.

Additionally, involving members of the interdisciplinary team who have expertise in family dynamics and communication skills may also facilitate an open discussion of such difficult topics and decision making.

CHALLENGES TO PROVIDING PALLIATIVE CARE IN LONG-TERM CARE SETTINGS

Nearly 1 of every 4 deaths in the United States occurs in a long-term care setting. These deaths are associated with brief lengths of stay, high rates of burdensome treatments and hospitalization, underuse of effective symptom management therapies, and low utilization of hospice and palliative care services. There are numerous challenges to improving end-of-life care in long-term care, including a high prevalence of comorbid conditions among residents, which complicates any diagnostic or therapeutic management plan. Alzheimer disease and other progressive neurodegenerative conditions are common, limiting the ability for residents to report symptoms and making it difficult for health care providers to assess for them. Prognostic ambiguity and poor communication between physicians, staff and family members can delay the transition from a restorative approach to care to one focused on comfort and quality of life. A lack of physician or midlevel providers, and limitations to timely diagnostic testing, increase the odds that residents will be transferred to an acute care facility instead of being managed in the resident's current setting. Additionally, high staff turnover decreases the effectiveness of palliative care training among nursing home staff and has been associated with lower quality of care.

▶ Symptom Management

A. Pain

The assessment of pain in older adults begins with patient report. Patient report is the "gold standard" for assessment and should be attempted in all patients independent of cognitive status, as those with moderate to severe dementia may be able to communicate the presence and severity of pain. However, self-report alone is often insufficient for in individuals with cognitive impairment. It is, therefore, important to use a combination of patient report, caregiver report and direct observation of the patient to inform a clinical assessment. Verbal descriptor scales, the pain thermometer, or Faces Pain Scales can be used as alternatives to verbal numeric rating scales or visual analogue scales, which may be difficult to use for individuals with diminished cognitive status. Observational signs of distress may include changes in facial expressions, vocalizations, body movements, social interactions, activity patterns, and mental status. Several observational scales have been developed to assess for pain, including the Pain Assessment in Advanced Dementia (PAINAD) and the Pain Assessment Checklist for Seniors with Limited Ability to Communicate (PACSLAC).

The choice of an analgesic medication should be made based on the severity of pain, previous responses to analgesic medications, possible interactions of the analgesic with comorbid conditions or other medications, care setting and support services. Acetaminophen should be considered the first line of therapy for mild pain, although care should be taken not to exceed a total daily dose of 3 g in most older adults. Acetaminophen should also be considered with new dementia-related behavior changes even when the presence of pain is uncertain, as there is evidence that its use may decrease these behaviors, as well as improve activity levels and social engagement. Nonsteroidal antiinflammatory drugs (NSAIDs) should generally be used with caution in older adults because of the high risk of side effects, such as renal failure, gastrointestinal irritation, and worsening heart failure.

Opioids are primarily used for moderate to severe pain, although nonopioid therapies, such as corticosteroids, antiepileptics, antidepressants, and topical agents, such as capsaicin and lidocaine patches, remain important adjunct therapies to control pain. Table 11–1 lists commonly used opioids, with estimated conversions when going from one drug, or route of administration, to another. One opioid that should be avoided for all older adults is meperidine, as its metabolites often lead to neuroexcitatory adverse effects such as delirium. In addition, morphine and codeine should be avoided with patients who have a history of renal insufficiency. Long-acting opioids, such as extended-release

morphine or transdermal fentanyl patches, are useful when pain is persistent to ensure continuous pain relief throughout the day, with an additional short-acting immediate-release opioid to provide as-needed breakthrough pain relief. An effective and safe dose for a breakthrough opioid is approximately 10% of the total 24-hour standing dose.

Health care providers are often hesitant to use opioids in older adults because of a concern that they may exacerbate comorbid illnesses or precipitate adverse effects such as delirium. However, there is good evidence that undertreatment of pain is a greater risk factor for the development of delirium than the use of opioids. In long-term care settings in particular, the undertreatment of pain is of serious concern. This is partly because when orders are written for "PRN" (as needed) pain medications, they are rarely given—not even when there is evidence of patient discomfort. Clinicians should be especially specific when drafting orders for patients in long-term care. For example, to evaluate and treat breakthrough pain, an order might state: "Observe patient every 2 hours. If patient exhibits behaviors consistent with physical discomfort (eg, grimacing, guarding, moaning), administer morphine 5 mg oral solution." or "Ask patient to rate pain every 2 hours. If patient reports a pain level of 5 or higher on a 0 to 10 scale, administer 5 mg of oral morphine." If opioids are prescribed, constipation should be aggressively managed with a stimulant laxative, such as senna. Methylnaltrexone, a multireceptor antagonist that does not effectively cross the blood–brain barrier, can be given subcutaneously as a second-line agent to reverse refractory opioid-induced constipation. (See Chapter 54, "Managing Persistent Pain in Older Adults," for more detailed approaches to chronic pain management in the older adult.)

B. Dyspnea

Dyspnea is a common symptom among older palliative care patients, particularly those with chronic obstructive pulmonary disease (COPD), congestive heart failure (CHF), end-stage pulmonary disease, and lung cancer. Dyspnea is characterized by rapid, labored, or shallow breathing—and may be underdiagnosed and undertreated because of the patient's diminished capacity to communicate during advanced illness. Use of the Visual Numeric Scale or the Modified Borg Scale may facilitate assessment and assist with monitoring treatment efficacy.

Treatment focused on the underlying cause of dyspnea is preferred if it is consistent with the resident's goals of care. This may include antibiotics for pneumonia or furosemide for a heart failure exacerbation. There is an increase in the body of evidence supporting use of opioids to relieve the sensation of breathlessness. In opioid-naive patients, it is recommended that clinicians start at low doses of opioids (ie, 2 mg of immediate-release oral morphine) and titrate up as needed to achieve adequate symptom control. Supplemental oxygen often provides significant relief of dyspnea for individuals who are hypoxemic, although there does not seem to be

Table 11–1. Common opioids and equivalent potency conversions.

Opioid	Oral (mg)	IV (mg)
Morphine	30	10
Hydrocodone	30	–
Oxycodone	20	–
Hydromorphone	7.5	1.5
Fentanyl[a]	–	0.1 mg (100 mcg)

[a]A 25 mcg/hour fentanyl patch is equivalent to approximately 50 mg of oral morphine.

similar benefit in nonhypoxic individuals with life-limiting illness.

Simple environmental changes may help patients breathe easier. For example, directing a bedside fan toward the patient's face and elevating the head of the bed can relieve feelings of breathlessness. Clinicians should note that lengthy discussions with the patient may exacerbate breathlessness. Close-ended questions, providing a nonverbal means of communication (eg, pen and paper), or relying on proxy informants can help reduce the burden of prolonged patient interviews. Shortness of breath may also be linked to anxiety or spiritual distress thus warranting judicious involvement of the interdisciplinary team.

C. Nausea and Vomiting

Nausea and vomiting are prevalent symptoms near the end of life, and may result from both disease processes and iatrogenic adverse effects. Identifying the likely cause of nausea is critical to developing an effective therapy. Medication and constipation-induced nausea should always be considered as possible contributors to nausea. Medications commonly associated with nausea in older populations include opioids, antibiotics, antineoplastic agents, vitamins (zinc, iron), and acetylcholinesterase inhibitors. Antiemetic medications can deliver symptomatic relief for nausea. Different antiemetic medications can be used to target specific neurotransmitters to effectively treat common cause of nausea and vomiting (Table 11–2).

Table 11–2. Common causes of nausea and their pharmacologic treatments.

Cause	Preferred Class of Antiemetic	Examples
Gut inflammation	Serotonin receptor antagonist	Ondansetron, granisetron
Toxic/metabolic (including opioid-induced)	Dopamine antagonist	Prochlorperazine, metoclopramide, haloperidol
Chemotherapy	Serotonin receptor antagonist	Ondansetron, granisetron
Malignant bowel obstruction	Dopamine antagonist + glucocorticoids + octreotide	Metoclopramide, haloperidol; dexamethasone; octreotide
Anticipatory	Benzodiazepine	Lorazepam
Constipation	Laxatives	Stimulant (senna, bisacodyl), osmotic (lactulose)
Motion-induced/labyrinthitis	Anticholinergic	Scopolamine, promethazine
Increased intracranial pressure	Glucocorticoids	Dexamethasone

D. Delirium

The approach to delirium for patients with a life-limiting illness is similar to the approach for those who are not at the end of life. However, diagnostic tests and subsequent interventions need to be tailored to an individual's preferences and goals for care. The assessment of delirium at the end of life should focus on consideration of reversible causes, such as pain, adverse medication effect, urine retention, or fecal impaction. Nonpharmacologic strategies to prevent delirium remain important, including frequent reorientation, promoting daytime activity and a quiet nighttime environment, and avoidance agents that may precipitate delirium, including anticholinergic medications. Small doses of antipsychotics (eg, haloperidol 0.5 mg) are often effective in decreasing agitation at the end of life. Treatment using benzodiazepines is less effective as they may cause worsening agitation in some individuals.

E. Grief and Depression

Patients receiving palliative care may exhibit signs of grief or depression; however, it can be difficult to differentiate between the two. Grief is an adaptive, universal, and highly personalized emotional response to the multiple losses that occur at the end of life. This response is often intense early on after a loss, but the impact of grief on daily life generally decreases over time without clinical intervention. Major depression, however, is neither universal nor adaptive, although it is common among persons with advanced illness. Feelings of pervasive hopelessness, helplessness, worthlessness, guilt, lack of pleasure, and suicidal ideation are key in distinguishing depression from grief. Both cognitive therapy and antidepressant medications are effective treatments in reducing distressing symptoms and improving quality of life for those with depression. Clinicians may also consider psychostimulants, such as methylphenidate, for those depressed patients with a prognosis of only days to weeks.

F. Fatigue and Somnolence

Fatigue is both underrecognized and poorly treated by physicians and yet it is considered the most distressing symptom among patients other than pain. Assessment is focused on identifying correctable causes and determining the impact of fatigue on patients and their family members. Common causes include direct effects from the advanced illness and/or its treatments, anemia, hypoxemia, deconditioning, sedating medications, psychological issues including depression. Trials of moderate exercise have demonstrated significant benefits in patients with cancer. Improvements have been shown to include less fatigue, decreased sleep disturbance, improved functional capacity, and better quality of life. The psychostimulant methylphenidate has some evidence for its effectiveness to treat fatigue in advance illness, although trials have been small. Nondrug treatments, such as prioritizing one's activities, may also be of benefit.

G. Advanced Dementia

Hospice care for individuals with advanced dementia improves patient and caregiver outcomes, including better symptom management, fewer unmet needs, decreased hospitalizations during the last 30 days of life, and higher caregiver satisfaction with end-of-life care, compared to those receiving usual care. Unfortunately, hospice is underutilized in advanced dementia, in part because of the difficulty of predicting death within 6 months using current hospice eligibility criteria. Hospice should at least be considered for any nursing home patient with advanced dementia who develops a pneumonia, febrile episode, or eating problem, as these are markers of a poor 6-month prognosis (see Chapter 3, "Goals of Care & Consideration of Prognosis," for more information).

Many individuals with advanced dementia will develop feeding and eating difficulties. Unfortunately, patient preferences regarding artificial nutrition and hydration are often not documented until it is too late in the disease to have the discussion. Family members are then faced with the decision to administer food and fluids via a percutaneous endoscopic gastrostomy (PEG) tube, often during a hospitalization for pneumonia. There is no evidence that PEG tubes improve survival, prevent aspiration pneumonia, decrease the risk for pressure ulcers, improve patient comfort, or prolong life. Significant harms are associated with use of PEG tubes in advanced dementia including the likelihood of less caregiver contact during the mealtime and high rates of physical and chemical restraint use to prevent the feeding tube displacement. Alternatives to PEG placement include careful hand feeding and proper oral care. Patients who are imminently dying may require little to no intake in the final days of life.

CARING FOR FAMILY MEMBERS: GRIEF AND BEREAVEMENT

When caring for older patients who are dying, consideration must also be given to the health and well-being of their family members, both before and after the death. Losing someone through death can be an emotionally intense, stressful, and often overwhelming experience, impacting both physical and mental health. The suffering associated with this type of loss is most intense in the first 6 months, and is usually associated with feelings of disbelief, yearning, anger, and depressed mood, that gradually resolve. Intense distress generally peaks by 6 months into bereavement, but occasional spikes in distress may linger for years beyond the death. Most people successfully cope with their feelings of grief without medical intervention and by relying on their own inner resources, families, friends, spiritual community, and other sources of support. It is also common for family caregivers to feel a pervasive sense of guilt after the death; however, this alone is not an indicator of a pathologic grief response.

For 10% to 20% of bereaved individuals, grief can become complicated, prolonged, and have a significant detrimental impact on their ability to function. Clinicians can recognize and treat complicated grief early on, thereby preventing psychiatric morbidity, suicidal ideation, functional disability, and poor quality of life. The symptoms of complicated or prolonged grief are distinct from normal grief, bereavement related depression, and anxiety disorders. Key features include unusually intense separation distress with persistent yearning and longing for the deceased, as well as dysfunctional thoughts, feelings, or behaviors related to the loss. Several psychotherapeutic treatments have been shown to be beneficial including cognitive behavioral therapy and complicated grief treatment.

A growing body of evidence suggests that aggressive care at the end of life is associated with worse bereavement outcomes for family members. Improving physician communication with families can enhance clinical outcomes for critically ill patients, including decreasing ICU length of stay, lowering the rate of resuscitation attempts, and earlier hospice enrollment. Information about bereavement and counseling resources has been shown to improve family members' bereavement outcomes in terminally ill ICU patients.

Abernethy AP, McDonald CF, Frith PA, et al. Effect of palliative oxygen versus room air in relief of breathlessness in patients with refractory dyspnoea: a double-blind, randomised controlled trial. *Lancet.* 2010;376(9743):784-793.

Baile WF, Buckman R, Lenzi R, Glober G, Beale EA, Kudelka AP. SPIKES—a six-step protocol for delivering bad news: application to the patient with cancer. *Oncologist.* 2000;5(4):302-311.

Bernabei R, Gambassi G, Lapane K, et al. Management of pain in elderly patients with cancer. SAGE Study Group. Systematic assessment of geriatric drug use via epidemiology. *JAMA.* 1998;279(23):1877-1882.

Center to Advance Palliative Care. *Improving Palliative Care in Nursing Homes.* New York, NY: Mount Sinai School of Medicine; 2008 [cited November 24, 2009]. Available from: http://www.capc.org/capc-resources/capc_publications/nursing_home_report.pdf

Center to Advance Palliative Care (2012). *Palliative Care Tools, Training, & Technical Assistance.* Retrieved on January 12, 2012. Available from: www.CAPC.org

Hanson LC, Eckert KJ, Dobbs D, et al. Symptom experience of dying long-term care residents. *J Am Geriatr Soc.* 2008;56(1):91-98.

Husebo BS, Ballard C, Sandvik R, Nilsen OB, Aarsland D. Efficacy of treating pain to reduce behavioural disturbances in residents of nursing homes with dementia: cluster randomised clinical trial. *BMJ.* 2011;343:d4065.

Jennings AL, Davies AN, Higgins JP, Gibbs JS, Broadley KE. A systematic review of the use of opioids in the management of dyspnoea. Thorax 2002;57(11):939-944.

Kehl KA. Moving toward peace: an analysis of the concept of a good death. *Am J Hosp Palliat Care.* 2006;23(4):277-286.

Meier DE, Lim B, Carlson MD. Raising the standard: palliative care in nursing homes. *Health Aff (Millwood).* 2010;29(1):136-140.

Mitchell SL, Teno JM, Kiely DK, et al. The clinical course of advanced dementia. *N Engl J Med.* 2009;361(16):1529-1538.

Mitchell SL, Teno JM, Miller SC, Mor V. A national study of the location of death for older persons with dementia. *J Am Geriatr Soc.* 2005;53(2):299-305.

Shear K, Frank E, Houck PR, Reynolds CF III. Treatment of complicated grief: a randomized controlled trial. *JAMA.* 2005;293(21):2601-2608.

Steinhauser KE, Christakis NA, Clipp EC, McNeilly M, McIntyre L, Tulsky JA. Factors considered important at the end of life by patients, family, physicians, and other care providers. *JAMA.* 2000;284(19):2476-2482.

White DB, Braddock CH III, Bereknyei S, Curtis JR. Toward shared decision making at the end of life in intensive care units: opportunities for improvement. *Arch Intern Med.* 2007;167(5):461-467.

USEFUL WEBSITES

Pain Assessment Checklist for Seniors with Limited Ability to Communicate (PACSLAC). http://www.geriatricpain.org/Content/Assessment/Impaired/Pages/PACSLAC.aspx

Pain Assessment in Advanced Dementia (PAINAD). http://web.missouri.edu/~proste/tool/cog/painad.pdf

Ethics & Informed Decision Making

12

Alexander K. Smith, MD, MS, MPH

Bernard Lo, MD

Case Vignette

You are in clinic seeing a longstanding patient, an 87-year-old woman with diabetes, congestive heart failure, hypertension, and mild cognitive impairment. She ambulates using a cane. The patient's adult daughter accompanies her on this visit. The daughter lives several towns away, and prior to today had not visited for several months. The daughter reports being shocked at the deteriorating condition of her mother's home. She describes a cluttered house, with trip hazards everywhere and stinking piles of garbage in the kitchen. The patient herself says she has some recent difficulty with her vision, but other than that believes she is doing fine. On examination, her blood pressure is 180/82 and her score on the Montreal Cognitive Assessment (MOCA) is 23/30. Laboratory tests show a HbA1c (glycosylated hemoglobin) of 12.5. A visit by a home nurse confirms the daughter's concerns about the living situation, also noting that the patient's medications have been removed from their bottles and placed together in a jar on the dresser. When you meet the patient next you explain your concerns about her living situation and ability to care for herself. She responds that she's doing "just fine," and, "I won't move into a nursing home!"

ETHICAL ISSUES IN THE CARE OF OLDER ADULTS

The high prevalence of cognitive impairment, dementia, and functional dependence raise ethical issues in the everyday care of older adults. These tensions require that clinicians be familiar with ethical issues that are central to the care of older adults. These issues are often cast as principles (central guiding concepts) or virtues (qualities of the good clinician). Tables 12–1 and 12–2 provide descriptions of the major principles and virtues, with examples of how these might operate in the daily practice of caring for older adults.

As illustrated by this case, a central tension that commonly arises in the care of older adults is the balancing of autonomy and beneficence concerns. We have a duty to protect those who cannot care for themselves, but also a duty to

respect those who still have capacity and make choices that put them at some medical risk. Determination of decision-making capacity is the essential first step in such situations.

DECISION-MAKING CAPACITY AND INFORMED DECISION MAKING

Given the burden of cognitive impairment in older adults, determination of decision-making capacity is a critical skill for care of older adults. Outline below is a practical approach to assessing decision-making capacity in older adults. The core features of determining decision-making capacity are as follows:

1. The patient must make a decision.
2. The patient must explain the reasons behind the decision.
3. The decision cannot result from delusions or hallucinations.
4. The patient must demonstrate understanding of the medical situation and the risks, benefits, and alternatives of the decision, and alternatives to the decision.
5. The decision must be consistent with the patients values and preferences over time.

Several features of this strategy for assessing capacity are worth greater explanation. First, decision-making capacity is specific to the decision at hand. Some decisions are relatively straightforward and simple, such as timing of meals, whereas others are complex, such as the decision about safety in the home illustrated in the case. Second, as in the case, tests of mental status such as the Mini Mental Status Exam (MMSE) and the Montreal Cognitive Assessment (MOCA) may inform a decision, but are not determinative. Even a patient with moderate dementia, suggested by an MMSE or MOCA in the teens, may be able to make simple decisions but lack the capacity for complex decisions making. Conversely,

Table 12–1. Ethical principles.

Principle	What This Principle Means	Example Issues and Questions That Illustrate the Ethical Principle in the Context of the Case
Respect for autonomy	Autonomy is Greek for "self rule." We should respect people's right to shape their own lives and make medical care decisions according to their values. Several ethical concepts follow from this principle, including informed consent, freedom from interference/control by others, and freedom from unwanted bodily intrusion (including surgery or life-sustaining treatment). Advance directives are an extension of autonomy, as is substituted judgment by surrogate decision makers. Clinicians can enhance patient's autonomy by making sure that they understand their options and consequences. *Respect for persons* is a related principle, and includes treating people as worthy of respect, dignity, and compassion, even if they lack the decision making capacity necessary to form autonomous preferences.	Goals and values discussions—"When you think about where you want to live going forward, what factors are most important to you?" Priority setting—"There are a number of health issues we could discuss today, including your blood pressure management, preventing falls, your diabetes, and home safety. Which of these is most important to discuss today?"
Best interests (nonmaleficence and beneficence)	*Nonmaleficence* ("do no harm") and the related concept *beneficence* are guidelines that forbid physicians from providing therapy that on balance does more harm than good, that is ineffective, or stems from malicious or selfish acts. Physicians, as a profession with special training, skills, and knowledge, have a fiduciary duty ("held in trust") to patients to act in their best interests. Clinicians have an obligation to promote well-being of those who cannot look out for themselves.	Balancing harms, risks, and benefits—"It doesn't make sense to aim for really tight blood sugar control anymore—you would be at risk for the harms of low levels like fainting or falling, and you're unlikely to benefit given your health condition." Concern about living environment—"I worry about you continuing to live in your home. I know maintaining your independence is important to you, but if you fall at home or suffer a stroke you will almost certainly end up in a hospital and skilled nursing facility for a long time—things you also want to avoid."
Justice	Resources are not unlimited, and should be apportioned fairly—people should get what they deserve. Clinicians have an obligation to be prudent stewards of scarce health care resources. The meaning of "fair" is debatable: Does it mean to each according to their efforts? According to their needs? This also includes the principle that physicians should treat similarly situated patients equally and consistently.	The clinician may feel that he/she is not reimbursed fairly for the hard work of caring for this frail older patient.

Table 12–2. Virtues-based ethical concerns.

Virtue	What This Virtue Means	Example in the Context of the Case
Compassion	An active regard for another's welfare with sympathy, tenderness, and discomfort at suffering.	Caring enough to make time for this patient and her daughter, time to really understand why she so deeply wants to remain at home and fears of institutionalization.
Discernment	Bringing insight, judgment, and understanding to a clinical situation. "Practical wisdom."	Sorting through the long list of chronic conditions and medications to focus on what is most important to the patient's health and well-being.
Trustworthiness	Essential in medical care where patients place themselves in the doctor's care. Being trustworthy means meriting confidence in one's character and conduct.	Keeping up to date with diabetes guidelines and treatments in older adults so clinical advice is sound. Keeping promises to patients and caregivers, while also acknowledging the limits of those promises.
Fidelity	Being faithful to the patient's interests, even if they do not align with the interests of the clinician.	Spending time talking with patients and families even if not reimbursed well. Not ordering remunerative tests that don't help the patient or pose risk.

a patient with paranoid schizophrenia may have a perfect cognitive test but completely lack capacity for complex decisions. Third, patients may be unable to speak (eg, dysarthria from stroke) yet still be able to participate in decision making by communicating using other methods. Finally, capacity is assessed clinically, and does not require specialized input from psychologists or psychiatrists. Such specialized opinions may be sought in particular cases where psychiatric or neuropsychiatric issues are a major concern, but in general most capacity questions should be answerable by generalist clinicians. Competency, in contrast to capacity, is a legal status determined by the courts, and is generally based on the patient's ability to provide for food, clothing, and shelter.

Case Vignette (*continued*)

You reiterate your concerns about the home environment. You say to her, "to make sure I've done a good job explaining my concerns, can you tell me what I'm worried about?" In her response, she clearly indicates understanding, acknowledging that her home environment is full of fall hazards and that she needs assistance with her medications. However, she reiterates her long-held preference for remaining in her home despite these risks. You decide that she has the capacity to make this decision. She agrees to a family meeting with her daughter and a social worker to discuss how she might receive more support at home.

How much knowledge of the risks and benefits of treatment and the alternatives must a patient demonstrate? The answer to this question has practical implications not only for the clinician's assessment but for the amount and manner in which they communicate information to the patient. While the extent of what constitutes an "informed" decision is a subject of some debate, we advocate that clinicians consider the following points when deciding how much information to provide.

1. The risks of providing too much information (so-called information dumping). Patients do not need a mini-medical school curriculum to make an informed decision. The major concerns relative to the patient's circumstances should be discussed.

2. Prognosis is a critical component of informed decision-making with older adults. Clinicians should routinely offer to discuss prognosis (see Chapter 3, "Goals of Care & Consideration of Prognosis").

3. The manner of presentation of information may influence the decision. In one study, for example, subjects who were told the risks of a surgical intervention in terms of the likelihood of dying were less likely to choose that intervention than those who were presented the same risks as likelihood of survival. Consider the possibility that framing the information may introduce bias, and

offer alternative presentations of the risks and benefits to minimize such bias.

4. Disclosure of information is different from informed decision making: what the patient understands or believes may differ from what is disclosed. Check in with the patient about the patient's understanding in a nonjudgmental way, using the teachback method illustrated in the case.

ADVANCE CARE PLANNING AND ADVANCE DIRECTIVES

Advance care planning is the process of a patient talking with the patient's loved ones, often in conjunction with a health care clinician, about plans and preferences for future care. These plans may be codified in official forms called *advance directives* or *living wills*. These official documents may include designation of a surrogate decision maker (see below) and preferences for future care. Physician orders for life-sustaining treatment (POLST) are specific orders that are valid across settings (eg, homes, nursing homes, first responders to 911 calls, hospitals). A majority of states now have or are developing POLST programs. Advance directives and surrogate decision making allow for a form of "extended" autonomy.

Early excitement about advance directives was blunted by data showing directives were rarely completed, rarely followed, and that surrogates perform no better than chance at anticipating patient preferences. Emphasis has since shifted from completion of the advance directive documents themselves to preparation for "in-the-moment" decision making. This preparation encourages patients to think about their values and goals for future care and communicate these clearly to surrogates and clinicians. Completion of an advance directive may stimulate these discussions, but it is the conversation, not the directive that should take center stage.

SURROGATE DECISION MAKING

When patients lack capacity, clinicians turn to surrogate decision makers for assistance. The ideal surrogate decision maker is someone selected by the patient, in advance, who has extensive knowledge of the patient's values, preferences, and goals. The legal term for the surrogate varies by state, and may be the "health care proxy" in some states and the "durable power of attorney for health care decision making" in others. In some states, the surrogate decision maker, if not designated, is determined by law (eg, spouse, then adult children, then siblings, then parents). Conservators are court-appointed surrogates.

A general approach to surrogate decision making for incapacitated patients is outlined in Figure 12–1. This approach is generally accepted in the ethics and clinical communities, and has strong value as a starting point. It is not without controversy, however. The simplicity of the "hierarchical"

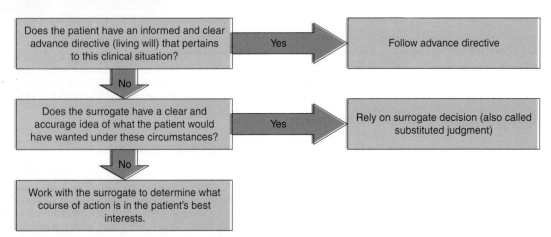

▲ **Figure 12–1.** A general approach to decision making for incapacitated patients. (*Note:* If no advance directive or surrogate is available, skip the middle step and act according to the patient's best interests.)

approach belies some of the ethical complexities encountered in attempting to follow this algorithm in clinical practice. Sulmasy and Snyder suggested that the hierarchical approach emphasizes information over empathy, emphasizes preferences that are ultimately unknowable in advance over values, and places an unfair burden on surrogate decision makers to choose from a menu of options. They argue for a "substituted interests and best judgments" approach in which the surrogate and clinician work together to determine the best course of action based on the patients values rather than preferences.

BALANCING PROMOTION OF INDEPENDENCE AND PATIENT SAFETY

> ### Case Vignette (*continued*)
>
> After a family meeting with you, a social worker, the patient, and her daughter, the patient enrolls in a Program of All-Inclusive Care for the Elderly (PACE). This PACE program allows her to live at home at night and receive comprehensive service at a day center. A home health aide visits her weekly and the daughter pays for a housecleaner.

In ordinary care of older adults, clinicians must balance competing demands of respect for persons and promotion of independence on the one hand, and patient safety and health interests of the older adult on the other. As in the case, maximizing a sense of self control or independence is central to the quality of life of many older adults, including those who reside in the community and institutional settings. In many cases, patients make choices that conflict with the clinician's sense of what is in their best interests—as, for example, in the case, choosing to reside in an unclean and possibly dangerous

environment and taking poor care of one's health. This tension is evident in other common issues in geriatrics, in preventing falls, for example, the tension between patient safety and independence.

The challenge for the clinician is to work with the patient to maximize independence while minimizing the risk of harms. In this case, a possible solution was to recognize that the underlying value was not a refusal of assistance, but a preference to reside at home. This allowed the patient, caregiver, and clinical team to come up with a plan to provide supportive services in the form of a PACE program for nursing home eligible older adults (for more on PACE, see Chapter 14, "Ambulatory Care & the Patient-Centered Medical Home"). Recognizing that clinicians have a duty to provide care for those who cannot provide for themselves, the clinician in this case should have seriously considered reporting a case of elder self-neglect to the appropriate local agency. Like the clinician, these agencies ideally work with the patient to maximize independence and minimize harm.

Even when patients have capacity for complex decision making, as in this case, family members and other caregivers often play a strong role in terms of providing and arranging services, and helping the patient make decisions. In each case, the physician should look to the patient for guidance as to how involved family should be in these issues. Physicians need to be respectful of older adults who want to maintain independence in decision making, as well as those who prefer a more family-centered decision-making style. For the latter, the physician's duty to promote an informed understanding of the options and consequences of treatments and alternatives extends to the larger family unit.

This case also highlights how virtue ethics work in conjunction with a principles-based approach. The time the clinician spent discussing the issue with the patient and her daughter, deliberating, setting up visiting nurses, and writing referrals to agencies is unlikely to be reimbursed in proportion to the effort involved. This issue is one that exemplifies the ethical principle of justice and needs to be addressed at the level of our society. From an individual perspective, however, the clinician in this case acted out of a sense of caring and fidelity. This is "good doctoring," and gratifying in its own right.

Ahalt C, Walter LC, Yourman L, Eng C, Perez-Stable EJ, Smith AK. "Knowing is Better": preferences of diverse older adults for discussing prognosis. *J Gen Intern Med.* 2011;27(5):568-575.

Beauchamp TL, Childress JF. *Principles of Biomedical Ethics.* 6th ed. New York, NY: Oxford University Press; 2009.

Castillo LS, Williams BA, Hooper SM, Sabatino CP, Weithorn LA, Sudore RL. Lost in translation: the unintended consequences of advance directive law on clinical care. *Ann Intern Med.* 2011;154(2):121-128.

Fagerlin A, Schneider CE. Enough. The failure of the living will. *Hastings Cent Rep.* 2004;34(2):30-42.

Lo B. *Resolving Ethical Dilemmas: A Guide for Clinicians.* 4th ed. Baltimore, MD: Lippincott Williams & Wilkins; 2009.

Meier DE, Beresford L. POLST offers next stage in honoring patient preferences. *J Palliat Med.* 2009;12(4):291-295.

Moody HR. *Ethics in an Aging Society.* Baltimore, MD: Johns Hopkins; 1992.

POLST. Last accessed Sept 30, 2013. http://www.polst.org/programs-in-your-state/

Prendergast TJ. Advance care planning: pitfalls, progress, promise. *Crit Care Med.* 2001;29(2 Suppl):N34-N39.

Smith AK, Williams BA, Lo B. Discussing overall prognosis with the very elderly. *N Engl J Med.* 2011;365(23):2149-2151.

Sudore RL, Fried TR. Redefining the "planning" in advance care planning: preparing for end-of-life decision making. *Ann Intern Med.* 2010;153(4):256-261.

Sulmasy DP, Snyder L. Substituted interests and best judgments: an integrated model of surrogate decision making. *JAMA.* 2010;304(17):1946-1947.

Tulsky JA. Beyond advance directives: importance of communication skills at the end of life. *JAMA.* 2005;294(3):359-365.

Transitions and Continuity of Care

Lynn A. Flint, MD

13

GENERAL PRINCIPLES IN OLDER ADULTS

Older adults with chronic illnesses are frequently in contact with the health care system. They periodically require hospitalization for acute exacerbations of chronic illness, falls, infections, and other problems. For these patients, hospitalization often marks the beginning of a journey through a series of disconnected settings and providers. Because of this lack of connection, the journey is not smooth. Mishaps along the way are sometimes insignificant, sometimes even undetected, but others are life altering. The discussion here focuses on how this journey became so complex, the risks of the journey, and the best practices and innovations aimed at minimizing these risks.

DEFINITIONS

The term *care transition* refers the transfer of a patient's care from one team of health care providers to another. Transitions usually occur when a patient physically moves between sites of care. Care transitions can be grouped into 3 broad categories. The first category, perhaps the most studied, includes community dwellers discharging from the hospital. For example, an older adult may develop a chronic condition for which he receives care from his primary care physician. Exacerbation of the chronic condition might prompt hospitalization, where hospital-based physicians, nurses, and therapists care for the patient. The patient may then move to a skilled nursing facility (SNF) for rehabilitation and/or nursing care and in that setting encounter an entirely new care team. When rehabilitation goals are achieved, the patient may return home, resume care with his primary care physician and may also receive home care from a new team to complete any remaining tasks in recovering from the original exacerbation. In this example, the patient underwent 3 separate transitions in care: primary care provider to hospital provider, hospital to SNF, SNF provider back to primary care provider

and to a new home health care team. The second category includes nursing home residents transitioning to and from the hospital. Although many of the problems seen in these transitions are the same as those encountered for community dwellers, additional challenges exist in transitions for these frail, functionally, and often cognitively, impaired patients. Finally, the third category includes patients who are facing the end of life. They often experience multiple transitions in providers in the moves between home, emergency room, and hospital with disease progression. For these patients, again, transitions carry the same risks as those for the community dwellers with chronic diseases, but also special problems come up for those near the end of life. *Transitional care* broadly refers to time-limited care processes aimed at ensuring safe and minimally disruptive transfers of care between different sites and providers.

BACKGROUND

The frequency of care transitions may be in part a consequence of changes in the structure and financing of the health care system over the past 30 years. In 1983, faced with ever-increasing costs, Medicare adopted a prospective payment scheme, whereby hospitals were no longer paid individual fees for individual services provided. Instead, hospitals received predetermined diagnosis-based fees for entire hospitalizations. Thus, hospitals had a financial incentive to increase efficiency and shorten length of stay. Indeed, length of stay decreased with the new legislation, but patients were not only discharged "quicker," they were also discharged "sicker." The "sicker" patients were more likely to be transferred to SNFs for rehabilitation and continued skilled nursing care prior to discharge home. Concurrently, fast-paced advances in hospital medicine coupled with the push to improve efficiency prompted physicians to restrict their practice to single sites (ie, clinic or hospital). Fewer primary care physicians continued to follow their patients while hospitalized. This shift in practice patterns meant that patients would routinely transfer care from one provider to another when moving from one setting to another.

Finances may also subtly encourage transfers of nursing home residents to the hospital. Medicare certified nursing facilities often provide temporary skilled rehabilitation and nursing services to their residents returning from the hospital. Reimbursement for skilled services is higher than the rate paid, often by Medicaid, for room, board, and custodial care. Medicare will only pay nursing homes for skilled services if patients have a preceding qualifying hospital stay. Thus, transfers to the hospital can be financially beneficial to nursing homes. Furthermore, nursing home residents using their Medicare Skilled Nursing Facility benefit can rarely simultaneously access their Medicare Hospice benefit, thus increasing the possibility of potentially avoidable end-of-life transitions.

For patients at the end of life, new symptoms and eventual functional decline prompt many care transitions. Because there are few comprehensive home care programs for people with life-limiting illnesses still seeking disease-directed therapies, patients with new symptoms often need to access care through the emergency room. Although functional decline is expected late in the course of life-limiting illness, often there is not time or staffing to develop plans for increased care when needed.

ADVERSE EVENTS DURING TRANSITIONS

Systems factors have contributed to the frequency of care transitions, and many factors inherent to the system increase the risk of negative outcomes during transitions. Transitions provide opportunities for new providers to reevaluate unresolved problems and refine care plans, but transitions are also fraught with risk. Older patients and those with multiple chronic illnesses—those who are most likely to experience multiple transitions—are particularly vulnerable to the risk of adverse events.

Studies describing the adverse events associated with transitions have focused on the transition of community dwelling adults from hospital to home or other facility and the transfer of nursing home residents from hospital to nursing home and back. A growing body of research describes transitions at the end of life. A prospective observational study of hospitalized adults showed that one in five discharged patients experienced an adverse event associated with discharge. The adverse events were most frequently related to medications but also included nosocomial infections, falls, and complications of procedures. Half of the adverse medication events were felt to preventable or at least "ameliorable." In a retrospective analysis of Medicare claims data, nearly one-fifth of beneficiaries who were hospitalized were readmitted within 30 days. Ninety percent of these rehospitalizations were considered "unplanned"; that is, *not* for follow-up treatments or procedures. In a study

of Medicare claims in nursing home resident decedents, nearly one-fifth had at least one "burdensome transition" in the last 90 days of life. "Burdensome transitions" were defined as hospitalization in the last 3 days of life, or multiple hospitalizations, or residing in different nursing home facilities in those last 90 days. In another study, geographic areas with greater rates of care transitions among nursing home residents also had greater rates of feeding tube placement in patients with severe cognitive impairment, a group that is unlikely to benefit from this invasive procedure. Transfers of nursing home residents have also been associated with drug regimen changes and adverse medication effects. Smith et al found that 50% of Medicare decedents visited emergency departments in the last month of life, 77% of these were admitted to the hospital and 68% of those admitted died there, despite the fact that several studies document that a majority of people would prefer to die at home. These findings suggest that patients' goals of care can be lost in transitions. Moreover, transitions seem to promote overuse of health care services, thereby contributing to ever-increasing health care spending. The goal of transitions research has been to identify the factors that contribute to these adverse events, particularly those that lead to readmission, and to design interventions to decrease the rate of readmissions and, ultimately, to better integrate health care across settings.

BARRIERS TO SUCCESSFUL CARE TRANSITIONS

A successful care transition is one in which providers have timely, complete information about the hospitalization and patients have the same information, as well as easy access to answers and support when problems arise. Coleman groups barriers to successful care transitions into 3 levels: systems, provider, and patient. Our health care system is composed of many autonomous health care facilities and networks of facilities. Communication and collaboration across sites and between networks is challenging for many reasons—from simple lack of readily available contact information for providers at different sites to laws protecting confidentiality. Information systems are often not shared between different systems, thereby slowing down the transfer of key data. Although the Health Insurance Portability and Accountability Act (HIPPA) has a provision allowing transfer of information between providers for the purpose of continuing care, many health care workers and staff are not familiar with that provision. Furthermore different institutions have different drug formularies based on contractual relationships with pharmaceutical companies, leading to medication substitutions with each transition. Another systems barrier has been the lack of incentives to ensure the quality of care transitions. However, Medicare's contracted Quality Improvement Organizations were tasked improving transitions in selected areas in with the 9th Scope of Work in 2008 and 10th Scope of Work in 2011; additionally, the Affordable Care Act proposes a pilot program using bundled payments for entire episodes of care across sites (ie, hospital and postacute SNF care), as an incentive to reduce readmissions.

Provider-level barriers stem from communication difficulties. The increasing prevalence of site-specific providers generates inpatient–outpatient physician discontinuity. Communication between inpatient and outpatient providers is most frequently accomplished via discharge summaries, but these often do not arrive in the receiving physician's office in a timely manner, if at all. Discharge summaries have also been shown to omit key information, such as which test results are pending and which follow-up appointments have been scheduled. Other forms of direct communication between inpatient and outpatient providers, such as telephone calls or e-mails, are infrequent.

Patient-level barriers include limitations in health literacy and self-efficacy. Patients may not know the details of their health history, or even the names and dosages of their medications, leading to the possibility of inaccurate medication prescription in the hospital. Additionally, with shorter inpatient stays, patients are generally still recovering and perhaps facing new diagnoses at the time of discharge. Thus, they are likely to have new self-care responsibilities, including monitoring of symptoms and signs, taking new medications, and keeping follow-up appointments either on their own or with the help of family or friends. Providers frequently overestimate patients and families' abilities (physically, socially, and cognitively) to manage their medical conditions. All of these problems can be traced back to the limitations in provider–patient communication. Discordance between physician explanations and patient understanding has been well documented. Communication can be even less effective when patients have low functional literacy or primarily speak a language other than English.

OVERCOMING THE BARRIERS: BEST PRACTICES

Excellent transitional care is associated with reduced rates of readmission to the hospital, cost savings and greater patient satisfaction. Readmissions can be avoided if inpatient and outpatient providers communicate effectively, medications are carefully reconciled at multiple key time points, and patients and families are educated about monitoring and care needs after discharge or transfer. The Joint Commission Guidelines for discharge summaries recommend that the following information be included: diagnoses, abnormal physical findings, important test results, discharge medications including reasons for changes, follow-up appointments, education provided to patient and family, and tasks to be completed (Table 13–1). For older adults, documentation of cognitive and functional status, skin condition including description of any pressure ulcers, nutritional status, goals of care, and surrogate decision makers are also important. Detailed medication reconciliation, with the assistance of a

Table 13–1. Key information to include in hospital and nursing facility discharge summaries for older adults.

Admission diagnosis
Comorbidities
Abnormal physical findings on admission
Cognitive status on admission
Significant test results
Discharge condition, including cognitive and functional status, pain level, nutritional status, and notable physical exam findings, including the presence or absence of pressure ulcers
Follow-up appointments
Tests still pending at discharge
Discharge medication list, with emphasis on new medications or doses, including explanation of why medications were started, changed or discontinued
Overall goals of care
Presence or absence of advance directive and/or living will
Name and phone number of surrogate decision maker
Home care services arranged

clinical pharmacist for patients with complex regimens, is essential to reducing adverse drug events. For patients with cognitive or functional disabilities or psychosocial challenges, a multidisciplinary team including social workers, nurse discharge planners, physical and occupational therapists is essential. Finally, using clear language and a trained interpreter if needed, discharging teams should counsel patients and families about medication changes, outpatient appointments, self-care and "red flags" signaling a call to the doctor or return to the hospital. For the patient transferring to an intermediate site of care, counseling should include a description of what to expect in the next site of care. If there have been major changes in goals of care and treatment limitations, a Physician Order for Life-Sustaining Treatment (POLST) form increases the likelihood that patients will have orders consistent with their wishes in the next setting. Finally, because written discharge summaries do not capture every detail, direct discussion between transferring and accepting providers can be helpful in complicated situations.

The transition from one setting to another is often a good time to review overall goals of care. This type of discussion could include the patient and family's understanding of the hospitalization and what they are expecting in the next setting. Eliciting specific hopes of future therapies can help discharging providers set realistic goals with the patient and initiate discussion of alternate plans in case those goals are not met.

EVIDENCE-BASED INTERVENTIONS

Coordination between different disciplines to accomplish all these tasks is key for effective transitional care. Naylor and colleagues designed an intervention utilizing advanced practice nurses for hospitalized elders at risk of poor postdischarge outcomes. The nurses provided personalized care coordination during the hospitalization, as well as follow-up visits and calls after discharge. They followed patients beginning at the time of hospital admission through 3 months after discharge. In a randomized trial, intervention patients were significantly less likely to be readmitted to the hospital within 24 weeks of the original discharge. Moreover, the intervention group incurred roughly half the health care costs of the control group in those 24 weeks.

Beyond care coordination, qualitative studies suggest that patient activation and self-management are also important to reducing adverse events associated with care transitions. The Care Transitions Intervention utilized a "transition coach," an advance practice nurse who worked with hospitalized older adults during the admission and for 4 weeks after discharge. The aim of the intervention was to empower patients to be more involved in their own self-management. Thus, rather than act as another provider, the transition coaches helped patients and caregivers take more active roles in their care. A second component of the intervention was a personal health record, carried by patients between settings, containing key information including diagnoses, medications, allergies, and advance directives. The intervention was studied in 2 randomized, controlled trials, 1 with patients enrolled in Medicare managed care plans, and 1 with patients using traditional fee-for-service Medicare. In both studies, intervention patients had lower rates of hospital readmission at 30, 90, and 180 days.

Other studies have focused on improving transitions for nursing home residents. Many hospitalizations for this population are considered avoidable, given a high prevalence of preventable admission diagnoses and significant geographic variation in readmission rates. Thus, many interventions designed to improve transitions for nursing home residents have focused simply on preventing hospitalizations. Berkowitz and colleagues studied the use of an admission template and automatic palliative care consultation for patients living in a SNF who had 3 or more hospitalizations in the 6 months preceding admission to the facility. A second component of the study was a regular meeting of the interdisciplinary team to examine root causes for rehospitalization events. Disposition was studied in the year prior to the intervention and after 1 year of implementation. Rehospitalization rates declined, home discharges increased, discharges to long-term care decreased and death on the unit increased (all deaths were felt to be expected). The Interventions to Reduce Acute Care Transfers (INTERACT) is a set of tools designed to help nursing home staff detect, evaluate and communicate early changes in resident status. A quality improvement project implementing these tools in multiple facilities showed a significant decline in rehospitalization, as compared with facilities not using the tools.

INNOVATIONS

Beyond making changes to care processes as described above, novel methods of information transfer and reimbursement for services have been proposed. These include improvement in accessibility of patient information across multiple sites of care. Options include universally accessible computer-based records and portable records that could be taken by patients themselves from site to site. Additionally, financial incentives for improving transitional care are being introduced, such as the development of Accountable Care Organizations that will receive bundled payments for entire episodes of care across several settings. Also part of the Affordable Care Act, the Community Based Care Transitions program will fund hospitals and community organizations to use proven interventions to integrate care for Medicare beneficiaries who are at high risk of hospital readmissions.

CONCLUSION

Older adults with complex medical conditions are at risk of adverse events as they traverse the various sites within the health care system. A number of interventions have been shown to improve post-discharge outcomes and reduce readmissions. Comprehensive changes at the patient, provider, institution and overall system levels are needed to improve transitional care as the population ages.

Bell CM, Schnipper JL, Auerbach AD, et al. Association of communication between hospital-based physicians and primary care providers with patients outcomes. *J Gen Intern Med.* 2008;24(3):381-386.

Berkowitz RE, Jones RN, Rieder R, et al. Improving disposition outcomes or patients in a geriatric skilled nursing facility. *J Am Geriatr Soc.* 2011;59(6):1130-1136.

Boockvar K, Fishman E, Kyriacou CK, Monias A, Gavi S, Cortes T. Adverse events due to discontinuation in drug use and dose changes in patients transferred between acute and long-term care facilities. *Arch Intern Med.* 2004;164(5):545-550.

Bookvar K, Vladek BC. Improving the quality of transitional care for persons with complex care needs. *J Am Geriatr Soc.* 2004;52(5):855-856.

Coleman EA. Falling through the cracks: challenges and opportunities for improving transitional care for persons with continuous complex care needs. *J Am Geriatr Soc.* 2003;51(4):549-555.

Coleman EA, Parry C, Chalmers S, Min SJ. The care transitions intervention: results of a randomized controlled trial. *Arch Intern Med.* 2006;166(17):1822-1828.

Forster AJ, Murff HJ, Peterson JF, Gandhi TK, Bates DW. The incidence and severity of adverse events affecting patients after discharge from the hospital. *Ann Intern Med.* 2003;138(3):161-167.

Gozalo P, Teno JM, Mitchell SL, et al. End-of-life transitions among nursing home residents with cognitive issues. *N Engl J Med.* 2011;365(13):1212-1221.

Hickman SE, Nelson CA, Perrin NA, Moss AH, Hammers BJ, Tolle SW. A comparison of methods to communicate treatment preferences in nursing facilities: traditional practices versus the physician orders for life sustaining treatment program. *J Am Geriatr Soc.* 2010;58(7):1241-1248.

Jenks SF, Williams MV, Coleman EA. Rehospitalizations among patients in the Medicare fee-for-services program. *N Engl J Med.* 2009;360(14):1418-1428.

Kahn KL, Keeler EB, Sherwood MJ, et al. Comparing outcomes of care before and after implementation of the DRG-based prospective payment system. *JAMA.* 1990;264(15):1984-1988.

Kripalani S, Jackson AT, Schnipper JL, Coleman EA. Promoting effective transitions of care at hospital discharge: a review of key issues for hospitalists. *J Hosp Med.* 2007;2(5):314-323.

Kosecoff J, Kahn KL, Rogers WH, et al. Prospective payment system and impairment at discharge: the 'quicker-and-sicker' story revisited. *JAMA.* 1990;264(15):1980-1983.

Naylor MD, Brooten D, Campbell R, et al. Comprehensive discharge planning and home follow-up of hospitalized elders: a randomized clinical trial. *JAMA.* 1999;281(7):613-620.

Naylor MD, Brooten DA, Campbell RL, Maislin G, McCauley KM, Schwartz JS. Transitional care of older adults with heart failure: a randomized, controlled trial. *J Am Geriatr Soc.* 2004;52(5):675-684.

Naylor M, Kurtzman ET, Grabowski DC, Harrington C, McClellan M, Reinhard SC. Unintended consequences of steps to cut readmissions and reform payment may threaten care of vulnerable older adults. *Health Aff (Millwood).* 2012;31(7):1623-1632.

Ouslander JG, Lamb G, Tappen R, et al. Interventions to reduce hospitalizations from nursing homes: evaluation of the INTERACT II collaborative quality improvement project. *J Am Geriatr Soc.* 2011;59(4):745-753.

Parry C, Min S, Chugh A, Chalmers S, Coleman EA. Further application of the care transitions intervention: results of a randomized controlled trial conducted in a fee-for-service setting. *Home Health Care Serv Q.* 2009;28(2-3):84-99.

Smith AK, McCarthy E, Weber E, et al. Half of older Americans seen in emergency department in last month of life; most admitted to hospital, and many die there. *Health Aff (Millwood).* 2012 Jun;31(6):1277-1285.

Teno JM, Mitchell SL, Skinner J, et al. Churning: the association between health care transitions and feeding tube insertion for nursing home resident with advanced cognitive impairment. *J Palliat Med.* 2009;12(4):359-362.

Van Walraven C, Seth R, Austin PC, Laupacis A. Effect of discharge summary availability during post-discharge visits on hospital readmission. *J Gen Intern Med.* 2002;17(3):186-192.

Wachter RM. The state of hospital medicine in 2008. *Med Clin North Am.* 2008;92(2):265-273.

Were MC, Li X, Kesterson J, et al. Adequacy of hospital discharge summaries in documenting tests with pending results and outpatient follow-up providers. *J Gen Intern Med.* 2009;24(9):1002-1006.

White HL, Glazier RH. Do hospitalist physicians improve the quality of inpatient care delivery? A systematic review of process, efficiency and outcome measures. *BMC Med.* 2011;9:58.

USEFUL WEBSITES

Interventions to Reduce Acute Care Transfers (Interact II). http://interact2.net

Society of Hospital Medicine. Project BOOST (Better Outcomes for Older adults through Safe Transitions). http://www.hospitalmedicine.org/ResourceRoomRedesign/RR_CareTransitions/CT_Home.cfm

The Care Transitions Project (Coleman, et al). http://www.caretransitions.org/

Transitional Care Model (Naylor, et al). http://www.transitionalcare.info

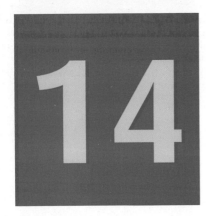

Ambulatory Care & the Patient-Centered Medical Home

Helen Kao, MD

GENERAL PRINCIPLES IN OLDER ADULTS

The vast changes occurring in medicine today are most prominent in ambulatory care. With the *Patient Protection and Affordable Care Act* passed in 2010, and growing urgency to curtail the rising costs of health care, ambulatory care has seen rapid changes to practice. The patient-centered medical home (PCMH) is one of the most widely adopted models of ambulatory health care that has been disseminated across the United States in recent years. The Centers for Medicare and Medicaid Services and the Veterans Affairs (VA), have both been implementing PCMH models at community health centers and VA medical centers around the country; private insurers and health plans are also redesigning their practices into PCMH models.

Why is PCMH being so strongly promoted as the ideal model of ambulatory care? PCMH is an approach to providing comprehensive, cost-effective primary care for patients of all ages. It aims to improve the delivery and experience of care for patients and clinicians through team-based coordinated care rather than the more ubiquitous fragmented health care norm that most patients have experienced for decades. Geriatric medicine is particularly well-suited to the PCMH approach to care because the principles of geriatrics ambulatory care (such as strong patient–provider relationships that recognize the role of family and caregivers, interprofessional team-based care, and continuous care throughout life stages and health care settings) are aligned with PCMH principles. Additionally, geriatrics-trained providers have specific skills that apply to many of the processes that comprise PCMH care.

Originally described by the American Academy of Pediatrics (AAP) in 1967, PCMH was adapted to patients of all ages by the American Academy of Family Physicians (AAFP, 2004) and the American College of Physicians (ACP, 2006), prior to a joint statement of principles in 2007 by AAP, AAFP, ACP, and the American Osteopathic Association. To date, 19 additional physician organizations support the PCMH model of care. PCMH aims to organize all care around the patient through an interprofessional team led by the patient's personal physician, with coordination and health tracking longitudinally over time to provide best outcomes. The National Committee for Quality Assurance is the organization that lays out specific standards for practices seeking to develop into and be recognized as a PCMH.

There are 7 core principles of PCMH of which the first 6 are aligned with geriatric medicine principles. The seventh principle, on appropriate payment systems to recognize the value of care provided by a PCMH, is also one that those caring for older adults are unified behind. This chapter highlights the shared goals between geriatrics ambulatory care and the first 6 PCMH principles to demonstrate ways in which both geriatric medicine values and the PCMH model of care can enhance the care of older adults.

PERSONAL PHYSICIAN

Each patient has a relationship with a personal physician who provides continuous and comprehensive care.

Continuous and comprehensive care carries significantly more weight for older patient populations than younger populations. Older adults have more chronic illnesses than younger adults, and are more likely to transition through multiple care settings and services (hospital and nursing home care, home health and hospice services, in addition to ambulatory clinic-based care). Geriatrics clinicians are uniquely trained in the care of patients in all of these care settings. With the increasing frailty that often accompanies aging with chronic conditions, older adults benefit from personal relationships with primary care providers who understand and can lead team care across the spectrum of settings, from enrollment in the primary care clinic through end-of-life stages. Providing coordinated transitional care, home-based, and palliative care are hallmarks of geriatrics ambulatory care which align with PCMH's principle for continuous and comprehensive care.

PHYSICIAN DIRECTED MEDICAL PRACTICE

The personal physician leads a team of individuals at the practice level who collectively take responsibility for the ongoing care of patients.

A core principle in the care of older adults has long been interprofessional team-based care (see Chapter 5, "The Interprofessional Team"). Geriatricians have been drivers for team-based care and education since the 1970s. Successful and sustained examples of physician-led team care include the VA Home-Based Primary Care (HBPC) and the Program for All-Inclusive Care of the Elderly (PACE). HBPC was founded in 1972 to provide skilled, interprofessional, and coordinated care to chronically ill home-bound aging veterans. They were an early example of how interprofessional team care improves outcomes for adults with chronic conditions. PACE, a medical-social care model founded in 1978, has been one of the most successful early models of a medical home for frail, nursing-home eligible clients. In PACE, all team members from physician to physical therapist to van driver, are engaged in a patient's care. In both models, a physician-led (and often geriatrician-led) team actively coordinates care and services across disciplines—working together to identify and address problems comprehensively, as well as to provide age-appropriate preventive care consistent with the older adult's goals of care. Older adults with multiple chronic conditions are especially well-served by PCMH team-based care as their illnesses and physical or cognitive impairments are too complex to be adequately addressed by a primary care provider alone.

WHOLE-PERSON ORIENTATION

The personal physician is responsible for providing for all the patient's health care needs or taking responsibility for appropriately arranging care with other qualified professionals. This includes care for all stages of life; acute care; chronic care; preventive services; and end-of-life care.

Caring for older adults requires clinicians to be attuned to whole-person care across an individual's life spectrum, and from wellness to debility. Geriatrics professionals contribute skills and knowledge of the effect of interactions between complex conditions (medical, cognitive, and affective); functional impairments; and possible mismatches between a patient's needs and the patient's financial, caregiving, and environmental situations on that individual's care. Attention to these multidirectional interactions by a geriatrician-led interprofessional team can highlight the needs of older adults with multiple comorbidities for whom "whole-person" care carries greater import than for younger, healthier patients.

In addition to whole-person care of complex conditions, geriatric medicine is the only field for which postgraduate medical education requires physicians to have clinical training in ambulatory care, acute hospital care, nursing home care, rehabilitative care, hospice, and noninstitutional long-term care settings (assisted living, day care, residential care, and home care). A comprehensive understanding of patient care through these various stages and settings enables geriatrics-trained clinicians to competently address older adults' health care needs not only from a medical perspective but from a medical-social-environmental perspective, drawing upon appropriate community resources to allow aging adults to remain living at home.

CARE COORDINATION AND INTEGRATION

Care is coordinated and/or integrated across all elements of the complex health care system (eg, subspecialty care, hospitals, home health agencies, nursing homes) and the patient's community (eg, family, public and private community-based services). Care is facilitated by registries, information technology, health information exchange and other means to assure that patients get the indicated care when and where they need and want it in a culturally and linguistically appropriate manner.

Clinicians caring for older adults need to have a keen understanding of the importance of integrating medical and social care, in particular the benefits of collaboration with community services. PCMH can draw from models of coordinated or integrated geriatrics care that have been shown to be effective: System of Integrated Care for Older Persons (SIPA, developed in Canada), Geriatrics Resources for Assessment and Care of Elders (GRACE), and Guided Care. All 3 models have demonstrated that integration of medical and social care—attending to the psychosocial, caregiving, and environmental needs of older adults, among other needs—improves patient outcomes. PCMH models serving disabled and older adults should develop robust means of linking appropriate patients to private and public community services so that their needs may be met in culturally and linguistically appropriate ways.

QUALITY AND SAFETY

Quality and safety are hallmarks of PCMH (such as evidence-based medicine, clinical decision support tools, continuous quality improvement, information technology).

PCMH presents the ideal opportunity to incorporate quality indicators specific to the care of older adults into primary care settings. Quality metrics to improve the care of older adults have been developed and available since 2000 (Assessing Care for Vulnerable Elders [ACOVE]), with updated revisions published in 2007. They include quality indicators for older adults based on geriatric syndromes (eg, falls, urinary incontinence, polypharmacy) for which treatments and thoughtful care plans can effectively improve an older patient's well-being. Screening and treatment for conditions included in the ACOVE quality indicators can be implemented. However, geriatric syndromes are still underdiagnosed. ACOVE can complement the preventive care and disease-oriented chronic condition quality indicators that currently dominate PCMH models of care.

ENHANCED ACCESS

Enhanced access to care is available through systems such as open scheduling, expanded hours and new options for communication between patients, their personal physician, and practice staff.

Enhanced access to care for practices taking care of the full spectrum of adults must not only implement systems changes as listed in this PCMH principle, but also provide care for patients who are or become too disabled to access their clinic-based providers. The ability to deploy PCMH clinicians to patients' places of residence in the community is a critical component to comprehensive care for patients across all stages of life.

Implementation of the PCMH model of care is an opportunity to bring the medical home to the homes of many patients who have become homebound. There is no more person-centered way to provide for "all the patient's health care needs" than by bringing care to the patient's home as the patient becomes more frail. A geriatrics house call can identify more problems with potentially serious consequences than routine office visits. The geriatrics tradition of housecalls to patients unable to reach clinic-based care, gives true meaning to a patient-centered medical "home."

SUMMARY

With increasing numbers of clinical practices adopting PCMH principles and growing attention to patient-centered quality care, geriatrics principles and the experience of multiple care models for older adults can contribute positively to the outcomes pursued by ambulatory care clinicians around the country. By having formal standards which practices must meet to be considered a PCMH, the National Committee for Quality Assurance has inherently brought formal recognition to many of the longstanding processes and workflows of geriatrics clinical practices. The PCMH movement generates many opportunities for practices to develop the care processes which will optimize outcomes for older adults, especially those with multiple chronic conditions and disability. As we look forward, advancements in team-based models of care and medical informatics will generate further advances in the care of older adults.

Beland F, Bergman H, Lebel P, et al. A system of integrated care for older persons with disabilities in Canada: results from a randomized controlled trial. *J Gerontol A Biol Sci Med Sci.* 2006;61(4):367-373.

Counsell SC, Callahan CM, Clark DO, et al. Geriatric care management for low-income seniors: randomized controlled trial. *JAMA.* 2007;298(22):2623-2633.

Landers S, Suter P, Hennessey B. Bringing home the "medical home" for older adults. *Cleve Clin J Med.* 2010;77(10):661-675.

Ramsdell JW, Swart JA, Jackson JE, Renvall M. The yield of a home visit in the assessment of geriatric patients. *J Am Geriatr Soc.* 1989;37(1):17-24.

Wenger NS, Solomon DH, Roth CP, et al. The quality of medical care provided to vulnerable community-dwelling older patients. *Ann Intern Med.* 2003;139(9):740-747.

Wenger NS, Roth CP, Shekelle P; ACOVE Investigators. Introduction to the assessing care of vulnerable olders—3 quality indicator measurement set. *J Am Geriatr Soc.* 2007;55 Suppl 2: S247-S252.

Wenger NS, Roth CP, Shekelle PG, et al. A practice-based intervention to improve primary care for falls, urinary incontinence, and dementia. *J Am Geriatr Soc.* 2009;57(3):547-555.

Wolff JL, Rand-Giovanetti E, Palmer S, et al. Caregiving and chronic care: the guided care program for family and friends. *J Gerontol A Biol Sci Med Sci.* 2009;64(7):785-791.

Providing Quality Care to Older Adults in the Emergency Department

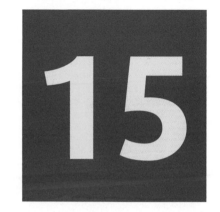

Gallane D. Abraham, MD
Corita R. Grudzen, MD, MSHS, FACEP

GENERAL PRINCIPLES

Adults age 65 years and older comprise 13% of the population, and are projected to grow to approximately 20% by 2030. Although older adults represent 25% of all emergency department (ED) visits, they account for almost half of all ED admissions and 60% of those that are considered preventable. They are more likely to present with urgent and emergent medical conditions, and are 5 times more likely to be admitted. This demographic shift and utilization pattern imply the number of ED visits by older adults will only increase. Models of emergency care must adapt to meet the special needs of this growing population.

Due to the medical and psychosocial complexity of many older adults, the ED is often an appropriate setting for care. However, presentations to the ED are often confounded by atypical features or vague symptoms, multiple comorbidities, and polypharmacy. For this reason, older adults are at high risk for adverse medication events or side effects, cognitive and functional decline, delirium, and falls during and subsequent to their ED visit and/or hospitalization. These clinical factors put older adults at risk for delays in diagnosis, inappropriate and insufficient treatment plans, ED revisit and rehospitalization. Structural aspects of the ED and hospital environment may also increase these risks. In addition, the often complex psychosocial needs require early intensive multidisciplinary case management to improve patient outcomes (Table 15–1). Older adults are often discharged from the ED with unrecognized illness or unmet social needs, and 20% experience a change in the ability to care for themselves after an acute illness or injury. Complications commonly ensue, with an often rapid decrease in functioning and quality of life; not surprisingly, 27% will experience ED revisit, hospitalization, or death within 3 months. This chapter addresses the complex needs of the older adult presenting to the ED and suggests key models of care, structural enhancements, financing, and clinical care protocols to improve quality care for older adults.

The current model of emergency care is designed to rapidly treat the acutely ill and injured, as opposed to managing older adults with complex and atypical presentations, multiple comorbidities, and acute exacerbations of chronic disease. To identify and address older persons' complex medical and psychosocial needs, emergency providers must account for baseline cognitive and functional limitations, obtain history from and collaborate with multiple sources, and develop a broad differential. Such an intensive case management approach will allow emergency providers to develop appropriate care plans that place older adults' needs in context.

MODELS OF EMERGENCY CARE

Models of geriatric emergency care are already being implemented. While their shared goal is to adapt the ED environment and care plans to the needs of older adults, the way the models are implemented will clearly differ. Elements currently include geriatric-friendly structural modifications such as diurnal lighting and noise reduction, universal screening and risk assessment, such as with the Identification of Seniors at Risk and the Timed Up & Go fall risk assessment, enhanced care coordination between ED and community health care providers, and linkages to community resources. No outcome data yet exists for such models of care, and no one approach has been standardized or described as superior. Most ED models of geriatric emergency care adapt these elements from other care settings, and almost all utilize a case-management approach, a collaborative assessment, planning, and care coordination process to improve outcomes for older adults.

In a 2011 systematic review of ED-based case management for older adults, Sinha et al identified 8 operational components that can inform the development of a comprehensive geriatric emergency care model. Key operational components include: 'implementation of an evidence based practice model; universal screening with validated risk assessment

Table 15–1. Geriatric emergency medicine high-yield facts.

1. Older adults have atypical and complex presentations of common diseases.
2. Comorbid conditions confound presentations, disposition, and disease course.
3. Polypharmacy and adverse medication effects are ubiquitous.
4. Cognitive and functional limitations are frequently present. Knowledge of baseline status is essential to evaluate new complaints.
5. Diagnostic tests may have normal values.
6. Patients have decreased functional reserve capacity to recover from an acute illness or injury.
7. Social and caregiver support must be evaluated to avoid poor outcomes.
8. Psychosocial context must be accounted for to improve outcomes, such as social support and mental health.

tools; nursing or midlevel clinician-directed geriatric case management; focused geriatric assessments to identify clinical and nonclinical factors that may impact care planning and future health care utilization; ED initiation of care and disposition planning; interprofessional and multidisciplinary work practices between the ED providers, hospital, primary care, and community health care providers; follow-up after discharge to maintain and facilitate care plans; and evaluation and monitoring of outcome measures for continuous quality improvement.' Furthermore, capacity building through the training of existing providers in geriatric competencies can also enhance care of older adults. This evidence base provides a framework to redesign emergency care for the older adult.

STRUCTURAL ENHANCEMENTS

The environment of the ED itself places older adults at risk for iatrogenic complications. The ED is a high-risk setting that can precipitate delirium, disorientation, anxiety, agitation, falls, disrupt the sleep–wake cycle, and impair communication in the visual and hearing-impaired. ED structural modifications can improve patient outcomes and safety. The ideal ED for older adults would feature diurnal lighting and noise reduction to preserve the sleep–wake cycle, as well as appropriate environmental stimuli and cognitive activities to prevent delirium. EDs can also modify flooring, add handrails, and develop appropriate signage to improve safety.

FINANCING

Comprehensive geriatric emergency care offers potential cost-savings for EDs, hospitals, and health systems. Accurate assessment of the value of reducing falls, delirium, and adverse medication events on the cost of prolonged hospitalization, ED revisit, and rehospitalization is essential to make

an evidence-based case to support financing a comprehensive geriatric ED. Collaboration with existing hospital and community health care partners to maximize available resources can improve cost savings and make financing geriatric ED interventions feasible.

CLINICAL CARE

Emergency care for the older adult involves treating both acute illnesses and injuries, as well as exacerbations of chronic disease. The most common reasons older adults present to the ED include falls, chest pain, adverse medication effects, neuropsychiatric disorders, alcohol and substance abuse, elder abuse and neglect, abdominal pain, and infections. The older adult will often present with vague symptoms, atypical presentations of common diseases, multiple acute conditions, and confounding medical comorbidities. Additionally, up to 40% of older adults will have cognitive impairment that is not readily apparent to emergency providers, further complicating their medical and psychosocial evaluation and disposition. For this reason, innovative approaches are necessary to deliver optimal care to this population.

▶ Universal Screening

Validated screening tools are used in other care settings and can rapidly identify those at high risk for poor outcomes. The Identification of Seniors at Risk (ISAR) (Table 15–2) is one such screening tool useful in the ED. It is comprised of 6 questions that identify older adults who are at high risk for poor health outcomes and intense health care resource utilization. Patients self-report functional capacity, need for assistance, visual acuity, memory, and recent hospitalization, and number of medications. If positive, the ISAR would then be followed by targeted interventions to address patients' needs.

▶ Falls

Approximately 33% of all older adults will fall annually, and 10% of such falls will result in major injuries. Falls are the leading cause of injury and injury-related death resulting in significant morbidity, disability, and decreased independence and quality of life. ED screening with the Timed Up & Go Test (see Table 15–2) is a simple means to rapidly identify patients at risk for falls with minimal equipment, training, or professional expertise. Identifying risk factors that contribute to falls, such as gait instability and environmental hazards, is important to create safe discharge plans for older adults.

▶ Delirium

Delirium is an emergency medical condition that affects 10% of older adults in the ED and independently carries a high morbidity and mortality. Delirium can prolong hospital

Table 15–2. Adapted universal screening and risk assessment.

High risk for poor health outcomes, high utilization	**Identification of Seniors At Risk (ISAR)** *Scoring: 0–6 (positive score shown in parentheses = 1 point)* 1. Before the illness or injury that brought you to the Emergency, did you need someone to help you on a regular basis? (yes) 2. Since the illness or injury that brought you to the Emergency, have you needed more help than usual to take care of yourself? (yes) 3. Have you been hospitalized for 1 or more nights during the past 6 months (excluding a stay in the Emergency Department)? (yes) 4. In general, do you see well? (no) 5. In general, do you have serious problems with your memory? (yes) 6. Do you take more than three different medications every day? (yes) Scoring: ISAR >2 = High Risk
Fall Risk	**Timed Up and Go** Stand from chair Walk 10 feet Turn around Walk back 10 feet Sit in chair Scoring: <10 seconds = Normal 10–29 seconds = Below Normal, Variable Mobility >30 seconds = Impaired Mobility
Delirium	**Confusion Assessment Method** Acute onset/fluctuating course Inattention *and either* Disorganized thinking or Altered consciousness

length of stay, increase dependence, and is independently associated with poor health outcomes. It is underrecognized and undertreated in the ED. The Confusion Assessment Method (CAM) (see Table 15–2) is a validated tool that has been adapted for use in the ED. CAM-rated delirium is associated with falls resulting in injuries, inadequate pain control, and increased sedative or restraint use, all of which can result in prolonged hospitalization, poor functional outcomes, institutionalization, and increased mortality. This 5-minute test can differentiate delirium from dementia by the presence of mental status changes that are acute in onset and fluctuating in course, characterized by inattention, disorganized thinking, and an altered level of alertness. Older adults identified as having delirium often require admission. If discharged, they are often non-compliant with medications and unable to recall discharge instructions, placing them at risk for ED revisit and rehospitalization.

▶ Cognitive Impairment

Between 16% and 40% of older adults presenting to the ED will have some form of cognitive impairment. In one study,

70% of those discharged home with cognitive impairment had no prior history of dementia and were less likely to have assistance with home care. Thus, the cognitively impaired will require focused ED assessment and multidisciplinary case management to ensure their cognitive limitations do not result in poor health outcomes.

FUTURE OF EMERGENCY CARE

Emergency care will continue to evolve to meet the demographic changes of the 21st century, and is necessary to improve the quality and decrease the costs of health care for older adults. Goals of geriatric emergency care remain the same as for all emergency patients: to provide appropriate, timely, and comprehensive emergency care for acute illnesses and injuries and exacerbations of chronic disease. Universal screening in the ED will evolve and help identify older adults who are at high-risk for falls, delirium, and subsequent functional or cognitive impairment. This, in turn, may improve outcomes and decrease the harms associated with health care utilization. Future goals include improving pain management, access to ED-based palliative care services, and linkages to geriatric primary care, home care, and community resources. Finding alternatives to the use of chemical sedation and restraints will further improve emergency care for older adults. Structural modifications will allow EDs to adapt to the special needs of older adults. An intensive and multidisciplinary case management approach will help emergency providers develop care plans that meet not only older adults' goals of care but also their psychosocial needs.

Adams JG, Gerson LW. A new model for emergency care of geriatric patients. *Acad Emerg Med.* 2003;10(3):271-274.

AfHRa, Quality. HCUP Nationwide Inpatient Sample (NIS). *Healthcare Cost and Utilization Project (HCUP)* 2006; 2000.

Elie M, Rousseau F, Cole M, Primeau F, McCusker J, Bellavance F. Prevalence and detection of delirium in elderly emergency department patients. *CMAJ.* 2000;163(8):977-981.

Fitzgerald RT. American College of Emergency Physicians White Paper. The future of geriatric care in our Nation's emergency departments: impact and implications; 2008.

Friedmann PD, Jin L, Karrison TG, et al. Early revisit, hospitalization, or death among older persons discharged from the ED. *Am J Emerg Med.* 2001;19(2):125-129.

Gerson LW, Counsell SR, Fontanarosa PB, Smucker WD. Case finding for cognitive impairment in elderly emergency department patients. *Ann Emerg Med.* 1994;23(4):813-817.

Grayson VK, Velkoff VA. The next four decades: the older population in the United States: 2010 to 2050. No. 1138. US Department of Commerce, Economics and Statistics Administration, US Census Bureau; 2010.

Han JH, Shintani A, Eden S, et al. Delirium in the emergency department: an independent predictor of death within 6 months. *Ann Emerg Med.* 2010;56(3):244-252e1.

Hickman L, Newton P, Halcomb EJ, Chang E, Davidson P. Best practice interventions to improve the management of older people in acute care settings: a literature review. *J Adv Nurs.* 2007;60(2):113-126.

Hoogerduijn JG, Schuurmans MJ, Korevaar JC, Buurman BM, de Rooij SE. Identification of older hospitalised patients at risk for functional decline, a study to compare the predictive values of three screening instruments. *J Clin Nurs.* 2010;19(9-10):1219-1225.

Hustey FM, Meldon SW. The prevalence and documentation of impaired mental status in elderly emergency department patients. *Ann Emerg Med.* 2002;39(3):248-253.

Hustey FM, Meldon SW, Smith MD, Lex CK. The effect of mental status screening on the care of elderly emergency department patients. *Ann Emerg Med.* 2003;41(5):678-684.

Hwang U, Morrison RS. The geriatric emergency department. *J Am Geriatr Soc.* 2007;55(11):1873-1876.

Inouye SK. Delirium in older persons. *N Engl J Med.* 2006; 354(11):1157-1165.

Inouye SK, Bogardus ST Jr, Charpentier PA, et al. A multicomponent intervention to prevent delirium in hospitalized older patients. *N Engl J Med.* 1999;340(9):669-676.

Inouye SK, van Dyck CH, Alessi CA, Balkin S, Siegal AP, Horwitz RI. Clarifying confusion: the confusion assessment method. A new method for detection of delirium. *Ann Intern Med.* 1990;113(12):941-948.

Johnston CB, Harper GM, Landefeld CS. Chapter 4. Geriatric disorders. In: McPhee SJ, Papadakis MA, Rabow MW, eds. *CURRENT Medical Diagnosis & Treatment 2012.* New York: McGraw-Hill; 2012.

Keim SM, Sanders AB. Geriatric emergency department use and care. In: *Geriatric Emergency Medicine.* New York: The McGraw-Hill Companies, Inc.; 2004:1-3.

Mathias S, Nayak US, Isaacs B. Balance in elderly patients: the "get-up and go" test. *Arch Phys Med Rehabil.* 1986;67(6): 387-389.

McCusker J, Bellavance F, Cardin S, Trepanier S. Screening for geriatric problems in the emergency department: reliability and validity. Identification of Seniors at Risk (ISAR) Steering Committee. *Acad Emerg Med.* 1998;5(9):883-893.

McCusker J, Dendukuri N, Tousignant P, Verdon J, Poulin de Courval L, Belzile E. Rapid two-stage emergency department intervention for seniors: impact on continuity of care. *Acad Emerg Med.* 2003;10(3):233-243.

McCusker J, Healey E, Bellavance F, Connolly B. Predictors of repeat emergency department visits by elders. *Acad Emerg Med.* 1997;4(6):581-588.

McCusker J, Verdon J, Tousignant P, de Courval LP, Dendukuri N, Belzile E. Rapid emergency department intervention for older people reduces risk of functional decline: results of a multicenter randomized trial. *J Am Geriatr Soc.* 2001;49(10):1272-1281.

Morley JE, Miller DK. Old and vulnerable in the emergency department. *Acad Emerg Med.* 1995;2(8):667-669.

Podsiadlo D, Richardson S. The timed "up & go": a test of basic functional mobility for frail elderly persons. *J Am Geriatr Soc.* 1991;39(2):142-148.

Richard N, Bhuiya F, Xu J. National hospital ambulatory medical care survey: 2007 emergency department summary. *Natl Health Stat Rep.* 2010;26(26):1-31.

Roberts DC, McKay MP, Shaffer A. Increasing rates of emergency department visits for elderly patients in the United States, 1993 to 2003. *Ann Emerg Med.* 2008;51(6):769-774.

Samaras N, Chevalley T, Samaras D, Gold G. Older patients in the emergency department: a review. *Ann Emerg Med.* 2010; 56(3):261-269.

Siebens H. The domain management model—a tool for teaching and management of older adults in emergency departments. *Acad Emerg Med.* 2005;12(2):162-168.

Sinha SK, Bessman ES, Flomenbaum N, Leff B. A systematic review and qualitative analysis to inform the development of a new emergency department-based geriatric case management model. *Ann Emerg Med.* 2011;57(6):672-682.

Strange GR, Chen EH, Sanders AB. Use of emergency departments by elderly patients: projections from a multicenter data base. *Ann Emerg Med.* 1992;21(7):819-824.

Wei LA, Fearing MA, Sternberg EJ, Inouye SK. The confusion assessment method: a systematic review of current usage. *J Am Geriatr Soc.* 2008;56(5):823-830.

Hospital Care

Kathryn J. Eubank, MD
Edgar Pierluissi, MD
C. Seth Landefeld, MD

GENERAL PRINCIPLES IN OLDER ADULTS: HAZARDS OF HOSPITALIZATION

Almost 20% of people 65 years of age or older are hospitalized each year in the United States, a rate nearly 4 times that of the general population. Those 65 years of age or older account for approximately 38% of all hospital admissions, 47% of inpatient care days, and 45% of hospital expenditures. Older adults account for 74% of all in-hospital deaths and have more discharges to places other than home. Many are frail and experience disability and comorbid illnesses. Because of their medical complexity, older patients typically require services from multiple health care providers, most of whom have no formal training in geriatric medicine.

Hospitalization is a critical time for older patients, and heralds a period of high risk that extends beyond discharge, especially for the frail and the very old. The landmark Harvard Medical Practice Study (HMPS) demonstrated that adverse events occured in approximately 4% of hospitalizations. Because older adults make up almost half of all inpatient care days, they are at a disproportionate risk for hospital adverse events. For example, in the HMPS, patients age 65 years or older accounted for only 27% of the hospitalized population, but experienced 43% of all adverse events.

Hospitalization-associated disability is a common and feared complication of hospitalization for older adults. New activities of daily living (ADL) deficits occur in as many as 30% of patients 70 years of age or older who are admitted to an acute care hospital from the community, and hospitalization accounts for approximately 50% of new disability that community-dwelling older adults experience. Hospital processes of care and environment contribute both to failure to recover from functional loss that occurred before admission as well as new decline during the hospitalization (Figure 16–1).

There are a number of factors that contribute to the hostile environment of hospitals. Bed rest and low mobility are major contributors to functional decline. Even short periods of bed rest can result in significant loss of muscle mass and strength in older adults. There are many reasons that bed rest occurs even when not explicitly written for, including crowded hospital rooms; beds that are difficult to transfer in and out of either because of height or rails; hallways that are cluttered and polished, slick floors that present a hazard to an older patient trying to navigate in unfamiliar territory; and lack of adaptive devices that the patient may use at home to overcome deficiencies such as raised toilet seats or shower chairs. Patients are frequently attached to peripheral devices such as IV poles, oxygen tubing, urinary catheters, cardiac monitors or other tethers that inhibit mobility. Concerns about falls often result in inappropriate confinement to bed. Studies show that most patients will not ambulate on their own unless explicitly told to do so, yet clinicians rarely discuss exercise in the hospital with patients. In addition, older adults may experience enforced dependence when nursing staff and concerned families assist patients with ADLs regardless of the patient's underlying ability to perform independently. Undernutrition is another factor that contributes to functional decline. Up to a quarter of hospitalized older adults receive less than 50% of required daily protein-energy intake either because of nothing by mouth (NPO) status, poor appetite, or eating an unfamiliar and unappetizing diet. Older adults are also at high risk for adverse drug events as a result of more comorbidities and polypharmacy, with approximately 10% to 15% experiencing an in-house adverse drug event. Singly or in combination, all of these factors can result in disability, falls, delirium, depression, pressure ulcers, bowel and bladder dysfunction, and increase the risk for the loss of independence and need for institutional rehabilitation.

Despite this grim situation, hospital care can be improved for older patients. Focused efforts have improved treatment of specific conditions such as myocardial infarction, congestive heart failure, and pneumonia. Moreover, reengineering the microsystem of care (eg, how care is delivered on a hospital ward or how hospital care is linked to posthospital care) has been shown to improve outcomes in this vulnerable population.

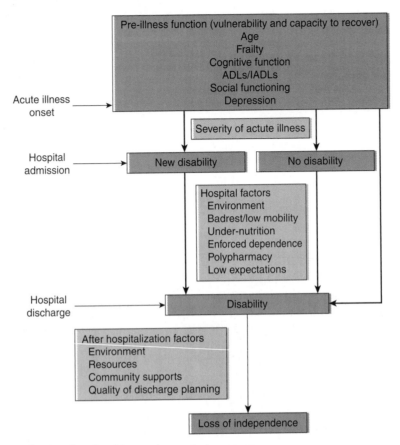

▲ Figure 16–1. Hospitalization, functional loss and capacity to recover.

SUCCESSFUL MODELS OF CARE

A number of interventions that target older patients who are at high risk for hospital-associated complications have been developed to address the challenges above. Successful care models focus on goals of care, comprehensive geriatric assessment, and interprofessional, team-based care. Attention is given to the physical environment, processes of care, and prevention of specific hospital associated complications that are common in vulnerable older patients. These models include Acute Care for Elders (ACE) units, the Hospital Elder Life Program (HELP), clinical pathways and care maps, and geriatrician–surgical comanagement.

ACE units were developed with the explicit goal to prevent functional decline and improve the quality of care for older adults during acute hospitalization. ACE units utilize comprehensive geriatric assessment and interprofessional team-based care to align care plans with patient goals and to prevent common complications of hospitalization, such as deconditioning, cognitive and nutrition decline, and polypharmacy, rather than correcting them after they develop.

ACE units include a prepared environment that promotes mobility (raised toilet seats, low beds, carpeted hallways, handrails, and assistive devices) and orientation (clocks, calendars, rooms for group meals to increase socialization). Nursing protocols are deployed to promote continence, enhance sleep via nonpharmacologic means, maintain good nutrition, promote skin integrity, and provide frequent reorientation and inclusion of patients in plans of care. Emphasis is placed on discharge planning early in hospitalization with the explicit goal of returning home to independent living. In addition, medical care plans are reviewed to prevent polypharmacy as well as minimize unnecessary procedures. In randomized trials, ACE units have been shown to improve or maintain ADLs, decrease discharges to long-term care, increase provider and patient satisfaction, and, in some studies, showed decreased length of stay and decreased cost even after accounting for capital costs of unit modification.

HELP is another multicomponent intervention. It was developed to prevent delirium in older hospitalized adults using hospital volunteers implementing its protocols on general medical wards throughout the hospital. The interventions were aimed at patients who were at medium to high risk for developing delirium based on predetermined risk factors and were aimed to address the specific risk factors of individual patients. For example, sleep deprivation can lead to delirium and measures were initiated to promote quiet environments (turning beepers to vibrate and keeping hallways quiet) and nonpharmacologic sleep protocols (warm milk and back rub for insomnia). Other risk factors addressed included immobility, visual and hearing impairment, cognitive impairment, and dehydration. Randomized trials showed a reduction in incident delirium of one-third compared to control groups, as well as improvements in duration and severity. Similar results have been obtained on nonmedicine services such as reductions in delirium following implementation of protocols in hip fracture patients on surgical wards.

Clinical pathways or care maps are methods for improving standardization of care across various providers and units. Clinical pathways or care maps are problem-specific management plans that delineate standardized key steps along an optimal timeline to achieve specific goals. For example, a care map for total knee replacement might include nursing-initiated pain protocols, automatic discontinuation of Foley catheters within hours postoperatively when certain predetermined criteria are met, and automatic ambulation on postoperative day 1. The Institute for Healthcare Improvement has identified standardization as a first step in developing more reliable systems independent of individual providers or unit assignment. Care maps have been shown to decrease lengths of stay for postsurgical care (knee arthroplasty, transurethral prostate resection, carotid endarterectomy), to decrease postoperative complications (cardiac surgery, femoral neck fracture), to increase physical function and ambulation at discharge (hip fracture), to decrease inpatient mortality (community-acquired pneumonia, congestive heart failure), and to improve pain assessment and end-of-life care (inpatient hospice, acute oncology unit). Each care map or clinical pathway is problem specific and ideally developed around evidence-based care shown to improve outcomes in the vulnerable older adult.

Geriatrician comanagement with surgical services is another promising model in which geriatricians manage the patients' medical and geriatric issues while the surgeons focus on surgical and perioperative care. Geriatrician–orthopedist comanagement of the patient with hip fracture repair, as well as elective joint replacement, is the most common comanagement model. These services have protocols in place to optimize rapid preoperative assessment, decrease time from admission to surgery, and focus on many of the issues common to the other models above. Most use care maps to standardize care such as thrombosis prophylaxes or time to ambulation. Trials show decreased lengths of stays, decreased postoperative complications, improved mobility, decreased inpatient mortality, and improved nursing and surgeon satisfaction.

APPROACH TO THE HOSPITALIZED OLDER ADULT

▶ Goals of Care

The successful management of the hospitalized older adult will incorporate features of effective models of care described above. A common feature of these models is the recognition that the care plan must be consistent with the patient's goals of care. Failure to understand a patient's goals of care is common, and can lead to frustration and dissatisfaction on the parts of patients, family members, and caregivers.

The goals of hospital care should be established upon admission for each patient. For older persons, these can vary widely and may include prolonging survival, relieving specific symptoms, maintaining or regaining ability to walk or care for oneself, getting help taking care of oneself, avoiding institutionalization, being reassured during a frightful experience, and providing comfort and peace while dying. Family members may share these goals but may also have additional goals, such as getting help caring for the patient, facilitating a transition in care from home to long-term care, or being protected from a frightening situation. Physicians and other professionals involved in the care of the patient may share these goals and also aim to achieve quality, efficiency, and patient satisfaction measures for inpatients, reduce hospital costs, and avoid adverse events.

Such discussions may be initiated with open-ended requests, such as: "Different patients have different goals when they are admitted to the hospital. Can you tell me about what you would like us to accomplish while you are in the hospital?" Discussions of goals of care are broader than simply cataloging do-not-resuscitate (DNR) decisions or reviewing options for specific therapeutic interventions. In fact, DNR and other decisions may be ill-informed without discussion of the goals of care. Explicit articulation of goals of care will sometimes identify disagreements or unreasonable expectations, which should be recognized and usually addressed.

▶ Comprehensive Geriatric Assessment

A second feature of these models is the addition of a comprehensive assessment of a patient's physical, cognitive, psychological, and social functioning to the problem-focused assessment (Table 16–1). The problem-focused assessment will identify and address the reason for admission. The comprehensive assessment of key functional domains will ensure that an appropriate care plan is implemented. Just as the underlying reasons for the hospitalization of an older adult may be multifactorial, the care plan must address these multiple factors.

Functional assessment determines the patient's ability to walk and to perform basic ADLs (eg, bathing, dressing, transferring from a bed to a chair, using the toilet, self-feeding) both at baseline, before onset of the acute illness, and on

Table 16–1. Geriatric assessment on admission.

What to Assess	How to Assess	Why it Matters	What to Do with Findings
Physical Function			
Ask about:			
ADLs	Before you became ill, were you able to bathe, toilet, dress, eat, and transfer from bed to a chair, without assistance? Currently, are you able to bathe, toilet, dress, eat, and transfer from bed to a chair, without assistance?	The patient may not be getting sufficient assistance at home at baseline or may have experienced a hospitalization-associated decline in function requiring additional assistance after discharge to ensure that all ADLs can be met.	Work with family, friends, hospital social worker, and community-based case manager to ensure patient has sufficient support that matches their functional abilities after discharge. If new onset, refer to appropriate therapy service for retraining (physical therapy/occupational therapy). Implement strategies to prevent further decline while inpatient.
Mobility	Are you able to ambulate? Do you need to use assistive devices?	Ability to ambulate safely is important to maintain independence.	Refer to physical therapy for gait assessment and education regarding safe use of assistive devices if indicated. Implement strategies to prevent decline.
Falls	Have you fallen in the past year?	Having fallen in past year is a strong risk factor for future falls.	Work with primary care clinician, therapy and home safety evaluators to ensure that appropriate interventions to reduce falls are implemented.
Cognitive Function			
Ask about:			
Orientation	Can you tell me why you are here? The name of this place? What city/state are we in? What is today's day, date, month, year? I want you to repeat and then remember 3 words I am about to say. I will ask you to say them again in 1 minute. (3-Item Recall) Please repeat these numbers: 4, 9, 2, 1, 7. (Attention)	Dementia significantly increases the risk for delirium, increases the burdens and morbidity of treatment, increases risk for rehospitalization and affects planning for safe discharge, and raises concern for decision-making capacity. For patients with dementia, assess caregivers for burnout or stress. Delirium is present in ~15% of patients on admission and develops in another 15% during hospital stay.	Consider further testing with the Montreal Cognitive Assessment (MOCA) or neuropsychological evaluation, occupational therapy consultation for a Kaufmann Evaluation of Living Skills (KELS) test. If dementia, consider referral as outpatient to memory or geriatrics clinic and referral of caregivers to Alzheimer's Association and to Family Caregiver Alliance. If delirium is present, diagnose and address underlying etiologies.
Psychological Function			
Ask about:			
Symptoms of Depression	Over the last 2 weeks, have you felt down, depressed, or hopeless? Lost interest in or pleasure in doing things?	Depression and depressive symptoms are common and often underdiagnosed in the hospital, especially among patients with stroke. Depressive symptoms, especially those that persist after discharge are associated with worse physical function and mortality after hospital discharge.	If positive, further testing can be performed using the PHQ-9 or geriatric depression scales (GDS). Evaluate for medical causes for depression such as thyroid, cardiac, neurologic, and endocrine diseases. Encourage exercise in the hospital and afterwards, discuss findings with primary provider and coordinate plan for starting treatment in the outpatient setting.
Social Function			
Ask about:			
Social Circumstances	Where do you live? Do you live with anyone? Is anyone coming into your home to help you with cooking, cleaning, shopping (IADLs)? Are you satisfied with the help you are getting? Do you have to go up steps to get home? Do you feel safe there? Do you wish to return to where you live?	Knowledge of a patient's social situation is necessary for developing an effective home discharge plan. Any evidence of elder abuse should be reported to a local adult protective services agency.	Coordinate discharge resources with social worker, rehabilitation staff, and primary provider. Resources might include in-home supportive services, Meals on Wheels, visiting nurses, case management services. Any evidence of elder neglect or abuse should be reported to a local adult protective services agency.

admission. For some patients, an unmet need for assistance with ADLs at baseline may be a contributing factor to the hospitalization. Patients who are dependent in an activity of daily living on admission have longer hospitalizations, higher risk for additional ADL dependence at discharge, and higher risk for death on average than otherwise similar patients who are independent in ADL. Patients dependent in ADLs at discharge are at increased risk for nursing home placement, loss of additional ADLs after discharge, and for death during the next year. Past history of falls is also important to elicit on admission and address during the hospitalization and in collaboration with the primary care provider after discharge.

Cognitive and psychological assessment should include assessment of mental status and affect. Among hospitalized older medical patients, ≥20% have dementia, ≥15% are delirious on admission, and another 15% experience delirium during hospitalization. Symptoms of depression are common, and 33% of hospitalized older medical patients have major or minor depression.

Neuropsychiatric assessment begins on meeting the patient. Stop to consider the possibility of dementia, delirium, and depression: They are frequently present but infrequently reported. To whom are you speaking? If you are obtaining the history from a surrogate rather than the patient, cognitive impairment from dementia or delirium or both is likely. Serious cognitive impairment is indicated by an inability to recall any of 3 items; it is largely ruled out by recall of 3 items and ability to draw the face of a clock as in the Mini-Cog. Listen for evidence of any change in mental status or behavior, and watch for signs of impaired thinking, speech, or judgment. The presence of fluctuating mental state, impaired attention, and/or consciousness or disorganized thinking suggests a delirium. Evidence of inattention includes difficulty focusing, being easily distracted, or failure to repeat 5 digits. The Confusion Assessment Method (CAM) is a highly sensitive and specific screening tool for delirium in hospitalized older adults. As a simple screen for depression, ask the patient whether he or she has felt sad, depressed, or hopeless over the last month.

It is critical for the attending physician, along with other members of the interprofessional team, to understand the patient's social context in order to develop an effective after hospital care plan. Social isolation, loneliness, and lack of social supports are common in hospitalized older adults. This will affect the amount of in-home supportive services, meals and transportation assistance, and assistive devices a patient may require. Any hesitations or concerns should be explored further for evidence of elder neglect or abuse. The prevalence of elder abuse is higher in hospitalized settings (~14%) than in the general community (~3% to 4%). Ask about how the patient manages his or her finances to explore for evidence of financial abuse. Concerns about abuse should be discussed with a social worker and reported to the local adult protective services agency.

In addition to completing a functional, cognitive, psychological, and social assessment on every older adult admitted to the hospital, a geriatrics-focused review of systems may identify conditions that are commonly considered geriatric syndromes, including incontinence, falls, sensory impairment, undernutrition, and social isolation. Each of these conditions can and should be addressed specifically. In addition, however, it is important to recognize that frequently 2 or more geriatric syndromes occur synchronously in frail patients, and that the burden of this frailty on patients, families, and professionals is substantial.

▶ Interprofessional Care

The third common feature of many successful models of care for older adults is an interprofessional approach that addresses the multiple factors that may contribute to hospitalization. In most cases, designing and implementing strategies to achieve the goals of care requires the physician's expertise and the expertise of a team of other experts. For example, consider the situation of an 83-year-old widow with chronic obstructive pulmonary disease (COPD) and mild cognitive impairment who lives alone, has declined over the past month in her ability to take care of her home and her affairs, is admitted with hypoxia and hypercarbia attributed to a COPD exacerbation, and wishes to live in her home until she dies. Although the physician may have the expertise to treat the COPD exacerbation, nursing, social work, and occupational therapy expertise is also required to promote the patient's independent function at home after discharge.

THERAPY

In general, the treatment of disease should not differ according to age. Treatment should be selected on the basis of the goals of care for a particular patient and on the basis of evidence that a particular treatment regimen will achieve the specified goal.

Older patients may differ from younger patients according to their goals. For example, treatment directed primarily at amelioration of symptoms and dysfunction rather than prolongation of survival may be desired more often by patients in their 90s than by those in their 60s. Also, insofar as these choices are influenced by prognosis, which is determined in part by age, patients should be informed accurately when they desire this information. Nonetheless, the goals of care differ between patients of the same age and should be determined individually.

Evidence of the efficacy of a treatment regimen in achieving a specific goal should be sought. In some situations, treatment efficacy may differ by age. For example, thrombolytic therapy of acute myocardial infarction is less efficacious in prolonging survival in persons age 75 years and older than in younger persons, and acute coronary revascularization may be more efficacious in these patients. Doses of therapies often need to be titrated to reflect renal or hepatic function, which often decline with age. The risk of side effects from many drugs and procedures also increases with age, and these risks should be considered in estimating the net benefit of a specific treatment strategy.

Unfortunately, most evidence about the efficacy of many therapies is based on studies of younger persons, and specific evidence about the efficacy of those therapies in persons age 75 years or older is inadequate. In these situations, it is reasonable to extrapolate from evidence in younger patients, taking into account age-related differences in hepatic and renal function and risks of side effects when deciding on and implementing a specific treatment regimen.

PREVENTION

To prevent iatrogenic complications common in hospitalized older adults, additional assessments on admission and throughout the hospital stay are required (Table 16–2).

Table 16–2. Prevention strategies for common hazards experienced by older adults in the hospital.

Hazard	How to Assess	When to Assess	How to Prevent
Disability	Ask the patient or the nurse if the patient is getting out of bed for every meal and walking 3-4 times daily.	Daily	Promote mobility: Order physical therapy consultation, avoid bedrest orders, remove unnecessary catheters, write for patient to be out of bed for all meals and to ambulate at 3-4 times daily.
Delirium	Look for signs of inattentiveness, disorganized thinking or changes in consciousness.	Daily	Promote mobility. Provide patient with eyeglasses, hearing aids, frequent orientation with calendars and clocks. Avoid sedating medications, restraints, unnecessary catheters.
Depression	Over the last 2 weeks, have you felt down, depressed, or hopeless? Lost interest in or pleasure in doing things?	At discharge	Promote mobility. Avoid sedating medications. Avoid anticholinergic medications.
Falls	Have you fallen in the past 6 months?	At admission	Promote mobility. Provide patient with eyeglasses, hearing aids, frequent orientation with calendars and clocks. Avoid sedating medications, restraints, unnecessary catheters. Address incontinence.
Incontinence	Do you have trouble controlling your urine, feces? Have you had accidents in the past 6 months?	At admission and during hospitalization for prolonged hospitalizations.	Promote mobility. Avoid anticholinergic medications and bladder catheterization. Use scheduled voiding while awake.
Constipation	When was your last bowel movement? Review nursing documentation regarding last bowel movement.	Daily	Promote mobility. Maintain hydration. Provide fiber in diet. Provide laxatives such as senna for patients receiving opiates for pain.
Pressure Ulcers	Skin examination.	Daily	Promote mobility. Frequent position changes (every 2 hours) for patients that are bedbound. Maintain nutritional state. Keep skin dry. Consider pressure reducing mattress.
Infection	Is bladder catheter or IV catheter present?	Daily	Promote mobility to stimulate deeper breathing. Remove unnecessary bladder and intravenous catheters.
Inappropriate prescribing	Review all medications for polypharmacy, drug–drug interactions, and appropriate dosages.	Daily	Review all medications for efficacy and appropriateness in older adults, considering prognosis, goals of care, and need for monitoring.
Undernutrition	See chapter for useful nutritional screening tools.	Daily	Avoid unnecessary NPO orders; ask caregiver to bring in dentures; provide a diet that is the least restrictive possible, of the proper consistency, and that is culturally appropriate; provide nutritional supplementation for patients that are undernourished on admission.

Functional decline is a feared, but all too common, adverse outcome of hospitalization. Many complications can be prevented through a dedicated effort to maintain mobility in the hospital. Clinicians should set walking expectations early for each patient and assess compliance daily. Although symptoms and fear of injury may limit some patients, most are motivated by avoiding functional decline and simply being asked to walk. Clinicians should also treat pain that may be inhibiting in-hospital walking; ensure assistive devices are available with appropriate rehabilitation therapy training; and remove unnecessary tethers such as bladder and intravenous catheters, oxygen lines, and cardiac monitoring. Unnecessary bladder catheters, in addition to causing iatrogenic infection and limiting mobility, are associated with increased functional decline and mortality after hospital discharge.

In addition, hospitalization provides an opportunity for the assessment and implementation of routine preventive maneuvers in older patients: Maneuvers that should be considered in every older hospitalized patient include:

- Deep venous thrombosis prophylaxis

- Influenza vaccination.

- Pneumococcal vaccination.

- Determination of smoking status and counseling about smoking cessation.

- Screening for alcoholism and seeking counseling when indicated.

- Screening for undernutrition, including vitamin D deficiency

TRANSITIONING FROM HOSPITAL TO HOME

It is increasingly recognized that transitions between care providers and across settings are common and fraught with hazards. Older adults, especially, express confusion regarding self-management after hospitalization. These hazards and confusion have led to a new focus of care called "transitional care" (see Chapter 13, "Transitions and Continuity of Care"). There are numerous interventions aimed at improving the transitional care of older adults leaving the hospital. While these multicomponent interventions differ, they all have several key components in common. All implement strategies to improve patient and caregiver engagement in the process starting at the time of admission. All seek early identification of postdischarge care needs and use interprofessional teams to properly address those needs throughout the hospitalization, as well as after discharge. All invest a considerable amount of time and resources into improving patient understanding about the reasons for admission, what is required to manage their health at discharge, appropriate signs and symptoms that signal a need for early intervention, and who they should contact for questions or help. All give special attention to medication reconciliation, patient instruction, and cross-site communication of medication changes. All also improve communication between inpatient and outpatient clinicians via phone calls and improved discharge summary communication. Table 16–3 is a checklist for improving care at the time of transition from hospital to next site of care.

In addition to the topics common to the interventions above, inpatient clinicians caring for older adults need an

Table 16–3. Transitional care checklist.

Patient and Family Education	☐	Have the patient, caregivers, and all members of the care team been included in the planning process and agree with the care plan?
	☐	Have the patient and caregiver been adequately educated about their condition including what makes it better or worse, signs/symptoms to watch for, and when to seek medical attention?
Medications	☐	Do the patient and caregiver understand how and when to take their medications and side effects to watch for? Is proper monitoring in place for high risk medications?
	☐	Has the medication list been properly reconciled to avoid polypharmacy and inappropriate medications?
Functional Status/Home Environment Alignment	☐	What is the patient's functional status? Does the patient need referral to therapy services or will the patient require more supervision at discharge?
Cognitive Status/Home Environment Alignment	☐	What is the patient's cognitive status? Has there been a change? Does the patient require increased assistance or supervision after discharge?
Medical equipment	☐	Are there specific services that need to be in place prior to leaving the hospital? For example, has oxygen been delivered to the home? Durable medical equipment? Supplies?
Follow-up and Communication with Primary Provider	☐	Is follow up arranged and occurring in a timely manner? Are the patient and caregiver aware and in agreement with needed follow-up and referrals?
	☐	Is there a plan and direct responsibility for following up on any pending labs/studies?
	☐	Is the discharge summary completed and has it been sent to the primary care, specialist, and receiving clinicians? If going to another facility, is the discharge summary ready and being sent with the patient and does it include who can be contacted for questions?

understanding of the multiple postdischarge sites of care available for this population. Will the patient require rehabilitation for deconditioning? If so, will the patient meet requirements for intensive rehabilitation hospitals versus skilled nursing facilities (SNFs)? Is there a skilled need that requires home services after discharge or inpatient SNF services, (often this depends on the availability of a caregiver)? Has the patient declined in physical or cognitive function such that 24-hour supervision will be required at discharge? Can 24-hour supervision be done at home or will nursing home placement be required? Is the patient nearing the end-of-life with goals more consistent with hospice care? Should hospice care be arranged prior to discharge? Most patients prefer to stay in their homes as long as possible and good transitional care can help them achieve that goal by optimizing care at home if possible, and putting plans in place to regain and optimize functional status.

Baztán JJ, Suárez-García FM, López-Arrieta J, Rodríguez-Mañas L, Rodríguez-Artalejo F. Effectiveness of acute geriatric units on functional decline, living at home, and case fatality among older patients admitted to hospital for acute medical disorders: meta-analysis. *BMJ.* 2009;338:b50.

Covinsky KE, Pierluissi E, Johnston CB. Hospitalization-associated disability: "She was probably able to ambulate, but I'm not sure." *JAMA.* 2011;306(16):1782-1793.

Creditor M. Hazards of hospitalization of the elderly. *Ann Intern Med.* 1993;118(3):219-223.

Forster AJ, Clark HD, Menard A, et al. Adverse events among medical patients after discharge from hospital. *CMAJ.* 2004;170(3):345-349.

Fried TR, Bradley EH, Towle VR, Allore H. Understanding the treatment preferences of seriously ill patients. *N Engl J Med.* 2002;346(14):1061-1066.

Friedman SM, Mendelson DA, Kates SL, McCann RM. Geriatric comanagement of proximal femur fractures: total quality management and protocol-driven care result in better outcomes for a frail patient population. *J Am Geriatr Soc.* 2008;56(7): 1349-1356.

Rotter T, Kinsman L, James EL, et al. Clinical pathways: effects on professional practice, patient outcomes, length of stay and hospital costs. *Cochrane Database Syst Rev.* 2010;(3): CD006632.

USEFUL WEBSITES

Estimating Prognosis for Elders http://www.eprognosis.org

The Hospital Elder Life Program (HELP). http://www.hospitalelderlifeprogram.org/public/public-main.php

Perioperative Care in Older Surgical Patients

17

Lawrence Oresanya, MD

Emily Finlayson, MD, MS

GENERAL PRINCIPLES IN OLDER ADULTS

More than a third of all surgical procedures are performed in individuals older than age 65 years and one-third of older adults undergo a surgical procedure in the last year of life. In 2007, more than 4 million major operations were performed on older adults. Use of less-invasive procedures is also increasing. With advancements in technology, coronary angioplasty and lower-extremity endovascular procedures have surpassed rates of coronary artery bypass grafting and lower-extremity bypass. These minimally invasive approaches broaden the scope of illness that can be treated and together with the aging of the population is contributing to an increase in the number of older patients undergoing surgical interventions.

SURGICAL RISK IN THE OLDER ADULT

Caring for the older surgical patient presents unique problems: older individuals present with more advanced disease, have more comorbidities and suffer more complications than younger patients. Appropriate patient selection and perioperative care is essential for optimizing surgical outcomes in this population. The benefits of the most commonly performed surgical procedures are well established. Colon resections increase colorectal cancer-free survival, and hip replacements significantly improve joint pain and functional ability. These benefits, however, must be weighed against the risk of mortality, morbidity, and decreased quality of life that sometimes follow these operations.

Nationally representative large cohort studies provide the most realistic information about surgical risk in older adults. In a national sample of patients undergoing high-risk cancer operations, patients older than age 80 years who were undergoing esophageal resections had an operative mortality of 20% with only 19% of patients experiencing long-term survival beyond 5 years. Morbidity after surgery in older adults is also high. Bentrem et al found that medical complications, such as strokes, myocardial infarction, pneumonia, and renal failure, occur at much higher rates in older adults. These severe medical complications are the proximal cause of the high perioperative mortality seen in older patients. Surgical complications, such as wound infections, bleeding, and need for reoperation, are not more frequent, but the occurrence of nonfatal postoperative complications is independently associated with decreased long-term survival.

Major operations may also result in a diminished quality of life by causing postoperative cognitive and functional decline. The risk of postoperative cognitive dysfunction following cardiac surgery is well studied, and there is now increasing evidence that postoperative cognitive dysfunction also occurs after noncardiac procedures. Up to 10% of patients older than age 60 years suffer from memory problems 3 months out from noncardiac surgery. It is unclear whether it is acute illness, anesthesia, or surgery that is the primary contributor to this condition. Functional changes following surgery can also be prolonged and irreversible. More than half of patients undergoing abdominal operations experience significant functional decline that persists for up to a year after surgery. A recent study assessing functional status following colectomy in nursing home residents found that the most active patients suffer the greatest decline as they have the most to lose. These findings emphasize the importance of addressing the risk of functional decline in all older patients, even the most active. For some patients, loss of independence weighs heavier than mortality when deciding whether to undergo a high-risk operation. Awareness of these risks is essential for appropriate patient selection. It also allows clinicians to offer a realistic expectation of outcomes, which, in turn, informs decision making by the older individual and their families.

CLINICAL CARE

▶ Preoperative Assessment

A. Cognition

Older individuals' cognitive capacity, decision-making capacity, and risk for postoperative delirium should be assessed preoperatively. For patients without a known history of dementia, a cognitive assessment using the Mini-Cog test (see Chapter 6, "Geriatric Assessment") should be performed. The Mini-Cog is a 3-item recall and clock draw test that efficiently screens for cognitive impairment. One point is awarded for each item recalled and 2 points for a normal-appearing clock. A score of 0–2 points indicates a positive screen for dementia. This screening is the initial step in identifying patients that may lack the capacity to make medical decisions and who are at high risk for delirium. When initial evaluation identifies cognitive impairment, assessment of decision-making capacity is essential. For patients lacking capacity advance directives or a surrogate decision maker should be used (see Chapter 12, "Ethics & Informed Decision Making"). Older adults who are at risk for delirium should be identified preoperatively. Major risk factors for delirium are dementia, hearing impairment, depression, preoperative narcotic use, medical comorbidities, electrolyte abnormalities, malnutrition, and poor functional status. Identifying patients who are at risk for delirium is crucial as a number of measures implemented early in the patient's hospital course can reduce this risk. Comanagement by a geriatrician, appropriate use of analgesics and prophylactic use of atypical antipsychotics have been evaluated in clinical trials and found to significantly decrease the incidence and severity of delirium.

B. Cardiovascular

Cardiovascular complications are associated with high operative mortality rates. To identify and help reduce this risk, the American College of Cardiology and the American Heart Association (ACC/AHA) has developed recommendations for cardiac evaluation and care for non-cardiac surgery. For older adults with active cardiac disease or coronary artery disease (CAD) risk factors and poor functional status who are about to undergo elective intermediate or high-risk surgery, strong consideration should be given to non invasive preoperative cardiac testing and evaluation by a cardiologist (Table 17–1).

C. Pulmonary

Prolonged intubation (>48 hours), pneumonia, atelectasis and bronchospasm occur after surgery in more than 15% of patients older than age 70 years. Risk factors for these complications include active pulmonary disease, current cigarette smoking, congestive heart failure, chronic renal failure, cognitive disorders, and functional dependence.

Table 17–1. Postoperative management of the older patient.

Mobilize the patient by postoperative day #1
Perform pain assessments with each set of vital signs
Institute a pain management plan for pain score >5
Dentures, hearing aids, and corrective lenses should be made readily accessible
Provide chest physical therapy with incentive spirometry or deep breathing exercises
Institute aspiration precautions (head of bed elevation with repositioning; sit upright during meals)
Monitor fluid status for at least the first 5 days (ins and outs, daily weights)
Consider blood transfusion for hemoglobin level ≤8 or hematocrit ≤24
Administer appropriate deep venous thrombosis prophylaxis
Perform daily assessment of all central lines and reevaluate their indications for use
Remove Foley catheters by postoperative day #3
If temperature >38°C after postoperative day #2 obtain urinalysis and urine culture, examine wound and line sites, blood cultures and chest radiograph
Maintain serum glucose less than 200 mg/dL by postoperative day #1

Reproduced with permission from McGory ML, Kao KK, Shekelle PG, et al. Developing quality indicators for elderly surgical patients. *Ann Surg.* 2009;250(2):338-347.

Routine pulmonary testing beyond assessment for these risk factors on history and physical should be based on clinical criteria. Preoperative chest x-ray is recommended for older individuals undergoing major surgery who have cardiopulmonary disease and have not had a chest x-ray in the last 6 months. It may also be obtained as a baseline for patients requiring ICU admission postoperatively. Pulmonary function tests are rarely required and are mainly reserved for those undergoing lung resections and patients with severe chronic obstructive pulmonary disease (COPD). To decrease the risk of pulmonary complications smoking cessation should be initiated at least 2 months prior to elective surgery and active pulmonary diseases should be adequately treated.

D. Functional Status

Functional dependence is an independent predictor of mortality following surgery in older adults. Robinson et al recently reported that dependence with even 1 activity of daily living significantly increased the risk of 6-month mortality (odds ratio [OR] 13.9; 95% confidence interval [CI] 2.9, 65.5). The ability to perform activities of daily living (ADLs) and instrumental activities of daily living (IADLs) should be assessed preoperatively. This identifies older adults who will benefit from occupational and physical therapy in the postoperative period.

E. Nutritional Status

Older patients with functional dependence are at high risk of malnutrition. Fourteen percent of nursing home residents, 39% of inpatients, and 50.5% of individuals in rehabilitation are malnourished. All older patients should be screened for malnutrition preoperatively. Patients with unintentional weight loss of >10% to 15% of the last 6 months, body mass index (BMI) <18.5 and serum albumin <3 g/dL are described as being at severe nutritional risk. Preoperative nutritional support should be provided to these patients. Enteral nutrition is the preferred route for nutritional support; when this option is not available secondary to gastrointestinal conditions, parenteral nutrition should be used.

F. Frailty

Evaluation of frailty is emerging as an important means of preoperative risk assessment in older adults. Using the "eyeball test" physicians have long tried to predict which older patients were at high risk of complications following surgery. Assessments of frailty now quantify these previously intuitive assumptions. Frail patients have been found to have over twice the odds of postoperative complications as compared to nonfrail patients and are more likely to be discharged to a nursing facility. Current measures of frailty remain primarily research tools; work is ongoing to validate frailty measures that are easy to use in clinical settings.

▶ Postoperative Care

The aim of postoperative care is to return older patients to a high level of functioning as quickly as possible. This goal is achieved with measures that promote recovery and prevent complications. Through a review of the literature and expert interviews, McGory et al have compiled measures that constitute the basic level of postoperative care that should be provided to older patients undergoing any kind of surgery. Table 17–1 is adapted from this work and highlights important aspects of routine postoperative care for older adults.

When possible, patients should be out of bed and walking by the first postoperative day. Physical therapy and occupational therapy consultation should be obtained for patients with functional impairment. Early ambulation along with chest physiotherapy using incentive spirometers decreases the risk of pulmonary complications. Appropriate fluid resuscitation should be provided and fluid balance should be monitored through documentation of intake, output and daily weights. Oral or enteral nutrition should be resumed as soon as the gastrointestinal tract is functional. To prevent infectious complications, aspiration precautions should be instituted, Foley catheters should be removed within 48 hours and the need for central lines and drains should be reviewed daily and removed once no longer needed.

A. Management of Common Postoperative Issues in Older adults

1. Pain—Older patients are at higher risk of undertreated pain. Inadequate treatment of pain impedes recovery, prevents the patient from participating in activities and can lead to delirium, depression and pulmonary complications. To avoid these complications, pain levels should be assessed frequently and a pain management plan that delivers adequate analgesia while avoiding untoward effects of the analgesics should be implemented. The numeric rating scale is the preferred pain-intensity rating scale for use in older adults. Postoperative pain is best managed with regional anesthesia. For patients undergoing major surgery, epidural regional analgesia with opioids and local anesthetic agents initiated intraoperatively provides the most effective pain control. Intravenous and oral analgesics such as opioids, acetaminophen and nonsteroidal antiinflammatory drugs (NSAIDs) also provide effective pain relief. They may be used as supplements to regional anesthesia or as the primary analgesics for less-invasive operations. These medications are best delivered as patient-controlled analgesics (PCAs) or on a scheduled dose. This is preferred over as-needed doses of medication, because patients spend less time in pain. Although effective pain control is important, providers need to be vigilant for side effects of analgesics. Older patients are at increased risk of hypotension, respiratory depression, over sedation and constipation than can occur as a side effect of analgesics. Use of regional analgesics; short-acting agents; smaller, less-frequent doses; and frequent patient assessment can decrease the risk of these complications.

2. Delirium—Delirium occurs in between 15% and 50% of older patients postoperatively. It is associated with increased mortality and medical complications. The physiologic conditions most commonly responsible for delirium in the postoperative setting are pain, hypoxia, hypoglycemia, electrolyte imbalance, and infection. The initial evaluation of the delirious patient should be focused on identifying these disorders. Pain should be adequately treated, serum electrolytes and glucose should be checked, an infectious work-up should be performed and other postoperative complications ruled out. Further measures in the prevention and management of delirium include optimization of environmental stimuli and a review of current medications. Older patients should have their eyeglasses and hearing aids made readily available. The Beers criteria identifies a number of potentially inappropriate medications for older patients. Avoiding anticholinergics, antihistamines and benzodiazepines may help decrease the incidence of delirium in older patients. For patients with agitated delirium who at risk of injury, frequent reorientation is required, this may be provided by family members or a sitter; restraints should be avoided. When these measures are unsuccessful low doses of antipsychotics such as quetiapine or Haldol can be prescribed. Their use, however, remains controversial and they should be used with caution.

3. Cardiac Complications—Cardiac complications occur frequently in older patients. The most common postoperative cardiac complications requiring urgent treatment are atrial fibrillation and myocardial infarction. Atrial fibrillation can occur as a result of the increased sympathetic tone associated with the stress of surgery, volume overload, hypoxia/hypercarbia, electrolyte abnormalities, or as a result of underlying heart disease. Management of new-onset atrial fibrillation begins with an assessment of hemodynamic stability and rate control. In patients with hemodynamic instability emergent cardioversion is required. Rate control is achieved using either β blockers or diltiazem. Intravenous amiodarone may be used when the first-line drugs are ineffective. Most cases of new-onset atrial fibrillation spontaneously revert to sinus rhythm. However, atrial fibrillation persists for more than 24–48 hours; anticoagulation should be considered to reduce the risk of stroke.

Perioperative myocardial infarction occurs mainly as a result of prolonged myocardial oxygen supply–demand imbalance and only rarely as a result of acute coronary syndrome (ACS). It is diagnosed based on a rise and fall of troponins in the setting of myocardial ischemia as evidenced by electrocardiogram (ECG) changes, imaging findings or cardiac symptoms. Tachycardia, tachyarrythmias, hypertension, anemia and hypoxia all contribute to myocardial oxygen supply–demand imbalance and can result in non–ST-segment elevation myocardial infarction (NSTEMI) in the perioperative period. When NSTEMI is suspected, management begins with heart rate and blood pressure control with β blockers and appropriate pain control. For patients with ST-segment elevation and suspected ACS, immediate cardiology consultation should be obtained.

MODELS OF SURGICAL CARE

Prehabilitation, enhanced recovery programs (ERPs), and geriatric comanagement are some of the innovative models being implemented to improve the outcomes of surgical care for older patients. In prehabilitation programs, older adults participate in structured exercise programs in the weeks prior to elective surgery. These programs have been found to significantly improve older patients' preoperative functional status and may enhance postoperative recovery. Current research on prehabilitation is focused on identifying the optimal exercise regimen and on improving compliance with the programs. ERPs are another model aimed at promoting early physiologic and physical recovery after surgery. These programs use structured evidence based protocols to optimize preoperative patient preparation, minimize the surgical stress response and encourage early postoperative nutrition and mobilization. ERPs decrease hospital lengths of stay and complication rates in older patients. Lastly, models in which surgeons and geriatricians work closely together to care for the older surgical patient are being developed. Collaboration should begin at the time of patient and procedure selection and continue through the recovery period. This model will certainly improve the quality of surgical care received by the older adult.

Bentrem DJ, Cohen ME, Hynes DM, Ko CY, Bilimoria KY. Identification of specific quality improvement opportunities for the elderly undergoing gastrointestinal surgery. *Arch Surg.* 2009;144(11):1013-1020.

Finlayson E, Fan Z, Birkmeyer JD. Outcomes in octogenarians undergoing high-risk cancer operation: a national study. *J Am Coll Surg.* 2007;205(6):729-734.

Fleisher LA, Beckman JA, Brown KA, et al. ACC/AHA 2007 guidelines on Perioperative cardiovascular evaluation and care for noncardiac surgery: executive summary. *J Am Coll Cardiol.* 2007;50(17):1707-1732.

Flinn DR, Diehl KM, Seyfried LS, Malani PN. Prevention, diagnosis, and management of postoperative delirium in older adults. *J Am Coll Surg.* 2009;209(2):261-268.

Fried T, Bradley E, Towle V, Allore H. Understanding the treatment preferences of seriously ill patients. *N Engl J Med.* 2002;346(14):1061-1066.

Khuri SF, Henderson WG, DePalma RG, et al. Determinants of long-term survival after major surgery and the adverse effect of postoperative complications. *Ann Surg.* 2005;242(3):326-341; discussion 341-343.

Kwok AC, Semel ME, Lipsitz SR, et al. The intensity and variation of surgical care at the end of life: a retrospective cohort study. *Lancet.* 2011;378(9800):1408-1413.

Lawrence V, Hazuda H, Cornell J, et al. Functional independence after abdominal surgery in the elderly. *J Am Coll Surg.* 2004;199(5):762-772.

Makary MA, Segev DL, Pronovost PJ, et al. Frailty as a predictor of surgical outcomes in older patients. *J Am Coll Surg.* 2010;210(6):901-908.

Mayo NE, Feldman L, Scott S, et al. Impact of preoperative change in physical function on postoperative recovery: argument supporting prehabilitation for colorectal surgery. *Surgery.* 2011;150(3):505-514.

McGory ML, Kao KK, Shekelle PG, et al. Developing quality indicators for elderly surgical patients. *Ann Surg.* 2009;250(2):338-347.

Robinson TN, Raeburn CD, Tran ZV, Angles EM, Brenner LA, Moss M. Postoperative delirium in the elderly risk factors and outcomes. *Ann Surg.* 2009;249(1):173-178.

Terrando N, Brzezinski M, Degos V, et al. Perioperative cognitive decline in the aging population. *Mayo Clin Proc.* 2011;86(9): 885-893.

Long-Term Care, Nursing Home, & Rehabilitation

18

Theresa A. Allison, MD, PhD

GENERAL PRINCIPLES IN OLDER ADULTS

Older adults, more than any other age group, reside in a variety of settings. Particularly as physical and cognitive function decline, older adults require increasing levels of assistance for their care. In addition, functional decline following serious illness or injury affects the ability of older adults to return directly from hospital to home, leading to a need for institutional rehabilitation prior to return to the community. This chapter describes the variety of living situations available to older adults, including both short-term and long-term nursing home care (Figure 18–1).

LONG-TERM CARE IN THE COMMUNITY

The overwhelming majority of caregiving takes place in the community, with more than 7 million individuals receiving agency home health care and an estimated 10.9 million who need assistance. Although the nursing home census has now risen to 1.8 million, most older adults continue to live at home throughout their lives, with family members and friends providing care as needed. Within the community, elders can receive services ranging from custodial care (assistance with activities of daily living and light household chores) to the Hospital at Home model.

▶ Models

Models of care range from single-family dwellings, to apartments, to "intentional communities," to the Residential Care Facility for Elders (RCFE), also known in many states as the Assisted Living Facility (ALF) or Board and Care Home. Unlike nursing homes, ALFs are considered social models of care, regulated by a variety of state agencies across the United States, and providing a range of services. In the most basic Board and Care Home, an elder can expect to receive help with laundry, housekeeping, and meal preparation. In the

larger ALFs, there may be assistance with medication administration, and even dementia special care units. Some ALFs are built adjacent to nursing homes and marketed as continuing care communities. At all of these residential settings, older adults may be able to receive the following:

- *Home medical care:* Medical services from clinicians who make house calls
- *Home health agency care:* Skilled nursing, social work, rehabilitation services and, assuming the ALF has a hospice waiver, interdisciplinary home hospice services
- *In-home social services:* Custodial assistance with activities of daily living (bathing, toileting, transferring, feeding), light housekeeping, shopping, and food preparation (also called *Home Health Aid and Attendance*)
- *Private case management services*

In addition, home-dwelling elders have the option of attending adult day health centers (ADHCs), where they can participate in activities and receive limited amounts of nursing, medication administration, exercise, and physical and occupational therapy.

In contrast, the Program for All-Inclusive Care of the Elderly (PACE) is open to nursing home-eligible adults who are attempting to live at home but who require more resources than they and their families can provide. PACE model programs provide complete medical, nursing, rehabilitative and social services within the context of an adult day health center that has a fully staffed clinic on site. This integrated model provides care for patients while at home and contracts with local hospitals if an elder becomes too sick to remain safely in the community.

▶ Financing

Neither Medicare nor Medicaid cover long-term care in the community setting, so financing derives from either personal

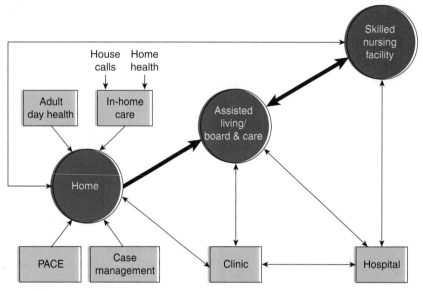

▲ **Figure 18–1.** Sites of long-term care. A diagrammatic representation of the locations in which elders live (*circles*), with *thick arrows* showing the directions in which elders move from location to location. The *thin arrows* identify those medical services available to elders living in different sites and the medical/service centers to which elders travel (*squares*).

resources or optional long-term care insurance programs, all of which are highly variable. Although Medicare reimburses a limited amount of skilled home health nursing and rehabilitation, the only long-term home health option covered by Medicare is the Medicare Hospice benefit, intended to last for 6 months or less. Medicaid programs in different states cover limited in-home social services (long-term, nonskilled custodial care), adult day health care, transportation, and housing subsidies. State and local governments similarly provide home-delivered meals, home attendant care, homemaker services, and transportation that vary from place to place. The PACE model operates as a capitated, "dual-medi" (Medicare/Medicaid-enrolled participant) system, which makes it cost-effective for low-income elders and unaffordable for much of the middle class. The Department of Veterans Affairs (VA) is the largest single-payer system to cover long-term care in the community, but access to services is locale dependent. In addition, VA long-term care benefits are dependent upon the degree of service connection of the chronic illness or disability and the financial status of the veteran.

▶ Clinical Care

Of all of the outpatient models in geriatrics, only PACE includes total clinical care, with onsite physicians, nurses, and therapists. ADHCs and skilled home care agencies have nursing, rehabilitation and social work services. ALFs and the community-based portions of continuing care communities may have a licensed vocational nurse on site, but they are predicated upon a social,

rather than a medical model of care. The focus in such congregant living environments is on social support, not clinical assessment. It is essential for clinicians to clarify if their patients live in a nursing home or assisted-living situation, because the latter include no skilled monitoring of patients outside of the skilled home services ordered by the physician.

INSTITUTIONAL LONG-TERM CARE

The skilled nursing facility (SNF) or nursing home is not a popular institution in the United States. In an often-quoted study, 30% of surveyed hospital patients stated that they would "rather die" than be transferred to an SNF. This is sobering when we consider that 43% of Americans over the age of 65 are likely to spend time in nursing homes. Although nursing homes continue to operate under a medical model of care, there is a growing movement to change the "culture" of nursing homes so that they are less institutional and more homelike. For example, "homelike" nursing homes encourage their inhabitants to eat, sleep, and wake up when they wish, and to visit with pets, children, friends, and family. This section primarily addresses the regulatory requirements of nursing homes.

▶ Models

SNF care is often divided into the categories of short-term and long-term care, yet the regulatory requirements remain the same for both types. When a nursing home is used as a site for short-term rehabilitation (physical, occupational, and speech therapy), the institution is reimbursed only for 720 minutes of skilled rehabilitation per week. In contrast, the acute rehabilitation center (ARC) is a high-acuity, posthospital institution designed to provide a minimum of 2 hours of intensive rehabilitation each day. The ARC is not covered in this chapter partly because its exercise requirements are not tolerated by most older adults, and partly because Medicare rarely reimburses for more than a few weeks of care, making it a site of almost exclusively short-term care. It is important, however, to be aware of the difference between acute rehabilitation (ARC) and subacute rehabilitation (SNF) in the context of stroke, because aggressive, early rehabilitation leads to earlier improvements in functional status. An older adult who would benefit from ARC but who cannot yet tolerate the minimum requirements may be admitted temporarily to a nursing home and then transferred to an acute rehabilitation setting with the goal of return to long-term institutional or home care.

In terms of long-term care, the nursing home is the most well known, but not the only form of institutional care. The "culture change" movement has given rise to newer, more home-like forms, the most well-studied of which is the Greenhouse model. A Greenhouse is home to 10 or 12 nursing-home eligible older adults with caregivers who function outside of the conventional roles of nursing. In a Greenhouse, caregivers, or *Shahbazim*, are as likely to be found cooking or gardening with residents as to be found providing traditional bed and body care.

▶ Financing

The financial structure of the nursing home is currently undergoing a shift as a consequence of decreases in Medicaid reimbursement. Medicare part A continues pay for posthospital care only. A Medicare-qualifying stay at a nursing home occurs within 30 days of a 3-day hospital stay and requires either skilled nursing (typically IV medications or daily wound care) or rehabilitation 5 days a week. The Medicare part A benefit can be invoked even if the patient is initially discharged home, or after discharge from a skilled nursing facility, if that patient suffers a functional decline within the first 30 days of return to home. Medicare part A can also be invoked for a hospice patient who suffers a nonrelated illness or injury, such as a cancer patient who fractures a femur. Medicare covers the cost of care for the first 20 days and then requires that the patient pay a copayment for the remaining 100 days of coverage. Once this benefit has been exhausted, the patient must remain out of hospital for 3 months before a new benefit period can be invoked. Long-term care costs, in contrast, are not reimbursed by Medicare. Adults who lack adequate long-term care private insurance are required to "spend down" until they qualify for Medicaid. Severe cuts in Medicaid funding in states such as California are resulting in long-term care bed crises, in which it is becoming increasingly difficult for older adults to find institutional homes. Alternate payor sources include private long-term care insurance, VA coverage for certain service-connected veterans, and the resident elders and their families.

▶ Clinical Care

The clinical structure of the nursing home is rigidly defined, even though the federal regulations themselves are relatively vague. The creation of the Minimum Data Set (MDS) has led to improvement in the quality of care without creating parallel improvements in quality of life. Care is managed through an interdisciplinary team consisting of the following members:

- *Nursing:* Registered nurses (RNs) provide nursing assessments as well as pass medications, manage intravenous access and provide skilled treatments. Licensed vocational nurses (LVNs), with 2-year training, are licensed to pass medications and provide some treatments, but do not receive the formal training in clinical assessment of RNs. Certified nursing assistants (CNAs or NAs) have completed a 40-hour certification program, and provide almost all of the activities of daily living (ADLs) care required by elders living in the home.

- *Rehabilitation:* Physical therapists (PTs) provide gait and balance training and much of the work involved in strengthening the body after a debilitating episode. Physical therapy assistants, who lack the formal training of the PT, work with patients on established workout routines. Occupational therapists (OTs) provide therapy around ADLs and instrumental activities of daily living (IADLs). They often focus on the small motor skills of the hands, and their work is highly dependent upon the functional status of the patient. Occupational therapy assistants can similarly work as OT extenders to help patients complete established exercise sets. Speech and language pathologists, or speech therapists (STs), focus on deficits in both speech and swallowing, and represent a crucial part of acute stroke rehabilitation, as well as in the slower neurodegenerative diseases found commonly in nursing homes. Most short-term care rehabilitation units do not have respiratory therapists working on site, unless they specialize in the care of ventilator-dependent patients.

- *Nutrition:* SNFs are required to provide at least 1 registered dietitian for their residents. The nutritionist provides recommendations for nutritional supplementation as well as individual education and recommendations. In some facilities, the nutritionists partner with the kitchen to develop healthy menus, but this is not one of the federal regulatory requirements.

- *Pharmacy:* Nursing homes require the presence of a pharmacist, but not a pharmacy. Although larger nursing homes may elect to have an onsite dispensing pharmacy, many smaller facilities contract out with local pharmacies that are willing to deliver medications, sometimes urgently or after hours. The pharmacist is required to complete drug regimen reviews in order to prevent polypharmacy complications and to reduce the rate of medication errors.

- *Social services:* The social services at a nursing home can be highly variable and include 2 completely separate sets of professionals. Licensed clinical social workers assist with social, financial, and other systems-based issues, and may provide counseling, depending upon the setting. In contrast, Title 42 also mandates that the nursing home provide "meaningful activities," and these are done through the work of either recreation therapists or activities staff members. At some nursing homes, there is also chaplaincy support for the spiritual care of the residents.

- *Medical services:* Medical services are mandated in nursing homes, but onsite medical care is highly variable. Physicians are required to provide the nursing home with their call schedule, but they are not required to establish set hours in which to provide face-to-face care. Reimbursement involves a fee-for-service model in most practices. The notable exceptions are some large Health Management Organizations and the VA, in which the physicians work for a salary. Unlike the outpatient setting, the SNF is tightly regulated under both the federal and state governments. Medicare requires that physicians see and admit patients within 72 hours of their arrival at the nursing home, and then every 30 days for the next 3 months. After this period, federal regulations dictate that they must see the patient every 60 days. State regulations vary, with certain states requiring a physician admission exam within 48 hours of patient arrival or requiring monthly visits, only some of which may be performed by a nurse practitioner in a comanaged process.

This interdisciplinary team (IDT), augmented by administrators, housekeepers, kitchen staff, family, and any other appropriate members, meet together quarterly and annually to discuss the overall health and well-being of each elder residing in the nursing home. These meetings are documented and an individual plan of care created. The care plan determines not only the clinical and social treatment of the patient, but also the Medicare or Medicaid reimbursement.

In 1987, a major reform was enacted on the federal level. Part of an Omnibus Budget Reconciliation Act, OBRA 87 became the basis for the MDS collected on each patient and as a mechanism for improving quality of care. As part of this regulatory process, nursing homes are subject to annual, unannounced surveys by the state in which they are located. State surveys, which may take place during or after business hours, result in a report that must be posted at the nursing home. In addition, results are converted to a "5 star" rating system that is reported publicly at http://www.medicare.gov/NursingHomeCompare. Along with site-wide health and safety assessments, surveyors examine resident plans of care

Table 18–1. Illnesses/conditions that trigger a Resident Assessment Protocol (RAP).

Delirium
Cognitive loss
Visual function
Communication
ADL functional/rehabilitation potential
Urinary incontinence and indwelling catheter
Psychosocial well-being
Mood state
Behavioral symptoms
Activities
Falls
Nutritional status
Feeding tubes
Dehydration/fluid maintenance
Dental care
Pressure ulcers
Psychotropic drug use
Physical restraints

(POCs, or care plans). For specific areas of concern, Resident Assessment Protocols (RAPs) are required as well (Table 18–1).

These problems, when identified, must be addressed by the IDT and incorporated into the POC. Care must be taken to explain why it is that a patient is suffering from one of these 18 conditions, as the surveyors will look closely at charts flagged with them. Reporting of every scratch and bruise on nursing home residents is mandated, and intended to prevent elder abuse and ensure that an important injury is not left unnoticed. The Centers for Medicare and Medicaid Services (CMS) has the right to penalize nursing homes including through fines, temporary denial of payment, assigned oversight, or even the removal of nursing home certification to provide care CMS beneficiaries (which effectively forces the nursing home to close). Table 18–2 categorizes the deficiencies.

HOSPICE AND END-OF-LIFE CARE

The long-term care nursing home bed is intended to be the final resting place of the person who resides in it. Nursing home residents have the right to be offered hospice care, and the Medicare hospice benefit can be invoked in a nursing home. It covers, as in the outpatient setting, a visiting hospice agency, but does not cover room, board, or 24-hour-a-day custodial care. Some nursing homes have dedicated hospice rooms and others incorporate palliative care training into their continuing education programs. Unlike the ALFs, the nursing homes do not require a hospice waiver. Instead, they require physician documentation of end-of-life treatment preferences. To improve the likelihood that do-not-resuscitate (DNR) and do-not-intubate (DNI) orders will

Table 18–2. Nursing home health inspection score.

Severity	Scope of Deficiency		
	Isolated Incident	Pattern of Incidents	Widespread Occurrence
Immediate jeopardy to health or safety	J	K	L
Actual harm without immediate jeopardy	G	H	I
No actual harm but with potential for greater than minimal harm	D	E	F
No actual harm but with potential for minimal harm	A	B	C

Reproduced with permission from Centers for Medicare and Medicaid Services website: http://www.cms.gov

be respected upon transfer to a local emergency room, both nursing homes and home hospice providers are beginning to adopt new, legally binding advance directive orders. Called Physician Orders for Life-Sustaining Treatment (POLST) on the West Coast and Medical Orders for Life-Sustaining Treatment (MOLST) on the East Coast, these are legally binding medical orders when signed by both patient and physician. They specify code status, hospitalization or do-not-transfer status, the patient's preferences for artificial nutrition, and the patient's designated proxy.

Angelelli J. Promising models for transforming long-term care. *Gerontologist.* 2006;46(4):428-430.

Baker B. *Old Age in a New Age: The Promise of Transformative Nursing Homes.* Nashville, TN: Vanderbilt University Press; 2007.

Bodenheimer T. Long-term care for frail elderly people—the On Lok model. *N Engl J Med.* 1999;341(17):1324-1328.

Boult C, Green AF, Boult LB, Pacala JT, Snyder C, Leff B. Successful models of comprehensive care for older adults with chronic conditions: evidence for the Institute of Medicine's "retooling for an aging America" report. *J Am Geriatr Soc.* 2009;57(12): 2328-2337.

Castle NG. Turnover begets turnover. *Gerontologist.* 2005;45(2): 186-195.

Castle NG. Measuring staff turnover in nursing homes. *Gerontologist.* 2006;46(2):210-219.

Code of Federal Regulations, Title 42, Volume 3, Part 483 (rev. 2000). *Requirements for States and Long-Term Care Facilities.* Washington, DC: U.S. Government Printing Office.

High KP, Bradley SF, Gravenstein S, et al. Clinical practice guideline for the evaluation of fever and infection in older adult residents of long-term care facilities: 2008 update by the Infectious Diseases Society of America. *J Am Geriatr Soc.* 2009;57(3): 375-394.

Kaye HS, Harrington C, LaPlante MP. Long-term care: Who gets it, who provides it, who pays, and how much? *Health Aff.* 2010;29(1):11-21.

Kemper P, Murtaugh CM. Lifetime use of nursing home care. *N Engl J Med.* 1991;324(9):595-600.

Leff B, Burton L, Mader SL, et al. Hospital at home: feasibility and outcomes of a program to provide hospital-level care at home for acutely ill older patients. *Ann Intern Med.* 2005;143(11): 798-808.

Mattimore TJ, Wenger NS, Desbiens NA, et al. Surrogate and physician understanding of patients' preferences for living permanently in a nursing home. *J Am Geriatr Soc.* 1997;45(7):818-824.

Ng T, Harrington C, Kitchener M. Medicare and Medicaid in long-term care. *Health Aff.* 2010;29(1):22-28.

Rabig J, Thomas W, Kane RA, Cutler LJ, McAlilly S. Radical redesign of nursing homes: applying the green house concept in Tupelo, Mississippi. *Gerontologist.* 2006;46(4):533-539.

Rahman AN, Applebaum RA. The nursing home minimum data set assessment instrument: Manifest functions and unintended consequences—past, present, and future. *Gerontologist.* 2009;49(6):727-735.

Ramsdell JW, ed. *Medical Management of the Home Care Patient: Guidelines for Physicians.* 3rd ed. American Medical Association and American Academy of Home Care Physicians; 2007.

Stafford PB. *Elderburbia: Aging with a Sense of Place.* Santa Barbara, CA: ABC Clio, LLC; 2009.

Unwin BK, Porvaznik MD. Nursing home care: part I. Principles and pitfalls of practice. *Am Fam Physician.* 2010;81(10):1219-1227.

Unwin BK, Porvaznik M, Spoelhof GD. Nursing home care: part II. Clinical aspects. *Am Fam Physician.* 2010;81(10):1229-1237.

Weiner AS, Ronch JL. *Culture Change in Long-Term Care.* Binghamton, NY: The Haworth Social Work Practice Press; 2003.

Weiner JM, Freiman MP, Brown D. *Nursing Home Care Quality: Twenty Years after the Omnibus Budget Reconciliation act of 1987.* Menlo Park, CA: The Henry J. Kaiser Family Foundation; 2007.

USEFUL WEBSITES

Family Caregiver Alliance (a clearinghouse of resources for caregivers which includes support groups, educational materials and opportunities for advocacy). http://www.caregiver.org

National clearinghouse for elder care services (including area agencies on aging, abuse and assistance organizations, and caregiver materials). http://www.eldercare.gov

Nursing Home Compare feature at the Centers for Medicare and Medicaid Services (CMS) (ranks all skilled nursing facilities in the US based upon their most recent state survey results). http://www.medicare.gov/nursinghomecompare

The Alzheimer's Association (the largest dementia research, advocacy, and support organization in America). http://alz.org

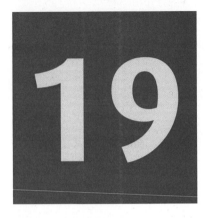

19

Home-Based Care

Jessica L. Colburn, MD
Jennifer L. Hayashi, MD
Bruce Leff, MD

▼ HOME-CARE MODELS

Specific home-care models have proven effective at providing high-quality care to vulnerable older adults. These models include preventive home-care programs and medical house calls that integrate medical and social supportive services focusing on the care of chronically disabled persons, home geriatric assessment, posthospital case management/transitional care models, home rehabilitation, and hospital at home.

PREVENTIVE HOME CARE/GERIATRIC ASSESSMENT

Many models of preventive home care for older adults at risk of functional decline have been described and evaluated. Models differ in their target populations, intensity and degree of geriatric assessment, and follow-up. Results of these studies are varied, but overall, programs that target high-risk patients and provide multidimensional assessment and multiple follow-up visits have demonstrated reduction in nursing home admission, improvement in functional status, and reduction in mortality. The high initial cost currently makes this model rare in practice.

MEDICAL HOUSE CALLS

Medical house calls are visits to provide ongoing longitudinal medical care within the patient's home environment. House call visits may be done by a physician alone, or patients may receive primary health care from a team, such as in the Home-Based Primary Care Program through Veteran's Affairs facilities. In the house call team model, patients are cared for by a multidisciplinary team of physicians and other health care professionals, including, but not limited to nurses, home health aides, social workers, and physical and occupational therapists. Some programs include pharmacists and mental health professionals on their teams. The team meets on a regular basis, manages the care of active patients carefully, and integrates medical and social supportive services. Such programs have demonstrated improvement in function, reduced costs, decreased medication use, improved satisfaction, improved end-of-life care, and fewer nursing home admissions and outpatient visits.

POSTHOSPITALIZATION CASE MANAGEMENT & TRANSITIONAL CARE MODELS

Specific home-based case management strategies, especially those that are focused on conditions associated with complex management issues and high rates of early hospital readmission (eg, congestive heart failure), are associated with a significant reduction in the number of acute hospital readmissions.

HOME REHABILITATION

Home rehabilitation (specifically after a stroke or a major joint replacement) has proved to be feasible, acceptable to patients and caregivers, and as effective as hospital-based rehabilitation.

HOSPITAL AT HOME

Hospital at home models that provide hospital-level services in the home setting as a substitute for a needed hospital admission have been developed and have demonstrated comparable clinical outcomes, reduced length of stay, decreased readmission rates, increased patient and caregiver satisfaction, and reductions in important geriatric complications, such as delirium.

MEDICARE HOME HEALTH SERVICES

ELIGIBILITY REQUIREMENTS

Medicare will pay for certain home care services. Physicians who care for older patients need to be familiar with the basic entry criteria for these services. Medicare was designed as an acute illness benefit rather than insurance to pay for the long-term care of older persons with chronic conditions. Thus, Medicare home health benefits are linked to transitions from acute care settings and to what Medicare refers to as a "skilled need." Home health care services for Medicare patients are covered by Medicare Part A. Physicians and approved home health agencies are reimbursed for services as long as certain criteria are met. The basic requirements for Medicare to reimburse home health expenses are as follows: the physician certifies that the patient is homebound, the patient has a skilled need, the skilled need is reasonable and necessary, the rendered service is intermittent or part time, the physician completes the face-to-face encounter form, and the physician signs Form CMS-485, which is the plan of care.

1. Homebound Requirement

To qualify as "homebound," a patient must have a condition resulting from illness or injury that makes it a "considerable and taxing effort to leave the home" without the aid of supportive devices such as crutches, canes, wheelchairs or walkers, special transportation, or another person or if leaving the home is medically contraindicated. However, a person does not have to be bedridden or absolutely homebound. Absences from the home must be infrequent, of short duration, or for medically relevant services. Examples of nonmedical reasons for leaving the home are attending religious services or taking a stroll or drive. No specific definitions of "short duration" or "infrequent" are provided in the Medicare guidelines. Illnesses or injuries that result in a person's confinement to the home include stroke, blindness, dementia, amputation, or a psychiatric problem in which the patient refuses to leave the home or would be unsafe leaving the home unattended.

2. Skilled Need Requirement

A skilled need is required for a home care agency to receive reimbursement from Medicare for home health services. Skilled needs are those that require special training and certification to administer to be safe and effective, such as those provided by nurses or therapists. An example of a skilled need is the monitoring of a patient with a complex medical condition that requires adjustment of medicines and reevaluation by a skilled nurse. Other examples include wound care treatment, catheter care, physical therapy, training of patients or caregivers to manage medical conditions such as diabetes or wound treatment, and education and monitoring of new medications such as warfarin. Single home visits by a skilled

nurse for the sole purpose of obtaining a blood specimen do not qualify as a skilled need. Once a person has home health services for a skilled need, other covered Medicare home health services such as social work, occupational therapy, and home health aide can also be obtained. Thus, the skilled nursing or physical therapy need unlocks the Medicare home health benefit for the patient, and a broad range of services may be used as appropriate for the care of the patient. Services can be provided as long as the skilled need exists.

Not all skilled needs are reimbursable. For example, if a patient has been managing his or her diabetes with injections without difficulty and the glucose is well controlled, training would not be appropriate, and payment would be denied. If the patient had been taking oral medications, however, and the physician adds insulin to the medical regimen, it would be appropriate to request nursing services to train the patient to manage diabetes with the new insulin regimen.

3. Reasonable and Necessary Skilled Needs

Skilled needs must be reasonable and necessary. Documentation should be provided on the plan of care (Form CMS-485) and any supplementary forms. If appropriate medical information is not present, the medical record will be reviewed by a regional intermediary designated by the Center for Medicare and Medicaid Services (CMS) to determine whether the services are reasonable and necessary. One example of a reasonable and necessary skilled need is that of the patient discharged home after hospitalization with heart failure. However, this person's need would not qualify as reasonable and necessary if there were no documentation of changes to the medical regimen and Form CMS-485 documented the patient as having stable vital signs and no functional impairments. Another example provided in the *Home Health Agency Manual* is a patient who was discharged from the hospital after a hip fracture, and home health services were requested solely for monthly vitamin B_{12} injections. Although the injection is a skilled need, if there is no documentation of approved conditions for the administration of vitamin B_{12}, there is no evidence that the injection is medically necessary or reasonable, and the claim would be denied.

Centers for Medicare & Medicaid Services. *Home Health Agency Manual.* https://www.cms.gov/manuals/downloads/bp102c07.pdf

4. Face-to-Face Encounter Requirement

A face-to-face encounter requirement for certification of eligibility for home health services was established in Section 6407 of the Affordable Care Act of 2010. It requires a physician to document that the physician, or a nonphysician practitioner working with the physician, had a face-to-face encounter visit with the patient within 90 days prior to the start of care, or 30 days after the start of care. The encounter must be related to the reason for referring the patient to home health services. This face-to-face encounter form is also required for recertification of hospice services (Table 19–1).

Table 19–1. Face-to-face encounter form.

Encounter must occur within 90 days prior to start of treatment or within 30 days after start of treatment, and must be related to the reason for the home care referral.
Must be an encounter with a physician or a nonphysician provider working with the physician.
Form must include: • Patient's name, date of face-to-face encounter.   • Name of the provider who performed the encounter.   • Medical reason for the patient's homebound status.   • Patient's clinical condition when seen.   • How that clinical condition supports the need for medically necessary skilled home care services.   • Physician's signature, and the date of the physician's signature. Must be an original signature, can be a faxed copy of the signed face-to-face encounter form.

5. Part-Time or Intermittent Service

"Intermittent" means skilled nursing care that is provided fewer than 7 days per week or less than 8 hours per day over a period of 21 days or less for a medical condition that is expected to require skilled services at least once every 60 days. Therefore, a one-time intravenous infusion (eg, the condition is not expected to recur and will not require intermittent service) would not qualify for reimbursement. Exceptions to the time limit may be made on an individual basis if appropriate documentation is provided.

6. Plan of Care

Form CMS-485 is the comprehensive plan of care for each patient. This form lists diagnoses, medications, diet, activities, and services needed, such as wound treatments, in addition to other information. The patient must be under the care of a physician qualified to sign the physician certification at the time of enrollment into home health, and the physician must review and sign the form at least every 60 days. Additional state requirements regarding timing of signatures may also exist. Physicians can bill Medicare for certifying the plan of care.

PAYMENT DENIALS

Single visits are common reasons for payment denial for nonphysician home health services. If a patient complained of urinary symptoms, Medicare would not pay for a home health nurse to make a single visit to obtain a urinary specimen, even if the patient was diagnosed and treated with antibiotics for an infection. However, if the home health agency plans to follow up for re-evaluation of a skilled need, but a patient is hospitalized, placed in hospice, or dies after a single visit, the agency would be reimbursed for that visit.

Another common reason for denial is the determination of non-acute events (eg, when physical therapy is ordered for frail patients with medically stable diseases or with gradual progressive disability). Since its inception, Medicare has operated based on an acute care model, and reimbursements are primarily for acute events with a foreseeable period of recovery. In most cases, there must be a clear end point before services will be approved. Before home health services are requested, the physician should consider whether the service is expected to improve the patient's condition.

Other common reasons for denial are failure of physicians to complete the face-to-face encounter form and failure to sign Form CMS-485. The plan of care should be reviewed at least every 60 days, updated, if needed, and signed.

INNOVATIONS IN CARE DELIVERY

▶ Independence at Home

The Independence at Home Demonstration was authorized by Section 3024 of the Affordable Care Act of 2010. In the Demonstration, the CMS Innovation Center will work with home-based primary care practices to test the hypothesis that comprehensive home-based interdisciplinary teams can provide high-quality care and save money for the Medicare system on care provided to high-cost Medicare beneficiaries with multiple chronic conditions and functional impairment. Quality indicators will include reduced hospitalization, improved patient and caregiver satisfaction, and improved health outcomes, among others. Practices will be rewarded financially for providing high-quality care at reduced cost through a shared-savings mechanism between CMS and the participating practices. This Demonstration program began in 2012.

▶ Medicare Advantage Plans

Medicare Advantage plans have also developed models of care to improve quality and cost for patients with multiple chronic conditions who frequently utilize high cost care, such as emergency room visits and frequent hospitalizations. INSPIRIS is one company that partners with Medicare Advantage Plans to provide comprehensive care management for the 5% to 10% of plan members with the most complex health care needs and highest costs, and they have been shown to reduce health care utilization and readmissions, and to improve outcomes and patient satisfaction.

▶ Program of All-Inclusive Care for the Elderly

The Program of All-Inclusive Care for the Elderly (PACE) is a model of care that is focused on keeping chronically ill adults in their community for as long as possible. To be eligible to participate in PACE, an individual must be older than age 55 years, certified by the state to qualify for nursing home placement, in a situation where the patient is able to continue living safely in the community, and living within a PACE service area. For individuals enrolled in PACE who are Medicare and Medicaid (dual) eligible, the program receives set funding from Medicare and Medicaid for each participant enrolled in the program. For participants who are not eligible for Medicaid, the participant may pay the Medicaid portion out of pocket. Services include physician and nursing care, an adult day program, transportation, home health aides, social work, complete prescription drug coverage, respite care, and physical and occupational therapy.

▼ ADDITIONAL RESOURCES

MEDICAID

Medicare recipients may also receive Medicaid ("dual eligible") if they meet the income and wealth requirements.

Medicaid provides reimbursement for many home health services for which Medicare does not. In addition, several states have launched Medicaid waiver programs to provide home care services for Medicare patients who are Medicaid and nursing home eligible in hopes of reducing nursing home admissions. States must assure CMS that the cost of providing these services in the home or community will not exceed that of placing individuals in an institution. Some of the services provided include personal care, respite care, and other needed assistance in the home.

AREA AGENCIES ON AGING

Area Agencies on Aging (AAAs) were established in 1973 under the Older Americans Act to provide resources for older adults. Local AAAs provide several types of assistance: information and access services, community-based services, in-home services, housing services, and elder rights services.

Information and access services include providing information and referrals for services outside the AAA, caregiver support, and retirement planning and education. Community-based services include employment services such as skill assessment, testing, and job placement. They also offer information on senior centers, congregate meals, adult day care, and volunteer opportunities. In-home services may consist of Meals on Wheels, assistance with personal care, shopping and housekeeping, telephone calls and personal visits for homebound adults, personal emergency response devices, financial assistance with gas and electric bills for low-income individuals, and respite care for caregivers. AAAs help older adults find alternative housing as they transition from independent living to varying levels of need for assistance, usually in an attempt to avoid nursing home placement. Senior housing facilities, group homes, assisted-living facilities, and adult

foster care are options that AAAs help individuals to explore. AAAs can also provide information on nursing home placement. Finally, AAAs provide legal assistance and investigate elder abuse charges and neglect, including self-neglect both in the community and within long-term care facilities.

▼ THE PHYSICIAN'S ROLE IN HOME CARE

A physician may provide home care at several distinct levels: posthospitalization and rehabilitation care, acute home care, assessment visits, and home-based primary care. In providing such care, the physician often works in conjunction with the resources of a home health agency, including skilled nursing care, home health aide care, physical and occupational therapists, and social workers.

One inference to be drawn from the description of these categories is the importance of selecting appropriate patients for home care. Patient selection requires an understanding of the patient's medical condition, suitability of the patient's environment, including the level of available caregiver support, and ability of the home health agency to support the patient's particular needs.

POSTACUTE HOSPITALIZATION & HOME REHABILITATION CARE

In posthospitalization care and home rehabilitation care, the focus is on restoring function and completing the management of medical problems. The interdisciplinary care team provides much of the care in this setting, with a physician providing medical oversight and supervision.

HOME CARE & ASSESSMENTS

In acute home care, the physician is actively involved in management of acute illness. Physician home visits, home health agency involvement, and close coordination of the interdisciplinary care team are crucial to assess and manage the patient. In addition, assessment home visits, which may be performed on a one-time basis, allow a physician to evaluate the impact of the home environment, caregiver, or functional disability on the patient's health, including nonadherence, difficult diagnoses, and excessive use of health services.

HOUSE CALLS & HOME-BASED PRIMARY CARE

In addition to the usual components of a patient encounter (ie, the history and physical examination and counseling), the house call permits and encourages functional, social, caregiver, and environmental assessments. Inspecting the home environment with patient/family permission (eg, clutter and obstacles, adaptive equipment, lighting, bathroom setup, kitchen setup, refrigerator contents, medication setup) can

Table 19–2. Home care equipment.

Essential	Optional
Sphygmomanometer	Oto-/ophthalmoscope
Stethoscope	Ear wax removal equipment
Phlebotomy equipment	Dictaphone
Thermometer	Glucometer
Specimen cups for urine, sputum, stool	Point of care monitors (eg, INR monitoring)
Gloves	Digital camera
Reflex hammer	Laptop computer/electronic medical record
Vibration fork	
Occult blood cards and developer	Pulse oximeter
Lubricating jelly	Wound care kit
Toenail clippers	Gynecological speculum
Tongue depressors	Peak flowmeter
Prescription pad	Scale
Sharps container	Portable electrocardiograph

INR, international normalized ratio.

help the physician understand functional and medical issues. Also, observations of patient–caregiver interactions in the home are often remarkably different from those observed in the office setting and can provide valuable insight into management issues. Physicians may choose to do a single house call to assess particular aspects of a patient's home environment or care needs, or a physician may provide primary care in the home setting. In some cases, physicians work with an interdisciplinary care team, including nurse practitioners, nurses, social workers, and home health aides, in a house call practice providing home-based primary care. Table 19–2 lists recommended equipment for house calls.

▶ Billing for Medicare Physician Care Plan Oversight

Medicare Part B pays for physician house calls. Home visits are billed using codes 99341-99350. Visits to domiciliary care facilities are billed using CPT codes 99324-99337. In addition, Medicare Part B pays for care plan oversight (CPO) using CMS common practice coding system code G0181. Separate codes must be used for initial home health certification (G0180), recertification (G0179), and CPO (G0181). Physicians can be reimbursed for a minimum of 30 minutes per calendar month spent on home care orders and communication with home-care providers. It may also include time spent reviewing records or coordinating care with other

disciplines. CPO does not include time spent in discussion with pharmacists for the purpose of calling in prescriptions, nor does it include time spent in discussions with patients or family members. Medicare Part B reimbursements are subject to 20% copayments, for which the Medicare beneficiary is responsible.

Boling PA. Care transitions and home health care. *Clin Geriatr Med.* 2009;25(1):135-148, viii.

Boling PA. Preface. Home care, from origins to present day. *Clin Geriatr Med.* 2009;25(1):xi-xiii.

DeJonge KE, Taler G, Boling PA. Independence at home: community-based care for older adults with severe chronic illness. *Clin Geriatr Med.* 2009;25(1):155-169, ix.

Huss A, Stuck AE, Rubenstein LZ, Egger M, Clough-Gorr KM. Multidimensional preventive home visit programs for community-dwelling older adults: a systematic review and meta-analysis of randomized controlled trials. *J Gerontol A Biol Sci Med Sci.* 2008;63(3):298-307. Erratum in: *J Gerontol A Biol Sci Med Sci.* 2009;64(2):318.

Leff B, Burton JR. The future history of home care and physician house calls in the United States. *J Gerontol A Biol Sci Med Sci.* 2001;56(10):M603-M608.

McCall N, Komisar HL, Petersons A, Moore S. Medicare home health before and after the BBA. *Health Aff (Millwood).* 2001;20(3):189-198.

Shepperd S, Doll H, Angus RM, et al. Avoiding hospital admission through provision of hospital care at home: a systematic review and meta-analysis of individual patient data. *CMAJ.* 2009;180(2):175-82.

Stuck AE, Kane RL. Whom do preventive home visits help? *J Am Geriatr Soc.* 2008;56(3):561-563.

USEFUL WEBSITES

American Academy of Homecare Physicians (this organization is an excellent source of information on home care as it relates to physician practice in home care and the Independence at Home model). http://aahcp.org

Center for Medicare and Medicaid Services (various sites have excellent information on the Medicare home health and hospice program and the Independence at Home Demonstration). http://www.cms.gov

National Association for Home Care & Hospice (this site, although for a trade group that represents home care agencies, hospices, home care aide organizations, and medical equipment suppliers, provides general information and links related to the home care industry). http://www.nahc.org

National Association of Area Agencies on Aging (this site has a number of helpful links to find local services). http://www.n4a.org

The Aging Traveler

Gerald Charles, MD

GENERAL PRINCIPLES IN OLDER ADULTS

1. Older adults, because of their diminished physiologic reserve, are more vulnerable to most of the hazards facing any traveler.

2. Because exacerbation of chronic illness is a major risk for any traveler, focusing on "disease management and education" in advance of travel is particularly important for older travelers.

3. Any form of travel increases the risk of venous thromboembolism, which can be more serious in older adults.

4. A prior knowledge of resources available to health professionals called to help in a medical emergency during air travel may be lifesaving.

OVERVIEW OF TRAVEL PROBLEMS

"Wandering reestablishes the original harmony which once existed between man and the universe."

Anatole France

Travel is enjoyed by many and tolerated by some, but is simply a part of modern life. Everyone who travels, however, is subject to certain "risks" inherent in travel. Among them are exposures to unfamiliar climates, foods, illnesses, language and customs, hazards caused by "relaxed" public safety standards, lack of handicap access, crime in unfamiliar settings and risks specific to a particular mode of travel. Problems for elders also increase when stressed by dehydration, temperature extremes, acute illness or exacerbation of chronic illnesses and increased falls risk as a result of such factors as lack of handrails, uneven surfaces or even an unfamiliar hotel room in the middle of the night. Older adults are also affected more by jet lag and this condition, when coupled with confusion in a person with even mild cognitive impairment in an unfamiliar setting can be a formula for adverse events. Anyone who has ever been confused in a busy airport while worrying about how to get to the correct airport gate in time for their flight will realize that any underlying confusion will likely make travel even more stressful. Thus, almost all of the factors that contribute to travel risk are amplified in elder travelers.

Robust data about the demographics of the medical problems of travel are lacking. There are some surveillance systems in place, such as the *GeoSentinal Surveillance Network,* which aggregates data about infectious diseases worldwide from a network of travel and tropical-medicine clinics on 6 continents. This network may be useful in assessing the likely causes of febrile illness in a returning traveler or understanding infectious disease travel risks based on the location of travel. There are, however, really no comparable entities collecting data about other problems related to travel. Nations usually do not keep information about victims of crime or accidents in formats that allow aggregation of those data and there are many problems assembling international statistics. Many travel-related health problems are never reported and institutions such as hotels and airlines are not in the business of collecting this kind of information. What data we do have indicate that common infections (upper respiratory infections and gastroenteritis) are common and motor vehicle accidents are the most likely traumatic event followed by falls and pedestrian accidents. Less common are health problems resulting from crime, unusual problems resulting from "adventuring," and incidents arising from civil unrest. The principle that "common things occur commonly" certainly pertains to travel.

RISK OF VENOUS THROMBOEMBOLISM DUE TO TRAVEL

Deep venous thrombosis (DVT) and venous thromboembolism (VTE) are common illnesses with an estimated frequency of 1–2 per 1000 individuals. The estimated 28-day mortality for a first episode of VTE in ambulatory persons is around 11%, illustrating the serious nature of this problem. Among the numerous recognized risk factors for DVT and VTE are hypercoagulable states, immobility, cancer, orthopedic problems, and other surgical procedures, but advancing age is an *independent* risk factor for DVT and VTE. Although it has been recognized for some time, the risk of DVT and VTE incident to travel has been somewhat difficult to quantify. Early studies of "the economy-class syndrome" offered conflicting conclusions about the risk. A recent meta-analysis concluded that the pooled relative risk for VTE in travelers is 2.0 (95% confidence interval [CI], 1.5–2.7). By excluding studies with control participants who were referred for VTE evaluation which led to "referral bias" in the control group, the relative risk for any form of travel was determined to be 2.8 (CI 2.2–3.7). A dose–response relationship was identified with an 18% higher risk of VTE for each 2-hour increase in duration of travel. Of particular interest was a 26% higher risk for every 2 hours of air travel. When we consider the ease and frequency of long distance air travel in today's world and the factors known to be associated with increased VTE risk without travel, we see that the known increased risk of VTE while travelling should be an important consideration in preparing an older adult for travel. It is appropriate for the clinician to assess the magnitude of the risk in individual patients with the goal of deciding whether a pretravel risk-reduction intervention is warranted. All older travelers will benefit from particular attention to attenuating the modifiable risks of travel such as dehydration, immobility and combating lower extremity venous stasis. Treatment with various forms of anticoagulation should be considered for those at greatest risk. Suggestions include:

1. Low risk (eg, age only, obesity, active inflammation, recent nonorthopedic surgery): encourage frequent ambulation, hydration and perhaps compression stockings.

2. Moderate risk (eg, prior DVT, known venous disease): above plus low-dose aspirin if no contraindications.

3. High risk (eg, recurrent DVT/VTE, hypercoagulable state, malignancy, etc): above plus consideration of low-molecular-weight heparin or the newer oral anticoagulants, such as factor Xa or thrombin inhibitors.

Because advancing age is an independent risk factor for DVT and VTE, many older travelers will likely fall into at least the moderate-risk group.

RESOURCES ABOUT TRAVEL RISKS

A number of resources are available to any traveler and to the health professional providing advice to an elder traveler. The U.S. Department of State maintains an excellent website devoted to international travel (http://www.travel.

Table 20–1. Checklist for travelers.

1. Is there any reason I should not travel?
   Who to ask? Primary Provider and/or Travel Clinic
2. Do I need any vaccines ("shots")?
   Who to ask? Primary Provider and/or Travel Clinic
   Web: http://wwwnc.cdc.gov/travel/page/vaccinations.htm
3. How to prevent blood clots while traveling.
   Who to ask? Primary Provider
   Web: http://wwwnc.cdc.gov/travel/new-announcements.htm
4. Medical information to carry with you:
   Medical Problem List,   Medication List (doses and
   frequency)   Known Allergies   Copy of Recent Electrocardiogram
   (EKG),   Insurance Card (other than Medicare)
5. Any medication schedule changes for time zone changes?
   Who to ask: Primary Provider or Pharmacist

Web Resources for International Travel:
Health Questions: http://wwwnc.cdc.gov/travel/page/yellowbook-2012-home.htm
Ship Travel (sanitation): http://wwwn.cdc.gov/inspectionquerytool/inspectiongreensheetrpt.aspx
International Travel Safety: http://www.travel.state.gov

state.gov) focusing on advice about handling difficulties encountered while travelling internationally and highlights areas in the world with particular risks. The Centers for Disease Control and Prevention maintains a website devoted primarily to illness related to and vaccines recommended for international travel (http://wwwnc.cdc.gov/travel), including the well-known "Yellow Book." The CDC also maintains the very useful "Green Sheet" report from the Vessel Sanitation Program, which lists most international cruise ships and the results of sanitary inspections of those ships (http://wwwn.cdc.gov/inspectionquerytool/inspection-greensheetrpt.aspx).

It is important for health professionals providing travel advice for older adults to also encourage the traveler to carry with them a listing of their chronic medical problems, a list of their current medications and should ideally include a copy of a recent electrocardiogram. Anyone who has been asked to provide medical care to a confused traveler who is unable to clearly state what their medical problems are or what medications they take will realize the usefulness of this information. Finally, older travelers should be reminded that Medicare does not provide coverage in other countries and that additional health insurance coverage should be encouraged. A suggested "checklist" for patients contemplating travel is shown in Table 20–1.

SHIP TRAVEL

Cruise ships are a very popular vacation mode for elders. Recent publicity aside, ship travel as a mode of transportation is not very risky short of gross navigational miscalculation. Events such as collisions, running aground, or pirate attacks are highly publicized but are actually relatively infrequent. The principal risks to ship travelers actually involve the hazards of shore travel (eg, vehicle accidents, pedestrian accidents, and falls) which account for the vast majority of the traumatic medical problems while "cruising." Although shipboard epidemics attributable to viral gastroenteritis caused by *norovirus* or viral upper respiratory infections are relatively uncommon occurrences, their appearance on a ship will be amplified by the contained environment. Although many viral illnesses are highly contagious when spread by ship's staff, such as food handlers, or by other travelers who are infected, good epidemiologic surveillance is effective in limiting shipboard epidemics. Ships registered in countries with rigorous public health standards enforced by government agencies (eg, the United States and the United Kingdom) may be less likely than ships of some other countries to present infectious disease risks to travelers. Data about individual cruise lines and individual ships are readily available from the Centers for Disease Control and Management in the form of the "Green Sheet" previously mentioned. Most larger cruise ships have a medical department aboard that can provide initial care for minor illness or injury and can help in arranging medical evacuation in more serious situations.

AIR TRAVEL

"If there is a physician on board, could you please identify yourself to a flight attendant?" Some estimates suggest that 60% to 70% of physicians have been involved in some sort of in-flight medical emergency. While in-flight medical emergencies are haphazardly recorded and there is little follow up among the airlines, it is estimated that in-flight emergencies occur between 0.4 and 3.4 per 100,000 passenger trips. One study of in-flight emergencies showed approximately 3% were sudden death and some 13% were "significant" cardiovascular problems, including myocardial infarctions and cerebrovascular accidents. Given the number of worldwide flights daily, estimates are that there are approximately 30 in-flight emergencies each day.

The nature and estimated frequencies of in-flight emergencies are shown in Table 20–2. It is clear that older adults will be at greater risk of in-flight emergencies from some, but not all, of these causes. They will have a greater probability of having coronary artery disease (either known or unknown), chronic obstructive pulmonary disease, syncope because of autonomic dysregulation, and perhaps more confusion from various causes such as underlying cognitive impairment or adverse medication side effects. Because the health professional facing an in-flight emergency involving an older adult does not have the diagnostic support to make more than a "best guess" about the cause of the distress, consideration

Table 20–2. Nature of in-flight emergencies.

Category (% of All Emergencies)	Problem (% of Category)
Neurologic (16.7%)	Syncope/loss consciousness (50%) Seizure (33%)
Cardiac (15.9%)	Suspected infarct (50%) Angina (33%)
Psychiatric (14.9%)	Anxiety (33%) Alcohol related (33%) Panic (33%)
Gastrointestinal (10.9%)	Gastroenteritis (50%) Abdominal pain (33%) Airsickness (33%)
ENT (8.9%)	Otic barotrauma (50%) Sinus barotrauma (10%)
Pulmonary (6.9%)	Asthma (50%) COPD (20%) Dyspnea (20%)
Trauma (3.9%)	Turbulence (50%) Alcohol related (50%)
Diabetes and hypoglycemia (3.7%)	Almost all is hypoglycemia
Symptoms only (8.9%)	Chest pain most common

COPD, chronic obstructive pulmonary disease; ENT, ear, nose, throat.

must be given to the illness frequencies shown in Table 20–2 that might account for the observed problem.

The health professional can benefit from knowledge about what resources are available in the event of an emergency and a recounting of those resources is in order.

1. Flight attendants are experienced, trained in emergency procedures, and have some training in emergency first aid. Many have "been there and done that" during in-flight medical emergencies, so consult them early and often!

2. Most U.S. carriers have an experienced physician trained in emergency medicine and aerospace medicine available for consultation by air-to-ground communication. As a general rule, any emergency where diverting the aircraft for an unscheduled landing is being considered will require approval from this "on-call flight surgeon" as well as the Captain of the aircraft.

3. All U.S. aircraft having one or more flight attendants will have an automatic external defibrillator (AED) on board. The flight attendants will be trained in its operation. An AED can indicate the cardiac rhythm and will not administer a shock unless the rhythm is one that may respond to the shock.

4. Most major carriers and all U.S. airlines except "commuter airlines" must have an "Enhanced On-Board Emergency Medical Kit." This kit contains diagnostic

equipment (blood pressure cuff, stethoscope, etc), oropharyngeal airways, intravenous infusion equipment, oral medications, injectables, inhalers and resuscitation equipment including an Ambu bag, laryngoscope and airways. Table 20–3 is a more complete enumeration of the contents.

5. Larger jet aircraft carry medical oxygen in "walk around" tanks and the number of tanks varies with the size of the aircraft. Each tank supplies approximately thirty minutes of oxygen so extended hours of oxygen support will not be possible. "Commuter airlines" aircraft are not required to carry medical oxygen and will usually not have the "Enhanced Emergency Medical Kit." Commuter aircraft will, however, have an AED onboard if the aircraft has at least 1 flight attendant.

Some older adults have such severe medical problems that flying is not advised. The most common contraindication to air travel is pulmonary insufficiency with chronic obstructive pulmonary disease (COPD) being the most common diagnosis. A PaO_2 (partial pressure of arterial oxygen) of less than 70 mm Hg at rest is usually a contraindication to air travel. In essence, any medical condition requiring supplemental oxygen at rest should be carefully evaluated to see if the stress of flying at a cabin pressure altitude of 6000 to 8000 feet can be tolerated. Supplemental oxygen can be arranged on-board and the duration of the oxygen administration is not constrained by the limited amount of emergency medical oxygen on board. Prior arrangements with the airline must be made and consultation with the medical department of the airline must be completed so the appropriate flow rate of the oxygen at altitude can be determined in advance. As a general rule, passengers may not take their personal oxygen tanks on board the aircraft and only certain types of concentrators are approved by the Federal Aviation Administration for use on board. Other medical problems that are contraindications to flying include unstable coronary disease or a recent myocardial infarction (usually said to be 3 weeks prior), recent surgery (2–3 weeks for ear, nose, and throat [ENT], ocular, or gastrointestinal surgery, and several more weeks for orthopedic surgery where DVT risk is increased), significant neurologic disability or recent stroke and behavioral issues caused by cognitive impairment or psychiatric problems.

The question of liability in responding to an on-board medical emergency was somewhat clarified in the United States in 1998 by the passage of the Aviation Medical Assistance Act (Public Law 105-170) which provides some "good samaritan" protection to health professionals rendering aid in a medical emergency in flight. To be covered by this law, the health professional must render care in good faith, be "medically qualified," be a volunteer and must not accept monetary payment for services rendered. The medical care rendered "must be similar to the care that others with similar training would provide under such circumstances." The United States, Canada, and the United Kingdom do not require health professionals to volunteer to provide care in an emergency, but many European countries and Australia do. The flag of the airline determines whether health professionals are or are not "required" to provide care. It is clear that enforcement of the "must volunteer" provision is problematic. Some uncertainty about legal jurisdiction in the case of international flights or even domestic flights over various states remains unsettled by case law as few lawsuits against health professionals providing care in medical emergencies in flight are on record. In-flight emergencies are best handled if the provider is aware of the treatment resources available on board the aircraft, is prepared to render care in the face of considerable uncertainty because of the lack of diagnostic information, provides care only "within the scope of a person with similar training," and understands that, in the final analysis, clinical decisions made at 35,000 feet are often "your best guess."

Some understanding of the risks of travel by older adults, resources for planning in advance of travel and what resources are available to health professionals in the event of being called to help in a medical emergency will better prepare both the elder traveler and the responding health professional when that "dreaded call" comes over the public address system in the midst of a journey.

Table 20–3. Contents of an enhanced on-board emergency medical kit.

Prefilled Syringes	Other
Atropine	500 mL IV saline
Dextrose	IV tubing
Diazepam	IV catheter
Epinephrine	Three endotracheal tubes
Epinephrine autoinjector	Two laryngoscopes
Lidocaine	Three oropharyngeal airways
Sodium bicarbonate	Gloves, sponges, tape
Ampules & Vials	**Monitoring**
Diphenhydramine	Sphygmomanometer
Epinephrine	Stethoscope
Furosemide	AHA Algorithm Book
Digoxin	**Syringes & Needles**
Nalbuphine	**Drugs—Miscellaneous**
Naloxone	Albuterol inhaler
Procainamide	Ammonia inhalants
Promethazine	Aspirin tablets
Solu-Cortef	Clonidine tablets
	Nitroglycerine tablets

Chandra D, Parisini E, Mozaffarian D. Meta-analysis: travel and risk for venous thromboembolism. *Ann Intern Med.* 2009;151(3):180-190.

Gendreau MA, DeJohn C. Responding to medical events during commercial airline flights. *N Engl J Med.* 2002;346(14):1067-1073.

Leder K, Torresi J, Libman MD, et al. GeoSentinal surveillance of illness in returned travelers, 2007-2011. *Ann Intern Med.* 2013;150(6):456-468.

Peterson DC, Martin-Gill C, Guyette FX, et al. Outcomes of medical emergencies on commercial airline flights. *N Engl J Med.* 2013;368(22):2075-2083.

Ross AGP, Olds GR, Cripps AW, et al. Enteropathogens and chronic illness in returning travelers. *N Engl J Med.* 2013;368(19):1817-1825.

Sack RL. Clinical practice: jet lag. *N Engl J Med.* 2010;362(5):440-447.

Delirium

21

Tammy Ting Hshieh, MD
Sharon K. Inouye, MD, MPH

ESSENTIALS OF DIAGNOSIS

▶ Clinical diagnosis based on detailed history, cognitive assessment, and physical and neurologic examination.

▶ The pathognomonic feature is an acute change in baseline mental status developing over hours to days.

▶ Other key features include fluctuating course with an increase or decrease in symptoms over a 24-hour period; inattention, with difficulty focusing attention; and either disorganized thinking, such as rambling or incoherent speech, or altered level of consciousness (vigilant or lethargic).

▶ Perceptual disturbances, such as hallucinations, or paranoid delusions present in approximately 15% to 40% of cases.

▶ Search for organic or physiologic causes (eg, illness, drug related, or metabolic derangement).

▶ Delirium is often misdiagnosed as dementia, depression, or psychosis.

▶ Accepted delirium criteria provided by Confusion Assessment Method.

General Principles in Older Adults

Delirium is an acute disorder of attention and cognitive function that may arise at any point in the course of an illness. It is often the only sign of a serious underlying medical condition, especially in older persons who are frail or who have underlying dementia.

The prevalence of delirium on admission can range from 10% to 40%. During hospitalization, it may affect an additional 25% to 50%. The rates of postoperative delirium are estimated at 10% to 52%. Even higher rates (70% to 87%) are seen in ICUs. In addition, 80% of terminally ill patients become delirious before death.

Three forms of delirium have been recognized: the hyperactive, hyperalert form; the hypoactive, hypoalert, lethargic form; and the mixed form, which combines elements of both. The hypoactive form is often unrecognized but more common among older hospitalized patients; it is associated with a poorer overall prognosis.

Delirium as a geriatric syndrome is inherently multifactorial and develops as a result of interactions between predisposing risk factors and noxious insults or precipitants. Thus, it is imperative that clinicians identify and address all potential factors and observe patients closely for resolution.

▶ Prevention

The major predisposing risk factor for delirium is preexisting cognitive impairment, specifically dementia, which increases the risk of delirium 2- to 5-fold. Virtually all chronic medical illnesses can predispose older persons to delirium, as can specific neurological and metabolic disorders. A full list of risk factors is included in Table 21–1.

The foremost precipitating factor is medications, which contribute to more than 40% of cases of delirium. The medications most frequently associated with delirium are those with known psychoactive effects, such as sedative hypnotics, opiates, H_2 blockers, and anticholinergic drugs. The American Geriatrics Society published a list of potentially inappropriate medications for older adults, known as the *2012 Revised Beers Criteria*, which encompasses some of these delirium-provoking medications. In addition, delirium risk increases in direct proportion to the number of medications prescribed. Herbal therapies are being increasingly recognized as causing or contributing to delirium, especially when taken concurrently with a psychoactive medication. This is particularly true for psychoactive herbs, such as St. John's wort, kava kava, and valerian root. Table 21–1 lists other precipitating factors, including intercurrent illness, environmental, and surgery.

Table 21–1. Risk factors and precipitating factors for delirium.

Risk Factors	Precipitating Factors
Cognitive Status • Dementia/cognitive impairment • Depression • History of delirium **Coexisting Medical Conditions** • Severe/terminal illness • Multiple comorbidities • Neurologic disease (including history of stroke, intracranial bleeding, meningitis, encephalitis, Parkinson disease) • Metabolic derangements (including hyper/hyponatremia, hyper/hypoglycemia, hypercalcemia, thyroid or adrenal dysfunctions, and acid–base disorders) • Fracture or trauma • Anemia • Low serum albumin • Infection with HIV **Functional Status** • Functional dependence • Immobility • Low level of activity • History of falls, gait instability **Sensory Impairment** • Visual • Hearing **Decreased Oral Intake** • Dehydration • Malnutrition **Demographic** • Age 65 years or older • Male sex • Lower educational attainment	**Drugs** • All tricyclic antidepressants • Anticholinergic drugs • Benzodiazepines • Corticosteroids • H_2-receptor antagonists • Narcotics • Polypharmacy • Alcohol **Intercurrent Illnesses** • Infection • Hypoxia • Shock • Fever/hypothermia • Withdrawal • Low serum albumin • Metabolic derangements (including hyper/hyponatremia, hyper/hypoglycemia, hypercalcemia, thyroid or adrenal dysfunctions, and acid–base disorders) **Environmental** • Admission to ICU • Physical restraints • Bladder catheterization • Pain • Emotional stress • Multiple procedures • Prolonged sleep deprivation **Surgery** • Orthopedic • Cardiac • Prolonged cardiopulmonary bypass

American Geriatrics Society 2012 Beers Criteria Update Expert Panel. Updated Beers criteria for potentially inappropriate medication use in older adults. *J Am Geriatr Soc.* 2012;60(4):616-631. (Systematic review and grading of evidence on 53 medications and medication classes with potential for drug-related problems or adverse drug events in older patients.)

Fong, TG , Tulebaev SR, Inouye SK. Delirium in elderly adults: diagnosis, prevention and treatment. *Nat Rev Neurol.* 2009;5(4):210-220. (Review of current clinical practice in delirium, with a focus on neurologic pathophysiology, and includes discussion on diagnosis, treatment, outcomes, economic impact, and future directions.)

Inouye SK. Delirium in older persons. *N Engl J Med.* 2006;354(11):1157-1165. (Comprehensive review on current clinical practices in delirium – including epidemiology, diagnosis, prevalence, management, link with dementia; identifies areas of controversy and highlights need for future research.)

Table 21–2 shows targeted preventive interventions, most of which can also be nonpharmacologic treatments for delirium. Prevention of delirium by targeting vulnerable patients with predisposing risk factors or precipitating factors has been shown to be effective. In addition, proactive geriatrics consultation (daily geriatrician visits and targeted recommendations based on a structured protocol) is effective in vulnerable patients with preexisting dementia or functional impairments.

Pharmacologic prevention of delirium has demonstrated conflicting results in a number of randomized controlled trials examining joint surgeries and postoperative delirium. Olanzapine has been found to lower incidence but increase duration and severity of delirium while haloperidol decreased duration, severity, and length of stay but had no effect on incidence. In general, the use of antipsychotics

Table 21–2. Nonpharmacologic and pharmacologic treatments for delirium.

Nonpharmacologic (By Risk/Precipitating Factor)	Targeted Intervention	Pharmacologic	Targeted Intervention
		Neuroleptics	
Sleep deprivation	Sleep protocol (back massage, relaxation techniques, soothing music, decreased light/noise, warm milk or caffeine-free herbal tea, private room, minimizing of vital sign checks/procedures/medication administration overnight) Avoid using sedatives, especially diphenhydramine Maintain sleep–wake cycle	**Typical**	
		Haloperidol (Haldol)	• *Pros:* Proven/tested, IV/intramuscular/oral formulations, oral formulation theoretically has less QTc prolonging effects, pharmacokinetically optimal • *Cons:* Sedation, hypotension, acute dystonia, extrapyramidal symptoms, anticholinergic side effects (dry mouth, constipation, urinary retention, confusion), worsens Parkinson disease rigidity • *Loading dose:* 0.25–1 mg every 20–30 minutes until patient manageable. Maximum daily dose of 3–5 mg. Peak effect in 4–6 hours (oral), 20 minutes (intramuscular/intravenous) • *Maintenance dose:* Divide loading dose by 2, give every 12 hours; taper over 2–3 days • *Caveats:* D_2 dopaminergic receptors are saturated at low doses. Thus, >5 mg/24 hours has no clinical benefit, only increases harm
Dehydration	Recognition of volume depletion and replenishment of fluids		
Hearing Loss	Proper hearing aids or amplifiers available and in use		
Vision Loss	Provision of proper visual aids (patient's own glasses, magnifying lenses, or adaptive equipment)		
Immobility	Ambulate as soon as possible (assistance or supervision when needed) Out of bed to chair with meals Active range-of-motion exercises if confined to bed Involve in self-care (toileting, hair brushing, dressing) Minimize lines and drains (telemetry, intravenous access, bladder catheters)		
		Atypical	
Cognitive impairment	Frequent orientation to person, place, time Large updated board, calendars, clocks Family presence, private room, close to nursing station Involve patients in decisions and daily toileting Eye contact during interactions	Olanzapine (Zyprexa, Zydis)	• *Pros:* Less extrapyramidal symptoms, dissolvable tablet formulation • *Cons:* Increased anticholinergic side effects can worsen confusion, potential QTc prolongation • *Starting dose:* 2.5–5 mg. Repeat in 20 minutes if needed
		Quetiapine (Seroquel)	• *Pros:* Sedating effect helps maintain sleep–wake cycle • *Cons:* Oral formulation only, QTc prolongation • *Starting dose:* 6.25–12.5 mg
Medications (sedating or psychoactive)	Use alternative and less harmful medications Avoid those with long half-lives Allow for impaired kidney and liver function Use lowest dose possible Taper and discontinue unnecessary medications American Geriatrics Society 2012 Beers Criteria: • All tricyclic antidepressants • Anticholinergics • Benzodiazepines • Corticosteroids • H_2-receptor antagonists • Sedative hypnotics • Meperidine/chlorpromazine/thioridazine	Risperidone (Risperdal)/Ziprasidone (Geodon)	• *Pros:* Sedating effect helps maintain sleep–wake cycle, oral and intramuscular formulations • *Cons:* Can be very sedating, QTc prolongation, tardive dyskinesia
		Benzodiazepines	• *Pros:* Used for alcohol/sedative withdrawal; lorazepam (Ativan) is benzodiazepine of choice because of decreased half-life, no active metabolite, intravenous version • *Cons:* Generally not recommended because oversedating, worsens confusion • *Starting dose:* 0.25–0.5 mg

prophylactically in delirium prevention is not recommended since no study successfully prevented delirium or demonstrated decreased morbidity. Sedation depth during surgery has been correlated with postoperative delirium. Light sedation has been associated with decreased rates of delirium, suggesting a role for lighter sedation in older surgical patients, to prevent delirium.

Inouye SK, Bogardus ST Jr, Baker DI, Leo-Summers L, Cooney LM Jr. The Hospital Elder Life Program: a model of care to prevent cognitive and functional decline in older hospitalized patients. *J Am Geriatr Soc.* 2000;48(12):1697-1706. (The practical implementation of a multicomponent targeted program to improve cognitive and functional outcomes in older hospitalized patients.)

Inouye SK, Bogardus ST Jr, Charpentier PA, et al. A multicomponent intervention to prevent delirium in hospitalized older patients. *N Engl J Med.* 1999;340(9): 669-676. (Successful clinical trial of a multiple risk factor reduction strategy for the prevention of delirium in hospitalized older medical patients with 40% reduction in delirium.)

Marcantonio ER, Flacker JM, Wright RJ, Resnick NM. Reducing delirium after hip fracture: a randomized trial. *J Am Geriatr Soc.* 2001;49(5):516-522. (Randomized controlled trial of proactive geriatric consultation, which successfully reduced occurrence of delirium in hip fracture patients by 36%.)

Siddiqi N, Stockdale R, Britton AM, Holmes J. Interventions for preventing delirium in hospitalized patients. *Cochrane Database Syst Rev.* 2007;(2):CD005563. (Sparse evidence on effectiveness of interventions to prevent delirium; proactive geriatric consultation may reduce delirium incidence and severity, and prophylactic low-dose haloperidol may reduce delirium duration and severity.)

Sieber FE, Zakriya KJ, Gottschalk A, et al. Sedation depth during spinal anesthesia and the development of postoperative delirium in elderly patients undergoing hip fracture repair. *Mayo Clin Proc.* 2010;85(1):18-26. (Light propofol sedation decreased prevalence of postoperative delirium by 50%, as compared with deep sedation, making it a simple, safe and cost-effective means of preventing postoperative delirium.)

▶ Clinical Findings

A. Symptoms & Signs

Initial evaluation of delirium is largely based on establishing a patient's baseline cognitive functioning and the clinical course of any cognitive change. Thus, a detailed history from a reliable informant, such as a spouse, child, or caregiver, is most important. The history should seek to clarify the acuity of any mental status changes and seek clues to the underlying cause.

The cardinal historical features of delirium are acute onset and fluctuating course, in which symptoms tend to come and go or increase and decrease in severity over a 24-hour period. This is the major feature distinguishing delirium from dementia, which usually develops gradually and progressively over months to years.

1. Cognitive changes—Usually determined through cognitive testing and, most importantly, close clinical observation of the quality of the patient's response. For example, a person may score correctly on a particular cognitive task but during the task may demonstrate fluctuating attention, easy distractibility, rambling speech or lethargy.

2. Inattention—Decreased ability to focus, maintain and shift one's attention. For example, patients will demonstrate difficulty maintaining or following a conversation, perseverate on a previous answer, require repetition of instructions or struggle to follow instructions on cognitive tasks (simple repetition, digit span, backward recitation of months/days).

3. Disorganized thinking—Manifested as rambling and, at its extreme, incoherent speech. Problems with memory, disorientation, or language are frequent.

4. Altered level of consciousness—Ranges from agitated, vigilant states to lethargic or stuporous states.

5. Other features—Not essential for diagnosis but commonly seen are psychomotor agitation or retardation, perceptual disturbances (eg, hallucinations, illusions), paranoid delusions, emotional lability, and sleep-wake cycle disturbances.

B. Laboratory Findings and Imaging

The algorithm in Figure 21–1 provides a systematic approach to the diagnosis and evaluation of delirium in the older person. No specific laboratory tests exist that positively identify delirium. Current research has focused on specific biomarkers that have been promising, but all require further investigation: S-100 beta, insulin-like growth factor-1, neuron specific enolase and inflammatory markers including cytokines interleukin (IL)-8, tumor necrosis factor (TNF)-alpha, monocyte chemoattractant protein (MCP)-1, procalcitonin, and cortisol.

Laboratory tests in the evaluation of delirious patients should include complete blood count, electrolytes (including calcium), kidney and liver function, glucose, and oxygen saturation. Furthermore, in searching for occult infection, blood cultures, urinalysis/urine culture, chest x-ray may be considered. Other laboratory tests may be pursued if specific contributing factors have not been identified in a particular patient. These include thyroid function tests, arterial blood gas, vitamin B_{12} levels, drug levels, toxicology screens, cortisol levels, and evaluation of the cerebrospinal fluid.

Brain imaging with CT or MRI are indicated by a history or signs of recent fall or head trauma, fever of unknown origin, new focal neurologic symptoms, or no obvious cause has been identified. An electroencephalogram may be indicated to evaluate for occult seizure activity. It can also be used in differentiating delirium from nonorganic psychiatric disorders.

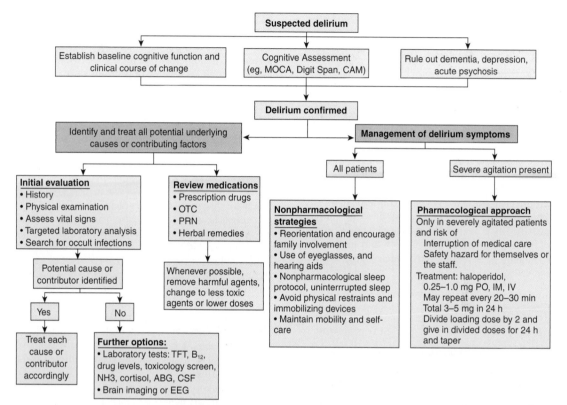

▲ **Figure 21–1.** Algorithm for the evaluation of suspected delirium in the older adult. ABG, arterial blood gas; B$_{12}$, vitamin B$_{12}$; CAM, Confusion Assessment Method; CSF, cerebrospinal fluid; EEG, electroencephalogram; IM, intramuscular; IV, intravenous; MOCA, Montreal Cognitive Assessment; NH$_3$, ammonia level; OTC, over-the-counter; PO, oral; PRN, as needed; TFT, thyroid function tests. (Adapted and reproduced with permission from Goldman L, Schafer AI. *Goldman's Cecil Medicine*. 24th ed. Philadelphia, PA: Elsevier Saunders; 2012.)

American Psychiatric Association. *Diagnostic and Statistical Manual of Mental Disorders*. 5th ed. Washington, DC: American Psychiatric Association; 2013. (Reference standard for definition of and diagnostic criteria for delirium.)

Inouye SK, van Dyck CH, Alessi CA, Balkin S, Siegal AP, Horwitz RI. Clarifying confusion: the confusion assessment method. A new method for the detection of delirium. *Ann Intern Med*. 1990;113(12):941-948. (Validation study for the CAM instrument in hospitalized elderly and a subset of persons with dementia.)

Khan BA, Zawahiri M, Campbell NL, Boustani MA. Biomarkers for delirium—a review. *J Am Geriatr Soc*. 2011;59 Suppl 2:S256-S261. (Literature review of potential biomarkers for delirium shows promise with S-100 beta, insulin-like growth factor 1, and inflammatory markers.)

Wei LA, Fearing MA, Sternberg EJ, Inouye SK. The Confusion Assessment Method: a systematic review of current usage. *J Am Geriatr Soc*. 2008;56(5):823-830. (CAM improves identification of delirium and is optimally used when scored based on observations made during formal cognitive testing and after training in the use of the instrument.)

Wong CL, Holroyd-Leduc J, Simel DL, Straus SE. Does this patient have delirium? Value of bedside instruments. *JAMA*. 2010;304(7):779-786. (Eleven instruments for diagnosis of delirium were evaluated and best evidence supports use of the CAM which takes approximately 5 minutes to administer.)

C. Physical Examination

Detailed physical examination is essential for evaluation of delirium. Delirium may often be the initial manifestation of serious underlying disease in an older person; thus, astute attention to early localizing signs on physical examination may allow early diagnosis of a precipitating insult. A careful search for evidence of occult infections should be performed, including signs of pneumonia, urinary tract infection, acute abdominal processes, joint infections, or new cardiac murmur. A detailed neurologic examination with attention to focal or lateralizing signs is also crucial.

D. Special Tests

1. Diagnostic and Statistical Manual of Mental Disorders IV-Text Revision (DSM-5)—The American Psychiatric Association DSM-5 guidelines were developed based on expert opinion and remain the current standard for definition and diagnostic criteria for delirium.

2. Confusion Assessment Method—Simple, validated tool currently in widespread use (Table 21–3). It has sensitivity of 94% to 100%, specificity of 90% to 100%, and negative predictive value of 90% to 100% for delirium. It has also been validated in patients with dementia. In the intensive care setting, it is feasible to perform cognitive evaluation and screen for delirium using the CAM-ICU, a modification of the CAM for use in mechanically ventilated, restrained, or nonverbal patients. CAM-ICU has not, however, been found to perform as well, with sensitivity of 64% to 73% and negative predictive value of 83%; among verbal patients, the sensitivity drops to <50%.

3. Other instruments—Instruments developed and validated for use in identification of delirium include the Nursing Delirium Screening Scale (NuDesc), Delirium Symptom Interview, NEECHAM Confusion Scale, Delirium Observation Screening Scale, and Intensive Care Delirium Screening Checklist. Instruments developed and validated for use in determining severity of delirium, once it is identified, include the Memorial Delirium Assessment Scale, Clinical Global Impression Scale, and Delirium Severity Index. Other instruments that both diagnose and determine severity of delirium include the Delirium Rating Scale-98 and Cognitive Test for Delirium.

▶ Differential Diagnosis

The main diagnostic dilemma facing the clinician is differentiating delirium from dementia. This is especially difficult when knowledge of baseline cognitive function is missing or when there are known cognitive deficits and one must determine whether the current condition is caused by underlying chronic cognitive impairment or to delirium. Thus, it is crucial to obtain a reliable history about baseline status from an informant. Inattention and altered level of consciousness are usually not features of mild to moderate dementia, and their presence supports the diagnosis of delirium. In patients with known dementia, a history that includes worsening confusion over and above the baseline cognitive impairment also suggests delirium.

Other important diagnoses that must be differentiated from delirium are depression, mania, and other nonorganic psychotic disorders, such as schizophrenia. These diseases do not typically arise in the context of a medical illness. Again, the history and clinical course can assist in providing important clues in differentiating these syndromes. Altered level of consciousness is not prominent in these other diseases. At times, the differential diagnosis can be quite difficult as a result of subtle symptoms or an uncooperative patient. Because of the potential life-threatening nature of delirium, one should err on the side of treating the patient as delirious until further information is available.

Table 21–3. CAM diagnostic criteria for delirium.[a]

1. **Acute onset and fluctuating course.** This feature is based on evidence from a family member or nurse of a positive response to the following questions: Is there evidence of an acute change in mental status from the patient's baseline? Did the (abnormal) behavior fluctuate during the day; that is, tend to come and go, or increase or decrease in severity?
2. **Inattention.** This feature is based on the observation of the presence of difficulty focusing attention (eg, being easily distracted, or having difficulty keeping track of what was being said).
3. **Disorganized thinking.** This feature is based on the observation of the presence of disorganized thinking or incoherent speech, such as rambling or irrelevant conversation, unclear or illogical flow of ideas, or unpredictable switching from subject to subject.
4. **Altered level of consciousness.** This feature is based on the observation of the presence of a level of consciousness other than "alert." This altered level of consciousness can be either vigilant (hyperalert) or various levels of hypoalert states, such as lethargy (drowsy, easily arousable), stupor (difficulty to arouse), or coma (unarousable).

CAM, Confusion Assessment Method.

[a]The diagnosis of delirium requires the presence of features 1 and 2, and either 3 or 4. The ratings for the CAM should be completed after review of the medical chart, discussion with a family member or nurse, and a brief cognitive assessment of the patient (eg, using a brief cognitive screen, such as orientation, word recall, and the Digit Span test).

Adapted and reproduced with permission from Inouye SK, van Dyck CH, Alessi CA, Balkin S, Siegal AP, Horwitz RI. Clarifying confusion: the confusion assessment method. A new method for detection of delirium. *Ann Intern Med.* 1990;113(12):941-948.

Delirium: diagnosis, prevention and management (Clinical Guideline 103). National Institute for Health and Clinical Excellence 2010. Publicly available at http://guidance.nice.org.uk/cg103. (Up-to-date and comprehensive source of evidence based medical practice for the prevention and treatment of delirium.)

Greer N, Rossom R, Anderson P, et al. *Delirium: Screening, Prevention, and Diagnosis—a Systematic Review of the Evidence.* VA-ESP Project #09-009 2011. Washington, DC: Department of Veterans Affairs; 2011. Publicly available at http://www.ncbi.nlm.nih.gov/books/NBK82554/. (Up-to-date review of prevention and diagnosis of delirium with discussion of areas where future research is needed.)

Fick D, Foreman M. Consequences of not recognizing delirium superimposed on dementia in hospitalized elderly individuals. *J Gerontol Nurs.* 2000;26(1):30-40. (Delirium was less likely to be recognized in patients with dementia. These cases were also more likely to be readmitted to the hospital.)

Inouye SK, Foreman MD, Mion LC, Katz KH, Cooney LM Jr. Nurses' recognition of delirium and its symptoms: comparison of nurse and researcher ratings. *Arch Intern Med.* 2001;161(20):2467-2473. (Prospective study of nurse recognition of delirium: Nurses often missed delirium when present—70% of cases missed—but rarely identified delirium when absent. Risk factor for underrecognition included older age, vision impairment, dementia, and hypoactive delirium.)

Complications

Delirium is associated with adverse hospital outcomes, including increased morbidity, mortality, functional decline, and immobility and its attendant complications (aspiration pneumonia, pressure ulcers, deep venous thrombosis, pulmonary emboli, urinary tract infections). Moreover, delirium is associated with complications related to its underlying causes. All of these factors contribute to the poor long-term prognosis for delirium in older patients. Delirium is also independently associated with long-term problems, such as poor long-term functioning, mortality, increased length of stay, need for formal home health care rehabilitation services, new institutionalization, and increased costs of care.

Cole MG, Ciampi A, Belzile E, Zhong L. Persistent delirium in older hospital patients: a systematic review of frequency and prognosis. *Age Ageing.* 2009;38(1):19-26. (Persistent delirium is more prevalent than previously recognized and is associated with adverse outcomes, poorer prognosis.)

Inouye SK, Schlesinger MJ, Lydon TJ. Delirium: a symptom of how hospital care is failing older persons and a window to improve quality of hospital care. *Am J Med.* 1999;106(5):565-573. (Considers delirium as a quality of care measure given the frequency of delirium and the correctable deficiencies in hospital care that can be implemented to reduce delirium. Provides in-depth discussion of the approaches to improving quality of care for hospitalized older persons.)

Marcantonio ER: In the clinic. Delirium. *Ann Intern Med.* 2011;154(11):ITC6-1-ITC6-16. (Review that provides clinical overview and interactive resources on delirium, focusing on prevention, diagnosis, treatment, practice improvement and patient education.)

Witlox J, Eurelings LS, de Jonghe JF, Kalisvaart KJ, Eikelenboom P, van Gool WA. Delirium in elderly patients and the risk of postdischarge mortality, institutionalization, and dementia: a meta-analysis. *JAMA.* 2010;304(4):443-451. (Meta-analysis of the current literature on delirium and its complications suggest poor outcomes, even independent of other co-morbidities and confounders.)

Treatment

Three concurrent approaches are involved in the treatment of delirium (see Figure 21–1): (a) identification and treatment of the underlying medical cause; (b) eradication or minimization of contributing factors of delirium; and (c) management of delirium symptoms.

Complete review of the medication history (including prescription, over-the-counter, as needed, and herbal medications) is needed to identify potentially contributing medications. Drug interactions should be evaluated. Current kidney and liver function status should be assessed and medication dosage/frequency adjusted accordingly. A complete history and physical (including neurological) examination should be performed, along with selected laboratory and radiologic screening tests. Occult infection should be evaluated.

If no identifiable cause or contributor is identified, further testing should be pursued, as shown in Figure 21–1.

A. Nonpharmacologic Strategies

In general, nonpharmacologic strategies should be used in all delirious patients. Table 21–2 details a number of the strategies utilized to prevent or treat delirium, including reorientation, environment optimization, sensory deficit correction, avoiding restraints, mobility/self-care, and sleep hygiene.

B. Pharmacologic Strategies

Pharmacologic therapy for delirium should be reserved for severely agitated individuals whose behavior threatens medically necessary care (such as mechanical ventilation) or poses a safety hazard. All medications used in the treatment of delirium can also cause or worsen confusion; thus, a general principle is to use the lowest dose possible for the shortest period of time. The end point should be an awake and manageable patient, not a sedated patient. All too often, a medication is started for management of agitated delirium but continued indefinitely, obscuring the ability to follow mental status on serial evaluation and putting the patient at significant risk for adverse drug reactions.

Acetylcholine deficiency has been recognized as a contributing factor in the etiology of delirium. Cholinesterase inhibitors, however, have not been beneficial in the management of delirium, despite previous hopes. Small trials of donepezil and rivastigmine did not demonstrate benefits in delirium and in one trial, may have been associated with increased mortality. Table 21–2 covers the classes of medications currently recommended for the treatment and management of delirious patients.

American Psychiatric Association. Guideline watch: Practice guideline for the treatment of patients with delirium. *Am J Psychiatry.* 2004; DOI:10.1176/appi.books. 9780890423363.147844 (Clinical practice guidelines based on review of the literature and expert opinion.)

Lonergan E, Luxenberg J, Areosa Sastre A, Wyller TB. Benzodiazepines for delirium. *Cochrane Database Syst Rev.* 2009;(1):CD006379. (No controlled trials support the use of benzodiazepines in nonalcohol withdrawal delirium.)

Lonergan E, Britton AM, Luxenberg J, Wyller T. Antipsychotics for delirium. *Cochrane Database Syst Rev.* 2008;(2):CD005594. (Low-dose haloperidol has similar efficacy in delirium as atypical antipsychotics such as olanzapine and risperidone. High-dose haloperidol has increased side effects.)

Milisen K, Foreman MD, Abraham IL, et al. A nurse-led interdisciplinary intervention program for delirium in elderly hip-fracture patients. *J Am Geriatr Soc.* 2001;49(5):523-532. (Intervention focused on education of nursing staff, systematic cognitive screening, and geriatric assessment reduced the duration and severity of delirium after hip fracture. No effect was noted on incidence of delirium.)

▶ Prognosis

Delirium has traditionally been described as a reversible syndrome, implying that patients invariably return to their baseline cognitive and functional state. Clinically, however, delirium is not always transient, and can result in long-term cognitive and functional deficits. After delirium, some patients develop subjective memory complaints, and demonstrate reduced performance on cognitive tests. These research findings suggest that the pathologic processes associated with delirium may be associated with direct and persistent neurologic damage.

Furthermore, patients who develop delirium have been found more likely to be diagnosed with dementia at a later date. It appears that delirium increases the risk of developing dementia and may accelerate the rate of progression to dementia. Thus, delirium can in fact alter the trajectory of cognitive decline for older persons.

Fong TG, Jones RN, Shi P, et al. Delirium accelerates cognitive decline in Alzheimer disease. *Neurology.* 2009;72(18):1570-1575. (Delirium accelerates trajectory of cognitive decline in Alzheimer disease.)

Girard TD, Pandharipande PP, Ely EW. Delirium in the intensive care unit. *Crit Care.* 2008;12 Suppl 3. (Delirium was independently associated with increased hospital stays, lower 6-month survival and persistent cognitive impairment in adult ICU patients.)

McCusker J, Cole M, Abrahamowicz M, Primeau F, Belzile E. Delirium predicts 12-month mortality. *Arch Intern Med.* 2002;162(4):457-463. (This prospective case-control study confirmed that delirium was an independent marker of increased mortality in older hospitalized patients.)

USEFUL WEBSITES

American Psychiatric Association guidelines. http://psychiatryonline.org/guidelines.aspx

Hospital Elder Life Program. http://www.hospitalelderlifeprogram.org/public/public-main.php

National Institute for Health and Clinical Excellence (NICE) guidelines for delirium. http://guidance.nice.org.uk/cg103

Systematic Reviews of delirium studies by Martin Cole and colleagues in the Cochrane Library, Database of Abstracts of Reviews of Effectiveness. http://www.cochranelibrary.com

Veteran Affairs guidelines for delirium. http://www.hsrd.research.va.gov/publications/esp/delirium.cfm

Cognitive Impairment & Dementia

22

Kaycee M. Sink, MD, MAS
Kristine Yaffe, MD

ESSENTIALS OF DIAGNOSIS

- ▶ Impairment in at least 2 of the following cognitive domains: memory, executive function, language, visuo-spatial function, and personality/behavior.
- ▶ Significant impairment in social or occupational functioning.
- ▶ Significant decline from previous level of function.
- ▶ Deficits not occurring solely in the presence of delirium or accounted for by major psychiatric disorder.

▶ General Principles in Older Adults

The prevalence of dementia approximately doubles every 5 years after age 60 years. Among community-dwelling elders older than age 85 years, the prevalence is estimated to be 25% to 45%. Prevalence is even higher in nursing homes (>50%). Approximately 60% to 70% of dementia cases are attributable to Alzheimer' disease (AD); Lewy body dementia (DLB) and vascular dementia (VaD) are the other more common forms. In addition, a significant percentage of patients have mixed disease (AD and VaD or AD and DLB). Frontotemporal dementia (FTD) is a more recently recognized form whose prevalence is uncertain.

Cognitive function in older adults is considered a spectrum and ranges from cognitive changes seen in normal aging to mild cognitive impairment (MCI) to dementia. Compared with younger adults, older adults often perform more slowly on timed tasks and have slower reaction times. Mild memory impairment may be present with subjective problems such as difficulty recalling names or where an object was placed. In the case of normal aging, however, the person usually remembers the information later, has intact learning, and any deficits in memory function are subtle, relatively stable over time, and do not cause functional impairment.

MCI is a disorder in which cognitive function is below normal limits for that patient's age and education but is not severe enough to qualify as dementia. MCI is characterized by subjective cognitive complaints, preferably corroborated by someone else; evidence of objective cognitive impairment in 1 or more cognitive domains (memory, language, executive function, etc); and intact functional status. When MCI involves memory (amnestic MCI), it is associated with an increased risk of AD and may actually represent a form of very early AD. Among patients with amnestic MCI, 10% to 15% per year convert to AD compared with 1% to 2% of age-matched controls. Although many patients with MCI will progress to AD with time, it is a clinically heterogeneous group, with some patients progressing to other types of dementias and others remaining cognitively stable. The most severe type of cognitive impairment is dementia. This diagnosis requires deficits in multiple domains of cognitive functioning (at least 2) that represent a significant change from baseline and that are severe enough to cause impairment in daily functioning (see "Essentials of Diagnosis" above).

Dementia often goes undiagnosed or undocumented in primary care settings, especially early in the course of the disease. Cognitive impairment and dementia should be detected as early as possible in older patients so that secondary causes of cognitive impairment can be identified. Drug therapy for AD remains symptomatic (not disease modifying) and may improve a patient's quality of life, extend the period of relatively good function, and delay nursing home placement. In addition, early diagnosis allows patients and caregivers to plan future needs and for primary practitioners to adjust medication regimens and assess treatment goals.

McKhann GM, Knopman DS, Chertkow H, et al. The diagnosis of dementia due to Alzheimer's disease: Recommendations from the National Institute on Aging-Alzheimer's Association workgroups on diagnostic guidelines for Alzheimer's disease. *Alzheimers Dement.* 2011;7(3):263-269.

▶ Prevention

At this time, there are no proven strategies to prevent MCI or dementia. However, control of vascular risk factors such as hypertension, hyperlipidemia, and diabetes may reduce the risk of both AD and VaD. In addition, evidence is accumulating that regular physical activity (including walking) may be an important behavioral strategy for reducing the risk of cognitive impairment and dementia. Cognitive activity, such as mental exercises, moderate alcohol intake, and nutritional strategies, may also reduce risk, but more data is needed. Both depression and smoking are linked to increased risk of dementia and they should be screened for in older adults. Gingko biloba, nonsteroidal antiinflammatory drugs (NSAIDs), statins, estrogens, and vitamin E are *not* recommended for prevention because they have failed to delay or prevent dementia in large clinical trials and in some cases, may cause harm.

Daviglus ML, Bell CC, Berrettini W, et al. NIH state-of-the-science conference statement: Preventing Alzheimer's disease and cognitive decline. Ann Intern Med. 2010;153(3):176-181.

▶ Clinical Findings

A. Patient History

The history is the most important part of the evaluation of a patient with possible cognitive impairment or dementia. Although it may be unreliable, eliciting the history first from the patient can be very informative and useful. Allowing patients to give their version of the history also enables assessment of recent and remote memory. Questions about their medical and surgical history as well as current medications may help to assess both recent and remote memory. For example, if a patient has denied any medical or surgical history, the discovery of a large abdominal surgical scar on examination is very informative.

Because the history from a patient with cognitive impairment can be incomplete and incorrect, it is crucial to also obtain history from a family member, caregiver, or other source. The history should focus on how long the symptoms have been present, whether they began gradually or abruptly, and the rate and nature (stepwise vs. continual decline) of their progression. Specific areas on which to focus include the patient's ability to learn new things (eg, use of a microwave or a remote control), language problems (eg, word-finding difficulties or absence of content), trouble with complex tasks (eg, balancing the checkbook, preparing a meal), spatial ability (eg, getting lost in familiar places), and personality changes, behavioral problems, or psychiatric symptoms (eg, delusions, hallucinations, paranoia). Obtaining a good functional assessment will help to determine the severity of impairment and the need for caregiver support or, in patients without caregivers, the need for more supervised placement.

This should include an assessment of the activities of daily living (ADLs) and instrumental activities of daily living (IADLs; eg, cooking, cleaning, shopping, managing finances, using the telephone, managing medications, and driving or arranging transportation). In addition, the clinician should assess the patient's family and social situation because information obtained may be instrumental in developing a treatment plan.

It is important to obtain a detailed medication history and history of comorbid conditions, including symptoms of depression and alcohol and other substance use. Although potentially reversible causes of dementia account for <1% of cases, a large part of the work-up is directed toward identifying and treating these causes. Table 22–1 summarizes the key elements of the history and physical examination.

B. Symptoms & Signs

Early signs and symptoms of dementia are often missed by both physicians and families, especially in AD, in which social graces are often retained until moderate stages of the disease. Subtle hints of early dementia or MCI may include

Table 22–1. Key elements of the history and physical examination.

History
Duration of symptoms and nature of progression of symptoms
Presence of specific symptoms related to
• Memory (recent and remote) and learning
• Language (word-finding problems, difficulty expressing self)
• Visuospatial skills (getting lost)
• Executive functioning (calculations, planning, carrying out multistep tasks)
• Apraxia (not able to do previously learned motor tasks, eg, slicing a loaf of bread)
• Behavior or personality changes
• Psychiatric symptoms (apathy, hallucinations, delusions, paranoia)
Functional assessment (ADLs and IADLs)
Social support assessment
Medical history, comorbidities
Thorough medication review, including over-the-counter medications, herbal products
Family history
Review of systems, including screening for depression and alcohol/substance abuse

Physical Examination
Cognitive examination
General physical examination with special attention to
• Neurologic examination, looking for focal findings, extrapyramidal signs, gait and balance assessment
• Cardiovascular examination
• Signs of abuse or neglect
Screen for impairments in hearing and vision

ADLs, activities of daily living; IADLs, instrumental ADLs.

frequent repetition of the same questions or stories, reduced participation in former hobbies, increased accidents, and missed appointments. Poorly controlled chronic conditions may suggest lack of adherence to medication prescriptions because of memory problems, especially if these conditions were previously well controlled. Self-neglect, difficulty handling money, and getting lost are more obvious signs.

1. Alzheimer disease—The classic triad of findings in AD is memory impairment manifested by difficulty learning and recalling information (especially new information), visuospatial problems, and language impairment, which, in combination, are severe enough to interfere with social or occupational functioning. Classically, AD patients have little or no insight into their deficits, which may be a result of their compromised executive functioning (planning, insight, and judgment). Early in the course of disease, patients with AD retain their social functioning and ability to accomplish overlearned, familiar tasks, but often have difficulty with more complicated tasks, such as balancing a checkbook or making complex decisions. Because symptoms are insidious and family members often dismiss the short-term memory loss as normal aging, several years may pass before the patient receives medical attention. Disorientation is common among patients with AD and typically begins with disorientation to time, then place, and ultimately to person. Patients develop a progressive language disorder that begins with subtle anomic aphasia and ultimately progresses to fluent aphasia and then to mutism at the end stages of the disease. They have difficulty with visuospatial tasks and may be prone to getting lost, even in familiar surroundings. The disease is slowly progressive, and patients show continual decline in their ability to remain independent.

Behavioral changes are common in AD, as in all dementia subtypes, and no neuropsychiatric symptom or behavioral disturbance is pathognomonic. Early changes may be manifested by apathy and irritability (≤70% of patients) and depression (30% to 50% of patients). Agitation becomes more common as the disease progresses and may be especially notable regarding issues of grooming and dressing. Psychotic symptoms, such as delusions, hallucinations, and paranoia, are also common, affecting up to 50% of patients in moderate to advanced stages.

2. Dementia with Lewy bodies—DLB is the second most common form of dementia after AD, affecting up to 20% to 30% of patients with dementia. The core features of DLB are parkinsonism, fluctuation in cognitive impairment, and visual hallucinations. The presence of 1 of these features suggests possible DLB, and the presence of 2–3 suggests probable DLB. Rapid eye movement (REM) sleep behavior disorder and severe sensitivity to antipsychotics are suggestive of DLB and autonomic insufficiency, syncope, and depression are supportive features. These symptoms should occur in the absence of other factors that could explain them. The parkinsonism in patients with DLB generally presents after, or

concurrent with, the onset of the dementia. This is in contrast to the Parkinson disease (PD)-related dementia, which generally occurs late in the disease. Parkinsonism in DLB is manifested primarily by rigidity and bradykinesia; tremor is less common (<10% to 25% of patients in large series). The development of parkinsonism late in the stages of a dementia is not specific for DLB because many patients with advanced AD also develop increased tone, bradykinesia, and tremor.

Like AD, DLB is insidious in onset and progressive, although it classically has a fluctuating quality on a day-to-day basis. The fluctuation is seen in the level of alertness, cognitive functioning, and functional status. Early in the course, memory and language deficits are less prominent than in AD. In contrast, visuospatial abilities, problem solving, and processing speed are more significantly impaired than in AD at the same stage. Visual hallucinations occur in 60% to 85% of autopsy confirmed DLB patients compared with 11% to 28% of autopsy confirmed AD patients. They are classically very vivid and often are of animals, people, or mystical things. Unlike true psychosis, most patients with DLB can distinguish hallucinations from reality and, early on, tend not to be disturbed by them. Caution is advised in the use of antipsychotic medications because patients with DLB are exquisitely sensitive to neuroleptics, and a dramatic worsening of extrapyramidal symptoms may occur. Neuroleptics should not be given as a diagnostic test because deaths have been reported among those with DLB.

3. Vascular dementia—In general, the diagnosis is based on the presence of clinical or radiographic evidence of cerebrovascular disease in a patient with dementia. Sudden onset of dementia after a stroke or stepwise, rather than continuous, decline is supportive of the diagnosis in the context of cortical strokes and focal neurologic findings on examination. However, because a considerable percentage of patients have subcortical vascular disease, the course may appear to be more gradual. In addition, many patients have mixed AD and VaD and mild, progressive, non-VaD may suddenly be unmasked by the occurrence of a stroke.

Memory impairments in VaD are often less severe than in AD. Patients with VaD have impaired recall but tend to have better recognition and benefit from cueing in contrast to AD patients. On formal neuropsychiatric testing, "patchy" deficits may be found, often with difficulty on speeded tasks and tests of executive function. As in AD, behavioral and psychological symptoms are common. Depression may be more severe in patients with VaD.

4. Frontotemporal dementia—FTD develops at a relatively young age (mean age of onset is in the 50s). It is estimated that FTD accounts for approximately 25% of presenile dementias. There is a behavioral variant (formerly known as Picks disease), and a language variant that includes primary progressive aphasia and semantic dementia.

Behavioral variant FTD (bvFTD) is characterized by early changes in personality and behavior with relative sparing of memory and is often misdiagnosed as a psychiatric disorder. However, some symptoms are highly specific for bvFTD (97% to 100%; eg, hyperorality, early changes in personality and behavior, early loss of social awareness [disinhibition], compulsive or repetitive behaviors, progressive reduction in speech [early], and sparing of visuospatial abilities) and reliably distinguish it from AD. The hyperorality may be manifested by marked changes in food preference (often toward junk food and carbohydrates) or simply excessive eating. Another interesting phenomenon is that some patients with FTD develop new artistic talents without having had any prior interest.

Cognitive testing in patients with FTD may reveal normal mini-mental state examination (MMSE) scores early in the disease. More formal neuropsychiatric testing reveals deficits in frontal systems tasks such as verbal fluency, abstraction, and executive functioning, and these deficits are seen earlier than in a typical patient with AD. In contrast to patients with AD, FTD patients tend to show preserved visuospatial abilities and relatively preserved memory, especially recognition memory.

5. Other dementias—Many other diseases are associated with cognitive impairment and dementia, such as PD and its related disorders, Huntington disease (HD), HIV, and alcoholism. Approximately 30% of patients with PD develop dementia. This generally occurs late in the course of PD, and is characterized by slowing of mental processing, impaired recall (but usually preserved recognition memory), executive dysfunction, and visuospatial problems. HD is a rare autosomal dominant disorder characterized by motor (chorea, dystonia), behavioral, and cognitive impairments. With the advances in HIV care and the increasing numbers of long-term survivors, HIV-associated neurocognitive disorder (HAND) should be considered in the differential diagnosis of cognitive impairment. With the use of highly active antiretroviral therapy, the prevalence of HIV-associated dementia has declined, but up to 40% of HIV-infected persons may suffer from cognitive impairment. Although chronic alcohol abuse impairs cognitive functioning, there is controversy as to whether a true dementia syndrome related to alcohol exists (separate from thiamine deficiency and head trauma), partly because there have been no large-scale studies.

6. Advanced & end-stage disease—The advanced symptoms of most dementias appear similar, and, in late stages, it is nearly impossible to distinguish between different types of dementia. In advanced dementia (typically with a score <10 on the MMSE), language skills are significantly impaired. There may be very little meaningful speech, and comprehension is very impaired. Some patients will progress to the point of mutism. Patients with advanced dementia have progressive difficulty with even the most basic ADLs, such as feeding themselves, and may progress to the point at which they are incontinent of bowel and bladder and are completely dependent in all ADLs. Symptoms of parkinsonism such as rigidity

are common. Gait is impaired and, ultimately, patients may stop walking, leading to a bed-bound state. Seizures are occasionally seen in end-stage dementia patients. Patients who do not die of other comorbidities tend to develop concomitant complications (eg, malnutrition, pressure ulcers, recurrent infections). The most common cause of death in advanced dementia is pneumonia.

Cardarelli R, Kertesz A, Knebl JA. Frontotemporal dementia: a review for primary care physicians. *Am Fam Physician.* 2010;82(11):1372-1377.

McKhann GM, Knopman DS, Chertkow H, et al. The diagnosis of dementia due to Alzheimer's disease: recommendations from the National Institute on Aging-Alzheimer's Association workgroups on diagnostic guidelines for Alzheimer's disease. *Alzheimers Dement.* 2011;7(3):263-269.

McKieth IG, Dickson DW, Lowe J, et al. Diagnosis and management of dementia with Lewy bodies. Third report of the DLB consortium. *Neurology.* 2005;65(12):1863-1872.

C. Physical & Mental Status Examination

The physical examination of a patient with cognitive impairment or dementia focuses on identifying clues to the cause of the dementia, comorbid conditions, conditions that may exacerbate the cognitive impairment (eg, sensory impairment or alcoholism), and signs of abuse or neglect. The neurologic examination should be directed at identifying evidence of prior strokes, such as focal signs, and of parkinsonism, such as rigidity, bradykinesia, or tremor, keeping in mind that late in the course of dementia increased tone and brisk reflexes are nonspecific. Gait and balance are an important part of the examination and should be assessed routinely. A careful cardiovascular evaluation, including measurement of blood pressure and examination for carotid disease and peripheral vascular disease, may help in supporting the diagnosis of VaD. Some patients without dementia who have significant hearing or visual impairments may demonstrate behavior that suggests dementia and have a low score on mental status testing. Therefore, it is important to identify and correct, if possible, sensory impairments before making a diagnosis of dementia.

D. Screening Tests

The effectiveness of screening asymptomatic patients for dementia is controversial. However, for patients with a high risk of dementia (eg, patients age 80 years and older) or for those who report memory impairment, screening with a standardized and validated tool is recommended.

1. Mini-Mental State Examination—The MMSE, a 30-point tool that tests orientation, immediate recall, delayed recall, concentration/calculation, language, and visuospatial domains, has been the most widely used screening test of cognition. However, the MMSE is copyright protected and forms should be purchased from Psychological Assessment Resources. The MMSE, like many screening tests, is a culturally and language-biased test, and adjustments should be made for age and level of education. When scores are adjusted for age and education, the MMSE has a high sensitivity and specificity for detecting dementia (82% and 99%, respectively). Because it is administered verbally and patients are asked to write and draw, hearing, visual, or other physical impairments may make the scoring less valid. A patient with early cognitive impairment may score within normal limits for age and education; however, if the test is repeated every 6–12 months, the MMSE can detect cognitive decline and suggest a diagnosis of MCI or dementia. Among patients with AD, MMSE scores decline an average of 3 points per year, whereas for those with MCI, 1 point per year is more typical. In patients who are aging normally, MMSE scores should not decline much from year to year. As a general guideline, scores above 26 are normal, scores of 24–26 may indicate MCI, and a score <24 is consistent with dementia. However, it is best to compare each patient's score with age and education adjusted median scores and to monitor for change in addition to assessing for functional decline.

2. Montreal Cognitive Assessment—The Montreal Cognitive Assessment (MOCA) is gaining favor as a screening test for cognitive impairment. Similar to the MMSE, it is a 30-point screening test that assesses a variety of cognitive domains including memory (with a 5-word recall task), orientation, visuospatial function, concentration, calculation, attention, abstraction, language, and executive function (which is not represented on the MMSE). It is more sensitive than the MMSE, particularly for detecting MCI. The test and directions can be downloaded for free at www.mocatest.org in multiple languages, as well as for the blind. The form shows a cutoff score of 26 (25 and below indicating impairment), but this value is likely too high for most U.S. populations. For example, in a large, ethnically diverse sample of adults in the Dallas Heart Study, the mean score for a 70-year-old with high school education is about 20.5. Test scores are highly influenced by education level. Normative data is accumulating and providers should consult the literature for tables that provide age and education stratified means and standard deviations for populations similar to the patient being tested. Longitudinal data on the MOCA is needed.

3. Mini-Cog—Attempts have been made to create brief, focused, screening tools that are less time-consuming than the MMSE and are freely available. Two commonly used tests are the Clock Draw Test (CDT) and the 3-Item Recall; when used together, this is called the "Mini-Cog." In the Mini-Cog, the patient is asked to draw a clock face with the hands set at a designated time. Several CDTs are available, each with a different scoring system. However, evidence suggests that a simple dichotomy between normal and abnormal clocks has a relatively good sensitivity (approximately 80%) for detecting dementia, even for inexperienced raters. Normal clocks

have all the numbers in the correct position and the hands correctly placed to display the requested time. Using the Mini-Cog is quick and easy, and if both are normal, it essentially rules out dementia. The Mini-Cog may be particularly useful in poorly educated or non–English-speaking patients for whom the MMSE is not so helpful.

E. Cognitive Assessment

The cognitive assessment of a patient with cognitive impairment or dementia should be paired with the physical examination. Patients are less likely to be threatened or offended by questions about cognitive abilities if the questions are framed as part of the physical examination. In addition to administering a standardized assessment tool such as the MMSE or MOCA, providers should also assess domains of cognitive functioning that are not well represented in the MMSE or MOCA, such as judgment and insight. The diagnosis of dementia requires that there be impairment in 2 or more cognitive functions such as memory, language, visuospatial function, and executive functioning. Language can be assessed by simply listening for a lack of content in the patient's dialogue or the use of vague terms to replace nouns, such as "thing" or "it." Asking the patient to name common things in the room may be helpful if the language seems normal. Evidence of impaired executive functioning is often discovered in the history and can be assessed during the examination as well. For example, if the patient is not able to describe a complex function that the patient may normally do (or used to do) in fine detail, there may be a problem with executive functioning.

Borson S, Scanlan J, Brush M, Vitaliano P, Dokmak A. The mini-cog: a cognitive "vital signs" measure for dementia screening the multilingual elderly. *Int J Geriatr Psychiatry.* 2000;15(11): 1021-1027.

Nasreddine ZS, Phillips NA, Bédirian V, et al. The Montreal Cognitive Assessment, MoCA: a brief tool for mild cognitive impairment. *J Am Geriatr Soc.* 2005;53(4):695-699.

Rossetti HC, Lacritz LH, Cullum CM, Weiner MF. Normative data for the Montreal Cognitive Assessment (MoCA) in a population-based sample. *Neurology.* 2011;77(13):1272-1275.

F. Laboratory Findings

In the evaluation of a patient with cognitive impairment or newly diagnosed dementia, laboratory studies are generally used to rule out potentially treatable causes of dementia (Table 22–2). Vitamin B_{12} deficiency and hypothyroidism are common in older adults and can affect cognitive functioning. Treatment of these conditions is warranted, although few cases of dementia are actually caused by (or improved with treatment of) vitamin B_{12} deficiency or hypothyroidism. Most clinicians will also perform complete blood count, electrolytes, creatinine, glucose, calcium, and liver function

Table 22–2. Potentially "reversible"/treatable causes of cognitive impairment.

B$_{12}$ deficiency	Subdural hematoma
Thyroid disease	Normal pressure hydrocephalus
Hypercalcemia	Central nervous system neoplasms
Depression	Drug effects
Alcoholism	Heavy metals

tests. One should screen for latent syphilis and HIV if there is a high index of suspicion of these conditions.

G. Imaging

Routine CT or MRI scanning in the evaluation of patients with dementia remains controversial, but it is generally recommended that 1 noncontrast CT or noncontrast MRI be obtained in the evaluation of cognitive impairment to rule out treatable causes of dementias, such as subdural hematoma, normal pressure hydrocephalus, and tumor. In addition to looking for structural lesions, imaging may be helpful in the diagnosis of the particular type of non-AD dementia. MRI is more sensitive for vascular changes and measures of hippocampal volume. Neuroimaging is likely to be of low yield in patients with a typical clinical appearance of AD and symptoms that have been present for more than 1–2 years. Advantages and disadvantages of neuroimaging can be discussed with patients and families.

Imaging studies for VaD are also nonspecific. This is because many older patients will have some degree of small vessel ischemic disease on CT or MRI. In fact, by age 85 years, nearly 100% of patients will have white matter hyperintensities on imaging studies. Therefore, simply seeing evidence of vascular disease does not warrant diagnosis of VaD. If, however, there is extensive disease, multiple infarcts, or infarcts in key anatomical locations (eg, thalamus) in a patient with a history or neuropsychological findings consistent with VaD, it is probable that the imaging findings are clinically relevant. In FTD, there is classically asymmetric volume loss of the frontal or anterior temporal lobes in comparison to the overall atrophy seen in AD.

Fluorodeoxyglucose positron emission tomography (FDG-PET) scans measure glucose metabolism in specific areas of the brain and may be helpful in distinguishing early AD from FTD or DLB. Although FDG-PET has been shown to improve diagnostic accuracy of pathologically confirmed AD, it is not considered standard in the work up of AD and is generally not needed to make a diagnosis. In addition, Medicare currently only pays for FDG-PET when used to distinguish AD from FTD. Amyloid-binding PET tracers (such as AV-45) have recently become clinically available. However, as of the writing of this chapter, amyloid PET imaging is not covered by Medicare and the role of its use in the clinical diagnosis of AD is yet to be determined. It is not recommended as a screening test for asymptomatic individuals in part because up to 30% of cognitively "normal" older adults test positive for brain amyloid, and because there is currently no treatment that will delay or prevent onset of symptoms.

Hort J, O'Brien JT, Gainotti G, et al. EFNS guidelines for the diagnosis and management of Alzheimer's disease. *Eur J Neurol.* 2010;17(10):1236–1248.

Knopman DS, DeKosky ST, Cummings JL, et al. Practice parameter: diagnosis of dementia (an evidence-based review). Report of the quality standards subcommittee of the American Academy of Neurology. *Neurology.* 2001;56(9):1143-1153.

H. Special Tests/Examinations

1. Neuropsychological testing—Neuropsychological testing is generally performed by neuropsychologists and consists of an in-depth battery of standardized examinations that test multiple cognitive domains, including intelligence, memory, language, visuospatial abilities, attention, reasoning, and problem solving, as well as other measures of executive function. The diagnosis of dementia can generally be made by obtaining a detailed history and physical examination (including a brief cognitive evaluation) and does not require neuropsychological testing. However, there are instances in which referral for formal neuropsychological testing can be particularly helpful (eg, when patients have early or mild symptoms, especially if they have high premorbid intelligence and are performing "normally" on tools such as the MMSE). Neuropsychological testing can also be helpful in patients with low intelligence or education and in those with depression, schizophrenia, or other psychiatric illness in which it may be hard to determine how much the condition is contributing to the apparent cognitive deficits. Likewise, in patients with atypical features, such as early language impairment, neuropsychological testing may be helpful in the differential diagnosis of an unusual type of dementia. In addition, a more thorough cognitive battery can identify relative strengths that may be important to patients and their caregivers and may be useful for establishing a baseline from which to reassess.

2. Kohlman Evaluation of Living Skills—A Kohlman Evaluation of Living Skills (KELS), generally performed by occupational therapists, assesses a patient's ability to perform tasks required for safe independent living. For example, a patient is asked to write a check for a mock bill, use the telephone, or identify dangerous situations in pictures and state what he or she would do. This evaluation may be helpful when a patient with known or suspected dementia is living alone and there is concern about whether the patient needs to be moved to a more supervised setting such as assisted living.

3. Genetic Testing—Tremendous advances have been made in elucidating the genetics of AD. Two categories of genetic defects have been defined: those that cause early onset AD and those involved in late-onset AD. Early onset familial AD is rare and accounts for approximately 5% of all AD cases. Patients with early onset AD usually develop dementia in their 40s to 50s and almost always before age 65 years. Because early onset AD is often familial, it is important to obtain a detailed family history of dementia. It is inherited in an autosomal dominant fashion. Mutations that cause early onset AD have been identified in 3 genes thus far: presenilin 1 (*PSEN1*), presenilin 2 (*PSEN2*), and amyloid precursor protein (*APP*) on chromosomes 14, 1, and 21, respectively. A mutation in *PSEN1* is the most common. Testing for genetic mutations in a patient with early onset AD is not clinically useful for that patient because it will not alter the management of the disease. However, if the patient has children who wish to know whether they have inherited the gene, the family should be referred for genetic counseling. In addition, genetic testing of patients with early onset AD may be valuable for research.

In contrast to early onset AD, late-onset AD (age >60–65 years) is associated with genes that increase the risk of AD but not in an autosomal dominant fashion. Physicians may be asked by patients or family members for the "Alzheimer blood test," most likely referring to apolipoprotein E (*APOE*) genotyping. The association between *APOE* and risk of AD is well established. The presence of one ε4 allele increases the risk of AD by about 2–3 times, whereas the ε2 allele may be protective. It is important to keep in mind that *APOE*–ε4 is only a genetic risk factor for AD; therefore, the absence of an ε4 allele does not rule out the diagnosis nor does the presence of homozygous ε4/ε4 rule it in. In fact, most patients with AD do not carry the ε4 allele. There is broad consensus that *APOE* testing be reserved for research purposes only.

Pinsky LE, Burke W, Bird TD. Why should primary care physicians know about the genetics of dementia? *West J Med.* 2001;175(6):412-416.

▶ Differential Diagnosis

The differential diagnosis of dementia includes the potentially treatable causes of dementia listed in Table 22–2, among them metabolic abnormalities, structural brain lesions, medications, alcoholism, and depression. The differential diagnosis also includes delirium, uncorrected sensory deficits, amnestic disorders, and other psychiatric conditions.

A. Depression

Depression commonly coexists with dementia (up to 30% to 50% of patients), but it may also be the only cause for cognitive deficits and, therefore, must be ruled out or treated before a diagnosis of dementia can be made. A patient's memory complaints that are disproportional to objective deficits should alert a provider to the possibility of depression. This is in contrast to dementia, in which patients tend to minimize their deficits. It is important to keep in mind that older patients who develop reversible cognitive impairments while depressed are at high risk for dementia over the next few years.

B. Delirium

Delirium is a common cause of confusion in older adults, particularly in those who are hospitalized, and may be incorrectly labeled as dementia. In contrast to dementia, delirium is characterized by abrupt onset of altered cognition and consciousness, decreased attention, perceptual disturbances (commonly visual hallucinations), and impressive fluctuations in symptoms. Table 52–3 in Chapter 52, "Evaluating Confusion in Older Adults," contrasts delirium, depression, and dementia. If delirium is suspected, underlying causes should be sought and treated. Dementia is one of the key risk factors for delirium. If cognitive deficits persist after the resolution of delirium, further work-up for dementia should be pursued.

C. Medications & Sensory Deficits

Medications are commonly associated with confusion in older adults. Many classes of drugs have been implicated, including opiates, benzodiazepines, neuroleptics, anticholinergic drugs (many unsuspected medications have significant anticholinergic properties), H_2 blockers, and corticosteroids. Clinicians should ask patients or caregivers to bring in all medications, including nonprescription medicines, for review. Drug–drug interactions and appropriateness of doses should be assessed. In addition, any nonessential medications should be discontinued. Reassessment of the patient may reveal marked improvement in cognition and function. Similarly, correction of sensory deficits (visual or hearing impairments) in patients who have been misidentified as having dementia can be equally rewarding.

D. Alcohol Abuse

Patients with cognitive impairment, disorganization, frequent accidents, or failure at home or work should be screened for alcohol abuse. Years of heavy alcohol use may contribute to permanent cognitive impairment, possibly through direct toxic effects on the brain or thiamine deficiency or from complications of alcohol abuse such as head trauma related to falls or violence. However, alcohol abuse may also be responsible for more acute declines in a patient's level of function; improvement in cognition and function may be seen on cessation of drinking.

E. Other Psychiatric Conditions

Chronic psychiatric conditions such as schizophrenia or bipolar affective disorder may also be included in the differential diagnosis of dementia, especially when behavioral changes and psychiatric symptoms such as delusions and hallucinations predominate. In addition, older patients with chronic schizophrenia are more likely to develop dementia than unaffected adults. The pattern of cognitive deficits seen in geriatric schizophrenia patients is distinct from AD, and autopsy series confirm that AD does not account for the cognitive impairments.

Complications

A. Delirium

Delirium, as well as being considered in the differential diagnosis of dementia, is also a major complication of dementia. Risk factors for delirium include cognitive impairment, severe medical illness, elevated blood urea nitrogen (BUN)-to-creatinine ratio, and visual impairment, among others. When patients with dementia are hospitalized, it is critical to be aware of their high risk for delirium and to take measures to avoid precipitating factors, such as the use of physical restraints and bladder catheters, malnutrition, and use of multiple new medications.

B. Behavioral & Psychological Disturbances

Behavioral and psychological symptoms of dementia (BPSD) are very common, affecting up to 80% of patients with dementia. These symptoms, which are associated with worse prognosis, earlier nursing home referral, greater costs, and increased caregiver burden, include the following:

- Agitation and aggression
- Disruptive vocalizations
- Psychotic features (delusions, hallucinations, paranoia)
- Depressive symptoms
- Apathy
- Sleep disturbances
- Wandering or pacing
- Resistance to personal care (bathing and grooming)

Although agitation and psychosis are common in dementia, especially as the disease progresses, any new behavioral symptoms should be evaluated before being attributed solely to the dementia. Precipitating causes of new agitation may include delirium, untreated pain, fecal impaction, urinary retention, new medications, sensory impairment, and environmental causes (eg, new environment, excessive stimulation).

The delusions seen in patients with AD are usually not as complex or bizarre as those of schizophrenia. Table 22–3 lists some common delusions of dementia. In addition, hallucinations, if present, tend to be visual compared with the

Table 22–3. Common delusions in patients with dementia.

Paranoid Delusions	Misidentifications
People are stealing things	Misidentifies familiar people (eg, believes daughter is wife)
Accusations of infidelity	Current home is not their home
Belief that someone is trying to harm them	Impersonation (eg, spouse is an impersonator)

auditory hallucinations common in schizophrenia. More than 50% of patients with AD will have psychosis at some point, occasionally requiring drug therapy. However, in many patients the psychosis is self-limited. Thus, it is important to attempt periodically to withdraw any drug therapies being used to manage agitation or psychosis. In fact, federal regulations require an attempt to withdraw (or decrease the dose of) such medications every 6 months in patients residing in nursing homes.

C. Complications Related to Caregiver Stress

Informal caregivers provide the majority of care to patients with dementia at considerable financial and personal costs. The risk of caregiver stress rises with the patient's advancing severity of dementia, increased dependence in ADLs, and the presence of problem behaviors. Clinicians should assess caregivers for stress because stress is associated with poor outcomes for both patients and caregivers, including increased risk of placement in a nursing home, increased risk of patient neglect or abuse, and increased risk of depression among caregivers (reported to affect 30% to 50%). Stress can be reduced with therapeutic interventions such as respite care and caregiver support.

Treatment

In the management of patients with cognitive impairment or dementia, the goals are to preserve function and autonomy for as long as possible and to maintain quality of life for both the patient and the caregivers. The medications currently available offer modest symptomatic benefit. There are currently no disease-modifying drugs on the market.

A. Cognitive Impairment

1. Cholinesterase inhibitors—Cholinesterase inhibitors (ChEIs) are currently the mainstay of treatment for AD of any severity (mild to severe): donepezil, rivastigmine, and galantamine. All have been shown to modestly improve cognitive function and delay functional decline in mild to moderate AD and are likely of benefit even in moderate to severe dementia. Use of ChEIs in MCI is common, especially for the amnestic type, but not FDA approved. Clinical trials indicate that there may be some symptomatic benefit in MCI, although they do not prevent progression to AD. In addition, although the ChEIs are FDA approved only for AD and PD dementia, benefit has also been shown in patients with DLB, and mixed AD plus VaD. All of the ChEIs have the same relative efficacy in AD and generally differ only in their half-lives (and, therefore, dosing regimen) and specificity for receptors (rivastigmine also inhibit butyrylcholinesterase, but the clinical significance is still unknown). Gastrointestinal side effects, including nausea, vomiting, and diarrhea, are a class effect and are the most common reason for discontinuation. These side effects can usually be ameliorated by slow titration of the drug over 8–12 weeks. Sleep disturbance and nightmares are also reported. In addition, ChEIs appear to increase the risk of syncope. Caution should be used when prescribing to patients with bradycardia. Table 22–4 lists the recommended initial doses and target doses for each of the ChEIs. Donepezil 23 mg is not recommended over 10 mg dosing because there are increased side effects and lack of clinical benefit.

Assessing effectiveness of therapy with ChEIs in individual patients has not been formally standardized for clinical practice. Effect sizes are modest in clinical trials, with only 40% to 50% of patients showing evidence of improvement on measures of cognitive functioning, ADL scores, or subjective clinician ratings. Stable or improved MMSE or MOCA scores over 6–12 months suggests the drug may be effective. Although switching ChEIs because of lack of efficacy or intolerable side effects may be beneficial for some patients, there is little evidence to support doing so.

The appropriate length of treatment with ChEIs is still unknown, but many experts recommend that therapy be continued indefinitely (or until there is no function left to lose) if improvement or stabilization is noted. Clinicians and caregivers may notice a decline in function if ChEIs are discontinued.

2. Memantine—Memantine, an *N*-methyl-D-aspartate (NMDA) antagonist, is FDA approved for the treatment of moderate to severe AD. It is often added to ChEI therapy when the dementia reaches moderate severity. Memantine is generally well tolerated. Headache is the only side effect reported in controlled clinical trials that occurred in at least 5% of patients and at twice the placebo rate (6% with memantine compared to 3% in placebo group). Dizziness, confusion, and constipation may also be reported infrequently.

3. Other treatments—There has been interest in antioxidants, such as ginkgo biloba and vitamin E (α-tocopherol), for the treatment of dementia because they have a plausible mechanism of action. Studies of ginkgo suggest it may be of mild benefit in dementia, but the evidence is inconsistent. Large-scale, high-quality, randomized controlled trials have found that neither ginkgo biloba nor vitamin E are effective for prevention of dementia in older adults with normal cognition or MCI.

Although NSAIDs, statins, and estrogen looked promising as treatments for AD in observational studies, randomized controlled trials have failed to show benefit of these agents for the treatment of AD.

Schwartz LM, Woloshin S. How the FDA forgot the evidence: the case of donepezil 23 mg. *BMJ*. 2012;344:e1086.

B. Vascular Dementia

No drug therapies have been specifically approved for the treatment of VaD. The principles of treatment of VaD rely on the treatment of stroke risk factors such as smoking, diabetes and hyperlipidemia. Treatment of hypertension (HTN) is somewhat controversial. Although controlling HTN may help reduce the incidence of dementia, some observational data suggest that, once dementia is present, permissive mild HTN (up to systolic blood pressures in the 150s) may be better for cognitive function than lower blood pressures. ChEIs and memantine may be of benefit in VaD.

Kaviragan H, Schneider LS. Efficacy and adverse effects of cholinesterase inhibitors and memantine in vascular dementia: a meta-analysis of randomized controlled trials. *Lancet Neurol*. 2007;6(9):782-792.

C. Problem Behaviors

1. Nonpharmacologic approaches—Because BPSD are common and may adversely affect both patient and caregiver quality of life, it is important to manage them as dutifully as the cognitive symptoms. Once precipitating causes

Table 22–4. Cholinesterase inhibitors.

Drug	Starting Dosage	Target Dose
Donepezil[a]	2.5-5.0 mg daily	10 mg daily (increase q 4 weeks)[b]
Rivastigmine[c]	1.5 mg BID	6 mg BID (increase by 1.5 mg BID q 2 weeks)[d]
Galantamine[e]	4 mg BID	8-12 mg BID (increase q 4 weeks)

[a]Also available in orally dissolving tablets.
[b]Donepezil 23 mg has not been shown to be more effective than 10 mg and risk of side effects is greater.
[c]Also available in a patch. Starting dose is 4.6 mg/24 hours. Increase to 9.5 mg after 4 weeks.
[d]Retitrate from 1.5 mg BID (oral) or 4.6 mg (patch) if treatment is interrupted for more than several days.
[e]Also available in extended release form for once daily dosing. Start at 8 mg daily, increase by 8 mg every 4 weeks to max of 16–24 mg daily.

Table 22–5. Dementia related difficult behaviors: practical tips for caregivers and medical providers.

Maintain familiarity and routines as much as possible.
Any change in the routine can produce anxiety and distress for patients with dementia. Changes in living arrangement, going on vacation, or being hospitalized may provoke agitation and other undesirable behaviors.

Decrease number of choices.
Patients with dementia may become overwhelmed with too many choices and become frustrated by their inability to sort things out. Limiting choices may be helpful. A good example is the case of a patient who resists changing clothes or insists on wearing the same clothes every day. In this case, it might be helpful for the caregiver to lay out only 1 outfit or to give the patient 2 choices: eg, "Would you like to wear the blue blouse or the red blouse?" Similarly, simplifying conversation and environment is also important. Too much input is often overwhelming or misinterpreted.

Tell, don't ask.
At first glance, this recommendation may seem uncomfortable to some. However, with the apathy that is commonly associated with dementia, it may be a struggle to get patients with dementia to agree to do anything. Instead of asking "Do you want to go to dinner now?," which may often result in a "no" answer followed by an argument, it may be more effective to say, "It is time to go to dinner now." Similarly, patients may be more agreeable if things are framed in positive rather than negative terms. For example, use "come with me" rather then "don't go there."

Understand that they *can't*, rather than they *won't*.
Family members and caregivers often believe that the patient with dementia is being stubborn and willfully making things difficult. Caregivers can waste much time and energy trying to "teach" something to patients who cannot learn. Helping caregivers understand the limitations of their loved one may improve quality of life for both.

Don't try logic or reason.
Because of the executive dysfunction that accompanies dementia, there is a relatively early loss of the ability to reason and use logic, which becomes more profound as the illness progresses. Trying to rationalize with a demented person often leads to frustration on the part of both parties. This is particularly true for delusions. If the patient has a nonthreatening delusion, arguing with the patient and trying to get the patient to see that it does not make sense is often fruitless and frustrating for both parties.

Always keep the goals in mind.
Is it really important if grandma thinks it is 1954, or that her daughter is her sorority sister? Why can't she wear that raincoat in the house if she wants to? By keeping the goals and "big picture" in mind, some conflict may be avoided. It is also important for caregivers and physicians to remember that most behaviors do not last indefinitely but are rather temporary stages.

(eg, delirium, pain, fecal impaction, broken hearing aids) of new behavioral problems have been ruled out, it is critical to try to identify what the behavior may represent. When patients are agitated or displaying other problem behaviors, it is often because they do not have the language skills to express their needs. Providers and caregivers should try to learn what the behaviors for a patient with dementia may represent and then attempt to address underlying needs. Keeping a behavior log may be useful. Federal regulation requires that the least-restrictive methods for behavior problems be tried first for nursing home residents. Nonpharmacologic treatments should be attempted before initiating drug therapies.

A few strategies that may be helpful in reducing agitation in patients with dementia include music, reminiscence therapy, exposure to pets, outdoor walks, and bright light exposure. One of the unifying themes in many of these strategies is that the therapy works best if it is tailored to the patient. For example, with music therapy, playing music that is consistent with patients' prior preferences seems to be superior to playing a standard tape for everyone. One study confirmed an intuitive assumption that providing intensive education and training on understanding and treating BPSD for nursing assistants or care providers also significantly

decreases agitation among patients with dementia in nursing home settings.

Table 22–5 presents less evidence-based, but more practical tips for both caregivers and medical providers of patients with dementia-related difficult behaviors.

2. Pharmacologic approaches—If nonpharmacologic approaches fail, it may become necessary to add drug therapy. However, there are no approved pharmacologic therapies for BPSD and modest benefits must be weighed against potential harms. Several classes of drugs are used for BPSD, including antipsychotics, antidepressants, mood stabilizers, and ChEIs. Table 22–6 lists drugs and doses commonly used to treat BPSD.

Antipsychotics: The atypical antipsychotics olanzapine and risperidone have the best evidence for effectiveness (which is modest), but side effects should be considered and weighed against potential benefits. There is a black box warning on all atypical antipsychotics for increased risk of mortality and cerebrovascular events when used in patients with dementia. A discussion with the patient's decision maker about the risks and benefits of using antipsychotics should be documented. In addition to stroke and mortality, side effects to consider are extrapyramidal symptoms and tardive

Table 22–6. Pharmacotherapy for behavioral and psychological symptoms of dementia.

Drug	Starting Dosage	Max Recommended Dosage[a]
Haloperidol[b]	0.25-0.5 mg daily	2-3 mg/day
Risperidone[c]	0.25 mg bid	1.5 mg/day
Olanzapine[d]	2.5 mg daily	5-10 mg/day
Trazodone	25 mg qhs	50-100 mg qhs
SSRIs (eg, citalopram)	10 mg daily	20-40 mg/day
Carbamazepine	100 mg daily	300-400 mg/day
Divalproex sodium[e]	125 mg bid	~1000 mg/day

SSRI, selective serotonin reuptake inhibitor.

[a]Use the lowest dose that achieves benefit.
[c]Also available in IV formulations.
[d]Also available in liquid form (do not mix with cola or tea) and orally dissolving tablets.
[e]Also available intramuscularly and in orally dissolving tablets.
[f]Also available in sprinkles.

dyskinesia (at higher doses), sedation, weight gain, diabetes mellitus, and hyperprolactinemia. Low-dose typical antipsychotics (such as haloperidol) may be used in the acute care setting, but should be avoided as a chronic medication due to the risk of irreversible tardive dyskinesia. In one study, even low-dose oral haloperidol (1.5 mg/day) resulted in tardive dyskinesia in 30% of older patients at 1 year and >60% of patients at 3 years.

Mood stabilizers: Mood stabilizers such as carbamazepine and valproic acid have shown benefit for some secondary outcomes in small trials. However, because of side effects, drug–drug interactions, and necessary blood test monitoring, these agents are not recommended as first-line treatments. If attempts at nonpharmacologic approaches and use of more common drug classes have failed, referral to a geriatrician or geropsychiatrist should be considered. Benzodiazepines are not recommended for the chronic management of BPSD. They have not been found to be more efficacious than other classes of drugs. In addition, adverse effects associated with benzodiazepine use, such as increased risk of falls, sedation, withdrawal, and occasionally paradoxical excitation, make them a particularly poor choice.

Schneider LS, Tariot PN, Dagerman KS, et al. Effectiveness of atypical antipsychotic drugs in patients with Alzheimer's disease. *N Engl J Med.* 2006;355(15):1525-1538.

Sink KM, Holden KF, Yaffe K. Pharmacological treatment of neuropsychiatric symptoms of dementia: a review of the evidence. *JAMA.* 2005;293(5):596-608.

► Management

A. Advance Directives

Establishing advance directives and having the patient appoint a durable power of attorney (DPOA) for health care should be a part of the management plan of patients with dementia. It is particularly important to have this discussion as early as possible so that patients can participate in decisions to direct their end-of-life care. Even patients with moderate dementia are able to consistently state preferences and choices, including the appointment of a DPOA. In addition to preferences regarding resuscitation, specific interventions such as the use of artificial hydration and nutrition should be addressed and included. Patients may also want to appoint a DPOA for finances. Consultation with an elder law attorney or estate planner may be helpful.

B. Safety Issues

1. Driving—Cognitive impairment has been shown to adversely affect driving ability, even among patients with mild dementia. Some states require reporting of AD and "related conditions" to the department of public health or the state's department of motor vehicles. Primary care providers should familiarize themselves with their state's law on reporting. If a patient with dementia is involved in a motor vehicle accident, the physician may be held liable if required reporting has not been done.

2. Home safety—Home safety should be assessed by interviewing a reliable informant or, preferably, by a home visit from a visiting nurse or occupational therapist. Specific safety measures to consider implementing include grab bars in the bathrooms, good lighting, clear pathways through the house, reducing clutter, and disabling stoves if there is concern for potential kitchen fires. If there is any indication that a patient may not be safe in the home or there is evidence of self-neglect or concern about elder abuse by others, the provider should contact adult protective services, which has a variety of resources and can quickly develop a plan for ensuring patient safety.

3. Wandering—Patients with dementia may wander and become lost. Some form of identification (eg, sewn in clothing, identification bracelet) is recommended. The Alzheimer's Association has a program called Safe Return. When registered, patients receive identification products, including wallet cards, jewelry, and clothing labels. The Safe Return program maintains a national photo/information database and 24-hour toll-free emergency crisis line for help in locating missing patients. Registration can be done through the Alzheimer's Association for a nominal cost.

4. Caregiver assistance—Caring for a patient with dementia can be exhausting and stressful and can lead to physical and mental health problems in the caregiver and the risk of abuse to the patient. Immediately on making a diagnosis of dementia, the primary care provider should make a referral to a knowledgeable social worker or office on aging for a list of resources to assist the caregiver. Such resources could include provision of educational materials and referrals to the Alzheimer's Association, the Caregiver Alliance, or other support and educational organizations. Proactive use of in-home or institutional respite or adult day care services should be considered for all caregivers. In addition, the use of privately hired case managers who specialize in elder care or dementia care can be very helpful in relieving some of the caregiver burden. Primary care providers should make an assessment of caregivers at each follow-up appointment. If caregiver stress is detected, caregivers should be asked about their use of resources and provided additional referrals as needed. If caregiver stress is severe, referral to a 24-hour respite program (either nursing home or assisted-living facility) may be helpful.

Dubinsky RM, Stein AC, Lyons K. Practice parameter: Risk of driving and Alzheimer's disease (an evidence-based review). *Neurology.* 2000;54(12):2205-2211.

Feinberg LF, Whitlatch CJ. Are persons with cognitive impairment able to state consistent choices? *Gerontologist.* 2001;41(3):374-382.

▶ Prognosis

The prognosis of dementia is variable depending on the cause and presence of comorbid conditions. Estimates of survival from time of onset or diagnosis of AD have been broad. Median life expectancy is 3–15 years. Patients with earlier ages of onset tend to have longer survival, and patients with VaD may have slightly shorter survival. Death is commonly a result of terminal pneumonia in the degenerative dementias and to cardiovascular events in VaD. It may be useful to use a staging scale such as the Functional Assessment Staging (FAST staging) for AD to help families understand the progression of the disease. There are 7 stages in the FAST staging system, with 7 being end-stage dementia. This scale is widely available online and the Alzheimer's Association website features it for patients and families. When patients reach stage 7, referral for hospice may be indicated.

As many as 90% of patients with dementia are eventually institutionalized. The median time to nursing home placement is 3–6 years from diagnosis. Dementia severity, dependence in ADLs, difficult behaviors, and caregiver age and burden are significant risk factors for placement. Interventions that include caregiver support and education in managing difficult behaviors may extend time to nursing home placement.

USEFUL WEBSITES

Alzheimer's Association (extensive informational materials for patients and caregivers as well as a link to clinical trials in your area). www.alz.org

Alzheimer's Disease Education and Referral Center (of the National Institutes of Health and National Institute on Aging). www.nia.nih.gov

Family Caregiver Alliance (provides information, support, and guidance for family and professional caregivers. Includes topic-specific newsletters, information on care facilities and legal issues, and online discussion lists). www.caregiver.org

Montreal Cognitive Assessment (download the MOCA test form and directions in many languages for free). www.mocatest.org

Cerebrovascular Disease

23

Daniel Antoniello, MD

ESSENTIALS OF DIAGNOSIS

▶ Stroke presents as a neurologic deficit or headache of abrupt onset.

▶ Hemorrhagic strokes can be intracerebral or subarachnoid.

▶ Urgent neuroimaging studies are essential for diagnosis.

▶ General Principles in Older Adults

Stroke recently declined from the third to the fourth leading cause of death in the United States, which is testament to a half century of progress in cerebrovascular disease prevention and acute care. It remains, however, a leading cause of disability, with up to half of all patients who survive a stroke failing to regain independence and needing long-term health care. Stroke primarily affects the elderly, and for each successive decade after the age of 55 years, the stroke rate doubles for both men and women.

The majority of strokes (80% of cases) result from insufficient blood flow to the brain (ischemic stroke), whereas bleeding that destroys and compresses the brain parenchyma accounts for 15% (intracerebral hemorrhage [ICH]). Bleeding that occurs in the subarachnoid space (subarachnoid hemorrhage) accounts for 5% of strokes.

▶ Clinical Findings

A. Signs & Symptoms

A stroke presents as an acute neurologic deficit. The neurologic impairment reflects the area of the brain affected. Although the presenting focal neurologic symptoms are variable, 80% of patients present with unilateral weakness; 90% have a speech and/or motor deficit. In addition, deficits in sensation, vision, language, cognition and balance may occur.

Older patients have more severe stroke deficits at presentation than do younger patients. After the onset of symptoms, timely evaluation and diagnosis are paramount. This is because the effect of thrombolysis is time dependent. Thus, neurologic screening tools like the Cincinnati Stroke Scale (Table 23–1) can be useful in early triage.

B. Special Tests

In patients suspected of stroke, diagnostics occur in 2 phases: (a) acute triage and (b) investigations into etiology after stroke is established as the diagnosis.

In the acute triage phase, several tests should be performed routinely in all patients with suspected stroke. This is to establish a diagnosis, identify systemic conditions that may mimic or cause stroke, and identify conditions that influence therapeutic options. Immediate diagnostic studies in all patients should include noncontrast brain CT, blood glucose, serum electrolytes/renal function tests, electrocardiogram (ECG) markers of cardiac ischemia, complete blood count including platelet count, prothrombin time/international normalized ratio (INR), activated partial thromboplastin, oxygen saturation.

Given the clinical history and examination, additional acute tests may be indicated. These include hepatic function tests, toxicology screen, blood alcohol level, arterial blood gas (if hypoxia is suspected), and chest radiography (if lung disease is suspected). For those patients in which diagnostic uncertainty remains, lumbar puncture may be performed (if subarachnoid hemorrhage is suspected and CT scan is negative for blood) or an electroencephalogram (EEG) may be necessary (if seizures are suspected as the cause of their neurologic symptoms).

▶ Differential Diagnosis

The diagnosis of stroke can be firmly established with history, examination and advanced imaging techniques. Intracerebral

Table 23–1. Cincinnati stroke scale.

Facial Droop
　Normal: Both sides of face move equally
　Abnormal: One side of face does not move at all
Arm Drift
　Normal: Both arms move equally or not at all
　Abnormal: One arm drifts compared to the other
Speech
　Normal: Patient uses correct words with no slurring
　Abnormal: Slurred or inappropriate words or mute
Interpretation:
　If any 1 of these 3 signs is abnormal, the probability of a stroke is 72%

hemorrhage is visible immediately on CT (Figure 23–1). Diffusion-weighted imaging (DWI) MRI sequences are approximately 90% sensitive in detecting cerebral infarction (Figure 23–2). Therefore, once the diagnosis of stroke is made, the differential diagnosis lies with investigating the etiology of the stroke (Table 23–2).

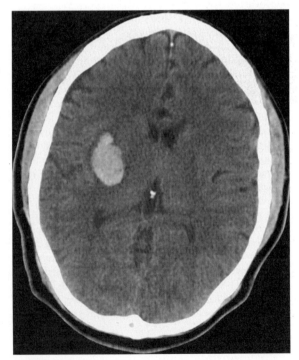

▲ **Figure 23–1.** CT scan of a patient with sudden onset left hemiplegia shows an intracerebral hemorrhage in the right basal ganglia.

Whether an ischemic stroke or intracerebral hemorrhage is diagnosed, etiology needs to be established to determine the most effective secondary stroke prevention measures. For ischemic stroke the work-up should aim to establish the stroke subtype: (a) large artery atherosclerosis (ie, carotid or intracranial vessel stenosis), (b) cardioembolism (ie, atrial fibrillation), (c) small vessel occlusion (ie, lacunar stroke), (d) stroke of other determined cause (ie, arterial dissection), or (e) stroke of an undetermined cause (ie, cryptogenic).

For the majority of primary intracerebral hemorrhages, the underlying etiology is hypertension (hypertensive vasculopathy), cerebral amyloid angiopathy, or anticoagulation-related hemorrhage.

▶ Complications

Following stroke onset, some patients may deteriorate neurologically over the next few hours or days. Clinical manifestation may take the form of decreased level in consciousness, an exacerbation of the previous neurological deficit, or the appearance of a new deficit. Both neurologic and nonneurologic causes of deterioration are often treatable if recognized promptly.

Common neurologic causes of deterioration are progressive stroke, brain swelling, recurrent ischemic stroke, hemorrhagic transformation, and, less commonly, seizures. Large strokes of the cerebral hemisphere or cerebellum are at the highest risk for complicating brain edema and increased intracranial pressure. Swelling in cerebellar strokes may cause obstructive hydrocephalus requiring acute neurosurgical intervention.

Medical complications are a common and an important problem after acute stroke as they can be barriers to optimal recovery. During hospital admission infection is common. Urinary tract infection or pneumonia may occur in up to one-quarter of patients, and both are associated with increasing age. The appearance of fever after stroke should prompt a search for pneumonia, as it is an important cause of death. The risk of deep venous thrombosis and pulmonary embolism is highest among immobilized and older patients with severe stroke. Pain, falls, and depression are all common during hospitalization and after discharge.

▶ Treatment

A. Initial Management & Acute Ancillary Care

The acute care of patients with ischemic stroke should include: (a) stabilization and initial assessment, (b) decision making regarding thrombolysis with the only approved treatment in the United States—intravenous tissue plasminogen activator (t-PA), (c) consideration of endovascular therapies, and (d) effective communication with patients and families.

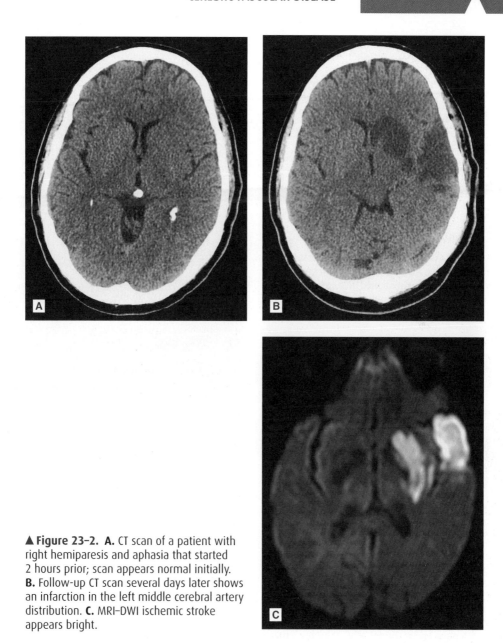

▲ **Figure 23–2. A.** CT scan of a patient with right hemiparesis and aphasia that started 2 hours prior; scan appears normal initially. **B.** Follow-up CT scan several days later shows an infarction in the left middle cerebral artery distribution. **C.** MRI–DWI ischemic stroke appears bright.

As in any other emergency, the management of acute stroke starts with assessment of the "ABCs": *A*irway, *B*reathing, *C*irculation. Most stroke patients do not require intubation; however, those with a depressed level of consciousness are at the highest risk of requiring ventilator support. Acute assessment of the circulatory status includes ECG, blood pressure monitoring, and cardiac enzyme determination.

Most patients with acute ischemic stroke have an elevated blood pressure. This elevation is usually transient and helps maintain perfusion to ischemic brain tissue, therefore rapid reduction should be avoided. No treatment is recommended unless the mean arterial pressure is >130 mm Hg or systolic pressure is >220 mm Hg. Exceptions to this rule involves IV thrombolytic therapy, which requires a blood pressure <185/110 mm Hg.

After initial emergency room management, patients should be admitted to stroke units, as specialized care improves survival and functional outcome, regardless of age.

Table 23–2. Common etiologies of ischemic stroke and intracerebral hemorrhage in elderly.

Ischemic Stroke
Cardioembolic (atrial fibrillation)
Large artery atherosclerosis (carotid or intracranial vessel stenosis)
Small vessel occlusion (lacunar stroke)

Intracerebral Hemorrhage
Hypertensive vasculopathy
Cerebral amyloid angiopathy
Anticoagulation related

B. Specific Therapies

1. Acute ischemic stroke—Reperfusion of the ischemic brain is the most effective therapy for acute ischemic stroke. By restoring blood flow to threatened tissues before they progress to infarction, reperfusion therapies salvage viable brain tissue (the ischemic penumbra) and improve clinical outcomes.

The association between thrombolysis treatment and improved outcome is maintained in all age groups, even very elderly people. Thus, age alone should not be a barrier to treatment. Regarding the risk of intracerebral hemorrhage in older individuals, studies have varied. A recent meta-analysis of pooled thrombolysis data concluded that the risk of symptomatic intracerebral hemorrhage did not increase among elderly patients, despite less-favorable outcomes, which were attributed to comorbidities.

The benefit of thrombolytic therapy is strongly time dependent: the more rapid the treatment, the more favorable the outcome. Patients are candidates for IV t-PA if the medicine is administered within 3 hours of symptom onset, and there are no contraindications. A recent European study (ECASS III) showed that benefit could be extended to the 3–4.5-hour window, but this is only available in patients younger than 80 years of age. Patients and families should be given an explanation of the risks and benefits of t-PA.

Endovascular treatment, including intraarterial thrombolysis and mechanical thrombectomy, is a promising alternative treatment that can be used as isolated therapy or in combination with intravenous thrombolysis ("bridging therapy"). In carefully selected patients with large vessel occlusions (ie, middle cerebral artery), such techniques have been shown to be safe and effective. Limited data exist regarding the benefits of endovascular therapies in the oldest old population, >80 years of age.

2. Intracerebral hemorrhage—ICH remains the least-treatable form of stroke. Apart from management in a specialized stroke or neurologic intensive care unit, no specific therapies have been shown to improve outcome after ICH. Age is an independent predictor of outcome after ICH, with age >80 years associated with 30-day mortality.

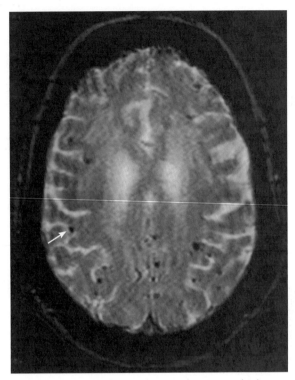

▲ **Figure 23–3.** Gradient-echo MRI showing multiple chronic "clinically silent" hemorrhages (dark punctuate lesions) in cortical and cortical-subcortical regions characteristic of cerebral amyloid angiopathy.

For the majority of elderly patients with intracerebral hemorrhages, the underlying etiology is (a) hypertension (hypertensive vasculopathy), (b) anticoagulation-related hemorrhage, or (c) cerebral amyloid angiopathy. Longstanding hypertension causes weakening of the small, deep-penetrating arteries that can rupture causing hemorrhage into the deep structures of the brain. Anticoagulation with warfarin increases the risk of ICH and worsens the severity of hemorrhage, doubling its mortality. Cerebral amyloid angiopathy (CAA), defined as amyloid deposition in the cerebral vessel walls, may cause large and symptomatic hemorrhage or small and clinically silent hemorrhage (Figure 23–3). Severe CAA is present in 12% of patients >85 years of age, and patients with symptomatic hemorrhages should be taken off of all antithrombotics.

C. Secondary Prevention Strategies

The successful prevention of a recurrent ischemic stroke hinges upon a comprehensive approach. This involves the identification and treatment of stroke risk factors, such as hypertension, diabetes, and hyperlipidemia. Of equal if not greater importance is the modification of life styles that increase the risk of a stroke, such as diet, exercise, and smoking cessation.

Antihypertensive therapy forms the cornerstone of secondary stroke prevention. A recent meta-analysis of several large trials of blood pressure reduction for secondary stroke prevention found a 24% relative risk reduction. It is generally recommended that blood pressure reduction begin after 24 hours of a stroke if the patient is neurologically and hemodynamically stable.

Although few trials have included the very old, there is convincing evidence that lowering low-density lipoprotein with statins reduces vascular events, including ischemic stroke.

Antiplatelet agents are the first choice to prevent recurrent strokes in patients with noncardioembolic strokes. Available alternatives are aspirin, aspirin and dipyridamole, and clopidogrel. The combination of aspirin and clopidogrel should be avoided, as it is associated with major bleeding events.

1. Atrial fibrillation—Atrial fibrillation dramatically increases in prevalence with age, and is associated with a nearly 5-fold increase in stroke risk. Cardioembolic stroke related to atrial fibrillation is the most frequently encountered stroke subtype in very old patients. Warfarin reduces the stroke risk by 68%. Despite this, many physicians assume that a combination of warfarin therapy and head trauma from falls leads to a substantially high risk of subdural hemorrhage and they decide not to anticoagulate their elderly patients whom they believe are prone to falling. Evidence contrary to this practice shows that the risk of this complication is outweighed by the benefit of stroke protection provided by warfarin.

Urgent anticoagulation (heparin infusion) with the goal of preventing early recurrent stroke is not recommended because of the risk of hemorrhage. Typically, patients are placed on aspirin during the acute phase as a "bridge" to eventual oral anticoagulation with warfarin. Anticoagulation should be initiated within 2 weeks.

New oral anticoagulants dabigatran, rivaroxaban, and apixaban have become available. They are at least as effective as warfarin in the prevention of stroke in patients with atrial fibrillation. These agents share common properties such as high fixed oral dosing, no interaction with food, no need for anticoagulation monitoring, and rapid onset and offset of action. However, the safety of these newer agents in elderly patients with low body weight and impaired renal function has yet to be rigorously determined.

2. Carotid stenosis—Carotid artery stenosis is another major risk factor for ischemic stroke in the elderly. Evidence is clear that carotid endarterectomy (CEA) is more effective than medical therapy for preventing recurrent stroke in patients with symptomatic carotid stenosis (those who have had a recent stroke or transient ischemic attack), particularly in those with severe (70% to 99%) stenosis. CEA is also efficacious in patients with moderate (50% to 69%) symptomatic carotid stenosis, although the efficacy is less dramatic.

Early surgery in symptomatic patients (within 2 weeks if possible) is recommended as the risk of a recurrent stroke is front-loaded. Recent studies show that CEA is safer than carotid artery stenting for older patients.

3. Transient ischemic attack—In the era of advanced neuroimaging, transient ischemic attack (TIA) has been redefined from a time based diagnosis (<24 hours) to a brain tissue-based diagnosis. The new definition is as follows: "A TIA is a brief episode of neurologic dysfunction caused by focal brain or retinal ischemia, with clinical symptoms typically lasting less than 1 hour, and without evidence of acute infarction. The corollary is that persistent clinical signs or characteristic imaging abnormalities define infarction—that is, stroke."

After having a TIA, the short-term risk of having a stroke is high: 10% of patients have a stroke within 90 days, with half of those occurring in the first 2 days. Thus, TIA should trigger the same prompt evaluation and work-up as a persistent neurologic deficit (ie, stroke) and requires the implementation of proven interventions to reduce this substantial short term stroke risk.

▶ Prognosis

Advanced age increases the risk of mortality after a stroke and is also a risk factor for recurrence. Compared with younger patients, older stroke survivors recover more slowly and have more severe deficits. The severity of stroke and prestroke medical condition heavily influence the outcome. Of those patients >80 years of age who receive thrombolysis, 20% end up with no significant disability and are eventually discharged home.

Adams HP Jr, Bendixen BH, Kappelle LJ, et al. Classification of subtype of acute ischemic stroke. Definitions for use in a multicenter clinical trial. TOAST. Trial of Org 10172 in acute stroke treatment. *Stroke.* 1993;24(1):35-41.

Adams HP Jr, del Zoppo G, Alberts MJ, et al. Guidelines for the early management of adults with ischemic stroke. *Stroke.* 2007;38(5):1655-1711.

Albers GW, Caplan LR, Easton JD, et al. TIA Working Group. Transient ischemic attack—proposal for a new definition. *N Engl J Med.* 2002;347(21):1713-1716.

Alshekhlee A, Mohammadi A, Mehta S, et al. Is thrombolysis safe in the elderly?: analysis of a national database. *Stroke.* 2010;41(10):2259-2264.

Barnett HJ, Taylor DW, Eliasziw M, et al. Benefit of carotid endarterectomy in patients with symptomatic moderate or severe stenosis. North American Symptomatic Carotid Endarterectomy Trial Collaborators. *N Engl J Med.* 1998;339(20):1415-1425.

Brott TG, Hobson RW 2nd, Howard G, et al. Stenting versus endarterectomy for treatment of carotid-artery stenosis. *N Engl J Med.* 2010;363(1):11-23.

Chen RL, Balami JS, Esiri MM, Chen LK, Buchan AM. Ischemic stroke in the elderly: an overview of evidence. *Nat Rev Neurol.* 2010;6(5):256-265.

Diener HC, Weber R, Lip GY, Hohnloser SH. Stroke prevention in atrial fibrillation: do we still need warfarin? *Curr Opin Neurol.* 2012;25(1):27-35.

Furie KL, Kasner SE, Adams RJ, et al. Guidelines for the prevention of stroke in patients with stroke or transient ischemic attack: a guideline for healthcare professionals from the American Heart Association/American Stroke Association. *Stroke.* 2011;42(1):227-276.

Furlan A, Higashida R, Wechsler L, et al. Intra-arterial prourokinase for acute ischemic stroke. The PROACT II study: a randomized controlled trial. Prolyse in acute cerebral thromboembolism. *JAMA.* 1999;282(21):2003-2011.

Hacke W, Donnan G, Fieschi C, et al. Association of outcome with early stroke treatment: pooled analysis of ATLANTIS, ECASS, and NINDS rt-PA stroke trials. *Lancet.* 2004;363(9411):768-774.

Hacke W, Kaste M, Bluhmki E, et al; ECASS Investigators. Thrombolysis with alteplase 3 to 4.5 hours after acute ischemic stroke. *N Engl J Med.* 2008;359(13):1317-1329.

Hacke W, Kaste M, Fieschi C, et al. Intravenous thrombolysis with recombinant tissue plasminogen activator for acute hemispheric stroke. The European Cooperative Acute Stroke Study (ECASS). *JAMA.* 1995;274(13):1017-1025.

Hacke W, Kaste M, Fieschi C, et al. Randomised double-blind placebo-controlled trial of thrombolytic therapy with intravenous alteplase in acute ischaemic stroke (ECASS II). *Lancet.* 1998;352(9136):1245-1251.

Herman B, Leyten AC, van Luijk JH, Frenken CW, Op de Coul AA, Schulte BP. Epidemiology of stroke in Tilburg, the Netherlands. The population-based stroke incidence register: 2. Incidence, initial clinical picture and medical care, and three-week case fatality. *Stroke.* 1982;13(5):629-634.

Indredavik B, Bakke F, Slordahl SA, Rokseth R, Håheim LL. Stroke unit treatment. 10-year follow up. *Stroke.* 1999;30(8):1524-1527.

Johnston SC, Gress DR, Browner WS, Sidney S. Short-term prognosis after emergency department diagnosis of TIA. *JAMA.* 2000;284(22):2901-2906.

Kammersgaard LP, Jørgensen HS, Reith J, et al. Copenhagen Stroke Study. Short- and long-term prognosis for very old stroke patients. The Copenhagen Stroke Study. *Age Ageing.* 2004;33(2):149-154.

Kothari RU, Pancioli A, Liu T, Brott T, Broderick J. Cincinnati Prehospital Stroke Scale: reproducibility and validity. *Ann Emerg Med.* 1999;33(4):373-378.

Langhorne P, Stott DJ, Robertson L, et al. Medical complications after stroke: a multicenter study. *Stroke.* 2000;31(6):1223-1229.

Man-Son-Hing M, Nichol G, Lau A, Laupacis A. Choosing antithrombotic therapy for elderly patients with atrial fibrillation who are at risk for falls. *Arch Intern Med.* 1999;159(7):677-685.

Mishra NK, Ahmed N, Andersen G, et al; VISTA collaborators; SITS collaborators. Thrombolysis in very elderly people: controlled comparison of SITS International Stroke Thrombolysis Registry and Virtual International Stroke Trials Archive. *BMJ.* 2010;341:c6040.

Mohr JP, Thompson JL, Lazar RM, et al. A comparison of warfarin and aspirin for the prevention of recurrent ischemic stroke. *N Engl J Med.* 2001;345(20):1444-1451.

Rashid P, Leonardi-Bee J, Bath P. Blood pressure reduction and secondary prevention of stroke and other vascular events: a systematic review. *Stroke.* 2003;34(11):2741-2748.

Rincon F, Mayer SA. Current treatment options for intracerebral hemorrhage. *Curr Treat Options Cardiovasc Med.* 2008; 10(3):229-240.

Sacco RL, Wolf PA, Kannel WB, McNamara PM. Survival and recurrence following stroke. The Framingham Study. *Stroke.* 1982;13(3):290-295.

Sanossian N, Ovbiagele B. Prevention and management of stroke in very elderly patients. *Lancet Neurol.* 2009;8(11):1031-1041.

Tissue plasminogen activator for acute ischemic stroke. The National Institute of Neurological Disorders and Stroke rt-PA Stroke Study Group. *N Engl J Med.* 1995;333(24):1581-1587.

Towfighi A, Saver JL. Stroke declines from third to fourth leading cause of death in the United States: historical perspective and challenges ahead. *Stroke.* 2011;42(8):2351-2355.

Towfighi A, Greenberg SM, Rosand J. Treatment and prevention of primary intracerebral hemorrhage. *Semin Neurol.* 2005;25(4): 445-452.

Parkinson Disease & Essential Tremor

24

Nicholas B. Galifianakis, MD, MPH
A. Ghazinouri, MD

PARKINSON DISEASE

ESSENTIALS OF DIAGNOSIS

▶ Any combination of resting tremor, bradykinesia, rigidity, and postural instability (late feature). Bradykinesia is a required feature for diagnosis.

▶ Asymmetric onset is the norm.

▶ Responds well to levodopa in most cases.

▶ Diagnostic accuracy improves with observation over time.

▶ General Principles in Older Adults

Parkinson disease (PD) is the second most common chronic progressive neurodegenerative disorder, after Alzheimer disease. It affects an estimated 1% of people older than age 65 years and up to 3% older than age 85 years, or approximately 1.5 million people in the United States and more than 5 million people worldwide. With the aging of the world's population, and with age being the strongest risk factor for PD, incidence is expected to rise dramatically in coming decades. By 2050, some researchers project more than 2.5 million cases in the United States.

PD is generally considered a disease of the older adult, but it can affect younger age groups. The mean age of onset is about age 60–65 years. Several key points should be emphasized about the care of older PD patients. The differential diagnosis of parkinsonian symptoms in patients older than the age of 75 years is mostly limited to either idiopathic PD or secondary parkinsonism, as onset of atypical etiologies is rare in this age group. Older PD patients often present with an akinetic-rigid syndrome, more nonmotor symptoms, and less tremor. Levodopa is the drug of choice in patients older than age 70 years, as dopamine agonists (such as pramipexole

and ropinirole), amantadine, and anticholinergics are poorly tolerated in this age group.

▶ Pathogenesis

The clinical presentation of PD was first described by James Parkinson in his 1817 "Essay on Shaking Palsy." It was not until the 20th century that the pathologic hallmarks of PD, α-synuclein-positive Lewy bodies and dopaminergic cell loss of the substantia nigra, were described. It is estimated that by the time the first symptoms emerge, 60% of substantia nigra neurons have already died. Neurochemically, this results in dopamine depletion in the nigrostriatal pathway. Physiologically, this leads to inhibition of the thalamus and reduced excitation of the motor cortex, manifesting as the cardinal motor features of PD (bradykinesia and rigidity).

A fundamental shift in our understanding of PD pathology has occurred in recent years. It has long been known that the pathology spreads beyond the substantia nigra as PD progresses, which explains much of the disabling nonmotor features of advanced PD, such as dementia, depression, and autonomic failure. However, we now know that even before any motor symptoms occur, pathology has spread through specific areas of the olfactory system, lower brainstem, and peripheral nervous system. This "premotor" phase of PD can manifest as hyposmia, sleep disorders, mood disorders, and constipation. In summary, from the earliest to the most advanced stages, PD pathology occurs in a much wider distribution of the central and peripheral nervous systems than previously thought, making PD much more than just a movement disorder.

The mechanisms of neurodegeneration in idiopathic PD are not well understood but likely include complex interactions between environmental factors and genetic predisposition. Environmental risk factors remain elusive, although exposure to pesticides, agricultural occupation, and rural place of residence are known to be risk factors. Cigarette smoking and coffee consumption are possible protective factors.

Genetics play a role. There are now up to 18 genes or loci (designated as the PARK loci) that cause or predispose people to PD. Although some of these genes account for the 5% to 10% of PD that seems to be inherited in a mendelian pattern, some also contribute to a higher percentage of "sporadic" PD that has more complex modes of inheritance. Perhaps more importantly, discovering the function of these genes in neurons has helped elucidate several important mechanisms of pathogenesis in PD overall.

▶ Clinical Findings

PD has an insidious onset and gradually progresses, leading to increasing disability over time. The cardinal motor features include resting tremor, bradykinesia, rigidity, and gait impairment/postural instability, although the latter usually arises later in the disease. Nonmotor features are also prominent, and increasingly become the main source of disability as the disease progresses.

PD remains a clinical diagnosis. Bradykinesia plus 1 of the other cardinal manifestations must be present to diagnose idiopathic PD. Other clinical features that are supportive of the diagnosis are asymmetric presentation and a strong response to dopaminergic medications. Approximately 20% of PD cases present without tremor. Diagnostic accuracy increases to over 90% in patients followed by movement disorders specialists.

A. Symptoms & Signs

Rest tremor is the most common presenting symptom of PD. It usually attenuates with use of the affected limb. However, *action tremor* is fairly common and should not steer the clinician away from a PD diagnosis if other parkinsonian features are present. In early stages, the tremor may only appear when the patient is distracted (while talking or walking) and the patient may even be able to suppress it with concentration. With progression, tremor becomes more constant, more common with actions, and higher in amplitude, impairing many activities of daily living (ADLs). On examination, tremor is a rhythmic, oscillatory, involuntary movement. Parkinsonian tremor is asymmetric, relatively slow (frequency 3–6 Hz), and tends to have a prominent pronation–supination component to it (as opposed to flexion–extension), frequently giving the tremor a "pill-rolling" quality. Examiners should observe tremor at rest, with different postures and actions, including handwriting and drawing spirals. If there is no obvious tremor, distracting tasks should be given to patients to elicit mild tremor.

Bradykinesia is defined as a slowness or lack of movement. It manifests as loss of dexterity and difficulty initiating and maintaining the amplitude and velocity of movement. ADLs, like eating and dressing, will take more time to complete. It is often described by patient as "weakness," although strength is actually intact. Many of the common complaints of the PD patient are direct manifestations of bradykinesia including small handwriting (micrographia), loss of facial expression (hypomimia), quiet monotone speech (hypophonia), and slower walking with shorter steps. To elicit bradykinesia, the examiner asks the patient to perform rapid repetitive movements (such as finger taps, hand openings and closings, and heel stomps), as quickly and largely as possible. Examining handwriting and having the patient draw spirals can reveal micrographia. It is also important to take note of lack of spontaneous movements, such as blink rate, expression in speech, hand gestures while speaking, or the amount of shifting one's position.

Rigidity is subjectively experienced by the patient as "stiffness," and when severe enough, can lead to painful aching or cramping. Patients may experience musculoskeletal complaints (such as painful, frozen shoulder), and it is common for a patient to seek care from an orthopedic surgeon or rheumatologist before a neurologist. Rigidity is defined as the increased resistance that is felt as the examiner passively moves a body part about a joint to assess muscle tone. The increase in tone should be constant, independent of the speed or direction of the passive movement. This even increase in tone has been termed *lead pipe* rigidity, as opposed to the variable resistance felt when examining spasticity. When tremor is superimposed on rigidity, a ratcheting sensation can be sensed, giving the rigidity a "cogwheeling" component.

Postural instability and gait dysfunction are less prominent at presentation. In early PD, mild gait impairment can manifest as subtly shortened stride length, decreased arm swing, and stooped posture. In moderate PD, the gait becomes more shuffling, posture stooped, and patients turn en bloc, requiring several steps to make a turn. In advanced PD, festination (a sense that the body wants to hasten forward) or freezing of gait (the inability to take effective steps) can occur. Freezing of gait is especially sensitive to anything that requires more attention of the patient, including initiating gait, narrow spaces or doorways, turns, or even carrying something. Postural instability can be assessed with the "pull test." More than 3 corrective steps backward is considered abnormal. This should be done only by experienced examiners with caution, as patients can have surprising lack of postural reflexes, and may even need to be caught by the examiner. Gait dysfunction is not as responsive to treatment, can lead to falls and loss of mobility, and many patients end up wheelchair-bound.

A diverse range of *nonmotor symptoms* are increasingly being recognized as characteristic of PD. Patients frequently describe hyposmia, constipation, dream enactment, and mood symptoms years before the appearance of any movement disorder. However, as the disease progresses to moderate and advanced stages, additional nonmotor problems lead to significant disability. In fact, nonmotor symptoms most strongly correlate with decreased quality of life (QOL) in PD.

Cognitive and behavioral impairment is almost universal in PD, with earlier stages showing mild impairment in attention, visual–spatial, and executive function. Memory and language are relatively spared. In advanced stages, dementia and psychosis (especially visual hallucinations and delusions) are common. A majority of patients with PD have depression and anxiety at some point. The autonomic nervous system is greatly affected in PD, with constipation, gastroparesis, orthostatic hypotension, urinary urgency, erectile dysfunction, and sweating dysregulation. With the exception of constipation, autonomic complaints usually do not become prominent or disabling until later in the course, when incontinence and severe orthostatic hypotension can lead to severe disability. Sleep can be disturbed with dream enactment, insomnia and sleep apnea, contributing to excessive daytime sleepiness and fatigue.

B. Patient Examination

The physical examination should include a complete neurologic examination. Extraocular eye movements, motor strength, sensory, and cerebellar examinations should be normal. The extrapyramidal examination is the central focus of the examination of a PD patient. Part III of the Unified PD Rating Scale (UPDRS) is the best validated, standardized, objective tool that the clinician can routinely use in examining a patient. In using the UPDRS, the clinician carefully examines facial expression, speech, tremor, rapid repetitive tasks, muscle tone, gait, and balance. Details about the objective findings related to the cardinal features of PD are discussed in the section above.

C. Laboratory Findings

At this time, there are no laboratory tests or imaging studies that can confirm the diagnosis of PD. However, PD is not a diagnosis of exclusion. To the contrary, only when certain red flags come to the attention of the clinician (especially lack of response to dopaminergic therapy) is it necessary to rule out atypical and secondary causes of parkinsonism. Genetic testing is commercially available for certain PARK gene mutations. Routine testing for these genes is not yet recommended, and for the most part, clinical use of genetic testing remains restricted to settings where there is a strong family history, or when onset occurs before the age of 40 years.

D. Imaging Tests

The FDA has approved the use of DaTSCAN (^{123}I-ioflupane, a ligand that uses single-photon emission computed tomography [SPECT] imaging to detect presynaptic dopamine transporters) in trying to distinguish PD from essential tremor. PD patients (but also some atypical parkinsonism patients) will have a decreased DaT signal in the basal ganglia. However, DaTSCAN should not be considered a routine test, as it is no more sensitive or specific than examination

by a movement disorders neurologist. Advanced functional imaging techniques remain a research tool for the vast majority of situations. Routine MRI of the brain is usually normal in early stages of PD. Only in settings when the diagnosis remains in question is an MRI ordered to investigate secondary or atypical parkinsonism.

▶ Differential Diagnosis

Idiopathic PD is the most common cause of parkinsonism. It is important to think of secondary or atypical causes when certain red flags are seen; namely symmetric presentation, lack of tremor, and the presence of atypical features that are rarely seen early in PD. The strongest alert is a lack of response to higher doses of dopaminergic medications (more than 1000–1500 mg/day of levodopa).

The 2 most common etiologies of secondary parkinsonism are vascular and drug induced. These are especially important to consider in older adults, as atypical parkinsonian syndromes rarely have onset after the age of 75 years. In fact, when exposure to dopamine-blocking drugs can be ruled out by history, idiopathic PD and vascular parkinsonism account for the vast majority of cases in older patients.

Vascular parkinsonism can result from chronic ischemic damage or multiple infarcts in the brain. Patients often present with a symmetric akinetic-rigid syndrome. Findings tend to be more severe in the legs, and gait is prominently affected. Vascular parkinsonism occasionally responds to dopaminergic medications, but not as robustly as with PD.

Drug-induced parkinsonism results from exposure to dopamine receptor blocking agents, most commonly antiemetics and antipsychotics (both typical and atypical) or dopamine depleters (such as reserpine or tetrabenazine). In older adults, parkinsonian features can persist for months after the offending dopamine receptor blocking agent has been discontinued. Other secondary causes of parkinsonism are more rare (Table 24–1).

Atypical parkinsonism results from neurodegenerative disorders that lead to parkinsonism. They are also termed "Parkinson Plus" syndrome as they are associated with disabling features, such as autonomic failure, early falls, and early dementia, not usually seen in early PD. These early disabling atypical features, the lack of response to medications, and the rapid progression of these illnesses combine to give these diseases a poor prognosis. Table 24–2 lists the signs for these disorders.

A common challenge in the differential diagnosis is distinguishing between the tremor of PD and that of essential tremor (ET). The action tremor of ET tends to be more symmetric, higher frequency, and more extension–flexion as opposed to the asymmetric lower frequency, pronation–supination tremor of PD. The diagnosis can be especially difficult when one considers that a minor amount of rigidity and bradykinesia can occasionally be seen in ET. ET patients

Table 24–1. Secondary causes of parkinsonism and tremor.

Vascular Parkinsonism
Toxin-induced (pesticides, methylphenyltetrahydropyridine [MPTP] manganese, carbon monoxide, cyanide, methanol)
Structural brain lesions (hydrocephalus, tumor, trauma)
Metabolic disorders (Wilson disease, hypoparathyroidism)
Infectious (AIDS, syphilis, Creutzfeldt-Jakob disease)
Postencephalitic parkinsonism (von Economo encephalitis lethargica)
Drug-Induced Parkinsonism
• Dopamine receptor blocking agents (antipsychotics and antiemetics)
• Dopamine depletors (reserpine and tetrabenazine)
Drug-Induced Tremor
• Amphetamines
• Antidepressants
• Antipsychotics
• β-Agonists
• Corticosteroids
• Lithium
• Amiodarone
• Methylxanthines (including coffee and tea)
• Thyroid hormone
• Valproic acid

should not have the anosmia, rapid eye movement (REM) sleep behavior disorder, and more significant parkinsonism seen in PD.

▶ Complications

PD, historically viewed as a movement disorder, is now recognized as a complex condition with diverse clinical manifestations, including neuropsychiatric and other nonmotor

Table 24–2. Atypical neurodegenerative causes of parkinsonism.

Condition	Red Flags
Multiple systems atrophy (MSA)	Early autonomic failure with erectile dysfunction, urinary incontinence, syncope, cerebellar signs, spasticity or other upper motor neuron signs
Progressive supranuclear palsy (PSP)	Prominent axial features, such as oculomotor abnormalities, especially vertical gaze impairment, early falls and dysphagia, upright posture
Corticobasal degeneration (CBD)	Persistent asymmetry, cortical sensory signs, neglect, alien limb, severe early dystonia, aphasia
Lewy body dementia (DLB)	Early dementia, visual hallucinations, delusions, fluctuating level of consciousness/cognition, extreme neuroleptic sensitivity

features. As PD progresses, it can affect many parts of the central and peripheral nervous system, leading to diverse complications. Autonomic dysfunction can lead to drooling, bloating, gastroparesis, constipation, urinary dysfunction, incontinence, erectile dysfunction, temperature dysregulation and orthostatic hypotension which can lead to syncope. Two major sources of morbidity and mortality are dysphagia and gait dysfunction. Dysphagia can lead to aspiration or choking. Postural instability and freezing of gait can lead to injurious falls or the many complications associated with immobility. Sleep dysfunction, somnolence, and fatigue are extremely common in PD. When prominent, cognitive–behavioral dysfunction is a major source of disability and are the PD symptoms most associated with poor QOL. Furthermore, patients with advanced PD experience complications from its treatment as well.

A. Motor Fluctuations and Dyskinesia

Complications of dopaminergic therapy are significant sources of disability in moderate stage PD patients. "Wearing off" is managed in two ways; shortening the interval between doses, or adding a catechol-*O*-methyltransferase (COMT) or monoamine oxidase (MAO) inhibitor. Dyskinesia can be managed either by slightly reducing the amount of levodopa at each dose or by adding amantadine. If the patient is taking a long-acting (controlled-release) formulation of levodopa multiple times a day, an unpredictable "stacking effect" may contribute to dyskinesia, and conversion to a short-acting levodopa regimen should be considered. Deep brain stimulation (DBS), especially globus pallidus interna (GPi)-DBS, can have a robust antidyskinetic effect. Because management of complications is complex, and because DBS can alleviate both problems in some patients, prompt referral to a neurologist is strongly recommended for advanced treatment options.

B. Dementia and Psychosis

Dementia occurs in a majority of patients with advanced PD. First, look for medications that contribute to sedation and/or confusion (eg, dopamine agonists, amantadine, muscle relaxants, pain medications, and anticholinergic medications for tremor and bladder symptoms). Cholinesterase inhibitors (eg, donepezil, galantamine, rivastigmine) can be beneficial for attention, bradyphrenia, and psychotic features like visual hallucinations. To treat psychosis, address medications first (eg, lowering dopaminergic medications or consider using quetiapine and clozapine). All other typical and atypical antipsychotics are contraindicated in PD, especially in older adults. Always rule out general medical issues, such as infections, especially if there is a component of delirium.

C. Depression

Selective serotonin reuptake inhibitors (SSRIs) are first-line agents for depression in PD, but serotonin-norepinephrine reuptake inhibitors (SNRIs) may address a broader spectrum of neurotransmitter deficits in PD. However, few clinical trials provide evidence for the choice among antidepressants in PD. Care should be taken to avoid drug interactions with MAO inhibitors like selegiline.

D. Orthostatic Hypotension

Medications that contribute to orthostatic hypotension should be reduced if possible. Consider antihypertensives, which are frequently no longer needed as PD progresses. Dopaminergic drugs can also exacerbate hypotension. Salt in the diet can be liberalized, and water intake encouraged. The head of the bed should be raised above 30 degrees. Eating small, frequent meals can avoid splanchnic dilatation. Hot weather, hot liquids, and hot showers should be avoided. Pharmacotherapy, such as fludrocortisone and/or midodrine is sometimes used when the above measures fail, but cause complications in older patients and should be used with caution.

E. Gastrointestinal Complications/Constipation

Dysphagia must be monitored closely and patients should be promptly referred for swallowing evaluation when present. Drooling can respond to careful administration of botulinum toxin to the salivary glands. Constipation is practically universal in PD. Hydration, exercise, and a healthy, high-fiber diet should be encouraged. Stool softeners and laxative agents (eg, docusate and Senokot) should be taken daily.

F. Falls

Falls are a major source of injury, morbidity, and mortality in PD, and patients with postural instability need to be closely monitored for falls and referred promptly to physical therapy for gait and balance evaluation and management.

G. Referral Guidelines

Consider referring patients to a neurologist or movement disorders specialist when: (a) the diagnosis is in question; (b) a patient is not responding to standard therapies; (c) the patient has unacceptable side effects; (d) complications occur from PD or its treatments; or (e) surgical interventions are considered.

▶ Treatment

A. Nonpharmacologic Therapy

Care of the PD patient requires a multidisciplinary team approach, including important aspects such as patient education, exercise, diet, and rehabilitation services. Patients and their families should be educated about the natural history of PD and available treatments and resources. Support

groups are particularly valuable. As the disease progresses and new symptoms and complications arise, treatment regimens can become complex. Patients will need to learn to differentiate among symptoms related to PD, medication side effects, or other conditions. Exercise improves mood, strength, balance, flexibility, and mobility. A combination of aerobic, strengthening, and flexibility exercises can maintain functional status. A well-balanced healthy diet and adequate hydration can prevent constipation and orthostatic hypotension. Furthermore, protein restriction may be necessary in some patients, as amino acids compete with levodopa for absorption, thus blocking its therapeutic effect. Involving a nutritionist may be vital, especially as weight loss and disuse atrophy can occur and are associated with poor outcomes. Physical, occupational, speech, and swallowing rehabilitation therapies aimed at improving daily function and QOL can be effective at all stages. Emotional and psychological needs of the patient and family should also be addressed through counseling of a chaplain, psychiatrist, psychologist, or other mental health provider.

B. Pharmacotherapy

PD is an incurable illness, with no treatments proven to slow disease progression. However, PD is somewhat unique among neurodegenerative disorders in that it benefits from a diverse range of effective symptomatic treatments such as dopaminergic medications. The primary goal of pharmacotherapy is to reduce symptoms to maintain independence, functional status, and QOL and reduce disability. A common misconception among patients (and clinicians) is that medications will "only last for so long" once started. This now discredited belief has led to an all-too-common practice of delaying treatment as long as possible. Treatment should be initiated and tailored to adequately reduce symptoms whenever patients are bothered by their symptoms, and certainly when functional status, independence or mobility is threatened. Many PD patients, especially young-onset and tremor/motor-predominant patients, can lead highly functional lives for many years with optimized treatment regimens. However, as the disease progresses, complications of dopaminergic medications, such as dyskinesia and motor fluctuations, occur and regimens can become complex. Especially in older adults, medications can exacerbate nonmotor symptoms, such as visual hallucinations, behavioral problems, orthostasis, and somnolence, and reductions may be necessary at the cost of decreased motor benefit.

1. Levodopa—Levodopa is the most effective and well-established drug in the treatment of PD. Converted by DOPA-decarboxylase into dopamine, it provides dopaminergic replacement. It ameliorates tremor, bradykinesia and rigidity, thus reducing morbidity and disability. Axial features of PD such as speech and gait impairment are frequently less responsive to levodopa and other dopaminergic medications.

Furthermore, in advanced PD, postural instability, speech impairment, autonomic dysfunction, dementia and psychiatric problems are not responsive to levodopa. Although levodopa does not slow the progression of PD pathology, life expectancy in PD has drastically improved today compared to the prelevodopa era.

Levodopa provides a robust and consistent improvement of motor features, and keeps patients highly functional for years. However, the vast majority of advanced patients will eventually experience motor complications, namely motor fluctuations and dyskinesia, manifest as inconsistent response to levodopa. In the earlier stages, patients experience "wearing off," where the duration of effect of each levodopa dose progressively shortens, and requires shorter intervals between doses. Later on, more unpredictability occurs, with some doses completely failing to "kick in," and others abruptly losing effect. Dyskinesias are involuntary hyperkinetic movements that occur at "peak-dose" levodopa levels. They are most commonly choreiform (abnormal twisting, writhing, dance-like movements) but can also be dystonic (pulling into more sustained and often painful postures).

Other side effects of levodopa include nausea, vomiting, lightheadedness, dizziness, somnolence, and, in more advanced patients, hallucinations and confusion. Peripheral decarboxylase inhibitors, such as carbidopa are always included in formulations of levodopa to reduce the gastrointestinal side effects by preventing peripheral conversion of levodopa to dopamine. Isolated carbidopa can be added to prevent the nausea experienced with standard levodopa formulations. Levodopa is generally a well-tolerated medication and most side effects can be avoided if started slowly and gradually titrated up to an effective dose. It should be taken on empty stomach at least 30–45 minutes before or after meals, to avoid protein blocking of absorption of levodopa. Long-acting formulations of levodopa (eg, Sinemet CR) are helpful for bedtime dosing as they can reduce nocturnal return of PD symptoms, but daytime use of these formulations can exacerbate complications.

2. Dopamine agonists—Dopamine agonists directly stimulate dopamine receptors in the striatum (the postsynaptic target of nigral neurons). The older ergot derivatives such as bromocriptine and pergolide are not used in clinical practice because of serious side effects such as heart valve damage. Newer nonergot agonists, such as pramipexole, ropinirole, and transdermal rotigotine, have replaced them. Dopamine agonists are effective as monotherapy in reducing cardinal motor features of PD. However, within 2–5 years, most patients will require the addition of levodopa. Dopamine agonists are also used as adjunctive therapy with levodopa when motor complications occur. As they are longer-acting, they can reduce the severity of "wearing off," and as they cause less dyskinesia than levodopa, they are sometimes used in order to attempt a decreased levodopa dose.

Dopamine agonists are poorly tolerated in older adults. Although side effects are similar to levodopa (nausea, vomiting, orthostatic hypotension, somnolence, dizziness, psychiatric symptoms, hallucinations), they occur more commonly and more severely, especially in older adults. Serious consideration should be given before starting a dopamine agonist in patients older than 70 years of age because of the side effects of somnolence, cognitive impairment, and psychosis. Dopamine agonists also have additional side effects, including impulse control disorder, that are rarely seen with levodopa. Patients on dopamine agonists should be educated about and frequently screened for compulsive gambling, eating, and shopping, hypersexuality, and other impulsive behaviors.

3. Other pharmacotherapies—Levodopa and dopamine agonists are the 2 main drug classes used as monotherapy in PD. Other PD drugs have minimal symptomatic benefits when used alone and serve as adjunctive therapy when motor complications occur. As most patients require these medications when they have entered the more complicated moderate to advanced stage of PD, one should consider consulting a neurologist before initiating these agents. COMT inhibitors (entacapone and tolcapone) and MAO-B inhibitors (selegiline and rasagiline) block the enzymatic breakdown of levodopa and are used to decrease motor fluctuations ("wearing off") by extending the duration of benefit of each dose of levodopa. Amantadine is the only medication with proven effectiveness for reducing dyskinesia. It reduces tremor and freezing of gait in some patients as well. Amantadine has dopamine agonist and anticholinergic properties, commonly exacerbates somnolence, cognitive impairment and psychosis, and has limited use in older adults. Similarly, anticholinergic medications like trihexyphenidyl can be effective at reducing tremor, dyskinesia, and dystonia, but older patients have low tolerance for their cognitive and autonomic impairment. These drugs should not be considered options in the geriatric population.

C. Surgical Therapies

In many patients, medications become progressively less effective in relieving PD symptoms consistently, especially after the onset motor fluctuations or dyskinesia. Some of these patients may benefit from surgical therapies. Candidacy for these interventions is complex. The ideal candidate is a patient who has a clear diagnosis of PD, continued good response to medications in the "on" state, suffers from disabling motor complications despite optimal medical management, is healthy enough to tolerate a neurosurgical intervention, has relatively intact cognition and does not suffer from a significant or uncontrolled mood disorder. There is no firm age-limit, but patients older than age 70 years are generally considered higher risk, and those older than age 80 years are rarely operated on.

1. Stereotactic lesioning—Pallidotomy (lesioning of the GPi) is effective in treating the cardinal features of PD and can drastically reduce levodopa-induced dyskinesias. Similarly, thalamotomy can reduce tremor. However, these lesioning procedures are irreversible, not adjustable, and bilateral procedures that are associated with dysphagia, dysarthria, and cognitive impairment. Consequently, today these procedures are mostly used only in situations where DBS is not feasible.

2. Deep brain stimulation—DBS of subthalamic nucleus (STN) or GPi has mostly replaced stereotactic lesioning procedures. Although more expensive, DBS has the advantages of being nondestructive, reversible, and programmable. Bilateral procedures are better tolerated. The DBS system is a 4-contact lead implanted into each hemisphere of the brain by stereotactic technique. The leads are connected to a pulse generator in the chest wall by subcutaneous extension wires. Clinicians program the device for optimal benefit to avoid side effects by adjusting the amplitude, pulse width, frequency and polarity of stimulation, and by changing the configuration of active contacts on each lead. Patients can also make some adjustments at home.

DBS of both targets can alleviate the cardinal features of PD, motor fluctuations, and dyskinesia. Both targets are effective at treating tremor, rigidity, and bradykinesia, especially in the limbs. However, as with medications, axial symptoms such as gait and speech are less responsive to DBS. In fact, DBS can make speech, falls, cognition, and behavioral symptoms worse, especially in high-risk patients. It is important to have extensive discussion with patients and their families before surgery to make sure that the symptoms that bother them the most (ie, their goals of treatment) match those that can be reliably alleviated by DBS. The largest recent randomized clinical trial found these 2 targets to have similar effectiveness and safety. However, STN-DBS has higher risk of falls and cognitive and mood side effects.

DBS has higher risk of infection and hardware problems than ablative procedures. Some side effects, such as speech impairment, spasticity, and mood changes, can result from stimulation of neighboring structures in the brain. Adjusting stimulation parameters often alleviates these stimulation-induced side effects.

▶ Prognosis

Caring for patients with advanced PD presents many challenges, and the prospect of having a chronic progressive debilitating disease is frightening. Patients can benefit from PD treatments for years and become disabled by nonmotor symptoms without effective treatments. Furthermore, PD drug doses frequently need to be lowered because of exacerbation of nonmotor symptoms, worsening, in turn, their motor symptoms.

A palliative care approach can be beneficial and is underutilized in advanced PD. PD has a variable, slow, and prolonged course, making accurate prognosis difficult. However, some trends predict an unfavorable prognosis. Onset of PD in older age, prominent nonmotor features, and prominent akinetic-rigid syndrome with gait dysfunction are associated with more rapid progression and poor outcomes; whereas younger-onset PD, lack of nonmotor features, and tremor predominance are associated with slower progression.

Palliative care, unlike hospice, is not limited to a particular prognosis. PD causes disability, suffering, and caregiver strain. Applying palliative care principles at every stage is important.

Addressing advanced directives and involving an attorney or estate planner for financial and legal issues (eg, establishing power of attorney) is important. Although it may be difficult to initiate end-of-life discussions, it is important to hear a PD patient's wishes, when they are still able to share them. A palliative care approach does not preclude life-prolonging therapies, but proactively focuses on relief of suffering from pain, depression, anxiety, and other psychosocial stressors for both patients and caregivers.

Ahlskog JE. Diagnosis and differential diagnosis of Parkinson's disease and parkinsonism. *Parkinsonism Relat Disord.* 2000;7(1): 63-70.

Braak H, Del Tredici K, Bratzke H, Hamm-Clement J, Sandmann-Keil D, Rüb U. Staging of the intracerebral inclusion body pathology associated with idiopathic Parkinson's disease (preclinical and clinical stages). *J Neurol.* 2002;249 Suppl 3:III/1-III/5. Review. PMID: 12528692

Follett KA, Weaver FM, Stern M, et al; CSP 468 Study Group. Pallidal versus subthalamic deep-brain stimulation for Parkinson's disease. *N Engl J Med.* 2010;362(22):2077-2091.

Hallett M, Litvan I. Evaluation of surgery for Parkinson's disease: a report of the Therapeutics and Technology Assessment Subcommittee of the American Academy of Neurology. *Neurology.* 1999;53(9):1910-1921.

Hoehn MM, Yahr MD. Parkinsonism: onset, progression, mortality. *Neurology.* 1967;17(5):427-442.

Langston, JW. The Parkinson's complex: parkinsonism is just the tip of the iceberg. *Ann Neurol.* 2006;59(4):591-596.

Stern MB, Lang A, Poewe W. Toward a redefinition of Parkinson's disease. *Mov Disord.* 2012;27(1):54-60.

USEFUL WEBSITES

Family Caregiver Alliance (provides information on support groups, hiring caregivers, and issues of long-term care). http://www.caregiver.org

National Parkinson Foundation, Inc. (provides information on educational programs, support groups, treatment options, and publications). http://www.parkinson.org

"We Move" Foundation (a useful central information resource). http://www.wemove.org

Unified Parkinson's Disease Rating Scale (UPDRS). http://www.mdvu.org/library/ratingscales/pd/updrs.pdf

ESSENTIAL TREMOR

ESSENTIALS OF DIAGNOSIS

▶ Characterized by a bilateral action tremor of the hands and forearms and possibly the head, voice, and trunk.

▶ Other neurologic signs are absent.

▶ Positive family history in about half of cases.

General Principles in Older Adults

ET is the most common movement disorder, affecting 4% of adults 40 years of age and older. Age and family history are the strongest risk factors. It has been referred to as familial tremor, but a significant percentage of ET patients do not have a family history. The term "benign" ET, used to differentiate it from tremors associated with PD and other neurodegenerative diseases, has fallen out of use, as the tremor itself can be quite disabling. There is also recent controversy regarding considering ET as a neurodegenerative disorder or a condition of normal aging of the nervous system.

Clinical Findings

ET is characterized by a postural-kinetic tremor, although rest tremor can occur. It often involves the arms, but commonly involves the head and voice as well. It is unusual for ET to be prominent in the legs, lips or chin. Bilateral involvement is the general rule but it can be asymmetric. An isolated head tremor can occur, but these cases are considered variants of cervical dystonia. ET progresses slowly and remains mild in majority of cases. In fact, some estimate that less than 10% of people with ET seek medical attention. ET worsens with anxiety, stress and caffeine intake, and is frequently reduced by alcohol, although this can be true for all forms of tremor.

ET is a clinical diagnosis, usually made by a thorough history and examination. Other than the tremor, neurologic examination should be normal, except for possible subtle findings such as hearing loss and subtle cerebellar signs.

Differential Diagnosis

The differential diagnosis includes parkinsonism, with a resting tremor and other signs. Action tremors are also found in dystonia and Wilson disease, but these conditions are associated with other neurologic abnormalities and occur in a younger population. Secondary causes of postural and kinetic tremor should only be considered with unusual presentations of tremor. Tobacco and caffeine use, as well as certain medications (see Table 24–1), may result in an enhanced

physiologic tremor that can closely mimic ET. Tremor can be seen with alcohol or sedative withdrawal, and can occur as part of a somatoform disorder or conversion disorder. Psychogenic tremors are usually interrupted on examination by distracting the patient.

Complications

ET can result in significant functional impairment and social embarrassment. ET has significant effects on functional status, especially on ADLs and IADLs, like feeding, dressing, manual work, and household chores. Furthermore, ET can have significant psychological impact as it worsens in social situations and can result in early retirement, social isolation, and increased level of care. Tremor is not the only neurologic manifestation of ET. Recent studies show patients with additional findings, such as subtle cerebellar dysfunction (difficulty with tandem gait, slight incoordination), mild cognitive deficits, anxiety, and hearing loss. ET is also associated with a higher risk of PD and may be associated with an increased risk of dementia.

Treatment

All current treatments for ET are solely symptomatic. The goal of treatment is not to eradicate all tremor, but to improve function and reduce social embarrassment. If the tremor is mild and nondisabling, treatment may not be required. Stress reduction and caffeine avoidance can ameliorate tremor, and can be sufficient in mild ET. Alcohol may reduce tremor, but regular use is not recommended because of rebound tremor and long-term effects, including a higher rate of alcoholism in ET patients. Occupational therapists can provide adaptive utensils and devices that can improve QOL. All medications for tremor can cause side effects and should be started at low doses and gradually increased until satisfactory control or intolerable side effects occur. Severe, refractory or atypical cases should be referred to a specialist for management including consideration for DBS.

A. Pharmacotherapy

1. First-line agents—Propranolol and primidone have the most evidence of efficacy in treating ET, reducing tremor by approximately 50% to 70% of patients. Propranolol is a nonselective β-blocker that crosses the blood–brain barrier, and the only agent approved by the FDA for ET. The average effective dose is 120 mg/day, up to 320 mg if tolerated. Mild ET can be treated with as-needed doses. Sustained-release preparations are equally effective. Potential side effects include bronchoconstriction, bradycardia, hypotension, lightheadedness, fatigue, impotence, and depression. Other β blockers are less effective than propranolol. Primidone is structurally similar to barbiturates. Most patients respond to about 250 mg daily.

Adverse effects include sedation, dizziness, ataxia, confusion, and depression. Response to treatment and side effects guide dose adjustments. Combining propranolol and primidone may provide additive benefit.

2. Second-line agents—Gabapentin or topiramate are antiseizure drugs that can be added to first-line agents if tremor control is unsatisfactory. Gabapentin is well tolerated, with typical effective dose around 1200 mg daily. Common side effects include sedation, dizziness, and unsteadiness. Topiramate is effective at doses above 100 mg twice daily. Its use is limited because of cognitive side effects, reduced appetite, weight loss, and paresthesia. Zonisamide is an alternative to topiramate, and is better tolerated and dosed daily. Benzodiazepines are occasionally used to control tremor, but common side effects (eg, sedation, cognitive dysfunction, hypotension, respiratory inhibition and abuse potential) limit their use. Calcium-channel blockers, theophylline, carbonic anhydrase inhibitors, isoniazid, clonidine, and phenobarbital have yielded contradictory results and are not recommended as first- or second-line agents.

3. Other pharmacotherapies—The use of botulinum toxin type A to treat limb tremor has been disappointing, and its use should only be considered in rare refractory cases. However, neck injections can be quite effective in reducing head tremor. A high risk of dysphagia limits its use for voice tremor.

B. Surgical Therapies

There is extensive evidence that unilateral thalamotomy or thalamic (ventral intermediate [VIM]) DBS is effective in treating patients with disabling, medication-refractory ET. Dysarthria, dysequilibrium, and cognitive impairment may occur after thalamotomy. DBS appears to be associated with fewer adverse events and bilateral intervention is better tolerated. The decision to use either procedure depends on individual patient circumstance, perioperative risks, and access availability to ongoing stimulator monitoring and adjustments.

Koller WC, Hristova A, Brin M. Pharmacologic treatment of essential tremor. *Neurology.* 2000;54(11 Suppl 4):S30-S38.

Louis ED. Essential tremor. *N Engl J Med.* 2001;345(12):887-891.

Louis ED, Ottman R, Hauser WA. How common is the most common adult movement disorder? Estimates of the prevalence of essential tremor throughout the world. *Mov Disord.* 1998;13(1):5-10.

Zesiewicz TA, Elble R, Louis ED, et al. Practice parameter: therapies for essential tremor: report of the Quality Standards Subcommittee of the American Academy of Neurology. *Neurology.* 2005;64(12):2008-2020.

Zesiewicz TA, Elble RJ, Louis ED, et al. Evidence-based guideline update: treatment of essential tremor: report of the Quality Standards subcommittee of the American Academy of Neurology. *Neurology.* 2011;77(19):1752-1755.

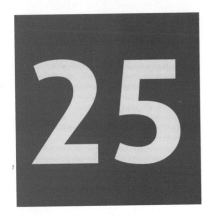

Falls & Mobility Disorders

Deborah M. Kado, MD, MS

Daniel Slater, MD, FAAFP

ESSENTIALS OF DIAGNOSIS

► Older adults who report >1 fall in the past year or a single fall with injury or gait and balance problems are at increased risk for future falls and injuries.

► Acute factors (infectious, toxic, metabolic, ischemic, or iatrogenic) may contribute to falls and mobility disorders.

► Medications, particularly psychotropic drugs, increase the risk for falls.

► Common modifiable fall risk factors important to consider include visual acuity, home environmental hazards, and footwear.

▶ General Principles in Older Adults

As people age, their risk of falling increases. Approximately 30% of people older than the age of 65 years and 50% of people older than age 80 years fall each year. Almost 60% of those with a history of falls in the previous year will suffer from a subsequent fall. Up to 50% of falls result in some type of injury, the most serious of which include hip, head trauma, and cervical spine fractures. Injuries that occur as a result of a falls contribute to a rate of accident-related deaths that rank seventh as a cause of death in the United States. Multiple risk factors account for the increased rate of falls observed in older persons and as such, falls are considered a geriatric syndrome.

One major risk factor for falls includes problems with mobility. As is true with falls, the risk for developing a mobility disorder increases with age. Mobility disorders range from subclinical to obvious and within this range, fall risk is elevated. Because the risk for mobility disorders and falls are increased in older persons, clinicians should be particularly aware of factors important in preventing and treating both. This chapter discusses falls and associated mobility disorders with regards to the background, epidemiology, risk factors, clinical evaluation, prevention, treatment, and prognosis of older persons who may be at risk or who have already developed mobility problems and recurrent falls.

A fall is defined as "inadvertently coming to rest on the ground or other lower level with or without loss of consciousness" (Close, 1999). Most falls do not result in serious physical injury, but those who fall become at increased risk for recurrent falls. In addition, many who experience an initial fall develop a fear of falling that itself can lead to an increased fall risk. Thus, it is particularly important to query about a history of falls when evaluating an older patient so that an appropriate evaluation and recommendations for prevention and treatment can be made before a significant injury occurs.

Mobility disorders refer to any deviation from normal walking. To walk normally, control of balance and posture both at rest and with movement is necessary. Thus, normal gait requires a complex integration of adequate strength, sensation, and coordination. For a normal healthy adult, walking is almost automatic, but in fact, the control of gait and posture is both complex and multifactorial, and a defect at any level can result in mobility problems.

The incidence and health impact of falls vary depending on age, sex, and living status. As stated earlier, the incidence increases with age with about a third of the population older than age 65 years and half of the population older than age 80 years reporting a fall in the previous year. Men and women tend to fall in equal proportions, but women are more likely to suffer from an injury. Similar to those older than age 80 years, approximately 50% of residents in long-term care settings fall each year. Of the 5% to 10% of falls that result in serious injury, the most common complications include major lacerations, head trauma, and fractures.

Fall-related injuries are the major reason that clinicians need to be acutely aware of this widespread problem that affects older patients. Although the majority of falls do not result in serious physical injury, in those age 65 years and older, falls account for 62% of nonfatal injuries leading to U.S. emergency department visits, and approximately 5%

lead to hospitalization. Patients who suffer from fall-related injuries are more likely to experience a decline in functional status and an increase in medical service utilization. In addition, they have an increased likelihood of long-term nursing home placement.

Special mention of hip fractures is deserved because they are amongst the most common and costly of fall-related injuries in older adults. More than 90% of all hip fractures occur as a result of a fall. Falls resulting in hip fracture are known to roughly double the 1-year mortality rate compared to matched seniors without hip fractures. The 1-year mortality rate ranges from 12% to 37%, and approximately half of those who fall and fracture a hip are unable to regain the ability to live independently.

Like falls, mobility disorders affect approximately 15% of those age 60 years and older and 80% of those age 85 years and older. One simple measure of mobility is to assess walking speed; in 1 observational study of about 900 older men and women (average age: 75 years; range: 71–82), gait speed averaged 1.2 m/s, and declined approximately 5% over 3 years. In general, slower gait speed is a risk factor for falls among older adults, but there is a U-shaped relationship in that those with faster walking speeds (≥1.3 m/s) also experience an increased rate of falls. Approximately 17% of falls in older persons can be attributed to balance, leg weakness, or gait problems. Of those with mobility problems, the causes are multifactorial in nature, with sensory deficits, myelopathy, and multiple infarcts being among the top 3 categories reported in the literature.

▶ Prevention

Fall prevention strategies appear to work in both institutional and community settings according to recent comprehensive systematic reviews published by the Cochrane Collaboration. Single and multifactorial intervention randomized controlled trials have been conducted, and while not uniformly in agreement, the preponderance of evidence demonstrate some positive benefit with fall rate declines. In addition, if these fall prevention strategies can be implemented in populations at risk for injurious falls, society on the whole will enjoy cost savings.

Thus, many organizations have taken on falls as a preventable health condition, and resources have been put towards implementing fall prevention programs. In the United States since 2004, the National Council on Aging (NCOA) has been leading the Falls Free Initiative to address the growing public health problem of falls and fall-related injuries among older adults by collaborative leadership. Initially, representatives from 58 national organizations, professional associations, and federal agencies got together to develop a blueprint for reducing falls and fall-related injuries that included 36 strategies. Since its inception, NCOA has developed coalition workgroups, 1 of which was responsible for having the U.S. Senate delegate the first day

of fall as National Fall Prevention Awareness Day, initially established in 2009. That same year, the American Geriatrics Society (AGS) and British Geriatrics Society (BGS) expert panel on fall prevention provided updated recommendations that health care providers follow a step-by-step process of decision making and intervention to manage falls among older persons assessed to be at high fall risk (see algorithm, Figure 25–1).

For preventive strategies to be most cost-effective, they should target those who are at highest risk for developing the outcome. Multiple studies have shown that the strongest risk factors for falling include: (a) previous falls; (b) decreased muscle strength; (c) gait and balance impairment; and (d) specific medication use. With the exception of previous falls, theoretically, muscle strength, gait and balance, and medication use could be potentially modifiable risk factors. Other potentially modifiable risk factors include visual impairment, depression, pain, and dizziness. Hard to modify or nonmodifiable fall risk factors are age, female sex, activities of daily living disabilities, low body mass index, urinary incontinence, cognitive impairment, arthritis, and diabetes.

Although advanced age is a risk factor for developing mobility disorders in general, there are no particular risk factors to highlight as the root cause of disabling gait disorders are most often unknown and/or multifactorial in etiology. As an example, weakness leading to mobility problems could stem from upper motor neuron (dysfunction of the cord and/or higher central motor pathways), lower motor neuron (problems with spinal motor neurons or peripheral nervous system), or primary myopathic problems. Some of the most disabling gait disorders result from serious neurologic disease and are beyond the scope of this chapter. However, because each of these diseases are also associated with an increased fall risk, they are listed for completeness: (a) extrapyramidal disorders (eg, Parkinson disease); (b) cerebellar ataxia (eg, cerebrovascular disease); (c) vestibular dysfunction (eg, acoustic neuroma); and (d) frontal lobe dysfunction (eg, normal pressure hydrocephalus).

Besides aging and/or deconditioning leading to muscle weakness and mobility problems, there are other nonneurologic medical problems that can lead to mobility disorders. Examples of these include visual loss, morbid obesity, orthopedic problems, rheumatologic disorders, pain, medications, and cardiorespiratory problems. Thus, in doing a clinical evaluation of an older patient, it is important to keep in mind these underlying systemic medical conditions that can adversely affect mobility, and hence lead to an unwanted fall.

▶ Clinical Findings

A. Symptoms & Signs

In the clinical evaluation of a geriatric patient, it is important to keep in mind identified independent risk factors for falling (Table 25–1). In addition, more often than not, falls in older

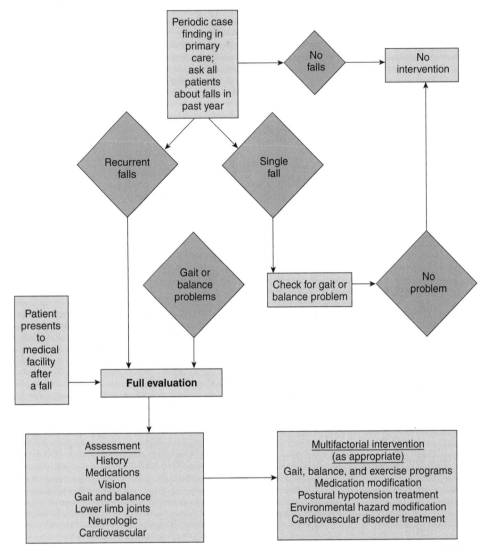

▲ **Figure 25–1.** Fall Prevention Algorithm. (Reproduced with permission from Panel on Prevention of Falls in Older Persons, American Geriatrics Society and British Geriatrics Society. Summary of the updated American Geriatrics Society/British Geriatrics Society clinical practice guideline for prevention of falls in older persons. *J Am Geriatr Soc.* 2011;59(1):148-157.)

adults are not owing to a single cause, but occur when there is an additional stress, such as an acute illness, new medication, or an environmental hazard, that makes an older person unable to compensate as well as a younger person, and thus more likely to fall. The activity profile of the older person also will affect their risk for falling. Sedentary individuals may have multiple risk factors for falling, but not be at danger because they modify their behavior to avoid the opportunity for falls. More active older adults may be less cautious and therefore be at increased risk for falling, because they may not

be able to compensate as well as a younger person to threats against postural stability.

To help prevent falls in older persons, multifactorial risk assessments have been advocated by the AGS/BGS and other organizations. These assessments begin with a basic falls history that inquires whether the patient experienced any fall in the past year. If a fall is reported, important details with regards to the activity that lead to the fall, any prodromal symptoms (eg, lightheadedness, imbalance), and where and when the fall occurred should be obtained. Patients should

Table 25–1. Independent risk factors for falling among community-dwelling older adults.

Risk Factor	Modifiable
Previous falls	No
Balance impairment	Yes
Decreased muscle strength	Yes
Visual impairment	Maybe
>4 Medications or psychoactive medication use	Yes
Gait impairment or walking difficulty	Maybe
Depression	Maybe
Dizziness or orthostasis	Maybe
Functional limitations (ADL disabilities)	Unlikely
Age >80 years	No
Female	No
Low body mass index	Unlikely
Urinary incontinence	Maybe
Cognitive impairment	Unlikely
Arthritis	Maybe
Diabetes	Unlikely
Pain	Maybe

ADLs, activities of daily living.

Data from Tinetti ME, Kumar C. The patient who falls. "It's always a trade-off." *JAMA*. 2010;303(3):258-266.

be asked about the number of falls in the past year, whether any injuries were sustained from any of the falls, and if they suffer from a fear of falling. Finally, patients should be asked if they suffer from any difficulties with walking or balance. All of the above questions are important because a "yes" answer to any would indicate a high likelihood of sustaining a future fall.

When inquiring about a specific fall, if there was an associated loss of consciousness, then orthostatic hypotension, or underlying cardiac or neurologic causes should be considered as precipitating factors. Other chronic medical conditions associated with an increased fall risk should be considered and include cognitive impairment, dementia, chronic musculoskeletal pain, knee osteoarthritis, urinary incontinence, stroke, Parkinson disease, and diabetes. Another crucial part of the medical history for an older person who might be at increased risk for falling includes a functional assessment of the activity of daily living skills, including use of adaptive equipment and mobility aids. In a patient who reports multiple falls, an inquiry into alcohol

use is warranted as most patients would not volunteer this information freely, and frequent alcohol consumption could increase fall risk. Finally, physicians should perform an up-to-date and careful review of the patient's medication list that should include current prescriptions and over-the-counter medications. One large observational study of 4260 older community-dwelling men demonstrated that 82.3% of participants reported inappropriate medication use (eg, polypharmacy, inappropriate medicine consumption, underutilization). And both polypharmacy (≥5 medications) and taking 1 or more potentially inappropriate medications were associated with having had a fall in the past year, highlighting the importance of addressing inappropriate use of medications as modifiable fall risk factor.

Once the history is obtained, clinicians should make sure that orthostatic vital signs, visual acuity, cognitive status, and cardiac system be included in a basic physical exam. Of vital importance is the evaluation of gait and balance. There are quite a few balance and mobility assessments that are effective at assessing fall risk, but are not practical in a busy clinical setting. Such tests include the Performance-Oriented Mobility Assessment (POMA; Table 25–2), Short Physical Performance Battery (SPPB), Berg balance test, and Safety Functional Motion test. However, there are 2 other tests, the Get Up and Go and the Functional Reach tests, that are more frequently used because they each take less than a minute to administer. For the Get Up and Go test, the physician should ask the patient to rise from a standard arm chair (without the use of arms if possible), walk a fixed distance across the room (3 meters), turn, walk back to the chair and sit down. Besides observing the patient for unsteadiness, if it takes >13.5 seconds to complete this task, the patient would be considered to be at increased risk for future falls. The functional reach test requires using a yardstick mounted on a wall at shoulder height. The patient is asked to stand close to the wall at comfortable stance with an outstretched arm with the shoulders perpendicular to the yardstick. The patient is then instructed to extend the arm forward as far as possible without taking a step or losing balance; the functional reach is measured along the yardstick in inches, and if <10 inches in men, there has been reported a 2 times greater risk for falling.

Finally, also important to the physical exam is the examination of the feet and footwear. High-heels, floppy slippers, shoes with slick soles can predispose people to trip and fall. Ill-fitting footwear that is too big, without sufficient grip or too much friction, and/or without proper fixation (untied or loosely tied shoes) will also contribute to increasing someone's fall risk. When selecting shoes, the upper shoe should be soft and flexible with smooth lining. The toe box should be deep enough to allow for toe wiggle room. The sole should be strong and flexible for good grip. The heel should provide a broad base for stability and be no higher than 4 cm. Finally, the fastening should provide a stable fit with some flexibility to allow for unusually shaped feet or swelling.

Table 25–2. Performance-oriented assessment of balance.[a]

Maneuver	Response		
	Normal	**Adaptive**	**Abnormal**
Sitting balance	Steady, stable	Holds onto chair to keep upright	Leans, slides down in chair
Arising from chair	Able to arise in a single movement without using arms	Uses arms (on chair or walking aid) to pull or push up; and/or moves forward in chair before attempting to arise	Multiple attempts required or unable without human assistance
Immediate standing balance (first 3–5 s)	Steady without holding onto walking aid or other objects for support	Steady, but uses walking aid or other object for support	Any sign of unsteadiness[b]
Standing balance	Steady, able to stand with feet together without holding object for support	Steady, but cannot put feet together	Any sign of unsteadiness regardless of stance or holds onto object
Balance with eyes closed (with feet as close together as possible)	Steady without holding onto any object with feet together	Steady with feet apart	Any sign of unsteadiness or needs to hold onto an object
Turning balance (360 degrees)	No grabbing or staggering; no need to hold onto any objects; steps are continuous (turn is a flowing movement)	Steps are discontinuous (patient puts one foot completely on floor before raising other foot)	Any sign of unsteadiness or holds onto an object
Nudge on sternum (patient standing with feet as close together as possible, examiner pushes with light even pressure over sternum 3 times; reflects ability to withstand displacement)	Steady, able to withstand pressure	Needs to move feet, but able to maintain balance	Begins to fall, or examiner has to help maintain balance
Neck turning (patient asked to turn head side to side and look up while standing with feet as close together as possible)	Able to turn head at least half way side to side and be able to bend head back to look at ceiling; no staggering, grabbing, or symptoms of lightheadedness, unsteadiness, or pain	Decreased ability to turn side to side to extend neck, but no staggering, grabbing, or symptoms of lightheadedness, unsteadiness, or pain	Any sign of unsteadiness or symptoms when turning head or extending neck
One-leg standing balance	Able to stand on one leg for 5 s without holding object for support		Unable
Back extension (ask patient to lean back as far as possible, without holding onto object if possible)	Good extension without holding object or staggering	Tries to extend, but decreased range of motion (compared with other patients of same age) or needs to hold object to attempt extension	Will not attempt or no extension seen or staggers
Reaching up (have patient attempt to remove an object from a shelf high enough to require stretching or standing on toes)	Able to take down object without needing to hold onto other object for support and without becoming unsteady	Able to get object but needs to steady self by holding on to something for support	Unable or unsteady
Bending down (patient is asked to pick up small objects, such as pen, from the floor)	Able to bend down and pick up the object and is able to get up easily in single attempt without needing to pull self up with arms	Able to get object and get upright in single attempt but needs to pull self up with arms or hold onto something for support	Unable to bend down or unable to get upright after bending down or takes multiple attempts to upright
Sitting down	Able to sit down in one smooth movement	Needs to use arms to guide self into chair or not a smooth movement	Falls into chair, misjudges distances (lands off center)

[a]The patient begins this assessment seated in a hard, straight-backed, armless chair.
[b]Unsteadiness defined as grabbing at objects for support, staggering, moving feet, or more than minimal trunk sway.

Reproduced with permission from Tinetti ME. Performance-oriented assessment of mobility problems in elderly patients. *J Am Geriatr Soc.* 1986;34(2):119-126.

B. Diagnostic Tests

In completing a work up for an older patient with falls or determined to be at increased risk for falling, other than a general medical work up, there is no standard diagnostic evaluation. However, laboratory tests for hemoglobin to rule out clinically significant anemia, a chemistry panel to rule electrolyte disorders, and/or hyper or hypo-osmolar states, thyroid-stimulating hormone (TSH) to rule out hypothyroidism, vitamin B_{12} level to rule out B_{12} deficiency (linked to proprioceptive problems), and serum 25-hydroxyvitamin D levels to rule out vitamin D deficiency (linked to falls and fractures) could be considered appropriate. In addition, falling can be a sign of medical illness and it is not uncommon for older patients to present with a fall to the emergency room, and later be diagnosed with an underlying urinary tract infection or pneumonia. A standard urinalysis and chest radiograph might be appropriate depending on the clinical scenario, especially if the patient suffers from significant cognitive impairment or dementia.

Fewer than 10% of falls are caused by a loss of consciousness, but when there is a history of such, a different approach to evaluation and prevention might be indicated. An electrocardiogram to evaluate for significant cardiac pathology should be included; routine Holter monitoring has not been shown to be effective. However, on cardiac exam if a crescendo–decrescendo systolic murmur is appreciated at the right upper sternal border, then echocardiogram would be indicated to rule out clinically significant aortic stenosis that when critical, can present with syncope. Carotid sinus sensitivity has also been linked to falls, and pacemaker placement might be considered in patients who experience carotid sinus massage-induced heart rate pauses of >3 seconds. Contraindications to carotid sinus massage include presence of carotid bruits, recent myocardial or cerebral ischemia, or previous ventricular tachyarrhythmias.

In patients who present with falls who have new or unexplained neurologic findings on examination, imaging with head CT or MRI may be indicated to rule out stroke, mass, normal pressure hydrocephalus, or other structural abnormality. If the patient has significant gait abnormalities, then spine radiographs or even MRI imaging may help exclude cervical spondylosis or lumbar stenosis as a cause of falls. Clinical signs consistent with cervical spinal spondylosis include neck stiffness, deep aching neck, arm and shoulder pain, and possibly stiffness or clumsiness while walking. If the condition is chronically progressive, there may be significant associated muscle atrophy. The hallmark symptom of cervical spondylotic myelopathy is weakness or stiffness in the legs and patients may present with gait instability; characteristically, there should be evidence of hyperreflexia, and a stiff or spastic gait would be expected in advanced cases. Lumbar spinal stenosis usually presents with pain, muscle weakness and tingling of the legs in the L4-S1 distribution with classic symptoms of pseudoclaudication, more recently referred to as neurogenic claudication (pain improves with sitting, worsens with standing or walking).

▶ Treatment

There are multiple interventions that can be implemented to decrease a patient's fall risk, and each needs to be tailored to the particular patient's needs. Overall, a multifactorial approach should be taken as modifiable factors, both intrinsic and extrinsic to the patient, have been shown to decrease fall rates. Of the interventions, medication reduction, physical therapy, and home safety modifications have demonstrated the best efficacy in fall prevention.

Starting with intrinsic modifiable fall risk factors (Table 25–3), visual impairment should be corrected if possible. The evidence supporting treatment of visual problems is not conclusive as a single intervention, but cataracts commonly affect older patients, and correction of vision may not only help to decrease the risk of falls, but improve quality of life. In patients with cardioinhibitory carotid sinus hypersensitivity who experience recurrent falls, dual chamber pacemaker placement is probably indicated. In all patients, but particularly in patients with postural hypotension, careful review of medications should be done. A goal should be to reduce the total number of medications and/or dose of individual medications. Psychoactive medications that include sedative hypnotics, anxiolytics, antidepressants and antipsychotic medications should be minimized and appropriately tapered and withdrawn if possible. If after discontinuation of predisposing medications a patient still has postural hypotension, then recommendations for adequate hydration, advice to slowly change positions, and the addition of a medication such as fludrocortisone may be considered. Finally, there is deemed to be sufficient evidence with regards to vitamin D and reducing the risk of falls that the AGS/BGS guidelines now recommend 800 IU of vitamin D daily for all older adults who are at risk for falling.

Extrinsic modifiable factors include checking the home environment to remove obvious fall hazards and ensuring that proper footwear is worn. In evaluating the home environment, removal of clutter to minimize tripping hazards, making sure there is adequate lighting, and installation of safety measures like shower bars and/or raised toilet seats are helpful to decrease fall risk. In assessing the footwear, foot problems can also be screened for and patients referred for treatment if necessary. Patients should be advised that they should wear well-fitting shoes of low heel height and high surface area.

In addition to reviewing and treating the intrinsic and extrinsic modifiable fall risk factors, patient education and information programs are helpful in falls prevention. For example, simple advice, such as a removal of multifocal lenses while walking or on stairs, can reduce the risk of falls. Perhaps most important is education and recommendations

Table 25–3. Recommended treatment of modifiable risk factors.

Risk Factors	Management
Intrinsic	
Vision	Check acuity and for cataracts, refer to ophthalmology if indicated; advise to avoid multifocal lenses while walking
Postural hypotension	Reduce medications, rule out dehydration, advise to change positions slowly, consider fludrocortisone if above 3 interventions don't work
Cardiovascular	Medical management, consider dual chamber cardiac pacing if carotid induced hypersensitivity >3-second pauses
Neurologic	Consider neuroimaging with MRI/CT, medical management as indicated
Arthritis	Medical management, consider physical therapy/occupational therapy referral, assistive devices as appropriate
Balance or gait impairment	Referral to physical and/or occupational therapy for progressive strength, balance and gait training
Vitamin D insufficiency/deficiency	Replete vitamin D with a minimum of 800 IU daily
Other medical conditions (cognitive impairment, depression, etc)	Medical management as indicated
Psychoactive medications	Eliminate or reduce dose of as many sedatives, antidepressants, anxiolytics, and antipsychotics as possible as these are associated with an increased fall risk
Other medications	Eliminate or reduce dose of as many medications as possible, paying close attention to: (a) antihypertensives that can lead to orthostasis/lightheadedness; and (b) antihistamines, anticonvulsants, opioids that can lead to confusion or impaired alertness
Extrinsic	
Home environmental hazards	Ideally, physical therapy/occupational therapy referral can assess home safety and make recommendations for safety improvements (eg, grab bars in shower, reaching devices, adequate lighting)
Footwear	Advise to wear well-fitting shoes with low heel height and high surface contact area

regarding physical activity. Although there is a lot of information available to the general public with regards to proper diet and exercise and good health, many probably do not link this beneficial information directly to fall risk reduction. Therefore, clinicians should make a specified recommendation regarding exercise and fall risk reduction as it has the best-associated evidence for reducing fall rates.

If during the clinical evaluation the patient demonstrates balance or gait instability, referral to physical therapy is warranted. Physical therapy should consist of progressive standing balance and strength exercise, transfer practice, and gait interventions, including use of appropriate assistive devices. Patients should also be trained on how to get up from the floor after a fall. Once mastering of these skills is accomplished, focusing on maintenance and building endurance should be encouraged. For all community-dwelling older patients, clinicians should recommend an individually tailored exercise program to maintain function, possibly increase endurance, and decrease their risk for falls. In the most recent systematic review on the topic, 43 trials tested the effect of exercise on falls. In trials of exercise classes that employed gait training, balance, and strengthening, there was a 17% risk reduction

in falling (n = 14 trials, 2364 participants, 95% confidence interval 0.72–0.97). There were 4 trials that examined the effects of Tai Chi on the risk and rate of falls, and the risk reduction was perhaps even more impressive at 37% (95% confidence interval 0.51–0.82).

Separate mention of treatment in acute and long-term care settings is warranted because this patient population clearly would be expected to be at an increased fall risk, and yet studied interventions in these patients have not demonstrated clear benefit. In particular, the use of bedrails, restraints, fall-alert bracelets, and bed alarms have not been shown to decrease fall rates, and may potentially increase fall risk. Even so, the AGS/BGS still provides the recommendation that multifactorial/multicomponent interventions should be considered in the long-term care setting; within this recommendation, exercise programs are also suggested, but to be implemented with caution due to risk of injury in frail persons. The AGS/BGS also recommends that vitamin D supplements of at least 800 IU daily should be provided to older persons residing in long-term care settings with: (a) proven or suspected vitamin D insufficiency (vitamin D 25-OH <30 ng/mL); (b) abnormal gait or balance; and/or (c) an increased risk for falls.

Prognosis

There is significant morbidity and mortality associated with falls in seniors. The prognosis for a single fall is not as severe as for an older person with repeated falls. Those who had fallen one or more times at home in the preceding 3 months were more than 3 times as likely as nonfallers to require institutional care within the subsequent year. Fallers had an overall 3-fold increase in subsequent fracture, with recurrent fallers age 60–74 years having an 8-fold increased risk of subsequent fracture. Additionally, recurrent fallers older than age 60 years had an overall risk of death about twice that of nonfallers. This was not simply a function of subsequent risk of fracture. In fact, recurrent fallers age 60–74 years had a 5-fold increased mortality independent of fracture.

Besides recurrent falls, inability to get up from a fall also portends a poor prognosis. Among 1103 community-dwelling residents in New Haven, Connecticut, there were 313 uninjured fallers, of whom 47% were unable to get up on their own. Even when they were not injured as a result of a fall, those unable to get up without help were more likely to suffer lasting decline in activities of daily living (35% vs. 26%). Not surprisingly, over an average follow-up of 16 months, compared with nonfallers, these individuals were also more likely to be hospitalized.

Older adults who fall also suffer from worse quality of life. Confusion and sadness are 4 times more common in recurrent fallers than nonfallers, and it appears that decisions to enter institutional care are often driven by fear of future falls and being unable to get up, rather than actual demonstrated disability. The negative impact of fear of falling should not be underestimated. Another study reported that compared with falls and fractures, fear of falling had the largest negative effect on health-related quality of life.

Although recurrent falls, inability to get up after a fall, and psychological implications following falls all are associated with poor prognosis, each is potentially modifiable. Careful attention should be made to underlying medical disorders that may contribute to an individual's fall risk. In 1 randomized controlled trial, a focused history and physical assessment by nurse practitioners following a fall lead to identification of modifiable medical conditions and decreased hospitalization rates over 2 years of follow-up.

In this chapter, we discussed the underlying predisposing risk factors, clinical evaluation, prevention, and treatment of falls in older persons. Although chronologic aging is inevitable, successful aging is not. The astute practitioner who is aware of fall risk factors, takes the time to do a proper assessment, and is knowledgeable about treatment can help our older population avoid falling and its associated ill health consequences.

Beattie BL. The National Falls Free Initiative, working collaboratively to affect change. *J Safety Res.* 2011;42(6):521-523.

Beer C, Hyde Z, Almeida OP, et al. Quality use of medicines and health outcomes among a cohort of community dwelling older men: an observational study. *Br J Clin Pharmacol.* 2011;71(4): 592-599.

Cameron ID, Muarray GR, Gillespie LD, et al. Interventions for preventive falls in older people in nursing care facilities and hospitals. *Cochrane Database Syst Rev.* 2010;(1):CD005465.

Close J, Ellis M, Hooper R, Glucksman E, Jackson S, Swift C. Prevention of falls in the elderly trial (PROFET): a randomized controlled trial. *Lancet.* 1999;353(9147):93-97.

Coussement J, De Paepe L, Schwendimann R, Denhaerynck K, Dejaeger E, Milisen K. Interventions for preventing falls in acute- and chronic-care hospitals: a systemic review meta-analysis. *J Am Geriatr Soc.* 2008;56(1):29-36.

Davis JC, Robertson MC, Ashe MC, Liu-Ambrose T, Khan KM, Marra CA. Does a home-based strength and balance programme in people aged > 80 years provide the best value for money to prevent falls? A systematic review of economic evaluations of falls prevention interventions. *Br J Sports Med.* 2010;44(2):80-89.

Delbaere K, Crombez G, Vanderstraeten G, Willems T, Cambier D. Fear-related avoidance of activities, falls and physical frailty. A prospective community-based cohort study. *Age Ageing.* 2004;33(4):368-373.

Donald IP, Bulpitt CJ. The prognosis of falls in elderly people living at home. *Age Ageing.* 1999;28(2):121-125.

Duncan PW, Studenski S, Chandler J, Prescott B. Functional reach: predictive validity in a sample of elderly male veterans. *J Gerontol.* 1992;47(3):M93-M98.

Gillespie LD, Robertson MC, Gillespie WJ, et al. Interventions for preventing falls in older people living in the community. *Cochrane Database Syst Rev.* 2009;(2):CD007146.

Gribbin J, Hubbard R, Smith C, Gladman J, Lewis S. Incidence and mortality of falls amongst older people in primary care in the United Kingdom. *QJM.* 2009;102(7):477-483.

Guralnick J, Simonsick E, Ferrucci L, et al. A short physical performance batter assessing lower extremity function: association with self-reported disability and prediction of mortality and nursing home admission. *J Gerontol.* 1994;49(2): M85-M94.

Iglesias CP, Manca A, Torgerson DJ. The health-related quality of life and cost implications of falls in elderly women. *Osteoporos Int.* 2009;20(6):869-878.

Kenny RAM, Richardson DA, Steen N, Bexton RS, Shaw FE, Bond J. Carotid sinus syndrome: a modifiable risk factor for nonaccidental falls in older adults (SAFE PACE). *J Am Coll Cardiol.* 2011;38(5):1491-1496.

MacIntyre NJ, Stavness CL, Adachi JD. The safe functional motion test is reliable for assessment of functional movements in individuals at risk for osteoporotic fracture. *Clin Rheumatol.* 2010;29(2):143-150.

Morrison RS, Chassin MR, Siu AL. The medical consultant's role in caring for patients with hip fracture. *Ann Intern Med.* 1998;128(12 Pt 1):1010-1020.

Panel on Prevention of Falls in Older Persons, American Geriatrics Society and British Geriatrics Society. Summary of the updated American Geriatrics Society/British Geriatrics Society clinical practice guideline for prevention of falls in older persons. *J Am Geriatr Soc.* 2011;59(1):148-157.

Quach L, Galica AM, Jones RN, et al. The nonlinear relationship between gait speed and falls: the maintenance of balance, independent living, intellect, and zest in the Elderly of Boston Study. *J Am Geriatr Soc.* 2011;59(6):1069-1073.

Rosado JA, Rubenstein LZ, Robbins AS, Heng MK, Schulman BL, Josephson KR. The value of Holter monitoring in evaluating the elderly patient who falls. *J Am Geriatr Soc.* 1989:37(5):430-434.

Rubenstein LZ, Robbins AS, Josephson KR, Schulman BL, Osterweil D. The value of assessing falls in an elderly population. A randomized clinical trial. *Ann Intern Med.* 1990;113(4):308-316.

Shumway-Cook A, Brauer S, Woollacott M. Predicting the probability for falls in community-dwelling older adults using the Timed Up & Go Test. *Phys Ther.* 2000;80(9):896-903.

Sudarsky L, Ronthal M. Gait disorders among elderly patients. A survey study of 50 patients. *Arch Neurol.* 1983;40(12):740.

Tinetti ME. Performance-oriented assessment of mobility problems in elderly patients. *J Am Geriatr Soc.* 1986;34(2):199-126.

Tinetti ME, Kumar C. The patient who falls. "It's always a trade-off." *JAMA.* 2010;303(3):258-266.

Tinetti ME, Liu WL, Claus EB. Predictors and prognosis of inability to get up after falls among elderly persons. *JAMA.* 1993;269(1):65-70.

Tolea MI, Costa PT Jr, Terracciano A, et al. Associations of openness and conscientiousness with walking speed decline: findings from the Health, Aging, and Body Composition Study. *J Gerontol B Psychol Sci Soc Sci.* 2012;67(6):705-711.

Osteoarthritis

26

C. Kent Kwoh, MD

Yong Gil Hwang, MD

ESSENTIALS OF DIAGNOSIS

- ► History suggests mechanical pain (ie, worse with activity, better with rest).
- ► Examination suggests joint line tenderness and boney enlargement.
- ► Radiographs demonstrate joint space narrowing, osteophytes, sclerosis, and bone cysts.

► General Principles in Older Adults

Osteoarthritis (OA) is the most common disease of the joints and is one of the leading causes of disability among older adults in the United States. Older age is the greatest risk factor for OA; the prevalence of symptomatic knee OA was 12.1% among adults age ≥60 years. OA is a complex disorder with multiple risk factors that range from genetic, demographic, metabolic, and biomechanical factors to congenital or developmental deformities of the joint. The diagnosis is based on history (ie, symptoms of joint pain, often with transient morning stiffness), physical examination (ie, crepitus, bony tenderness and bony enlargement) and characteristic radiographic features (ie, joint space narrowing with osteophytes). The multidisciplinary team approach used in geriatric medicine clearly applies to managing the OA patient. Nonpharmacologic measures are critically important in the management of OA in older adults and include aerobic, aquatic, and/or resistance exercises, as well as weight loss for overweight patients. Patient education and psychosocial support are as important as medical therapy, particularly in older adults. Pain relief is the primary indication for the use of pharmacologic agents in patients with OA who do not respond to nonpharmacologic interventions. Because of its efficacy–toxicity profile,

acetaminophen is often the initial therapy, and nonsteroidal antiinflammatory drugs (NSAIDs) may be prescribed for those who have inadequate response to acetaminophen. Oral NSAIDs should be used with great caution in older adults given the increased risk of side effects, with topical NSAIDs offering a better efficacy–toxicity profile. Other pharmacologic modalities, including tramadol, intraarticular corticosteroid injections, intraarticular hyaluronate injections, duloxetine, and opioids, are conditionally recommended in patients who have had an inadequate response to initial therapy. Surgical interventions are generally reserved for those who have failed medical therapy, and thus have persistent pain and marked limitations in activities of daily living. The natural course and prognosis of OA largely depends on the joints involved, the underlying risk factors, the presence of symptoms, and the severity of the condition. Recent studies show an increased mortality among persons with OA compared with the general population. Therefore, management of older patients with OA should also focus on effective treatment of cardiovascular risk factors and comorbidities, as well as on increasing physical activity.

► Prevention

The best treatment for OA is prevention. However, OA is often diagnosed in its later stages, and there are no proven therapies that can prevent the progression of joint damage caused by OA. Advances in imaging modalities, especially MRI, and innovations in molecular biology have greatly advanced our knowledge of OA, and efforts are ongoing to identify preclinical biochemical and imaging biomarkers that will provide opportunities to diagnose and treat OA earlier so as to prevent further progression of the disease and increased disability.

▶ Clinical Findings

A. Symptoms & Signs

1. Epidemiology of osteoarthritis—OA is the most common type of arthritis that involves the entire joint, characterized by changes in articular cartilage (thinning and fissuring), and associated changes in subchondral bone, synovium, ligaments, joint capsule, and/or periarticular muscles. Symptomatic OA is defined by the presence of frequent pain and radiographic evidence of OA in that joint. The Kellgren-Lawrence scale is often used to characterize the radiographic severity of OA. Furthermore, prevalence of radiographic OA varies by the joint involved and differs considerably depending on the inclusion criteria for radiologic severity for OA. Table 26–1 summarizes the prevalence data from 3 recent U.S. population-based studies (the National Health and Nutritional Examination Surveys [NHANES] III,

the Framingham Osteoarthritis Study, and the Johnston County Osteoarthritis Project). Hand and knee OA is more common among women, especially after age 50 years, and is also more common among African Americans. OA of the hip is more common in individuals of European descent compared to those of Asian or African descent.

2. Health impact—OA is the reason for an estimated 30% of ambulatory care visits and is 1 of the leading causes of disability among older adults in the United States. OA disables approximately 10% of people who are older than age 60 years and compromises the quality of life of more than 20 million Americans. As such, OA costs the United States economy nearly $81 billion per year in direct medical care (eg, physician visits, laboratory tests, medications, surgical procedures), with indirect expenses (eg, lost wages, home care, lost wage-earning opportunities) of an estimated $47 billion per year. Given the aging of the population and increases in the prevalence of major OA risk factors (eg, obesity), the burden of OA is increasing exponentially in both human and economic terms.

3. Risk factors—Epidemiologic studies have revealed several risk factors that may influence the development of OA and its subsequent progression. The influence of these risk factors upon the onset of OA differs considerably depending on the joint involved. As noted above, demographic characteristics, such as advancing age, sex, and race, are directly related to prevalence of OA. Genetic risk factors likely play a role as well, but they are probably polygenic and complex in nature. Potentially modifiable risk factors include obesity and biomechanical factors such as repetitive or isolated traumatic injury, malalignment (varus or valgus deformity), overload, joint instability caused by muscle weakness, and ligamentous laxity. These risk factors are particularly important in weight-bearing joints and may influence incidence more than radiographic progression. After age, obesity is the strongest risk factor for knee OA, particularly in women, and this risk applies across the age spectrum. A significantly elevated prevalence of knee OA from overuse has been demonstrated in farm workers, coal miners and construction workers. Long distance running or recreational activity itself is not related to the incidence of OA, barring the presence of joint injury. Age-related increase in obesity, varus/valgus laxity and decrease in muscle strength, and proprioception may also contribute to the development of OA with age.

4. Pathophysiology—Given the strong relationship of OA to age, OA has long been considered a "wear and tear" degenerative disease, an inevitable consequence of aging. However, OA can be best defined as failed repair of joint damage that has been caused by abnormal intra- and extraarticular processes involving a combination of biomechanical, biochemical, and genetic factors mediated by a variety of pathways, rather than a degenerative process. Microinjury from excessive mechanical stress is likely to contribute to or trigger the

Table 26–1. Prevalence of symptomatic OA.

Anatomic site, age, years	Source (ref.)	Percent (%) with Symptomatic OA		
		Male	Female	Total
Hands, >26	Framingham OA study (6)	3.8	9.2	6.8
71–74		18.2	17.2	
75–79		47.7	39.4	
80–84		20.6	24.9	
≥85		13.6	18.6	
Knees				
>26	Framingham OA study (5)	4.6	4.9	4.9
>45	Framingham OA study (5)	5.9	7.2	6.7
>45	Johnston County OA Project (7)	13.5	18.7	16.7
>60	NHANES III (4)	10	13.6	12.1
Hips, >45	Johnston County OA Project (10)	8.7	9.3	9.2

Symptoms and radiographic changes of OA in the symptomatic joint in the hands, knees, and hips, by age and sex, from 3 recent U.S. population-based studies: the NHANES III, the Framingham Osteoarthritis Study, and the Johnston County Osteoarthritis Project. The Framingham Osteoarthritis Study was a survey of knee and hand OA in 2400 adults age 26 years from suburban Boston, Massachusetts. The Johnston County Osteoarthritis Project was a study of hip and knee OA in 3000 African American and white adults age 45 years in a rural county in North Carolina.

Adapted and reproduced with permission from Lawrence RC, Felson DT, Helmick CG, et al; National Arthritis Data Workgroup. Estimates of the prevalence of arthritis and other rheumatic conditions in the United States. Part II. *Arthritis Rheum.* 2008;58(1):26-35.

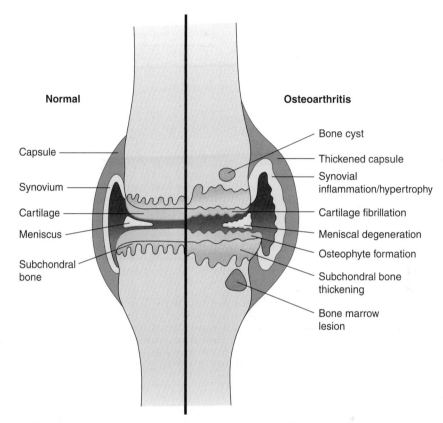

Normal

Capsule

Synovium

Cartilage

Meniscus

Subchondral
bone

Osteoarthritis

Bone cyst

Thickened capsule

Synovial
inflammation/hypertrophy

Cartilage fibrillation

Meniscal degeneration

Osteophyte formation

Subchondral bone
thickening

Bone marrow
lesion

▲ **Figure 26–1.** Pathology of osteoarthritis. The osteoarthritic joint is characterized by degradation and loss of the articular cartilage, thickening of the subchondral bone accompanied by formation of bone marrow lesions and cysts, osteophytes at the joint margins, variable degrees of synovitis with synovial hypertrophy, meniscal degeneration (knee), and thickening of the joint capsule. (Reproduced with permission from Loeser RF. Age-related changes in the musculoskeletal system and the development of osteoarthritis. *Clin Geriatr Med.* 2010;26(3):371-386.)

cascade of events that results in the characteristic pathologic features of OA (Figure 26–1). Further damage of articular cartilage is mediated by proinflammatory cytokines and other catabolic factors, causing collagen and proteoglycan degradation. Age-related changes such as chondrocyte senescence and aging changes in the matrix may contribute to development of OA. There are also age-related periarticular changes such as sarcopenia, causing decreased ability of the bridging muscles to act as internal shock absorbers to absorb the forces transmitted to the subchondral bone and cartilage.

a. Clinical features of OA—The most common symptom of OA is joint pain. Most patients complain of "mechanical" pain, which tends to worsen with activity and be relieved by rest. The onset of the symptoms of OA is usually insidious, beginning in only 1 or a few joints. Patients with hip or knee OA described 2 distinct types of pain: a dull, aching pain, which became more constant over time, and a less frequent

but more intense, often unpredictable pain, which resulted in significant avoidance of social and recreational activities. Any episodic increases in pain and joint swelling should raise suspicion of synovitis caused by crystalline disease, such as gout or pseudogout. With more advanced disease, pain may be noted with progressively less activity, eventually occurring even at rest and at night. The origin of pain in OA is rarely clear and is likely to be heterogeneous. Etiology of pain can be attributed to anatomic changes in the joint, but there are also a number of patient-specific factors that may modify pain perception and pain reporting. Pain is not caused directly by cartilage damage as cartilage is aneural, but subchondral bone, the periosteum, osteophyte, periarticular ligaments, periarticular muscle, synovium, and the joint capsule can all be sources of nociceptive pain in OA as a result of the rich innervation around them. According to a recent systematic review of MRI findings of knee OA, only the presence of bone marrow lesions and synovitis/effusion were significantly associated with the presence of knee pain. Nociceptor pain can become persistent, and persistent pain is often associated with central neurogenic sensitization, thereby establishing a peripherally stimulated, but centrally mediated, chronic pain syndrome. OA can cause morning stiffness, but this typically resolves less than 30 minutes after a patient awakens. Joint stiffness may recur following periods of inactivity, a phenomenon termed *gelling*. Prolonged morning stiffness lasting more than an hour, nighttime pain that keeps the patient from sleeping, and persistent joint swelling should suggest other potential diagnoses such as an inflammatory arthritis. Patients may also report joint locking or joint instability. In addition to chronic pain and disability, sleep disturbance, fatigue and depression are also prominent features of OA in the older population. Physical examination of the patient with OA may reveal joint-line tenderness, crepitus or grating sensation, and osteophytes, particularly in the hands at the distal interphalangeal (DIP) joints and the proximal interphalangeal (PIP) joints. A varying amount of joint effusion and/or soft-tissue swelling can be present, but tends to be intermittent without warmth. As OA progresses, range of joint motion becomes diminished, and joint deformity and/or joint laxity may develop.

b. Classification of OA—Although almost any joint can be involved, OA is often asymmetric and does not affect all joints equally. The joints most commonly affected are the hands, knees, hips, and spine; other joints, such as the shoulder, temporomandibular, sacroiliac, ankle, and elbow, are less commonly involved. OA has been classified as either primary (idiopathic) or secondary to known causes, but, as noted above, there has been much progress in the identification of risk factors for the development of OA. In the past, OA has been considered the prototype of noninflammatory arthritis; however, recent studies show that most types of OA have evidence of synovitis on MRI and/or in pathologic studies. For example, erosive hand OA has marked evidence of synovitis on gadolinium-enhanced MRI. OA has also been classified based on the site of involvement. The term *nodal-generalized OA* is characterized by polyarticular finger involvement (principally DIP and often PIP), OA of the first carpometacarpal (CMC), and a predisposition to OA of the knee, hip, and spine. It is most common in middle-aged women, typically with a strong family history among first-degree relatives and peak onset around the menopause. Patients complain of a symptomatic inflammatory component in the early stage and have mild functional disability in their hands. Their offspring have a significantly younger age of disease onset (both nodal and large joint OA) and often similar or more severe and extensive disease than their parents. Erosive hand OA shows marked subchondral change, a more florid and prolonged inflammatory component, and a tendency to intraarticular osseous fusion and prominent erosive, destructive changes, especially in the finger joints. It has a substantial impact on hand pain and disability. Systemic

Table 26–2. Classification of osteoarthritis.

Primary	Secondary
Nodal generalized OA	Trauma
Erosive OA	Inflammatory arthritis
Large joint OA	Metabolic/Endocrine
• Knee	• Hemochromatosis
• Hip	• Acromegaly
• Shoulder	• Hyperparathyroidism
Spinal OA	• Ochronosis
Inflammatory OA	Crystal deposition disease
Noninflammatory OA	• Calcium pyrophosphate
• Monoarticular	• Uric acid
• Pauciarticular	• Hydroxyapatite
• Polyarticular	Neuropathic disorders
	• Diabetes mellitus
	Anatomical abnormalities
	• Bone dysplasia

inflammatory signs and other typical features of rheumatoid arthritis (RA) (eg, nodules, extraarticular features, rheumatoid factor) are absent. Radiographically, central erosions and the "gull-wing" deformity characterize the disorder.

Certain systemic diseases are associated with the development of "secondary" OA. These include trauma, anatomical abnormalities, metabolic/endocrine disease, postinfectious arthritis, neuropathic disease, and abnormal structure and function of hyaline cartilage (Table 26–2).

5. Characteristics of specific joint involvement

Many of the characteristic clinical manifestations of OA are related to involvement of specific joints.

a. Hand OA—The hands are commonly involved in OA in the population over 50 years of age. The DIP joints and the first CMC joint are commonly affected areas. Enlargement of the first CMC joint can result in a squared appearance to the hand. Prominent palpable osteophytes in the DIPs and the PIPs are known as Heberden nodes and Bouchard's nodes, respectively. Among United States adults aged ≥60, 58% had DIP, 29.9% had PIP, and 18.2% had first carpal-metacarpal deformities. Symptomatic hand OA was associated with self-reported difficulty in lifting 10 lb, dressing and eating. Women and the very old (≥80 years) are especially vulnerable to the effect of hand problems on their daily activities.

b. Knee—Nearly half of adults will develop symptomatic knee OA by age 85 years. Patients with chronic, frequent knee pain most often report localized (69%) knee pain followed by regional (14%) or diffuse (10%) knee pain. Patients with advanced knee OA often experience knee buckling or instability ("giving way"). Of those who experienced buckling, 12.6% fell during an episode. Persons with knee buckling had worse physical function than those without buckling. Common findings of knee OA include crepitus on active motion of the knee, bony tenderness, osteophytes, effusion without palpable warmth, and limitation of range of motion. A joint effusion can lead to flexion of the knee, and synovial fluid may migrate into the semimembranosus bursa posteriorly, creating a fluctuant swelling along the posterior aspect of the knee (ie, popliteal or "Baker's" cyst).

c. Hip—Although anterior or inguinal pain and tenderness typically indicate true involvement of the hip joint, pain from hip OA may be felt in the trochanter, referred to the knee, or along the tensor fascia lata (meralgia paresthetica). Pain around the hip may be caused by pain referred to the hip area from other structures, such as the trochanter bursae, lumbosacral spine, or damaged sciatic nerve. An assessment of the range of motion of the hip and knee joint, tenderness over the greater trochanter (for bursitis), pain in the posterior hip or buttocks (for sciatic nerve damage associated with lumbar radiculopathy) and lower lumbar spine will help determine whether hip pain is referred from these other joint areas. The pain from bursitis is felt laterally and usually does not limit motion. Patients may complain of difficulty walking stairs or lying on their side at night. By comparison, OA of the hip is associated with pain and limited range of motion, particularly with extension and internal rotation. The patient develops a characteristic gait in which they shift weight to the contralateral uninvolved hip (antalgic gait). The extremity shortens as the femoral head migrates superiorly in the acetabulum. Radiographic findings include osteophytes (femoral or acetabular) and joint space narrowing (superior, axial or medial).

d. Spine OA—A continuum of clinical and radiologic findings including intervertebral disc narrowing, osteophytes arising from the margins of the vertebral body, and facet joint changes is often termed degenerative disease of the spine ("spondylosis"). Radiographic evidence of degenerative disease in the spine is almost universal in older people, but the correlation with the presence and severity of pain is very poor. Cervical spondylosis can cause neck pain, occipital headaches, upper extremity radicular pain, shoulder pain, and loss of dexterity of hands. In the cervical spine, although not common, large osteophytes may compromise the spinal canal, causing lower-extremity spasticity and gait disturbance. Anterior cervical osteophytes can impair movement, often related to diffuse idiopathic skeletal hyperostosis (DISH), and can cause pharyngeal stage dysphagia in older adults. Discogenic pain by disc herniation into the spinal canal or into the foramen is often characterized by low back and referred buttock/posterior thigh pain (radicular pain), aggravated by movement and sitting. Pain from facet joint OA is often aggravated by extension of the spine. Lumbar facet joint osteophytes can lead to lumbar canal stenosis from facet enlargement encroaching into the intervertebral foramina and/or spinal canal. The symptoms of spinal stenosis are often relieved by bending slightly forward, since the spinal canal dimensions increase in this position. Spinal stenosis can be related to neurogenic claudication, a pain in the legs or buttocks that worsens with prolonged standing and is relieved by sitting. Spondylolisthesis, a slipping of one vertebral body on another, is often associated with aching in the back and posterior thighs after standing. Nocturnal spine pain should raise concerns about a more ominous process, such as a malignancy. Osteoporosis-related compression fracture should be considered for the sudden onset of severe back pain.

▶ Differential Diagnosis

The clinical diagnosis of OA is based on history, physical examination, and, sometimes, characteristic radiographic features. Before making a clinical diagnosis of OA in older adults, other disorders should be excluded, as physical or radiographic finding of OA is quite common in older adults without accompanying symptoms. When an older patient presents with less-typical features or has unusual joint involvement, confirming the presence of OA unequivocally can be particularly difficult. The physician must distinguish OA from referred pain, other inflammatory joint diseases such as RA, gout or pseudogout (ie, calcium pyrophosphate disease [CPPD]), and soft-tissue processes such as periarticular bursitis (eg, pes anserine bursitis mimicking knee OA, greater trochanteric bursitis simulating hip OA). Such patients will benefit from imaging studies of affected joints in combination with selected laboratory tests, although most patients do not need imaging studies for the diagnosis of OA. The characteristic radiographic features of OA include joint space narrowing, subchondral sclerosis, osteophytes, subchondral cysts, and altered bone contours. The presence of articular cartilage calcification (chondrocalcinosis) may be a clue to the presence of CPPD or secondary OA from an endocrine, metabolic, or heritable disorder that predisposes OA. Ultrasonography may be useful to demonstrate underlying inflammatory process such as synovitis or bursitis. Laboratory studies are not helpful in diagnosing OA, but may be required to help rule out other disorders (eg, gout, RA, or septic arthritis) or to diagnose an underlying disorder causing secondary OA, particularly among those with knee, hip, or atypical joint involvement. Inflammatory markers, such as erythrocyte sedimentation rate (ESR) and C-reactive protein (CRP) level, and immunologic tests, such as antinuclear antibodies and rheumatoid factor, should not be ordered routinely in older adults unless there are signs and symptoms of inflammatory arthritis or systemic autoimmune diseases. A uric acid level is recommended only if gout is suspected. Because these immunologic tests or serum urate levels often yield false-positive results in older adults, performing them may only add unnecessary diagnostic confusion when the pretest probability is low. When a patient presents with acute joint pain with synovial effusion, joint aspiration and synovial fluid analysis should be performed to rule out infectious etiology or crystalline disease. Synovial fluid findings in OA

Table 26–3. Summary of American College of Rheumatology 2012 recommendations for the use of nonpharmacologic and pharmacologic therapies in osteoarthritis of the hand, hip, and knee.

	Nonpharmacologic Recommendations	Pharmacologic Recommendations
Strong	Cardiovascular (aerobic) and/or resistance land-based exercise Aquatic exercise Lose weight in case of overweight	No strong recommendations were made for the initial pharmacologic management of knee OA[a]
Conditional	Self-management programs Manual therapy in combination with supervised exercise Psychosocial interventions Medially directed patellar taping[c] Medially wedged insoles in case of lateral compartment OA[c] Laterally wedged subtalar strapped insoles in case of medial compartment OA[c] Thermal agents[c] Walking aids, as needed Tai chi programs Traditional Chinese acupuncture[a] Transcutaneous electrical stimulation[a]	Acetaminophen Oral NSAIDs Topical NSAIDs Tramadol Intraarticular corticosteroid injections[a] Topical capsaicin[b] Conditionally not recommended: Chondroitin sulfate Glucosamine
No recommendations	Balance exercises, either alone or in combination with strengthening exercises Laterally wedged insoles Manual therapy alone Knee braces Laterally directed patellar taping	Intraarticular hyaluronates, duloxetine, and opioid analgesics

A strong recommendation for using a modality required high-quality evidence and evidence of a large gradient of difference between desirable and undesirable effects of the treatment. A conditional recommendation for using a modality was based on absence of high-quality evidence and/or evidence of only a small gradient of difference between desirable and undesirable effects of the treatment. The lack of data from appropriate randomized controlled trials resulted in either not making a recommendation or making a recommendation not to use a modality, depending on the harms of the modality in other conditions and/or the values and preferences of Technical Expert Panel members.

[a]Intraarticular corticosteroid injections conditionally recommended for knee/hip OA, conditionally not recommended for hand OA.
[b]Topical capsaicin conditionally recommended for hand OA only, conditionally not recommended for knee OA.
[c]Conditionally recommended only for knee OA.

Adapted and reproduced with permission from Hochberg MC, Altman RD, April KT, et al; American College of Rheumatology. American College of Rheumatology 2012 recommendations for the use of nonpharmacologic and pharmacologic therapies in osteoarthritis of the hand, hip, and knee. *Arthritis Care Res (Hoboken)*. 2012;64(4):455-474.

usually suggest a minimally inflammatory (white blood cell count <2000/mm³) or noninflammatory process. A number of biochemical markers are under investigation to help with diagnosis and to determine risk of progression or response to therapy.

▶ **Treatment**

A. Goals of Treatment

Patients with OA seek medical attention because of pain. In addition to pain, OA is accompanied by structural changes not only within the joint, including cartilage loss and formation of osteophytes, but also changes in muscle, bone, tendons, ligaments, menisci, synovium, and the joint capsule. These changes result in altered joint mechanics and muscle weakness, causing decreased physical function and disability.

Therefore, functional improvement is as important as pain management in OA, particularly in the geriatric population. The multidisciplinary team approach often used in geriatric medicine clearly applies to managing the OA patient. The Osteoarthritis Research Society International (OARSI) and European League Against Rheumatism (EULAR) have developed guidelines for the management of OA of the hand, hip, or knee. Table 26–3 summarizes the most recent American College of Rheumatology (ACR) guidelines on the treatment of OA.

B. Nonpharmacologic Therapy

The nonpharmacologic program is critically important and needs to become a part of an OA patient's lifestyle. It should be used prior to or in conjunction with pharmacologic treatments. Nonpharmacologic modalities strongly recommended for the management of knee OA include aerobic, aquatic, and/or resistance exercises, as well as weight loss for overweight patients.

1. Exercise—Exercise is integral in reducing impairment, improving function, and preventing disability. A systematic review and meta-analysis for exercise therapy and OA of the hip or knee concluded that strength training or aerobic exercise regimens for patients with OA led to improved physical health and symptoms of OA. There was no significant difference in terms of reducing arthritis-related symptoms and disability in OA patients between aerobic and resistance training. For patients with advanced OA, range of motion and isometric strengthening exercise can initially be prescribed, and an exercise regimen may progress sequentially through isotonic strengthening, aerobic exercises, and, ultimately, to recreational exercise. Extra attention is needed for the older patient to enhance both safety and compliance with an exercise program; indeed, interventions such as supervised or individualized exercise therapy and self-management techniques may enhance exercise adherence. Tai Chi exercises specifically designed for patients with arthritis may also offer some symptomatic relief and are conditionally recommended by the ACR. Water exercises are of value for those with severe arthritis and marked deconditioning. In addition, elliptical training, cycling, and upper body exercise may help in such cases.

2. Weight loss—A 2007 meta-analysis of weight reduction and knee OA showed that physical disability diminished after a moderate weight reduction regime, with weight loss of >5% from the baseline to be achieved within a 20-week period; that is, 0.25% per week. In addition, pain and physical disability were reduced if the patient lost more than 6 kg (13.2 lb). The combination of diet and modest exercise in older adults with knee OA has been known to be most effective in weight control. However, weight loss in the overweight, inactive older patient is a particular problem as weight loss without exercise can cause inadvertent decrease in muscle mass (sarcopenia).

3. Other nonpharmacologic modalities—Other nonpharmacologic modalities conditionally recommended for knee OA include medial wedge insoles for valgus knee OA, subtalar strapped lateral insoles for varus knee OA, medially directed patellar taping, manual therapy, walking aids, thermal agents, self- management programs, and psychosocial interventions. Knee bracing was recommended by EULAR, but ACR has no recommendation because of conflicting data on efficacy. Patients may benefit from using a cane in one hand for OA of the contralateral hip or knee, but it needs to be properly fitted (ie, when standing, the elbow should be bent to approximately 20 degrees). When disability is more severe, a walker may be needed to maintain function. Physiotherapeutic measures include therapeutic ultrasound, manual therapy, application of heat and/or cold modalities, stretching/traction, and transcutaneous electrical nerve

stimulation (TENS). Patient education and psychosocial support are as important as medical therapy, particularly in older adults. The patient needs to be educated on the nature of OA and its impact on their physical activity. Therapeutic options and the risks and benefits of the different approaches to management should be provided in depth. The initial patient evaluation should include an assessment of symptoms of depression and specific coping strategies that may limit future compliance to therapeutic recommendations. Lifestyle modifications are an integral part of the nonpharmacologic program. A patient with lumbar spine, hip, or knee OA should avoid deep chairs and recliners from which posture is poor and rising is difficult. Resting the affected joint can ease pain short-term, but prolonged rest may lead to muscle atrophy and decreased joint mobility.

C. Pharmacologic Therapy

Pharmacologic therapy is added when the nonpharmacologic program does not provide adequate relief of pain. Pharmacologic modalities conditionally recommended for the initial management of patients with knee OA include acetaminophen, oral and topical NSAIDs, tramadol, intraarticular corticosteroid injections, intraarticular hyaluronate injections, and duloxetine. Opioids were conditionally recommended in patients who had an inadequate response to initial therapy, but opioids should be used with caution in older adults.

1. Analgesics—Acetaminophen is the initial therapy for mild OA because it is inexpensive, relatively safe, and effective. Although most patients have tried acetaminophen prior to visiting the physician, they rarely have tried the maximum recommended dose (4 g/day). It is important to review the patient's medications exhaustively, including combination products with opioid analgesics and nonprescription medications, when the physician considers initiating acetaminophen in the full dosage. Hepatotoxicity can occur, but, at the therapeutic range, is primarily seen mainly in patients with concurrent alcohol abuse or in conjunction with other hepatotoxic medications. In OA subjects with moderate-to-severe levels of pain, NSAIDs appear to be more effective than acetaminophen. When acetaminophen fails to control symptoms, the use of NSAIDs or intraarticular corticosteroid injections is recommended. There is no convincing evidence that any of the available NSAIDs is more effective than any other for OA of the knee or hip, and patients' responses to the different agents in terms of both efficacy and toxicity are unpredictable. Thus, low-cost products with a short half-life, such as ibuprofen or naproxen, may be an appropriate initial choice. If 2 to 4 weeks of low-dose therapy does not yield adequate control of pain, the dose should be gradually increased toward the maximum of that medication, taking into account the patient's other comorbid conditions. Patients should be well informed of adverse effects, including peptic ulcer, gastrointestinal bleeding, renal dysfunction, edema, abnormal liver function tests, elevated blood pressure, and the potential cardiovascular risk when the therapy is initiated. Presence of multiple comorbidities and the risk of NSAID-associated gastrointestinal (GI) side effects limit their use in older patients, those on aspirin or anticoagulants, and those on concomitant use of glucocorticoids. The risk of GI side effects is greatest in the first month of use. Central nervous system dysfunction in older adults can occur even with the standard dosages, particularly with indomethacin. Nephrotoxicity is more likely to occur in patients with preexisting diabetes mellitus, congestive heart failure, liver cirrhosis, diuretic therapy, or chronic kidney disease while using an NSAID. The nonacetylated salicylates, sulindac, and nabumetone appear to be less toxic to the kidney. Short-acting NSAIDs, such as ibuprofen, interfere with the desirable antiplatelet effects of low-dose aspirin and should not be administered within 3 hours of aspirin. The risk of GI bleeding can be lessened by use of a cyclooxygenase-2 selective inhibitors (eg, celecoxib or meloxicam) or concomitant use of a proton pump inhibitor or misoprostol. However, gastroprotective agents are not protective below the ligament of Treitz and lower GI bleeding risk, which is common with NSAID use in older adults, remains high even with use of these agents. The potential reduction in GI risks cannot justify the use of cyclooxygenase inhibitors as an initial agent, given concerns about the increased risk of cardiovascular events and their cost. Furthermore, in the presence of low-dose aspirin, reduction of GI adverse effects may not be maintained. Topical NSAIDs use is also conditionally recommended for the hip or knee OA. Topical NSAIDs are safer but may be less efficacious than oral NSAIDs. Topical capsaicin or other salicylate-containing topical agents (eg, trolamine salicylate, hydroxyethylsalicylate, diethylamine salicylate) can relieve OA pain. ACR guidelines supports the use of topical capsaicin only for hand OA. Tramadol is a dual-acting weak mu-receptor inhibitor with serotonin reuptake inhibition. It has been shown to have an additive effect with acetaminophen. Side effects of tramadol include nausea, vomiting, lightheadedness, dizziness or headache. Because of frequent central nervous system-induced side effects in older people, the initial dose should be lowered, or avoided if possible, in the geriatric population. Although the ACR and EULAR guidelines on treatment of knee OA support the use of opioids when other treatments have failed or are not appropriate, they are poorly tolerated in older patients because of increased sensitivity to adverse side effects, particularly sedation, confusion, and constipation. The lowest dose of opioids should be used, whenever possible. Increased risk of falls from opioids use is of great concern for those who are already vulnerable to falls as a result of underlying joint failure. Opioid analgesics may be beneficial in older patients who were either not willing to undergo or had contraindications for total joint arthroplasty after having failed all other nonpharmacologic and pharmacologic therapies. Oral administration of a serotonin and norepinephrine reuptake inhibitor (eg, duloxetine) shows promise in the treatment of OA.

Intraarticular glucocorticoid injections help to relieve pain and increase joint flexibility for variable periods of time. They may be of greater value when synovial effusions or signs of inflammation are present and in patients with 1 or a few joints that are painful despite the use of an NSAID. Intraarticular glucocorticoid injections are recommended to be limited to less than 5 times a year in any given joint. With proper use of aseptic technique, septic arthritis is a very rare complication. Steroid injections should be used with caution in diabetic patients. Hip joint injection requires ultrasonographic or fluoroscopic guidance, and efficacy of glucocorticoid injections at sites other than the knee or hip is less certain. Hyaluronic acid is a simple, conserved long-chain high-molecular-weight disaccharide that is a natural secretion of the synovium in a normal joint. However, hyaluronic acid in the joints of OA patients is most often of low molecular weight, losing its biomechanical and antiinflammatory properties. Intraarticular injection of moderate to high-molecular-weight hyaluronan preparations, also known as viscosupplementation, are widely used to treat OA of the knee, but there is still some uncertainty about whether the injections are superior to placebo, oral NSAIDs, or intraarticular glucocorticoids. Significant pain reduction is often not achieved until weeks following the initial injection. The injections are generally well tolerated but there is a risk of postinjection reactive inflammatory synovitis and a small risk of joint infection.

2. Nutraceuticals—Nutraceuticals are natural substances used to promote health and prevent disease. There are several nutraceuticals that are used for treatment of OA. The use of glucosamine and chondroitin for OA has been controversial, and results of randomized trials have varied. The balance of evidence from high-quality trials has shown little to no evidence of clinically meaningful benefit. ACR experts conditionally recommend that patients with knee or hip OA should not use the chondroitin sulfate or glucosamine. Other nutraceuticals that have been tried in the management of OA include flavocoxid, S-adenosylmethionine (SAM-e), Boswellia, collagen hydrolysate, Avocado-soybean, curcuma (tumeric), ginger, and evening primrose oil, but each of these have very limited evidence of efficacy.

3. Other agents—Colchicine has been tried in patients who have inflammatory OA that is refractory to NSAIDs and/or intraarticular glucocorticoids and who have evidence of CPPD crystals. Hydroxychloroquine has also been tried anecdotally in patients with inflammatory or erosive OA that has been unresponsive to NSAIDs.

D. Complementary and Alternative Treatment

Acupuncture is conditionally recommended only for patients with refractory symptoms who desire nontraditional therapies or who cannot undergo surgical interventions. According to a recent meta-analysis on the effectiveness of acupuncture for OA of the knee, acupuncture seems to provide improvement in function and pain relief as an adjunctive therapy for OA of the knee when compared with credible sham acupuncture and education control groups.

Recommendations for hip OA are similar to those for the management of knee OA.

Modalities conditionally recommended for the management of hand OA include instruction in joint protection techniques, provision of assistive devices, use of thermal modalities and trapeziometacarpal joint splints, and use of oral and topical NSAIDs, tramadol, and topical capsaicin.

E. Surgery

1. Arthroscopic surgery—Randomized trials have shown that arthroscopic surgery is no better than placebo for symptomatic benefit in knee OA. Recent epidemiologic studies have shown that meniscal damage is common in individuals with knee OA and may often be asymptomatic. Meniscectomy for traumatic injuries is associated with increased risk of developing knee OA. Therefore, the benefits of partial meniscectomy in knee OA is also unclear.

2. Total joint arthroplasty—Although there are no clear criteria for surgical indication, surgical interventions are generally reserved for individuals with severe symptomatic OA who have marked limitations in function, such as performing the activities of daily living, and who have failed nonpharmacologic and pharmacologic therapies. Potential surgical candidates should have had an adequate trial of exercise and physical therapy. The primary goals of joint replacement are pain relief and functional improvement. Total joint arthroplasty is usually selected for OA of the hip, knee, and shoulder, and arthrodesis (fusion) is usually preferred for the wrist, ankle, and first metatarsophalangeal (MTP) joint. Hemiarthroplasty may be beneficial in joint replacement surgery for hip and knee OA and is successful in all age groups, showing excellent outcomes, even in the presence of obesity; however, there is an increased risk of mortality in older adults, and older age is related to worse function, particularly in women. In selected patients, corrective osteotomy and joint resurfacing can be considered instead of total arthroplasty. Various surgical interventions have been used to treat pain and dysfunction arising from OA at the base of the thumb (CMC or trapeziometacarpal joint OA). Patients who fail to respond to more conservative treatment may be candidates for trapeziectomy or CMC joint replacement.

▶ Prognosis

The natural course and prognosis of OA largely depends on the joints involved, underlying risk factors, presence of symptoms, and the severity of the condition. OA is generally slowly progressive but stable, responding well to medical management. A subset of patients, however, follows a progressive trajectory and eventually requires surgical therapy.

There are several factors associated with relatively rapid progression of disease, but risk factors for progression vary according to the joints involved. There are no FDA-approved disease-modifying drugs for OA, and current therapeutics mainly focus on relief of pain and functional improvement. Although a multidisciplinary approach and joint replacement surgery have altered the severity of OA's impact, patients with OA still experience varying degrees of physical disability. A coping strategy of pain avoidance with limitation of activity may play a role in causing muscle weakness and joint instability and thus, contribute to physical disability. Therefore, patient education and psychosocial support are as important as medical therapy, particularly in older adults, to prevent disability. Recent studies have shown moderate evidence of increased mortality among persons with OA compared with the general population. History of diabetes, cancer, or cardiovascular disease, and the presence of walking disability were major risk factors for premature mortality. Possible explanations for the excess mortality include reduced levels of physical activity among persons with OA as a result of involvement of lower-limb joints and presence of comorbid conditions, as well as adverse effects of medications used to treat symptomatic OA, particularly NSAIDs. Therefore, management of patients with OA and walking disability should focus on effective treatment of cardiovascular risk factors and comorbidities, as well as on increasing physical activity.

Altman RD. Early management of osteoarthritis. *Am J Manag Care.* 2010;16 Suppl Management:S41-S47.

Altman RD. Osteoarthritis in the elderly population. In Nakasato Y, Yung RL, eds. *Geriatric Rheumatology: A Comprehensive Approach.* 1st ed. New York, NY: Springer Publishing; 2011:187-196.

Anderson AS, Loeser RF. Why is osteoarthritis an age-related disease? *Best Pract Res Clin Rheumatol.* 2010;24(1):15-26.

Brouwer RW, Raaij van TM, Bierma-Zeinstra SM, Verhagen AP, Jakma TS, Verhaar JA. Osteotomy for treating knee osteoarthritis. *Cochrane Database Syst Rev.* 2007;(3):CD004019.

Buckwalter JA, Saltzman C, Brown T. The impact of osteoarthritis: implications for research. *Clin Orthop Relat Res.* 2004;(427 Suppl):S6-15.

Cooper C, Snow S, McAlindon TE, et al. Risk factors for the incidence and progression of radiographic knee osteoarthritis. *Arthritis Rheum.* 2000;43(5):995-1000.

Dziedzic K, Thomas E, Hill S, Wilkie R, Peat G, Croft PR. The impact of musculoskeletal hand problems in older adults: findings from the North Staffordshire Osteoarthritis Project (NorStOP). *Rheumatology (Oxford).* 2007;46(6):963-967.

Ehrlich GE. Erosive osteoarthritis: presentation, clinical pearls, and therapy. *Curr Rheumatol Rep.* 2001;3(6):484-488.

Felson DT, Niu J, McClennan C, et al. Knee buckling: prevalence, risk factors, and associated limitations in function. *Ann Intern Med.* 2007;147(8):534-540.

Felson DT, Niu J, Clancy M, Sack B, Aliabadi P, Zhang Y. Effect of recreational physical activities on the development of knee osteoarthritis in older adults of different weights: the Framingham Study. *Arthritis Rheum.* 2007;57(1):6-12.

Fitzcharles MA, Shir Y. New concepts in rheumatic pain. *Rheum Dis Clin North Am.* 2008;34(2):267-283.

Hart LE, Haaland DA, Baribeau DA, Mukovozov IM, Sabljic TF. The relationship between exercise and osteoarthritis in the elderly. *Clin J Sport Med.* 2008;18(6):508-521.

Hochberg MC. Prognosis of osteoarthritis. *Ann Rheum Dis.* 1996;55(9):685-688.

Hochberg MC. Mortality in osteoarthritis. *Clin Exp Rheumatol.* 2008;26(5 Suppl 51):S120-S124.

Hochberg MC, Altman RD, April KT, et al; American College of Rheumatology. American College of Rheumatology 2012 recommendations for the use of nonpharmacologic and pharmacologic therapies in osteoarthritis of the hand, hip, and knee. *Arthritis Care Res (Hoboken).* 2012;64(4): 455-474.

Kirwan JR, Elson CJ. Is the progression of osteoarthritis phasic? Evidence and implications. *J Rheumatol.* 2000;27(4): 834-836.

Lawrence RC, Felson DT, Helmick CG, et al. Estimates of the prevalence of arthritis and other rheumatic conditions in the United States. Part II. *Arthritis Rheum.* 2008;58(1):26-35.

Loeser RF. Aging and osteoarthritis. *Curr Opin Rheumatol.* 2011;23(5):492-496.

Loeser RF. Age-related changes in the musculoskeletal system and the development of osteoarthritis. *Clin Geriatr Med.* 2010;26(3):371-386.

Loeser RF Jr. Aging and the etiopathogenesis and treatment of osteoarthritis. *Rheum Dis Clin North Am.* 2000;26(3):547-567.

Loeser RF, Goldring SR, Scanzello CR, Goldring MB. Osteoarthritis: a disease of the joint as an organ. *Arthritis Rheum.* 2012;64(6):1697-1707.

Manheimer E, Linde K, Lao L, Bouter LM, Berman BM. Meta-analysis: acupuncture for osteoarthritis of the knee. *Ann Intern Med.* 2007;146(12):868-877.

McAlindon TE, Wilson PW, Aliabadi P, Weissman B, Felson DT. Level of physical activity and the risk of radiographic and symptomatic knee osteoarthritis in the elderly: the Framingham study. *Am J Med.* 1999;106(2):151-157.

Messier SP, Loeser RF, Miller GD, et al. Exercise and dietary weight loss in overweight and obese older adults with knee osteoarthritis: the Arthritis, Diet, and Activity Promotion Trial. *Arthritis Rheum.* 2004;50(5):1501-1510.

Nuesch E, Dieppe P, Reichenbach S, Williams S, Iff S, Juni P. All cause and disease specific mortality in patients with knee or hip osteoarthritis: population based cohort study. *BMJ.* 2011;342:d1165.

Sale JE, Gignac M, Hawker G. The relationship between disease symptoms, life events, coping and treatment, and depression among older adults with osteoarthritis. *J Rheumatol.* 2008;35(2):335-342.

Sinusas K. Osteoarthritis: diagnosis and treatment. *Am Fam Physician.* 2012;85(1):49-56.

Towheed TE, Maxwell L, Judd MG, Catton M, Hochberg MC, Wells G. Acetaminophen for osteoarthritis. *Cochrane Database Syst Rev.* 2006;(1):CD004257.

van Baar ME, Assendelft WJ, Dekker J, Oostendorp RA, Bijlsma JW. Effectiveness of exercise therapy in patients with osteoarthritis of the hip or knee: a systematic review of randomized clinical trials. *Arthritis Rheum.* 1999;42(7):1361-1369.

van Gerwen M, Shaerf DA, Veen RM. Hip resurfacing arthroplasty. *Acta Orthop.* 2010;81(6):680-683.

Zhang W, Moskowitz RW, Nuki G, et al. OARSI recommendations for the management of hip and knee osteoarthritis, part II: OARSI evidence-based, expert consensus guidelines. *Osteoarthritis Cartilage.* 2008;16(2):137-162.

Zhang Y, Niu J, Kelly-Hayes M, Chaisson CE, Aliabadi P, Felson DT. Prevalence of symptomatic hand osteoarthritis and its impact on functional status among the elderly: The Framingham Study. *Am J Epidemiol.* 2002;156(11):1021-1027.

Osteoporosis & Hip Fractures

27

Rubina A. Malik, MD, MSc

ESSENTIALS OF DIAGNOSIS

▶ Osteoporosis is a systemic skeletal disease characterized by low bone mass and microarchitectural deterioration of the bone tissue, with a consequent increase in bone fragility and susceptibility to fracture.

▶ Osteoporosis is more common in women than in men, although the incidence among men is increasing.

▶ The prevalence of osteoporosis and osteoporotic fractures increases with age.

▶ General Principles in Older Adults

Osteoporosis is a skeletal disorder characterized by compromised bone strength, resulting in bone fragility and susceptibility to fractures. Bone strength is a function of bone mineral density (BMD) and bone quality. Bone quality refers to the architecture, bone turnover, damage accumulation, and mineralization occurring at the bony matrix. Bone mass is assessed with the use of bone density measurements; ie, dual x-ray absorptiometry (DXA), but currently there is no way to measure bone quality in a quantitative and comparable way.

Osteoporosis is a disease with its origin in childhood. Although genetic factors primarily account for peak bone mass, environmental factors such as nutrition and exercise can alter the genetically determined pattern of skeletal growth. At present, not enough is known about the genetics of osteoporosis to influence clinical decision making. However, it is known that illness and medications during a person's lifetime can impact the accrual of peak mass such that individuals start at a lower peak bone mass. Modulation of peak bone mass can even occur during intrauterine life and is affected by maternal nutrition, smoking, and level of exercise. During adulthood, bone tends to have a steady

state of formation and resorption with a stable bone mass. For women, menopause marks the start of increased bone resorption. For most older adults bone resorption exceeds bone formation, with acceleration of the process caused by medical illness and medications.

Older adults are particularly susceptible to the adverse outcomes attributed to osteoporosis. Comorobidities, such as cognitive and gait impairments, which are more prevalent as a patient gets older, predisposes the individual to falls and the development of fragility fractures.

According to the National Osteoporosis Foundation, the United States has some 52 million individuals with low bone mass: 9 million with osteoporosis and 43 million with osteopenia. The prevalence of osteoporosis and osteopenia increases with age for both men and women. With the growth in the geriatric population as a consequence of the coming of age of the baby boomers, the prevalence of osteoporosis and fractures is expected to increase exponentially.

An estimated 1.5 million fragility fractures occur in the United States each year. Approximately 50% of women and 20% of men older than age 50 years will have a fragility fracture in their remaining lifetime, with potentially devastating results. In general, osteoporotic fragility fractures involve the hip, vertebral, and wrist fractures. However, the effect of osteoporosis on the skeleton is systemic and there is an increased risk of almost all types of fractures in patients with low bone mass. It is estimated that the annual U.S. health care cost of fractures is approximately $20 billion, most of it attributed to acute care hospitalization followed by subacute rehabilitation. Although the overall prevalence of fragility fractures is higher in women, men generally have a higher rate of fracture-related mortality because of associated comorbidities. Even though vertebral fractures are the most prevalent of all fragility fractures, hip fractures contribute more to significant health care expenditure and are associated with the most serious outcomes.

Pathogenesis

Primary osteoporosis defines bone loss associated with the normal aging process; this occurs in both men and women. At the cellular level osteoblasts and osteoclasts work synergistically at a bone resorption pit to maintain bone homeostasis. Many proteins and hormones have been implicated in the pathogenesis including estrogen, vitamin D, and parathyroid hormone (PTH), all of which either increase bone resorption or reduce bone formation, such that the bone remodeling unit in a patient with osteoporosis has incomplete filling of the resorption pits. The primary regulator of bone remodeling is now recognized to be the receptor activator of nuclear factor kappa-B ligand (RANKL) produced by osteoblasts. RANKL binds to RANK receptors on osteoclast precursors and induces maturation as well as activity. Osteoblasts also produce osteoprotegerin (OPG) which blocks RANKL, thereby inhibiting osteoclast activity and maintaining bone homeostasis. This bone remodeling process serves to maintain calcium balance and to repair damage at the bony matrix.

Secondary osteoporosis is bone loss caused by a variety of diseases, conditions, or drugs. In the ambulatory and nursing home geriatric population, secondary hyperparathyroidism (caused by vitamin D deficiency) accounts for approximately 20% of secondary causes. With age there is decreased absorption of intestinal calcium and decreased renal calcium conservation, with a resultant increase in bone resorption as a result of increased PTH; thus calcium and vitamin D must be replaced aggressive in older adults. In 50–60% of men with osteoporosis, there is often a secondary cause—such as hypogonadal states during adolescence or adulthood; or the use of steroids or alcohol. Fifty percent of perimenopausal women also have secondary causes attributed to hypogonadal states or the use of medications such as steriods, thyroid therapy or anticonvulsant therapy.

Clinical Findings

A. Symptoms & Signs

Osteoporosis is generally a silent disease with no clinical manifestations until there is a fracture. Risk factors, the FRAX algorithm, a physical exam assessment, laboratory assessment, and imaging can potentially identify a patient who is at risk for osteoporosis.

1. Risk factors—Several important common clinical risk factors for osteoporosis and falls have been identified through epidemiologic studies and indicate how closely each of the entities are codependent (Table 27–1). Approximately 95% of hip fractures are caused by falls and so risk factors for falls have to be considered.

2. Fracture risk assessment tool—The FRAX algorithm, a fracture risk assessment tool developed by the World Health Organization, uses some of the above clinical risk factors,

Table 27–1. Risk factors.

Osteoporosis/Fracture	Falls
Women >65 years of age	Advanced age
Men >70 years of age	Dementia
White or Asian race	Previous falls
Low body weight (<127 lb or body mass index <20)	Low body weight
Family history of osteoporosis[a]	Low muscle strength
Personal history of fragility fracture[a]	Poor nutrition
Fragility fracture in first-degree relative	Polypharmacy
Long-term use of glucocorticoids	Use of long-acting benzodiazepines
Alcohol >2-3 drinks per day[a]	Poor vision
Estrogen deficiency <45 years	Self-rated poor health
Testosterone deficiency	Difficulty in rising out of chair
Low calcium intake	Resting tachycardia
Vitamin D deficiency	Vitamin D deficiency
Sedentary lifestyle	Sedentary lifestyle
Current tobacco use[a]	

[a]Nine validated risk factors for fracture—age; sex; personal history of fracture; low body mass index; use of oral glucocorticoid therapy; osteoporosis secondary to another condition; parental history of hip fracture; current smoking; and alcohol intake of 3 or more drinks per day—are used in the FRAX algorithm.

BMD measurements, and country-specific fracture data to calculate a patient's 10-year probability of a fragility fracture. FRAX was developed to be applicable to both postmenopausal women and men ages 40 to 90 years. It is validated to be used in untreated patients only. The algorithm is accessible online for physicians to use in a primary care setting at www.sheffield.ac.uk/FRAX. The National Osteoporosis Foundation Clinician's Guide recommends treating patients when they have a FRAX 10-year probability of hip fracture ≥3% or a 10-year probability of other major osteoporosis-related fracture ≥20%.

A literature review by Green and colleagues found no single physical examination finding or combination of findings sufficient to rule in osteoporosis or spinal fracture without further testing. Several examination findings including low body weight (<51 kg), inability to place the back of the head against a wall when standing upright, low tooth count (<20 count), self-reported humped back, and rib–pelvis distance ≤2 fingerbreadths can significantly increase the likelihood of osteoporosis or spinal fracture and identify additional women who would benefit from earlier screening. Height loss resulting from vertebral compression fractures can be measured in the clinic over time or using the patient's recalled maximal adult height, can be potentially useful tool but the studies were not all in agreement as to its predictive value. Nevertheless, most experts would agree that a loss of height >3 cm should warrant further testing such as a lateral spine film or DXA scan.

Other pertinent physical exam findings should focus on secondary causes of osteoporosis, which will depend on the clinical history and identified risk factors. In the geriatric population, a comprehensive review of all used medications is essential.

B. Imaging Studies

Imaging studies are critical in osteoporosis not only to identify patients at risk, but also to monitor the effect of pharmacotherapy.

1. Chest and bone radiographs—Osteoporosis is most commonly diagnosed by simple radiographs but the bone loss has to be >30% in order to be detected. The main radiographic features are radiolucency, cortical thinning, and occult fractures. Vertebral fractures are frequently asymptomatic and may easily be missed on radiographs that are obtained for other indications. Many studies have noted that vertebral fractures are inadequately reported and thus few of these patients receive appropriate osteoporosis-specific pharmacotherapy. Also during the past decade a number of publications have identified insufficiency fractures, especially at the medial femoral condyle of the knee and femoral head, which are frequent findings in older individuals and indicate increased fragility of the skeleton.

Patients on antiresorptive therapy who complain of bone pain should have radiographs of the affected site. Recently atypical subtrochanteric and femoral shaft fractures have been identified in older individuals and associated with long-term bisphosphonate therapy. These fractures have typical features that help to identify them, including location in the subtrochanteric region and femoral shaft, transverse or short oblique orientation, minimal or no associated trauma, a medial spike when the fracture is complete, absence of comminution, cortical thickening, and a periosteal reaction of the lateral cortex.

2. Dual x-ray absorptiometry—DXA measurement remains the gold standard to determine bone density, estimate fracture risk, identify candidates for intervention, and to assess changes in bone mass over time in treated and untreated patients. DXA is indicated in women age 65 years and older, as well as in younger and perimenopausal women with risk factors for fragility fractures. Medicare covers the cost in all older women (>65 years) for initial diagnosis and for follow-up after 2 years.

The International Society of Clinical Densitometry (ISCD) recommends BMD testing in all men age 70 years and older, and in men younger than age 70 years with clinical risk factors for fracture, including a prior history of a fragility fracture, a disease or condition associated with low bone mass or bone loss, and if taking medications associated with low bone mass or bone loss. The American College of Physicians (ACP) recommends that clinicians periodically perform assessment of risk factors for osteoporosis in older men, and that clinicians obtain DXA scans for men who are at increased risk for osteoporosis and are candidates for drug therapy.

The routine DXA examination includes results for the hip, spine, and wrist; BMD measurement at central sites (spine and hip); and provides reproducible values at important sites of osteoporosis-associated fractures. Peripheral sites can also identify patients with low bone mass and predict fracture risk.

Bone density data are reported as T scores and Z scores. In 1994, the World Health Organization (WHO) used T scores to classify and define BMD measurements (Table 27–2). The definitions, originally only for postmenopausal women, have been adapted by the ISCD to classify BMD in premenopausal women, men, and children. Each standard deviation change in the BMD increases fracture risk by 2–2.5 times.

Annual losses of bone mass normally seen with aging are in the range of 1% per year, the precision error of current instruments (approximately 1% to 2% with DXA) means that the interval between scans should be at least 2 years. Patient with high-dose steroid therapy can have rapid bone loss in a shorter interval and annual scans should be obtained.

DXA has some disadvantages. It is a 2-dimensional measurement, which only measures density/area and not the volumetric density. Areal BMD is influenced by bone size and will overestimate fracture risk in individuals with small body frame, who will have lower BMD. Spine and hip DXA are also sensitive to degenerative changes, and individuals with considerable degenerative disease will have increased density, suggesting a lower fracture risk than is actually present. All structures overlying the spine, such as aortic calcifications, or morphologic abnormalities, such as after laminectomy, will affect BMD measurements and thus need to be considered when reviewing DXA results.

Table 27–2. World Health Organization diagnostic categories.

Category	Definition by Bone Density
Normal	BMD is within 1 standard deviation (SD) of a young normal adult (T score is greater than −1.0)
Osteopenia	BMD is between 1 and 2.5 SD below a young normal adult (T score is −1 to −2.5)
Osteoporosis	BMD is 2.5 SD or more below a young normal adult (T score is less than −2.5)
Severe or established osteoporosis	BMD is 2.5 SD or more below a young adult with 1 or more fragility fractures

Table 27–3. Assessment for secondary causes of osteoporosis.

Hypogonadism	Serum testosterone, prolactin
Primary hyperparathyroidism	PTH, ionized calcium
Secondary hyperparathyroidism	25-Hydroxy vitamin D, PTH
Multiple myeloma	Serum and urine protein electrophoresis
Hyperthyroidism	Thyroid-stimulating hormone, thyroxine (T_4)

C. Laboratory Evaluation

Laboratory testing in patients with presumed osteoporosis are usually undertaken to rule out or find common secondary causes of osteoporosis. Preliminary testing should include basic chemistry panel; a complete blood count; and liver function panel. Patients who have Z scores less than −2 standard deviations (SD) from their age-matched cohorts or who have physical findings, should be assessed for more specific secondary causes of osteoporosis (Table 27–3). It is important to note in the geriatric population secondary hyperparathyroidism caused by vitamin D deficiency is prevalent and all older patients should have a 25-hydroxy vitamin D and PTH assessment.

1. Bone turnover markers—Additional laboratory testing includes bone turnover markers (BTMs), which are traditionally categorized as bone formation or bone resorption markers (Table 27–4). Their routine use in clinical practice remains a challenge because of their wide biologic and analytical variability. It should be noted that resorption markers must be measured in the morning on the second void urine because there is a large diurnal variation.

The best established clinical use for BTMs is in monitoring treatment efficacy and compliance. Antiresorptive agents rapidly decrease BTMs. On average, BTMs change by 50%

Table 27–4. Bone turnover markers.

Bone Formation Markers (Produced by Osteoblast Activity)	Bone Resorption Markers (Produced by Osteoclast Activity)
Procollagen type I N propeptide (PINP)[a]	Tartrate resistant acid phosphatase[a]
Procollagen type I C propeptide (PICP)[a]	C-terminal telopeptides (CTX)[b]
Osteocalcin[b]	N-terminal telopeptides (NTX)[b]
Alkaline phosphatase (bone specific)[a]	

[a]Marker is measured in the serum.
[b]Marker is measured in the serum or urine.

following antifracture treatment, making it easier to use in monitoring treatment efficacy within months compared to BMD changes, which take years. The resorption markers are also independent risk factors for fracture.

▶ Complications

Osteoporosis results in massive costs both to the individual and to society through associated fragility fractures. A fracture is considered to be osteoporotic (fragility fracture) if it is a result of relatively low trauma, such as a fall from standing height or less, or use of a force that in a young healthy adult would not be expected to cause a fracture. The most common sites of fragility fractures are the hip, spine, and distal forearm. The presence of 1 or more low-impact fragility fractures is considered as a sign of severe osteoporosis and often the BMD measured may be in the normal or osteopenic range.

A. Hip Fracture

Hip fracture incidence increases with age and typically peaks after age 85 years. With increasing life expectancy, and hip fracture incidence rates rising exponentially with age, this will result in an emergent number of hip fractures. In 2004, there were approximately 329,000 hip fractures in the United States and about one-third occurred in men.

In general, men have poorer outcomes after hip fracture than women. Mortality rates are doubled in men, with approximately 32% of men dying within a year of a hip fracture. This disparity in mortality may be attributed to increased comorbidities and more postoperative complications in men. Men also have poorer functional recovery in physical activities 1 year after the hip fracture. Of those who were not institutionalized before fracture, 25% remain in an institution a year or longer after fracture.

Hip fractures are classified by the area of femur affected and by whether displacement is present. The types of hip fracture are intracapsular fractures, intertrochanteric fractures, and subtrochanteric fractures. The injured leg is often shortened, externally rotated and abducted when the patient is lying flat. Plain radiographs are diagnostic, but in a few instances of a negative radiograph, obtaining a MRI is helpful to evaluate for an occult fracture.

Surgery remains the main therapeutic option and provides the best opportunity for functional recovery. Conservative therapy can be considered in a patient with a nondisplaced femoral neck fracture or for patients too ill to undergo surgery. A displaced intracapsular fracture is likely to have vascular compromise to the head of the femur, resulting in non-union and osteonecrosis, and thus often require hemiarthroplasty. Intertrochanteric and subtrochanteric fractures can be treated with internal fixation with sliding screws or nails.

B. Vertebral Fracture

The incidence of all vertebral fractures has been estimated to be 3 times that of hip fracture. Both the prevalence and incidence of radiographic vertebral fractures increase with age. Among white women, the prevalence of vertebral fractures increases from 5% to 10% between the ages of 50 and 59 years and to >30% at 80 years of age or older.

Multiple vertebral fractures can lead to increased thoracic kyphosis with height loss and development of "dowager's hump"; protuberant abdomen as internal organs are contained in a smaller compartment; complaints of pain in the muscles of the neck because patients must extend the neck to look forward; reduction in the distance between the bottom of the rib cage and the top of the iliac crests, which may be associated with dyspnea and gastrointestinal complaints (eg, early satiety and constipation); functional and physical limitation because of chronic pain, which leads to anxiety, depression, and loss of self-esteem and self-image.

Lateral thoracic and lumbar spine radiographs are the standard tool for assessment. Differential diagnoses for vertebral deformities are malignancy; metabolic bone diseases; degenerative disease; Scheuermann disease; Paget disease; hemangioma; infection; and dysplastic changes.

Data from randomized, controlled trials (RCTs) evaluating the efficacy of pain medications for acute vertebral fracture are lacking. Nonsteroidal antiinflammatory drugs, analgesics (including narcotics and tramadol), transdermal lidocaine, and tricyclic antidepressants are commonly used. Although the pain typically subsides over several weeks, narcotics are often required to facilitate mobility and avoid prolonged bed rest. Calcitonin has been found to modestly reduce pain associated with an acute vertebral fracture. Limited evidence also supports the use of therapeutic exercise programs to reduce pain and improve strength, balance, functional status, and quality of life.

Two recent procedures being performed on patients with acute vertebral fractures to relieve pain are kyphoplasty (inflating a small balloon at the site of a compression deformity to reduce the pressure) and vertebroplasty (placing cement at the site of a compression deformity). Often the 2 procedures are performed consecutively to minimize extravasation of the cement material. Observational studies noted reduced pain, disability and length of hospital stay; however, a RCT with a sham procedure showed no benefit.

C. Wrist Fracture

Wrist fractures show a pattern of occurrence that differs from that of hip and vertebral deformities. The incidence of this type of fracture increases in white women from the age of 45 to 60 years, followed by a plateau. Wrists fractures are generally associated with a fall from an outstretched arm.

A recent review article summarized that having had a previous hip fracture was likely to increase the risk of another fracture 3-fold, and of a hip fracture nearly 4-fold, and the lifetime risk of another vertebral fracture was 4-fold higher. Thus, secondary prevention after any fragility fracture should focus on fall prevention and treatment for osteoporosis since further fragility fractures are likely to occur.

▶ Prevention

Effective therapies for prevention of osteoporosis and fractures are now available.

A. Peak Bone Mass

Attainment of peak bone mass is primary in preventing osteoporosis and fractures in adulthood. This includes modification of general lifestyle factors, such as a balanced diet containing calcium and vitamin D, regular exercise, smoking cessation and avoidance of heavy alcohol use.

B. Exercise

A Cochrane analysis noted that aerobics, weight-bearing, and resistance exercises were all effective on the BMD of the spine. Walking was also found to be effective on both BMD of the spine and the hip and should be encouraged. Long-term studies to determine fracture data are required.

The positive implications of exercising in the geriatric population extend far beyond improvements in BMD: prevention of falls through improvements in muscle strength, balance and posture control; increase in fitness and quality of life; and decrease in pain intensity and frequency at the spine.

C. Fall Prevention

Falls prevention is integral in fracture prevention (see Chapter 25, "Falls & Mobility Disorders").

D. Hip Protectors

Hip protectors consist of a hard or soft shell with a soft padding that covers the area over the greater trochanter of the hip. Their use should be encouraged for patients at increased risk, especially those in a nursing home. Compliance remains an issue.

E. Calcium Supplementation

The Institute of Medicine (IOM) recommends a total daily elemental calcium intake of 1000 mg for all adults 19–50 years old, including pregnant and lactating women, 1000 mg for men 51–70 years old, and 1200 mg for women >50 years old and men >70 years old.

Calcium supplements are available as salts with varying concentrations of elemental calcium. Calcium citrate does not require acid for absorption, can be taken with or without food, and is preferred in patients taking proton pump inhibitors or H_2-receptor antagonists, or in those with achlorhydria.

Calcium carbonate should be taken with food and in divided doses to enhance absorption.

Calcium supplements are generally well tolerated but constipation, intestinal bloating and excess gas can occur. A slightly higher risk of kidney stones has been reported. Some reports suggest that calcium supplementation increases the risk of cardiovascular disease, but the data is inconsistent with most prospective studies *not* depicting an increased risk. Calcium supplementation can increase BMD in children and adolescents, and reduce bone loss in postmenopausal women and older men.

F. Vitamin D Supplementation

Vitamin D is necessary for optimal absorption of calcium. Older adults often do not produce adequate amounts through cutaneous production or from the diet. Vitamin D deficiency is associated with muscle weakness, and can predispose a person to falls.

Vitamin D status can be evaluated by measuring serum 25-hydroxy vitamin D (25-OH-D); a level of ≥30 ng/mL is considered acceptable; ≤10 ng/mL is considered severe deficiency or osteomalacia; and a range between 10 and 30 ng/mL is considered an insufficiency when accompanied by a notable rise in serum PTH. The IOM recommends a dietary allowance of vitamin D of 600 IU daily for people up to 70 years old and 800 IU daily for those ≥71 years old. Hypercalciuria and hypercalcemia can be seen with vitamin D toxicity.

The Women's Health Initiative (WHI) reported a reduction in fractures among the women who were adherent to calcium and vitamin D supplementation. The antifracture effect of vitamin D is more pronounced in the institutionalized and involves its effect on muscle strength and falls prevention.

▶ Treatment

Guidelines by the National Osteoporosis Foundation (NOF) recommend osteoporosis treatment in postmenopausal women or men age 50 years and older with a T-score of less than −2.5 at the femoral neck, hip, or spine; patients with low bone mass (T-score between −1.0 and −2.5) and a 10-year probability of hip fracture of ≥3% or a 10-year probability of major osteoporosis-related fracture of ≥20%, as determined by FRAX; and in patients with a fragility fracture.

Current osteoporosis therapy are divided into antiresorptive and anabolic agents (Table 27–5). Antiresorptive therapy available in the United States are bisphosphonates, hormone replacement therapy (HRT), selective estrogen receptor modulators (SERMs), denosumab, and calcitonin. Parathyroid hormone is the only anabolic agent available in the United States.

A. Bisphosphonates

Bisphosphonates are potent antiresorptive agents that bind hydroxyapatite crystals on bone surfaces and permanently

Table 27–5. FDA approved agents for osteoporosis.

Agent	Efficacy	Side Effects	Dosing	Delivery
Bisphosphonates: *Alendronate* *Risedronate* *Ibandronate* *Zoledronic acid*	Reduced vertebral, hip, and nonvertebral fractures (no data on ibandronate for hip fracture)	Gastrointestinal side effects Arthralgia/myalgia Renal toxicity Atypical fractures Osteonecrosis of the jaw	5-10 mg oral daily, 70 mg oral weekly 5 mg oral daily, 35 mg oral weekly, 　150 mg oral monthly 2.5 mg oral daily, 150 mg oral monthly, 　3 mg IV every 3 months 5 mg IV every 12 months	
Hormone Replacement Therapy	Reduced vertebral, hip, and nonvertebral fractures	Increased thromboembolic events, cholelithiasis, irregular uterine bleeding	Multiple oral and transdermal formulations	
Raloxifene (selective estrogen receptor modulator)	Reduced vertebral fractures	Increased thromboembolic events, hot flashes, leg cramps	60 mg oral daily	
Calcitonin	Reduced vertebral fractures	Nausea (injectable form)	200 IU	Nasal spray daily (alternate each side of nostril)
		Rhinitis, epistaxis (nasal form)	100 IU	Subcutaneous or intramuscular every other day
Denosumab	Reduced vertebral, hip and nonvertebral fractures	Eczema, dermatitis, rash, cellulitis	60 mg	Subcutaneously every 6 months
Teriparatide	Reduced vertebral, hip and nonvertebral fractures	Nausea, headache, dizziness, and leg cramps	20 mcg	Daily subcutaneous injections for 24 months

inhibit osteoclast function. FDA-approved agents are alendronate, risedronate, ibandronate and zoledronic acid.

Bisphosphonates may be given orally on a daily (alendronate, risedronate), weekly (alendronate, risedronate), or monthly (risedronate, ibandronate) schedule or intravenously every 3 months (ibandronate) or intravenously once yearly (zoledronic acid). Oral bisphosphonates must be taken on an empty stomach because of their poor absorption and bioavailability. Patients must sit upright and fast for 30 minutes (with alendronate and risedronate) to 60 minutes (with ibandronate) after ingestion. Prior to the initiation of any bisphosphonates therapy, calcium and vitamin D must be adequately repleted because of the possibility of inducing hypocalcemia, especially in older adults.

Oral bisphosphonates are commonly associated with gastrointestinal side effects, including dyspepsia, heartburn, indigestion, and pain while swallowing. More serious gastrointestinal effects include erosive esophagitis and esophageal ulcerations; thus patients are reminded to take a full glass of water (6–8 oz) and remain upright after the dose. Acute phase reactions (fever, myalgia, arthralgia, headache, and flu-like symptoms) have been reported with both oral and intravenous bisphosphonates. Intravenous zoledronic acid has been associated with acute renal failure and should be used with caution in patients with renal impairment. Alendronate should also be used with caution in patients with severe renal insufficiency (creatinine clearance <35 mL/min). Long-term effects, including osteonecrosis of the jaw and atypical fracture, are rare and benefits from fracture reduction outweigh the harms.

All bisphosphonates have been shown to significantly improve BMD of the spine and reduce risk of vertebral and hip fractures. There are no published data for hip fracture reductions with ibandronate in randomized clinical trials. There are no studies of comparative efficacy of the bisphosphonates with each other.

The duration of bisphosphonate therapy is not yet clear. Seven-year follow-up of patients using alendronate showed that spinal BMD continued to increase through 7 years of treatment and remained stable. After the withdrawal of treatment, there was a small increase in biochemical markers of bone turnover. It appears that skeletal benefits may be preserved for at least 1–2 years after cessation, but long-term follow-up studies are needed.

B. Hormone Replacement Therapy

Hormone replacement therapy (HRT) is approved for the prevention of osteoporosis in postmenopausal women, although the primary indication is for the treatment of moderate-to-severe menopausal symptoms. The exact mechanism of HRT on bone remodeling has not been elucidated, however it is clear that the loss of estrogen during menopause results in an acceleration of bone resorption in most women.

Combined estrogen and progesterone therapy have produced a 1.4% to 3.9% increase in BMD at skeletal sites. Studies have shown that estrogen reduces the risk for vertebral and hip fracture, as well as the risk of nonvertebral fracture. In the WHI trial, treatment of postmenopausal women with combined therapy reduced the risk of hip fracture by 33%.

The timing of initiation and duration of HRT remains unclear. It is suggested that women start estrogen within 2–7 years of menopause. Several studies have shown that HRT begun before 60 years of age prevents nonvertebral, hip, and wrist fractures, but there is insufficient evidence that fracture risk is reduced when HRT is begun after age 60 years. Estrogen begun and continued after age 60 years appears to maintain BMD. The duration of therapy necessary to protect women against fragility fractures is indefinite. HRT can be administered as an oral or transdermal formulation. It may be given on a continuous basis, with no interruption in therapy, or as a cyclical regimen.

Compliance with HRT is typically poor because of common side effects and concern about increased incidence of breast or endometrial cancer. Women who have not undergone hysterectomy should have progestin added to the estrogen regimen to prevent endometrial hyperplasia. Low-dose HRT can reduce the amount of uterine bleeding, fluid retention, mastalgia, and headaches, making estrogen therapy much easier to tolerate.

Safety results from the WHI study showed an increased risk of coronary heart disease, pulmonary embolism, and stroke associated with the use of combined hormonal therapy in women with an intact uterus. As a result, HRT is considered second line therapy for only prevention of osteoporosis in young perimenopausal women with menopausal symptoms.

C. Selective Estrogen Receptor Modulators

SERMs are compounds that bind to and activate estrogen receptors but have agonist/antagonist properties at different tissue sites. Raloxifene is approved for the prevention and treatment of postmenopausal osteoporosis and indicated for the reduction of invasive breast cancer.

Raloxifene at 60 mg per day has been shown to increase BMD by 2% and reduce the risk of new vertebral fracture by 40% after 2 years. However, raloxifene has not demonstrated a protective effect on nonvertebral or hip fracture risk.

D. Calcitonin

Calcitonin, an endogenous hormone secreted by the parafollicular C cells of the thyroid gland, which helps to maintain calcium homeostasis. Calcitonin acts directly on osteoclasts, with inhibitory effects on bone resorption. Calcitonin is approved for the treatment of postmenopausal osteoporosis. Calcitonin nasal spray has been shown to have modest effects on spine BMD (1.5% increase) and significantly reduce the risk of new vertebral fractures by 33% in women with prevalent vertebral fractures. There was no significant effect on hip or nonvertebral fracture risk. Calcitonin is an option for women who cannot tolerate bisphosphonates or SERMs. In some patients, calcitonin has an analgesic effect, making it suitable for patients with acute vertebral fracture. Calcitonin nasal spray is generally administered once per day, alternating nostrils daily. Injectable calcitonin can be administered subcutaneously or intramuscularly.

E. Denosumab

Denosumab is a human monoclonal antibody with a high affinity and specificity for RANKL. When denosumab binds to RANKL, it prevents RANKL–RANK interaction resulting in a decrease in osteoclastic bone resorption.

Denosumab is approved for osteoporosis treatment. Results from phase 3 study in women with osteoporosis showed that treatment with denosumab increased lumbar spine BMD by 6.5%, and significantly reduced the risk of vertebral (68%) and hip (40%) fractures compared with placebo. Prior to starting denosumab, patients with preexisting hypocalcemia must have this condition corrected because it could worsen with treatment. Denosumab may be given to patients with renal impairment without dose adjustment.

F. Parathyroid Hormone

Teriparatide is an FDA-approved anabolic agent that is synthetic PTH. It stimulates bone remodeling, preferentially increasing formation over resorption, and reduces the risk of new vertebral fractures (65% reduction) and nonvertebral fractures (35%) with significant improvements in BMD of 10% to 14%.

Teriparatide is administered as daily subcutaneous injections. Eleven percent of patients developed mild hypercalcemia. Osteosarcomas have been induced in rats given teriparatide. However, an independent oncology advisory board concluded that the rat carcinogenicity data are very unlikely to have clinical relevance in humans being treated with teriparatide for a relatively short duration (it is approved for only 2 years' use).

Upon termination of teriparatide treatment, sequential therapy with an oral or IV bisphosphonate may strengthen the beneficial effects of teriparatide. Concurrent therapy with teriparatide and oral bisphosphonates has been avoided because oral bisphosphonates have been shown to reduce the positive effects of teriparatide on bone turnover.

In summary, given a choice of pharmacotherapy, clinical risk factors for fracture and comorbidities should be taken into account when tailoring therapy for osteoporosis. Risk factors such as age and previous fracture are critical to choosing an optimal treatment strategy. Clinicians need to be aware of the safety concerns associated with each drug and treatment should be made on an individual basis taking into account the relative benefits and risks in different patient population.

Bauer DC, Glüer CC, Cauley JA, et al. Broadband ultrasound attenuation predicts fractures strongly and independently of densitometry in older women: a prospective study. Study of Osteoporotic Fractures Research Group. *Arch Intern Med.* 1997;157(6):629-634.

Bonaiuti D, Shea B, Iovine R, et al. Exercise for preventing and treating osteoporosis in postmenopausal women. *Cochrane Database Syst Rev.* 2002;(3):CD000333.

Burge R, Dawson-Hughes B, Solomon DH, Wong JB, King A, Tosteson A. Incidence and economic burden of osteoporosis-related fractures in the United States, 2005-2025. *J Bone Miner Res.* 2007;22(3):465-475.

Cauley JA, Robbins J, Chen Z, et al. Effects of estrogen plus progestin on risk of fracture and bone mineral density. *JAMA.* 2003;290(13):1729-1738.

Consensus development conference: diagnosis, prophylaxis and treatment of osteoporosis. *Am J Med.* 1993;94(6):646-650.

Ensrud KE, Schousboe JT. Clinical practice. Vertebral fractures. *N Engl J Med.* 2011;364(17):1634-1642.

Gillespie LD, Robertson MC, Gillespie WJ, et al. Interventions for preventing falls in older people living in the community. *Cochrane Database Syst Rev.* 2009;(2):CD007146.

Gillespie WJ, Gillespie LD, Parker MJ. Hip protectors for preventing hip fractures in older people. *Cochrane Database Syst Rev.* 2010;(10):CD001255.

Green AD, Colón-Emeric CS, Bastian L, Drake MT, Lyles KW. Does this woman have osteoporosis? *JAMA.* 2004;292(23):2890-2900.

Guglielmi G, Muscarella S, Bazzocchi A. Integreated imaging approach to osteoporosis: state of the art review and update. *Radiographics.* 2011;31(5):1343-1364.

Hamerman D. Bone health across the generations: a primer for health providers concerned with osteoporosis prevention. *Maturitas.* 2005;50(1):1-7.

Harvey N, Dennison E, Cooper C. Osteoporosis: impact on health and economics. *Nat Rev Rheumatol.* 2010;6(2):99-105.

Kanis JA, Johansson H, Oden A, Dawson-Hughes B, Melton LJ 3rd, McCloskey EV. The effects of a FRAX revision for the USA. *Osteoporosis Int.* 2010;21(1):35-40.

Kanis JA, McCloskey EV, Johansson H, Oden A, Ström O, Borgström F. Development and use of FRAX in osteoporosis. *Osteoporosis Int.* 2010;21 Suppl 2:S407-S413.

Kanis JA, Oden A, Johansson H, Borgström F, Ström O, McCloskey E. FRAX and its applications to clinical practice. *Bone.* 2009;44(5):734-743.

Kanis J. Diagnosis of osteoporosis and assessment of fracture risk. *Lancet.* 2002;359(9321):1929-1936.

Lewiecki EM, Bilezikian JP. Denosumab for the treatment of osteoporosis and cancer related conditions. *Clin Pharmacol Ther.* 2012;91(1):123-133.

Link TM. Osteoporosis imaging: state of the art and advanced imaging. *Radiology.* 2012;263(1):3-17.

Link TM, Guglielmi G, van Kuijk C, Adams JE. Radiologic assessment of osteoporotic vertebral fractures: diagnostic and prognostic implications. *Eur Radiol.* 2005;15(8):1521-1532.

Liu H, Paige NM, Goldzweig CL, et al. Screening for osteoporosis in men: a systematic review for an American College of Physicians guideline. *Ann Intern Med.* 2008;148(9):685-701.

Marshall D, Johnell O, Wedel H. Meta-analysis of how well measures of bone mineral density predict occurrence of osteoporotic fractures. *BMJ.* 1996;312(704):1254-1259.

Melton LJ 3rd, Atkinson EJ, Cooper C, O'Fallon WM, Riggs BL. Vertebral fractures predict subsequent fractures. *Osteoporosis Int.* 1999;10(3):214-221.

National Osteoporosis Foundation. NOF releases updated data and national breakdown of adults age 50 and older affected by osteoporosis and low bone mass. Washington, DC. NOF Press Release, Nov 1, 2013. Available from: http://nof.org/news/1648.

NIH Consensus Development Panel on Osteoporosis Prevention, Diagnosis, and Therapy. Osteoporosis prevention, diagnosis, and therapy. *JAMA.* 2001;285(6):785-795.

Oot, S. ed. *Bone Health and Osteoporosis: A Report of the Surgeon-General.* Rockville, MD: US Department of Health and Human Services; 2004.

Orwig DL, Chiles N, Jones M, Hochberg MC. Osteoporosis in men: update 2011. *Rheum Dis Clin North Am.* 2011;37(3):401-414.

Richards JB, Kavvoura FK, Rivadeneira F, et al. Collaborative meta-analysis: associations of 150 candidate genes with osteoporosis and osteoporotic fracture. *Ann Intern Med.* 2009;151(8):528-537.

Sambrook P, Cooper C. Osteoporosis. *Lancet.* 2006;367(9527):2010-2018.

Schmitt NM, Schmitt J, Dören M. The role of physical activity in the prevention of osteoporosis in postmenopausal women. An update. *Maturitas.* 2009;63(1):34-38.

Shane E, Burr D, Ebeling PR, et al. Atypical subtrochanteric and diaphyseal femoral fractures: report of a task force of the American Society for Bone and Mineral Research. *J Bone Miner Res.* 2010;25(11):2267-2294.

Silverman S, Christiansen C. Individualizing osteoporosis therapy. *Osteoporosis Int.* 2012;23(3):797-809.

Siris ES, Baim S, Nattiv A. Primary care use of FRAX: absolute fracture risk assessment in postmenopausal women and older men. *Postgrad Med.* 2010;122(1):82-90.

Siris ES, Miller PD, Barrett-Connor E, et al. Identification and fracture outcomes of undiagnosed low bone mineral density in postmenopausal women: results from the National Osteoporosis Risk Assessment. *JAMA.* 2001;286(22):2815-2822.

Vasikaran S, Eastell R, Bruyère O, et al. Markers of bone turnover for the prediction of fracture risk and monitoring of osteoporosis treatment: a need for international reference standards. *Osteoporos Int.* 2011;22(2):391-420.

Wang L, Manson JE, Sesso HD. Calcium intake and risk of cardiovascular disease: a review of prospective studies and randomized clinical trials. *Am J Cardiovasc Drugs.* 2012;12(2):105-116.

Warriner AH, Patkar NM, Yun H, Delzell E. Minor, major, low-trauma, and high-trauma fractures: what are the subsequent fracture risks and how do they vary? *Curr Osteoporos Rep.* 2011;9(3):122-128.

Winsloe C, Earl S, Dennison EM, Cooper C, Harvey NC. Early life factors in pathogenesis of osteoporosis. *Curr Osteoporos Rep.* 2009;7:140-144.

World Health Organization. *Techinical Report: Assessment of Fracture Risk and Its Application to Screening for Postmenopausal Osteoporsis: A Report of a WHO Study Group.* Geneva, Switzerland: World Health Organiation; 1994.

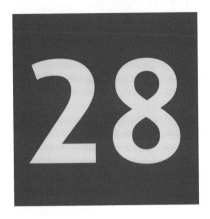

Coronary Disease

Sanket Dhruva, MD

Melvin Cheitlin, MD

ESSENTIALS OF DIAGNOSIS

▶ Chest discomfort or dyspnea provoked by exertion and subsiding with rest or nitroglycerin.

▶ Presence of risk factors (hypertension, dyslipidemia, smoking, diabetes, renal disease, male, older age) accompanying symptoms.

▶ Electrocardiographic changes: ST elevation, ST depression, T-wave changes, new Q waves.

▶ Exercise or pharmacologic stress test evidence of myocardial ischemia.

▶ Angiographic evidence of coronary stenosis.

▶ Older adults with coronary disease often have atypical or non-specific symptoms such as abdominal pain, dizziness, confusion, or fatigue instead of more classic symptoms.

▶ General Principles in Older Adults

The prevalence of cardiovascular disease (CVD) and especially coronary artery disease (CAD) is increasing. In the United States, 82.6 million people have CVD, and of these, 40.4 million are older than age 60 years. Among people free of CVD at age 50 years, there is a lifetime risk for developing it of 51.7% for men and 39.2% for women. The good news is that the overall rate of death attributable to CVD has declined 30.6% from 1998 to 2008 and the actual number of patients dying in the same period decreased by 14.1%. A large percentage of this decrease is related to better therapy for patients with acute coronary syndromes (ACSs) and chronic stable angina.

Analysis of National Health and Nutrition Examination Survey (NHANES) data comparing death rates attributable to CAD between 1980 and 2000 found that approximately 47% of the decrease in coronary deaths was attributable to medical and surgical treatments and approximately 44% to changes in coronary risk factors. Unfortunately, these decreases in risk factors were partially offset by increases in obesity and type II diabetes.

Increasing age is a major factor in the increasing incidence of CVD, including aortic stenosis and CAD. In the age group 85 to 94 years, the average annual rate of first cardiovascular events is 24 times that of those in the age group 35 to 44 years. For women, comparable rates occur about 10 years later in life, with the difference narrowing with advancing age. Older adults also have a greater number of comorbidities. At least partly for this reason, they also have fewer surgical and interventional procedures, more adverse events from medication, more polypharmacy, are less frequently referred for cardiac rehabilitation and have a higher morbidity and mortality than younger patients with similar CVD. Congestive heart failure is the most common diagnosis on hospital discharge and the majority of these patients are age 65 years or older. Finally, approximately 80% of people who die are ≥65 years of age and most die with CAD.

A. Cardiovascular Changes with Normal Aging

With normal aging there are a number of changes seen in the heart and other organs that alter function and are precursors to a variety of diseases seen in older adults (Table 28–1). These changes occur in everyone as they age and must be distinguished from changes related to diseases such as CAD and other vascular diseases. These normal changes associated with aging also do not occur at the same rate in everyone, so physiologic aging and chronologic aging differ from person to person.

Table 28–1 lists the consequences of these changes. The practical effect of these aging changes on cardiac function is no change in cardiac output at rest or with moderate exercise and no change in left ventricular ejection fraction

Table 28–1. Cardiovascular changes with aging and their consequences.

Change	Consequences
Decrease in arterial elasticity, increase in arterial stiffness	Increased afterload on the left ventricle (LV), systolic hypertension and the development of left ventricular hypertrophy (LVH) and increased size of myocardial cells.
Changes in the LV wall decreasing LV compliance	Prolongation of diastolic relaxation. This is possibly related to an increase in the magnitude of the L-type Ca^{++} current that may be important in maintaining myocardial contraction and a slowing of inactivation of the L-type Ca^{++} current prolonging Ca^{++} influx with each heartbeat. Increased intracellular Ca^{++} can result in calcium-dependent arrhythmias.
Noncompliant LV	End-diastolic LV stiffness increases the importance of atrial systole to the filling of the LV and maintaining stroke volume. With a stiff LV, the development of atrial fibrillation can result in a marked drop in stroke volume. Increased LV stiffness is responsible for an S_4. With extensive LV decreased compliance, diastolic heart failure can occur.
Dropout of atrial pacemaker cells	Apoptosis of myocardial cells, including a loss of 50% to 75% of atrial pacemaker cells by age 50 years, slows the intrinsic heart rate. Can result in sick sinus syndrome.
Fibrosis of the cardiac skeleton	Fibrosis of the annular valve rings and the fibrous trigones can result in various degrees of atrioventricular block because the His bundle passes through the right fibrous trigone. Fibrosis and calcification of the aortic ring can be the first stage of aortic stenosis. Fifty percent of older patients have grades I–II systolic ejection murmurs.
Decreased responsiveness to β-adrenergic receptor stimulus and decreased reactivity of baro- and chemoreceptors	Slowing of response to position change with decreased sympathetic reflexes and postural hypotension.

or stroke volume. With stress (eg, trauma, disease, surgery) that requires an increase in cardiac output and increase in O_2 demand, there is less ability to meet this increased demand as a result of the decrease in cardiac reserve.

B. Cardiovascular Risk Factors

Risk factors for vascular disease, including CAD, have been identified for decades. Because their effect on the development of vascular disease is a function of the number of risk factors present, the concentration of the factors and the duration of exposure and cumulative damage, the risk factors are as important—if not more so—in the older patient. Whether a risk factor will affect the development of vascular disease is also partially genetically determined. For instance, everyone who smokes does not develop CAD. In addition, in older adults we do not have evidence that elimination of a particular risk factor will result in a decrease in the incidence of cardiovascular events. For some risk factors, for instance, hypertension, the evidence that controlling the blood pressure reduces cardiac events is excellent, including in older patients. Patients older than age 65 years with systolic blood pressure greater than 180 mm Hg have a 3–4-fold increase in CAD compared to those with a systolic blood pressure less than 120 mm Hg. Treating hypertension in patients older than age 70 years has resulted in a decrease in the incidence of stroke and reduced cardiac events. The Hypertension in the Very Elderly Trial (HYVET), which included almost 4000 patients older than age 80 years, showed that with blood-pressure-lowering treatment, the incidence of stroke was decreased by 30% and cardiac death by 23%.

In older adults, the prevalence of smoking decreases. In 2007 to 2009, among people ≥65 years of age, 9.3% of men and 8.6% of women were current smokers. Older smokers are less likely to quit smoking than younger smokers, but the older smokers, if quitting is attempted, are more likely to succeed. Absolute rates of disease incidence and mortality as a result of smoking increase steadily as age and duration of smoking increases. There is no evidence that the disease consequences of smoking decrease in older adults. The proportional benefits of smoking cessation are somewhat less among older adults because of the cumulative damage of a long duration of smoking and possibly because patients susceptible to the increased risk of coronary disease from smoking have died at a younger age, leaving those less susceptible. However, cessation is the only way to alter smoke-related disease risk.

Hyperlipidemia as a cardiac risk factor is more complex. Serum cholesterol concentration increases progressively until age 50 years in men and age 65 years in women, and then begins to decline. Age-related changes in the concentration of cholesterol are mainly caused by increases in low-density lipoprotein (LDL) cholesterol. High-density lipoprotein (HDL) level remains relatively stable with age and is approximately 10 mg/dL higher in women than in men. A high level of LDL cholesterol and low level of HDL cholesterol remain predictors for the development of CAD in older adults. Clinical trial data indicate that in older patients with established CAD, LDL-lowering therapy is beneficial and it is standard therapy for older patients who are at higher risk and otherwise in good health to be given LDL-lowering therapy.

Between 2005 and 2006 the prevalence of diabetes mellitus in adults ≥65 years of age was 17%. The prevalence of diabetes mellitus in the United States is projected to more than double from 2005 to 2050, with the largest increases in the oldest age groups, increasing by 220% in those ages 65–74 years and by 449% in those age ≥75 years. The presence of type II diabetes in the older age group doubles the risk of CAD, and when combined with hyperlipidemia, increases the risk 15-fold. At least 68% of people age 65 years or older with diabetes die of some form of heart disease; 16% die from stroke. Older adults are at increased cardiac risk from the constellation of signs known as the metabolic syndrome: central obesity, insulin resistance, dyslipidemia, and hypertension. The presence of the metabolic syndrome leads to an increased risk of CVD and renal events.

Physical inactivity in patients older than age 75 years is frequent, with 38% of men and 51% of women reporting no leisure-time physical activity. In patients 60–80 years old, frequent exercise raises HDL cholesterol, controls obesity, lowers blood pressure, and reduces insulin resistance, all protective effects against vascular disease.

Bechtold M, Palmer J, Valtos J, Iasiello C, Sowers J. Metabolic syndrome in the elderly. *Curr Diab Rep.* 2006;6(1):64-71.

Burns DM. Cigarette smoking among the elderly: disease consequences and the benefits of cessation. *Am J Health Promot.* 2000;14(6):357-361.

National Cholesterol Education Program (NCEP) Expert Panel on Detection, Evaluation, and Treatment of High Blood Cholesterol in Adults (Adult Treatment Panel III). Third Report of the National Cholesterol Education Program (NCEP) Expert Panel on Detection, Evaluation, and Treatment of High Blood Cholesterol in Adults (Adult Treatment Panel III) final report. *Circulation.* 2002;106(25):3143-421.

Pearson TA, Blair SN, Daniels SR, et al. AHA Guidelines for Primary Prevention of Cardiovascular Disease and Stroke: 2002 Update: Consensus Panel Guide to Comprehensive Risk Reduction for Adult Patients Without Coronary or Other Atherosclerotic Vascular Diseases. *Circulation.* 2002;106(3):388-391.

Roger VL, Go AS, Lloyd-Jones DM, et al. Heart disease and stroke statistics—2012 update: a report from the American heart Association. *Circulation.* 2012;125(1):e2-e220.

Aronow WS, Fleg JL, Pepine CJ, et al. ACCF/AHA 2011 expert consensus document on hypertension in the elderly: a report of the American College of Cardiology Foundation Task Force on Clinical Expert Consensus documents developed in collaboration with the American Academy of Neurology, American Geriatrics Society, American Society for Preventive Cardiology, American Society of Hypertension, American Society of Nephrology, Association of Black Cardiologists, and European Society of Hypertension. *J Am Coll Cardiol.* 2011.;57(20):2037-2114.

ACUTE CORONARY SYNDROME

▶ General Principles in Older Adults

ACS has 3 components: ST-segment elevation myocardial infarction (STEMI), non–ST-segment elevation myocardial infarction (NSTEMI), and unstable angina (UA). All 3 share a common pathophysiologic origin related to progression of coronary plaque, instability, and rupture. STEMI refers to the elevation of the ST segment in at least 2 contiguous leads along with either biomarker evidence (troponin I or T; creatine kinase, myocardial bound [CK-MB]; myoglobin) of myocardial necrosis or symptoms consistent with ischemia. NSTEMI has a similar definition, but without elevation of the ST segment in at least 2 contiguous leads. UA is chest pain or discomfort that is accelerating in frequency or severity and can occur at rest, but does not result in myocardial damage as noted by negative cardiac biomarkers. Patients with UA are at increased risk for progression to myocardial infarction (MI). The percentage of ACS composed of STEMI varies from 29% to 47% but has been decreasing over time.

Of the estimated 1.2 million MIs or fatal coronary heart disease (CHD) events occurring annually in the United States, 67% occur in persons older than age 65 years and 44% occur in persons older than age 75 years. Older patients are more likely to have NSTEMI than STEMI. Case fatality rates increase markedly with age; 80% of all MI deaths occur in persons older than age 65 years. Although the incidence of MI is higher in men than in women at all ages, the total number of MIs or fatal CHD events is greater in women than men older than age 75 years, reflecting the fact that the proportion of women in the surviving population increases with age. The prevalence of silent or clinically unrecognized MI increases with age and prevalence may be twice as high as recognized MI in older adults. The long-term prognosis after clinically unrecognized MI is similar to that of recognized MI in older adults.

▶ Prevention

Despite the high prevalence of CHD and ACS in industrialized countries, these disorders are potentially preventable or can be delayed through early and aggressive management of risk factors as discussed above. Although some risk factors, such as age, sex, and genetics, cannot be modified, lifelong adherence to behavior modification, including regular physical exercise; maintenance of desirable body weight; a diet rich in fruits, vegetables, and whole-grains but low in trans and saturated fats; and avoidance of tobacco products, can significantly reduce this risk.

Aspirin, adenosine diphosphatase (ADP) receptor antagonists, β-blockers, angiotensin-converting enzyme inhibitors, angiotensin receptor blockers, and statins have been shown to improve post-ACS prognosis. In addition, cardiac rehabilitation programs also reduce mortality and rehospitalizations after ACS.

Clinical Findings

A. Symptoms & Signs

The proportion of MI patients who have chest pain declines with age; <50% of MI patients older than 80 years complain of chest pain. Likewise, diaphoresis occurs less frequently in older patients with acute MI. Dyspnea is often the presenting manifestation of acute MI in older adults and is the most common initial symptom in persons older than 80 years. The prevalence of atypical symptoms (eg, gastrointestinal disturbances, overwhelming fatigue, dizziness, syncope, confusion, stroke) also increases with age, and up to 20% of patients older than 85 years with acute MI have neurologic complaints (see Chapter 63, "Addressing Chest Pain in Older Adults").

Physical findings associated with ACS are nonspecific but may include signs of acute heart failure, occurring in up to 40% of older patients with MI. These signs include an S_3 or S_4 gallop, new mitral regurgitation murmur, or signs of pulmonary or systemic venous congestion, such as pulmonary rales or elevated jugular venous pressure (JVP). In patients with right ventricular infarction, the Kussmaul sign (rise in JVP with inspiration) may be present.

1. Electrocardiography—Classic electrocardiographic features of a STEMI are ST-segment elevation of at least 1 mm in 2 or more contiguous leads corresponding to the anatomical distribution of a coronary artery (eg, leads II, III, avF), often with subsequent evolution to pathologic Q waves or new left bundle-branch block. ST elevation is not present in NSTEMI or UA, but there can be ST-segment depression or T-wave inversion, or both. Electrocardiographic changes often resolve with resolution of chest pain, so a nondiagnostic or even normal electrocardiogram (ECG) taken when the patient is free of symptoms does not exclude ischemia. However, the initial ECG is often nondiagnostic in older adults because of preexisting conduction system disease (eg, left bundle-branch block), presence of a ventricular pacemaker, prior infarct, left ventricular hypertrophy, metabolic abnormalities, or drug effects (eg, hypokalemia, digoxin), and the high prevalence of NSTEMI.

Atypical symptoms and physical findings, coupled with the high prevalence of nondiagnostic ECGs, often lead to delayed presentation and recognition of ACS. This time lag increases the risk of complications and reduces the window of opportunity for timely and effective intervention. Clinicians should maintain a high index of suspicion for ACS in all older patients with a wide range of unexplained symptoms and/or significant physical distress.

2. Cardiac biomarkers—Definitive diagnosis of STEMI or NSTEMI requires abnormal cardiac biomarker elevation. Troponins I and T have become the gold standard for diagnosis because of their greater sensitivity and specificity compared with the CK-MB isoenzyme. Serial measures of biomarkers that exceed the normal range and exhibit a typical rise-and-fall pattern in a patient with clinical and/or electrocardiographic features of cardiac ischemia are diagnostic of MI. In the absence of recurrent ischemia, CK-MB levels rise within 4–6 hours, peak at approximately 24 hours after MI onset and return to normal within 36–48 hours. Troponin levels rise within 2–3 hours of onset of symptoms, peak at 24–72 hours, and may remain elevated for up to 10–14 days, especially in large infarctions.

Differential Diagnosis

The differential diagnosis of ACS in older adults includes other cardiovascular conditions as well as pulmonary, gastrointestinal, musculoskeletal, and neurologic disorders. Important cardiovascular conditions that should be considered include aortic dissection, pericarditis, myocarditis, acute pulmonary edema resulting from cardiomyopathy, valvular heart disease, and arrhythmia. Pulmonary disorders include pneumonia, pulmonary embolus, pneumothorax, pleurisy, and pleural effusion. Gastrointestinal disorders include esophagitis, esophageal spasm, esophageal rupture, gastroesophageal reflux, peptic ulcer disease, cholelithiasis, and pancreatitis. Musculoskeletal disorders include muscular strains, costochondritis, injuries involving the cervical or thoracic spine, disorders of the shoulder joint, and chest wall trauma. Neurologic conditions include stroke or transient ischemic attack, radiculopathy, and altered sensorium or delirium. Psychogenic conditions, including anxiety and hyperventilation syndrome, may also mimic the ACS symptoms.

Complications

Major MI complications include acute heart failure, conduction disturbances (eg bundle branch block, advanced atrioventricular [AV] block), atrial fibrillation, myocardial rupture, sudden death and cardiogenic shock. Each complication is associated with worse prognosis and occurs 2–4 times more frequently in older patients.

Treatment

Table 28–2 lists the major therapeutic options for ACS. Management of STEMI and NSTEMI differs with respect to the use of early reperfusion therapy but is otherwise similar. For UA, the primary goals of therapy are symptom relief and preventing progression to NSTEMI or STEMI. Guidelines recommend that older patients receive the same treatment as younger patients with close monitoring for adverse events and with the caution that their general health, comorbidities, cognitive status, and life expectancy be taken into account and that increased sensitivity to hypotension-inducing drugs and possible altered pharmacokinetics be considered.

Table 28–2. Management of acute myocardial infarction.

General measures
Oxygen to maintain arterial saturation ≥90%
Morphine for pain and dyspnea
Nitroglycerin for ischemia and heart failure
Reperfusion therapy
Fibrinolysis
Primary angioplasty/stenting
Antithrombotic therapy
Aspirin
Heparin/low-molecular-weight heparin
Glycoprotein IIb/IIIa inhibitors
Clopidogrel
β-Blockers
Angiotensin-converting enzyme inhibitors
Other agents
Nitrates
Angiotensin receptor blockers
Calcium channel blockers
Lipid-lowering agents
Antiarrhythmic agents
Magnesium

A. General Measures

Maintenance of adequate arterial oxygenation and relief of chest discomfort are important goals. Intravenous morphine should be administered every 5–30 minutes as needed for relief of chest pain, monitoring closely for signs of respiratory depression, bradycardia, hypotension, and impaired sensorium, all of which are more common in older adults. Sublingual nitroglycerin should be administered acutely for the treatment of ischemic chest pain or dyspnea.

Patients with persistent chest pain or signs of pulmonary congestion should receive topical nitroglycerin ointment or an intravenous nitroglycerin infusion, titrated to control symptoms while avoiding excessive blood pressure (BP) reduction. In patients with signs of right ventricular infarction (ST elevation or depression in right precordial or inferior leads with elevated JVP and Kussmaul sign), nitroglycerin should be avoided as it may precipitate severe hypotension.

B. Reperfusion Therapy

Recanalization of the involved coronary artery as quickly as possible reduces mortality and morbid MI complications. Reperfusion can be achieved either pharmacologically with fibrinolytics or mechanically with percutaneous coronary intervention (PCI) with stent implantation. In general, mechanical reperfusion is more effective than fibrinolysis if it can be achieved in a timely manner. The recommended time from hospital presentation to reperfusion is 90 minutes.

Mechanical reperfusion has a lower risk of intracranial hemorrhage, particularly in patients older than 75 years, in whom the risk of intracranial bleeding is 1% to 2% with fibrinolysis. Mechanical reperfusion benefits patients with both STEMI and NSTEMI, whereas fibrinolytic therapy is only effective in STEMI and is contraindicated in treatment of NSTEMI.

Patients with UA who have severe or recurrent symptoms or electrocardiographic abnormalities should undergo coronary angiography followed by percutaneous or surgical revascularization based on anatomic findings. Patients who respond to medical therapy and have no further symptoms should undergo a symptom-limited stress test for risk stratification. Patients with severe ischemia, ischemia at low cardiac workload, or ischemia in association with reduced left ventricle (LV) systolic function should proceed to angiography and possibly revascularization. Those with less-severe ischemia or a normal stress test may be managed medically.

1. Fibrinolytics—The 5 fibrinolytic agents approved for intravenous use for the treatment of STEMI in the United States are streptokinase, alteplase, anistreplase, reteplase, and tenecteplase. Use of fibrinolytic agents should be restricted to those who fulfill criteria for fibrinolysis and can be treated within 6 hours of symptom onset (Table 28–3). In-hospital mortality increases with increasing age along with the risk of intracranial hemorrhage and ventricular free wall rupture in older patients receiving fibrinolytics.

2. PCI—Mechanical reperfusion (ie, PCI with or without stenting) is associated with improved outcomes in

Table 28–3. Criteria for fibrinolytic therapy in older adults.

Indications	Contraindications
Symptoms of acute MI within 6–12 hours of onset[a]	Absolute
ST elevation ≥1 mm in 2 or more contiguous limb leads or ≥2 mm in 2 or more contiguous precordial leads or left bundle-branch block not known to be present previously	Previous hemorrhagic stroke at any time
	Any stroke or cerebrovascular event within 1 year
	Known intracranial neoplasm
	Suspected aortic dissection or acute pericarditis
	Relative
	Blood pressure ≥180/110 mm Hg on presentation, not readily controlled
	Known bleeding disorder
	Recent major trauma or internal bleeding (within 2-4 weeks)
	Noncompressible vascular puncture (eg, subclavian intravenous catheter)
	Active peptic ulcer disease

[a]Within 6 hours in patients ≥75 years old.

patients of all ages and is superior to fibrinolysis in older patients. Either bare metal stents or drug-eluting stents may be implanted. The latter are generally preferred, given the lower risk of restenosis, although they require a longer duration of treatment with dual antiplatelet agents. Early angiography and coronary intervention is associated with improved short- and long-term outcomes in patients with either STEMI or NSTEMI. In STEMI patients, the target door-to-balloon time is 90 minutes. Mechanical reperfusion, if available, is the preferred strategy in older patients with documented ACS, although used less often than in younger patients. Older patients do have a lower rate of angiographic success and less ST-segment resolution and more postinfarction complications.

C. Antithrombotic Therapy

1. Aspirin—Aspirin is indicated for all patients with ACS. It is effective in older adults and should be continued indefinitely in all patients with documented CHD. The recommended dosage in the acute setting of ACS is 325 mg daily; dosages of 75–325 mg daily are suitable for long-term use.

2. Anticoagulation—Anticoagulation is indicated in patients with NSTEMI and UA, although the benefits in STEMI are less well-established. Its benefit is even greater in ACS complicated by recurrent ischemia or atrial fibrillation. Anticoagulation is also indicated in patients receiving a short-acting fibrinolytic agent (eg, recombinant tissue-type plasminogen activator) and those receiving a glycoprotein IIb/IIIa inhibitor.

Anticoagulant options include unfractionated heparin (UFH), bivalirudin, low-molecular-weight heparin (LMWH) agents such as enoxaparin and dalteparin, and fondaparinux. LMWH provides more stable anticoagulation than UFH and offers the advantage of subcutaneous administration without the need to monitor activated partial thromboplastin time (aPTT). In addition, LMWHs have been associated with improved clinical outcomes although they are contraindicated in renal failure and have been associated with increased bleeding in older adults, which may be due to decreased creatinine clearance.

3. Antiplatelet therapy—Antiplatelet agents that block the ADP receptor have been shown to reduce repeat major cardiac events after percutaneous coronary stent implantation in ACS patients. In addition, these agents reduce cardiovascular mortality, nonfatal MI, and nonfatal stroke by approximately 20% compared with aspirin alone during long-term therapy after NSTEMI. Currently available agents include clopidogrel, prasugrel, and ticagrelor. Prasugrel is more potent than clopidogrel but is not recommended in patients older than 75 years because of the bleeding risk. Clopidogrel recently became generic and is the most commonly used ADP receptor antagonist. The initial dosage is 300–600 mg orally followed by 75 mg daily.

4. Glycoprotein IIb/IIIa inhibitors—These potent antiplatelet agents block the final pathway leading to platelet aggregation. Available agents include abciximab, eptifibatide, and tirofiban. Most data for these agents came prior to the routine use of ADP receptor antagonists, where they were shown to reduce the risk of recurrent ischemic events and improve clinical outcomes in patients with documented MI, particularly those undergoing percutaneous coronary revascularization. These agents similarly benefit younger and older patients, although the risk of bleeding is higher in those who are older; dosage adjustment may be necessary in patients with impaired renal function.

D. β Blockers

Early administration of intravenous β blockers reduces mortality partly because of reduced sudden cardiac death, recurrent ischemic events, and both supraventricular and ventricular tachyarrhythmias in appropriately selected ACS patients. Intravenous β-blocker therapy should be initiated as soon as possible in all patients with suspected ACS in the absence of contraindications (ie, heart rate <50 beats/min, systolic BP <90–100 mm Hg, PR interval ≥240 milliseconds, heart block greater than first degree, moderate or severe pulmonary congestion, or active bronchospasm).

Cardioselective β blockers are preferred, and intravenous metoprolol and atenolol have been approved for treatment of ACS. Patients receiving intravenous β blockers should be carefully observed for bradyarrhythmias, hypotension, dyspnea, and bronchospasm. It is prudent to use lower dosages and a slower dose titration schedule in patients older than 75 years and in those with multiple comorbidities or unstable hemodynamics. Dose adjustment is necessary for atenolol in renal impairment.

E. Angiotensin-Converting Enzyme Inhibitors & Angiotensin Receptor Blockers

Angiotensin-converting enzyme (ACE) inhibitors and angiotensin receptor blockers (ARBs) are beneficial in patients 65–74 years of age, but there is no clear evidence of benefit in patients older than age 75 years. Data suggest that ACE inhibitors are particularly beneficial in patients with anterior STEMIs and MIs complicated by clinical heart failure or significant LV systolic dysfunction (LV ejection fraction <40%). Contraindications to ACE inhibitors include systolic BP <90–100 mm Hg, advanced renal insufficiency—especially if worsening renal function is evident, bilateral renal artery stenosis, and hyperkalemia. ACE inhibitor therapy can be initiated with captopril 6.25 mg 3 times a day or enalapril 2.5 mg twice daily. Once the maintenance dose has been achieved, changing to a once-daily agent at equivalent dosage (eg, lisinopril 20–40 mg) is appropriate. Throughout the initiation and titration phase of ACE inhibitor therapy, BP, serum creatinine, and potassium should be carefully monitored. ARBs are generally used for patients who do not tolerate ACE inhibitors because of cough.

F. Lipid-Lowering Agents

3-Hydroxy-3-methylglutaryl-coenzyme A (HMG CoA) reductase inhibitors (statins) should be initiated early in the course of ACS at high doses (eg, atorvastatin 80 mg) and continued indefinitely. These agents have been shown to decrease mortality and recurrent ischemic events after NSTEMI and STEMI.

G. Nitrates

Nitrate preparations are effective in controlling ischemia, treating heart failure, and managing hypertension in patients with ACS. As noted above, the options include sublingual nitroglycerin, topical nitroglycerin ointment, and intravenous nitroglycerin infusion. Nitrate tolerance generally occurs within about 24 hours.

H. Calcium Channel Blockers

Calcium channel blockers have not been shown to improve mortality in ACS patients, and the use of short-acting dihydropyridines (eg, nifedipine) is contraindicated, as are the nondihydropyridines (eg, verapamil and diltiazem) in patients with heart failure and LV dysfunction.

I. Potassium & Magnesium

Potassium should be maintained within a range of 3.5–4.5 mEq/L and magnesium above 2.0 mEq/L.

▶ Prognosis

Approximately 15% to 20% of patients with STEMI die before reaching the hospital, a proportion that likely increases with advancing age. Among patients with recognized ACS, both short- and long-term mortality increase progressively with age. Other factors associated with increased mortality include anterior MI, clinical heart failure, impaired LV systolic function, atrial fibrillation, complex ventricular arrhythmias, poor functional status, diabetes mellitus, and lack of guideline-based treatment. Although short-term prognosis is more favorable in NSTEMI than in STEMI, mortality rates at 2 years are similar.

Anderson JL, Adams CD, Antman EM, et al. ACC/AHA 2007 guidelines for the management of patients with unstable angina/non-ST-Elevation myocardial infarction: a report of the American College of Cardiology/American Heart Association Task Force on Practice Guidelines (Writing Committee to Revise the 2002 Guidelines for the Management of Patients With Unstable Angina/Non-ST-Elevation Myocardial Infarction) developed in collaboration with the American College of Emergency Physicians, the Society for Cardiovascular Angiography and Interventions, and the Society of Thoracic Surgeons endorsed by the American Association of Cardiovascular and Pulmonary Rehabilitation and the Society for Academic Emergency Medicine. J Am Coll Cardiol. 2007;50(7):e1-157.

Antman EM, McCabe CH, Gurfinkel EP, et al. Enoxaparin prevents death and cardiac ischemic events in unstable angina/non-Q-wave MI. Results of the thrombolysis in myocardial infarction (TIMI) IIB trial. Circulation. 1999;100(15):1593-1601.

Antman EM, Hand M, Armstrong PW, et al. 2007 Focused Update of the ACC/AHA 2004 Guidelines for the Management of Patients With ST-Elevation Myocardial Infarction: a report of the American College of Cardiology/American Heart Association Task Force on Practice Guidelines: developed in collaboration With the Canadian Cardiovascular Society endorsed by the American Academy of Family Physicians: 2007 Writing Group to Review New Evidence and Update the ACC/AHA 2004 Guidelines for the Management of Patients With ST-Elevation Myocardial Infarction, Writing on Behalf of the 2004 Writing Committee. J Am Coll Cardiol. 2008;51(2):210-247.

Berger AK, Schulman KA, Gersh BJ, et al. Primary coronary angioplasty vs. thrombolysis for the management of acute myocardial infarction in elderly patients. JAMA. 1999;282(4):341-348.

de Boer MJ, Ottervanger JP, van 't Hof AW, et al. Reperfusion therapy in elderly patients with acute myocardial infarction: a randomized comparison of primary angioplasty and thrombolytic therapy. J Am Coll Cardiol. 2002;39(11):1723-1728.

Fox KA, Poole-Wilson PA, Henderson RA, et al. Interventional versus conservative treatment for patients with unstable angina or non-ST-elevation myocardial infarction. The British Heart Foundation RITA 3 randomised trial. Randomized Intervention Trial of Unstable Angina. Lancet. 2002;360(9335):743-751.

Indications for ACE inhibitors in the early treatment of acute myocardial infarction: systematic overview of individual data from 100,000 patients in randomized trials. ACE Inhibitor Myocardial Infarction Collaborative Group. Circulation. 1998;97(22):2202-2212.

Indications for fibrinolytic therapy in suspected acute myocardial infarction: collaborative overview of early mortality and major morbidity results from all randomised trials of more than 1000 patients. Fibrinolytic Therapy Trialists' (FTT) Collaborative Group. Lancet. 1994;343(8893):311-322.

Krumholz HM, Hennen J, Ridker PM, et al: Use and effectiveness of intravenous heparin therapy for treatment of acute myocardial infarction in the elderly. J Am Coll Cardiol. 1998;31(5):973-979.

Montalescot G, Dallongeville J, Van Belle E, et al; OPERA Investigators. STEMI and NSTEMI: are they so different? 1 year outcomes in acute myocardial infarction as defined by the ESC/ACC definition (the OPERA registry). Eur Heart J. 2007;28(12):1409-1417.

Schwartz GG, Olsson AG, Ezekowitz MD, et al; Myocardial Ischemia Reduction with Aggressive Cholesterol Lowering (MIRACL) Study Investigators. Effects of atorvastatin on early recurrent ischemic events in acute coronary syndromes: the MIRACL study: a randomized controlled trial. JAMA. 2001;285(13):1711-1718.

Smith SC Jr, Blair SN, Bonow RO, et al: AHA/ACC guidelines for preventing heart attack and death in patients with atherosclerotic cardiovascular disease: 2001 update. A statement for healthcare professionals from the American Heart Association and the American College of Cardiology. J Am Coll Cardiol. 2001;38(5):1581-1583.

Thiemann DR, Coresh J, Schulman SP, Gerstenblith G, Oetgen WJ, Powe NR. Lack of benefit for intravenous thrombolysis in patients with myocardial infarction who are older than 75 years. Circulation. 2000;101(19):2239-2246.

Williams MA, Fleg JL, Ades PA, et al; American Heart Association Council on Clinical Cardiology Subcommittee on Exercise,

Cardiac Rehabilitation, and Prevention. Secondary prevention of coronary heart disease in the elderly (with emphasis on patients > or =75 years of age): an American Heart Association scientific statement from the Council on Clinical Cardiology Subcommittee on Exercise, Cardiac Rehabilitation, and Prevention. *Circulation.* 2002;105(14):1735-1743.

Yusuf S, Zhao F, Mehta SR, Chrolavicius S, Tognoni G, Fox KK; Clopidogrel in Unstable Angina to Prevent Recurrent Events Trial Investigators. Effects of clopidogrel in addition to aspirin in patients with acute coronary syndromes without ST-segment elevation. *N Engl J Med.* 2001;345(7):494-502.

CHRONIC CORONARY HEART DISEASE

▶ General Principles in Older Adults

CHD is the leading cause of death in the United States in both men and women. Chronic stable angina is the most common form of CHD and is the initial form of presentation in 80% of patients. Although the incidence and prevalence of CHD are both higher in men than in women, the rates for women increase progressively after menopause, and the greater longevity of women compared with men results in a slight predominance of women in the total number of CHD cases. The prevalence of CHD increases progressively with age, affecting 16.1% of women and 18.6% of men older than 75 years.

▶ Prevention

Primary prevention of CHD may be achieved through lifelong avoidance of tobacco products, participation in regular physical exercise, maintenance of desirable body weight, consumption of a diet rich in fruits, vegetables, and whole-grain foods, and limited consumption of foods high in trans and saturated fats and cholesterol. Early identification and aggressive treatment of risk factors as discussed above is essential.

▶ Clinical Findings

A. Symptoms & Signs

The most common symptom of chronic CHD is central chest discomfort, often described as pressure, tightness, or heaviness, typically brought on by physical exertion or emotional stress and relieved by rest or nitroglycerin. The discomfort may radiate to or primarily be in the jaw, left or both arms, back or epigastrium. The discomfort typically lasts longer than a few minutes and up to 20 minutes. If longer than 20 minutes, ACS should be ruled out. Taking a breath, moving arms or body or coughing does not affect the discomfort. However, many older adults with CHD, including those with prior MI or UA, manifest atypical symptoms, such as dyspnea, fatigue, weakness, dizziness, or abdominal discomfort, whereas others, particularly diabetics, are entirely asymptomatic, in part because of the high prevalence of physical inactivity at older age (see Chapter 63, "Addressing Chest Pain in Older Adults").

Table 28–4. Canadian Cardiovascular Society Classification of Angina.

Class I: No discomfort with ordinary activity, only with strenuous exertion.
Class II: Angina mildly limiting ordinary activity; ie, >2 blocks walking on level, >1 flight of stairs.
Class III: Angina markedly limiting ordinary activity; walking <2 blocks on the level, <1 flight of stairs.
Class IV: Angina with any activity or at rest.

Myocardial ischemia occurs when the myocardial O_2 demands are not met by an increase in myocardial blood supply. The earliest events are increased myocardial stiffness of the ischemic myocardium, followed by decreased contractility, metabolic alterations resulting in increased lactic acid formation, changes in electrical repolarization, and finally the discomfort we recognize as angina. The symptoms and events created can be angina, dyspnea, or the development of malignant ventricular arrhythmias, including sudden death. If the volume of ischemic myocardium is large, symptoms of shortness of breath, exercise intolerance and even heart failure may occur.

Angina is graded using the Canadian Cardiovascular Society Classification system based on the level of activity required to produce symptoms (Table 28–4).

The physical examination in patients with chronic CAD can be entirely normal. In other patients, physical findings are nonspecific but may include an S_3 or S_4 gallop, mitral regurgitation murmur, a laterally displaced or dyskinetic apical impulse (especially in patients with prior MI), or signs of heart failure (eg, pulmonary rales, elevated JVP, peripheral edema).

B. Special Tests

Basic laboratory tests can reveal factors that contribute to the pathophysiology of stable angina such as complete blood count (anemia), thyroid-stimulating hormone (TSH) (hyperthyroidism), and toxicology screen (cocaine or amphetamine use).

1. Electrocardiography—The ECG may demonstrate pathologic Q waves in patients with prior MI. Other ECG findings are nonspecific. The ECG is especially informative if done while the patient is experiencing chest discomfort. At such times, flat or down-sloping ST depression may be seen. If the patient is not experiencing angina at the time the ECG is done, it may be entirely normal.

2. Stress tests—The noninvasive procedure of choice for diagnosing CHD is an exercise test or pharmacologic stress test using adenosine, dipyridamole, regadenoson, or dobutamine, usually accompanied by echocardiographic or radionuclide imaging. Meta-analysis suggests that an ECG exercise test without imaging has a mean sensitivity of 68% and a specificity of 77%. However, because of selection bias, the sensitivity is nearer to 50% with a specificity of 85% to 90%. The ability of the older patient to achieve 85% of maximal estimated heart rate for age and sex is markedly reduced compared to younger patients. Also, an exercise ECG stress test can only be interpreted if the resting ECG is normal or has minor ST–T-wave changes. The presence of LVH, moderate ST–T-wave changes, Wolff-Parkinson-White syndrome, or left bundle-branch block makes changes in the exercise ECG non-interpretable.

The exercise ECG stress test provides 80% to 90% sensitivity and specificity for diagnosing CHD, although the predictive accuracy of the test is dependent on the pretest likelihood of CHD. In general, it is preferable to perform an exercise test if the patient is capable of doing so, as the duration of exercise is an independent powerful predictor of prognosis. However, because many older patients are limited by arthritis, neurologic conditions, or poor physical conditioning, it is often necessary to perform a pharmacologic stress test (eg, dobutamine echo, adenosine sestamibi).

3. Coronary angiography—Coronary angiography remains the gold standard for determining the presence, extent, and severity of CHD as well as the suitability for percutaneous or surgical revascularization. Older patients are more likely to have multivessel disease and left main CAD.

4. Other tests—Multidetector cardiac CT with coronary calcium quantification showing a high burden of coronary calcium is associated with extensive CAD and worse prognosis, but routine use of this technology is controversial. CT with contrast coronary angiography can also demonstrate proximal coronary disease and its severity. However, it requires special expertise and is not generally available.

▶ Differential Diagnosis

The differential diagnosis of chest pain includes:

1. **Cardiac:** coronary vasospasm, pericarditis, cardiomyopathy, arrhythmias, syndrome X or microvascular coronary artery dysfunction, cocaine or amphetamine vasospasm

2. **Vascular:** aortic dissection, arteritis

3. **Gastrointestinal:** esophageal reflux, esophageal spasm, duodenal ulcer, pancreatitis, cholecystitis

4. **Pulmonary:** pulmonary embolus, pneumothorax, pleurisy, pneumonia

5. **Neurologic:** shingles, neuropathy

6. **Musculoskeletal:** costochondritis, rib fracture, arthritis, muscle pain

7. **Psychogenic causes:** panic attacks, hyperventilation, anxiety

Angina as a result of myocardial ischemia can occur whenever there is an imbalance between myocardial O_2 demand and supply. Other diseases where angina is a symptom without epicardial CAD are valvular aortic stenosis, hypertrophic cardiomyopathy, and myocarditis. With nonobstructive coronary artery plaques, an unusual increase in myocardial O_2 demand can result in myocardial ischemia and angina: hyperthyroidism, arteriovenous fistulae, and excessive sympathetic stimulation. Patients with anemia, hypoxemia, and hyperviscosity can have decreased O_2 delivery resulting in angina.

▶ Complications

The major complications of chronic CHD are progression to ACS, development of heart failure because of the cumulative effects of myocardial injury or infarction (ischemic cardiomyopathy), and development of conduction abnormalities or arrhythmias, including ventricular tachycardia and ventricular fibrillation. Sudden cardiac death is the initial manifestation of CHD in up to 20% of cases.

A. Risk Stratification

The patients at highest risk are those with ACS. In patients with chronic CAD, the risk increases with higher Canadian Class, decreased LV function (LV ejection fraction), location, severity and extent of coronary artery stenosis, high-risk noninvasive stress test, general physical health, comorbidities, and uncontrolled vascular risk factors.

▶ Treatment

A. Goals of Treatment

The goals of therapy for chronic CHD are to control symptoms, prevent or slow progression and prevent major complications. Since myocardial ischemia is the basis for the symptoms, the factors involved in myocardial O_2 demand must be considered. The major requirements for myocardial O_2 demand are myocardial contractility and LV wall tension, the determinants of which are the systolic BP, the LV diastolic radius, the LV wall thickness, and the heart rate. The coronary blood flow to the myocardium depends on the degree of coronary artery obstruction and changes that effect patency determined by the severity of the atherosclerotic plaque, plaque rupture with platelet aggregation or thrombus, varying degrees of coronary vascular tone, and coronary spasm. The pharmacologic approach to therapy addresses these factors:

1. *Decrease in myocardial O_2 demand:* β blockers, ACE inhibitors, ARBs, treatment of hypertension, lowering of heart rate.

2. *Increase coronary blood flow:* nitrates, Ca^{++} channel blockers.

3. *Decrease factors causing obstruction:* nitrates, antiplatelet drugs.

4. *Open or bypass obstruction:* coronary bypass surgery, PCI with and without stenting.

5. *Optimal treatment:* involves lifestyle modifications, attention to risk factors, pharmacologic interventions, and, in selected patients, percutaneous or surgical revascularization.

B. Lifestyle Modifications

All patients with CHD should be strongly advised to discontinue all tobacco products. Gradual weight reduction through diet and regular exercise should be encouraged in overweight patients (body mass index >25–30 kg/m^2). Patients with CHD should eat a balanced diet rich in fruits, vegetables, and whole grains while limiting intake of trans and saturated fats (including partially hydrogenated oils) and cholesterol. Patients should also engage in a total of at least 20–30 minutes of moderate intensity physical activity on most days of the week unless limited by active cardiovascular symptoms or other medical conditions. Walking, stationary cycling, and swimming are suitable exercise modalities for older adults with mild functional impairments. When beginning an exercise program, patients should be instructed to start at a slow and comfortable pace, gradually increasing the duration of exercise over a period of weeks. Patients who have suffered an MI or who have had coronary bypass surgery should be strongly encouraged to participate in a formal cardiac rehabilitation program. Such programs have been associated with reduced mortality, improved exercise tolerance and quality of life, and enhanced mood and sense of well-being.

C. Pharmacotherapy

1. Aspirin—Long-term use of aspirin in CHD patients markedly reduces the risk of death, MI, and stroke. The absolute benefit is greatest in high-risk patients, including those older than 65 years. The optimal dose of aspirin is unknown, but 75 or 81 mg once daily provides benefits equivalent to higher doses with a lower risk of side effects, including bleeding. In patients intolerant to low-dose aspirin, clopidogrel 75 mg daily is an acceptable alternative.

2. β Blockers—β Blockers reduce the risk of death and reinfarction after MI. β Blockers are also highly effective antianginal agents and appear to reduce the incidence of coronary events in patients with chronic CHD. It is reasonable to start and continue β blockers indefinitely in all patients who have had ACS or have LV dysfunction with or without heart failure symptoms unless contraindicated. In patients without prior MI, the optimal dose of β blockers is unknown, but a rational therapeutic goal is to gradually increase the dose until the patient has no or minimal ischemic symptoms and the resting heart rate is <60 beats/min. Older patients may be less tolerant of β blockers because of the effects of aging on sinus node function and the presence of comorbidities (eg, pulmonary disease); dosages should, therefore, be adjusted accordingly and heart rate should be followed for bradycardia.

3. Nitrates—Sublingual nitroglycerin remains the drug of choice for treatment of an acute episode of angina. As a result

of drying of the oral mucosa in older adults, nitroglycerin spray may be more effective than tablets for older patients. Older patients may also be more likely to experience orthostatic hypotension with nitroglycerin; they should be advised to take the medication in a sitting or reclining position. Long-term nitrates, such as isosorbide mononitrate, are effective antianginal agents, but have not been shown to improve clinical outcomes. In addition, tolerance to nitrates develops rapidly, requiring a daily 6- to 8-hour nitrate-free interval. Several oral and transdermal nitrate preparations are available for chronic use. If the patient has taken a phosphodiesterase-5 (PDE-5) inhibitor within 48 hours, any organic nitrate is strictly contraindicated because of the possibility of excessive hypotension.

4. Calcium channel blockers—Calcium channel blockers are effective antihypertensive and antianginal agents, but they have not been shown to improve clinical outcomes in CHD patients. In addition, they may be associated with worsening heart failure and, with the exception of amlodipine and felodipine, should be avoided in patients with impaired LV systolic function. Verapamil and diltiazem slow the heart rate and conduction through the AV node, especially when used in combination with a β-blocker, thus increasing the risk of bradyarrhythmias and syncope in older patients with sinus node dysfunction (sick sinus syndrome) or impaired AV nodal conduction. Verapamil and, to a lesser extent, diltiazem also impair gastrointestinal motility and may lead to constipation or ileus.

5. Angiotensin-converting enzyme inhibitors—ACE inhibitors do not exert a direct antiischemic effect, but ramipril reduces mortality and major cardiovascular events in a broad range of patients with established vascular disease or diabetes. In addition, ACE inhibitors improve outcomes in patients with reduced LV systolic function with or without symptoms. ACE inhibitors should be given as first-line therapy in patients with CHD, especially those with hypertension, reduced LV function, diabetes and/or chronic renal disease. Thus, initiation of an ACE inhibitor should be strongly considered in all older adults with established CHD in the absence of contraindications.

6. Angiotensin receptor blockers—ARBs have been shown to improve outcomes in patients with diabetes and in hypertensive patients with LV hypertrophy; however, the value of these agents in patients with CHD is unproven. Both ACE inhibitors and ARBs have been shown in patients with coronary disease to improve endothelial function by increasing the availability of nitric oxide that should prove beneficial. A meta-analysis showed that compared to controls, ARBs reduce the risk of strokes, heart failure and new onset diabetes. Currently, routine use of an ARB in patients with CHD is not recommended, but they are an appropriate alternative in patients who require an ACE inhibitor but are intolerant of these agents because of cough.

7. Lipid-lowering agents—Statins reduce mortality and cardiovascular morbidity in patients with CHD, and the benefits extend to patients at least up to the age of 85. Statins have been shown to reduce adverse cardiovascular events even in patients who have LDL cholesterol below 100 mg/dL. This beneficial effect has been attributed to the cholesterol-independent pleiotropic effects of statins including improvement in endothelial function, enhancing the stability of atherosclerotic plaques, decreasing vascular oxidative stress and inflammation, and inhibiting the thrombogenic response. Therefore, all patients with CHD or diabetes should be on statins to lower LDL cholesterol to ≤70 mg/dL if not contraindicated. As with other medications, it is advisable to start with a lower dose and titrate the drug more slowly in patients older than 75 years.

8. Warfarin—Warfarin is indicated in patients with CHD complicated by atrial fibrillation or LV mural thrombus with embolization. Warfarin can also be used as an alternative to aspirin in aspirin-intolerant patients. Older patients are at increased risk for bleeding complications with warfarin, especially during concomitant treatment with nonsteroidal antiinflammatory drugs (NSAIDs).

9. Other therapies—Mainly for patients with angina refractory to maximal treatment with the above drugs are spinal cord stimulation and external counterpulsation, but there is not enough data to recommend these. A new antianginal drug is ranolazine, a partial fatty acid oxidation inhibitor that shifts adenosine triphosphate (ATP) production from fatty acids to more oxygen-efficient carbohydrate oxidation. However, it prolongs the QT interval. Because it does not affect heart rate or BP, it is useful in those patients who have not responded to maximally-tolerated other antianginal medications.

D. Revascularization

Patients with stable CAD who can perform ordinary activity without symptoms on optimal medical therapy and who have normal or only moderately depressed LV function can be managed medically. Supporting this recommendation is the COURAGE trial, where patients with stable angina, objective evidence of myocardial ischemia, and an LV ejection fraction ≥30% with coronary vessels suitable for PCI were randomized to optimal medical management or PCI with optimal medical management. In a follow-up of 2.5–7 years (median: 4.6 years), there was no difference between optimal medical management with or without PCI in the composite of MI, stroke, and death.

PCI and coronary artery bypass surgery are highly effective in improving symptoms and quality of life in older patients with CHD; >50% of all revascularization procedures in the United States are now performed in patients older than 65 years. On the other hand, both coronary angioplasty with and without stents and bypass surgery are associated with increased mortality and major complications in the very old, especially in patients older than age 80 years; thus, careful selection of candidates for revascularization procedures is of paramount importance. In general, percutaneous coronary revascularization is associated with lower mortality and major morbidity (including stroke, delirium) as well as much more rapid recovery compared with coronary bypass surgery in older patients. However, the need for repeat revascularization procedures is higher after angioplasty, and long-term outcomes are similar. Thus, both procedures represent suitable options for older patients with severe symptomatic CHD, and the choice of procedure should be based on anatomical considerations, prevalent comorbidities, and patient preferences. Up to 50% of older patients undergoing coronary bypass surgery may experience a decline in cognitive function in the perioperative period. Although these cognitive deficits are transient in many patients, a significant proportion may exhibit persistent cognitive impairment during long-term follow-up.

▶ Prognosis

The prognosis of chronic CHD is highly variable. Although some patients remain minimally symptomatic or asymptomatic for decades, others experience marked disability despite multiple therapeutic interventions. Still others succumb to the disease after suffering a large MI or fatal arrhythmia. Factors that adversely influence prognosis include older age, male gender, more severe CHD, more severe heart failure or LV systolic dysfunction (lower ejection fraction), more severe symptoms or functional limitations, presence of diabetes or atrial fibrillation, and presence of significant ventricular arrhythmias (Table 28–5).

Table 28–5. Impact of common comorbidities in older patients with heart failure.

Condition	Impact
Renal dysfunction	Exacerbated by diuretics, ACE inhibitors
Chronic lung disease	Diagnostic uncertainty, difficulty in assessing volume status
Cognitive dysfunction	Interferes with compliance and patient assessment
Depression, social isolation	Interferes with compliance, worsens prognosis
Postural hypotension, falls	Aggravated by vasodilators, β blockers, diuretics
Urinary incontinence	Aggravated by diuretics, ACE inhibitors (cough)
Sensory deprivation	Interferes with compliance
Nutritional disorders	Exacerbated by dietary restrictions
Polypharmacy	Increased drug interactions, decreased compliance
Frailty	Exacerbated by hospitalization, increased fall risk

Ades PA: Cardiac rehabilitation and secondary prevention of coronary heart disease. *N Engl J Med.* 2001;345(12):892-902.

American Diabetes Association. Standards of medical care for patients with diabetes mellitus. *Diabetes Care.* 2002;25(1): 213-229.

Bangalore S, Kumar S, Wetterslev J, Messerli FH. Angiotensin receptor blockers and risk of myocardial infarction: meta-analyses and trial sequential analyses of 147 020 patients from randomized trials. *BMJ.* 2011;342:d2234.

Boden WE, O'Rourke RA, Teo KK, et al. Optimal medical therapy with or without PCI for stable coronary disease. *Circulation.* 2007;356(15):1503-1516.

Dargie HJ. Effect of carvedilol on outcome after myocardial infarction in patients with left-ventricular dysfunction: the CAPRICORN randomized trial. *Lancet.* 2001;357(9266):1385-1390.

Dickstein K, Kjekshus J; OPTIMAAL Steering Committee of the OPTIMAAL Study Group. Effects of losartan and captopril on mortality and morbidity in high-risk patients after acute myocardial infarction: the OPTIMAAL randomized trial. *Lancet.* 2002;360(9335):752-760.

Expert Panel on Detection, Evaluation, and Treatment of High Blood Cholesterol in Adults: Executive summary of the third report of the National Cholesterol Education Program (NCEP) expert panel on detection, evaluation, and treatment of high blood cholesterol in adults (Adult Treatment Panel III). *JAMA.* 2001;285(19):2486-2497.

Liao JK. Effects of statins on 3-hydroxy-3-methylglutaryl coenzyme a reductase inhibition beyond low-density lipoprotein cholesterol. *Am J Cardiol.* 2005;96(5A):24F-33F.

Newman MF, Kirchner JL, Phillips-Bute B, et al; Neurological Outcome Research Group and the Cardiothoracic Anesthe-siology Research Endeavors Investigators. Longitudinal assessment of neurocognitive function after coronary-artery bypass surgery. *N Engl J Med.* 2001;344(6):395-402.

Patel MR, Dehmer GJ, Hirshfeld JW, Smith PK, Spertus JA. ACCF/SCAI/STS/AATS/AHA/ASNC/HFSA/SCCT 2012 Appropriate use criteria for coronary revascularization focused update: a report of the American College of Cardiology Foundation Appropriate Use Criteria Task Force, Society for Cardiovascular Angiography and Interventions, Society of Thoracic Surgeons, American Association for Thoracic Surgery, American Heart Association, American Society of Nuclear Cardiology, and the Society of Cardiovascular Computed Tomography. *J Am Coll Cardiol.* 2012;59(9):857-881.

Pearson TA, Blair SN, Daniels SR, et al. AHA guidelines for primary prevention of cardiovascular disease and stroke: 2002 update: consensus panel guide to comprehensive risk reduction for adult patients without coronary or other atherosclerotic vascular diseases. American Heart Association Science Advisory and Coordinating Committee. *Circulation.* 2002;106(3):388-391.

Williams MA, Fleg JL, Ades PA, et al; American Heart Association Council on Clinical Cardiology Subcommittee on Exercise, Cardiac Rehabilitation, and Prevention. Secondary prevention of coronary heart disease in the elderly (with emphasis on patients > or =75 years): an American Heart Association scientific statement from the Council on Clinical Cardiology Subcommittee on Exercise, Cardiac Rehabilitation, and Prevention. *Circulation.* 2002;105(14):1735-1743.

Yusuf S, Sleight P, Pogue J, Bosch J, Davies R, Dagenais G. Effects of an angiotensin-converting-enzyme inhibitor, ramipril, on cardiovascular events in high-risk patients. The Heart Outcomes Prevention Evaluation Study Investigators. *N Engl J Med.* 2000;342(3):145-153.

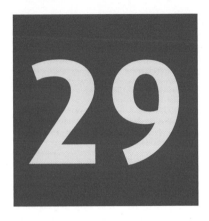

Heart Failure & Heart Rhythm Disorders

Susan M. Joseph, MD
Jane Chen, MD
Michael W. Rich, MD

HEART FAILURE

ESSENTIALS OF DIAGNOSIS

▶ Exertional dyspnea, fatigue, orthopnea, lower-extremity swelling.

▶ Pulmonary rales, elevated jugular venous pressure, peripheral edema.

▶ Echocardiography reveals left ventricle systolic or diastolic dysfunction.

General Principles in Older Adults

Incidence and prevalence of heart failure (HF) increase exponentially with age, reflecting the increasing prevalence of hypertension and coronary heart disease (CHD) at older age and the marked reduction in cardiovascular reserve that accompanies normative aging. There is a 4-fold increase in the incidence of HF between ages 65 and 85 years. Although the incidence of HF is higher in men than in women at all ages, women comprise slightly more than half of prevalent HF cases because of the higher proportion of women among older adults.

HF is currently the most common cause of hospitalization in the Medicare age group; more than 70% of the nearly 1 million annual hospitalizations for HF involve persons older than age 65 years. HF is also a major source of chronic disability in older adults, and is the most costly Medicare diagnosis-related group.

Prevention

Primary prevention of HF is feasible through aggressive treatment of the major conditions that cause HF (ie, hypertension and CHD). Antihypertensive therapy reduces the risk of incident HF by as much as 64% in older adults. The greatest benefit is seen in octogenarians with systolic hypertension. Similarly, treatment of other coronary risk factors may prevent or delay the onset of CHD, thus reducing the risk of HF.

Clinical Findings

A. Symptoms & Signs

Symptoms include exertional shortness of breath, effort intolerance, fatigue, cough, orthopnea, paroxysmal nocturnal dyspnea, and swelling of the feet and ankles. However, exertional symptoms are less prominent in older adults in part because of reduced physical activity. Conversely, altered sensorium, irritability, lethargy, anorexia, abdominal discomfort, and gastrointestinal disturbances are more common symptoms of HF in older adults (see Chapter 7, "Atypical Presentations of Illness in Older Adults").

Signs of HF include tachycardia, tachypnea, an S_3 or S_4 gallop, pulmonary rales, elevated jugular venous pressure, hepatojugular reflux, hepatomegaly, and dependent edema. In severe HF, the pulse pressure may be narrowed, and there may be signs of impaired tissue perfusion, such as diminished cognition. Depending on the cause of HF, additional findings may include severe hypertension, a dyskinetic apical impulse, a murmur of aortic or mitral origin, or peripheral signs of endocarditis. As with symptoms, the signs of HF in older adults are often nonspecific or atypical.

B. Special Tests

1. Chest radiography—The chest x-ray can assess for presence of pulmonary edema or cardiomegaly and rule out other causes of dyspnea (pneumonia, pneumothorax). Of note, up to 40% of HF patients with elevated pulmonary capillary wedge pressure have no radiographic evidence of congestion.

2. Electrocardiography—An electrocardiogram (ECG) may reveal dysrhythmias, left ventricular (LV) hypertrophy, left atrial enlargement, or signs of ischemia or infarction. Low voltage suggests infiltrative cardiomyopathy or pericardial effusion.

3. Echocardiography—Echocardiography is usually the preferred test for evaluating LV function. Echocardiography provides information about atrial and ventricular chamber size and wall thickness, valve function, LV diastolic function, and pericardial disorders. Less common alternatives to echocardiography include radionuclide angiography and magnetic resonance imaging in certain circumstances.

4. Stress test—A stress test should be considered if severe CHD is suspected.

5. Cardiac catheterization—Cardiac catheterization is not recommended in the routine diagnostic evaluation of patients with HF, but should be considered if there is suspicion for severe CHD. Cardiac catheterization is indicated prior to coronary revascularization or valve procedures.

▶ Differential Diagnosis

The diagnosis of HF is straightforward in patients with severe symptoms and overt signs of congestion but may be difficult in patients with less-severe HF and atypical symptoms. Other causes of dyspnea and fatigue in older individuals include acute and chronic pulmonary disease, obstructive sleep apnea, obesity, anemia, hypothyroidism, poor physical conditioning, and depression (see Chapter 64, "Addressing Dyspnea in Older Adults," for more in-depth discussion of work-up of dyspnea in older adults). Lower-extremity edema, in the absence of other signs of HF, may be caused by venous insufficiency, renal or hepatic disease, or medications (especially calcium channel blockers). An elevated BNP (B-type natriuretic peptide) level may be helpful in differentiating dyspnea of cardiac origin from that resulting from pulmonary or other causes. However, BNP levels increase with age, especially in women, so the specificity of elevated levels for diagnosing HF declines with age.

In addition to establishing a diagnosis of HF and determining etiology, it is important to identify factors that may contribute to worsening HF symptoms. Common precipitants of HF exacerbations in older adults include nonadherence to dietary restrictions or medications, myocardial ischemia or infarction, uncontrolled hypertension, arrhythmias (especially atrial fibrillation or flutter), anemia, systemic illness (pneumonia, sepsis), iatrogenesis (postoperative volume overload, blood transfusions), and adverse drug reactions (nonsteroidal antiinflammatory drugs).

▶ Complications

Complications include progressive symptoms and functional decline, recurrent hospital admissions, supraventricular and ventricular arrhythmias (which may lead to syncope or sudden death), cognitive impairment and worsening renal function caused by hypoperfusion, and deep vein thrombosis or mural thrombus with systemic embolization.

▶ Treatment

A. Goals of Treatment

The goals of HF therapy are to alleviate symptoms, improve functional capacity and quality of life, reduce hospitalizations, and maximize functional survival. Optimal management of the older patient involves identification and treatment of the underlying cause and precipitating factors, implementation of an effective pharmacotherapeutic regimen, and coordination of care through the use of an interprofessional team. Management of HF in older adults is often complicated by comorbid conditions that may influence both the clinical course and treatment (Table 29–1). Thus, it is essential that HF management be individualized, with due consideration given to concomitant illnesses, prognosis, goals of care, lifestyle, and therapeutic preferences (see Chapter 3, "Goals of Care & Consideration of Prognosis," for more on goals of care).

B. Interprofessional Care

HF is responsive to a team approach and interprofessional care (see Chapter 5, "The Interprofessional Team"). Common features of successful interventions include a nurse coordinator, intensive patient education and promotion of self-management skills (eg, daily weights), and close follow-up (especially after hospital discharge).

Table 29–1. Impact of common comorbidities in older patients with heart failure.

Condition	Impact
Renal dysfunction	Exacerbated by diuretics, ACE inhibitors
Chronic lung disease	Diagnostic uncertainty, difficulty in assessing volume status
Cognitive dysfunction	Interferes with compliance and patient assessment
Depression, social isolation	Interferes with compliance, worsens prognosis
Postural hypotension, falls	Aggravated by vasodilators, β blockers, diuretics
Urinary incontinence	Aggravated by diuretics, ACE inhibitors (cough)
Sensory deprivation	Interferes with compliance
Nutritional disorders	Exacerbated by dietary restrictions
Polypharmacy	Increased drug interactions, decreased compliance
Frailty	Exacerbated by hospitalization, increased fall risk

ACE, angiotensin-converting enzyme.

Table 29–2. Angiotensin-converting enzyme inhibitors for systolic heart failure.[a]

Agent	Starting Dose	Target Dose
Captopril	6.25 mg TID	50 mg TID
Enalapril	2.5 mg BID	10–20 mg BID
Lisinopril	2.5–5 mg QD	20–40 mg QD
Ramipril	1.25–2.5 mg QD	10 mg QD
Quinapril	10 mg BID	40 mg BID
Fosinopril	5–10 mg QD	40 mg QD
Trandolapril	1 mg QD	4 mg QD

[a]Agents approved by the FDA for the treatment of heart failure in the United States.

C. Systolic Heart Failure

Angiotensin-converting enzyme (ACE) inhibitors and β blockers are the cornerstone of therapy for patients with impaired LV systolic function, whether symptomatic or asymptomatic. Available evidence indicates that older patients treated with ACE inhibitors experience improved quality of life, fewer symptoms and hospitalizations, and decreased mortality. Table 29–2 lists the ACE inhibitors approved for treatment of HF in the United States. Potential adverse effects of ACE inhibitors include worsening renal function, hyperkalemia, and hypotension. Close monitoring of renal function, electrolytes, and blood pressure is warranted during initiation and titration of ACE-inhibitor therapy. Cough occurs in up to 20% of patients receiving ACE inhibitors and may be severe enough to require discontinuation in 5% to 10% of cases, but there is no evidence that this occurs more frequently in older adults. In patients who are unable to tolerate ACE inhibitors because of cough, ARBs (angiotensin receptor blockers) are an acceptable alternative.

β Blockers reduce mortality and hospitalizations in patients with HF and reduced LV systolic function. These agents are recommended for all patients with stable HF in the absence of contraindications. Major contraindications include resting heart rate <45 beats/min, systolic blood pressure (BP) <90–100 mm Hg, markedly prolonged PR interval or heart block greater than first degree, active bronchospasm, and decompensated HF. β Blockers approved for the treatment of HF in the United States include sustained-release metoprolol succinate and carvedilol. The starting dosage for metoprolol is 25 mg once daily; for carvedilol, it is 3.125 mg twice daily. The dose should be increased gradually to achieve daily dosages of 100–200 mg for metoprolol and 50 mg for carvedilol. With proper patient selection and dose titration, most HF patients tolerate β blockers. However, some may experience a transient increase in symptoms, and a small minority may require discontinuation because of severe side effects.

Digoxin is a mild inotropic agent that improves symptoms and reduces hospitalizations in patients with moderate HF but has no effect on mortality. The benefits of digoxin in octogenarians are similar to those in younger patients. Digoxin is recommended for HF patients who remain symptomatic despite other therapy. The volume of distribution and renal clearance of digoxin are reduced in older patients. As a result, a digoxin dosage of 0.125 mg daily is usually sufficient; patients with reduced renal function may require lower dosages. Serum digoxin levels of 0.5–1.0 ng/mL are therapeutic. Higher levels provide no additional benefit but increase the risk of toxicity. Routine monitoring of serum digoxin levels is not recommended, but a level should be obtained whenever toxicity is suspected. Because of the risk of potential side effects of digoxin—including bradycardia, heart block, supraventricular and ventricular arrhythmias, gastrointestinal disturbances, and central nervous system disorders (especially visual changes)—the risks and benefits of using digoxin in the individual older patient should be weighed carefully. Hypokalemia, hypomagnesemia, and hypercalcemia increase the risk of digoxin toxicity, and numerous medications, including quinidine, amiodarone, dronedarone, and verapamil, are associated with an increase in serum digoxin levels.

Diuretics, with the exception of spironolactone and eplerenone, have not been shown to improve clinical outcomes in HF patients, but they are essential for relieving congestion and edema and for maintaining an euvolemic state. Some patients with mild HF may respond to a thiazide diuretic, but most will require a more potent loop diuretic. Patients should be instructed to restrict dietary sodium intake to no more than 2 g/day, and the diuretic dosage should be adjusted to maintain euvolemia, as reflected by daily-recorded weights that are within 2 pounds of the patient's predetermined dry weight. Patients with more severe HF or refractory volume overload may benefit from the addition of metolazone 2.5–10 mg daily. Diuretics are commonly associated with potassium and magnesium loss, and older patients are at increased risk for diuretic-induced electrolyte disturbances. Serial monitoring of electrolytes is warranted, and supplements should be prescribed as needed. Overdiuresis may result in hypotension, fatigue, and worsening renal function.

Spironolactone reduces mortality by up to 30% in patients with advanced systolic HF. The dose of spironolactone is 12.5–25 mg daily. Spironolactone is contraindicated in patients with serum creatinine >2.5 mg/dL or serum potassium >5.0 mEq/L, and serum electrolytes and renal function should be assessed within 1–2 weeks after initiating therapy. Up to 10% of patients treated with spironolactone experience painful gynecomastia requiring discontinuation. Eplerenone, a selective aldosterone antagonist, has demonstrated benefit in patients with post-myocardial infarction (MI) LV dysfunction already taking an ACE inhibitor and β-blocker, and in patients with New York Heart Association (NYHA) Class II symptoms and LV ejection fraction ≤35%. Gynecomastia

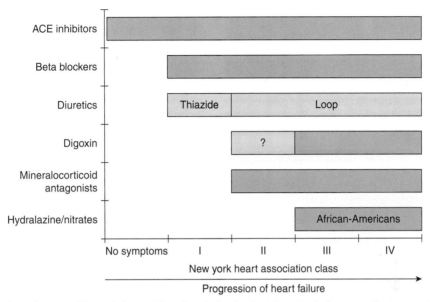

▲ **Figure 29–1.** Drug therapy of heart failure with reduced ejection fraction. Shaded areas reflect current recommendations based on the results of large randomized clinical trials (Class I, Level of Evidence A).

is less common with eplerenone than with spironolactone; other adverse effects are similar.

Figure 29–1 summarizes current pharmacotherapy of systolic HF. All patients with LV systolic dysfunction should receive an ACE inhibitor or ARB and β-blocker unless contraindicated. Diuretics should be prescribed and the dosage adjusted to maintain euvolemia. In patients unable to tolerate an ACE inhibitor or ARB, the combination of hydralazine and nitrates provides an alternative. Although this combination has not been studied extensively in older adults, it has demonstrated morbidity and mortality benefits in younger patients with systolic HF. The most common side effects are headache and dizziness. Digoxin can be added to the regimen of patients with persistent symptoms despite other therapeutic measures, and aldosterone blockade should be prescribed for patients with moderate-to-severe HF symptoms unless contraindicated.

1. Device therapy—Patients with systolic HF are at increased risk for sudden cardiac death (SCD) from malignant ventricular arrhythmias. Implantable cardioverter-defibrillators (ICDs) are efficacious in reducing SCD in high-risk patients with systolic dysfunction. However, the benefit of ICDs in reducing all-cause mortality appears to decline with age, in part because older patients are at increased risk for death from other causes, both cardiac and noncardiac. In addition, older adults are more likely to have procedure-related complications, and may be more likely to receive inappropriate shocks (eg, for atrial fibrillation), which can significantly worsen quality of life. Therefore,

the decision to pursue ICD therapy in older adults must be individualized.

D. Heart Failure with Preserved Ejection Fraction

The prevalence of heart failure with preserved ejection fraction (HFPEF) increases with age, especially among women. HFPEF is often associated with hypertension, chronic kidney disease, diabetes, concentric LV hypertrophy, vascular stiffness, and LV diastolic dysfunction. Primary therapy entails aggressive management of hypertension and CHD. BP should be treated in accordance with current guidelines, and CHD should be controlled with medications and percutaneous or surgical revascularization if appropriate. Older patients with impaired LV diastolic filling are at increased risk for atrial fibrillation (AF), and AF is a common precipitant of acute HF. In such cases, restoration and maintenance of sinus rhythm may be desirable. In patients with persistent AF, the ventricular rate should be controlled with β blockers, calcium channel blockers (diltiazem or verapamil), or digoxin.

Medical therapy for HFPEF focuses on treating hypertension, restricting sodium, and optimizing volume status. Diuretics are indicated to relieve congestion and volume overload. Overdiuresis should be avoided, as patients with HFPEF may be preload-dependent and insufficient LV preload may reduce cardiac output. Although ACE inhibitors, ARBs, β blockers, and aldosterone antagonists improve outcomes in systolic HF, there is currently no evidence of benefit in patients with HFPEF.

E. Advanced Heart Failure

Some HF patients have persistent severe symptoms and an unacceptable quality of life despite maximum medical therapy. Additional options for these patients may include cardiac resynchronization or surgical approaches.

1. Cardiac resynchronization therapy—In patients with severe HF symptoms despite optimal medical therapy, left ventricular ejection fraction (LVEF) ≤35%, and prolonged QRS duration on ECG, biventricular pacing or "cardiac resynchronization" may improve symptoms and cardiac hemodynamics. Although few patients older than age 75 years were enrolled in clinical trials testing cardiac resynchronization therapy (CRT), several small observational studies have demonstrated improvements in quality of life and exercise tolerance in patients ≥75–80 years of age. Therefore, CRT may be a reasonable therapeutic option in selected older adults with severe HF symptoms (ie NYHA class III or IV).

2. Surgical management

a. Left ventricular assist devices—Left ventricular assist devices (LVADs) are surgically implanted heart pumps that provide support to the LV to increase cardiac output and reduce congestion in patients with advanced systolic HF. Implantable LVADs are approved as "bridge to transplant" (BTT) or "destination therapy" (DT; permanent use without plans for transplantation) in individuals with advanced HF who are not candidates for a cardiac transplantation; as such, these devices are increasingly being used in older adults.

Randomized trials have demonstrated improved quality of life and survival in patients with refractory HF receiving LVADs as compared with medical management alone, including continuous intravenous inotropic therapy. However, there is considerable morbidity and mortality with LVAD therapy, especially in DT patients who tend to be older than BTT patients. The 1- and 2-year survival rates for participants in the HeartMate II DT trial were 68% and 58%, respectively, but more recent registry data following FDA approval show 1-year survival rates exceeding 70%. Most deaths occur in the first few months after implantation, with the most common modes of death being stroke, multiorgan failure, and HF. Older age increases the risk of complications, but age alone is not an exclusion criterion for LVAD therapy. In a retrospective single-center study, hospital length of stay, survival, adverse events, and quality of life were similar in patients younger or older than age 70 years who received an LVAD. Multidimensional preoperative assessment is performed to enhance patient selection and outcomes. This assessment should be combined with individualized decision making focused on goals, risks, and benefits to determine the best approach to care for each patient. With improved patient selection and technologic advances, perioperative morbidity and mortality will likely decline.

b. Heart transplantation—Heart transplantation provides definitive therapy for end-stage HF but is only available for a tiny fraction of patients because of a lack of donor availability. The annual number of heart transplants in the United States has plateaued at approximately 2200. Although there is not a firm age "cutoff" for transplantation, candidacy is based on the overall clinical picture, making it very uncommon in individuals older than age 70 years. Most centers consider advanced age a relative contraindication for transplantation. Other contraindications include severe pulmonary hypertension, active infection or malignancy, severe chronic lung disease, significant renal impairment, severe peripheral vascular disease or carotid disease, severe psychiatric disease, primary liver disease with coagulopathy, and diabetes with end-organ dysfunction.

Although older heart transplant recipients (age >60 years) are at increased risk for posttransplantation morbidity and death, survivors report better quality of life, psychological adjustment, and adherence than younger patients. Thus, heart transplantation may be considered in highly selected patients 65–75 years of age with advanced HF.

F. End-of-Life Care

In light of the exceptionally poor prognosis associated with established HF (worse than for most forms of cancer, see "Prognosis" below), end-of-life issues should be addressed in all HF patients. Information should be provided about the clinical course and prognosis, and patients should be encouraged to express their preferences for end-of-life care and should assign a durable power-of-attorney. In patients with end-stage HF and persistent severe symptoms despite optimal medical therapy, referral for palliative care or hospice should be considered.

▶ Prognosis

The prognosis for older patients with HF is poor, with 5-year survival rates of 20% to 40% in patients older than age 65 years and 2-year survival rates of 40% to 50% in those older than age 85 years. The long-term prognosis is similar in patients with either systolic HF or HFPEF. Factors associated with a worse prognosis include older age, male gender, more severe symptoms, lower LVEF, ischemic etiology, AF, diabetes, hyponatremia, renal insufficiency, anemia, and ventricular arrhythmias. Among patients with systolic HF, approximately 50% of deaths attributable to HF occur suddenly as a result of arrhythmia, while the remainder are attributable to progressive HF. In contrast, mortality in patients with HFPEF is often unrelated to HF and may occur as a complication of other acute illness (eg, pneumonia, hip fracture) or associated comorbid conditions (eg, dementia).

Adamson RM, Stahovich M, Chillcott S, et al: Clinical strategies and outcomes in advanced heart failure patients older than 70 years of age receiving the HeartMate II left ventricular assist device: a community hospital experience. *J Am Coll Cardiol.* 2011;57(25):2487-2495.

Brophy JM, Joseph L, Rouleau JL. Beta-blockers in congestive heart failure. A Bayesian meta-analysis. *Ann Intern Med.* 2001;134(7):550-560.

Cohn JN, Tognoni G; Valsartan Heart Failure Trial Investigators. A randomized trial of the angiotensin-receptor blocker valsartan in chronic heart failure. *N Engl J Med.* 2001;345(23):1667-1675.

Cutro R, Rich MW, Hauptman, PJ. Device therapy in patients with heart failure and advanced age: too much too late? *Int J Cardiol.* 2012;155(1):52-55.

Flather MD, Yusuf S, Køber L, et al. Long-term ACE-inhibitor therapy in patients with heart failure or left-ventricular dysfunction: a systematic overview of data from individual patients. ACE-Inhibitor Myocardial Infarction Collaborative Group. *Lancet.* 2000;355(9215):1575-1581.

Gottdiener JS, Arnold AM, Aurigemma GP, et al. Predictors of congestive heart failure in the elderly: the Cardiovascular Health Study. *J Am Coll Cardiol.* 2000;35(6):1628-1637.

Heiat A, Gross CP, Krumholz HM. Representation of the elderly, women, and minorities in heart failure clinical trials. *Arch Intern Med.* 2002;162(15):1682-1688.

Hunt SA, Abraham WT, Chin MH, et al; American College of Cardiology Foundation; American Heart Association. 2009 Focused update incorporated into the ACC/AHA 2005 Guidelines for the Diagnosis and Management of Heart Failure in Adults A Report of the American College of Cardiology Foundation/American Heart Association Task Force on Practice Guidelines Developed in Collaboration With the International Society for Heart and Lung Transplantation. *J Am Coll Cardiol.* 2009;53(15):e1-e90.

Kitzman DW, Gardin JM, Gottdiener JS, et al; Cardiovascular Health Study Research Group. Importance of heart failure with preserved systolic function in patients > or = 65 years. Cardiovascular Health Study. *Am J Cardiol.* 2001;87(4):413-419.

Maisel AS, Krishnaswamy P, Nowak RM, et al; Breathing Not Properly Multinational Study Investigators. Rapid measurement of B-type natriuretic peptide in the emergency diagnosis of heart failure. *N Engl J Med.* 2002;347(3):161-167.

McAlister FA, Lawson FM, Teo KK, Armstrong PW. A systematic review of randomized trials of disease management programs in heart failure. *Am J Med.* 2001;110(5):378-384.

Packer M, Coats AJ, Fowler MB, et al; Carvedilol Prospective Randomized Cumulative Survival Study Group. Effect of carvedilol on survival in severe chronic heart failure. *N Engl J Med.* 2001;344(22):1651-1658.

Pitt B, Zannad F, Remme WJ, et al. The effect of spironolactone on morbidity and mortality in patients with severe heart failure. *N Engl J Med.* 1999;341(10):709-717.

Rathore SS, Curtis JP, Wang Y, Bristow MR, Krumholz HM. Association of serum digoxin concentrations and outcomes in patients with heart failure. *JAMA.* 2003;289(7):871-878.

Rich MW. Device therapy in the elderly heart failure patient: what is the evidence? *Expert Rev Cardiovasc Ther.* 2010;8(9):1203-1205.

Rich MW. Pharmacotherapy of heart failure in the elderly: adverse events. *Heart Fail Rev.* 2012;17(4-5):589-595.

Rich MW, McSherry F, Williford WO, Yusuf S; Digitalis Investigation Group. Effect of age on mortality, hospitalizations and response to digoxin in patients with heart failure: the DIG study. *J Am Coll Cardiol.* 2001;38(3):806-813.

Santangeli P, Di Biase L, Dello Russo A, et al. Meta-analysis: age and effectiveness of prophylactic implantable cardioverter-defibrillators. *Ann Intern Med.* 2010;153(9):592-599.

Vitale CA, Chandekar R, Rodgers PE, Pagani FD, Malani PN. A call for guidance in the use of left ventricular assist devices in older adults. *J Am Geriatr Soc.* 2012;60(1):145-150.

Wolinsky FD, Overhage JM, Stump TE, Lubitz RM, Smith DM. The risk of hospitalization for congestive heart failure among older adults. *Med Care.* 1997;35(10):1031-1043.

Zile MR, Brutsaert DL. New concepts in diastolic dysfunction and diastolic heart failure: part II: causal mechanisms and treatment. *Circulation.* 2002;105(12):1503-1508.

USEFUL WEBSITES

American Heart Association (excellent source of materials for both practitioners and patients). www.americanheart.org

Heart Failure Society of America (source materials for physicians and patients). www.hfsa.org

HEART RHYTHM DISORDERS

BRADYARRHYTHMIAS

 ESSENTIALS OF DIAGNOSIS

▶ Exercise intolerance, shortness of breath, fatigue, palpitations, dizziness, syncope.

▶ Sinus bradycardia, sinus pauses, paroxysmal supraventricular tachyarrhythmias accompanied by bradyarrhythmias (tachybrady syndrome).

General Principles in Older Adults

Bradycardias in older adults are mainly caused by degenerative changes affecting impulse formation and conduction. Sinus node dysfunction includes sinus bradycardia, sinus pauses, chronotropic incompetence (inability to increase heart rate according to activity needs), and tachybrady syndrome (atrial fibrillation or atrial flutter alternating with sinus bradycardia). Pacemaker implantation is the only effective treatment for symptomatic bradycardia without reversible cause.

Prevention

Currently there are no known measures to prevent age-related sinus node dysfunction or conduction system disease.

Clinical Findings

A. Symptoms & Signs

Patients with sinus node dysfunction may have symptoms associated with bradycardia or tachycardia. The most common presentation of sinus bradycardia is fatigue. Patients with chronotropic incompetence may have no symptoms at rest but develop fatigue or shortness of breath with exercise. Sinus pauses may result in dizziness or syncope. In patients with tachybrady syndrome, the tachyarrhythmias may cause palpitations. Termination of the tachycardia may be associated with a prolonged pause and symptoms of dizziness or syncope.

Older patients often have delayed conduction in the atrioventricular (AV) node (first-degree AV block or Mobitz type I second-degree AV block), which is usually asymptomatic and benign. Mobitz type II AV block (infranodal block) is frequently asymptomatic, but associated with a high risk of progression to complete AV block. Complete heart block (CHB) can present with symptoms of fatigue, shortness of breath, or syncope. In older patients with CHB, stable escape rhythm, and minimal symptoms, the systolic BP is usually elevated.

Carotid hypersensitivity is a common cause of unexplained falls in older patients. Gentle carotid sinus massage, after careful auscultation to rule out bruits, may elicit sinus pauses of greater than 3 seconds in patients with carotid hypersensitivity. Pauses less than 3 seconds during carotid sinus massage are not considered abnormal.

B. Special Tests

1. Electrocardiography—Twelve-lead ECGs and rhythm strips may reveal sinus bradycardia, sinus pauses, AV-nodal conduction delay, or His-Purkinje system disease (left or right bundle-branch block, fascicular block).

2. Ambulatory monitoring—Documentation of a rhythm abnormality associated with symptoms is essential for determining therapy. Twenty-four- or 48-hour monitors are useful in patients with frequent symptoms, whereas 30-day monitors are preferable in those with less-frequent symptoms. In patients with rare but potentially serious symptoms (eg, syncope), an implantable loop recorder should be considered. In a study of patients 61–81 years of age with recurrent unexplained syncope, an implantable loop recorder established a diagnosis in 43% of cases, compared with conventional methods which were diagnostic in 6% of cases.

3. Other cardiac tests—Treadmill exercise testing can be useful in patients with suspected chronotropic incompetence. Exertional shortness of breath or fatigue associated with an inadequate increase in heart rate confirms the diagnosis. Exercise testing can also elicit Mobitz type II AV block or CHB in patients with advanced His-Purkinje system disease. Electrophysiology studies are not usually helpful in establishing an etiology for bradyarrhythmias, but markedly prolonged conduction from His bundle activation to ventricular depolarization (≥100 milliseconds) is an indication for pacemaker placement with or without symptoms.

▶ Differential Diagnosis

The symptoms of bradycardia are nonspecific and may be a result of a variety of other causes, both cardiac (HF, coronary artery disease, valvular heart disease) and noncardiac (chronic lung disease, anemia, hypothyroidism, deconditioning). Light-headedness or syncope may be caused by hypotension, autonomic dysfunction (eg, as a result of diabetes or parkinsonism), pulmonary embolism, or neurologic events. Many medications can cause symptoms that mimic those of bradycardia. Polypharmacy, decreased renal function, and systemic absorption of topical medications (eg, β-blocker eye drops) must all be considered as potential etiologies of bradycardia.

▶ Complications

Bradyarrhythmias may result in falls or syncope with potential for serious injuries, for example, hip fracture or intracranial hemorrhage, especially in patients receiving anticoagulation. Rarely, profound sinus arrest or CHB without an escape rhythm may be fatal.

▶ Treatment

Management of bradycardia begins with identification of potentially aggravating factors. Medications that can cause bradycardia should be discontinued, if feasible. Patients should be asked about herbal preparations that may cause bradycardia (eg, motherwort and valerian root). Evaluation and treatment for thyroid, lung, or other heart disease should be undertaken if indicated.

In patients with symptomatic bradycardia not from correctable causes, permanent pacemaker implantation is the only effective therapy. Pacemakers are also indicated in Mobitz type II block or CHB. Asymptomatic sinus bradycardia, first-degree AV block, and Mobitz type I second-degree AV block are not indications for pacemaker implantation.

▶ Prognosis

Pacemaker implantation does not affect survival but does reduce symptoms and improve quality of life in patients with symptomatic bradyarrhythmias. Patients with tachybrady syndrome have worse prognosis as a consequence of thromboembolism and other complications from atrial tachyarrhythmias.

TACHYARRHYTHMIAS—ATRIAL FIBRILLATION & ATRIAL FLUTTER

ESSENTIALS OF DIAGNOSIS

▶ Palpitations, shortness of breath, chest pain, dizziness.

▶ Rapid, irregular pulse (may be regular in atrial flutter).

▶ ECG demonstrates atrial fibrillation or atrial flutter.

General Principles in Older Adults

The prevalence of AF increases with age. Currently, there are approximately 3 million people in the United States with AF, and this number is projected to double by the year 2050, with 50% of affected individuals being older than the age of 80 years. AF is more common in men than in women at all ages. Atrial flutter (AFL) is closely related to AF, and patients frequently will have both arrhythmias at different times.

Prevention

In older adults, AF most commonly occurs in the setting of hypertension, coronary artery disease (CAD), valvular abnormalities, or HF. AF also occurs frequently in older patients with systemic illnesses, such as pneumonia, and following cardiac or noncardiac surgery. Hyperthyroidism (including subclinical hyperthyroidism), acute or chronic lung disease, sleep-disordered breathing, pulmonary embolism, and pericardial disease are additional precipitants of AF. Prevention and appropriate treatment of these conditions can reduce incident AF.

Clinical Findings

A. Symptoms & Signs

Symptoms associated with AF are highly variable. Palpitations caused by rapid ventricular rates are common, as are shortness of breath, fatigue, and dizziness. Many patients are asymptomatic or mildly symptomatic. Acute HF caused by tachycardia and loss of atrial contraction is a common presentation of AF in older patients, especially those with impaired diastolic function. Some patients have no cardiac symptoms but present with thromboembolic events, such as a transient ischemic attack or stroke. Rarely, asymptomatic patients with AF and rapid ventricular rates present with HF symptoms as a result of tachycardia-mediated cardiomyopathy.

The cardinal physical finding of AF is an irregularly irregular rhythm. AF can be very rapid, with ventricular rates of 130–180 beats/min In older patients with conduction disease, ventricular rates can be normal or even slow. AFL is often regular as a result of more organized atrial activity that conducts to the ventricle with 2:1, 3:1, or 4:1 AV block. An irregular rhythm caused by variable block is also common, and may be indistinguishable from AF based on physical examination alone. Signs of volume retention and HF may be seen in patients with diastolic or systolic ventricular dysfunction in whom the loss of atrial contraction diminishes cardiac output.

B. Special Tests

1. Electrocardiography—The ECG is diagnostic in patients with ongoing AF or AFL. AF is characterized by lack of organized atrial activity and irregular QRS intervals. AFL is more organized, and the most common finding is a "sawtooth" pattern best seen in the inferior leads (II, III, and aVF).

2. Echocardiography—Echocardiography is useful to assess underlying cardiac disease and chamber dimensions, and to rule out tachycardia-mediated cardiomyopathy. Increasing left atrial size is associated with greater risk for recurrent arrhythmias. Severe valvular disease, systolic dysfunction, and pulmonary hypertension are associated with reduced likelihood of restoring and maintaining sinus rhythm.

3. Cardiac catheterization—Cardiac catheterization is not routinely indicated in evaluation of AF, but may be considered for assessment of CAD, cardiomyopathy, or valvular abnormalities.

4. Other tests—Serum electrolytes and thyroid function tests should be measured in all patients with newly diagnosed AF or AFL. In patients with a permanent pacemaker or ICD, device interrogation can provide information about rate control and overall AF burden.

Differential Diagnosis

AF and AFL must be distinguished from other types of supraventricular arrhythmias. Frequent premature atrial complexes, paroxysmal atrial tachycardia, and multifocal atrial tachycardia (MAT) may present with similar symptoms and physical findings to those seen with AF or AFL, but in most cases the 12-lead ECG is sufficient to establish the correct diagnosis. Occasionally, vagal maneuvers or administration of adenosine may be necessary to distinguish AFL from other supraventricular arrhythmias. AF or AFL may also present as a wide complex tachycardia that may be difficult to distinguish from ventricular tachycardia.

Complications

AF and AFL are not immediately life-threatening but can result in significant complications if not properly treated. The most devastating complication is stroke. Stroke can occur in the presence or absence of AF; indeed, in 1 major study more than 60% of patients were in sinus rhythm at the time of stroke. Risk factors for stroke, as indicated by the CHADS$_2$ score, include congestive HF, hypertension, age 75 years or older, diabetes, and prior stroke or transient ischemic attack (TIA). CHADS$_2$ assigns 2 points for stroke and 1 point for each of the other risk factors. Patients with no risk factors have an annual stroke risk of less than 3%, whereas those with all 5 risk factors have an annual stroke risk of greater than 18%. A recent update of the CHADS$_2$ scoring system (CHA$_2$DS$_2$-VASc) assigns 2 points for age 75 years or older, 1 point for age 65–74 years, 1 point for vascular disease (coronary, aortic, or peripheral arterial disease), and 1 point for female sex. A CHADS$_2$ or CHA$_2$DS$_2$-VASc score of ≥2 is associated with an annual stroke risk of at least 4%. In addition to stroke and

TIA, thromboembolic events attributable to AF can affect circulation to the bowel, kidney, other organs, or limbs.

In patients with chronic AF and rapid ventricular rates, tachycardia-mediated cardiomyopathy can occur. HF and SCD may result from the cardiomyopathy. In older patients with LV hypertrophy and diastolic dysfunction, myocardial ischemia and non–ST-elevation MI can occur as a result of oxygen supply–demand mismatch.

▶ Treatment

A. Goals of Treatment

Management of patients with new-onset AF or AFL should begin with identification of possible precipitating causes (see above). The primary objectives of treatment include prevention of stroke and other thromboembolic events, controlling the ventricular rate, and alleviating symptoms.

B. Antithrombotic Therapy

The risks of thromboembolic events are not significantly different between AF and AFL, or between paroxysmal and persistent forms of AF. Stroke risk should be assessed using the $CHADS_2$ or CHA_2DS_2-VASc score. If the score is 2 or higher, long-term anticoagulation with warfarin or one of the newer agents is recommended. Note that under the CHA_2DS_2-VASc system, all men age 75 years or older and all women age 65 years or older are candidates for systemic anticoagulation, even in the absence of other risk factors. Furthermore because stroke risk increases progressively with age, older patients derive the greatest absolute benefit from anticoagulation.

The annual risk of serious bleeding on warfarin is estimated at 3%, and there is no evidence that older patients have higher incidences of significant bleeding as long as the dose is carefully adjusted to maintain the international normalized ratio (INR) between 2.0 and 3.0. (Exception: Patients with mechanical prosthetic valves require an INR from 2.5–3.5.) Foods high in vitamin K (eg, green leafy vegetables), antibiotics, and amiodarone can all affect INR levels. Older patients should be cautioned against concomitant use of warfarin and nonsteroidal antiinflammatory drugs because of increased risk of gastrointestinal bleeding. Patients with CAD are often treated with warfarin, aspirin, and another antiplatelet agent (eg, clopidogrel). To minimize the risk of bleeding, unnecessary agents should be discontinued when clinically appropriate (eg, clopidogrel 3–12 months after percutaneous coronary intervention).

Recently, 3 new anticoagulants became available with therapeutic effects comparable to warfarin. Rivaroxaban, apixaban (factor Xa inhibitors) and dabigatran (a direct thrombin inhibitor) have been shown to be as effective as warfarin in preventing thromboembolic events in patients with AF, without an increase in major bleeding and with reduced risk of intracranial hemorrhage (ICH). All have the advantage of a fixed-dose regimen without the need for INR monitoring. However, there are no available measures to acutely reverse the effects of these agents in patients with significant bleeding. In older patients with decreased creatinine clearance, lower doses are recommended, and the drugs are contraindicated in patients with creatinine clearances <15 mL/min. In addition, postmarketing data have raised concern that the risk of serious or life-threatening bleeding may be increased in patients older than 80 years of age who are receiving dabigatran.

In patients with absolute contraindications to warfarin and other anticoagulants, such as history of bleeding requiring blood transfusions or ICH, daily aspirin is reasonable. Combination therapy with clopidogrel and aspirin is more effective than aspirin alone in reducing stroke risk, but the risk of bleeding is similar to that of warfarin.

C. Rate Control

Effective control of ventricular rate during AF and AFL is a primary goal in both acute and chronic phases of management. Optimal rate control is traditionally defined as a resting heart rate (in AF) of 60–80 beats/min and a heart rate of 90–115 beats/min with activity. However, "lenient" rate control, defined as a resting heart rate of <110 beats/min, is associated with similar quality-of-life scores as stricter rate control. β Blockers are the drugs of choice in patients with CAD or reduced systolic function. Calcium channel blockers are not recommended in patients with depressed LV systolic function. Digoxin slows ventricular conduction through its effect on the parasympathetic nervous system but has limited efficacy in patients with high sympathetic tone, such as during physical exertion, in the immediate postoperative period, or in the setting of infection. In relatively sedentary patients, low-dose digoxin may provide adequate rate control, alone or in combination with β blockers or calcium channel blockers. In patients refractory to pharmacologic rate control, radiofrequency ablation of the AV node with permanent pacemaker implantation is an effective method of rate control and is associated with improved quality of life.

D. Rhythm Control

Restoration and maintenance of sinus rhythm is often necessary to alleviate symptoms. Rhythm control has not been shown to reduce mortality or strokes, and it does not circumvent the need for long-term anticoagulation in patients at high risk for thromboembolic events. Rhythm control is more difficult to achieve in patients with prolonged AF duration, depressed systolic function, severe diastolic dysfunction, or larger atrial size.

In patients who present with AF and rapid ventricular rate who are hemodynamically unstable, immediate electrical cardioversion is indicated. In stable patients, rate control with β blockers or calcium channel blockers should be initiated. In patients who remain symptomatic, electrical cardioversion may be performed with a low risk of thromboembolic events if the duration of AF is less than 48 hours or if the patient has been on warfarin with therapeutic INRs for at least 3 consecutive weeks. If the duration of AF is unknown, if the patient is not on long-term anticoagulation, or if recent INRs have been subtherapeutic, a transesophageal echocardiogram should be performed to rule out the presence of left atrial thrombus before cardioversion. Anticoagulation must be continued for a minimum of 1 month after cardioversion because of continuing risk of thrombus formation from atrial stunning after cardioversion. In patients with risk factors for stroke, anticoagulation should be continued indefinitely. Elective cardioversion with the new anticoagulants has not been well studied. Preliminary data suggest that continuous use of dabigatran for a minimum of 3 weeks before cardioversion is not associated with increased risk of stroke relative to warfarin.

Cardioversion may be performed either pharmacologically or electrically. Direct current cardioversion is more effective and safer than pharmacologic cardioversion. The only intravenous agent approved by the FDA for conversion of AF is ibutilide, but there is a risk of inducing prolonged QT interval and torsades de pointes ventricular tachycardia, especially in patients with HF. Although widely used, intravenous amiodarone is no more effective than placebo in the acute conversion of AF to sinus rhythm.

Long-term maintenance of sinus rhythm usually requires an oral antiarrhythmic agent. Quinidine and procainamide are rarely used because of limited efficacy and multiple side effects. Disopyramide is relatively contraindicated in older adults as a result of prominent anticholinergic side effects. Flecainide and propafenone are relatively effective for maintaining sinus rhythm but should not be used in patients with structural heart disease. Sotalol and dofetilide are renally cleared and can prolong the QT interval; consequently, these agents must be used cautiously, especially in older women (who tend to have longer QT intervals at baseline) with decreased creatinine clearance. Amiodarone is commonly used because of its effectiveness and relative lack of short-term side effects. However, thyroid, liver, neurologic, and lung toxicity may occur during long-term use, and routine monitoring of these organ systems is essential. Dronedarone is an agent similar to amiodarone without long-term organ toxicities, but rare cases of acute liver failure have been reported. Dronedarone is contraindicated in patients with active HF or persistent AF.

Radiofrequency ablation for typical "sawtooth" AFL is commonly performed with high success and low complication rates. Ablation of AF, which mainly involves electrical isolation of the pulmonary veins from the left atrium, has become a frequently performed and relatively effective procedure. The success rate, defined as freedom from recurrence of AF at 1 year, is approximately 70% for paroxysmal AF, but much lower for persistent or permanent AF. Major complications, including stroke, pulmonary hemorrhage, deep venous thrombosis, pulmonary embolism, cardiac perforation or tamponade, esophageal perforation, and death, occur in 3%

to 5% of cases. AF ablation has not been shown to reduce stroke risk, so it does not obviate the need for long-term anticoagulation in high-risk patients. Few studies have specifically examined the efficacy and safety of AF ablation in older patients, but limited retrospective data suggest that in selected octogenarians outcomes are similar to those in younger patients, although postprocedure hospitalization times are longer. A surgical approach for treatment of AF, the Cox-Maze procedure, has a success rate of greater than 90% for curing AF, and has been shown to reduce strokes. In patients with a history of AF who require valvular or bypass surgery, concomitant Coz-Maze procedure should be considered.

Prognosis

Untreated AF is associated with increased mortality mainly as a consequence of strokes and tachycardia-induced cardiomyopathy with resultant HF and increased risk of sudden death. With appropriate treatment, the long-term prognosis of AF and AFL is excellent, and survival rates are similar in patients managed with rate control or rhythm control. Hemodynamic instability or severe symptoms attributable to AF are associated with significant morbidity and high costs from recurrent hospitalizations, procedures, and antiarrhythmic medications.

VENTRICULAR ARRHYTHMIAS

General Principles in Older Adults

The prevalence of ventricular arrhythmias increases with age as a result of age-related changes in the ventricular myocardium coupled with the increasing prevalence of cardiac disease. Ventricular arrhythmias range from isolated ventricular ectopic beats or nonsustained ventricular tachycardia (NSVT), both of which are benign in patients with structurally normal hearts, to ventricular tachycardia and fibrillation, which may cause syncope or SCD.

Prevention

Because most serious ventricular arrhythmias are related to underlying cardiac disease, prevention and early treatment of MIs and other conditions that may cause cardiomyopathy, such as hypertension and diabetes, are crucial. Early detection of cardiomyopathy is important to prevent lethal ventricular arrhythmias.

Clinical Findings

A. Symptoms & Signs

Isolated premature ventricular complexes (PVCs) are usually asymptomatic. Occasionally patients may feel "skipped" heart beats or palpitations. NSVT is defined as 3 or more consecutive PVCs at a rate in excess of 100 per minute and lasting less than 30 seconds. NSVT is often asymptomatic but can cause palpitations, transient light-headedness, or syncope. Ventricular tachycardia (VT) may cause palpitations, light-headedness or syncope. Ventricular fibrillation (VF) is associated with hemodynamic collapse and results in syncope or SCD if not immediately treated.

Physical findings associated with PVCs include an intermittently irregular heart beat during auscultation that may be associated with lack of peripheral pulse. NSVT and VT are associated with rapid pulse and, in some cases, hypotension. VF is associated with lack of pulse or BP.

B. Special Tests

1. Electrocardiography—In patients with isolated PVCs, the ECG shows wide-complex beats of ventricular origin. VT manifests as consecutive wide-complex beats, which, if sustained, are usually regular. Torsades de pointes is a polymorphic VT with waxing and waning QRS amplitude that occurs in the setting of prolonged QT interval. VF is a chaotic rhythm without discreet QRS complexes. Baseline ECGs should be examined for prior MI or prolonged QT interval (eg, caused by medications or electrolyte abnormalities). A PVC burden of >25% of total heart beats may be associated with progression to cardiomyopathy.

2. Echocardiography, stress testing, and cardiac catheterization—These tests provide information about the presence and severity of underlying cardiac disease and the potential for serious ventricular arrhythmias. LVEF and the presence of severe ischemia are the main determinants of prognosis. Acute coronary ischemia may cause sustained VT or VF, for which emergent cardiac catheterization is indicated.

3. Electrophysiology study—The main role of an electrophysiology study (EPS) is for risk stratification of SCD in patients with structural heart disease and NSVT. In asymptomatic patients with CAD, an LVEF of 36% to 40%, and NSVT, induction of sustained VT during an EPS is associated with increased risk of SCD. In patients with syncope of unclear etiology, known CAD or a focal wall motion abnormality, and LVEF ≥40%, EPS may be considered to assess the possibility of ventricular arrhythmia as the cause of syncope. EPS is not useful for SCD risk stratification in patients with nonischemic cardiomyopathy.

▶ Differential Diagnosis

Wide-complex beats may be ventricular or supraventricular in origin. An isolated wide-complex beat preceded by a P wave suggests supraventricular origin with aberrant conduction. Wide-complex tachycardia with AV dissociation is ventricular in origin. Other diagnostic criteria for VT are the presence of fusion or capture beats (sudden narrow QRS among wide-complex beats) and left bundle-branch block morphology with right axis deviation. In older patients, baseline conduction abnormalities are common. Comparison of tachycardia morphology with baseline sinus beats may help differentiate supraventricular tachycardia with aberrancy from VT.

▶ Complications

The most important complication of ventricular arrhythmias is SCD, which often occurs without premonitory symptoms. Ventricular arrhythmias may also be associated with syncope, falls, chest pain, dyspnea, or acute HF.

▶ Treatment

Isolated PVCs generally do not require therapy. In highly symptomatic patients, β blockers are the agents of choice. Rarely, in patients with disabling symptoms unresponsive to β blockers, antiarrhythmic drugs are used. Radiofrequency ablation is helpful for reducing ectopy burden if a single source of PVCs can be identified.

The presence of NSVT is an indication for further investigation. In patients with normal LVEF, treatment is the same as for isolated PVCs. In patients with CAD, LVEF of 36% to 40%, and inducible monomorphic VT during EPS, an ICD is indicated to prevent SCD. Patients with LVEFs of 35% or less, regardless of etiology, are candidates for an ICD for primary prevention of SCD. Patients with unexplained syncope in the presence of cardiomyopathy have an indication for an ICD for secondary prevention (ie, an event likely attributable to serious ventricular arrhythmias) of SCD. Ablation of sustained VT may be performed to reduce ICD shocks in patients with recurrent arrhythmias not responsive to medical therapy.

The role of ICDs in patients older than 75 to 80 years of age is controversial. Meta-analysis of existing trials and retrospective studies have concluded that in patients age 75 years or older, ICDs do not convey significant overall mortality benefit, especially in patients with renal impairment. ICD implantation in patients in their eighth or ninth decade of life carries implications that must be communicated to patients and their families. ICD shocks are frequently painful, and effective treatment of ventricular arrhythmias may alter the mode of death from sudden to a more gradual process of living longer with reduced quality of life. Device disablement in the event of terminal illness or repetitive shocks should also be discussed prior to ICD implantation.

▶ Prognosis

The prognosis of ventricular arrhythmias is governed by the nature and severity of underlying cardiac disease. In the absence of structural heart disease or depressed LVEF, the prognosis of PVCs and NSVT is excellent. The presence of NSVT in patients with decreased systolic function is a marker for increased mortality, but there is no evidence that suppression of PVCs and NSVT improves survival. In patients with LVEF ≤35%, ICDs reduce mortality in younger patients, but the mortality benefit in older patients is unclear.

Andersen HR, Nielsen JC, Thomsen PE, et al. Long-term follow up of patients from a randomized trial of atrial versus ventricular pacing for sick sinus syndrome. *Lancet.* 1997;350(9086):1210-1216.

Bardy GH, Lee KL, Mark DB, et al; Sudden Cardiac Death in Heart Failure Trial (SCD-HeFT) Investigators. Amiodarone or an implantable cardioverter-defibrillator for congestive heart failure. *N Engl J Med.* 2005;352(3):225-237.

Bum Kim J, Suk Moon J, Yun SC, et al. Long term outcome of mechanical mitral valve replacement in patients with atrial fibrillation: impact of the maze procedure. *Circulation.* 2012;125(17):2071-2080.

Bunch JT, Weiss JP, Crandall BG, et al. Long-term clinical efficacy and risk of catheter ablation for atrial fibrillation in octogenarians. *Pacing Clin Electrophysiol.* 2010;33(2):146-152.

Buxton AE, Lee KL, Fisher JD, Josephson ME, Prystowsky EN, Hafley G. A randomized study of the prevention of sudden death in patients with coronary artery disease. *N Engl J Med.* 1999;341(25):1882-1890.

Damiano RJ Jr, Schwartz FH, Bailey MS, et al. The Cox maze IV procedure: predictors of late recurrence. *J Thorac Cardiovasc Surg.* 2011;141(1):113-121.

Epstein AE, DiMarco JP, Ellenbogen KA, et al; American College of Cardiology/American Heart Association Task Force on Practice Guidelines (Writing Committee to Revise the ACC/AHA/NASPE 2002 Guideline Update for Implantation of Cardiac Pacemakers and Antiarrhythmia Devices); American Association for Thoracic Surgery; Society of Thoracic Surgeons. ACC/AHA/HRS 2008 Guidelines for Device-Based Therapy of Cardiac Rhythm Abnormalities: a report of the American College of Cardiology/American Heart Association Task Force on Practice Guidelines (Writing Committee to Revise the ACC/AHA/NASPE 2002 Guideline Update for Implantation of Cardiac Pacemakers and Antiarrhythmia Devices): developed in collaboration with the American Association for Thoracic Surgery and Society of Thoracic Surgeons. *Circulation.* 2009;117(21):e350-e408.

Gage BF, Waterman AD, Shannon W, Boechler M, Rich MW, Radford MJ. Validation of clinical classification schemes for predicting stroke: results from the national registry of atrial fibrillation. *JAMA.* 2001;285(22):2864-2870.

Go AS, Hylek EM, Phillips KA, et al. Prevalence of diagnosed atrial fibrillation in adults: National implications for rhythm management and stroke prevention: the AnTicoagulation and Risk Factors in Atrial Fibrillation (ATRIA) Study. *JAMA.* 2001;285(18):2370-2375.

Kannel WB, Benjamin EJ. Current perceptions of the epidemiology of atrial fibrillation. *Cardiol Clin.* 2009;27(1):13-24.

Lampert R, Hayes DL, Annas GJ, et al; American College of Cardiology; American Geriatrics Society; American Academy of Hospice and Palliative Medicine, American Heart Association; European Heart Rhythm Association; Hospice and Palliative Nurses Association. HRS Expert Consensus Statement on the Management of Cardiovascular Implantable Electronic Devices (CIEDs) in patients nearing end of life or requesting withdrawal of therapy. *Heart Rhythm.* 2010;7(7):1008-1026.

Lip GY, Frison L, Halperin JL, Lane DA. Identifying patients at high risk for stroke despite anticoagulation: a comparison of contemporary stroke risk stratification schemes in an anticoagulated atrial fibrillation cohort. *Stroke.* 2010;41(12):2731-2738.

Moss AJ, Zareba W, Hall WJ, et al; Multicenter Automatic Defibrillator Implantation Trial II Investigators. Prophylactic implantation of a defibrillator in patients with myocardial infarction and reduced ejection fraction. *N Engl J Med.* 2002;346(12):877-883.

Ozcan C, Jahangir A, Friedman PA, et al. Long-term survival after ablation of atrioventricular node and implantation of a permanent pacemaker in patients with atrial fibrillation. *N Engl J Med.* 2001;344(14):1043-1051.

Parry SW, Matthews IG. Implantable loop recorders in the investigation of unexplained syncope: a state of the art review. *Heart.* 2010;96(20):1611-1616.

Smit MD, Crijns HJ, Tijssen JG, et al; RACE II Investigators. Effect of lenient versus strict rate control on cardiac remodeling in patients with atrial fibrillation data of the RACE II (RAte Control Efficacy in permanent atrial fibrillation II) study. *J Am Coll Cardiol.* 2011;58(9):942-949.

Yokokawa M, Kim HM, Good E, et al. Relation of symptoms and symptom duration to premature complex-induced cardiomyopathy. *Heart Rhythm.* 2012;9(1):92-95.

Wyse DG, Waldo AL, DiMarco JP, et al; Atrial Fibrillation Follow-up Investigation of Rhythm Management (AFFIRM) Investigators. A comparison of rate control and rhythm control in patients with atrial fibrillation. *N Engl J Med.* 2002;347(23):1825-1833.

USEFUL WEBSITES

American Heart Association (excellent source of materials for both practitioners and patients). www.americanheart.org

Heart Rhythm Society (source materials for physicians and patients). www.hrsonline.org

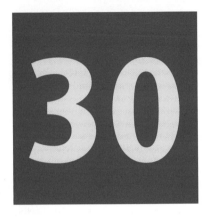

Hypertension

30

Quratulain Syed, MD

Barbara Messinger-Rapport, MD, PhD

► Diastolic hypertension in the absence of major risk factors and target organ damage is defined as diastolic blood pressure ≥90 mm Hg.

► Systolic hypertension in the absence of major risk factors and target organ damage is defined as systolic blood pressure ≥140 mm Hg.

► In the presence of normal diastolic blood pressure (<90 mm Hg), systolic hypertension is referred to as isolated systolic hypertension.

General Principles in Older Adults

Hypertension in older (and younger) adults is defined according to Joint National Committee on Prevention, Detection, Evaluation, and Treatment of High Blood Pressure VII (JNC 7) criteria as blood pressure (BP) >140/90 mm Hg based on the mean of two or more properly measured seated readings on each of two or more office visits.

Hypertension is very common among older adults. The prevalence of hypertension is as high as 63% in ages 60–79 years, and 74% in age ≥80 years. Hypertension is a major risk factor for cardiovascular and cerebrovascular morbidity and mortality. In 2008, 1 in 6 deaths were caused by heart disease and 1 in 18 deaths were caused by strokes in United States. Aging, higher body weight, smoking, reduced physical activity, and salt intake are major risk factors for hypertension.

In the presence of normal diastolic BP (<90 mm Hg), elevation in systolic BP is referred to as *isolated systolic hypertension* (ISH). Systolic pressure rises with age but diastolic pressure rises until about 55 years of age, and then gradually falls thereafter (Figure 30–1). Therefore, isolated diastolic hypertension is rare in the older adults. Diastolic hypertension, when present, usually occurs in combination with systolic hypertension in older adults (diastolic–systolic hypertension).

Elevated pulse pressure (PP), which is systolic pressure minus diastolic pressure, is increasingly being recognized as an important predictor of cerebrovascular and cardiac risk in older adults. PP increases with age in a manner parallel to the increase in systolic BP.

Pathogenesis

"Longevity is a vascular question, which has been well expressed in the axiom that man is only as old as his arteries. To a majority of men death comes primarily or secondarily through this portal. The onset of what may be called physiological arterio-sclerosis depends, in the first place, upon the quality of arterial tissue which the individual has inherited, and secondly upon the amount of wear and tear to which he has subjected it."

Sir William Osler, 1898

Hypertension in older adults is largely caused by increased arterial stiffness (collagen replacing elastin in the elastic lamina of the aorta), which accompanies aging. This leads to increased pulse wave velocity, causing late systolic blood pressure (SBP) augmentation and increasing myocardial oxygen demand. Reduction of forward flow also occurs, thus limiting organ perfusion. These undesirable alterations, combined with preexisting coronary stenosis or excessive drug-induced diastolic blood pressure (DBP) reduction, predisposes older adults to development of left ventricular hypertrophy and heart failure.

Endothelial dysfunction is another important contributor to BP elevation in older adults. Mechanical and inflammatory injury of aging arteries causes decreased availability of vasodilator nitric oxide (NO), which causes an unfavorable balance between vasodilators (such as NO), and vasoconstrictors (such as endothelin).

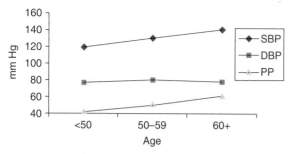

▲ **Figure 30–1.** Changes in systolic blood pressure (*SBP*), diastolic pressure (*DBP*), and pulse pressure (*PP*) with aging. SBP and PP increase with age. DBP plateaus or peaks at approximately 55 years. Plotted using data from Framingham Heart Study.

Autonomic dysregulation contributes to orthostatic hypotension (decrease in SBP >20 mm Hg and/or DBP >10 mm Hg after 3 minutes of standing), which is a risk factor for falls, syncope, and cardiovascular (CV) events. Autonomic dysregulation also leads to orthostatic hypertension, which is an increase in SBP upon assumption of upright posture, and is a risk factor for left ventricular hypertrophy (LVH), coronary artery disease (CAD), and silent cerebrovascular disease. There is no consensus definition for orthostatic hypertension, although studies have used the definition of a 20-mm Hg rise in SBP on standing up.

Age-related renal dysfunction, with glomerulosclerosis and interstitial fibrosis, is gradual and progressive. However, it can be hastened by acute insults or comorbid conditions. The resulting reduction in glomerular filtration rate (GFR) and other renal homeostatic mechanisms, such as membrane sodium/potassium–adenosine triphosphatase, results in increased intracellular sodium, reduced sodium–calcium exchange, volume expansion, and resultant hypertension. As reduced renal tubular mass provides fewer transport pathways for potassium excretion, older hypertensive patients are more prone to development of hyperkalemia.

Older adults exhibit increased sensitivity to salt, because of an age-related decrease in renal function and sodium/potassium–adenosine triphosphatase, with resultant inability of kidneys to excrete a sodium load.

▷ Differential Diagnosis

Most older adults with hypertension have primary, or essential, hypertension. Secondary hypertension refers to hypertension with an identifiable and treatable cause. Renovascular hypertension caused by renal artery stenosis is the most common cause of treatable secondary hypertension in older persons. Other causes, such as obstructive sleep apnea (OSA), primary aldosteronism, and thyroid disorders, should always

be considered in cases where BP remains above target despite 3 medications at moderate doses, and where history and physical exam suggest these disorders.

Obstructive sleep apnea is a strong and independent risk factor for development and progression of hypertension, especially treatment-resistant hypertension and its CV and renal complications. Volume overload and fluid shifts, as well as increases in sympathetic activation, oxidative stress, inflammation, and release of vasoactive substances secondary to intermittent hypoxemia, contribute to BP elevation in patients with OSA.

Chronic inflammatory burden from inflammatory disorders can lead to arterial stiffness and thus hypertension. Also, the nonsteroidal antiinflammatory drugs (NSAIDs) used to treat these disorders can cause elevation of BP. Other drugs, such as cyclooxygenase-2 inhibitors, glucocorticoids, erythropoietin analogs, some disease-modifying antirheumatic drugs (eg, leflunomide), immunosuppressants (eg, cyclosporine and tacrolimus), and antidepressants (eg, higher doses of venlafaxine), may increase BP. Saw palmetto, St. John's wort, licorice, ergotamine, and ergot-containing herbal preparations are associated with hypertension. Among street drugs, "herbal ecstasy," cocaine (and cocaine withdrawal), nicotine (and nicotine withdrawal), and stimulants (eg, methylphenidate), are also associated with hypertension.

Pheochromocytomas are rare tumors, responsible for 0.5% cases of secondary hypertension, that usually present between 30 and 60 years of age. Intracranial tumors in structures close to glossopharyngeal nerve can lead to baroreceptor failure, which can present as volatile hypertension (abrupt increase in BP, lasting minutes to hours, and tachycardia), hypertensive crisis (severe, unremitting hypertension, tachycardia, and headache) or orthostatic tachycardia (increase in heart rate [HR] by >30 beats/min from the supine to upright position).

▷ Special Situations

Four common conditions in older patients are associated with or complicate the diagnosis of hypertension: "white-coat" or "office" hypertension, postural or orthostatic hypotension, postprandial hypotension, and pseudohypertension.

White-coat hypertension is mild hypertension noted in the physician's office but with repeatedly normal measurements at home, at work, or by 24-hour ambulatory blood pressure monitoring (ABPM). End-organ disease, such as LVH, hypertensive retinopathy, or nephropathy, is notably absent. White-coat hypertension commonly coexists with metabolic risk factors such as hypercholesterolemia and hyperinsulinemia. However, the Syst-Eur trial and subgroup analysis of older patients in the IDACO study groups indicates that untreated individuals with white-coat hypertension had similar CV risk as individuals with normal BP.

Orthostatic hypotension is a 20-mm Hg drop in systolic BP or a 10-mm Hg drop in diastolic BP when rising from a sitting position. It is prevalent in approximately 20% of community-dwelling individuals >65 years of age, and in 30% of those >75 years of age. Orthostatic hypotension is associated with diabetes, hypertension, low body mass index, Parkinson disease, multiple system atrophy, Lewy body dementia, and medications. Among antihypertensives, α blockers, combined α and β-blockers, nitrates and diuretics can cause or aggravate orthostatic hypotension. In addition, antidepressants (such as paroxetine, sertraline, venlafaxine, and trazodone) and antipsychotics (such as risperidone, olanzapine, and quetiapine) can cause orthostatic hypotension. Diastolic orthostatic hypotension measured 1 minute after standing up and systolic orthostatic hypotension measured 3 minutes after standing up are predictive of a high vascular mortality in older home-dwelling persons. Orthostatic hypotension is also associated with increased risk of falls in older adults. Older adults should be screened for orthostatic hypotension on routine encounters. If symptomatic, culprit medications should be tapered or discontinued. Following prolonged bed rest or inactivity (eg, following hospitalization), patients should be instructed to stand up gradually to reduce excessive pooling of blood in the lower extremities. Activities that reduce venous return to the heart, such as coughing, straining, and prolonged standing, should be avoided, especially in hot weather. Knee-high compression stockings may be helpful in mild cases. Waist-high compression stockings with abdominal binders may be needed in more severe cases. In patients with autonomic failure and supine hypertension, raising the head of the bed by 10–20 degrees at night can reduce hypertension, prevent overnight volume loss, and help restore morning BP upon standing. Liberal intake of salt and water to achieve a 24-hour urine volume of 1.5–2 L may attenuate fluid loss commonly seen in autonomic insufficiency. In older adults with orthostatic hypotension caused by deconditioning, an exercise regimen comprising swimming, recumbent biking, or rowing can help with symptoms.

Postprandial hypotension has been defined as a 20-mm Hg decrease in SBP, or a decrease in SBP from >100 mm Hg to below 90 mm Hg within 2 hours after a meal. Falls, syncope, strokes, transient ischemic attacks, angina, and myocardial infarctions can result, and postprandial hypotension is an independent predictor of mortality. Postprandial hypotension occurs in 25% to 38% of institutionalized older adults. It appears to be a result of blunted sympathetic response to normal physiologic postmeal decrease in BP. It is more common among older adults with Parkinson's disease, diabetes, and essential hypertension. Polypharmacy, especially the use of diuretics and psychotropic medications, also appears to be a risk factor. Postprandial decreases in BP may be managed through a regimen of small frequent meals, limited dietary carbohydrates, and drinking water or coffee before meals. Among pharmacologic agents, α glucosidase inhibitors, guar gum, or premeal octreotide injections may aid in management.

Pseudohypertension is a significantly higher peripheral pressure (eg, brachial site) compared with a direct arterial measurement. Arterial rigidity from extensive atherosclerosis is considered to be responsible for this relatively rare phenomenon. Although it can be diagnosed by direct intraarterial measurement, this invasive technique is usually unnecessary. The presence of an Osler sign (a palpable radial artery when BP cuff is inflated above the systolic BP) is suggestive, but not diagnostic, of this condition. Pseudohypertension may be suspected in those who appear resistant to an adequate drug regimen, those who become very symptomatic to a gentle pharmacologic regimen, and those with very elevated BP but no clinical evidence of end-organ disease. Incidental radiographs of the distal extremities may reveal extensive arterial calcification.

▶ Clinical Findings

A. Symptoms & Signs

Most older adults with hypertension are asymptomatic. A minority may present with dizziness, palpitations, or headache. A morning headache, usually occipital, may be characteristic of stage III hypertension. End-organ damage, such as stroke, congestive heart failure (CHF), or renal failure, may be the initial presentation.

B. Patient History

A history suggesting postprandial or orthostatic hypotension may be elicited. These syndromes may reflect longstanding hypertension or the presence of associated problems that need to be considered in treating hypertension.

Patient history should be directed toward the possibility of secondary hypertension, focusing on recent weight gain, polyuria, polydipsia, muscle weakness, history of headaches, palpitations, diaphoresis, weight loss, anxiety, and sleep history (eg, daytime somnolence, loud snoring, and early morning headaches).

Symptoms suspicious for target organ damage include headache, transient weakness or blindness, claudication, chest pain, and shortness of breath. Comorbid conditions such as diabetes mellitus, CAD, heart failure, chronic obstructive pulmonary disease, gout, and sexual dysfunction are important to elicit because they will have an impact on coronary risk factor stratification and choice of initial therapy.

Medication history should include previous BP medications, current prescription drugs, over-the-counter drugs (especially NSAIDs and cold medicines), and herbal supplements (especially St. John's wort and saw palmetto). Lifestyle issues, including smoking, alcohol intake, drug use, regular exercise, and degree of physical activity, should be assessed. A dietary history targeting sodium (which can raise BP), fat intake (which can contribute to CV risk), and alcohol (which can raise BP if consumed in excessive amounts) is important as well.

C. Physical Examination

The physical examination focuses on the confirmation of hypertension and identification of possible secondary causes. Diagnosis of hypertension should be based on at least 3 different BP measurements on 2 or more separate office visits. Routine BP should be measured using an appropriate cuff size at heart level, while seated comfortably for at least 5 minutes. Orthostatic BP should be measured sitting, then standing after 1 then 3 minutes. It is advisable to check BP at least 1 hour after any consumption of alcohol, caffeine, or tobacco.

Home and 24-hour ambulatory BP monitoring may help differentiate truly resistant hypertension from white-coat hypertension.

Frail older nursing home residents may exhibit increased variability in BP readings during the day, where BP is likely elevated before breakfast and falls after breakfast. To avoid overaggressive treatments in this high-risk population, it is advisable to diagnose hypertension based on multiple readings, both before and after meals, as well as supine and standing.

D. Laboratory Tests

Complete blood count, renal and metabolic panel, lipid profile, thyroid-stimulating hormone (TSH), urinalysis (to quantify proteinuria), and 12-lead electrocardiogram are included in the initial evaluation.

Evidence should be sought for end-organ target disease (ie, ophthalmologic vascular changes, carotid bruits, distended neck veins, third or fourth heart sound, pulmonary rales, and reduced peripheral pulses). A cognitive evaluation (eg, the Montreal Cognitive Assessment or St. Louis University Mental Status Exam) is also helpful in tracking longitudinal cognitive changes in the older hypertensive patient. Secondary causes, including renal bruits (renal artery stenosis); moon face, buffalo hump, and abdominal striae (Cushing syndrome); tremor, hyperreflexia, and tachycardia (thyrotoxicosis) should be assessed.

▶ Complications

Older persons with hypertension have higher absolute risks of CV and cerebrovascular events. They are also more likely to have other comorbid conditions that worsen these outcomes. Thus, preventing target organ damage in older adults with hypertension is vital to reducing morbidity and mortality from hypertension. Target organ damage can occur overtly, in the form of stroke, acute myocardial infarction (MI), heart failure, or arrhythmia, or, more subtly, in the form of a neuropsychiatric deficit such as cognitive impairment. Atrial fibrillation is often a complication of hypertensive disease in older adults; 15% of strokes occur in people with atrial fibrillation. Diastolic dysfunction increases with age secondary to reduced vascular compliance and increased impedance to left ventricular ejection related to aging myocardium.

Other important complications include chronic renal insufficiency, end-stage renal disease, malignant hypertension, and encephalopathy. These disorders are most common with severe or poorly controlled hypertension.

Hypertension in mid-life (age 40–64 years) is a strong risk factor for cognitive impairment in late life (age >65 years). Hypertension is a known cause of vascular dementia (VaD) and studies have shown its effect on prevalence of Alzheimer dementia. However, there is no convincing evidence that lowering BP in late-life prevents the development of dementia or cognitive impairment in hypertensive patients without apparent prior cerebrovascular disease.

Thus, preventing organ damage in older adults is best accomplished by preventing and treating elevated BP in young and middle aged adults. As noted earlier, treatment of hypertension in older adults has substantial clinical benefit in stroke reduction. However, if life expectancy is less than 1 year, adapting targets to symptom reduction rather than stroke reduction may be considered.

▶ Treatment

A. Hypertension

The general objective of hypertension management for both community-dwelling and nursing home patients is to reduce morbidity and mortality by early diagnosis and treatment with the least-invasive and most cost-effective methods. Classification of hypertension, stratification for CV risks, and management strategies according to JNC 7 guidelines are shown in Table 30–1. Table 30–2 enumerates major risk

Table 30–1. Cardiovascular risk stratification.

Risk Factors	Target Organ Damage

Hypertension
  Tobacco
  BMI ≥30
  Abdominal obesity (waist circumference >102 cm in men and >88 cm in women)
  Physical Inactivity
  Dyslipidemia
	Heart
	  Left ventricular hypertrophy
	  Angina or prior myocardial infarction
	  Prior coronary revascularization
	  Heart failure

Diabetes
  Microalbuminuria or estimated GFR<60 ml/min
	Brain
	  Stroke or transient ischemic attack

Age (>55 years for men, >65 years for women)	Renal disease
	  Renal impairment
	  Diabetic nephropathy
	  Proteinuria >300 mg/24 hours

Family history of premature cardiovascular disease (age: men <55 years, women <65 years)	Peripheral arterial disease Retinopathy

Data from JNC 7 and the European Society of Hypertension (ESH) and European Society of Cardiology (ESC) 2007 guidelines.

Table 30–2. Medications.

Drug Group	Initial Dose	Typical Range	Indications in Addition to Hypertension	Side Effects/Comments
Diuretic				
HCTZ	12.5 mg/day	12.5–25 mg/day	Typical first-line therapy	Hypokalemia, hypercalcemia, hyperuricemia, hyponatremia, metabolic alkalosis, increased urinary frequency (all less likely at low doses)
Calcium channel blockers				
Dihydropyridines				
Amlodipine	2.5 mg/day	2.5–10 mg/day	Typical first-line therapy	Flush, headache, peripheral edema
Felodipine	2.5 mg/day	2.5–20 mg/day	Typical first-line therapy	Flush, headache, peripheral edema
Nondihydropyridines				
Verapamil	120 mg/day	120–240 mg/day–BID	Angina, arrhythmias	Constipation, AV block, CHF, transaminase elevation
Diltiazem (ER)	120–180 mg/day	240–480 mg/day	Angina	AV block, CHF, transaminase elevation
α-Blocker				
Terazosin	1–2 mg/day	1–5 mg/day	BPH, hypertension	Beers list 2012 PIM because of orthostatic hypotension; not recommended for routine treatment of hypertension
Doxazosin	1–2 mg/day	1–8 mg/day	BPH, hypertension	Same as for terazosin
Prazosin	1 mg BID	2–20 mg/day in divided doses 2–3 times/day	BPH, hypertension, PTSD-related nightmares (offlabel use)	Same as for terazosin
β-Blocker				
Bisoprolol	2.5–5 mg/day	2.5–20 mg/day	Systolic dysfunction	Chest pain, insomnia, diarrhea, bradycardia β-Blockers should be avoided as first line in treatment of hypertension in absence of preexisting CV disease
Metoprolol tartrate	25 mg BID	50–100 mg BID	CAD, systolic dysfunction	Bronchospasm, AV block, fatigue, insomnia; caution with diabetics, peripheral arterial disease; metoprolol is renally excreted
Carvedilol	3.125 mg BID	6.25–12.5 mg BID	CAD, systolic dysfunction	Bronchospasm, AV block, fatigue, insomnia; caution with diabetics, peripheral arterial disease; carvedilol is renally excreted
Atenolol	25 mg/day	25–50 mg/day	CAD, systolic dysfunction	Bronchospasm, AV block, fatigue, insomnia; caution with diabetics, peripheral arterial disease; atenolol is renally excreted, and has prolonged elimination half-life (15–35 hours) in ESRD
α$_2$-Adrenergic Agonist				
Clonidine oral	0.1 mg BID	0.1–2 mg BID–TID	Second- or third-line therapy or when unable to tolerate oral therapy (eg, patch)	Beers list 2012 PIM because of high risk of CNS adverse effects, bradycardia and orthostatic hypotension, not recommended for routine use in older adults
Clonidine patch (TTS)	0.1 mg/day (TTS-1)	0.1–0.2 mg/day (TTS-1 or 2)		
Direct Vasodilator				
Hydralazine	10 mg TID	50 mg BID–QID	Afterload reduction in CHF	Headache, tachycardia, lupus syndrome, fluid retention
Renin-Angiotensin System Inhibitors				
ACEIs				
Captopril	12.5–25 mg BID	25 mg–150 mg BID–TID	Diabetics, CHF, LV dysfunction after MI	Cough, rash, loss of taste, hyperkalemia; rarely leukopenia and angioedema
Enalapril	2.5 mg/day	5–20 mg/day	Diabetics, CHF, LV dysfunction after MI	Cough, rash, loss of taste, hyperkalemia; rarely leukopenia and angioedema
Lisinopril	5 mg/day	10–40 mg/day	Diabetics, CHF, LV dysfunction after MI	Cough, rash, loss of taste, hyperkalemia; rarely leukopenia and angioedema

(continued)

Table 30–2. Medications. (*continued*)

Drug Group	Initial Dose	Typical Range	Indications in Addition to Hypertension	Side Effects/Comments
ARBs				
Losartan	25 mg/day	50–100 mg/day	May be considered for diabetes, CHF if intolerant to ACEIs	Hyperkalemia, angioedema
Valsartan	80 mg/day	80–320 mg/day	May be considered for diabetes, CHF if intolerant to ACEIs	Hyperkalemia, angioedema
DRI				
Aliskiren	150 mg/day	150–300 mg/day		Rash, hyperkalemia, diarrhea, elevated creatinine and creatinine kinase, cough, angioedema

ACEIs, angiotensin-converting enzyme inhibitors; ARBs, angiotensin II receptor blockers; AV, atrioventricular; BID, twice daily; BPH, benign prostatic hypertrophy; CAD, coronary artery disease; CHF, congestive heart failure; CNS, central nervous system; CV, cardiovascular; DRI, direct renin inhibitors; ER, extended release; ESRD, end-stage renal disease; HCTZ, hydrochlorothiazide; LV, left ventricular; MI, myocardial infarction; PIM, potentially inappropriate medicines; PTSD, posttraumatic stress disorder; QID, 4 times daily; TID, 3 times daily.

factors. Little information is available to guide clinicians regarding hypertension management in octogenarians and nursing home residents, typically the frail, older adult group.

The National Institute for Health and Clinical Excellence (NICE) recommends aiming for a target BP below 140/90 mm Hg in people younger than 80 years of age with treated hypertension, and for a target clinic BP below 150/90 mm Hg in people age 80 years and older with treated hypertension. The American College of Cardiology Foundation and American Heart Association (ACCF/AHA) 2011 Expert Consensus recommends that an achieved SBP of 140–145 mm Hg, if tolerated, is acceptable in octogenarians. In patients with hypertension and chronic kidney disease (CKD) or diabetes mellitus (DM), JNC 7 recommends goal BP of <130/80 mm Hg irrespective of age, a target that may be too aggressive for most older adults.

The ACCORD-BP trial (age range: 40–79 years) failed to show any reduction in fatal and nonfatal major CV events with lowering SBP to <120 mm Hg, when compared with target SBP <140 mm Hg, in diabetics at high risk for CV events. These results were supported by the INVEST diabetes subgroup analysis, where mean age group was 66 years. In the AASK trial (age 18–70 years), lowering mean arterial pressure (MAP) to a goal of <92 mm Hg, didn't show any significant difference in all-cause mortality, CV death, or overall CV events, when compared to the usual MAP goal of 102–107 mm Hg, in African Americans with CKD. Consistent with difficulties in finding data for the oldest adults, the ACCORD-BP trial excluded those aged >79 years, whereas AASK trial excluded those aged >70 years. HYVET (Hypertension in the Very Elderly Trial), which targeted adults age >80 years and aimed reduction in BP to <150/80 mm Hg in the active treatment group, showed reduction in incidence of strokes, but a nonsignificant increase in all-cause mortality and CV

mortality in the active treatment group compared to placebo. In the INVEST substudy on outcomes of treatment of hypertension in individuals with CAD age >80 years when compared with individuals age <80 years, there was persistence of "J-curve" relationship between lower BP (especially DBP) and increased all-cause mortality, nonfatal MI and nonfatal strokes in individuals age >80 years (Figure 30–2). Keeping in view this data, it is expected that JNC 8 guidelines will have a fresh outlook on this issue.

Management of hypertension in frail older adults should be tailored while keeping in mind the individual's functional and cognitive status, and possible side effects of each management plan. The clinical benefit of treating hypertension in older adults appears within a year of treatment. Therefore, treatment of hypertension in older adults with limited life expectancy requires a review of benefits and risks of such therapy.

1. Nonpharmacologic Therapy—Lifestyle interventions may benefit older adults with hypertension and can include the following:

1. Dietary sodium

The USDA recommends reduction in dietary sodium intake to 2.3 g (6 g of sodium chloride) per day for adults 50 years or younger, and <1.5 g for adults >51 years, and those at high risk for vascular diseases. However, restricting sodium in frail elders may worsen or precipitate anorexia, malnutrition, sarcopenia and orthostatic hypotension. The TOHP and TONE trials which demonstrated long-term benefits of dietary salt reduction excluded very old subjects. The strongest evidence for dietary sodium recommendations for hypertension in older adults comes from the TONE trial, where there was clinical benefit to lowering dietary sodium to a mean of 2.3 g daily to adults

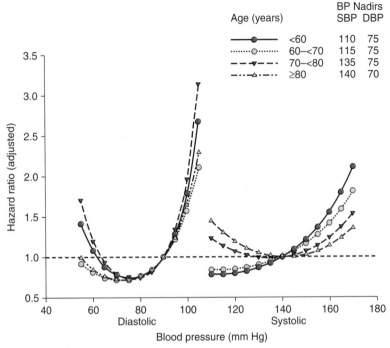

▲ **Figure 30–2.** Adjusted hazard ratio as a function of age (in 10-year increments), systolic and diastolic blood pressure. Reference systolic and diastolic blood pressure for hazard ratio:140 and 90 mm Hg, respectively. Blood pressures are the on-treatment average of all postbaseline recordings. The quadratic terms for both systolic and diastolic blood pressures were statistically significant in all age groups (all P _.001, except for diastolic blood pressure in 60-70-year-olds for whom P _0.006). The adjustment was based upon sex, race, history of myocardial infarction, heart failure, peripheral vascular disease, diabetes, stroke/transient ischemic attack, renal insufficiency, and smoking. (Reproduced with permission from American Journal of Medicine, Vol 123, No 8, Scott J. Denardo, Yan Gong, Wilmer W. Nichols, Franz H. Messerli, Anthony A. Bavry, Rhonda M. Cooper-DeHoff, Eileen M. Handberg, Annette Champion, Carl J. Pepine. Blood Pressure and Outcomes in Very Old Hypertensive Coronary Artery Disease Patients: An INVEST Substudy, Page No. 725, Copyright 2010.)

up to the age of 70 years. There are no data in older adults supporting a 1.5-g sodium restriction.

2. Diet plan

The Mediterranean diet has been shown to reduce all-cause mortality, and mortality as a result of cancer and CV disease in older adults. The Dietary Approaches to Stop Hypertension (DASH) diet includes whole grain products, fish, poultry, and nuts, with reduction in lean red meat, sweets, added sugars, and sugar-containing beverages. It is rich in potassium, magnesium, calcium, protein, and fiber. The DASH diet has shown reduction in BPs in short-term studies (with up to 8 weeks of follow-up) in middle-aged adults, but lacks long-term follow-up data in older adults.

3. Alcohol

Heavy alcohol intake (>300 mL/week or 34 g/day) is strongly, significantly, and independently related to elevation in SBP and DBP. It is also associated with higher risk of CV events, strokes, and all-cause mortality compared with occasional drinking. Aging is associated with a number of physiologic changes suggesting increased sensitivity to alcohol, which can additionally lead to increased cognitive impairment, functional decline, and falls in this population. Moderate alcohol consumption (1 standard drink, or 14 grams of pure alcohol, per day) is associated with reduced risk of CV disease. Therefore, the U.S. National Institute on Alcohol Abuse and Alcoholism (NIAAA) recommends that those age 65 years and older limit themselves to 1 alcoholic drink per day. However, further reduction may be considered in older adults experiencing cognitive impairment, falls, and functional decline, and for those who take prescription psychotropic medicines.

A standard drink is 12 oz of beer with 5% alcohol, 5 oz of wine with 12% alcohol, or 1.5 oz of hard liquor with 40% alcohol.

4. Exercise

Increasing physical activity to 30–45 minutes of aerobic activity 4 or more days per week. If this is not attainable, any increase in physical activity is likely to be beneficial.

5. Weight reduction

An obese older adult has a body mass index (BMI) >30 kg/m². The TONE trial showed reduction in BP with weight loss through physical exercise and dietary restrictions. However, it excluded individuals >80 years old and those with chronic diseases. Population data in older adults suggest that being underweight poses as great a threat to physical disability as being excessively obese. A 12-year follow-up of mortality data of the weight loss intervention group of TONE trial failed to show any mortality benefit over the non–weight-loss intervention group. Therefore, moderate weight loss should be encouraged in obese older adults, only if consistent with functional and nutritional goals.

6. Smoking cessation

Older adults should be encouraged to quit smoking, with the assistance of nicotine patches, gums, etc. Bupropion and varenicline may be prescribed while monitoring for adverse effects.

7. Polypharmacy

Medications that can potentially impair BP control (eg, venlafaxine, NSAIDs) should be stopped if clinically possible, weighing benefits and risks of such treatments.

8. Dark chocolate

Polyphenol-rich dark chocolate has been shown to lower BP in various studies. Clinical outcome data (eg, stroke reduction) are not available.

Use of nonpharmacologic measures to control hypertension in the nursing home setting may be limited because residents are often impaired in their activities of daily living, and unable to participate in moderate exercise. Also, weight loss is a problem rather than a goal for most nursing home residents. If their diet is restricted in salt or animal and dairy fat, they may lose weight, strength, muscle mass, bone density and essential nutrients.

2. Pharmacologic therapy—Antihypertensive medication improves CV and cerebrovascular outcomes in older adults with BP ≥160/90 mm Hg. The absolute benefit of hypertension treatment tends to be greater in men, in patients age 70 years or older, in those with previous CV complications, and in the presence of wider PP. The key to achieving maximal benefit and minimal risk in older adults is to "start low and go slow." Lower initial doses of antihypertensives minimize the risk of postural and postprandial hypotension as well as ischemic symptoms, especially in frail older adults. Choice of initial antihypertensive agent thus depends on comorbidities and side effects. If the baseline BP is more than 20/10 mm Hg

above goal or optimal reduction in BP is not achieved with one agent, a second agent can be added while weighing benefits and risks of such therapy on individual basis.

Special attention should be paid to frail patients and octogenarians when initiating a new antihypertensive medication. They should be seen frequently, with updated medical history and assessment for any new adverse effects, especially dizziness or falls. Standing BP should always be checked to identify excessive orthostatic decline. Although BP values below which vital organ perfusion is impaired in octogenarians are unknown, SBP <130 and DBP <65 mm Hg should be avoided.

Route of administration may be an issue in nursing home residents with dysphagia and those who are unwilling to take pills. A low dose clonidine or nitroglycerin patch may be beneficial in BP management in these situations, while monitoring for potential adverse effects, particularly from clonidine. Because orthostatic and postprandial hypotension may contribute to the risk of falling, it may be appropriate to titrate antihypertensives based on readings obtained in standing posture. Also, BP tends to be highest before breakfast in the nursing home resident, and falls after breakfast. So titration of antihypertensives should be done based on multiple readings during various times of the day.

Table 30–2 summarizes data on antihypertensive agents commonly used in older patients.

a. Diuretics—Thiazide and related diuretics are the preferred first-line treatment in older adults and have proved particularly effective in blacks and in salt-sensitive hypertensive patients. Diuretics have been shown to lower cerebrovascular and CV morbidity and mortality, decrease left ventricular mass, and prevent heart failure. Diuretics are a reasonable choice for diabetics based on findings of ALLHAT trial, which indicated that despite the slightly higher incidence of diabetes in the thiazide treatment group of the trial, there was no significant difference in clinical events in diabetic patients assigned to either diuretic, angiotensin-converting enzyme (ACE) inhibitor or calcium channel blocker regimen. In low doses, thiazides have advantages of low cost and possible preservation of bone mineral density in older women. Side effects of thiazides include increased insulin resistance, hypokalemia, hypomagnesemia, hyponatremia, hypercalcemia, orthostatic hypotension, urinary incontinence, sexual dysfunction, and exacerbation of gout. Thiazides may be ineffective in patients with a creatinine clearance of <30 mL/min and can be replaced by loop diuretics (eg, furosemide) when a diuretic agent is necessary.

b. Angiotensin-converting enzyme inhibitors & receptor blockers—Because of well-known renoprotective effects of ACE inhibitors and ACE receptor blockers (ARBs) in type 2 diabetes, current guidelines suggest using one of these agents as first-line drugs in older adults with both diabetes and hypertension. ACE inhibitors also appear to improve vascular outcomes in high-risk patients, including diabetics and those with established vascular disease. The LIFE study showed reduced CV mortality and incidence of stroke in individuals with ISH when treated with losartan (ARB) compared to atenolol (β-blocker). ARBs are also used when there is intolerance to ACE inhibitors (because of cough). There is no long-term data available on aliskiren, which is the only available drug in the class of direct renin inhibitors.

c. β Blockers—Older adults are less responsive than younger adults to β blockers and are less likely to have BP control with β-blocker as a sole agent. In addition, compared with diuretics, β blockers may offer less reduction in cerebrovascular and CV events in older antihypertensive patients. However, they are effective in older adults with CAD for secondary prevention of MI, for rate control with exercise in atrial fibrillation, and for reducing mortality and hospital readmission in patients with left ventricular systolic dysfunction.

d. Calcium channel blockers—Nitrendipine (not currently available in United States), a dihydropyridine calcium channel blocker (CCB) related to amlodipine and felodipine, significantly decreases the risk of cerebrovascular morbidity and mortality. Dihydropyridine CCBs are available in the United States and include nifedipine, amlodipine, and felodipine. The ACCOMPLISH trial showed that amlodipine-based regimen may be more effective than a thiazide-based regimen in reducing CV events in high-risk patients, including diabetics, and is a good alternative choice for diabetics. However, CCBs are a heterogeneous group, and the benefits of one class of CCBs may not necessarily be extrapolated to another. Diltiazem and verapamil, two commonly used nondihydropyridine CCBs, have negative inotropic and chronotropic effects on left ventricular systolic function compared with amlodipine or felodipine. They may be used as adjunctive agents in patients with renal parenchymal disease and resistant hypertension but should be used with caution in systolic dysfunction.

e. α Blockers—Low doses of selective α_1-adrenergic antagonists (eg, terazosin, doxazosin) may be useful for managing hypertension in the setting of benign prostatic hypertrophy. Their major side effects are orthostatic hypotension, reflex tachycardia, and headache. The findings of slightly increased risk of stroke and CV events and a doubled risk of CHF in the doxazosin arm compared with chlorthalidone in the ALLHAT trial, suggest that the α-antagonists should not be chosen as a first-line antihypertensive agent.

f. Aldosterone antagonists—Aldosterone antagonists (spironolactone and eplerenone) are often beneficial in resistant hypertension due to primary hyperaldosteronism and OSA, including in African Americans.

g. Combination drugs—JNC 7 recommends that combination drug therapy be initiated for stage II hypertension (SBP ≥160 or DBP ≥100 mm Hg). In the ALLHAT trial, approximately half of the high-risk older adults with hypertension required combination therapy. Participants on lisinopril and amlodipine were more likely to require combination therapy than those assigned chlorthalidone. This finding supports the JNC recommendation that a diuretic be a primary choice for an antihypertensive agent.

Combination drugs potentiate antihypertensive activity by acting at different sites simultaneously. Formulations that combine low doses of different classes of drugs improve BP control while minimizing the adverse effects of either drug. These drugs may, in some cases, be priced competitively with either of the combination agents, reducing the patient's out-of-pocket expenses as well. Lower cost, increased ease of compliance, and potential for fewer side effects make combination drugs attractive for use in older adults once the need for more than one agent is established.

B. Diabetes & Hypertension

Type 2 diabetes is 2.5 times more likely to develop in individuals with preexisting hypertension compared with those with normal BP and greatly increases CV risk. Treatment options are discussed in individual drug sections.

C. Hypertension in African Americans

The first-line agent in African Americans with uncomplicated hypertension should be a thiazide diuretic. CCBs effectively lower BP and decrease CV events, especially stroke in this population, and can be a good alternative or second choice. Renin-angiotensin-aldosterone system (RAAS) inhibitors appear less effective than other drug classes in decreasing BP in older African Americans, unless combined with diuretics or CCB.

D. Hypertension & Chronic Kidney Disease

Treatment with an ACE inhibitor or ARB is recommended in presence of proteinuria >300 mg/day or concomitant history of heart failure. However, the AASK trial failed to demonstrate any reduction in CV outcomes with β blocker versus ACE inhibitor versus amlodipine CCB regimen in treatment of hypertension in African American patients with CKD.

E. Hypertension & Heart Failure

Older adults with hypertension and systolic heart failure (HF) should be treated with a diuretic, β-blocker, ACE inhibitor, and aldosterone antagonist in absence of hyperkalemia or significant renal dysfunction. If a patient cannot tolerate ACE inhibitor, an ARB should be used. Older African American patients with hypertension and HF may also benefit from combination of hydralazine and isosorbide dinitrate. Hypertension and asymptomatic left ventricle dysfunction should be treated with β-blocker and ACE inhibitor. If HF is refractory to conventional therapy, work-up for renal artery stenosis should be pursued as renal revascularization may improve HF in hypertensive patients.

Diastolic HF is very common in the older adults. Fluid retention should be adequately treated with loop diuretics, hypertension should be controlled, and comorbidities should be treated. No specific drug class demonstrates superior clinical outcomes at this time.

F. Resistant Hypertension

Hypertension is considered resistant if BP cannot be reduced to goal with an appropriate triple-drug regimen, including a diuretic (plus ACE inhibitor, CCB, β-blocker, or ARB) and if each of the 3 drugs is at or near maximum recommended doses. With ISH in older adults, resistant hypertension is defined as the inability to lower systolic BP to <160 mm Hg with a similar regimen.

The common causes of resistant hypertension include patient nonadherence to the prescribed medications and diet, a suboptimal medication regimen, drug interaction, pseudotolerance (salt, water retention), and office hypertension. Secondary hypertension and pseudohypertension should also be considered.

In hypertensive patients with OSA who are overweight, the cornerstone of treatment is weight loss, which improves sleep efficiency and oxygenation and lowers BP. In the absence of dramatic reductions in etiologic factors for OSA, these patients generally require lifetime treatment with continuous positive airway pressure to reduce the number of hypoxemic events. Addition of the mineralocorticoid-receptor antagonist spironolactone to conventional antihypertensive-drug regimens has been shown to reduce the severity of OSA and to lower BP in patients with OSA and resistant hypertension.

A patient's adherence to dietary salt moderation can be estimated by obtaining a 24-hour urine collection for sodium. If the patient's hypertension remains resistant, other medications can be added to the triple therapy. Clonidine in tablet form or by transdermal patch, or another centrally acting sympatholytic agent, can be considered in low doses to avoid side effects of sedation and orthostatic hypotension. Minoxidil, reserpine, and hydralazine are used cautiously because of their high rates of side effects in older patients.

ACCORD Study Group, Cushman WC, Evans GW, et al. Effects of intensive blood-pressure control in type 2 diabetes mellitus. *N Engl J Med.* 2010;362(17):1575-1585.

ALLHAT Officers and Coordinators for the ALLHAT Collaborative Research Group. The Antihypertensive and Lipid-Lowering Treatment to Prevent Heart Attack Trial. Major outcomes in high-risk hypertensive patients randomized to angiotensin-converting enzyme inhibitor or calcium channel blocker vs diuretic: the antihypertensive and lipid-lowering treatment to prevent heart attack trial (ALLHAT). *JAMA.* 2002;288(23):2981-2997.

Almoosawi S, Fyfe L, Ho C, Al-Dujaili E. The effect of polyphenol-rich dark chocolate on fasting capillary whole blood glucose, total cholesterol, blood pressure and glucocorticoids in healthy overweight and obese subjects. *Br J Nutr.* 2010;103(6):842-850.

Aronow WS, Ahn C. Association of postprandial hypotension with incidence of falls, syncope, coronary events, stroke, and total mortality at 29-month follow-up in 499 older nursing home residents. *J Am Geriatr Soc.* 1997;45(9):1051-1053.

Aronow WS, Fleg JL, Pepine CJ, et al. ACCF/AHA 2011 expert consensus document on hypertension in the elderly: A report of the American College of Cardiology Foundation task force on clinical expert consensus documents developed in collaboration with the American Academy of Neurology, American Geriatrics Society, American Society for Preventive Cardiology, American Society of Hypertension, American Society of Nephrology, Association of Black Cardiologists, and European Society of Hypertension. *J Am Coll Cardiol.* 2011;57(20):2037-2114.

Beckett NS, Peters R, Fletcher AE, et al. Treatment of hypertension in patients 80 years of age or older. *N Engl J Med.* 2008;358(18):1887-1898.

Buddineni JP, Chauhan L, Ahsan ST, Whaley-Connell A. An emerging role for understanding orthostatic hypertension in the cardiorenal syndrome. *Cardiorenal Med.* 2011;1(2):113-122.

Chobanian AV, Bakris GL, Black HR, et al. The seventh report of the joint national committee on prevention, detection, evaluation, and treatment of high blood pressure: The JNC 7 report. *JAMA.* 2003;289(19):2560-2572.

Conlin PR, Chow D, Miller ER 3rd, et al. The effect of dietary patterns on blood pressure control in hypertensive patients: results from the dietary approaches to stop hypertension (DASH) trial. *Am J Hypertens.* 2000;13(9):949-955.

Cook NR, Cutler JA, Obarzanek E, et al. Long-term effects of dietary sodium reduction on cardiovascular disease outcomes: observational follow-up of the trials of hypertension prevention (TOHP). *BMJ.* 2007;334(7599):885-888.

Dahlof B, Lindholm LH, Hansson L, Schersten B, Ekbom T, Wester PO. Morbidity and mortality in the Swedish trial in old patients with hypertension (STOP-hypertension). *Lancet.* 1991;338(8778):1281-1285.

Daskalopoulou SS, Khan NA, Quinn RR, et al. The 2012 Canadian hypertension education program recommendations for the management of hypertension: Blood pressure measurement, diagnosis, assessment of risk, and therapy. *Can J Cardiol.* 2012;28(3):270-287.

Denardo SJ, Gong Y, Nichols WW, et al. Blood pressure and outcomes in very old hypertensive coronary artery disease patients: an INVEST substudy. *Am J Med.* 2010;123(8):719-726.

Emberson JR, Shaper AG, Wannamethee SG, Morris RW, Whincup PH. Alcohol intake in middle age and risk of cardiovascular disease and mortality: accounting for intake variation over time. *Am J Epidemiol.* 2005;161(9):856-863.

Fisher AA, Davis MW, Srikusalanukul W, Budge MM. Postprandial hypotension predicts all-cause mortality in older, low-level care residents. *J Am Geriatr Soc.* 2005;53(8):1313-1320.

Franklin SS, Thijs L, Hansen TW, et al. Significance of white-coat hypertension in older persons with isolated systolic hypertension: a meta-analysis using the international database on ambulatory blood pressure monitoring in relation to cardiovascular outcomes population. *Hypertension.* 2012;59(3):564-571.

Gangavati A, Hajjar I, Quach L, et al. Hypertension, orthostatic hypotension, and the risk of falls in a community-dwelling elderly population: the maintenance of balance, independent living, intellect, and zest in the elderly of Boston study. *J Am Geriatr Soc.* 2011;59(3):383-389.

Gaziano JM, Gaziano TA, Glynn RJ, et al. Light-to-moderate alcohol consumption and mortality in the physicians' health study enrollment cohort. *J Am Coll Cardiol.* 2000;35(1):96-105.

Intersalt: an international study of electrolyte excretion and blood pressure. Results for 24-hour urinary sodium and potassium excretion. Intersalt Cooperative Research Group. *BMJ*. 1988;297(6644):319-328.

Kjeldsen SE, Dahlof B, Devereux RB, et al. Effects of losartan on cardiovascular morbidity and mortality in patients with isolated systolic hypertension and left ventricular hypertrophy: a losartan intervention for endpoint reduction (LIFE) substudy. *JAMA*. 2002;288(12):1491-1498.

Knoops KT, de Groot LC, Kromhout D, et al. Mediterranean diet, lifestyle factors, and 10-year mortality in elderly European men and women: the HALE project. *JAMA*. 2004;292(12): 1433-1439.

Krause T, Lovibond K, Caulfield M, McCormack T, Williams B; Guideline Development Group. Management of hypertension: summary of NICE guidance. *BMJ*. 2011;343:d4891.

Norris K, Bourgoigne J, Gassman J, et al. Cardiovascular outcomes in the African American study of kidney disease and hypertension (AASK) trial. *Am J Kidney Dis*. 2006;48(5):739-751.

Pepine CJ, Handberg EM, Cooper-DeHoff RM, et al; INVEST Investigators. A calcium antagonist vs a non-calcium antagonist hypertension treatment strategy for patients with coronary artery disease. the international verapamil-trandolapril study (INVEST): a randomized controlled trial. *JAMA*. 2003;290(21):2805-2816.

Prevention of stroke by antihypertensive drug treatment in older persons with isolated systolic hypertension. final results of the systolic hypertension in the elderly program (SHEP). SHEP Cooperative Research Group. *JAMA*. 1991;265(24):3255-3264.

Puisieux F, Bulckaen H, Fauchais AL, Drumez S, Salomez-Granier F, Dewailly P. Ambulatory blood pressure monitoring and postprandial hypotension in elderly persons with falls or syncopes. *J Gerontol A Biol Sci Med Sci*. 2000;55(9):M535-M540.

Roger VL, Go AS, Lloyd-Jones DM, et al; American Heart Association Statistics Committee and Stroke Statistics Subcommittee. Heart disease and stroke statistics—2012 update: a report from the American Heart Association. *Circulation*. 2012;125(1):e2-e220.

Shah NS, Vidal JS, Masaki K, et al. Midlife blood pressure, plasma beta-amyloid, and the risk for Alzheimer disease: the Honolulu Asia Aging Study. *Hypertension*. 2012;59(4):780-786.

Shea MK, Nicklas BJ, Houston DK, et al. The effect of intentional weight loss on all-cause mortality in older adults: results of a randomized controlled weight-loss trial. *Am J Clin Nutr*. 2011;94(3):839-846.

Staessen JA, Fagard R, Thijs L, et al. Randomised double-blind comparison of placebo and active treatment for older patients with isolated systolic hypertension. The Systolic Hypertension in Europe (Syst-Eur) Trial Investigators. *Lancet*. 1997;350(9080):757-764.

USEFUL WEBSITES

American College of Cardiology. www.acc.org

American Heart Association. www.americanheart.org

American Society of Hypertension. www.ash-us.org

Cardiosource. www.cardiosource.com

Centers for Disease Control and Prevention. www.cdc.gov/nchs/fastats/hypertens.htm

Lifeclinic. www.bloodpressure.com

National Heart, Lung, and Blood Institute. www.nhlbi.nih.gov

National Institute of Alcohol Abuse and Alcoholism. *Module 1: Epidemiology of Alcohol Problems in the United States*. http://pubs.niaaa.nih.gov/publications/Social/Module1Epidemiology/Module1.html

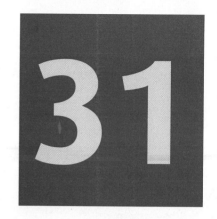

Valvular Disease

Margarita M. Sotelo, MD

Michael W. Rich, MD

G. Michael Harper, MD

General Principles in Older Adults

Degenerative valve disease is the most common form of valvular heart disease in the United States and as the population ages, clinicians will diagnose and manage more patients with this condition. Advances in surgical techniques have led to a greater number of older patients undergoing surgery for heart valve disease with improved morbidity and mortality risks. The decision to offer surgery to the older patient is complex. The patient's preference is foremost consideration after detailed discussion of risks, benefits, and goals of care. A multidisciplinary team approach with input from the cardiac surgeon, anesthesiologist, primary care clinician and cardiologist is key to achieving desired outcomes.

Weighing the projected benefit of surgery with the natural course of untreated disease is crucial. The patient's life-expectancy and quality of life regardless of the valve disease influence the potential benefit derived from surgery. Factors that should be weighed when considering surgery include a diagnosis of dementia, advanced cancer, severe pulmonary disease, significant frailty, symptomatic distress, and reluctance to undergo the procedure. Multivariable prognostic tools designed for older adults have been developed and validated and can provide clinicians more objectivity when estimating life expectancy (see Chapter 3, "Goals of Care & Consideration of Prognosis").

When deciding whether surgical treatment is indicated in older patients with aortic stenosis (AS), mitral stenosis (MS), mitral regurgitation (MR), or aortic insufficiency (AI), the presence of limiting symptoms referable to the valve disease is the clearest rationale. In asymptomatic patients with severe AI or severe primary MR, the American Heart Association (AHA) and American College of Cardiology (ACC) guidelines recommend operation when the left ventricular (LV) dimension and ejection fraction reach specific parameters. The goal is to prevent further deterioration. Preventive operations such as these are justified in the older patient when the perioperative risks of stroke, acute renal failure, cognitive dysfunction, and other complications that affect quality of life are low relative to the desired benefit. In general, older patients are at increased risk for major complications following valve surgery (both aortic and mitral) including atrial fibrillation (AF), heart failure (HF), prolonged mechanical ventilation, worsened renal function, bleeding, and delirium. As a result, length of stay tends to be longer and convalescence slower.

In-hospital mortality rates associated with valve surgery range from 4% to 8% in all comers. Emergency operations, age >79 years, end-stage renal disease, and ≥2 previous cardiac operations are all strongly predictive of higher risk. Concomitant coronary artery bypass graft (CABG), low body weight, female gender, mitral valve surgery, combined valve surgeries, preoperative arrhythmias, hypertension, diabetes, and LV ejection fraction <30% are other variables predictive of in-hospital mortality following aortic and/or mitral valve surgery.

AORTIC STENOSIS

 ESSENTIALS OF DIAGNOSIS

▶ Chest pain, shortness of breath, dizziness, syncope.
▶ Harsh systolic ejection murmur at the right upper sternal border radiating to the carotid arteries.
▶ Echocardiography demonstrates a calcified aortic valve with increased systolic velocities and reduced orifice area.

General Principles in Older Adults

The prevalence of AS increases with age, from 1.3% of 65–75-year-olds to 2.4% of 75–85-year-olds and 4% of those older than age 85 years. AS is the second most common indication for major cardiac surgery in older adults after coronary bypass surgery.

The most common cause of AS in the older adult is calcific valve disease. Aortic valve sclerosis represents an earlier stage of the disease. More than just a "wear-and-tear" process, evidence exists that calcific valve disease shares a common pathogenesis with atherosclerosis and common risk factors including age, male gender, hypertension, tobacco, lipoprotein (a), and low-density lipoprotein (LDL) cholesterol. Mechanical injury to the endothelium initiates the process that leads to lipid deposition, inflammation, neoangiogenesis, calcification, and sclerosis.

▶ **Prevention**

There are no effective strategies to prevent AS. The evidence supporting use of statins to delay AS progression is inconsistent. Statins are not currently recommended for the prevention or treatment of AS in the absence of other indications, such as coronary disease.

The renin-angiotensin system is thought to play a role in the pathogenesis of calcific aortic valve (AV) disease as in atherosclerosis, however, evidence that angiotensin-converting enzyme (ACE) inhibitors modify AS progression is lacking.

▶ **Clinical Findings**

A. Symptoms & Signs

AS is a progressive disease with a prolonged asymptomatic phase and a shorter symptomatic phase. Symptoms usually manifest in the sixth decade or later. The classic triad of symptoms associated with severe AS includes exertional angina, lightheadedness or syncope, and dyspnea or orthopnea. However, AS in the older adult is often occult until it reaches an advanced stage because sedentary older persons may experience few symptoms or may attribute their symptoms to another disease or to old age (see Chapter 7, "Atypical Presentations of Illness in Older Adults").

Significant AS is almost invariably associated with a grade II or greater systolic ejection murmur that is usually harsh and best heard in the right second intercostal space with radiation to the carotid arteries. The murmur may be difficult to hear in obese patients and in those with increased chest diameter because of chronic lung disease, whereas in others it may be heard best at the apex. Murmurs that peak in late systole tend to be associated with more severe AS, but the intensity of the murmur often diminishes in patients with severe LV failure. Other physical findings include an LV heave, S_4 gallop, and reduced intensity or absence of the A_2 component of the second heart sound. Classically, the carotid upstroke is delayed in patients with severe AS, but this finding may be masked in older patients with stiff, noncompliant vessels.

Table 31–1. Classification of AS severity.

AS Severity	Jet Velocity (m/sec)	Mean Gradient (mm Hg)	Valve Area (cm²)
Mild	<3	<25	>1.5–4
Moderate	3–4	25–40	1–1.5
Severe	>4	>40	<1

B. Special Tests

1. Electrocardiography and radiography—The electrocardiogram (ECG) often demonstrates LV hypertrophy, and the chest radiograph frequently reveals LV prominence.

2. Echocardiography—Echocardiography is the noninvasive procedure of choice for diagnosing AS. Typical echocardiographic features include a moderately or severely thickened and calcified valve with restricted opening. Doppler examination measures mean and peak velocities across the valve and allows for calculation of the effective aortic valve area. Table 31–1 classifies AS severity.

3. Cardiac catheterization—Because approximately 50% of older patients with severe AS have obstructive coronary artery disease (CAD), cardiac catheterization with coronary angiography is indicated for all patients in whom aortic valve replacement (AVR) is being considered. Catheterization can also provide definitive information about the severity of AS when the echocardiogram is nondiagnostic.

▶ **Differential Diagnosis**

The symptoms of AS may mimic many other cardiac and noncardiac diseases, including CAD, HF, arrhythmia, and chronic lung disease. Likewise, the physical findings, ECG, and chest radiograph are often nonspecific. Consequently, the clinician must maintain a high index of suspicion in patients with symptoms possibly attributable to AS in association with a systolic ejection murmur.

▶ **Treatment**

There is no effective medical therapy for severe AS. Because AS is generally a disease of older age, hypertension is a frequent comorbidity and contributes to the load on the LV. There are no clear recommendations for antihypertensive therapy in these patients. When used, vasodilators, including nitrates and ACE inhibitors, should be administered at a low dose and titrated cautiously in patients with moderate to severe AS because of the risk of hypotension.

Once symptoms develop, patients with severe AS should be referred for AVR because the prognosis is poor in the absence of definitive therapy. AVR is the procedure of choice for patients with severe symptomatic AS, and the results of valve replacement are excellent in properly selected candidates. Table 31–2 lists other class I indications for AV surgery. In patients older than 75 years, most cardiac surgeons will implant a bioprosthetic valve, which has acceptable durability in this group and obviates the need for long-term anticoagulation.

Age alone should not be a contraindication to surgery because several series have shown that older patients who underwent AVR for AS had quality-of-life outcomes during late follow up comparable to an age-matched general population.

AVR for symptomatic AS is associated with a 30-day survival of 86% to 94% in 75–85-year-old patients; 1-year survival of 85% to 89%; and 5-year survival of 60% to 69%. Factors predictive of operative mortality in octogenarians are urgent procedure, concurrent CABG, New York Heart

Association (NYHA) class IV HF, and prior percutaneous aortic valvuloplasty. In a group of octogenarians who underwent isolated AVR, nearly 75% survived at 5 years: 81% enjoyed favorable NYHA functional classes, 91% were free of angina, and 68% were living at home.

Reduced left ventricular ejection fraction (LVEF) <30% and low-gradient severe AS from LV systolic dysfunction and low transvalvular flow are factors associated with worse postoperative outcomes. A subgroup of patients, mostly older women, who develop excessive LV hypertrophy in response to AS are also at higher risk for operative mortality.

Aortic balloon valvotomy, a procedure where a balloon is placed across a stenotic AV and inflated, frequently results in a moderate reduction in transvalvular gradient and early symptom improvement. However, it is not recommended in older adults because of frequent acute complications, and restenosis occurs within 6–12 months in most patients.

Many older patients with severe symptomatic AS are considered inoperable because of high surgical risk. Transcatheter aortic valve replacement (TAVR) is an intervention that may be an alternative. TAVR is performed by following a balloon aortic valvotomy with deployment of a stented bioprosthetic valve into the aortic annulus transfemorally or through an alternative approach. When compared with standard care in older patients who are deemed unsuitable for surgery, TAVR was associated with lower 30-day all-cause mortality despite higher rates of strokes and vascular complications at 30 days. Furthermore, TAVR was associated with reduced severity of symptoms at 1 year. In high-risk patients who nevertheless were candidates for surgical treatment, TAVR and surgical AVR were associated with similar 1-year mortality rate, approximately 25%. TAVR patients had fewer ICU and total hospitalization days. They also had a more rapid improvement in NYHA class, a difference that was significant at 1 and 6 months, but not at 1 or 2 years. At 2 years, all-cause mortality was similar in both groups, approximately 34%. Strokes occurred more frequently in the TAVR group at 30 days, but did not differ significantly between the groups during the 2-year follow-up. Paravalvular regurgitation, which was associated with late mortality, was more frequent following TAVR.

Table 31–2. American College of Cardiology/American Heart Association guidelines.

Valvular Disease	Class I Indications for Valvular Surgery
Aortic stenosis	**Aortic valve replacement** • Symptomatic severe AS • Severe AS and LV ejection fraction of <0.5 • Severe AS and undergoing surgery on the aorta or other heart valves
Aortic insufficiency	**Aortic valve replacement** • Symptomatic severe AI irrespective of LV systolic function • Asymptomatic chronic severe AI and LVEF <0.5 at rest • Chronic severe AI and undergoing CABG or surgery on the aorta or other heart valves
Mitral regurgitation	**Mitral valve replacement or repair (preferred)** • Symptomatic (NYHA II-IV) chronic, severe MR, LVEF >30%, and LVESD <55 mm • Asymptomatic chronic severe MR, LVEF is 0.3-0.6, and/or LVESD ≥40 mm

Mitral stenosis	**Mitral Valve replacement or repair (preferred)**
	• Symptomatic (NYHA classes III-IV) moderate to severe MS when
	  1. PMBV is unavailable
	  2. PMBV is contraindicated because of left atrial thrombus despite anticoagulation
	  3. PMBV is contraindicated because of moderate to severe MR
	  4. PMBV contraindicated by unfavorable valve morphology

AI, Aortic insufficiency; CABG, coronary artery bypass grafting; LVEF, left ventricular ejection fraction; LVESD, left ventricular end systolic diameter; NYHA, New York Heart Association; PMBV, percutaneous mitral balloon valvotomy.

▶ Prognosis

Onset of symptoms secondary to AS heralds increased mortality risk. The average survival after the onset of angina or syncope is 3 years, 2 years after onset of dyspnea, and 1.5–2 years following onset of HF. In a more recent study, the 2-year survival rate after onset of symptoms was approximately 50%. HF was the cause of death in 50% to 60% and sudden cardiac death (SCD) in 15% to 20% of patients. SCD is rare in asymptomatic patients and is almost always preceded by symptoms. After AVR, survival is similar to that for persons of comparable age in the general population.

AORTIC INSUFFICIENCY

ESSENTIALS OF DIAGNOSIS

▶ Dyspnea, fatigue, palpitations, chest pain.

▶ Decrescendo diastolic murmur in the left third and fourth intercostal spaces.

▶ Echocardiography demonstrates AI.

General Principles in Older Adults

The prevalence of trace or greater AI in the Framingham Heart Study is 13% in men, 8.5% in women, and increases with age. Pure AI is uncommon in the older adult population; the majority with aortic valve disease have combined AS and AI. Hypertension is the most common cause of nonvalvular chronic AI. The most prevalent valvular cause is calcific valve disease.

Older patients develop symptoms or LV dysfunction earlier and suffer worse operative mortality. Concomitant CAD complicates the evaluation of symptoms, LV dysfunction, and indication for surgery.

Prevention

Therapies directed at preventing the various disorders that cause chronic AI may reduce its prevalence.

Clinical Findings

A. Symptoms & Signs

Patients with mild or moderate chronic AI are usually asymptomatic, and those with chronic severe AI report progressive exercise intolerance, shortness of breath, orthopnea, and fatigue.

In patients with mild-to-moderate chronic AI, a short, early diastolic decrescendo murmur is often the only physical finding. In those with chronic severe AI, the diastolic murmur becomes louder, occasionally reaching grade V or VI, and longer, often persisting throughout diastole with presystolic accentuation. The LV apical impulse is often diffuse and displaced laterally and inferiorly. An S_3 gallop is often present and may be palpable. Blood pressure is characterized by a widened pulse pressure and especially by a low diastolic pressure. Peripheral manifestations of severe chronic AI include bounding pulses, head bobbing, Quincke pulses (capillary pulsations), and femoral bruits with light compression of the artery.

B. Special Tests

1. Chest radiography—In patients with acute severe AI, the chest radiograph reveals pulmonary edema, often in association with a normal cardiac silhouette. In patients with chronic severe AI, the heart size is usually markedly increased.

2. Electrocardiography—Electrocardiographic findings are nonspecific, but LV hypertrophy may be evident in patients with severe chronic AI. Table 31–3 classifies AI severity.

3. Echocardiography—Transthoracic and transesophageal echocardiography, CT, and MRI are useful noninvasive techniques for evaluating AI. In most cases, transthoracic echocardiography is the initial procedure of choice. In mild-to-moderate chronic AI, the AI jet is visualized but the echocardiogram may be normal otherwise. In chronic severe AI, the left ventricle is usually dilated and there is a prominent AI jet. Echocardiography may also provide valuable insight into the cause of AI, such as infective endocarditis, flail aortic valve leaflet, or aortic root aneurysm or dissection.

4. Cardiac catheterization—In most cases, cardiac catheterization is not necessary to diagnose and quantify AI. Older patients who require surgery for AI should first undergo coronary angiography.

Differential Diagnosis

Other causes of chronic HF must be considered in the differential diagnosis of severe chronic AI.

Complications

The course of chronic severe AI is insidious and gradually progressive over many years, ultimately leading to severe HF. In asymptomatic patients with normal LVEF, the annual rate of progression to symptoms and/or LV dysfunction is <6%, 1.2% to asymptomatic LV dysfunction, and <0.2% to SCD.

Asymptomatic patients with LV dysfunction develop symptoms that indicate need for AVR within 2–3 years and are at greater risk of death.

The onset of angina, dyspnea, or HF heralds greater mortality, with annual rates of 10% in patients with angina and 20% in those with HF. Severity of HF symptoms correlate with mortality risk.

The annual risk of aortic dissection or rupture is approximately 7% in patients with aortic diameter of ≥6 cm.

Table 31–3. Classification of AI severity.

AI Severity	Regurgitant Volume (mL/beat)	Regurgitant Fraction (%)	Regurgitant Orifice (cm²)	LV Size
Mild	<30	<30	>0.10	Normal
Moderate	30–59	30–49	0.10–0.29	Normal
Severe	≥60	≥50	≥0.30	Dilated

Treatment

Mild chronic AI requires no additional treatment. Serial clinical evaluation and echocardiography are recommended at 2–3-year intervals. Annual echocardiography is recommended for patients with moderate to severe AI and minimal ventricular dilation. When the degree of ventricular enlargement approaches surgical indication, echocardiography is recommended every 6 months.

Chronic vasodilator therapy is recommended in patients with severe AI who are symptomatic or have LV dysfunction but are deemed inappropriate for surgery. Vasodilators may prolong the compensated phase of asymptomatic patients who have an enlarged LV but normal systolic function. In the absence of hypertension, vasodilators are not indicated in asymptomatic patients with mild to moderate AI and normal systolic function. In the presence of hypertension, blood pressure (BP) control with vasodilator therapy in asymptomatic AI patients is recommended to reduce wall stress, although systolic hypertension associated with severe AI is often difficult to lower. The goal is generally to lower BP to <150/90 mm Hg.

β Blockers are thought to worsen AI by prolonging diastolic regurgitation. However, based on observational data that β-blocker use is associated with improved survival in patients with chronic severe AI independent of comorbid hypertension and CAD, the use of this class of antihypertensive is not contraindicated and possibly beneficial as long as heart rate is >70 beats/min.

Table 31–2 lists class I indications for surgical treatment of AI. Patients with symptoms that improve with medical therapy remain at risk for dying and surgery relieves symptoms, is relatively low risk, and associated with long-term survival similar to expected rate. Severity and duration of AI and LV dysfunction, degree of symptoms and functional impairment, and degree of aortic enlargement are factors that affect postoperative survival and LV function. In older adults, symptoms should guide clinicians in deciding whether or not to recommend AVR, particularly in octogenarians. Older patients usually receive bioprosthetic valves.

MITRAL STENOSIS

ESSENTIALS OF DIAGNOSIS

▶ History of rheumatic fever or prior streptococcal infection.

▶ Exertional fatigue, hemoptysis, symptoms of HF.

▶ Opening snap and mid-diastolic rumbling murmur.

▶ Echocardiogram demonstrating thickened mitral valve with restricted motion and a diastolic pressure gradient between the left atrium and left ventricle.

General Principles in Older Adults

Based on pooled data from U.S. population-based studies, the prevalence of MS is 0.2% in those >65 years old.

MS is an obstruction to the LV inflow caused by a structurally abnormal mitral valve (MV). Normal valve area is 4–6 cm^2. Transvalvular pressure gradient rises when the area is reduced to <2 cm^2 and symptoms develop when <1.5 cm^2. The pathophysiology of MS is associated with the volume of flow through the valve and the duration of diastole. Consequently, patients with severe MS decompensate from conditions that result in tachycardia and increased flow, such as exercise, anemia, AF, and infection.

In developed nations, rheumatic fever has become rare, although it still accounts for the majority of MS cases. Degenerative etiology is common in developed countries. Mitral annular calcification (MAC) is a degenerative process characterized by the deposition of calcium along the valve annulus. It is reported to be more prevalent in older women and can cause functional MS by impairing the annular dilatation that normally occurs during diastole.

Prevention

Rheumatic MS can be prevented by prompt identification and treatment of group A β-hemolytic streptococcal infections. No interventions have been shown to prevent or delay the development of MAC.

Clinical Findings

A. Symptoms & Signs

The latency period from rheumatic fever episode to symptoms is 2–4 decades in developed countries and the mean age of presentation is in the fifth to sixth decades. Classic symptoms include exertional fatigue, a gradual decline in exercise tolerance, hemoptysis, dyspnea, and orthopnea.

Rheumatic MS is characterized by an opening snap in early diastole followed by a mid-diastolic rumbling murmur. The murmur is low pitched, best heard at the apex in left lateral decubitus position, and intensified by tachycardia. An earlier opening snap and longer duration of the diastolic murmur are associated with more severe stenosis. All of these features may be absent in patients with MS because of MAC. Additional findings associated with MS may include evidence for pulmonary hypertension (RV heave, augmented P2) and evidence for biventricular failure (pulmonary rales, elevated jugular vein pulse [JVP], and peripheral edema).

B. Special Tests

1. Chest radiography—The chest radiograph may demonstrate calcification in the region of the MV, evidence for left atrial or right ventricular enlargement, and increased vascular markings in the lower lung fields.

Table 31–4. Classification of MS severity.

MS Severity	Area (cm²)	Mean Gradient (mm Hg)	Pulmonary Artery Systolic Pressure (mm Hg)
Mild	>1.5-4.0	<5	<30
Moderate	1.0-1.5	5-10	30-50
Severe	<1.0	>10	>50

2. Electrocardiography—The ECG demonstrates left atrial enlargement or AF; right axis deviation and signs of right ventricular hypertrophy may also be present.

3. Echocardiography—Echocardiography is the diagnostic procedure of choice because it can reliably determine the presence of MS, assess disease severity, estimate left atrial size, and evaluate for rheumatic or calcific involvement of other valves. Transesophageal echocardiography allows better anatomic visualization, excludes left atrial clot, and is necessary before percutaneous mitral balloon valvotomy (PMBV). Table 31–4 classifies MS severity.

4. Cardiac catheterization—In older patients with severe MS who are being considered for cardiac surgery, coronary angiography is indicated to evaluate for obstructive CAD.

▶ Differential Diagnosis

Differential diagnosis includes other cardiac and pulmonary conditions that produce left- or right-sided HF, AF, or pulmonary hypertension.

▶ Complications

In minimally symptomatic patients, 10-year survival is >80%. Once limiting symptoms develop, the 10-year survival drops to 0% to 15%, and is inversely proportional to symptom severity.

After onset of severe pulmonary hypertension, the average survival is 3 years. Increased pulmonary arterial resistance may protect from pulmonary edema and allow patients to be asymptomatic for a prolonged period. Eventually, pulmonary hypertension leads to impaired right ventricular function and adversely affects prognosis.

Atrial fibrillation complicates one-third of symptomatic MS cases and affects older patients more frequently. Because atrial contraction helps maintain LV filling, the onset of AF reduces cardiac output, precipitates symptoms, and increases the risk of embolism (approaches 20% per year in the absence of anticoagulation).

Among untreated patients with severe MS, 60% to 70% die from progressive HF, 20% to 30% from systemic embolism, and 10% from pulmonary embolism.

▶ Treatment

Anticoagulation and rate control are indicated in AF (refer to Chapter 29, "Heart Failure & Heart Rhythm Disorders," for a discussion of AF management). Anticoagulation is also indicated in the setting of sinus rhythm with the presence of a left atrial thrombus or a history of embolism. Maintenance of sinus rhythm has been shown to improve exercise capacity; however, maintenance is difficult to achieve, even after valvotomy, particularly if duration of AF is >1 year and atrial diameter remains >45 mm. Anticoagulation should be continued in patients with persistent AF after valvotomy. Salt restriction and diuretics are useful to manage vascular congestion. Vasodilator therapy has not been shown to be beneficial in the absence of LV systolic dysfunction.

Percutaneous mitral balloon valvotomy (PMBV) involves placing a balloon across the valve and inflating it under pressure to split the fused commissures. While PMBV is the mainstay of treatment for MS in younger patients, most older adults are not suitable candidates for the procedure due to unfavorable valve morphology, such as calcified leaflets or commissures, fusion of subvalvular apparatus, or concomitant moderate or severe mitral regurgitation. Nonetheless, among older patients without contraindications, PMBV can be performed safely with salutary effects on symptoms. PMBV may also be considered as a palliative option in selected older adults who are not candidates for surgical treatment. Long-term outcomes after PMBV are less favorable in older compared to younger patients. In one study, 87% of those <40 years compared to 19% of those >70 years were in NYHA class I or II at 5-year follow-up, and mortality rates were 0% and 59%, respectively.

In patients with severe MS who are not candidates for open commissurotomy or PMBV, MV replacement offers the only viable therapeutic option. As with aortic valve replacement, mitral valve surgery in older patients is associated with increased morbidity and mortality. In the older patients with comorbid medical problems or pulmonary hypertension at systemic levels, perioperative mortality may be up to 10–20%.

MITRAL REGURGITATION

ESSENTIALS OF DIAGNOSIS

▶ Exertional dyspnea or fatigue, orthopnea, peripheral edema.

▶ Holosystolic murmur at the apex radiating to the axilla.

▶ Echocardiography demonstrates MR, increased left atrial size, and progressive ventricular dilation.

General Principles in Older Adults

The prevalence of mild or greater severity MR in the Framingham Heart Study is 19%. It is the most common valvular disorder in the older adult population and is the second most common reason for valve surgery in this population after AS.

Causes and mechanisms are distinct in MR; a specific cause can lead to MR through different mechanisms. The mechanisms are classified as primary and secondary. Primary MR results from intrinsic valve abnormalities causing incomplete coaptation of leaflets, backflow, and LV volume overload. Causes of primary MR include degenerative processes (eg, MV prolapse and annular calcification), ischemia (eg, chordal rupture), rheumatic fever, or endocarditis. In contrast, the valve structure is normal in secondary MR; LV remodeling secondary to myocardial infarction or other causes of dilated cardiomyopathy results in papillary muscle and leaflet displacement. Frequent causes of MR in older adults are degenerative processes, ischemia, and cardiomyopathy.

Prevention

Therapies directed at preventing the various disorders that cause acute or chronic MR may reduce the prevalence of this condition.

Clinical Findings

A. Symptoms & Signs

Chronic mild or moderate MR is usually asymptomatic, and chronic severe MR is often well tolerated as long as LV function is preserved. Once LV dysfunction develops, patients with severe chronic MR typically experience symptoms and signs of left-sided HF, including exertional dyspnea, orthopnea, an S_3 gallop, and pulmonary rales. As the disease progresses, signs of right-sided HF including elevated jugular venous pressure and peripheral edema, may ensue.

Chronic MR is characterized by an apical holosystolic murmur radiating to the axilla, back, or across the precordium. In patients with MV prolapse, a midsystolic click may be heard, followed by the MR murmur. In patients with severe chronic MR, the apical impulse is usually laterally displaced, and an S_3 gallop may be present.

B. Special Tests

1. Chest radiography—The most common finding is cardiomegaly from LV and left atrial enlargements. Annular calcification may be seen. In the absence of pulmonary hypertension, the right ventricle size is normal.

2. Electrocardiography—In chronic severe MR, the ECG reveals left atrial enlargement or AF; in advanced stages there may be evidence of right ventricle hypertrophy.

Table 31–5. Classification of MR severity.

MR Severity	Regurgitant Volume (mL/beat)	Regurgitant Fraction (%)	Regurgitant Orifice Area (cm²)
Mild	<30	<30	<0.20
Moderate	30-59	30-49	0.20-0.39
Severe	≥60	≥50	≥0.40

3. Echocardiography—Echocardiographic findings depend on the cause, chronicity, and severity of MR. A regurgitant MR jet is invariably present, and color Doppler techniques permit a qualitative assessment of MR severity. The preload is increased and afterload is reduced in MR resulting in a greater than normal LVEF. LV function may be hyperdynamic (eg, acute severe MR resulting from chordal rupture), normal (eg, moderate chronic MR), or impaired (eg, MR resulting from ischemic or dilated cardiomyopathy). The left atrial size is often normal in acute MR but becomes progressively dilated in severe chronic MR. The MV may appear structurally normal or there may be evidence of myxomatous degeneration, rheumatic involvement, endocarditis, or a flail leaflet. For patients in whom the cause or severity of MR remains in doubt after transthoracic echocardiography, the transesophageal approach provides excellent visualization of MV anatomy and function. Serial measurements of LV size and ejection fraction by echocardiography play a crucial role in management and timing of surgery.

4. Cardiac catheterization—Cardiac catheterization with left ventriculography is also helpful in assessing MR severity and determining LV function. However, the role of catheterization is principally limited to evaluating hemodynamics, pulmonary pressures, and coronary anatomy in patients with severe MR who are being considered for MV surgery. Table 31–5 classifies MR severity.

Differential Diagnosis

The differential diagnosis of MR includes numerous other conditions that may result in the clinical findings of left- or right-sided HF. Often, multiple such chronic conditions coexist in older patients, and it may be difficult to determine the extent to which the patient's symptoms are a result of MR or other causes.

Treatment

The mechanism of chronic MR influences outcomes with medical therapy. No medical therapy has been shown to delay the need for surgery in primary chronic MR with degenerative causes. Vasodilators are used in acute MR to increase forward flow, however, there are no conclusive studies of ACE inhibitors, angiotensin receptor blockers (ARBs), or other vasodilators for primary chronic MR, and they are not recommended for nonhypertensive asymptomatic patients.

Optimal medical therapy of systolic dysfunction HF reduces secondary MR (see Chapter 29, "Heart Failure & Heart Rhythm Disorders").

Chronic MR is the second most common indication for valve surgery in older adults. See Table 31–2 for ACC/AHA class I recommendations for surgery. Although surgery is recommended for young patients with asymptomatic MR and early LV dysfunction, the presence of symptoms is often the recommended surgical indication in octogenarians. However, MV surgery before onset of LV dysfunction has been associated with greater freedom from cardiovascular mortality and hospitalization in octogenarians with isolated, nonischemic, nonrheumatic MR disease. Observational evidence also exists that 7-year mortality is excellent and no different between younger and older patients with LVEF >40% who had surgery while in NYHA class I or II. Delay in surgery likely contributes to poor outcomes from MV surgery in the older adult population. Older patients with severe LV dysfunction or markedly dilated left ventricles respond poorly to surgery and should be managed medically.

The mechanism of chronic MR guides decision about surgical treatment. For primary MR, MV repair is the primary treatment to prevent LV dysfunction and should occur before LVEF decreases to <60% or left ventricular end-systolic diameter (LVESD) increases to ≥40 mm. Surgical treatment is less straightforward in secondary MR, which is primarily a ventricular, rather than a valve, problem. Outcome of surgery for secondary disease remains suboptimal with high operative and long-term mortality, recurrent MR, and HF rates.

Observational studies suggest that MV repair is preferred over replacement as treatment of primary MR because it:

1. preserves the native valve without prosthesis and in the absence of AF, obviates chronic anticoagulation,

2. preserves LV geometry and function, reducing risk of HF, and

3. is associated with improved survival.

Mitral repair also is associated with lower postoperative stroke and shorter ICU and hospital stay in patients age 75 years and older. However, because of unfavorable valve morphology and the concomitant need for other cardiac surgery, MV repair may be a more complicated procedure in older adults.

MV replacement is associated with worse short- and long-term mortality in patients with secondary ischemic MR. The benefit of any MV surgery for octogenarians with severe secondary ischemic MR is questionable; in one study fewer than half of patients who underwent either type of MV surgery were alive in 1 year.

Age, concomitant CAD, other valvular lesions, symptom severity, comorbidities, LV size, and LV function also influence operative outcomes following MV replacement. In 31,688 patients who underwent MV replacement alone or with concomitant CABG or tricuspid surgery, operative mortality increased from 4% in those aged <50 years to 17% in those aged >80 years and major operative complications increased from 13.5% to 35.5%, respectively. The volume of procedures performed in the institution is also a determinant of operative mortality in older adults, being as high as 20% in low-volume centers (<100 valve replacements/year).

Improvement in surgical techniques in recent years has yielded better outcomes in all age groups although it remains worse in the oldest group. Overall operative mortality declined from 16% in 1980 to 3% in 1995. Improvement in cardiac output and length of hospitalization were also observed in all age groups during this period. One reason proposed for the improvement in outcomes is the more frequent performance of MV repair. Patients older than 75 years who underwent MR surgery had more severe disease with NYHA class III or IV symptoms and more comorbidities, but experienced similar restoration in life expectancy compared with younger patients when adjusted to expected survival.

Percutaneously placed clips (MitraClip) that approximate the leaflets are now approved as treatment of MR. This procedure has been used to treat MR of primary degenerative and secondary functional causes. Commonly cited contraindications to the procedure are active endocarditis, MS, rheumatic valve disease, and leaflet anatomy that does not allow both leaflets to be grasped. Mean age of participants in published clinical trials ranged from 67 to 73 years. Short- and mid-term safety and efficacy as measured by in-hospital/procedural mortality, reduction in MR severity to ≤2+ at discharge and 12 months, and improvement in NYHA class appear favorable. Five- to 10-year durability of the clip is currently undetermined. The option of subsequent MV surgery is preserved in patients who had previously undergone this intervention.

Quality of life is frequently considered a better indicator of surgical success in older adults than survival. Two hundred twenty-five patients ≥70 years who underwent surgery for primary MR were surveyed at 3 years. Of those surveyed, 91% were alive, but greater than half had suboptimal quality-of-life scores. Increased age, preoperative AF, diabetes, renal disease, residual MR, and pulmonary hypertension predicted less-favorable scores.

Wall motion abnormalities often contribute to secondary MR. In selected patients with severe HF, LVEF <35%, and left bundle branch block and QRS duration ≥150 ms, cardiac resynchronization therapy (CRT) may improve MR, cardiac output, symptoms, and reverse remodeling long-term. One-year survival with improvement in NYHA class and without HF hospitalization in older persons who received CRT was comparable with patients younger than 75 years old. In addition, there was significant reduction in the presence of grade 2 or greater MR in both groups.

Prognosis

Complications of chronic severe MR include progressive LV failure eventually leading to AF, pulmonary hypertension, and death. Determinants of 5-year adverse events (death, congestive heart failure, new AF) in asymptomatic persons with primary MR are an effective regurgitant orifice >0.4 cm², increased age, diabetes mellitus, LV size, and LV function.

Patients with severe MR from flail leaflet frequently develop symptoms, LV dysfunction, or AF in 2–3 years, and mortality rate is estimated at 6% to 7% per year.

In older patients with secondary MR associated with systolic dysfunction HF, the degree of MR is independently and directly associated with 1-year mortality.

A. Prevention of Infective Endocarditis

High-velocity flow through abnormal heart valves is associated with damage to endothelium causing platelet-fibrin deposition which may serve as nidus for infective endocarditis (IE). The 2007 American Heart Association guidelines for prevention of infectious endocarditis include the following points:

1. Only a very few cases of IE is prevented by antibiotic prophylaxis, even if it is 100% effective.

2. Prophylaxis is reasonable for dental procedures in setting of valvular conditions at highest risk for adverse outcome from IE, namely, the presence of prosthetic heart valve, a history of IE, presence of cardiac valvulopathy after cardiac transplantation, and certain patients with congenital heart disease.

3. Dental procedures that involve manipulation of gingival, periapical region of teeth, or oral mucosa perforation warrant prophylaxis in the highest-risk persons listed above.

4. IE prophylaxis prior to genitourinary or gastrointestinal procedures is not recommended.

Bonow RO, Carabello BA, Chatterjee K, et al. 2006 Writing Committee Members; American College of Cardiology/American Heart Association Task Force. 2008 Focused update incorporated into the ACC/AHA 2006 guidelines for the management of patients with valvular heart disease: a report of the American College of Cardiology/American Heart Association Task Force on Practice Guidelines (Writing Committee to Revise the 1998 Guidelines for the Management of Patients With Valvular Heart Disease): endorsed by the Society of Cardiovascular Anesthesiologists, Society for Cardiovascular Angiography and Interventions, and Society of Thoracic Surgeons. *Circulation.* 2008;118(15):e523-e661.

Carabello BA. The current therapy for mitral regurgitation. *J Am Coll Cardiol.* 2008;52(5):319-326.

Carabello BA, Paulus WJ. Aortic stenosis. *Lancet.* 2009;373(9667):956-966.

Chikwe J, Goldstone AB, Passage J, et al. A propensity score-adjusted retrospective comparison of early-and mid-term results of mitral-valve repair versus replacement in octogenarians. *Eur Heart J.* 2011;32;618-626.

Conti V, Lick SD. Cardiac surgery in the elderly: indications and management options to optimize outcomes. *Clin Geriatr Med.* 2006;22(3):559-574.

Delnoy PP, Ottervanger JP, Luttikhuis HO, et al. Clinical response of cardiac resynchronization therapy in the elderly. *Am Heart J.* 2008;155(4):746-751.

Detaint D, Sundt TM, Nkomo VT, et al. Surgical correction of mitral regurgitation in the elderly: outcomes and recent improvements. *Circulation.* 2006;114(4):265-272.

Kodali SK, Williams MR, Smith CR, et al. Two-year outcomes after transcatheter or surgical aortic-valve replacement. *N Engl J Med.* 2012;366(18):1686-1695.

Kolh P, Kerzmann A, Honore C, Comte L, Limet R. Aortic valve surgery in octogenarians: predictive factors for operative and long-term results. *Eur J Cardiothorac Surg.* 2007;31(4):600-606.

Lee EM, Porter JN, Shapiro LM, Wells FC. Mitral valve surgery in the elderly. *J Heart Valve Dis.* 1997;6(1):22-31.

Leon MB, Smith CR, Mack M, et al; PARTNER Trial Investigators. Transcatheter aortic-valve implantation for aortic stenosis in patients who cannot undergo surgery. *N Engl J Med.* 2010;363(17):1597-1607.

Maisano F, Vigano G, Calabrese C, et al. Quality of life of elderly patients following valve surgery for chronic organic mitral regurgitation. *Eur J Cardiothorac Surg.* 2009;36(2):261-266.

Mehta RH, Eagle KA, Coombs LP, et al. Society of Thoracic Surgeons National Cardiac Registry. Influence of age on outcomes in patients undergoing mitral valve replacement. *Ann Thorac Surg.* 2002;74(5):1459-1467.

Rogers JH, Franzen O. Percutaneous edge-to-edge MitraClip therapy in the management of MR. *Eur Heart J.* 2011;32(19):2350-2357.

Shaw TRD, Sutaria N, Prendergast B. Clinical and haemodynamic profiles of young, middle aged, and elderly patients with mitral stenosis undergoing mitral balloon valvotomy. *Heart.* 2003;89(12):1430-1436.

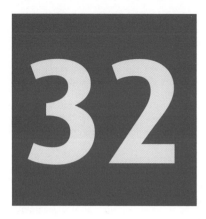

Peripheral Arterial Disease & Venous Thromboembolism

Teresa L. Carman, MD
Sik Kim Ang, MB, BCh, BAO

PERIPHERAL ARTERIAL DISEASE

ESSENTIALS OF DIAGNOSIS

► Common symptoms of leg discomfort with ambulation, rest pain, nonhealing ulcers, or gangrene.

► Abnormal pulse exam in most patients.

► Abnormal ankle-branchial index is diagnostic.

► Evidence of systemic atherosclerosis is common.

► History of diabetes mellitus, tobacco use, hypertension, or hyperlipidemia may be present.

► General Principles in Older Adults

Peripheral vascular disease broadly defines any vascular disease of the extracranial carotid arteries, the aorta and its branches, and the extremities. However, peripheral arterial disease (PAD) is usually used to refer to atherosclerotic disease of the lower extremities. Atherosclerotic PAD is the most common form of PAD in older adults. But, the differential diagnosis for arterial vascular disease is quite broad (Table 32–1).

The prevalence of PAD is >10% in individuals older than age 60 years and increases to >25% in people older than 75 years. Although PAD is associated with cardiovascular risk factors, a prevalence of approximately 9% has been documented in patients without traditional risk factors. Nontraditional risk factors, including ethnicity, also influence disease prevalence. Current guidelines call for screening all individuals who are older than age 65 years, patients older than age 50 years with a history of smoking or diabetes, and individuals with suspected PAD, including exertional leg symptoms and nonhealing wounds.

There are 2 management issues in patients with PAD. Both are important to successful patient care. First is the

need to adequately address underlying cardiovascular risk factors. Atherosclerosis is assumed to be a systemic process. Concomitant cerebrovascular or coronary disease has been demonstrated in up to 30% of patients. The second issue, which is usually more concerning to the patient, is the symptoms related to the vascular occlusive disease. Although most patients with PAD are asymptomatic or present with atypical lower-extremity symptoms, intermittent claudication, exertional muscle pain that is consistent in onset and rapidly relieved with rest, is the most common symptom clinically identified with PAD. A minority present with critical limb ischemia, including ulceration, tissue loss, or gangrene, and are at risk for limb loss.

► Clinical Findings

A. Signs & Symptoms

Intermittent claudication (IC) is recognized as the hallmark of PAD. However, it may be difficult for patients to adequately describe the symptoms of IC. IC is caused by the inability of the arterial supply to meet the metabolic demands of the muscles. Symptoms have been described as muscle pain, cramping, fatigue, tiredness or even weakness associated with exertion. The symptoms should be reproducible with a constant workload and resolve within 5–10 minutes of rest. Most importantly, the symptoms do not occur at rest or with standing alone.

Most patients with PAD do not have symptoms of IC. Most are asymptomatic, have nonspecific lower-extremity exertional symptoms, or even have resting symptoms that are difficult to relate to PAD. In many cases, patients are asymptomatic because they have altered their lifestyle becoming more sedentary and/or eliminated symptom producing activities. Others have nonspecific lower-extremity symptoms, both with exertion and at rest, potentially related to comorbid musculoskeletal or neuropathic conditions.

Table 32–1. Peripheral arterial disease.

Vascular etiology
- Atherosclerotic disease—including the carotid, renal, aortomesenteric, and extremities
- Embolic disease—including cardioembolic disease, paradoxical embolism and artery-to-artery embolism
- Dissection
- Thrombotic disease—related to inherited and acquired thrombophilic processes

Inflammatory
- Vasculitis—may affect any vessel, including large, medium, and small arteries
- Segmental medial arteriolysis—arteriopathy demonstrating necrosis of the media of unknown etiology

Infectious
- Mycotic aneurysm—syphilis, *Salmonella,* and multiple other organisms have been reported.

Neoplastic disease
- Primary arterial vascular neoplasm—angiosarcoma and similar malignancies
- Secondary thromboembolic disease—malignancy or myeloproliferative disease related

Drugs
- Culprit agents may include cocaine, amphetamine, ephedrine, intravenous immunoglobulin, "pressors," ergotamine, and heparin when associated with heparin-induced thrombocytopenia

Iatrogenic
- Closure devices
- Catheter-related arterial injury
- Small vessel atheroembolism following instrumentation

Traumatic
- Compression syndromes—popliteal artery entrapment and thoracic outlet syndrome
- Endoluminal iliac artery fibrosis
- Cystic adventitial disease
- Hypothenar hammer syndrome
- Vibration-induced injury

Environmental
- Raynaud disease
- Frost nip
- Frost bite
- Trench foot
- Thromboangiitis obliterans (Buerger disease)—usually in patients younger than age 50 years; related to tobacco, and occasionally to cannabis, use

Endocrine
- Calciphylaxis—may be uremic or nonuremic in nature

Critical limb ischemia, with rest pain, nonhealing ulcers or tissue loss, or gangrene, is the most severe presentation of PAD. These patients are at risk for limb loss. Patients may complain of coldness, numbness, or pain in the foot or toes. This is especially troubling at night when the limb is elevated—so-called nocturnal rest pain. These patients may prefer to sleep in a chair or hang the limb over the bed side in an effort to improve blood flow and reduce the symptoms.

Skin changes, including loss of hair elements and dystrophic nail changes, are common but nonspecific findings. Dependent rubor followed by pallor or blanching of the extremity with elevation may be easily assessed in the office. The feet should be regularly inspected at office visits for ulcers between the toes—so-called "kissing ulcers"—and ulcers related to ill-fitting footwear. Ulceration in PAD is a particularly ominous sign because many of these patients ultimately require revascularization for healing.

Pulse examination should include both palpation and grading of the peripheral pulses. Pulses are graded as absent (grade 0), present but diminished (grade 1), normal (grade 2) or bounding (grade 3). In addition to the routine palpation and inspection of the feet, patients should be examined for vascular disease involving other vascular beds. Blood pressure should be recorded in both arms. The higher of the 2 extremities should be used for monitoring hypertension and medication titration. The aorta, carotid and femoral arteries should be auscultated for the presence of bruits. The aorta should be palpated for the presence of an abdominal aortic aneurysm. However, the absence of a bruit or inability to palpate the aorta does not exclude disease. Coexistent compromise in cardiopulmonary function, neuropathy, arrhythmia, and severe anemia should be identified as these conditions may negatively impact PAD-related outcomes.

B. Laboratory Findings

There are no laboratory markers to identify patients with atherosclerotic PAD. Patients with PAD should have a fasting lipid profile to assist in the management of dyslipidemia. Fasting blood glucose or hemoglobin A1c monitoring for detection and treatment of diabetes should occur. Laboratory evaluation to exclude other nonatherosclerotic vascular disease (see Table 32–1) should be performed as indicated. This may include complete blood count (CBC), erythrocyte sedimentation rate (ESR), C-reactive protein (CRP), and a complete metabolic panel (CMP).

C. Diagnostic Testing

Along with pulse assessment, patients with a clinical suspicion of PAD should have baseline evaluation of their perfusion. The ankle-brachial index (ABI) can be used to determine the presence and severity of perfusion (Table 32–2). An ABI <0.91 is considered abnormal. The current American College of Cardiology and American Heart Association (ACC/AHA) guidelines recommend ABI measurement in patients with exertional leg symptoms suspicious for PAD, who have nonhealing wounds and are older than age 65 years. In patients with calcified arteries caused by advanced age, diabetes, renal disease, or other processes, the ABI will be inaccurate and the toe-brachial index (TBI) should be used. A TBI <0.7 is consistent with PAD.

The ABI is a ratio of systolic arterial pressures recorded in the upper and lower extremities. It can easily be performed

Table 32–2. Classification of the ankle-brachial index.

ABI	Clinical significance	Recommendations
>1.4	Consistent with calcified arteries	TBI should be used to determine presence of disease; PVR may be used to determine levels of disease
1.0–1.4	Normal	With high clinical suspicion for PAD based on symptoms consider treadmill exercise testing
0.91–0.99	Borderline	With high clinical suspicion for PAD based on symptoms consider exercise testing
0.71–0.9	Mild disease—many patients are asymptomatic but may present with claudication	PVR may be useful if there a need to determine level of disease
0.41–0.7	Moderate disease—usual claudication range	PVR may be useful if there a need to determine level of disease
<0.4	Severe disease Usually associated with poor would healing potential	Angiographic imaging is warranted for patients with nonhealing wounds or gangrene to determine reperfusion options

ABI, Ankle-brachial index; TBI, toe-brachial index; PAD, peripheral arterial disease; PVR, pulse volume recording.

in the office or by a vascular laboratory. The required equipment includes a continuous-wave handheld Doppler and a blood pressure cuff. To perform an ABI, the blood pressure cuff is placed sequentially over both upper extremities followed by both lower extremities. With the handheld Doppler positioned sequentially over the brachial, dorsalis pedis (DP) and posterior tibial (PT) arteries, the blood pressure cuff is inflated to suprasystolic pressure and then slowly deflated. The pressure at which the systolic signal is audible is recorded. The ABI is calculated by dividing the highest pressure of the limb, either the DP or PT, by the highest the brachial pressure.

Exercise ABI testing should be performed when patients have symptoms consistent with IC but a normal resting ABI. Standardized protocols are used and the patient must be able to safely walk on a treadmill without assistance. A history of significant cardiopulmonary disease, nonhealing ulcers or critical limb ischemia, and gait abnormalities are contraindications for exercise testing.

D. Additional Testing

When intervention is considered for lifestyle-limiting symptoms or for critical limb ischemia, additional testing to determine the anatomical level of disease and plan for revascularization is warranted. Segmental arterial limb pressures (SLP) and pulse volume recording (PVR) with or without exercise testing can localize disease as well as provide

hemodynamic information. Arterial duplex ultrasound may also be used to localize disease. Duplex imaging provides anatomic information regarding stenosis, occlusion, and calcification within the atherosclerotic lesions. The use of ultrasound avoids contrast and radiation associated with other angiographic imaging. Angiographic imaging, including computed tomographic angiography (CTA), magnetic resonance angiography (MRA), and conventional digital subtraction angiography (DSA), are not diagnostic tools but are used to determine the anatomic levels of disease and plan surgical or endovascular revascularization.

▶ Differential Diagnosis

Patients will not typically complain of lower-extremity pain with ambulation. Many patients attribute leg pain to arthritis or part of the aging process. The differential diagnosis of exertional leg symptoms may be quite broad, including a variety of musculoskeletal, neurogenic, and inflammatory conditions. A thorough history, including questions to determine the timing, onset, exacerbating and relieving factors, and a complete physical examination, can help distinguish PAD and IC from other vascular and nonvascular causes of lower-extremity exertional symptoms. It can be difficult to distinguish IC from pseudoclaudication or neurogenic claudication (Table 32–3). History demonstrating variability of the symptoms, symptom onset at rest or with standing, and the improvement when walking with a shopping cart or when bending forward, increases suspicion for neurogenic pseudoclaudication. PAD and other vascular disorders causing lower-extremity ischemia are included in the differential diagnosis of IC (see Table 32–1).

Table 32–3. Characteristics of intermittent claudication and pseudoclaudication.

Clinical Characteristic	Intermittent Claudication	Pseudoclaudication
Location	Typically calf; may be thigh or buttock with aortoiliac disease	May involve the thigh, buttock, or calf
Description	Aching, cramping, weakness, or fatigue of the muscle	Symptoms may be the same but also include burning, numbness, sharp shooting pain, or tingling
Exercise related	Onset and distance are reproducible	Variable in onset, duration, and reproducibility
Related to standing alone	Never	Frequently
Relief	Standing alone relieves the pain in 3–5 minutes	Usually required to sit or change position; pain may last for up to 30 minutes

▶ Treatment

A. General Considerations

Good skin and foot care should be recommended. Minor trauma may be associated with a limb or life-threatening event in patients with PAD. Diabetic patients should have routine podiatric nail care. Daily foot inspection should also be reinforced. Shoe gear and devices to offload pressure points and boney prominences are recommended. Patients who are hospitalized, in a nursing home, or otherwise immobile are prone to pressure injury and should be protected.

B. Cardiovascular Risk Reduction

The Reduction of Atherosclerosis for Continued Health (REACH) registry has confirmed the undertreatment of risk factors in PAD, as well as the risk for primary and recurrent cardiovascular events in this at-risk population. Aggressive cardiovascular risk factor modification is required to slow the progression of PAD and decrease future cardiovascular and cerebrovascular morbidity and mortality. Patients should be treated to achieve risk-reduction goals similar to patients with diagnosed coronary artery disease.

Patients should be advised to stop smoking, and offered counseling or pharmacologic therapy. Blood pressure should be treated to a target of <140/90 mm Hg or <130/80 mm Hg with diabetes or chronic kidney disease. β Blockers, angiotensin-converting enzyme (ACE) inhibitors, and diuretics should be included in the antihypertensive regimens. Diabetes should be managed to maintain a HbA1c (glycosylated hemoglobin) approximately 7% in an effort to reduce microvascular complications. Lipid-lowering regimens should include a "statin" to lower low-density lipoprotein (LDL) to <100 mg/dL. All patients should be on antiplatelet therapy. Aspirin 75–325 mg daily is recommended. In aspirin-intolerant individuals, clopidogrel 75 mg daily should be considered.

C. Exercise Therapy

A dedicated walking program can improve pain-free walking distance and maximal walking distance. Supervised exercise programs are more beneficial than self-directed programs. Unfortunately, these programs are not widely available or accessible. Motivated patients certainly benefit from self-directed walking programs. Patients should be instructed to perform a minimum of 3 walking sessions weekly. They should walk at a pace to induce symptoms within 5 minutes. After symptom onset, they should rest until the symptoms abate and then resume walking. Each exercise session should last for 30–45 minutes using walk-rest-walk cycles. Most patients will see improvement in their walking capacity within 4 to 8 weeks of participation and significant benefits are usually obtained by 12 to 26 weeks. Patients should be advised that acquired benefits are quickly lost once they stop exercising.

D. Pharmacotherapy

Two drugs are FDA approved for symptomatic patients with IC: cilostazol and pentoxifylline. Cilostazol is a phosphodiesterase 3 inhibitor. The mode by which it improves walking performance in IC is not well understood. The usual dose for cilostazol is 100 mg twice a day. Cilostazol is contraindicated in patients with a history of heart failure. Frequent side effects include headache, palpitations, feeling lightheaded or dizzy and gastrointestinal effects including nausea and diarrhea. These are more common in older adults. Most side effects are self-limited or are better tolerated by initiating therapy at a reduced dose and escalating to full therapy. A 50-mg tablet is available for dose reduction.

Pentoxifylline is a hemorrheologic agent thought to improved red blood cell distensibility. The usual dose is 400 mg 3 times daily. Although there are few side effects associated with pentoxifylline it also has not demonstrated consistent benefit for patients with IC.

For either drug, if clinical improvement is not realized after 26 weeks of therapy, the drug should be discontinued as polypharmacy may be a concern and several other drugs, such as statins, antiplatelet agents, and antihypertensives, are often prescribed concomitantly in this population. Neither cilostazol nor pentoxifylline affect the mortality associated with underlying cardiovascular risk.

E. Revascularization

Revascularization is indicated in patients with critical limb ischemia and may be considered in those limited by IC despite optimal medical therapy and participation in an exercise regimen. Angiography, MRA, or CTA is used to determine the optimal revascularization strategy. In patients with critical limb ischemia, including rest pain, ischemic ulceration, or gangrene, revascularization may be limb saving. For patients with IC, revascularization is generally elective.

A complete discussion of revascularization is beyond the scope of this chapter. The tools, strategies, and options for revascularization continue to evolve. Operators and patients alike usually prefer endovascular procedures to surgical management. Today, more patients are candidates for less-invasive procedures. The options and choice for revascularization should be individualized to each patient. Whether endovascular or surgical revascularization is planned, the risks, benefits, and alternatives for each procedure should be thoroughly and candidly discussed with the patient.

▶ Prognosis

As mentioned, the overwhelming risk to patients with PAD is the morbidity and mortality associated with secondary cardiovascular and cerebrovascular events. The overall limb prognosis in PAD is good. Approximately 75% of patients with IC remain stable or will improve under the influence of pharmacotherapy and exercise. Only approximately 25%

of patients will deteriorate with respect to walking capacity. A minority of these patients will require an intervention or surgery to improve walking capacity. Less than 4% of patients will suffer limb loss. Most of these patients will be diabetic or continue to smoke.

Bhatt DL, Eagle KA, Ohman EM, et al. Comparative determinants of 4-year cardiovascular event rates in stable outpatients at risk or with atherothrombosis. *JAMA*. 2010;304(12):1350-1357.

Cao P, Eckstein HH, De Rango P, et al. Chapter II: Diagnostic methods. *Eur J Vasc Endovasc Surg*. 2011;42(Suppl) 2:S13-S32.

Casillas JM, Troisgros O, Hannequin A, et al. Rehabilitation in patients with PAD. *Ann Phys Rehabil Med*. 2011;54(7):443-461.

Diehm C, Allenberg JR, Pittrow D, et al. Mortality and vascular, morbidity in older adults with asymptomatic versus symptomatic peripheral artery disease. *Circulation*. 2009;120(21):2053-2061.

Hirsch AT, Haskal ZJ, Hertzer NR, et al. ACC/AHA 2005 Practice guidelines for the management of patients with peripheral arterial disease (lower extremity, renal, mesenteric, and abdominal aortic). *Circulation*. 2006;113(11):e463-e654.

Mourad JJ, Cacoub P, Collet JP, et al. Screening of unrecognized peripheral arterial disease (PAD) using ankle-brachial index I high cardiovascular risk patients free from symptomatic PAD. *J Vasc Surg*. 2009;50(3):572-580.

Rooke TW, Hitsch AT, Misra S, et al. 2011 ACCF/AHA Focused update of the guideline for the management of patients with peripheral artery disease. *Circulation*. 2011;124(18):2020-2045.

VENOUS THROMBOEMBOLISM

 ESSENTIALS OF DIAGNOSIS

▶ Surgery (especially orthopedic), immobility, and malignancy are common risk factors.

▶ Typical complaints include acute limb pain and swelling for deep venous thrombosis; pleuritic chest pain and shortness of breath for pulmonary embolism.

▶ Physical findings are nonspecific and often absent.

▶ Confirmation with diagnostic imaging is required.

General Principles in Older Adults

Venous thromboembolism (VTE), including deep vein thrombosis (DVT) and pulmonary embolism (PE), is the third leading cause of cardiovascular death in the United States. More than 400,000 deaths annually are attributed to VTE. VTE risk increases with age. VTE risk for patients older than age 70 years is approximately 1% per year. Table 32–4 lists the inherited and acquired risk factors for VTE. Despite a known association between VTE and inherited thrombophilias, testing for these disorders is rarely indicated in geriatric patients. Patients with idiopathic VTE, without an identifiable etiology, should undergo age- and gender-appropriate cancer

Table 32–4. Risk factors for venous thromboembolism.

Commonly Identified VTE Risk Factors	Less-Commonly Recognized VTE Risk Factors
Inherited	Myeloproliferative disorders
Factor V Leiden	Chemotherapy drugs
Prothrombin gene mutation	Inflammatory bowel disease
Protein C deficiency	Multiple myeloma
Protein S deficiency	Infection/inflammation
Antithrombin deficiency	Sepsis
Hyperhomocystinemia	Paroxysmal nocturnal hemoglobinuria
Elevated lipoprotein (a)	Heparin-induced thrombocytopenia
	Vasculitis
Acquired	Factor VIII excess
Antiphospholipid antibodies	Nephrotic syndrome
Hyperhomocystinemia	Dysplasminogenemia
Malignancy	Dysfibrinogenemia
Obesity	
Travel	
Immobilization	
Surgery	
Trauma	
Prior venous thromboembolism	
Hormone therapy and oral contraceptives	
Indwelling lines and devices	

screening. Following a complete history, physical examination, and basic laboratory testing, additional testing using CT scans, bronchoscopy, bone marrow evaluation, and other evaluations are used to investigate underlying abnormalities.

▶ Clinical Findings

A. Signs & Symptoms

The signs and symptoms of VTE are nonspecific. Therefore, a clinical diagnosis is not acceptable. Patients may present with nonspecific constitutional, limb or cardiopulmonary complaints. High clinical suspicion and imaging is required to exclude VTE.

Up to 50% of DVTs are asymptomatic. Clinical symptoms include limb pain, swelling, erythema, and increased warmth. Superficial thrombophlebitis may present with localized erythema and tenderness associated with a palpable superficial venous cord. The Homan sign—pain on squeezing the calf or with passive dorsiflexion of the foot—is commonly referred to and noted on examination. However, it lacks sensitivity or specificity for diagnosing DVT and is unreliable for clinical diagnosis.

The symptoms of PE are equally nonspecific. Patients may present with tachycardia and tachypnea without associated complaints. When present, chest pain may be pleuritic in nature. Dyspnea, cough, near syncope, and palpitations are common. Hemoptysis is uncommon and usually associated with pulmonary infarction. Syncope is a common admitting complaint and PE is frequently overlooked in the differential diagnosis, leading to delays in diagnosis and management.

B. Laboratory Findings

No laboratory test is specific to diagnosis VTE. In the appropriate clinical setting, a negative D-dimer may be used to exclude VTE from the differential diagnosis. D-dimer is frequently positive following surgery, trauma, hospitalization, pregnancy, and in older adults. Therefore, it is best utilized in the outpatient ambulatory setting in patients at low-risk for VTE. A positive D-dimer is not helpful.

VTE patients should have CBC, CMP, and urinalysis performed to identify underlying disorders associated with VTE. Abnormalities on the initial laboratory testing should be used to direct additional testing or imaging that may be warranted. Antiphospholipid antibody testing may be helpful in the geriatric population. Testing for lupus anticoagulant and anticardiolipin antibodies may influence the duration of therapy and the choice of anticoagulation. Testing for other thrombophilias is less likely to be helpful. Protein C, protein S and antithrombin deficiency testing are virtually never warranted in older adults.

Patients with acute PE should have biomarker assessment, including troponin and BNP (B-type natriuretic peptide) or NT-proBNP (N-terminal pro brain natriuretic peptide), to look for evidence of myocardial injury. Both troponin and BNP, when normal, have a high negative predictive value for in-hospital and 30 days postdischarge mortality. When the biomarkers are normal they may be used to risk stratify patients for accelerated hospital discharge.

C. Diagnostic Testing

Venography is rarely required, but remains the gold standard for diagnosing DVT. Duplex ultrasound has become the test of choice to diagnose or exclude DVT. It is widely available, noninvasive, and well tolerated. Duplex ultrasound relies on the inability to completely compress the lumen of the vein using externally applied pressure. Intraluminal echogenicity is less specific for DVT. Secondary changes in the venous waveforms are also evaluated. Normal waveforms are phasic with respiration and augment with calf compression. The failure to augment or loss of phasicity, monophasic waveforms, may indicate proximal obstruction. Only venous segments that are adequately visualized can be assessed for DVT. This is a limitation that is frequently misunderstood. If a venous segment is not fully evaluated, DVT cannot be excluded. The sensitivity and specificity of duplex ultrasound for DVT diagnosis are approximately 98%. If there is negative testing but high clinical suspicion, especially for iliac, inferior vena cava (IVC), or calf vein DVT, repeat duplex imaging in 5–7 days is likely warranted.

Computed tomography venography (CTV) and magnetic resonance venography (MRV) may be used for diagnosis especially when imaging the IVC and pelvic veins. CTV can easily be added to CT PE imaging. This does not require additional contrast but the radiation exposure is significant. MRV does not use radiation and does not always require contrast. It may be helpful in evaluating patients with acute and chronic DVT. However, imaging may not be readily available and claustrophobia may limit some patient's ability to perform testing. CTV and MRV may be used as an alternative to venography to confirm the diagnosis of DVT when duplex imaging is nondiagnostic.

Up to 50% of patients with DVT may have clinically asymptomatic PE. Clinical suspicion for PE should prompt appropriate testing. Chest x-ray may be normal and is frequently nonspecific. When abnormal, findings of volume loss, atelectasis, effusions, or infiltrates predominate. Classically described Westermark sign (focal oligemia), Hampton hump (wedge-shaped pleural based density), and pulmonary artery enlargement are uncommon. Electrocardiogram findings are also frequently nonspecific. The most common finding is sinus tachycardia. The classically described $S_1Q_3T_3$ changes may be seen with large PE and right ventricular strain.

Computed tomography pulmonary angiogram (CTPA) is the most widely available and commonly used test for diagnosing PE. It is readily available and well tolerated. PE is diagnosed as an intraluminal filling defect within the pulmonary arteries. With advanced technology, scanners can complete imaging to the level of the subsegmental pulmonary arteries in a single breathhold. It requires contrast and may be limited in patients with renal insufficiency. Timing of the contrast bolus is essential, and in some patients may limit the sensitivity and specificity of the examination, especially for more peripheral emboli. CTPA can also be used to evaluate for radiographic signs of right heart strain associated with large PE. A right ventricle to left ventricle ratio >0.9 measured on a 4-chamber view is consistent with right-heart strain.

Ventilation-perfusion (V/Q) lung scanning is still used to diagnose of acute PE. However, in many centers availability is limited. The testing should be performed in the setting of a normal chest x-ray and when there is high clinical pretest probability for PE. Nondiagnostic intermediate or indeterminant scans are common. Only scans that are read as normal or near normal or high probability are helpful to exclude or diagnose PE.

Pulmonary angiography remains the gold standard for diagnosing PE, although it has been essentially replaced by CTPA imaging. The contrast and radiation exposure are similar and CTPA is less invasive. If CTPA imaging is nondiagnostic and there is a need to diagnose or exclude PE then angiography is the test of choice. Despite widely held beliefs that angiography is too invasive to use regularly, complications related to angiography are infrequent.

Echocardiography is not a diagnostic test for PE although echocardiographic information may be helpful to risk-stratify patients for thrombolytic therapy or for accelerated hospital discharge. Echocardiography is used to evaluate right-heart dysfunction. Right-heart strain portends a worse in-hospital outcome compared to patients without evidence for right ventricle volume overload. Findings on echocardiogram include right ventricle dilation, septal flattening or deviation toward the left ventricle, tricuspid regurgitation, and elevated right ventricle systolic pressure.

Differential Diagnosis

Unilateral leg pain, erythema and swelling are common symptoms. Within the differential diagnosis one must consider superficial thrombophlebitis, popliteal cyst with or without rupture, traumatic injury such as a sprain or ruptured calf muscle, cellulitis, and acute inflammation associated with chronic venous insufficiency (CVI). In patients with a low pretest clinical probability, a negative D-dimer excludes DVT and eliminates the need for additional testing.

The signs and symptoms associated with PE are also nonspecific. Other cardiopulmonary, vascular and inflammatory etiologies must be excluded. Included in the differential diagnosis are myocardial injury, pericarditis, congestive heart failure, pneumonia, pleuritis, pneumothorax, aortic dissection, and musculoskeletal sprain, strain, or contusion.

Complications

The risk of postthrombotic syndrome (PTS) after DVT is significant. Many patients develop symptoms within 2 years following the initial event. Extensive DVT and recurrent events increase PTS risk. The use of compression stockings for 2 years following DVT may decrease this risk by up to 50%. A minority of patients (<5%) will develop chronic thromboembolic disease (CTED) after PE. There are no clinical factors, biomarkers, or other strategies to determine which patients are at risk. Patients presenting with progressive dyspnea or right-heart dysfunction following PE should be evaluated for CTED.

Treatment

A. General Considerations

Anticoagulation is the mainstay of treatment for VTE. Appropriate therapy should be started when the diagnosis of VTE is considered. In patients at low risk for complications from anticoagulation, data collection and diagnostic testing should not delay the initiation of anticoagulation. Intravenous unfractionated heparin (UFH), low-molecular-weight heparin (LMWH), or fondaparinux are appropriate initial therapies for VTE.

Patients with DVT without signs or symptoms of PE can frequently be treated either solely or at least partially as an outpatient. Arranging home therapy, self-injection teaching and patient education required staff time and dedication but many patients are able to successfully perform the necessary tasks. Clinically stable patients with PE can frequently be assessed using echocardiography and biomarkers such as troponin and BNP. When normal, patients can be treated either inpatient or using an accelerated discharge plan. Close clinical follow up after discharge should be arranged for all VTE patients.

Patients with a contraindication to anticoagulation should be managed by IVC filter insertion. However, appropriate anticoagulation should be initiated once the anticoagulation risk has resolved.

B. Pharmacotherapy

UFH should be administered using weight-based bolus and infusion dosing. The activated partial thromboplastin time (aPTT) or anti-Xa assay should be titrated to keep the patient within the appropriate therapeutic range. It is important to recognize that the aPTT therapeutic range is institution specific and awareness of local protocols is necessary. In patients in whom thrombolysis may be considered, UFH is the drug of choice because of its short half-life and the ability to easily monitor therapy.

LMWHs provide the opportunity for once- or twice-daily dosing. Ease of administration also facilitates accelerated discharge or home therapy for appropriate patients. The available LMWHs are all renally excreted. Dose adjustment or avoidance is required with creatinine clearance <30 mL/min. Monitoring with LMWH specific anti-Xa assay may be prudent in patients with borderline renal function, with low body mass, or the morbidly obese. The assay must be drawn 4 hours after the dose. A target LMWH anti-Xa between 0.6 and 1.0 is appropriate for q 12 hour dosing, whereas a target of 1.0–2.0 is appropriate for daily dosing regimens. Patients who develop VTE in the setting of an underlying malignancy are best managed with LMWH monotherapy for the initial 3–6 months of treatment. Patients can then be reassessed for continuing LMWH or switching to warfarin therapy for the duration of their treatment.

Fondaparinux is a pentasaccharide molecule approved for treating both DVT and PE, when therapy is initiated in the hospital. Dosing is weight based. Patients who weigh <50 kg should receive 5 mg daily; who weigh 50–100 kg should be dosed at 7.5 mg daily; and who weigh >100 kg should receive 10 mg daily. Monitoring is not used. Fondaparinux is renally excreted. It should be used cautiously with renal insufficiency and is not appropriate with a creatinine clearance <30 mL/min. The half-life is approximately 17 hours. The drug should be avoided when there is a need for intervention or a high risk of bleeding. There is no antidote to reverse the effects of fondaparinux.

Warfarin remains the long-term drug of choice for most patients. In general, the first dose of warfarin may be started on the day of admission. Warfarin, a vitamin K antagonist, interrupts the terminal carboxylation of vitamin

K-dependent proteins. Therefore a minimum 4–5 day overlap between the parenteral drug and warfarin is required to ensure the premade vitamin K-dependent proteins have been adequately depleted. For most patients, the target international normalized ratio (INR) is 2.5, with an acceptable range being between 2 and 3. After the minimum 4–5-day overlap, the INR should be >2 on 2 consecutive days before stopping the parenteral drug and maintaining warfarin therapy.

An oral direct thrombin inhibitor, dabigatran, and oral anti-Xa agents, rivaroxaban and apixaban, have been studied in VTE, but are not yet approved. Potential advantages of these agents are the once- or twice-daily oral administration. These drugs do not require monitoring. The major disadvantage with these agents is a lack of an antidote for easy reversal.

C. Intervention

Patients with extensive DVT or massive PE who are unstable at the time of admission should be assessed for thrombolysis. The use of pharmacomechanical thrombolysis (PMT) or catheter-directed thrombolysis (CDT) are not confined to patients with phlegmasia cerulean dolens or venous gangrene. Patients with extensive DVT may benefit from PMT to help clear the thrombus in an effort to preserve valve function, improve mobility, and decrease symptoms associated with the acute DVT. PMT is not appropriate for all patients with DVT but especially with iliofemoral DVT consideration for PMT should be entertained.

Patients with massive unstable PE should also be considered for thrombolysis; either systemic infusion or catheter based therapies. Patients with submassive PE with significant cardiopulmonary dysfunction may be appropriate for thrombolytic therapy but the bleeding risks may outweigh the benefits in these patients. The risk for major bleeding in thrombolysis is approximately 15%. The risk for intracranial bleeding is often cited as 1% to 2%. Bleeding risk is increased in patients older than age 70 years. Recent surgery or trauma, gastrointestinal bleeding, uncontrolled hypertension, and recent stroke are contraindications to thrombolysis.

IVC filter insertion is appropriate in patients with a contraindication to anticoagulation or in whom anticoagulation is complicated by bleeding or thrombosis despite adequate therapeutic anticoagulation. Many IVC filters deployed today are used for relative indications, including underlying cardiopulmonary disease, significant PE, free floating DVT visualized on duplex ultrasound, and patients at high risk for noncompliance with anticoagulation. It is important to realize that IVC filters help manage patients with DVT and prevent massive PE. However, IVC filters do not treat DVT and anticoagulation is required to stop propagation of the DVT, prevent recurrent DVT as well as prevent embolism. Once the absolute or relative risk for anticoagulation has resolved appropriate anticoagulation should be initiated. Patients with an optionally retrievable IVC filter should be assessed for filter retrieval prior to stopping anticoagulation. There is sufficient data to suggest that retained filters may contribute to subsequent DVT. Once they are no longer required, they should be removed if possible.

D. Additional Considerations

Bed rest is frequently advised in DVT or PE; this is actually detrimental to recovery. Studies demonstrate that ambulation is not associated with increased risk for PE but does improve venous patency. Clinically stable patients should be encouraged to ambulate while hospitalized and return to normal activities after discharge.

Compression is recommended for patients with DVT. The risk of PTS approaches 70% following DVT. Ideally, patients should be prescribed knee-high stocking with a minimum of 20–30 mm Hg compression before discharge. For patients undergoing PMT or with extensive DVT and more severe symptoms, 30–40 mm Hg compression is recommended.

E. Duration of Therapy

The optimal duration of therapy for VTE is unknown. Decisions regard continuing or discontinuing anticoagulation should take into account the underlying etiology of the VTE, patient comorbidities, patient preference for anticoagulation, and the estimated risk for recurrence. In general, a situational event following surgery, hospitalization, or other limited risk factors should be treated a minimum of 3 months and until the attributable risk factor is no longer present. Patients with idiopathic VTE require a minimum of 6–12 months of initial anticoagulation. Patients with recurrent VTE, underlying high-risk thrombophilias, or cancer likely require indefinite therapy. However, to determine the optimal duration of therapy, the benefits of anticoagulation need to be weighed against the risk.

Almahameed A, Carman TL. Outpatient management of stable acute pulmonary embolism: proposed accelerated pathway for risk stratification. *Am J Med.* 2007;120(10Suppl):S18-S25.

Goldhaber SZ, Bounameaux H. Pulmonary embolism and deep vein thrombosis. *Lancet.* 2012;379(9828):1835-1846.

Kearon C, Akl EA, Comerota AJ, et al. American College of Chest Physicians. Antithrombotic therapy for VTE disease: Antithrombotic Therapy and Prevention of Thrombosis, 9th ed: American College of Chest Physicians Evidence-Based Clinical Practice Guidelines. *Chest.* 2012;141(2 Suppl):e419S-e494S.

Merli GJ. Pathophysiology of venous thromboembolism, thrombophilia and the diagnosis of deep vein thrombosis-pulmonary embolism in the elderly. *Clin Geriatr Med.* 2006;22(1):75-92.

Mos IC, Klok FA, Kroft LJ, et al. Safety of ruling out acute pulmonary embolism by normal computed tomography pulmonary angiogram in patients with an indication for computed tomography systematic review and meta-analysis. *J Thromb Haemost.* 2009;7(9):1491-1498.

Tripodi A, Palareti G. New anticoagulant drugs for the treatment of venous thromboembolism and stroke prevention in atrial fibrillation. *J Intern Med.* 2012;271(6):554-565.

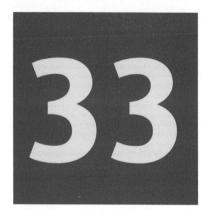

Chronic Venous Insufficiency & Lymphedema

Teresa L. Carman, MD

Sik Kim Ang, MB, BCh, BAO

CHRONIC VENOUS INSUFFICIENCY

ESSENTIALS OF DIAGNOSIS

▶ Pitting edema.

▶ Skin changes, including hyperpigmentation, lipodermatosclerosis, and varicose veins.

▶ Limb pain with prolonged standing.

▶ Chronic edema resulting in ulcer formation above the medial malleolus.

▶ Venous reflux may be identified on ultrasound imaging.

▶ General Principles in Older Adults

From epidemiologic studies, the prevalence of chronic venous insufficiency (CVI) is estimated to be between 5% and 30% in the general population. CVI is more common in women than in men, with a ratio of approximately 3:1. United States expenses related to CVI have been estimated at $1.9 billion to $2.5 billion annually.

The venous system is made up of deep veins within the subfascial, muscular compartment of the limbs, superficial veins, which are located in the epifascial, subcutaneous compartment and perforator veins, which communicate between the 2 compartments. Normal venous outflow depends on patency of the veins, intact venous valves, and a normal functioning calf muscle pump to return blood from the periphery to the right side of the heart.

CVI results venous hypertension or sustained venous pressure within the deep or superficial venous system. Venous hypertension may be related to failure of any of the required components: abnormal or damaged venous valves and reflux, venous outflow obstruction either as a result of intrinsic or extrinsic injury, or loss of the normal calf muscle

pump. Venous insufficiency may be primary or secondary. Risk factors for CVI include advancing age, obesity, pregnancy, history of lower-extremity injury, and prolong standing or dependency.

Patients with limited mobility, using walking aids, stroke, or using ankle-foot orthoses will frequently have decreased calf muscle pump and secondary CVI. Patients should always be questioned regarding sleeping habits. Chair or recliner sleeping is common in older adults because of back or joint pain, limited mobility, cardiopulmonary disease, or poor sleep habits.

Postthrombotic syndrome is 1 form of venous insufficiency related to valve damage or incomplete recanalization of the veins following deep vein thrombosis or phlebitis. Many venous thromboses are asymptomatic and the patient may not be aware of the risk for injury. This can be easily identified using duplex ultrasound.

▶ Clinical Findings

A. Signs & Symptoms

Patients with CVI may range from virtually asymptomatic to severe disease with the presence of venous ulceration. The clinical staging is best identified using the CEAP classification (Table 33–1). Symptoms associated with CVI include pain, itching, burning, aching, and heaviness or fatigue of the legs. Symptoms may improve dramatically with leg elevation, essentially relieving the venous hypertension.

The most prominent clinical finding in CVI is edema. Early in the disease, the edema is usually soft and pitting; however, as time progresses, many patients will develop thickening and fibrosis of the subcutaneous tissue termed *lipodermatosclerosis*. Unlike lymphedema, the edema of CVI usually involves the ankle and lower calf, but spares the dorsum of the foot. The edema is usually responsive to elevation. Patients will frequently report minimal swelling upon awakening but increasing edema as the day progresses.

Table 33–1. Clinical classification of venous disease.

C0	No visible sign of venous disease
C1	Telangiectasias (spider vein) or reticular veins
C2	Varicose vein
C3	Edema
C4	Trophic skin changes including pigmentation, eczema, lipodermatosclerosis, or atrophie blanche
C5	Healed venous ulcer
C6	Active venous stasis ulcer

Skin changes are also common. Patients may have dry, hyperkeratotic skin, inflammation or stasis dermatitis, hyperpigmentation or hemosiderin staining, atrophie blanche or white atrophic scarring of the subcutaneous tissue, or even venous ulceration. Venous ulceration may be differentiated from arterial ulceration by the characteristics of the ulcer (Table 33–2). Although mixed venous and arterial disease is common especially in older adults. Varicose veins are another prominent feature of CVI. Varicosities are typical of superficial vein involvement and may range from small venous telangiectasias or spider veins, to subdermal reticular veins that are 1–3 mm in size, to ropey, bulging varicosities.

B. Diagnostic Testing

History and physical examination are usually sufficient to make the diagnosis of CVI. However, both bedside and vascular laboratory testing may be used to confirm the diagnosis and to better localize the abnormality. The most basic office

Table 33–2. Differentiation between venous and arterial ulceration.

Characteristic	Venous	Arterial
Location	Medial malleolus or calf	Distal over the toes and foot
Base	Minimal fibrous slough Granular and healthy	Dry, fibrous or necrotic Punched out appearance
Pain	Usually absent or minimal	Painful, may require narcotic therapy
Associated findings	Warm limb Edema and fibrosis	Cool limb Edema from limb dependency
Color	Brown, violet, or blue from venous congestion	Erythematous from chronic dependency
Pulses	Usually normal	Absent
Treatment	Compression and elevation	Requires revascularization

assessment includes having the patient stand and examining the patient for bulging varicosities. Holding your hand over the groin at the saphenofemoral junction while the patient performs a Valsalva maneuver will confirm reflux if the veins pressurize. Photoplethysmography and air plethysmography are simple noninvasive tests that can evaluate for reflux, obstruction, and the calf muscle pump. However, testing is not widely performed.

Duplex ultrasonography for venous insufficiency is considered the "gold standard" for diagnosis venous insufficiency. Performed by the vascular laboratory, the testing is usually done standing or in deep Trendelenburg to augment valvular incompetency and reflux. Both Valsalva maneuvers and distal compression may be used to elicit reflux during imaging. The vascular laboratory should also be used to exclude peripheral arterial disease (PAD) in patients with absent or diminished pulses prior to commencing compression therapy. Patients with an ankle-brachial index (ABI) <0.7 require care and caution when using compression for managing edema or venous ulcer healing.

Varicosities that extend from the buttocks or are over the perineum or anterior abdominal wall may need further evaluation with magnetic resonance venography (MRV) to exclude pelvic reflux through the ovarian veins. Abdominal and pelvic CT imaging to exclude intrinsic or extrinsic injury to the inferior vena cava (IVC) from tumor or fibrosis should be considered with bilateral symmetrical swelling, especially if it is of recent onset or rapidly progressive.

▶ Differential Diagnosis

Most edema in older adults has multifactorial contributions from systemic illness, CVI or loss of the calf muscle pump, and medications. A thorough history and physical examination are required to exclude other secondary causes of edema apart from CVI or lymphedema. Systemic conditions related to heart failure, increased right-heart pressures from pulmonary hypertension or valvular heart disease, protein loss related to renal or enteric disease, decreased protein from cirrhosis, other liver disease or malnutrition, and endocrine disorders, such as Cushing disease, may cause swelling. Myxedema related to thyroid disease may also be confused with edema and should be excluded by biopsy.

Medications are a frequent cause for lower-extremity edema. Hormone therapy, steroids, dihydropyridine calcium channel blockers, thiazolidines, and nonsteroidal antiinflammatory agents are all associated with edema. In addition, gabapentin and pramipexole are common offenders.

▶ Complications

Pain, swelling, impaired mobility, and skin changes are the typical complications experienced with CVI. The most problematic complication is that of venous stasis ulceration.

Conservative estimates suggest that >20,000 patients are diagnosed with venous stasis ulcers annually. Ulcer care requires frequent office visits. Patients may experience pain associated with debridement. Some patients may feel isolated because of the appearance of the dressings or odor associated with active wounds. Bleeding from superficial varicosities, while dramatic, usually responds well to light compression and limb elevation. Secondary sclerotherapy may prevent recurrent bleeding.

▶ Treatment

A. General Considerations

The goals for treating CVI are to reduce edema, alleviate pain, and improve the overall condition of the skin. In patients with venous stasis ulcers, this translates further into wound healing and preventing recurrence. Conservative care for the skin is required. Water-based emollients will improve the skin texture and prevent dryness and cracking that may promote ulceration. Patients who develop venous eczema or stasis dermatitis may benefit from a low- or medium-potency topical corticosteroid for a short duration. If there is maceration and breakdown in the webspaces, an antifungal powder used twice daily should be recommended. Tinea pedis is a common source of cellulitis. For patients who develop wounds, standard wound care practices to keep the exudates well managed and the base of the wound moist should be used.

In addition to overall skin care, elevation and compression therapy are the mainstay of treatment for CVI. Patients should be questioned regarding sleeping habits as previously noted. Patients who are sleeping in a chair or recliner should be strongly advised to return to the bed. The opportunity to use elevation to provide passive decongestion of the legs cannot be underestimated. Elevation decreases the venous hypertension and reduces swelling and pain. Patients should be advised to elevate their legs several times a day. Elevation needs to be done with the legs above the level of the right atrium. In addition, patients should be encouraged to elevate the foot of their bed using a 3–4-inch brick under the bed posts. This will provide approximately 10 degrees of elevation of the foot of the bed and passive decongestion of their legs while they are sleeping. Elevating the ankles and legs with pillow is not as efficient as patients are required to maintain a still sleeping position on their back lest the pillows are kicked off the bed. Elevating the foot of the bed allows the patient to sleep comfortably in any position and maintain elevation. Unless the patient has significant esophageal reflux, most patients and spouses tolerate this change in sleeping position without too much difficulty.

B. Compression

Depending on the etiology of the CVI, the commitment to compression is generally a lifelong endeavor. Compression decreases venous capacitance, decreases capillary venous exudation, and improves the calf muscle pump function with respect to the ejection fraction and ejection volume with ambulation. The type of compression garment and the amount of compression or strength of the garment needs to be individually tailored to the patient. It is imperative that the compression is measured to fit appropriately. Most patients are sufficiently managed with a knee-high garment.

In general, patients with C1 to C2 or early C3 disease may be sufficiently managed with 15–20 mm Hg compression. Patients with C3 and C4 disease typically are best managed with 20–30 mm Hg compression. Patients with more severe disease including venous ulcers or healed ulceration, C5 and C6 disease, are best managed with 30–40 mm Hg compression. In reality, most older patients cannot apply stockings in excess of 20 mm Hg. Caregivers or family members may be required to assist with the stocking application. In addition, patients with moderate or severe PAD should also not be in higher grades of compression. The compression must be matched to the severity of the PAD.

Patients who are limited by osteoarthritis, limited mobility, prior hip replacement, or obesity frequently cannot reach their foot to apply the garments. Stocking donning aides may be helpful. In addition, using rubber gloves and a cotton-based stocking may be helpful for patients with arthritis of their hands. Patients should be advised to lose weight, if needed. Central obesity increases pressure in the venous system and further limits compliance with stockings. Exercise is helpful to increase venous return. If possible patients should walk on a regular basis to improve venous circulation. Pool exercise or walking may be helpful for patients with arthritis who find weight-bearing exercise uncomfortable. Regular foot and ankle exercises that augment the calf muscle pump action can be used to improve venous return.

C. Intervention

Patients who have persistent symptoms despite adequate conservative treatment or patients with recurrent superficial thrombophlebitis or venous stasis ulcers should be considered for intervention. For larger axial varicose veins venous stripping was historically used for most patients. Although still used, traditional venous stripping has been largely replaced by endovenous laser ablation therapy (EVLT) or radiofrequency ablation (RFA). These are catheter-based techniques that obliterate the vein from the lumen of the vessel using heat injury and thrombosis (endothermal ablation). Typically these procedures can be performed in an ambulatory setting and the patients experience little pain or bruising. Many patients return to normal activities the day after the procedure. Another technique, called *foam sclerotherapy*, is being used with increasing frequency, even for larger varicose veins. This is also performed in an office setting. Sclerosant foam is injected into the vein, typically using ultrasound guidance to injure the venous wall and facilitate scarring and closure of the vessel. Which procedure is best is determined by clinical factors and operator and patient preference. The surgeon or operator should choose the procedure likely to offer the best opportunity for successful venous closure. It is important to recognize that venous closure is not associated with improved venous ulcer healing but does decrease the rate of recurrence and, therefore, may be warranted after wound healing.

Reticular veins and venous telangiectasias may be managed by injection sclerotherapy. In many cases, this is considered cosmetic; however, when symptomatic, additional therapy may be considered. In similar fashion, symptomatic venous clusters and varicosities not related to the axial veins may benefit. Foam sclerotherapy or ambulatory phlebectomy can be used successfully for many of these cases. Again, the choice of therapy is operator dependent.

Bunke N, Brown K, Bergan J. Phlebolymphedema: usually unrecognized, often poorly treated. *Perspect Vasc Surg Endovasc Ther.* 2009;21(2):65-68.

Gloviczki P, Comerota AJ, Dalsing MC, et al. The care of patients with varicose veins and associated chronic venous disease: clinical practice guidelines of the Society for Vascular Surgery and the American Venous Forum. *J Vasc Surg.* 2011;53(5 Suppl): 2S-48S.

Meissner MH, Moneta G, Burnand K, et al. The hemodynamics and diagnosis of venous disease. *J Vasc Surg.* 2007;46(Suppl): 4S-24S.

Padberg FT, Johnston MV, Sisto SA. Structured exercise improves calf muscle pump function in chronic venous insufficiency: a randomized trial. *J Vasc Surg.* 2004;39(1):79-87.

LYMPHEDEMA

ESSENTIALS OF DIAGNOSIS

▶ Unilateral limb involvement (infrequently involves both limbs).

▶ Nonpitting edema involving the dorsum of the foot with squaring of the toes.

▶ History of cellulitis, malignancy, surgery, or trauma.

▶ Skin changes of CVI are usually absent.

General Principles in Older Adults

The lymphatic system is responsible for removing excess tissue fluid as well as proteinaceous debris and cellular matter from the tissues. Lymphedema is the pathologic accumulation of this protein rich fluid in the subcutaneous tissues. Lymphedema occurs when the lymphatics are either reduced in number, injured or destroyed, or malformed.

Lymphedema may be considered primary or secondary. Primary lymphedema is a result of the inherent absence or dysfunction of the lymphatics without a history of insult or injury. Primary congenital lymphedema is present at birth or within the first year of life. Lymphedema praecox begins in adolescence through the third decade of life. Lymphedema tarda has onset after age 40 years. These may be familial or sporadic in nature. Secondary lymphedema occurs as a result of injury or trauma that disrupts or obstructs lymphatic flow. The most common causes of secondary lymphedema are malignancy as a result of tumor infiltration, obstruction, or related to the therapies, including radiation or surgery; surgery, including lymph node dissection, vein harvest, or hernia repair; and repeated infection, including lymphangitis or cellulitis.

A more recently recognized phenomenon of phlebolymphedema is the result of the interaction between the venous system and the lymphatics. Phlebolymphedema has characteristics of both venous insufficiency and lymphedema. This occurs when chronic venous hypertension results in excess fluid filtration such that the lymphatic transport capacity is exceeded. Once the venous hypertension is relieved the lymphedema usually spontaneously regresses.

▶ Clinical Findings

A. Signs & Symptoms

It is important to distinguish among edema, venous insufficiency, and lymphedema. Each of these clinical conditions are distinct entities and managed using different modalities. Several clinical findings may be helpful to distinguish lymphedema from edema or venous insufficiency. Unlike venous insufficiency, which usually involves the ankles and distal calf, lymphedema begins distally, and the toes and foot are virtually always involved at the outset. Lymphedema is classically identified by the association of squared toes, a prominent dorsal foot hump, and a positive Stemmer sign. The Stemmer sign is the inability to pinch the skin at the base of the toes. It is not pathognomonic for lymphedema, but it is a common clinical finding. Ulceration is not common, but may be fairly difficult to manage given the fibrotic skin and excess exudates associated with skin injury.

Lymphedema is a chronic and progressive condition. It is graded in stages:

Stage 0: There are no observable clinical findings but the patient may be at risk as a result of lymphatic injury or insufficiency. This is latent or subclinical disease. This stage is usually unrecognized.

Stage 1: There is usually mild or intermittent swelling. The edema may still be pitting. Elevation may decrease the swelling. Skin findings such as thickening or fibrosis and pigmentation are not identified.

Stage 2: The swelling is usually persistent. Elevation typically has little effect on the swelling. The skin may be more fibrotic and hyperpigmentation may be noted.

Stage 3: This stage is consistent with elephantiasis or late-stage lymphedema. There is marked fibrosis of the skin. Hyperpigmentation may be pronounced. Secondary skin changes of hyperkeratosis and papillomatosis are common.

Within each stage of lymphedema, the degree of swelling can further be classified as mild (<20% increase in limb girth), moderate (20% to 40% increase in limb girth), or severe (>40% increase in limb girth).

B. Laboratory Findings

There are currently no laboratory markers to identify patients with lymphedema. When appropriate, laboratory evaluation to differentiate edema from lymphedema may be appropriate. This may include complete metabolic panel (CMP) to evaluate serum protein and albumin concentration. Urinalysis to exclude significant urinary protein losses may also be helpful.

C. Diagnostic Testing

Lymphedema is frequently diagnosed clinically based on the history and physical examination. Diagnostic imaging is fairly limited. Traditional contrast lymphangiography is rarely necessary or performed. In some centers, nuclear lymphoscintigraphy, sometimes also referred to as nuclear lymphangiography, is available and may be helpful. Lymphoscintigraphy uses a radiolabeled colloid to observe lymphatic uptake and transport from the point if a distal injection.

CT and MRI imaging will usually demonstrate soft-tissue swelling. Venous duplex ultrasound for deep vein thrombosis and to exclude significant deep or superficial venous reflux is included in the diagnostic algorithm. In patients with unilateral limb swelling, CT imaging of the chest, abdomen, or pelvis should be considered to exclude the presence of occult malignancy or obstruction of the lymphatics.

Differential Diagnosis

Edema is the accumulation of interstitial fluid. This may be from systemic causes such as cardiac or renal disease, medications, or protein maldistribution or losses. Venous insufficiency occurs when there is excess tissue fluid accumulation as a result of increased venous filtration or decreased venous reabsorption. In both cases, the interstitial fluid is mostly water with a lesser protein content. Lymphedema is a protein-rich fluid as a result of an inability of the lymphatic to reabsorb filtered fluid as well as protein. The differential diagnosis of extremity swelling is beyond the scope of this chapter. The differential diagnosis, clinical evaluation, and imaging should be individualized. In general, if the edema affects both of the upper or lower extremities, the differential should focus on systemic etiologies or a centrally obstructing process. If a single limb is involved, the pathology will usually be confined to a single body quadrant.

Lipedema is frequently confused with lymphedema. Lipedema is the accumulation of excess adipose subcutaneously. Patients may have fairly severe involvement of the extremities. One key differentiating feature is the foot-sparing associated with lipedema. Limb or muscular hypertrophy may also be confused for lymphedema. In these patients, MRI may be very helpful. The identification of hypertrophic musculature as opposed to the subcutaneous honeycombing of lymphedema can be readily identified. Klippel-Trenaunay and Parks-Weber syndromes are 2 other disorders associated with limb hypertrophy, usually in the absence of lymphedema.

Complications

Lymphedema is a chronic and disabling condition for many patients. It requires ongoing and aggressive care to prevent worsening of the disease process. Recurrent cellulites, lymphangitis, and wounds may also complicate the condition. Rarely, patients develop a lymphedema-associated arthropathy that can be painful and disabling. Even less common is the development of a lymphedema-associated angiosarcoma in the affected limb. However, patients who develop blue or purple skin lesions should be referred for biopsy and further evaluation.

Treatment

A. General Considerations

Prevention and education are key components to managing lymphedema. Education regarding the pathology and dysfunction of the lymphatics and their role in infection and injury modification is required. Patients need to be engaged in the long-term care because lymphedema will typically not improve, but certainly may worsen if care is not maintained.

Patients need to be advised of meticulous skin care to prevent minor injuries, ulceration, or trauma. Patients should moisturize their skin regularly. Keratolytic emollients or lactic-acid-based products may be recommended when there are extensive hyperkeratotic or papillomatous changes. Patient should see a podiatrist for nail care. Avoid trimming the cuticles or hangnails. Gloves are recommended for gardening, housework, and dishwashing. Early treatment of minor trauma or insect bites is recommended. Patients should be advised to use sunscreen and avoid sunburn or prolonged exposure. Avoid iatrogenic trauma, such as venipuncture, injections, and blood pressure measurement, in the affected extremity. The use of razors, hair waxing, or chemical hair removers is ill advised. Moderate exercise should be encouraged. Traditionally, patients have been advised to avoid vigorous exercise, but there are little data to support this recommendation. In contrast to venous insufficiency, elevation for passive decongestion of the limb has little effect in lymphedema.

B. Limb Decongestion

Treatment in lymphedema focuses on reducing and maintaining decongestion of the limb. Manual lymphatic drainage (MLD) is a physical therapy- or occupational therapy-directed program of limb and trunk massage and multilayered wrapping designed to decongest the lymphedematous limb. It is part of a program of complex decongestive therapy (CDT), which includes MLD, along with skin care, education, and exercises designed to decongest and maintain the condition of the limb. The MLD/CDT requires specialized training. The therapist should be specifically trained and certified in MLD.

In conjunction with MLD the use of pneumatic pumps may be helpful. The pumps may also be incorporated into a maintenance program and used at home on a regular basis. Newer pump designs are available that simulate MLD providing decongestion of the trunk as well as the extremity.

Once the limb is decongested, maintaining the gains of therapy is required. Most patients will use compression garments during the day. The daytime garment should provide continuous and graded compression. Compression of 30–40 mm Hg is usually recommended, but older patients may find this degree of compression difficult or impossible to apply. The use of the highest grade of compression that the patient can apply is likely to be the most helpful. Caregivers, family members, and other resources may also be required to assist with donning and doffing the garment. In addition, the compression much be matched to any degree of arterial insufficiency. A nighttime program with continued wrapping or the use of other devices may be recommended.

C. Pharmacotherapy

In general diuretics are of little benefit in lymphedema and are best avoided unless there are other indications for systemic diuretic therapy. Benzopyrenes including coumarin, rutoside, and bioflavonoids, are touted as beneficial for treating lymphedema. They are not available in the United States, and their exact roles in lymphedema are not well defined.

Antibiotics should be administered promptly for infections such as cellulitis or erysipelas in the setting of lymphedema. Injury related to the infection and inflammation can further damage the fragile lymphatics. If patients have more than 1 episode annually, consideration of preventive therapy may be appropriate. Many patients with lymphedema also have associated tinea pedis and use of antifungal powder to the webspaces is prudent. Secondary cutaneous fungal infections are also encountered, especially in stage 3 lymphedema. Aggressive and prolonged treatment may be required.

If patients develop wounds or persistent lymph drainage from skin fissure, they may have significant protein loss. Evaluation of their protein, albumin, and prealbumin may be warranted. Nutritional supplementation should be provided to optimize wound healing.

D. Surgical Therapy

Surgical advances in lymphedema have been disappointing. Microsurgical lymphatic bypass or anastomosis procedures typically do not have adequate durability in this progressive condition. In addition, few surgeons have the expertise or experience in these procedures. Debulking surgeries are rarely performed, except in cases of massive lymphedema. Again, few surgeons have experience with these techniques. Limb volume-reduction surgeries using liposuction are becoming more frequent. Patients with less fibrotic lymphedema may be surgical candidates. After the procedure, patients must be diligent with decongestive therapy, including MLD and compression.

International Society of Lymphology. The diagnosis and treatment of peripheral lymphedema. 2009 Consensus Document of the International Society of Lymphology. *Lymphology.* 2009;42(2):51-60.

Kerchner K, Fleischer A, Yosipovitch G. Lower extremity lymphedema. Update: pathophysiology, diagnosis, and treatment guidelines. *J Am Acad Dermatol.* 2008;59(2):423-331.

Murdaca G, Cagnati P, Gulli R, et al. Current views on diagnostic approach and treatment of lymphedema. *Am J Med.* 2012;125(2):134-140.

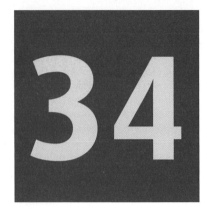

Chronic Obstructive Pulmonary Disease

Brooke Salzman, MD
Danielle Snyderman, MD

ESSENTIALS OF DIAGNOSIS

- Symptoms: dyspnea, cough, sputum production, and wheeze.
- Risk factors: tobacco smoke, air pollution.
- Spirometry: airflow obstruction that is not fully reversible.

General Principles in Older Adults

Chronic obstructive pulmonary disease (COPD) is a common pulmonary condition characterized by persistent airflow obstruction that is not fully reversible with bronchodilators. COPD is a major cause of morbidity and mortality in the United States and worldwide. In the United States, COPD affects 5% to 20% of the adult population, depending on the population studied. COPD is of special concern to older adults, as its prevalence rises steeply with age, affecting up to 10% of the older adult population. Over the past 30 years, mortality from COPD has increased substantially in the United States, and the number of women dying from COPD has surpassed the number for men. COPD is now the third leading cause of death in the United States, accounting for more than 126,000 deaths in 2005, and it is the fourth leading cause of death worldwide.

COPD represents a major public health challenge, as it is largely preventable and treatable, and, yet, it is the only common chronic illness where morbidity and mortality continue to climb. It is a significant cause of hospitalization, particularly in the older population. Rates of hospitalization for COPD increased more than 30% between 1992 and 2006. In 2006, COPD accounted for approximately 672,000 hospital discharges in the United States. The hospitalization rate for those 65 years of age and older was 4 times higher than for those in the 45–64 years of age group. According to the National Heart, Lung, and Blood Institute, the national projected annual cost for COPD in 2010 was $49.9 billion.

COPD is a more costly disease than asthma, and the majority of those costs are related to services associated with exacerbations. The burden of COPD is projected to increase in the coming decades as a result of continued exposure to COPD risk factors and the aging of the population.

COPD is defined as an inflammatory respiratory disease involving persistent airflow limitation that is incompletely reversible with bronchodilators. The airflow obstruction is usually progressive and associated with an abnormal chronic inflammatory response of the lungs to noxious particles or gases, primarily associated with cigarette smoking. Current definitions of COPD no longer include the terms "emphysema" and "chronic bronchitis," although such terms are still used clinically. Emphysema is defined pathologically and refers to the destruction of the alveoli, the gas-exchanging surfaces of the lung, resulting in the enlargement of the airspaces distal to the terminal bronchioles. Chronic bronchitis is a clinical term that is used to describe the presence of cough and sputum production for at least 3 months during each of 2 consecutive years.

Pathogenesis

Estimates of the prevalence of COPD depend on the definition and criteria used, and vary widely, ranging from 5.5% to >20%. In 2010, 14.8 million U.S. adults aged 18 years and older were estimated to have a clinical diagnosis of COPD. However, estimates may greatly underestimate the true prevalence of COPD because the disease is usually not diagnosed until it is clinically apparent and moderately advanced. It is estimated that at least an additional 12 million adults in the United States have COPD.

The prevalence of COPD, as well as mortality from COPD, rises considerably with age, with the highest prevalence among those older than age 65 years. Patients younger than age 35 years rarely have COPD, as the disease develops over years of inhalational exposure to a causative agent. In the past, studies showed that COPD prevalence and mortality were greater among men than women. However, this has generally been a consequence of differences in rates of smoking between men and women. Recent data suggest that women may be more susceptible to the effects of tobacco than men. Beginning in 2000, women have exceeded men in the number of deaths attributable to COPD in the United States.

Tobacco smoke is by far the most important risk factor for COPD, with an estimated 80% to 90% of COPD attributable to cigarette smoking. Smokers are 12–13 times more likely to die from COPD than nonsmokers. It is commonly stated that only 15% to 20% of smokers develop clinically significant COPD. However, experts propose that this statistic greatly underestimates the true burden of COPD. A 10-pack year history of smoking is considered to be the threshold for development of COPD. After 25 years of age, a nonsmoking adult's forced expiratory volume in 1 second (FEV_1) decreases by an average of 20–40 mL per year. In smokers who are susceptible to COPD, the FEV_1 decreases 2–5 times the normal rate of decline. Smoking cessation can give a former smoker the same average ongoing loss of lung function as a never-smoker.

Other risk factors for COPD include advancing age, secondhand smoke exposure, chronic exposure to environmental or occupational pollutants, α_1-antitrypsin deficiency, a childhood history of recurrent respiratory infections, a family history of COPD, and low socioeconomic status. Occupational pollutants associated with COPD include mineral dust from coal and hard rock mining, tunnel work, concrete manufacturing, and silica exposure; organic dust from cotton, flax, hemp, or other grains; and noxious gases, including sulfur dioxide, isocyanates, cadmium, and welding fumes. The percentage of COPD attributable to occupational exposures was estimated as 19.2% overall and 31.1 % in never-smokers.

α_1-Antitrypsin deficiency is a rare hereditary cause of COPD and accounts for only about 2% to 4% of cases. The deficiency is caused by a genetic anomaly of chromosome 14 that leads to premature hepatic and pulmonary disease because of increased tissue damage from neutrophil elastase. However, smoking significantly increases the risk for the progressive development of emphysema associated with α_1-antitrypsin deficiency. This rare recessive trait is most commonly seen in individuals of Northern European origin. Testing for the inherited deficiency is indicated for patients presenting at an early age for COPD, including those younger than age 45 years.

▶ Clinical Findings

A. Symptoms & Signs

The diagnosis of COPD should be suspected in any patient who has a history of tobacco use and any of the following: chronic cough, chronic sputum production, or dyspnea on exertion or rest. The presence of a productive cough is usually the initial presenting symptom of COPD. The cough associated with COPD is typically worse in the morning, but can be present throughout the day, while an isolated nocturnal cough is less consistent with COPD. Sputum production also initially occurs in the morning and tends to occur more frequently as the disease progresses. A change in sputum color or volume suggests an infectious exacerbation. Dyspnea is often associated with exertion or exercise early in the disease course and may be evaded by avoiding physical activities. However, dyspnea may develop at rest as the disease progresses. The Medical Research Council (MRC) dyspnea index is a validated tool for quantifying dyspnea and assessing the severity of COPD. Using the MRC, dyspnea can be graded on a 5-point scale with 1 being not being bothered by dyspnea except during strenuous activities, and 5 being too short of breath to leave the house or breathless with activities of daily living. Wheezing can also be the presenting symptom in patients with COPD. The relationship between the severity of symptoms related to COPD and the degree of airflow obstruction is highly variable. Some patients with advanced airflow limitation may be relatively asymptomatic. Less commonly reported symptoms associated with COPD include edema, chest tightness, weight loss, and increased nocturnal awakenings.

Important elements in the initial evaluation of COPD include assessing for risk factors, particularly smoking, prior medical history of asthma, allergies, or recurrent respiratory illnesses, and family history of COPD. Because COPD often coexists with other conditions such as coronary artery disease, heart failure, depression, and anxiety that may have a significant impact on symptoms as well as prognosis, clinicians should aim to identify and address comorbidities. For instance, approximately 30% of patients with COPD have congestive heart failure (CHF) and approximately 30% of patients with CHF have COPD. Each condition is commonly implicated for causing an exacerbation or acute flare of the other.

The physical examination may be unremarkable early in the disease. With more advanced disease, patients with COPD may have diminished or distant breath sounds and hyperresonance on percussion, and may demonstrate a prolonged expiratory phase and expiratory wheezing. Additional findings associated with COPD include an increased anteroposterior chest diameter or "barrel chest," use of accessory muscles of respiration including suprasternal retractions, and pursed lip breathing. The latter refers to learning forward and supporting oneself using the elbows to relieve dyspnea. The presence of jugular venous distension suggests elevated right heart pressures. Lower-extremity edema, central cyanosis, and a widened split second heart sound may indicate right-sided heart failure and cor pulmonale. Pulse oximetry at rest and with exertion should be performed to evaluate for hypoxemia and the need for supplemental oxygen.

COPD commonly manifests systemically, not only affecting the pulmonary system, often involving the cardiovascular, muscular, and immune systems, particularly in patients with severe disease. In addition, COPD is associated with chronic weight loss and may lead to cachexia, which is an independent predictor of mortality. Therefore, the BMI (body mass index) should be measured and monitored in patients with COPD. Other systemic findings include peripheral muscle wasting and weakness as a result of increased apoptosis and muscle disuse. Individuals with COPD have an increased likelihood of having osteoporosis, depression, chronic anemia, and cardiovascular disease.

B. Laboratory Findings

Suspected COPD should be confirmed by spirometry. Spirometry is a pulmonary function test that measures the presence and severity of airflow obstruction. The diagnosis of COPD is supported when spirometry demonstrates airflow obstruction that is not fully reversible with bronchodilators. The key spirometric measurements related to COPD are FEV_1 and forced vital capacity (FVC). The FEV_1 is the volume of air that a patient can expire in 1 second following a full inspiration. The FVC is the total maximum volume of air that a patient can exhale after a full inspiration. A postbronchodilator FEV_1-to-FVC ratio of less than 0.7 with less than 12% reversibility is diagnostic of airflow limitation and confirms the diagnosis of COPD.

Guidelines with recommendations for classifying COPD severity based on spirometry (Table 34–1) have been published. The USPSTF (U.S. Preventive Services Task Force) currently recommends against screening asymptomatic adults for COPD using spirometry because there is no evidence of benefit in this population regardless of a patient's age, smoking status, or family history of COPD. Furthermore, nonselective use of spirometry can lead to substantial overdiagnosis of COPD in "never smokers" older than age 70 years. Nor is it recommended to use periodic spirometry after initiation of therapy to routinely monitor disease status or to modify therapy. However, spirometry can be helpful to perform if there is a substantial change in symptoms or functional capacity.

Although spirometry is the major diagnostic test used to diagnose COPD, other tests may be helpful for ruling out other conditions or concomitant disease. A chest radiograph should be performed to evaluate for lung masses or nodules, interstitial or fibrotic changes, and pulmonary edema. A complete blood count should be performed to rule out anemia or polycythemia. An electrocardiogram and/or echocardiograph may be useful if there is suspicion for cardiac ischemia or CHF, or in patients with signs of cor pulmonale.

▶ Differential Diagnosis

The differential diagnosis of COPD includes asthma, health failure, bronchiectasis, bronchiolitis obliterans, lung cancer, interstitial lung disease, pulmonary fibrosis, sarcoidosis, cystic fibrosis, tuberculosis, and bronchopulmonary dysplasia. The clinical history, physical examination, and diagnostic testing such as spirometry, can help diagnose COPD. However, good evidence indicates that history and physical examination are

Table 34–1. Staging systems for COPD.

Stage: Degree of Airflow Limitation	Spirometric Findings	Symptoms	Therapy
Stage 1: Mild	FEV_1-to-FVC ratio <0.70 FEV_1 >80% of predicted	Chronic cough and sputum production may or may not be present. Patients often unaware of abnormal lung function.	Active reduction of risk factors including smoking cessation[a]; influenza and pneumococcal vaccinations[a]; short-acting bronchodilator as needed[a]
Stage II: Moderate	FEV_1-to-FVC ratio <0.70 FEV_1 between 50% and 80% of predicted	Dyspnea on exertion can develop. Cough and sputum production sometimes present.	Add regular treatment with single or combination of long-acting bronchodilators (β agonists and/or anticholinergics); Add pulmonary rehabilitation
State III: Severe	FEV_1-to-FVC ratio <0.70 FEV_1 between 30% and 50% of predicted	Greater dyspnea with exertion or at rest, wheeze and cough often prominent, reduced exercise capacity, fatigue, repeat exacerbations, greater impact on quality of life	Add inhaled corticosteroid inhalers if hospitalized for repeat exacerbations, oral steroid bursts for exacerbations
Stage IV: Very Severe	FEV_1-to-FVC ratio <0.70 FEV_1 <30% of predicted or FEV_1 <50% of predicted plus chronic respiratory failure	Shortness of breath at rest, increased functional impairment. Lung hyperinflation usual, hypoxemia and hypercapnia are common	Add long-term oxygen if chronic respiratory failure and hypoxic. Consider surgical treatments

[a]Applies to all stages of COPD severity.

not accurate predictors of airflow limitation. Studies suggest that the single best variable for identifying adults with COPD is a history of greater than 40 pack-years of smoking. A combination of all 3 of the following findings—greater than 55-pack-year history of smoking, wheezing on auscultation, and patient self-reported wheezing—is highly predictive of COPD. In contrast, the best combination of factors to exclude COPD is absence of a smoking history, no patient-reported wheezing, and no wheezing on physical examination.

▶ Treatment

The goals of COPD treatment are manifold and include reducing long-term decline in lung function, preventing and treating exacerbations, decreasing hospitalizations and mortality, relieving symptoms, improving exercise tolerance, and enhancing health-related quality of life. All patients diagnosed with COPD should receive immunizations, including pneumococcal vaccine and yearly influenza vaccinations. As smoking is usually the cause of COPD, smoking cessation is the most important component of therapy for patients who still smoke. Quitting smoking can prevent or delay the development of COPD, reduce its progression, and have a substantial impact on mortality. The rate of decline in lung function approaches that of a nonsmoker when a patient quits smoking. "Treating Tobacco Use and Dependence" is a comprehensive, evidence-based guideline published in 2008 by the U.S. Department of Health and Human Services.

Smoking cessation is paramount for patients with COPD at any age, and advanced age does not diminish the benefits of quitting smoking. Treatments shown to be effective for smoking cessation in the general population also have been shown to be effective in older smokers. Specifically, research has demonstrated the effectiveness of counseling interventions, physician advice, buddy support programs, age-tailored self-help materials, telephone counseling, and the nicotine patch in treating tobacco use in adults age 50 years and older. Unfortunately, smokers older than age 65 years may be less likely to receive smoking cessation medications.

Pharmacologic therapy for patients with COPD depends on the severity of symptoms, the degree of lung dysfunction, and response to, as well as tolerance of specific medications. A stepwise approach is often employed to provide symptomatic relief, improve exercise tolerance and quality of life, and possibly decrease mortality. However, none of the existing medications for COPD have been shown to conclusively modify the progressive decline in lung function that is characteristic of COPD. Therefore, pharmacotherapy for COPD is generally used to decrease symptoms and/or complications. Table 34–1 provides a summary of recommended treatment at each stage of COPD.

Evidence suggests that there is no benefit to treating asymptomatic persons with evidence of airflow obstruction on spirometry as there is no difference in the progression of lung dysfunction or development of symptoms in treated asymptomatic patients.

When treatment for COPD is delivered by an inhaled method, it is essential to train and evaluate patients regarding inhaler technique. Some older patients with COPD cannot effectively use a metered-dose inhaler (MDI) either because of difficulties with grip strength or coordination, or cognitive impairment, and may benefit from using a spacer or nebulizer. Use of a spacer or nebulizer can allow caregivers to more easily assist with medication administration. Some studies have shown dry powder inhalers (DPIs) to be easier to handle than MDIs but DPIs have not demonstrated superior health outcomes.

A. Bronchodilators

Bronchodilator medications are vital to the symptomatic management of COPD. They are generally used on an as-needed basis (short-acting) or on a regular basis (long-acting) to prevent or reduce symptoms and exacerbations. All categories of bronchodilators have been shown to increase exercise capacity in COPD without necessarily producing significant changes in FEV_1. Long-acting bronchodilators, including inhaled β agonists and anticholinergics, are more effective and convenient than treatment with short-acting bronchodilators. Monotherapy with a long-acting inhaled bronchodilator is the treatment of choice in patients with respiratory symptoms and an FEV_1 less than 60% of predicted, as these agents have been shown to reduce exacerbations and improve health-related quality of life. Data to support their use in symptomatic patients with an FEV_1 between 60% and 80% of predicted is limited, but individuals may have improvement in respiratory symptoms. Because there is insufficient evidence to favor 1 long-acting bronchodilator over others, the choice of agent should be based on patient preference, cost, and potential adverse effects.

1. β-Agonist bronchodilators—β-Agonist bronchodilators promote airway smooth-muscle relaxation by increasing cyclic adenosine monophosphate (AMP) within cells, and have demonstrated improvements in health status. Short-acting β agonists can be used as initial drug therapy for patients with mild intermittent symptoms as needed. Albuterol is recommended as the first-line treatment for patients with symptoms of mild COPD because the onset of action is more rapid than anticholinergic bronchodilators such as ipratropium. Oral therapy is slower in onset and has more side effects than inhaled treatment and generally not recommended.

Long-acting β agonists (LABAs) are indicated for patients with persistent symptoms at a dose of 1 or 2 puffs BID. LABAs prevent nocturnal bronchospasm, increase exercise endurance, reduce rates of exacerbations and hospitalizations, and improve quality of life.

β-Agonist bronchodilators stimulate adrenergic receptors and thereby can produce resting tachycardia, and have the potential to precipitate cardiac rhythm disturbances in susceptible patients. Other side effects include tremor, sleep disturbances, and hypokalemia.

2. Anticholinergic bronchodilators—Anticholinergic bronchodilators enhance smooth-muscle relaxation by blocking muscarinic receptors. Short-acting anticholinergic bronchodilators, including ipratropium bromide, can be used to alleviate symptoms as needed. The bronchodilating effect of short-acting inhaled anticholinergics lasts longer than that of short-acting β agonists and may extend up to 8 hours after administration. The long-acting tiotropium is considered a first-line agent for patients with persistent symptoms as it effectively prolongs bronchodilation for more than 24 hours and decreases hyperinflation. In addition, tiotropium has been shown to improve dyspnea, decrease exacerbations, and improve health-related quality of life when compared to placebo.

The main side effect of anticholinergic bronchodilators is dry mouth. Some patients have also reported a bitter, metallic taste. Closed-angle glaucoma is a very rare complication that has only been reported in individuals using a high dose of treatment with a nebulizer. A meta-analysis raised concerns for excessive cardiovascular morbidity associated with tiotropium; however, a large, randomized, controlled trial showed no evidence to support such concerns.

B. Methylxanthines

Theophylline is a xanthine derivative that acts as a nonspecific phosphodiesterase inhibitor and thereby increases intracellular cyclic AMP within airway smooth muscle. Bronchodilation tends to occur most effectively at high doses; however, high doses increase the risk for toxicity. The target range of 8–13 mg/dL is recommended, which is lower than prior recommendations, to achieve therapeutic value and avoid toxicity. Low-dose theophylline reduces exacerbations in patients with COPD but does not improve lung function. It is less effective and less-well tolerated than inhaled long-acting bronchodilators and is not recommended if those drugs are available and affordable. Toxic effects include the development of atrial and ventricular arrhythmias and grand mal convulsions. Other more common side effects include headaches, insomnia, nausea, and heartburn.

C. Glucocorticosteroids

The effects of oral and inhaled corticosteroids in COPD are much less dramatic than in asthma and their role is limited to specific indications. Most studies suggest that regular treatment with inhaled corticosteroids does not modify the progressive decline of FEV_1 or reduce overall mortality in patients with COPD. However, they have been shown to reduce the frequency of exacerbations and improve health status for symptomatic COPD patients with an FEV_1 <60% of predicted (stage III or IV), and in those with repeated exacerbations. Treatment with inhaled corticosteroids increases

the likelihood of pneumonia, and may be associated with decreased bone mineral density.

Chronic treatment with systemic corticosteroids should be avoided because of the multiple adverse effects and an unfavorable benefit-to-risk ratio. Adverse effects of systemic corticosteroids include, but are not limited to, steroid-induced osteoporosis, hypertension, hyperglycemia, myopathy, and delirium. However, short courses of systemic corticosteroids are utilized for COPD exacerbations, as they increase the time to subsequent exacerbation, decrease the rate of treatment failure, shorten hospital stays, and improve hypoxemia and FEV_1. A randomized, controlled trial (RCT) of patients with a COPD exacerbation compared 8 weeks and 2 weeks' worth of steroids to placebo. There were no significant differences between the 8-week and 2-week courses. A RCT comparing oral and intravenous steroids in equivalent dosages (60 mg daily) showed no difference in length of hospitalization and rates of early treatment failure.

D. Phosphodiesterase-4 Inhibitors

Phosphodiesterase-4 inhibitors, such as roflumilast, aim to reduce inflammation through inhibition of the breakdown of intracellular cyclic AMP. Roflumilast has been FDA approved for use in the United States. In patients with stage III or IV COPD and a history of exacerbations, this medication reduces exacerbations treated with oral steroids. Roflumilast cannot be given with theophylline. Adverse effects include nausea, anorexia, abdominal pain, diarrhea, sleep disturbances, and headache.

E. Combination Therapy

Symptomatic patients with COPD and a FEV_1 less than 60% of predicted may benefit from combination therapy, but it is not clear when combination therapy should be used instead of monotherapy. Several studies that have explored the value of combination therapy have shown significant improvements over single agents alone. For example, a combination of a short-acting β-agonist and an anticholinergic produces greater and more sustained improvements in FEV_1 than either drug alone. In addition, an inhaled corticosteroid combined with a long-acting β-agonist is more effective than the individual components in reducing exacerbations and improving lung function and health status in patients with moderate to very severe COPD. However, a recent Cochrane review concluded that the relative efficacy and safety of combination inhalers remains uncertain. Furthermore, combination therapy has been associated with a modest increase in the risk for adverse events.

F. Mucolytic Agents

These medications aim to decrease sputum viscosity and adhesiveness in order to facilitate expectoration. However, there is little evidence that documents objective and/or subjective improvements in pulmonary function and/or symptoms.

G. Antibiotics

The routine use of antibiotics is not recommended in the chronic management of COPD but they are utilized in the treatment of acute bacterial exacerbations of COPD. The use of antibiotics in moderately or severely ill patients with COPD exacerbations reduces the risk of treatment failure and death. The optimal choice of antibiotic and length of treatment are unclear.

H. Oxygen

Guidelines recommend that clinicians prescribe continuous oxygen therapy in patients with COPD who have severe resting hypoxemia (partial pressure arterial oxygen [PaO_2] <55 mm Hg or SpO_2 [oxygen saturation as measured using pulse oximetry] <88%). Studies have shown that the use of supplemental oxygen for 15 or more hours daily can help improve survival and quality of life in patients with COPD who have severe resting hypoxemia.

I. Lung Volume Reduction

Bullectomy, lung volume reductive surgery (LVRS), and lung transplantation have all been utilized to treat patients with COPD. However, research regarding use and benefit of these procedures for older adults is limited. Bullectomy can be used for a rare subset of patients with COPD who have giant bullous emphysema, where single or multiple large bullae encompass 30% or more of a hemithorax, Surgical resection of these bullae can restore significant pulmonary function and improve symptoms. LVRS is considered in patients with severe emphysema and disabling dyspnea who are refractory to optimal medical management. A variety of surgical approaches and reduction techniques have been utilized. Overall, LVRS has not demonstrated a survival benefit over medical therapy. LVRS has shown a survival advantage and improved quality of life only for a small subgroup of patients with upper lobe emphysema and low baseline exercise capacity. Unilateral or bilateral lung transplantation is a treatment option in highly selected patients with severe COPD. Studies demonstrate improvements in quality of life after lung transplantation; the effect on survival is less clear. However, age greater than 60 years is considered a relative contraindication for a double-lung transplant.

J. Pulmonary Rehabilitation

Pulmonary rehabilitation programs are effective in improving exercise capacity, quality of life, and perception of symptoms, regardless of age. Limited data suggest that benefits of pulmonary rehabilitation may also include reductions in the number of hospitalizations and improvements in survival. Pulmonary rehabilitation uses an interdisciplinary approach, including education and exercise training, and should be prescribed for symptomatic patients with an FEV_1 <50% of predicted and considered for COPD patients with less airflow obstruction if they have dyspnea, reduced exercise tolerance, a restriction in activities because of their condition, or impaired health status.

▶ Prognosis

As pharmacologic therapy has not been shown to slow or reverse the progressive loss of lung function that occurs, it remains difficult to prognosticate in COPD because of its variable history and individual heterogeneity. Data from both patients and their physicians demonstrate that advance care planning in COPD is rarely done well, if at all. Patients often have a poor understanding that COPD is a life-limiting illness. In the month prior to their death, less than one-third of patients with severe COPD, CHF, or cancer estimated their life expectancy to be less than 1 year. Clinicians themselves report their shortcomings when it comes to discussing end-of-life care with patients who have advanced COPD, often waiting until patients are too sick to make care decisions. The landmark study designed to improve end-of-life decision making, Study to Understand Prognoses and Preference for Outcomes and Risks of Treatments (SUPPORT), failed to influence end-of-life care. Specifically, SUPPORT showed that COPD patients who expressed a preference for care focused on comfort, rather than life-prolonging measures, were much more likely than patients with lung cancer to receive invasive mechanical ventilation, cardiopulmonary resuscitation, or tube feeding.

Although making a prognosis may be difficult, several tools have been developed to help clinicians stratify severity of disease. For example, the Global Initiatives for Chronic Obstructive Lung Disease (GOLD) Guidelines classifies stages of COPD from I-IV based on the degree of airflow obstruction as measured by spirometry. The GOLD Guidelines make accompanying treatment recommendations for each stage of severity. The GOLD Guidelines are limited because they only consider degree of airflow obstruction but do not take into account patients' individual symptoms or comorbidities. The BODE index, which includes BMI, exercise capacity, and subjective measures of dyspnea (Box 34–1), has been shown to predict mortality and may provide the clinician with a practical tool to classify how severity of disease may impact life expectancy. A higher BODE score corresponds with an increased risk of death.

Although the Bode Index has been helpful to predict survival over a 1–3-year period, it is not validated to predict a <6-month survival. The current National Hospice and Palliative Care Organization Criteria for hospice admission for COPD include disabling dyspnea at rest resulting in decreased functional capacity, and progression of end-stage pulmonary diseases, as evidenced by increasing visits to the emergency department or hospitalizations for pulmonary

Box 34–1. Bode Index

The MMRC (Modified Medical Research Council) Dyspnea Scale is a 5-point scale that allows patients to rate their level of dyspnea from 0-4. Zero correlates to breathlessness only with strenuous exercise and 4 correlates to breathlessness with minimal exertion (leaving the home, getting dressed). For more information, see Nishimura K, Izumi T, Tsukino M, Oga T. Dyspnea is a better predictor of 5-year survival than airway obstruction in patients with COPD. *Chest.* 2002;121(5):1434-1440. The 6-minute walk test is a simple test that measures the distance a patient can walk on a flat, hard surface in a 6-minute period of time. It has been used to measure outcomes to medical interventions in patients with moderate to severe heart and/or lung disease. For more information, see ATS Committee on Proficiency Standards for Clinical Pulmonary Function Laboratories. ATS statement: guidelines for the six-minute walk test. *Am J Respir Crit Care Med.* 2002;166(1):111-117.

Variable	Points on Bode Index			
	0	1	2	3
FEV_1 (% predicted)	≥65	50-64	36-49	≤35
6-Minute Walk Test (meters)	≥350	250-349	150-249	≤149
MMRC Dyspnea Scale	0-1	2	3	4
Body Mass Index	>21	≤21		

Bode Index Score	1-Year Mortality	2-Year Mortality	52-Month Mortality
0-2	2%	6%	19%
3-4	2%	8%	32%
5-6	2%	14%	40%
7-10	5%	31%	80%

infections and or respiratory failure. An FEV_1 <30% and/or a decrease of >40 mL/year provide objective evidence for disease progression, but are not necessary for certification. Additionally the presence of any of the follow support certification of the hospice benefit: hypoxemia pO_2 (partial pressure of oxygen) <55 mm Hg or Pox (pulse oximetry) <88% (on supplemental oxygen) or hypercapnia (pCO_2 [partial pressure of carbon dioxide] >55 mm Hg), right heart failure as a result of pulmonary disease (cor pulmonale), unintentional weight loss of >10% in the preceding 6 months, or resting tachycardia of >100/min. Certainly, these criteria serve as a rule of thumb that may guide clinicians to think more actively about increasing services available to patients with end-stage COPD, but studies show they have not been accurate in predicting survival time. Although epidemiologists and researchers have begun to identify characteristics of COPD patients who are most at risk to die in the next 6–12 months, perhaps a common sense approach is most practical when considering advance care planning for patients with COPD.

Factors associated with a poorer prognosis in COPD include FEV_1 <30% of predicted, declining performance status and emerging dependence in the activities of daily living, more than 1 acute hospitalization in the past year, additional comorbid illness, older age, depression, and single marital status. Clinicians' identification of many of these in their patients should prompt a discussion about advance care planning. Identification of a medical proxy is a meaningful first step. Ideally, an outpatient discussion between the clinician, patient, and designated proxy during a visit for this specific purpose could be scheduled. Topics that may be discussed at the meeting include the patient's understanding of their illness and its trajectory, discussion of patient preferences for initiation and termination of life prolonging measures including aggressive mechanical ventilation, and identification of the most appropriate setting (home vs. institutional) for end of life care. SUPPORT demonstrated preferences for life-sustaining treatments may change during the course of an illness; therefore, reassessments of patient preferences are particularly important after recent hospitalization, new decline in functional status, and/or new oxygen dependence.

With the chronic nature and severity of COPD, it has become clear that COPD is a major contributor to health care utilization and costs. The Center for Medicare and Medicaid Services (CMS) has begun to require health plans to conduct performance improvement initiatives focusing on reducing readmissions. Specifically, beginning in 2014, CMS will reduce payments to hospitals with high rates of COPD readmissions within 30 days of discharge. Performance improvement programs have focused on the medication management, discharge planning, and transitional care aspects of COPD management with the goal of reducing readmissions. Using GOLD Guidelines, an individualized medication regimen should be optimized with particular emphasis on teaching the correct administration of inhalers, medication reconciliation after hospitalization, and patient education about the purpose of each medication. In addition to proper medication reconciliation, discharge planning should focus on oxygen therapy when needed, coordination of follow-up appointments as needed, and pulmonary rehab. Transitional planning is essential for all chronic disease management and should focus on sound communication between health providers, family members, and home care agencies.

A controlled trial to improve care for seriously ill hospitalized patients. The study to understand prognoses and preferences for outcomes and risks of treatments (SUPPORT). The SUPPORT Principal Investigators. *JAMA.* 1995;274(20):1591-1598.

Adams SG, Smith PK, Allan PF, et al. Systematic review of the chronic care model in chronic obstructive pulmonary disease prevention and management. *Arch Intern Med.* 2007;167(6):551-561.

Almagro P, Barreiro B, Ochoa de Echaguen A, et al. Risk factors for hospital readmission in patients with chronic obstructive pulmonary disease. *Respiration.* 2006;73(3):311-317.

Barr RG, Bourbeau J, Camargo CA, Ram FS. Inhaled tiotropium for stable chronic obstructive pulmonary disease. *Cochrane Database Syst Rev*. 2005;(2):CD002876.

Calverley P, Pauwels R, Vestbo J, et al; TRial of Inhaled STeroids ANd long-acting beta2 agonists study group. Combined salmeterol and fluticasone in the treatment of chronic obstructive pulmonary disease: a randomized controlled trial. *Lancet*. 2003;361(9356):449-456.

Calverley PM, Anderson JA, Celli B, et al; TORCH investigators. Salmeterol and fluticasone propionate and survival in chronic obstructive pulmonary disease. *N Engl J Med*. 2007;356(8):775-789.

Calverley PM, Rabe KF, Goehring UM, Kristiansen S, Fabbri LM, Martinez FJ; M2-124 and M2-125 study groups. Roflumilast in symptomatic chronic obstructive pulmonary disease: two randomised clinical trials. *Lancet*. 2009;374(9691):685-694.

Celli BR, Cote CG, Marin JM, et al. The body-mass index, airflow obstruction, dyspnea, and exercise capacity index in chronic obstructive pulmonary disease. *N Engl J Med*. 2004;350(10):1005-1012.

Celli BR, Thomas NE, Anderson JA, et al. Effect of pharmacotherapy on rate of decline of lung function in chronic obstructive pulmonary disease: results from the TORCH study. *Am J Respir Crit Care Med*. 2008;178(4):332-338.

Claessens MT, Lynn J, Zhong Z, et al. Dying with lung cancer or chronic obstructive pulmonary disease: insights from SUPPORT. Study to Understand Prognoses and Preferences for Outcomes and Risks of Treatments. *J Am Geriatr Soc*. 2000; 48(5 Suppl):S146-S153.

De Jong YP, Uil SM, Grotjohan HP, Postma DS, Kerstjens HA, van den Berg JW. Oral or IV prednisolone in the treatment of COPD exacerbations: a randomized, controlled, double-blind study. *Chest*. 2007;132(6):1741-1747.

Fried TR, Bradley EH, O'Leary J. Changes in prognostic awareness among seriously ill older persons and their caregivers. *J Palliat Med*. 2006;9(1):61-69.

Halbert RJ, Natoli JL, Gano A, Badamgarav E, Buist AS, Mannino DM. Global burden of COPD: systematic review and meta-analysis. *Eur Respir J*. 2006;(28):523-532.

Institute for Clinical Systems Improvement. Diagnosis and Management of Chronic Obstructive Pulmonary Disease (COPD). 2011. https://www.icsi.org/_asset/yw83gh/COPD.pdf. Last accessed on October 24, 2013.

Janssen DJ, Engelberg RA, Wouters EF, Curtis JR. Advance care planning for patients with COPD: past present and future. *Patient Educ Couns*. 2012;86(1):19-24.

Littner MR. In the clinic: chronic obstructive pulmonary disease. *Ann Intern Med*. 2011;154(7):ITC4-1-ITC4-16.

Mahler DA, Wire P, Horstman D, et al. Effectiveness of fluticasone propionate and salmeterol combination delivered via the Diskus device in the treatment of chronic obstructive pulmonary disease. *Am J Respir Crit Care Med*. 2002;166(8):1084-1091.

National Institute of Clinical Excellence. *Management of Chronic Obstructive Pulmonary Disease in Primary and Secondary Care, 2010*. http://www.nice.org.uk/guidance/cg101. Accessed on July 2, 2012.

Qaseem A, Wilt TJ, Weinberger SE, et al; American College of Physicians; American College of Chest Physicians; American Thoracic Society; European Respiratory Society. Diagnosis and management of stable, chronic obstructive pulmonary disease: a clinical practice guideline update from the American College of Physicians, American College of Chest Physicians, American Thoracic Society, and European Respiratory Society. *Ann Intern Med*. 2011;155(3):179-191.

Ram FS, Rodriguez-Roisin R, Granados-Navarrete A, Garcia-Aymerich J, Barnes NC. Antibiotics for exacerbations of chronic obstructive pulmonary disease. *Cochrane Database Syst Rev*. 2006;(2):CD004403.

Singh S, Loke YK, Furberg CD. Inhaled anticholinergics and risk of major adverse cardiovascular events in patients with chronic obstructive pulmonary disease: a systematic review and meta-analysis, *JAMA*. 2009;301(12):1227-1230.

Tashkin DP, Celli B, Senn S, et al; UPLIFT Study Investigators. A 4-year trial of tiotropium in chronic obstructive pulmonary disease. *N Engl J Med*. 2008;359(15):1543-1554.

U.S. Preventive Services Task Force. Screening for chronic obstructive pulmonary disease using spirometry: U.S. Preventive Services Task Force recommendation statement. *Ann Intern Med*. 2008;148(7):529-534.

Welsh EJ, Cates CJ, Poole P. Combination inhaled steroid and long-acting beta2-agonist versus tiotropium for chronic obstructive pulmonary disease. *Cochrane Database Syst Rev*. 2010;(5):CD007891.

USEFUL WEBSITES

American Lung Association. *Chronic Obstructive Pulmonary Disease*. 2008. http://www.lung.org/assets/documents/publications/lung-disease-data/ldd08-chapters/LDD-08-COPD.pdf

Centers for Disease Control and Prevention. *Public Health Strategic Framework for COPD Prevention*. http://www.cdc.gov/copd/pdfs/Framework_for_COPD_Prevention.pdf

Global Initiative for Chronic Obstructive Lung Disease. *Global Strategy for the Diagnosis, Management, and Prevention of Chronic Obstructive Pulmonary Disease, 2013*. http://www.goldcopd.org/guidelines-global-strategy-for-diagnosis-management.html

National Heart Lung and Blood Institute. *Morbidity & Mortality: 2012 Chart Book on Cardiovascular, Lung, and Blood Diseases*. http://www.nhlbi.nih.gov/resources/docs/2012_ChartBook.pdf

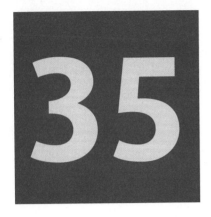

Gastrointestinal & Abdominal Complaints

Karen E. Hall, MD, PhD

General Principles in Older Adults

According to data from the U.S. Census Bureau in 2005, 45–50 million people older than age 65 years had at least 1 gastrointestinal (GI) complaint that impacted their daily life and that could result in a medical visit. GI symptoms are common in older adults and range from mild self-limited episodes of constipation or acid reflux to life-threatening episodes of infectious colitis or bowel ischemia. In addition to the increased prevalence of diseases such as diverticulitis and colon cancer in older patients, other common comorbidities, such as pain requiring nonsteroidal antiinflammatory drug use or atrial fibrillation requiring use of anticoagulants, increase the risk of GI complications such as ulceration or bleeding. Patients may present with unusual or subtle symptoms of serious GI disease caused by alterations in physiology with aging. An example of this is seen in older patients presenting with a GI perforation or colitis who do not have guarding or significant abdominal tenderness as a result of the decrease in visceral sensitivity that accompanies aging. Changes in the neuromuscular control of the colon with aging appear to predispose to constipation, thus explaining the increased prevalence of constipation and impaction developing with bed rest or use of constipating medications.

DISORDERS OF THE ESOPHAGUS

ESSENTIALS OF DIAGNOSIS

- ▶ Gastroesophageal reflux is experienced monthly by at least 40% of older persons and usually requires ongoing therapy.
- ▶ To maximize quality of life and minimize office visits, treatment of reflux can be started with a proton pump inhibitor along with initiation of lifestyle changes.

- ▶ Dysphagia may be oropharyngeal (mostly caused by neurologic disorders) or esophageal; the causes of esophageal dysphagia can generally be determined by history.
- ▶ Esophageal cancer usually presents in an advanced stage in older adults, with symptoms of progressive dysphagia and weight loss.

GASTROESOPHAGEAL REFLUX DISEASE

General Principles in Older Adults

Gastroesophageal reflux disease (GERD) is one of the more common GI disorders affecting older adults. Population studies indicate that more than 20% of adults older than age 65 years have heartburn at least weekly. This may actually underestimate the true prevalence of GERD because of the finding that, although symptoms appear to decrease in intensity with age, the severity of reflux and the risk of complications increases. Once symptoms develop, more than 50% of patients will have persistent symptoms and may require ongoing medical therapy.

Clinical Findings

A. Symptoms & Signs

GERD can be readily diagnosed if the patient complains of typical symptoms of pyrosis (substernal burning with radiation to the mouth and throat) and sour regurgitation, and if these symptoms improve with treatment. Pathophysiologic changes with aging outlined above may decrease symptoms of GERD, such that patients may present with atypical symptoms, such as a chronic cough, difficult-to-control asthma, laryngitis, or recurrent chest pain rather than heartburn.

B. Lab Findings

Patients with esophagitis may present with anemia and low iron levels. Esophagitis is a more common cause of anemia than has previously been recognized, and older patients presenting with anemia of unknown cause should have an esophagogastroduodenoscopy (EGD) exam to check for esophagitis and other upper GI tract sources of bleeding.

C. Diagnostic Studies

Upper endoscopy (EGD) should be performed in all patients with new-onset GERD who are older than 50 years of age, have persistent symptoms of reflux despite medical therapy, have a history of acid reflux longer than 5 years, and possibly have complications from acid reflux. EGD is safe to perform, even in the very old, frail patient. Patients thought to have atypical or extraintestinal manifestations of GERD should undergo ambulatory evaluation with a 24-hour pH probe after a negative work-up, including EGD and other tests for malignancy. Esophageal manometry is not routinely of benefit in the evaluation of older patients with GERD, unless antireflux surgery is being considered.

▶ Differential Diagnosis

In older patients with heartburn and dysphagia, malignancy in the esophagus and/or stomach must be considered and excluded as a cause. Patients presenting with chest pain or cough often must undergo evaluation to exclude acute coronary syndrome, aortic dissection, or pulmonary disease. Patients with hoarseness and cough may require evaluation to exclude oropharyngeal causes of dysphagia, such as stroke or malignancy.

▶ Complications

Complications that have been associated with GERD include esophagitis and esophageal ulceration, bleeding, strictures, Barrett esophagus, and esophageal adenocarcinoma, all of which are increased in patients older than 65 years of age. Risk factors shown in population studies for increased complications include age, male sex, white race, and presence of a hiatal hernia.

▶ Treatment

Treatment of GERD in older adults is essentially the same as that in younger patients. Although the "step-up" approach of lifestyle changes followed by acid-reducing drugs recommended in Table 35–1 may work, immediate initiation of a proton pump inhibitor (PPI) with lifestyle modifications usually results in fewer office visits, a reduction in procedures, improved patient satisfaction, and reduced overall costs. Cimetidine is generally not recommended in older patients

Table 35–1. Treatment of gastroesophageal reflux disease.

1. **Lifestyle modifications**
   Eat smaller, more frequent meals.
   Avoid chocolate, peppermint, and acidic foods (tomato juice, citrus juice) or foods that stimulate acid production (caffeine-containing foods).
   Do not eat 3-4 hours before going to bed.
   Minimize fats, alcohol, caffeine, and nicotine, especially at night.
   Sleep with head of bed elevated 6 in.
2. **Antacid liquids or tablets**
   Mylanta, Maalox, Gaviscon, Tums, Rolaids
3. **Histamine-2 receptor antagonists**
   Cimetidine (Tagamet; not routinely recommended in older patients because of increased incidence of drug interactions and delirium)
   Famotidine (Pepcid; 20 mg QD or BID)
   Nizatidine (Axid; 150 mg QD or BID)
   Ranitidine (Zantac; 150 mg QD or BID)
4. **Proton pump inhibitors**
   Esomeprazole (Nexium; 20-40 mg QD)
   Lansoprazole (Prevacid; 15-30 mg QD)
   Omeprazole (Prilosec; 20-40 mg QD)—available nonprescription as Prilosec 20 mg
   Pantoprazole (Protonix; 40 mg QD)
   Rabeprazole (AcipHex; 20 mg QD)
5. **Surgery**
   Laparoscopic fundoplication
   Nissen fundoplication

because of potential drug interactions and a higher incidence of adverse side effects compared with other histamine-2 receptor antagonists.

Persistent symptoms, or incomplete resolution of symptoms with treatment warrant evaluation with upper endoscopy. Although effective, chronic PPI use is associated with an increased relative risk of osteoporosis of 1.97 with long-term use of PPIs (>7 years). There have been reports of other concerns, such as decreased efficacy of clopidogrel anticoagulation for prophylaxis against coronary stent occlusion when clopidogrel is used in conjunction with PPIs (Table 35–2). For this

Table 35–2. Reported complications of PPIs.

1. Osteoporosis
2. Small intestinal bacterial overgrowth
3. Increased susceptibility to infection with enteric pathogens
   Traveler's diarrhea
   Clostridium difficile
4. Drug-drug interactions
   Cytochrome P450 interaction with clopidogrel
   Reduced absorption of Atazanavir
5. Increased susceptibility to aspiration pneumonia
6. Vitamin B_{12} and iron malabsorption
7. Increased risk of *Helicobacter pylori* gastritis
8. Acute interstitial nephritis

reason, it is recommended to reevaluate the need for PPIs in patients who have been taking them for longer than 6 months.

Antireflux surgery should be reserved for patients with severe refractory GERD with complications. Results from high-volume centers indicate that mortality and morbidity are not increased in older adults. However, as in younger patients undergoing reflux surgery, although there is an immediate decrease in patients with symptoms postsurgery to 10% to 15%, 60% of patients are taking acid-suppressive medications 5–15 years later. Endoscopic therapies for GERD such as the Enteryx and Stretta procedures have been withdrawn because of significant complications.

DYSPHAGIA

▶ General Principles in Older Adults

Dysphagia, or difficulty swallowing, is a common complaint in older adults. Dysphagia is classified as oropharyngeal (transfer) or esophageal (transit). Oropharyngeal dysphagia refers to impaired movement of liquids or solids from the oral cavity to the upper esophagus. Several changes with aging affect the ability to chew and swallow food, including painful or diseased teeth, xerostomia, poorly fitting dentures, and mandibular destruction. Transfer of food into the pharynx slows with aging, resulting in discoordination between the pharynx and delayed relaxation of the upper esophageal sphincter (UES). The result can be penetration of food into the area above the vocal cords, and possibly aspiration into the trachea. Studies of normal healthy adults older than age 85 years demonstrate that approximately 10% have silent aspiration documented on barium cinefluoroscopy. Causes include neuromuscular disorders affecting the tongue, soft palate, oropharynx, and UES, such as cerebrovascular disease, Parkinson disease, multiple sclerosis, Alzheimer disease, and upper motor neuron diseases. Other causes include muscular disorders such as myasthenia gravis, polymyositis, and amyloidosis. Finally, patients with a history of surgery or radiation to the oral cavity or neck are at risk for transfer dysphagia. Dysphagia occurring in the esophagus distal to the UES is transit dysphagia, and is even more common than transfer dysphagia. In a review of patients presenting with dysphagia in a primary care setting, the most common diagnoses were esophageal reflux (44%), benign strictures (36%), esophageal motility disorder (11%), neoplasm (6%), infectious esophagitis (2%), and achalasia (1%).

▶ Clinical Findings

A. Symptoms & Signs

Patients with oropharyngeal dysphagia typically cough, gag, choke, or aspirate their food during the initiation of a swallow. Patients may also complain of odynophagia, or painful

Table 35–3. Causes of odynophagia.

1. **Medications**
   Tetracycline
   Quinidine
   Doxycycline
   Alendronate
   Iron
   Nonsteroidal antiinflammatory drugs
   Acetylsalicylic acid
   Vitamin C
   Potassium chloride
2. **Infections**
   Viral (herpes simplex virus, cytomegalovirus, HIV, varicella-zoster virus)
   Bacterial (*Mycobacteria*)
   Fungal (*Candida, Aspergillus*)
3. **Acid reflux disease**
4. **Miscellaneous**
   Ischemia
   Chemotherapy
   Radiation
   Crohn disease
   Sarcoid

swallowing (Table 35–3). Those with transit dysphagia often complain of solid foods or liquids "sticking," "catching," or "hanging up" in their esophagus, and may point to their substernal area as the problem location. Using a series of questions and the algorithm outlined in Figure 35–1, the cause of esophageal (transit) dysphagia can be identified in nearly 90% of cases. Dysphagia to solids usually reflects an underlying mechanical obstruction, whereas dysphagia to both liquids and solids starting simultaneously usually reflects an underlying neuromuscular disorder. Patients with odynophagia may have underlying infection (such as candidal esophagitis) or obstruction. Globus (a persistent sensation of fullness in the throat that usually improves with eating) is a benign condition that may respond to passive esophageal dilation. History of smoking or heavy alcohol use is associated with increased risk of squamous cell esophageal cancer. The physician should look for evidence of anemia and unintentional weight loss as a result of an inability to eat, either of which could indicate a serious disorder such as malignancy. The nature of the dysphagia (solids or both solids and liquids) and the temporal nature of the swallowing disorder (intermittent or progressive in nature) are helpful in determining the likely cause. Finally, associated symptoms of chest pain or acid reflux should be elicited, as GERD is a risk for peptic strictures and development of Barrett esophagus and subsequent adenocarcinoma.

B. Diagnostic Studies

In older adults, a barium esophagogram is often ordered as the initial test to evaluate dysphagia, but an EGD should be

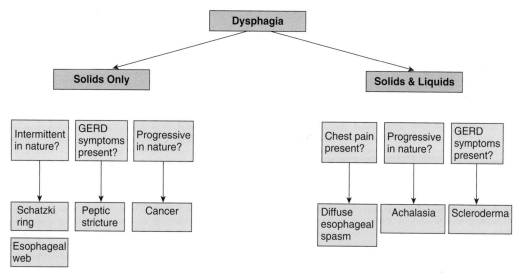

▲ **Figure 35–1.** Evaluation of dysphagia.

performed to check for malignancy and take biopsies. During EGD, the esophagus can be dilated if a stricture or mass is present. Patients with oropharyngeal symptoms of transit dysphagia should be evaluated by a speech language pathologist who can coordinate a swallowing study (modified barium swallow or videofluoroscopy) using thin, thick, and solid food materials. If upper endoscopy is normal and complaints of dysphagia persist, then esophageal manometry should be performed. This is a safe and readily performed procedure that can accurately identify neuromuscular disorders that cause dysphagia.

> ## Treatment

Treatment is directed toward the underlying disorder in addition to ensuring adequate nutrition and preventing aspiration. Patients with transfer dysphagia are taught which consistency of foods can be safely swallowed, proper swallowing techniques, and how to modify their posture to improve their swallowing. Medical therapy is not effective. Patients with transit dysphagia caused by increased contractility (achalasia and lower esophageal sphincter [LES] spasm) may benefit from LES dilation, botulinum toxin injection, or drugs that decrease smooth muscle contractions (anticholinergics, calcium antagonists, nitrates). Laparoscopic Heller myotomy has been performed in older patients with achalasia with reasonable safety and efficacy. If aspiration occurs or the nutritional status of the patient suffers, a feeding jejunostomy or gastrostomy should be considered if the patient has adequate ability to participate in the decision to use one. Use of feeding tubes in patients with dementia is controversial (see Chapter 68, "Defining Adequate Nutrition for Older Adults").

MOTILITY DISORDERS

> ## General Principles in Older Adults

Disorders of esophageal motility occur in older adults, and may be caused by underlying disease or by changes associated with aging.

> ## Clinical Findings

A. Signs & Symptoms

Presenting symptoms are usually dysphagia, chest pain, or other symptoms of persistent acid reflux disease. Common motility disorders that can occur in older adults include diffuse esophageal spasm, nutcracker esophagus, hypertensive LES, and ineffective esophageal motility. These conditions are diagnosed by esophageal manometry.

Achalasia is the most well-recognized motility disorder of the esophagus. Its prevalence increases with age; 7–12 in 100,000 older patients are affected. Treatment options include pneumatic dilatation, botulinum toxin injection of the LES, and surgery. Medical therapy (eg, nitrates, calcium channel blockers) is rarely effective; although these can be helpful in treatment of other motility disorders that cause dysphagia (see "Dysphagia" above). Pneumatic dilation produces significant relief of symptoms in many patients, but is associated with a 3% to 10% risk of perforation. For many older patients, initial treatment of achalasia can be approached using botulinum toxin injection. It is safe and effective and provides symptom relief in the majority of patients for up to 12 months. A second injection is often required; however, it is usually effective. Side effects are uncommon and include transient chest or abdominal pain, rash, or low-grade fever. Surgery should be reserved for patients who fail balloon dilation or botulinum toxin injection, and should be approached cautiously as the complication rate is higher.

▼ DISORDERS OF THE STOMACH

ESSENTIALS OF DIAGNOSIS

▶ Peptic ulcer disease is usually caused by nonsteroidal antiinflammatory drugs (NSAIDs) or *Helicobacter pylori.*

▶ Complications of peptic ulcer disease are more common in the elderly.

▶ Dyspepsia is a common complaint in the elderly and requires endoscopy to rule out ulcer or cancer.

▶ Symptoms of gastric cancer are nonspecific, and diagnosis is often delayed.

PEPTIC ULCER DISEASE

▶ General Principles in Older Adults

Peptic ulcer disease (PUD) refers to both gastric ulcers (GUs) and duodenal ulcers (DUs). Approximately 5 million cases of PUD will occur this year in the United States, and the demographics are shifting toward an older age of presentation. This may be a result of increased use of NSAIDs, *H. pylori* infection, and longer life span. Older adults are more likely to suffer complications of PUD, including hospitalization, need for blood transfusions, emergency surgery, and death. The 2 most common causes of PUD are NSAIDs and *H. pylori.*

▶ Clinical Findings

A. Symptoms & Signs

Patients may have hematemesis or coffee-ground emesis. Older patients are less likely to have epigastric pain with PUD than younger patients, with as many as 50% of patients without significant pain from either a GU or a DU. Because older patients may have little or no symptoms of significant ulceration, complications such as perforation are also more common in this age group. Chronic ulceration may present with symptoms of gastric outlet obstruction such as early satiety, nausea, and vomiting, as well as anemia.

B. Diagnostic Studies

In patients suspected of having PUD, a complete blood cell count (CBC), prothrombin time, blood urea nitrogen (BUN), and creatinine should be obtained and stool checked for occult blood. Patients should be asked about a history of PUD; their use of aspirin, NSAIDs, and warfarin; and previous diagnostic studies (upper GI series, testing for *H. pylori*). Upper endoscopy should be performed in older patients suspected of having PUD to identify the lesion, perform a biopsy in the stomach for *H. pylori*, rule out a malignancy, and initiate endoscopic therapy for a bleeding ulcer, if necessary.

▶ Complications

Hemorrhage and perforation are the most common complications of PUD and have been reported to occur in approximately 50% of patients older than 70 years. Morbidity and mortality of GI bleeding is higher in patients older than 70 years.

▶ Treatment

If an ulcer is found, therapy should be initiated with a PPI for at least 8 weeks to ensure healing. NSAIDs and aspirin should be stopped. Testing of biopsies for *H. pylori* urease production should be performed, and if the patient is found to be *H. pylori*-positive, double or triple antibiotic therapy should be started. In the case of a GU, healing should be documented 8–12 weeks later with follow-up EGD to make sure that the ulcer is not malignant. Patients with a prior history of PUD who require chronic NSAID or aspirin use should be treated concurrently with a PPI or misoprostol if they must have NSAIDs or acetylsalicylic acid (ASA). Both agents are effective in reducing the risk of PUD in chronic NSAID users, although, as a group, the PPIs are generally better tolerated than misoprostol. Patients with serious complications, such as hemorrhage or perforation, should avoid NSAIDs and ASA, as risk of recurrent bleeding is high, even with prophylaxis with PPIs or misoprostol.

DYSPEPSIA

▶ General Principles in Older Adults

Dyspepsia is defined as chronic or recurrent pain or discomfort in the upper abdomen, which is thought to arise in the upper GI tract. It is exceedingly common in clinical practice, affecting an estimated 20% to 30% of older adults.

▶ Clinical Findings

A. Symptoms & Signs

Patients may complain of upper abdominal pain, nausea, bloating, early satiety, or reflux symptoms. Dyspepsia traditionally has been classified as ulcer-like, reflux-like, or dysmotility-like; however, this classification has not been satisfactorily shown to improve either the evaluation or the treatment of patients with dyspepsia, suggesting that the symptoms are very nonspecific. However, it is important to distinguish patients with organic problems, such as an ulcer, from those with functional or nonulcer dyspepsia, because the treatment is dramatically different.

Evaluation of dyspepsia begins with a thorough history and physical examination to determine whether the pain or discomfort arises in the GI tract or elsewhere (heart, lungs, musculoskeletal system). Patients should be asked about unintentional weight loss, odynophagia, dysphagia, prior PUD, pancreatitis, biliary tract disease, bleeding, prior trauma, a family history of GI tract cancer, and evidence of blood loss or jaundice. *H. pylori* infection is a risk factor for PUD, and accounts for a significant number of cases of dyspepsia. Worldwide, more than 50% of patients older than age 60 years have *H. pylori* infection, although most are asymptomatic. Noninvasive tests for *H. pylori* include urease breath testing and stool antigen. These are more sensitive and specific than serum antibody for *H. pylori*. Patients undergoing endoscopy for dyspepsia should be tested for *H. pylori* with a rapid urease test of biopsy specimens, and, if positive, treated with a 14-day course of triple therapy (PPI + clarithromycin + amoxicillin).

B. Diagnostic Studies

Laboratory tests, including a CBC, erythrocyte sedimentation rate (ESR), liver function tests (LFTs), electrolytes, amylase, and lipase, should be performed. Older patients should be evaluated by upper endoscopy to rule out an ulcer or cancer. Initial testing with upper endoscopy has been shown to improve quality of life and lead to a reduction in dyspeptic symptoms. If endoscopy is normal and symptoms persist, a right upper quadrant (RUQ) ultrasonogram should be performed to check for evidence of cholecystitis (gallbladder wall thickening and fluid around the gallbladder). If this is normal and complaints persist, a solid-phase gastric emptying scan should be performed. In an older patient with persistent symptoms, concerns about occult malignancy should prompt a CT scan of the abdomen with both oral and intravenous contrast.

▶ Treatment

If the abdominal pain is caused by a specific disease, then treatment will be guided by the diagnosis. However, patients with persistent dyspeptic symptoms and a normal evaluation are categorized as having nonulcer dyspepsia. Treating this group of patients can be quite challenging. Few data support the routine use of antacids, antimuscarinic agents, or sucralfate. Routine treatment with histamine-2 receptor antagonists has shown a slight benefit, but better results have been obtained with the use of once- or twice-daily PPIs. It

is important to consider depression with somatization as a potential underlying cause, as recent studies have shown a correlation with chronic abdominal pain and depression. Older patients may have somatic manifestations of depression, such as chest pain, abdominal pain, nausea, and early satiety. There are no controlled, published studies to date on the use of selective serotonin reuptake inhibitors (SSRIs) in the treatment of dyspepsia; however, if the patient has other symptoms and signs of depression, use of SSRIs should be considered. Antidepressants that have been used to treat chronic pain include tricyclic antidepressants, fluoxetine, paroxetine, venlafaxine, and duloxetine. Anticonvulsants, such as gabapentin, carbamazepine, and lamotrigine, may provide safer pain relief in older patients who are not depressed.

▼ DISORDERS OF THE COLON

ESSENTIALS OF DIAGNOSIS

- ▶ Acute diarrhea is usually self-limited and caused by infections. Chronic diarrhea has many causes, and an extensive work-up may be needed.
- ▶ Diverticulosis increases with age. Complications include bleeding, diverticulitis, and perforation.
- ▶ Inflammatory bowel disease (IBD) may present for the first time in older people.

DIARRHEA

▶ General Principles in Older Adults

Patients with diarrhea most often complain of frequent stools (>3/day) or loose stools. However, other patients use the term *diarrhea* to describe fecal incontinence or fecal urgency. The etiology of acute diarrhea (lasting <2 weeks) in older adults is similar to that of younger adults, with a few exceptions. Most cases of acute diarrhea are related to viral or bacterial infections, but it can also be caused by medications, medication interactions, or dietary supplements. *Clostridium difficile* colitis is more prevalent in older adults because of more frequent hospitalizations, increased antibiotic use, and increased numbers of patients in institutional settings. *C. difficile* colonization in long-term care facilities has been estimated to be at least 50% in the United States. Chronic diarrhea, lasting longer than 2 weeks, may result from fecal impaction, medications, irritable bowel syndrome, IBD, obstruction from colon cancer, malabsorption, small bowel bacterial overgrowth, thyrotoxicosis, or lymphoma.

Small bowel bacterial overgrowth occurs when small bowel transit is slowed, or when the normal flora of the colon is altered with antibiotic treatment. The phenomenon causes premature fermentation of sugars by bacteria in the small bowel, leading to production of methane and/or hydrogen, which causes bloating and flatulence.

Lactase deficiency is common worldwide and is present in most individuals to some degree as they age, although it is less common in northern Europeans, North American Indians, and certain groups in Africa. Symptoms of bloating, abdominal distention, and loose stools usually begin in early adulthood, often worsening with age. Patients are usually aware that they are lactose intolerant; however, lactose intolerance can develop acutely after an episode of diarrhea because of other causes. This usually resolves, but may take several weeks or months in some patients. Celiac disease is an increasingly recognized cause of diarrhea and bloating in older adults. Whether this is occurring de novo in later life, or reflects chronic gluten intolerance is not clear. Uncommon causes of diarrhea include Whipple disease, jejunal diverticulosis, bowel ischemia, amyloidosis, lymphoma, and scleroderma with bacterial overgrowth.

▶ Clinical Findings

A. Symptoms & Signs

A complete history and physical examination, including a rectal examination, may provide information on cause and direct further evaluation. Medication history may reveal a causative agent for the diarrhea, and recent antibiotic use or hospitalization should trigger a work-up for *C. difficile*. A history of recent weight loss raises the concern for malignancy, IBD, microcytic colitis, malabsorption, or thyrotoxicosis. Fluid status should be assessed in all older patients with diarrhea because they are particularly susceptible to dehydration. Characteristic signs of bloating and gas may indicate small bowel overgrowth, or even underlying celiac disease.

B. Diagnostic Studies

Stool cultures should be obtained to exclude infection in patients with acute diarrhea. Routine stool cultures usually give a specific diagnosis in only 20% to 30% of cases, likely because most diarrheas are caused by viruses such as rotavirus and Norwalk agent. *C. difficile* toxin assay (toxin A and possibly toxin B) should be obtained if there is a history of recent antibiotic use. For chronic diarrhea, qualitative or quantitative stool fat should be checked to detect steatorrhea, and a thyroid-stimulating hormone (TSH) should be performed. In patients with *C. difficile* who fail sequential therapy with metronidazole first and then oral vancomycin, third line antibiotics such as rifaxamin or fidaxomin can be used. Colonoscopy is appropriate in patients with a history of weight loss, bloody diarrhea, and diarrhea lasting >4 weeks. If the colonoscopy appears grossly normal, biopsies should be obtained to rule out microscopic colitis, which has

a much higher prevalence in older adults. The mucosa may look normal, however biopsies demonstrate white cell infiltrates in the submucosa. Colonoscopy has a risk of causing perforation in patients with acute diarrhea caused by colitis, and should be used cautiously in patients with acute IBD or severe colitis. X-rays and CT scan of the abdomen may demonstrate bowel wall thickening with severe enteritis or colitis, and are also useful if complications such as perforation or abscess formation are suspected. In patients who are suspected to have small bowel bacterial overgrowth, a positive breath hydrogen/methane test will confirm early fermentation of ingested sugars in the small bowel. Serum antibodies to tissue transglutaminase (tTG), gliadin, and endomysial antigens are often positive in patients with celiac disease, with immunoglobulin (Ig) A tTG being the most sensitive and specific. The diagnosis is made on demonstration of villous damage and atrophy in small bowel biopsies performed during upper endoscopy.

▶ Treatment

Treatment of diarrhea is based on the underlying cause. In those with no evidence of acute infection and no blood in the stool, loperamide (≤8/day) is generally effective in treating symptoms. Bismuth subsalicylate, which has bactericidal action, can also be used. *C. difficile* is usually treated with metronidazole, and vancomycin is used for moderate-severe colitis or very ill patients. Older patients have a response to metronidazole that is less than that of younger patients (85% vs. 95%), and relapse of *C. difficile* diarrhea is more common in the older patient. Antidiarrhea agents should be avoided in *C. difficile* colitis because of the risk of precipitating ileus and megacolon. Care must be exercised in older adults with commonly used antimotility products, such as Lomotil, which contain atropine. In microscopic colitis, treatment is generally aimed at slowing colonic transit with the use of loperamide. Other alternatives include bismuth subsalicylate, prednisone, cholestyramine, or the 5-ASA products. Deodorized tincture of opium often improves symptoms in patients who fail to respond to other treatments. If small bowel overgrowth is present, then treatment with bismuth-containing medications may be helpful in mild cases. For severe small bowel overgrowth, treatment with 14–21 days of antibiotics to eradicate the bacteria is needed. A variety of antibiotics have been shown to be effective, including ciprofloxacin, neomycin, and rifaximin. If the underlying cause of slow intestinal transit is not addressed, or is not treatable, then overgrowth is likely to recur. Elimination of gluten is the treatment for celiac disease, and has become easier with the increase in gluten-free foods. Medication review is often helpful in patients with refractory celiac disease, as medications have been shown to be an unsuspected source of gluten. Web-based patient support groups are often a valuable resource for this kind of information.

DIVERTICULAR DISEASE

▶ General Principles in Older Adults

Diverticular disease has a higher incidence in industrialized nations and increases with age, such that >60% of those older than 70 years and nearly 80% of those older than 80 years have diverticular outpouchings of the colonic mucosa and submucosa. They are thought to develop because of increased colonic luminal pressures, particularly with constipation and straining. Diverticula are most commonly found on the left side of the colon; they are less common on the right side of the colon and are rarely, if ever, found in the cecum or rectum. The majority of patients who have diverticula are asymptomatic. They are commonly found during a barium enema, colonoscopy, or CT scan performed for some other reason. Approximately 15% to 20% of older adults who have diverticulosis will have a complication, among them diverticular bleeding or inflammation of a diverticulum (diverticulitis).

▶ Diverticular Bleeding

Diverticular bleeding is characterized by the sudden onset of painless hematochezia, sometimes in large volume. Although most diverticula are present on the left side of the colon, 70% of diverticular bleeding occurs on the right side. If an episode occurs and the patient is thermodynamically stable, colonoscopy can be scheduled urgently as an outpatient. Eighty percent of diverticular bleeding episodes stop spontaneously without requiring treatment. Patients should be hospitalized if bleeding persists, if they are hemodynamically unstable, or if blood loss compromises other organ systems. Older patients are at higher risk for poor outcomes with bleeding, and the threshold for hospitalization should be lower than in younger patients.

▶ Clinical Findings

A. Diagnostic Studies

Evaluation of lower GI diverticular bleeding usually involves colonoscopy to exclude sources of bleeding such as arteriovenous malformations (AVMs), ischemia, IBD, and cancer. Diverticular bleeding is often a diagnosis of exclusion in a patient with diverticula, significant bleeding and no other source found. If bleeding persists, a red blood cell scan or angiography should be performed, if necessary for intervention to control bleeding. In refractory cases, surgical resection of the bleeding area may be required.

In uncomplicated diverticulitis, patients have lower abdominal pain (usually on the left), fever, and an elevated white blood cell count. On physical examination, the patient does not appear hemodynamically unstable, and there

are no palpable abdominal masses or peritoneal signs. An abdominal radiograph should be performed to look for pneumoperitoneum. If there is no evidence of perforation or sepsis, treatment can be initiated in the outpatient setting with clear liquids for 2–3 days and oral antibiotics that should cover both anaerobes and Gram-negative organisms. Metronidazole and a fluoroquinolone or third-generation cephalosporin for 2 weeks is generally well tolerated and very effective. The patient should call the office in 24 hours and be seen 48–72 hours after the initial evaluation. If no improvement occurs, the patient should be hospitalized and a CT scan of the abdomen performed.

Diverticulitis becomes complicated if an abscess, stricture, or fistula develops. In addition to presenting with tachycardia or hypotension, older patients may present with lethargy or confusion. Abdominal examination may reveal a mass in the left lower quadrant, with or without peritonitis, or evidence of a draining fistula to the bladder, uterus, or skin. Patients with complicated diverticulitis require hospitalization. Patients should be given nothing by mouth and provided intravenous fluids. Blood cultures and an abdominal CT scan should be performed. Intravenous antibiotics should be initiated rapidly to cover both Gram-negative organisms and anaerobes. If no improvement is seen within 48–72 hours, an abdominal CT scan should be repeated, and consultation with surgery and interventional radiology should be pursued in case drainage or resection is required.

Patients with an episode of diverticulitis have approximately a 35% chance of a second episode occurring within the next 5 years. Patients with >2 episodes of diverticulitis in the same segment of colon should be referred to a surgeon for consideration of segmental resection.

INFLAMMATORY BOWEL DISEASE

▶ General Principles in Older Adults

Although the majority of patients with IBD are younger than age 65 years, approximately 10% to 15% of all newly diagnosed cases of Crohn disease and ulcerative colitis occur in patients older than age 65 years. Symptoms of Crohn disease are similar to those in a younger population, although older patients with Crohn disease may have fewer complaints of abdominal pain or cramps possibly because of reduced sensory thresholds or the concurrent use of multiple medications.

▶ Clinical Findings

A. Symptoms & Signs

Patients typically have a history of nonbloody diarrhea, unintentional weight loss, and fatigue. Evidence of anemia may be present (pallor, shortness of breath, reduced exercise tolerance). Extraintestinal manifestations of Crohn disease, including joint effusions, oral ulcers, painful nodular lesions on the extremities (erythema nodosum), uveitis, and back pain secondary to sacroiliitis, commonly occur. Although Crohn disease may develop anywhere from the mouth to the anus, it is less likely in older patients than in younger patients to involve large portions of the GI tract. The correct diagnosis is often delayed in older patients because symptoms of Crohn disease may mimic other diseases, including infectious diarrhea, ischemic colitis, lactose intolerance, medication-induced diarrhea, diverticulitis, celiac disease, microscopic colitis, and bacterial overgrowth.

Ulcerative colitis (UC) usually presents with tenesmus and frequent bloody bowel movements. Extraintestinal manifestations of UC are similar to those of Crohn disease and also include dermatologic manifestations, such as pyoderma gangrenosum (round or oval lesions on the shins and forearms). Older patients with UC are more likely than younger patients to have limited left-sided disease or proctitis. The first attack of UC in an older patient is generally more severe and more likely to require steroids than that in a younger patient. Of older patients with UC, approximately 15% will eventually require surgery.

B. Diagnostic Studies

The diagnosis of either UC or Crohn is made based on a thoughtful physical examination and history supplemented by appropriate laboratory studies and colonoscopy. Patients will require endoscopy for definitive diagnosis; however, this should be undertaken with caution in patients with severe colitis because of the risk of perforation. Limited examination with sigmoidoscopy using minimal insufflation may be adequate for diagnosis. Patients should be followed by a gastroenterologist with expertise in treating IBD.

▼ ANORECTAL DISORDERS

FECAL INCONTINENCE

▶ General Principles in Older Adults

Chronic fecal incontinence is the continuous or recurrent uncontrolled passage of fecal material for at least 1 month. Acute and chronic fecal incontinence occur commonly in older patients with comorbid conditions and are often a socially embarrassing and incapacitating problem. Despite its adverse effects on patients, fecal incontinence is underreported by older patients to physicians. The prevalence of fecal incontinence increases with age. Among community-residing people, the prevalence of fecal incontinence in older women is as high as 15%, and in older men 10%. The prevalence is nearly 50% in patients in long-term care. Fecal incontinence is now the second leading cause of nursing home placement in the United States. Up to 7% of the older population has incontinence of solid or liquid stool at least once each week. Fecal incontinence is closely associated with urinary incontinence and constipation (ie, the passage of infrequent, hard, or difficult-to-pass stools). Because overflow fecal incontinence with liquid stool is a common manifestation of constipation, the latter should always be considered in the work-up of fecal incontinence.

▶ Pathogenesis

Fecal incontinence is often a result of fecal impaction caused by constipation; it also can be caused by dysfunction of the internal or external anorectal sphincters. Factors that contribute to the risk of fecal incontinence include disordered muscle integrity, decreased rectal sensation or compliance, declining mental function, and loss of physical mobility. Rectal trauma, pudendal nerve injury, autonomic neuropathies, rectal prolapse, hyperosmolar diets, and fecal impaction are common physiologic factors contributing to incontinence. Aging is associated with neuronal loss and changes in neuromuscular function that may predispose patients to constipation and difficulty with anorectal control. Fecal incontinence can be classified as "passive," "urgency," or "fecal leakage." Patients with passive incontinence complain of leakage of small quantities of liquid or solid stool without awareness. Loss of external sphincter tone and leakage of liquid stool past an obstructing cancer or fecal impaction are common causes. Patients with urgency incontinence have frequent urgency to defecate, followed by passage of small quantities of liquid stool with or without mucus or blood. Urgency incontinence usually implies a loss of rectal compliance, which occurs with inflammatory, infectious, or radiation-induced colitis or stercoral rectal ulcers. Medications, especially opioids and anticholinergic agents, are common causes of constipation, impaction, and incontinence. Acute fecal incontinence may be seen in diarrheal states, and intermittent incontinence is often seen in patients with dementia, delirium, pelvic floor denervation, or excessive laxative use.

▶ Clinical Findings

A. Symptoms & Signs

The evaluation of fecal incontinence includes a careful review of the patient's cognitive status, a history of the circumstances of the incontinence episodes, abdominal and neurologic examination, and a rectal examination. Abdominal tenderness, bloating, or distention may indicate a fecal impaction. A careful rectal examination begins with visual inspection for skin irritation, the presence of fecal matter, rectal prolapse, or prolapsing hemorrhoids. The digital examination allows determination of internal and external anal sphincter tone. The rectal examination may occasionally detect structural defects (eg, rectal mass) that might contribute to overflow incontinence. The presence of hard stool in the rectal vault may suggest a fecal impaction; however, a negative rectal examination does not rule out a proximal fecal impaction. With high impactions, x-ray or CT scan of the abdomen may confirm feces. Mental status examination identifies the patient with dementia or delirium who may have lost self-toileting capacity. The absence of anal sphincter tone or anal wink may suggest denervation of the pudendal nerve (S2–4), resulting from a local or spinal cord lesion.

B. Diagnostic Studies

An abdominal plain film is helpful when fecal impaction is suspected. Acute onset of passive incontinence should prompt examination and spinal imaging to rule out cord compression. In select patients, but rarely in physically frail or bed-bound patients, a rigorous structural and functional evaluation of the anal sphincter with anorectal manometry, anal ultrasonography, defecography, pudendal nerve latency studies, or pelvic magnetic resonance imaging suggests a precise diagnosis. Other investigations performed by a gastroenterologist that may be helpful include flexible sigmoidoscopy or colonoscopy to look for a mechanical cause of incontinence such as a colonic mass or fistula. Anorectal manometry can objectively measure the resting pressure of the anal canal (predominantly from the internal anal sphincter), tone and contractile pressures of the external anal sphincter, and sensation within the anorectal area. Pudendal nerve testing may be required in some patients.

▶ Treatment

The treatment of fecal impaction includes disimpaction, bowel cleansing, modification of risk factors, and an effective maintenance regimen. Disimpaction should start with manual removal of stool and/or enemas, before administering a polyethylene glycol solution. Amounts of 1 to 2 L may be needed for initial treatment. Avoid magnesium citrate solutions and Fleet Phospho-Soda enemas in patients with underlying cardiac or renal disease, and do not use phosphate-containing oral solutions, as these have been linked to development of phosphate nephropathy. Prevention of recurrent impaction involves risk factor modification including mobilization, good hydration and nutrition, and minimizing use of constipating medications. Scheduled toileting after breakfast may decrease risk of impaction and fecal accidents in demented patients. Add fiber supplements when bowel function has been regularized to regulate bowel habits and prevent constipation. Regular use of a stimulant laxative such as senna or Dulcolax, or use of hyperosmolar solutions such as polyethylene glycol or lactulose, may prevent severe constipation or impaction in high-risk patients. Some high-risk patients require maintenance bowel cleansing with osmotic agents on a weekly basis. The role of diet in the prevention of impaction is unclear. Intermittent use of glycerin or bisacodyl suppositories is warranted if patients have infrequent episodes of constipation. The role of other agents, such as lubiprostone or probiotics, is not clear; however, these could be used as an alternative in patients who are unable to take other laxatives.

If a fissure is contributing to constipation and fecal impaction, conservative therapy with sitz baths, stool softeners, and fiber products usually leads to healing of an acute anal fissure over 1–2 weeks. Topical nitroglycerin, calcium channel blockers, or botulinum toxin injection can be used to treat nonhealing or chronic fissures. Surgical therapy, using lateral internal sphincterotomy, may be necessary in some patients; however, fecal incontinence may develop in 3% to 30% of patients.

COLONIC ISCHEMIA

▶ General Principles in Older Adults

The colon is more commonly affected by ischemia than the small bowel, because of the high prevalence of silent occlusion of the inferior mesenteric artery (IMA) in older patients (up to 10% of autopsies of persons older than age 80 years). The causes of colonic ischemia (CI) include acute and chronic mesenteric ischemia as a result of IMA thrombus or embolus, congestive heart failure (CHF), cardiac arrhythmias, shock, vasculitis, hematologic disorders, infections, medications (NSAIDs, digitalis, vasopressin, pseudoephedrine, sumatriptan, cocaine, amphetamines, gold), constipation, surgery, and trauma. Abdominal aortic aneurysm repair is a well-known risk for acute CI, with up to 3% of elective repairs and 14% of emergent repair developing CI, usually as a result of superior mesenteric artery (SMA) occlusion. The usual site of ischemic damage is the splenic flexure in the so-called watershed area of the colon primarily supplied by the IMA. Most cases of chronic CI do not have a definitive cause because of the insidious nature of the slow occlusion. The extent of injury can range from mild reversible colopathy to gangrene or fulminant colitis.

▶ Clinical Findings
A. Symptoms & Signs

Patients with acute CI usually present with crampy lower left quadrant pain and loose, bloody stools. Blood loss significant enough to lead to hemodynamic instability is atypical of CI and suggests other diagnoses. Physical examination often reveals abdominal tenderness of variable severity over the location of the affected portion of bowel. Peritoneal signs may be transiently present in reversible CI; the persistence of these signs for several hours suggests transmural infarction and mandates surgical exploration. Strictures, chronic colitis, gangrene resulting in perforation, and intraabdominal sepsis are complications of CI. Chronic CI may present with diarrhea, left-sided abdominal cramps, and gas or bloating as a result of dysmotility caused by the mismatch of blood supply to demand. Endoscopy may show mild inflammation in the left colon near the splenic flexure, but the mucosa can appear relatively normal if the ischemia is slowly developing. Many patients are asymptomatic and found to have IMA occlusion with extensive collateral blood supply to the affected colon.

B. Diagnostic Studies

Stool cultures should be obtained to exclude infectious colitis. The patient with suspected CI who does not have peritoneal signs should undergo a careful nonprepared colonoscopy within 48 hours of symptom onset. Patients with peritoneal signs should undergo urgent surgical exploration. CT scans are normal in up to 66% of patients with established CI, but may show colonic thickening, mucosal edema or pericolonic fluid and/or stranding suggestive of inflammation. Angiography using Doppler ultrasound may indicate a SMA occlusion; however, more invasive procedures, such as magnetic resonance angiogram or interventional angiography, often are required. The latter allows treatment with thrombolytics or angioplasty if required.

▶ Treatment

The patient with CI who does not have peritoneal signs should be treated with fluids, bowel rest, and broad-spectrum antibiotics. Underlying CHF or cardiac arrhythmias should be treated and vasoconstricting medications withdrawn. The patients should be monitored closely for fever, leukocytosis, or peritoneal signs. The persistence of peritoneal signs should prompt surgical exploration. Recurrence of CI occurs in only 3% to 10% of patients. Congenital or acquired thrombophilic states may account for a significant percentage of ambulatory patients presenting with CI, and should be tested.

ABDOMINAL PAIN

▶ General Principles in Older Adults

Obtaining a complete and accurate history may be difficult in older adults with abdominal pain because of cognitive impairment or sensory deficits that limit communication. At the same time, ability to mount a febrile response and the sensation of pain are limited in older patients in part because of age-related decreases in sensory function and increased use of medications, such as steroids and NSAIDs. Similarly, laboratory values may be spuriously normal in older patients despite the presence of considerable underlying disease. To prevent these factors from delaying diagnosis and treatment in older

patients, the physician must use great skill in the medical interview, physical examination, and diagnostic testing.

▶ Clinical Findings

A. Signs & Symptoms

The history should assess the chronology, character, location, and severity of the pain along with precipitating and alleviating factors. Chronology includes the onset, progression, and duration of pain. Pain of abrupt onset with rapid progression suggests a more aggressive cause. Characterization of the pain may help in diagnosis. Pain may be described as aching (appendicitis, diverticulitis, pelvic inflammatory disease), burning (GERD, perforated peptic ulcer), cramping (small bowel obstruction, biliary colic), boring (pancreatitis), excruciating (acute mesenteric ischemia), or tearing (ruptured abdominal aortic aneurysm). However, older patients may have limited pain or atypical presentations.

Location of the pain can also offer diagnostic clues. Epigastric pain and upper abdominal pain suggest a gastric, hepatobiliary, or pancreatic process. Gastric cancer can present with insidious epigastric pain or dyspepsia, and should be considered in the differential diagnosis of persistent abdominal pain. Liver disease can cause abdominal pain, usually in the RUQ, and in the case of parenchymal diseases such as viral hepatitis or nonalcoholic steatohepatitis (NASH), is a result of stretching of the liver capsule. Biliary disease, particularly gallstone obstruction, should be considered in sudden onset of RUQ pain and nausea. Acute and chronic pancreatitis can occur in older patients, and gallstones should always be looked for as a cause. Unfortunately, pancreatic cancer is also more prevalent in the geriatric age group, and may present with pain and jaundice late in the course of the disease. Midabdominal pain may represent an ileocecal process, whereas hypogastric pain suggests involvement of the colon or genitourinary structures. Shifting location of the pain may represent appendicitis or the development of peritonitis after visceral rupture. Subdiaphragmatic irritation is often referred to the shoulder. Because cardiac disease presents atypically in older adults, any complaints of upper abdominal discomfort by patients with appropriate risk factors should raise the suspicion of coronary disease.

Severe pain in the absence of commensurate physical findings should raise the suspicion of acute mesenteric ischemia. Postprandial pain suggests GUs, mesenteric ischemia, pancreatitis, cholecystitis, or biliary colic. Patients with DUs may report relief of pain with food.

A thorough medication history should be obtained. The use of NSAIDs, steroids, and anticoagulants should be noted. The possibility of drug-induced pancreatitis or hepatotoxicity should be considered.

Absence of fever in older patients should not diminish the suspicion for infection because older patients frequently do not mount an appropriate febrile response to infectious agents. The abdomen should be examined for distension, ecchymoses, abnormal masses, enlarged organs, hernias, and abnormal peristalsis. Hyperperistalsis suggests obstruction or enteritis, whereas hypoperistalsis supports the diagnosis of peritonitis. An abdominal bruit, although neither sensitive nor specific, supports the diagnosis of mesenteric ischemia. The absence of rebound tenderness in older adults should not exclude the possibility of peritonitis. Rectal and genital/pelvic examinations are an essential component of the evaluation.

B. Diagnostic Tests

A urinalysis and CBC with differential should be ordered with the caveat that older patients may have significant underlying infection with normal white blood cell counts. Serum chemistry analysis provides information regarding fluid status. Amylase, lipase, and a liver chemistry profile are appropriate in the setting of upper abdominal pain, and an abdominal ultrasound should be obtained to check for liver abnormalities, and biliary obstruction caused by stones or neoplasm. Diagnostic tests should be ordered based on the findings of the history, physical examination, and laboratory evaluation. A set of supine and upright plain abdominal films is useful in identifying obstruction, radiopaque gallstones, or a calcified pancreas. An upright chest x-ray film should be obtained to check for air under the diaphragm. Suspected hepatobiliary or pancreatic disease should be investigated by ultrasonography or CT scan. CT scanning is useful in demonstrating appendicitis, diverticulitis, bowel obstruction, retroperitoneal hemorrhage, and mesenteric lymph node enlargement, as well as hepatobiliary, pancreatic disease and cancer. Carcinoembryonic antigen (CEA) levels may be elevated in patients with GI cancer, although this is not sensitive enough to use as a screening test. Endoscopy should be performed, and biopsies of the stomach and colon taken to check for MALT (mucosal-associated lymphoid tissue) lymphoma and *H. pylori* infection. Patients suspected of having acute mesenteric ischemia should have prompt selective mesenteric angiography.

Affronti J. Biliary disease in the elderly patient. *Clin Geriatr Med.* 1999;15(3):571-578.

Becher A, Dent J. Systematic review: aging and gastro-oesophageal reflux disease symptoms, oesophageal function and reflux oesophagitis. *Aliment Pharmacol Ther.* 2011;33(4):442-454.

Arthurs ZM, Titus J, Bannazadeh M, et al. A comparison of endovascular revascularization with traditional therapy for the treatment of acute mesenteric ischemia. *J Vasc Surg.* 2011;53(3):698-705.

Brandt LJ, Boley SJ. AGA technical review on intestinal ischemia. *Gastroenterology.* 2000;118(5):954-968.

Desilets AR, Asal NJ, Dunican KC. Considerations for the use of proton pump inhibitors in older adults. *Consult Pharm.* 2012;27(2):114-120.

Esfandyari T, Potter JW, Vaezi MF. Dysphagia: a cost analysis of the diagnostic approach. *Am J Gastroenterol.* 2002:97(11): 2733-2777.

Farrell JJ, Friedman LS. Gastrointestinal bleeding in the elderly. *Gastroenterol Clin North Am.* 2001;30(2):377-407, viii.

Galmiche JP, Hatlebakk J, Attwood S, et al; LOTUS Trial Collaborators. Laparoscopic antireflux surgery vs esomeprazole treatment for chronic GERD: the LOTUS randomized clinical trial. *JAMA.* 2001;305(19):1969-1977.

Greenwald DA, Brandt LJ, Reinus JF. Ischemic bowel disease in the elderly. *Gastroenterol Clin North Am.* 2001;30(2):445-473.

Khuroo MS, Yattoo GN, Javid G, et al. A comparison of omeprazole and placebo for bleeding peptic ulcer. *N Engl J Med.* 1997;336(15):1054-1058.

Koutroubakis IE, Sfiridaki A, Theodoropoulou A, Kouroumalis EA. Role of acquired and hereditary thrombotic risk factors in colon ischemia of ambulatory patients. *Gastroenterology.* 2001;121(3):561-565.

Lau JY, Sung JJ, Lee KK, et al. Effect of intravenous omeprazole on recurrent bleeding after endoscopic treatment of peptic ulcers. *N Engl J Med.* 2000;343(5):310-316.

Lee J, Anggiansah A, Anggiansah R, Young A, Wong T, Fox M. Effects of age on the gastroesophageal junction, esophageal motility, and reflux disease. *Clin Gastroenterol Hepatol.* 2007;5(12): 1392-1398.

Martin SP, Ulrich CD 2nd. Pancreatic disease in the elderly. *Clin Geriatr Med.* 1999;15(3):579-605.

Morganstern B, Anandasabapathy S. GERD and Barrett's esophagus: diagnostic and management strategies in the geriatric population. *Geriatrics.* 2009;64(7):9-12.

Murad Y, Radi ZA, Murad M, Hall K. Inflammatory bowel disease in the geriatric population *Front Biosci (Elite Ed).* 2011;3: 945-954.

Regev A, Schiff ER. Liver disease in the elderly. *Gastroenterol Clin North Am.* 2001;30(2):547-563, x-xi.

Rolland Y, Dupuy C, Abellan van Kan G, Gillette S, Vellas B. Treatment strategies for sarcopenia and frailty. *Med Clin North Am.* 2011;95(3):427-438.

Ross SO, Forsmark CE. Pancreatic and biliary disorders in the elderly. *Gastroenterol Clin North Am.* 2001;30(2):531-545, x.

Ruotolo RA, Evans SR. Mesenteric ischemia in the elderly. *Clin Geriatr Med.* 1999;15(3):527-557.

Saif MW, Makrilia N, Zalonis A, Merikas M, Syrigos K. Gastric cancer in the elderly: an overview. *Eur J Surg Oncol.* 2010; 36(8):709-717.

Spira RM, Nissan A, Zamir O, Cohen T, Fields SI, Freund HR. Percutaneous transhepatic cholecystostomy and delayed laparoscopic cholecystectomy in critically ill patients with acute calculus cholecystitis. *Am J Surg.* 2002;183(1):62-66.

Stevens TK, Palmer RM. Fecal incontinence in long-term care patients. *Long-Term Care Interface.* 2007;8:35.

Tariq SH. Fecal incontinence in older adults. *Clin Geriatr Med.* 2007;23(4):857-869, vii.

Wang YR, Dempsey DT, Friedenberg FK, Richter JE. Trends of Heller myotomy hospitalizations for achalasia in the United States, 1993-2005: effect of surgery volume on perioperative outcomes. *Am J Gastroenterol.* 2008;103(10):2454-2464.

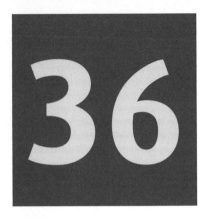

Constipation

Alayne Markland, DO, MSc

▶ Constipation is common in older adults and requires careful assessment to rule out mechanical causes.

▶ May present with other abdominal complaints, such as pain, bloating, and/or gas.

▶ May involve infrequent defecation, difficulty passing stool, or incomplete evacuation of stool.

▶ A diagnosis of chronic constipation requires the presence of symptoms for at least 12 weeks.

General Principles in Older Adults

Chronic constipation is one of the most frequent gastrointestinal disorders encountered among older adults in clinical practice. Constipation is often associated with other abdominal complaints (pain, bloating, and gas), as well as decreased overall well-being. It may involve infrequent defecation, difficulty in passing stool, or incomplete evacuation of stool. Physicians often define constipation as infrequent passage of stool; however, patients often define it as straining to defecate or sensation of incomplete evacuation. For chronic constipation to be diagnosed, symptoms should be present for at least 12 weeks.

Chronic constipation disproportionately affects older individuals with an estimated prevalence of 40% among people older than age 65 years. Women are also at increased risk, having 2–3 times more constipation than men. African Americans also exhibit increased risk. Many community-dwelling older adults commonly use nonprescription preparations, such as stimulant and bulking laxatives. Nearly 85% of physician visits for constipation result in a prescription for laxatives and more than $820 million are spent per year on nonprescription agents. Few resources are available to health care providers to guide them in an evidence-based approach to this common problem.

Clinical Findings

A. Symptoms & Signs

Symptoms of constipation reported by patients often differ from definitions and classification from clinical criteria. Patients often report symptoms related to bloating, fullness, and incomplete evacuation. However, clinicians often focus on stool frequency and consistency to define constipation. The Rome III criteria, published in 2006, define chronic constipation as symptoms that have persisted for the past 3 months with an onset at least 6 months prior to diagnosis, with the following 3 criteria being met:

1. Must include 2 or more of the following:
   a. Hard or lumpy stool in ≥25% of defecations
   b. Straining during ≥25% defecations
   c. Sensation of incomplete evacuation for at least 25% of defecations
   d. Sensation of anorectal obstruction or blockage for ≥25% of defecations
   e. Manual maneuvers to facilitate ≥25% of defecations (eg, digital evacuation, support of the pelvic floor)
   f. Fewer than 3 defecations per week
2. Loose stools are rarely present without use of laxatives
3. Insufficient criteria for irritable bowel syndrome (IBS)

Differentiating symptoms of chronic constipation from IBS with constipation (IBS-C) may not be as important in older adults, as age ≥50 years is associated with lower rates of IBS. However, management can differ between the 2 diagnoses. IBS-C is defined by recurrent abdominal pain or discomfort for at least 3 days per month in the previous 3 months (onset ≥6 months prior to the diagnosis) that is associated with at least 2 of the following:

1. Improvement of pain or discomfort upon defecation
2. Onset associated with change in frequency of stool
3. Onset associated with a change in form or appearance of stool

Symptoms of hematochezia, family history of colon cancer/inflammatory bowel disease, anemia, positive fecal occult blood test, unexplained weight loss ≥10 pounds, constipation that is refractory to treatment, and new-onset constipation without evidence of potential primary cause are all considered "alarm" symptoms and may necessitate further evaluation with more invasive testing, if indicated.

B. Diagnostic Studies

In most cases, patients with chronic constipation do not warrant extensive diagnostic evaluation. Older patients who have "alarm" symptoms should consider the benefits and risks of doing further evaluation with colonoscopy or other invasive testing.

The clinical evaluation should consist of a thorough history containing the above questions and an appropriate physical examination and laboratory testing. Physical examination should be performed, including a rectal exam, palpating for hard stool, assessing for masses, anal fissures, sphincter tone, prostatic hypertrophy in males, hemorrhoids, push effort during attempted defecation, and posterior vaginal masses in women. Laboratory testing should include a complete blood count, serum calcium, thyroid function tests, and fecal occult blood testing. It is also important to ask about stool frequency, consistency, and other associated symptoms, such as straining and fecal incontinence (see "Fecal Impaction" below). Radiologic examination with abdominal plain films may also detect significant stool retention in the colon and suggest the diagnosis of megacolon. Marker studies or colonic transit studies can be used in patients with infrequent defecation. A marker study involves ingestion of radiopaque markers with a subsequent abdominal radiograph to detect the markers in the right, left, or rectosigmoid colon. Other forms of transit time evaluation with radioactive tracers and wireless motility capsule technologies (that record data after ingestion) are also available.

▶ Differential Diagnosis

The causes of constipation can be categorized as primary (types of constipation) or secondary (eg, caused by a medical diagnosis or use of medications) in nature. Table 36–1 lists primary causes of constipation and Table 36–2 lists secondary causes.

Table 36–1. Primary pathophysiologic causes of chronic constipation.

Type	Characteristics
1. Normal transit constipation	Most common subtype Transit and stool frequency are within normal ranges but patients complain of constipation, bloating, and pain[a]
2. Slow-transit constipation	Increased intestinal transit time Reduced colonic motility Multiple etiologies—gut, cellular, and protein-level responses
3. Defecatory dysfunction	More common in older adults and women Structural problems seen on anorectal manometry and defecography Pelvic floor dyssynergia (failure to relax or inappropriate contraction of puborectalis muscle and external anal sphincter during defecation) Pathogenesis not well understood

[a]Presence of pain increases the likelihood of a diagnosis of IBS-C instead of chronic constipation.

Many prescription drugs have constipation and slowed colonic motility as side effects. Constipation-inducing medications in older adults include opioids, anabolic steroids, anticonvulsants, anticholinergic agents, antihypertensive agents, tricyclic antidepressants, antiparkinsonian agents, antipsychotics, diuretics, and sympathomimetic drugs. Nonprescription agents also implicated in causing constipation include antihistamines, calcium supplements, iron supplements, antidiarrheal agents, nonsteroidal antiinflammatory drugs (NSAIDs), and calcium- and aluminum-containing antacids.

Table 36–2. Secondary causes of chronic constipation in older adults.

- Malignancy
- Medications/polypharmacy (prescription and nonprescription drugs, including opioids)
- Endocrine/metabolic (diabetes mellitus, hypothyroidism, hypercalcemia, hypokalemia)
- Neurologic disorders (Parkinson disease, diabetic autonomic neuropathy, spinal cord injury, dementia, stroke)
- Rheumatologic disorders (systemic sclerosis and other connective tissue disorders)
- Psychological disorders (depression or eating disorders)
- Anatomic dysfunction (strictures, postsurgical abnormalities, anal fissures, megacolon, hemorrhoids)
- Decreased mobility/sedentary lifestyle

Treatment

Once secondary causes of constipation have been evaluated and addressed as possible, the management of constipation varies according to type. The treatment and prevention of slow-transit constipation includes patient education about bowel habits, dietary changes, and drug therapies. Management of dyssynergic defecation involves biofeedback, relaxation exercises, and suppository programs. Patients with slow-transit and dyssynergic defecation should receive treatment for the dyssynergia first before other measures are started.

A. Nonpharmacologic Therapy

Nonpharmacologic treatment options or lifestyle modifications involve diet, exercise, and biofeedback (if dyssynergic defecation is diagnosed). Very little clinical trial evidence exists to support dietary and exercise recommendations that are recommended to prevent or treat constipation, especially in older adults.

Dietary options include increasing fluid and fiber. In one study of 883 people >70 years of age, there was no association between estimated fluid intake and constipation; however, in 21,000 nursing home residents a weak association was found between decreased fluid intake and constipation. Adequate fluid intake may be an important general health recommendation and may also impact treatment of constipation, especially with fiber supplementation. The daily recommended amount of fiber is 20–35 g/day, but most Americans only consume 5–10 g/day. Increasing daily fiber intake through dietary measures is recommended. Information should be given on the fiber contained in common foods. Patients should increase fiber intake slowly—5 g/day at 1-week intervals—until the recommended intake is attained. Patients should be informed that an immediate response is not expected, and that flatus and bloating may occur, but are usually temporary. Increasing fiber intake gradually may help with some of these unwanted side effects.

Probiotics have also been tested for the treatment of constipation. *Lactobacillus* and *Bifidobacterium* are symbiotics flora in the large intestine that may promote colonic mucosal health. Low levels of both have been reported in individuals with chronic constipation. Although properly controlled trials are lacking, some prospective evidence does report efficacy of probiotics (*Lactobacillus*) improving constipation in nursing home residents. Survival and viability of these probiotic bacteria in a commercial form has not been standardized for these treatments to have high levels of evidence for clinical use.

Increased physical activity is associated with lower rates of constipation in older adults. Physical inactivity may also be associated with reduced colonic transit time. Exercise should be encouraged in older adults, when appropriate.

Biofeedback is an effective treatment for dyssynergic defecation, which is characterized by paradoxical contraction or failure to relax the pelvic floor muscles during defecation. Biofeedback can involve both sensory training and muscle contraction/relaxation techniques. In patients with dyssynergic defecation, biofeedback was consistently found to be more effective than continuous use of polyethylene glycol (PEG, MiraLAX), standard therapy (other types of stool softeners and laxatives), sham therapy (therapy aimed at overall body relaxation), or the use of diazepam in 4 randomized controlled trials. However, trials are needed to determine the efficacy of biofeedback in older adults.

Many people will have already tried fluids, fiber, and fitness, but often not in a sustained manner. Most Americans do not consume enough dietary fiber and increasing the intake of fiber and fluids may be enough to help prevent constipation in healthy older adults. Consideration may also involve nutritional expertise, physical therapy (when appropriate), and family/caregivers in making dietary and exercise changes for the treatment of constipation. Preventing and treating constipation with nonpharmacologic and pharmacologic treatments may be needed for older adults in specific situations—that is, in the postoperative period, during hospitalization, or other health care environments when decreased mobility is anticipated—and when using acute or chronic opioid medications.

B. Pharmacologic Therapy (Including Nonprescription Preparations)

The main categories of medications for prevention of constipation (nonprescription preparations) are bulking agents, stool softeners/emollients, and osmotic agents. The main categories for the treatment of chronic constipation are bulking agents, stool softeners/emollients, osmotic agents, stimulants, chloride change activators, 5-HT$_4$ receptor agonists, and guanylate cyclase-c receptor agonists. Table 36–3 lists the pharmacologic treatments for constipation based on existing evidence from the American College of Gastroenterology Chronic Constipation Task Force.

1. Bulking agents—Bulking agents expand with water to increase the bulk of the stool with the result of having softer stool. Patients may need to try different types of fiber to achieve the desired outcome, including minimization of side effects. Some patients may better tolerate soluble and synthetic bulking agents than insoluble agents. Adequate hydration with bulking agents may be necessary for the desired outcome. Patients taking fiber need to increase their fluid intake to 30 mL/kg of body weight daily to avoid worsening of constipation or impaction. Fiber may also inhibit the absorption of other drugs and should be taken 1 hour before or 2 hours after other medications. Bulking agents should also be increased slowly over weekly periods to avoid side effects, similar to increasing dietary fiber consumption. Bulking agents are considered to be first-line agents for constipation. However, many older adults may not be good candidates for

Table 36–3. Evidence-based pharmacologic management options for chronic constipation.

Therapy	Recommendations
Bulking agents	
Psyllium	Grade A
Calcium polycarbophil	Grade B
Methylcellulose	Grade B
Stool softeners/emollients	
Docusate calcium/sodium	Grade B
Mineral oil (linked with aspiration in older adults)	Grade C
Osmotic laxatives	
Lactulose	Grade A
Sorbitol	Grade B
PEG (polyethylene glycol)	Grade A
Magnesium hydroxide	Grade C
Stimulants	
Senna	Grade A
Bisacodyl	Grade A
5-HT$_4$ (serotonin) agonists	
Tegaserod maleate	Grade -[a]
Prucalopride (not available in U.S.)	Grade A
Chloride channel activator	
Lubiprostone	Grade A[b]
Guanylate cyclase-C receptor antagonists	
Linaclotide	Grade A

Grade A: evidence from ≥2 randomized, controlled trials (RCT) with adequate samples sizes, good design, and results at the p <0.05 level.
Grade B: evidence from a single, high-quality RCT as defined for Grade A, or recommendations based on evidence from ≥2 RCTs with conflicting evidence or inadequate sample sizes.
Grade C: no RCT data.

[a]Tegaserod was approved for the treatment of IBS-C in women <65 years old. The FDA removed it from the market in 2007 for increased risk of cardiovascular events.
[b]Data exist for adults >65 years of age without significant comorbid disorders.

using a bulking agent. Some examples of when bulking agents may not be the first-line agent for older adults with constipation include when taking high doses of narcotic medications, difficulty with swallowing or dysphagia (because of the consistency of certain types of fiber when mixed with water), anyone with surgical resection of the majority of the colon, patients who have a suspected rectal mass or possible bowel obstruction, and older adults who do not consume adequate amounts of fluid.

2. Stool softeners and emollients—Stool softeners and emollients are effective by having a detergent effect on the stool consistency. This class of medications for constipation is well tolerated and does not interfere with other medications. Although no placebo-controlled trials exist for the use of these medications, in a study in 170 patients, psyllium husk was as effective for softening stools and had similar overall efficacy as docusate. Mineral oil is also an emollient and may help lubricate the stool through the colon. Aspiration and lipoid pneumonia are known risks of using mineral oil in older adults. Stool softeners are often used when bulking agents do not work or are not preferred. Because of their mechanism of action as a detergent, stool softeners can also be used in combination with bulking agents. Like bulking agents, stool softeners alone are not good treatments for older adults on narcotic medications who have constipation.

3. Osmotic laxatives—Osmotic laxatives promote the secretion of water into the intestinal lumen by osmotic activity and the hyperosmolar nature of these medications. PEG has the best evidence of use and is now available over-the-counter as a treatment for occasional constipation. It improves stool frequency and consistency in patients with chronic constipation. Studies suggest that PEG can be dose adjusted or used every other day with efficacy. An open-label study with 117 participants, ≥65 years of age, using PEG over 12 months reported relatively few side effects and no serious adverse events related to the medication. A recent evidence-based review article concluded that PEG may be better for constipation symptoms than lactulose. Common use of PEG or magnesium hydroxide-containing preparations (milk of magnesia) in patients with congestive heart failure or chronic renal disease should be done with extreme caution as they can cause electrolyte imbalances, such as hypokalemia and diarrhea, further worsening fluid–electrolyte balances. Osmotic agents are useful when first-line bulking agents and/or stool softeners are not effective.

4. Stimulants—Stimulants, such as senna and bisacodyl-containing compounds, increase intestinal motility by increasing peristaltic contractions. Stimulants also decrease water absorption from the lumen. Patients usually report more unfavorable side effects from these medications: abdominal discomfort and cramping. Evidence exists for using bisacodyl given placebo-controlled studies. Evidence also exists for senna, although fewer clinical trials exist comparing senna to placebo than that for bisacodyl. There is no evidence to support that long-term use of stimulant laxatives damages the enteric nervous system. Stimulant laxatives have been associated with melanosis coli. The presence of melanosis coli (which may be seen on colonscopy) is a marker of chronic laxative use and may not indicate any other clinical consequences.

5. 5-HT$_4$ (serotonin) agonists—5-Hydroxytryptamine receptor subtype 4 (5-HT$_4$) receptors are found in the colon and mediate the release of other neurotransmitters that may initiate peristaltic action. These prokinetic agents enhance gastrointestinal motility by increasing intestinal contractions. These drugs are no longer marketed in the United States, and little data exist for use in older adults. Other prokinetic agents, such as metoclopramide and erythromycin, have not been formally evaluated for the treatment of constipation. Because of the side-effect profile in older adults, metoclopramide should not be used for chronic constipation.

6. Colonic secretagogues (increases intestinal fluid secretion)

a. Chloride channel activators—Lubiprostone is a chloride channel activator that improves motility in the intestine by increasing intestinal fluid secretion without altering serum electrolyte concentrations. Retrospective data from 3 pooled clinical trials of lubiprostone in older patients (n = 57) without significant comorbidities showed improvement in stool frequency, stool consistency, and decreased straining compared to patients taking placebo. The side effects of this medication include nausea, diarrhea, headache, abdominal distention, and abdominal pain, and are generally well-tolerated.

b. Guanylate cyclase C receptor antagonists—Linaclotide is another colonic secretagogue that stimulates intestinal fluid secretion and transit. Two large phase 3 trials have been performed in patients with chronic constipation, and the linaclotide-treated groups had significantly higher rates of 3 or more complete spontaneous bowel movements per week and in increase in 1 or more complete spontaneous bowel movements from baseline during at least 9 of 12 weeks compared with placebo. The most common adverse event was diarrhea, which led to discontinuation of treatment in approximately 4% of patients. The long-term risks and benefits of linaclotide in treating chronic constipation remain unknown.

c. Opioid antagonists—Two peripherally acting *mu* opioid receptor antagonists exist that may have some role in the treatment of opiate-induced constipation and paralytic ileus (alvimopan and methylnaltrexone). Data are lacking currently in older adults. These medications act peripherally and do not cross the blood brain barrier, thus not affecting the analgesic properties of opioids.

▶ Fecal Impaction

Constipation is an important factor in the development of fecal impaction in older adults, especially in those who have limited mobility in the community and in long-term care settings. Fecal impaction results from an individual's lack of ability to sense and respond to the presence of stool in the rectum. Mobility and decreased rectal sensation contribute to fecal impaction in older adults.

To diagnosis fecal impaction, a digital rectal examination is very important. Although impacted stool may not be a hard consistency, the key to diagnosis is finding a large amount of stool in the rectum. Fecal impaction can also occur in the proximal rectum or sigmoid colon, which would not be detected on digital rectal examination. If fecal impaction is suspected, obtaining an abdominal radiograph may help identify the area of impaction.

The management of fecal impaction involves disimpaction and colon evacuation, followed by a maintenance bowel regimen. Digital disimpaction can be used to fragment a large amount fecal material in the rectum. Following digital disimpaction, a warm-water enema with mineral oil may be used to soften the impaction and assist with emptying the stool from the impacted area. Very little evidence exists for guiding the treatment of fecal impaction. However, if conservative measures with digital disimpaction and enemas fail, local anesthesia to relax the anal canal along with abdominal massage may be useful. In rare cases, using a colonoscopy with a snare to fragment the fecal material in the distal colon may be needed. If at any time, abdominal tenderness or bleeding occurs, which may indicate bowel perforation or ischemia, surgery may be necessary.

Brandt LJ, Prather CM, Quigley EM, Schiller LR, Schoenfeld P, Talley NJ. Systematic review on the management of chronic constipation in North America. *Am J Gastroenterol.* 2005;100 Suppl 1:S5-S21.

Gallegos-Orozco JF, Foxx-Orenstein AE, Sterler SM, Stoa JM. Chronic constipation in the elderly. *Am J Gastroenterol.* 2012;107(1):18-25.

Higgins PDR, Johanson JF. Epidemiology of constipation in North America: a systematic review. *Am J Gastroenterol.* 2004;99(4):750-759.

Lee-Robichaud H, Thomas K, Morgan J, Nelson RL. Lactulose versus polyethylene glycol for chronic constipation. *Cochrane Database Syst Rev.* 2010;(7):CD007570.

Lembo A, Camilleri M. Chronic constipation. *N Engl J Med.* 2003;349(14):1360-1368.

Leung L, Riutta T, Lotecha J, Rosser W. Chronic constipation: an evidence-based review. *J Am Board Fam Med.* 2011;24(4):436-451.

Longstreth GF, Thompson WG, Chey WD, Houghton LA, Mearin F, Spiller RC. Functional bowel disorders. *Gastroenterology.* 2006;130(5):1480-1491.

Rao SS, Go JT. Update on the management of constipation in the elderly: new treatment options. *Clin Interv Aging.* 2010;5:163-171.

Wald A. Constipation in the primary care setting: current concepts and misconceptions. *Am J Med.* 2006;119(9):736-739.

USEFUL WEBSITES

National Digestive Diseases Information Clearinghouse. *Constipation*; http://digestive.niddk.nih.gov/ddiseases/pubs/constipation/

National Institute on Aging. *AgePage: Concerned About Constipation?* http://www.nia.nih.gov/health/publication/concerned-about-constipation

The Rome Foundation. http://romecriteria.org/

Fluid & Electrolyte Abnormalities

37

Mariko Koya Wong, MD
Kellie Hunter Campbell, MD, MA

ESSENTIALS OF DIAGNOSIS

- ▶ Hyponatremia is commonly defined as a serum sodium concentration less than 135 mEq/L (or 135 mmol/L).
- ▶ Hypernatremia is commonly defined as a serum sodium greater than 148 mEq/L (or 148 mmol/L).
- ▶ Hypokalemia is typically defined as a serum potassium concentration of less than 3.5 mEq/L.
- ▶ Hyperkalemia is typically defined as a serum potassium concentration greater than 5.0 mEq/L.
- ▶ Nocturnal polyuria is present when urine production during 8 hours of sleep is >33% of 24-hour urine production, nighttime urine production rate is >0.9 mL/min *or* 7 PM to 7 AM urine volume is >50% of total 24-hour volume.

General Principles in Older Adults

Fluid and electrolyte abnormalities are common among older adults as a consequence of age-related functional changes in the kidney, multiple comorbidities, and polypharmacy. This chapter discusses concepts of sodium disorders, potassium disorders, and nocturnal polyuria as they relate to older adults.

HYPONATREMIA

General Principles in Older Adults

Older adults are more vulnerable to developing sodium disorders as a result of age-related changes in water and sodium metabolism. Older adults may have an impaired ability to excrete water and to dilute urine because of reductions in the number of functioning nephrons and decreased renal blood

flow with age, predisposing them to water overload and possible hyponatremia. Geriatric patients also tend to be on multiple medications that are associated with sodium disorders, such as diuretics and psychotropic medications (Table 37–1). Reviewing all medications is an integral part of evaluating patients with sodium disorders.

Hyponatremia is commonly defined as a serum sodium concentration less than 135 mEq/L (or 135 mmol/L). This occurs in 7% to 11% of older patients and up to 50% of older hospitalized patients.

▶ Pathogenesis

A. Hypervolemic Hyponatremia

In older adults, the most common etiology of hyponatremia is increased intake and subsequent retention of water. This type of hyponatremia is commonly described as dilutional or hypervolemic hyponatremia. These patients typically will exhibit edematous states, resulting from conditions such as congestive heart failure, cirrhosis, or the nephrotic syndrome. These conditions decrease effective circulating blood volume, leading to increased antidiuretic hormone (ADH) secretion, which results in water retention. Dilutional hyponatremia can also be iatrogenic, as a result of administration of excess IV fluids, especially in hospitalized patients.

B. Hypovolemic Hyponatremia

Although less common, salt depletion with or without loss of extracellular fluid, can cause depletional or hypovolemic hyponatremia. Hypovolemic hyponatremia can be caused by renal losses (eg, diuretic use) or from extrarenal losses, such as vomiting, diarrhea, laxative abuse, ostomies, or the presence of large burns. A particular etiology to consider in geriatric patients is restricted sodium intake, especially in the setting of tube feeding.

Table 37–1. Medications associated with hyponatremia.

Class of Drug	Examples
Antipsychotics	Fluphenazine, thiothixene, phenothiazine, haloperidol
Antidepressants	TCAs, MAOIs, SSRIs (especially fluoxetine)
Anticonvulsants	Carbamazepine
Diuretics	Loop diuretics, thiazides
ACE inhibitors	Lisinopril, enalapril, ramipril
Chemotherapeutic agents	Vincristine, vinblastine, cyclophosphamide, cisplatin, methotrexate

ACE, Angiotensin-converting enzyme; MAOI, monoamine oxidase inhibitor; SSRI, selective serotonin reuptake inhibitor; TCA, tricyclic antidepressant.

Adapted with permission from Liamis G, Milionis H, Elisaf M. A review of drug-induced hyponatremia. *Am J Kidney Dis*. 2008 Jul;52(1): 144-153. © Elsevier.

C. Euvolemic Hyponatremia

The syndrome of inappropriate secretion of antidiuretic hormone (SIADH) is a disorder in which water excretion is partially impaired because of the inability to suppress secretion of ADH. Patients with SIADH will generally appear euvolemic. Many diseases that are common in older adults are associated with SIADH such as central nervous system disorders and malignancies (Table 37–2). In addition, although rare, older age itself may be a risk factor for SIADH. Medications (Table 37–1) are also an important cause of SIADH. As a result of multimorbidity, older adults are at

Table 37–2. Diseases associated with SIADH.

Central Nervous System Diseases	Stroke, Hemorrhage, Vasculitis, Tumor, Trauma, Infection
Malignancies	Small cell carcinoma of the lung (most commonly associated), cancers of the pancreas and bowel, lymphoma
Inflammatory lung diseases	Infection (such as pneumonia, lung abscesses, tuberculosis) bronchiectasis, atelectasis, acute respiratory failure, positive pressure ventilation
Endocrine	Hypothyroidism, adrenal insufficiency
Others	Acute psychosis, pain, postoperative state, severe hypokalemia
Idiopathic	Advanced age itself can be a risk factor for hyponatremia

Adapted with permission from Fried LF, Palevsky PM. Hyponatremia and hypernatremia. *Med Clin North Am*. 1997 May;81(3):585-609. © Elsevier.

higher risk for polypharmacy, typically defined as the use of 5 or more medications. In older patients, careful medication review is imperative. Other causes of euvolemic hyponatremia include hypothyroidism and adrenal insufficiency. An elevated serum potassium level in conjunction with hyponatremia should increase suspicion for adrenal insufficiency. Lastly, it is important to include pseudohyponatremia in the differential, which can occur in the setting of hyperlipidemia or hyperproteinemia.

▶ Clinical Findings

A. Symptoms & Signs

The primary symptoms for sodium disorders (hyper- or hyponatremia) are neurologic. Slow changes in serum sodium concentration (chronic hyponatremia) are more likely to be asymptomatic as the brain has had time to adapt to osmotic changes. Symptoms associated with hyponatremia include anorexia, nausea, vomiting, headache, weakness, loss of coordination, muscle cramps, agitation, tremors, disorientation, psychosis, delirium, seizures, and coma. Patients with chronic hyponatremia are more prone to have marked gait and attention impairments leading to increased risk of falls.

B. Evaluation of Volume Status

After obtaining the history, the next step in the work-up of a patient with hyponatremia is to evaluate the volume status. Patients who are hypovolemic may have dry mucous membranes, tachycardia, and/or relative or orthostatic hypotension. On the other hand, hypervolemic patients may have increased jugular vein pressures, crackles at lung bases, ascites, and/or peripheral edema.

C. Laboratory Findings

On laboratory exam, serum osmolality, urine osmolality, and urine sodium should be obtained. Hyponatremia secondary to pseudohyponatremia or hyperglycemia will have a normal serum osmolality while all other etiologies will demonstrate a low serum osmolality. Urine osmolality of more than 100 mOsm/kg is consistent with an inability to normally excrete water, which is generally caused by SIADH or low effective circulating volume depletion, such as true hypovolemia, heart failure, and cirrhosis. Urine sodium is useful in differentiating between the two. A urine sodium of less than 25 mEq/L suggests hypovolemia and more than 40 mEq/L suggests SIADH.

▶ Treatment

Treatment of hyponatremia is based on the presence of symptoms, the severity of symptoms when present, and the acuity of the condition.

A. Acute Hyponatremia

Asymptomatic patients with acute hyponatremia may be treated like those with chronic hyponatremia (see below). Otherwise, therapy is aimed at correcting the major symptomatic consequences of hyponatremia while avoiding induction of central pontine myelinolysis (CPM). In patients with severe hyponatremia (serum sodium below 120 mEq/L) with severe neurologic symptoms such as seizures, the use of 3% hypertonic IV saline is recommended. In the first 2–3 hours, the saline should be infused to increase the serum sodium by 1–2 mEq/L per hour. Then the infusion should be slowed to increase the serum sodium an additional 8–12 mEq/L over the next 24 hours. The rate of infusion for each patient based on the desired change in the serum sodium can be calculated using the following formula:

Change in serum sodium in older men
= (infusate Na – serum Na)/[(0.50 × body weight) + 1]

Change in serum sodium in older women
= (infusate Na – serum Na)/[(0.45 × body weight) + 1]

These equations have limitations and thus the actual change in serum sodium may differ. The equations should be used to guide the initial infusion rate, which should then be adjusted by obtaining frequent serum sodium levels to avoid rapid overcorrection, which can cause CPM. Symptoms of CPM include behavioral disturbances, movement disorders, and seizures, usually occurring several days after treatment. Furosemide can be used in conjunction with IV hypertonic saline to limit treatment-induced expansion of extracellular fluid volume.

B. Chronic Hyponatremia

The goal is to identify underlying causes and intervene appropriately. For example, patients who are hyponatremic because of volume depletion secondary to diuretic use should hold their diuretics and receive volume repletion, such as IV isotonic saline. In contrast, patients with SIADH will not benefit from IV isotonic saline as the infused salt will be excreted in the concentrated urine, resulting in net retention of water and worsening of their hyponatremia. In these patients, long-term water restriction may be needed. Use of demeclocycline in patients who do not respond to water restriction is also an option.

HYPERNATREMIA

▷ General Principles in Older Adults

Older adults have a decreased ability to concentrate urine and a reduced sensation of thirst, which, if combined with limited access to fluids, may predispose older adults to water depletion and hypernatremia. Hypernatremia is commonly defined as a serum sodium greater than 148 mEq/L (or 148 mmol/L).

Hypernatremia is associated with high mortality. In hospitalized patients 65 years and older, the prevalence is approximately 1%, and the mortality rate is 7 times that of age-matched hospitalized patients. In a study of patients with hypernatremia in short-term and long-term geriatric care units, the mortality was roughly 40%.

▷ Pathogenesis

There are 4 clinical conditions that can lead to hypernatremia in older patients. In many patients, there will be overlap of these conditions. Hypernatremia usually results from excessive loss of body water relative to the loss of sodium, and in older patients hypernatremia is most often associated with inadequate fluid intake. Hypernatremia secondary to excess salt intake is rare.

A. Insufficient Intake

There are multiple reasons why older adults may have inadequate fluid intake. Many older adults, have impaired thirst or hypodipsia. Cognitive impairment such as underlying dementia and decreased level of consciousness such as delirium especially in the hospital setting present barriers to adequate hydration. Another common cause of insufficient fluid intake in older adults is impaired mobility or dependence on caregivers for access to water. Older adults with dysphagia may also have inadequate fluid intake.

B. Loss of Water

This is seen with increased insensible losses (eg, from fever) and in diabetes insipidus. Diabetes insipidus (DI) is a syndrome characterized by hypotonic polyuria from either inadequate ADH secretion (central DI) or inadequate renal response to ADH (nephrogenic DI). Nephrogenic DI can be induced by drugs such as lithium and cisplatin. Patients with DI usually compensate by increasing their fluid intake; thus, when they have adequate access to water, most patients maintain normal sodium concentrations. It is when they have limited access to water or have inadequate intake, that they usually develop hypernatremia.

C. Water Deficiency in Excess of Salt Deficiency

This can be caused by gastrointestinal losses, such as vomiting and diarrhea; or renal losses, such as osmotic diuresis secondary to hyperglycemia, solute load with parenteral nutrition, tube feeding, or IV contrast. Diuretics can lead to excess renal loss as well. Skin losses can occur from burns and severe dermatitis.

D. Salt Excess

This is usually iatrogenic, for example, from the administration of excess saline or sodium bicarbonate.

▶ Clinical Findings

Symptoms of hypernatremia include confusion, restlessness, hyperreflexia, progressive obtundation, coma, and, in severe cases, death.

▶ Treatment

The main goal of treatment is to administer dilute fluids to replace the water deficit and to limit further water loss. The first step is calculation of the total body water deficit.

Water deficit in older men = body weight
$\times$ 0.50(Pna−140)/Pna

Water deficit in older women = body weight
$\times$ 0.45(Pna−140)/Pna

where Pna = sodium concentration in mEq/L, weight in kg.

The next step is to determine the rate at which to correct the hypernatremia. In general, efforts should be made to replace the total water deficit over a 48-hour period, with a decrease in serum sodium of no more than 0.5 mEq/L per hour. The serum sodium level should be monitored frequently. Replacement fluid should be similar in osmolality as that of the bodily fluid lost. In general, hypotonic fluids, usually 0.5% normal saline (NS), should be used for replacement. In the setting of asymptomatic or chronic hypernatremia, oral fluid replacement is preferred. However, because hypernatremia is usually a result of insufficient intake from impaired thirst or inability to respond to thirst, older patients more commonly require hospitalization and correction with IV fluids.

Treatment of DI differs in that (in addition to the correction of water deficit as above) efforts must be made to reduce the excessive urinary water loss. In central DI, intranasal or oral desmopressin is used. In nephrogenic DI, treatment includes sodium restriction and administration of a thiazide diuretic plus a prostaglandin synthesis inhibitor such as indomethacin or ibuprofen.

POTASSIUM DISORDERS

▶ General Principles in Older Adults

Although less common than disorders of sodium balance, disorders of potassium balance can have serious consequences for older adults. Older adults are susceptible to disorders of potassium balance for several reasons—underlying changes in the structure and function of the kidney that occur with aging, common chronic medical conditions that disrupt potassium homeostasis, and polypharmacy that affects potassium regulation.

HYPOKALEMIA

Hypokalemia is typically defined as a serum potassium concentration of <3.5 mEq/L.

▶ Pathogenesis

Hypokalemia is usually a result of depletion of serum potassium from extrarenal losses, intrarenal losses, or iatrogenic causes. Rarely, hypokalemia can result from an acute shift of potassium from the extracellular compartment into cells.

A. Extrarenal Losses

Extrarenal losses of potassium occur in the GI tract. Chronic diarrhea can cause a loss of serum potassium because of an increase in stool volume. Among older adults, diarrhea is associated with many commonly prescribed medications, including antibiotics, proton pump inhibitors, allopurinol, neuroleptics, serotonin reuptake inhibitors, and angiotensin II receptor blockers. More rarely, diarrhea may occur because of malabsorptive disorders or GI infections. Habitual laxative use can also result in loss of potassium. As many as one-third of older adults suffer from chronic constipation and resort to chronic use of laxatives.

Though not a cause of potassium depletion, decreased nutritional intake of potassium can potentiate the hypokalemia caused by extrarenal losses. Older adults may have limited nutrition because of impaired access as a result of financial constraints or institutionalization, or because of poor dentition or swallowing disorders.

B. Intrarenal Losses

Intrarenal losses of potassium occur as a result of conditions that directly affect the kidney. These include renal tubular acidosis (types I and II), vitamin D deficiency, malignancy, medications, acute kidney injury, postobstructive and osmotic diuresis (Table 37–3). Other conditions that may result in intrarenal losses of potassium, although less commonly in older adults, include diabetic ketoacidosis and ureterosigmoidectomy.

C. Iatrogenic Causes

The most common cause of hypokalemia among older adults is medications. Thiazide and loop diuretics are commonly prescribed to older adults for management of blood pressure, congestive heart failure, and edema. Mineralocorticoids and glucocorticoids may also affect potassium levels, although they do not exert direct effects on the kidney. Medications that cause transcellular shifts in potassium are generally transient with reversibility within several hours of administration. Selective β_2-sympathomimetic agonists such as pseudoepinephrine and albuterol, xanthines including theophylline, and high doses of calcium channel blockers such as verapamil can cause transient shifts of potassium into cells (Table 37–4).

▶ Clinical Findings

Although mild hypokalemia is generally asymptomatic, more severe hypokalemia (less than 3 mEq/L) can result

Table 37-3. Intrarenal causes of hypokalemia.

	Mechanism of Action	Etiology in Older Adults
Renal tubular acidosis type I	Distal effects on collecting tubules leading to inappropriate secretion of hydrogen into the urine	Obstructive uropathy from benign prostatic hyperplasia, prostate cancer Autoimmune disease
Renal tubular acidosis type II	Proximal tubules are affected resulting in failed bicarbonate reabsorption	Vitamin D deficiency Malignancy Medications such as carbonic anhydrase inhibitors
Acute kidney injury	Renal hypoperfusion or toxic injury Insufficient delivery of sodium and water within the nephron and decreased potassium excretion	Baseline reduction in kidney function Comorbidities such as hypertension and diabetes that predispose to chronic kidney disease
Postobstructive diuresis	Decreased ability to reabsorb sodium in the distal tubules; inability to concentrate urine; increased tubular transit flow that reduces the time for reabsorption of sodium and water	Hospitalized patients after treatment for obstructive uropathy

in neuromuscular weakness, including paralysis and respiratory muscle dysfunction, rhabdomyolysis, GI disruption including constipation and ileus, and cardiac dysregulation evidenced by electrocardiogram (ECG) changes and cardiac arrhythmias.

▶ Treatment

Because only a small portion of total-body potassium is present in the extracellular space, estimation of potassium deficiency from serum potassium levels is crude. In general, each 1 mEq/L decrease is equivalent to between 150 and 400 mEq/L in total-body potassium. For older adults with decreased muscle mass, the lower estimates are most appropriate.

Treatment of hypokalemia involves replacement of potassium. However, supplemental administration of potassium can be dangerous because of the high risk of severe hyperkalemia, particularly in hospitalized patients and those with underlying chronic kidney disease. Intravenous potassium is

associated with the highest risk of hyperkalemia and should be avoided if possible. Oral potassium supplementation is preferable. Generally potassium chloride is the preferred choice for potassium repletion because it effectively treats most causes of hypokalemia. Potassium phosphate may be used in situations where phosphate replacement is also required. Potassium bicarbonate may be used in the setting of metabolic acidosis. For older patients on diuretics, instruction in adequate potassium intake through the diet is important. Also combining a potassium-sparing diuretic (amiloride, triamterene, or spironolactone) may offset potassium loses from thiazide or loop diuretics. However, caution must be taken to avoid overcorrection that results in hyperkalemia.

HYPERKALEMIA

Hyperkalemia is typically defined as a serum potassium concentration >5 mEq/L.

▶ Pathogenesis

Hyperkalemia is the result of underlying physiologic and pathophysiologic changes that commonly occur in older adults which predispose to elevated potassium levels and is augmented by iatrogenic factors. Age-related changes in the kidney include the development of glomerulosclerosis and arteriosclerosis which lead to a gradual decline in glomerular filtration rate over time. Although these structural and functional changes do not cause hyperkalemia, they do predispose older adults to experience hyperkalemia if also affected by medical conditions or medications that disrupt potassium balance.

Older adults are more likely to experience pathologic changes to the kidney as a result of common comorbidities

Table 37-4. Medications associated with hypokalemia.

Medication Class	Mechanism of Action
Thiazide and loop diuretics	Increased sodium reabsorption and increased potassium secretion at collecting tubules
Mineralocorticoids and glucocorticoids	Increased filtration rate and increased distal sodium delivery with increased potassium secretion
β Agonists	Translocation of potassium into cells
Xanthines	Translocation of potassium into cells
Calcium channel blockers (high doses)	Translocation of potassium into cells

such as diabetes, hypertension, and urinary obstruction. These comorbidities can lead to disruptions in renin and aldosterone activity which impair renal tubular potassium secretion into the urine resulting in increased serum potassium levels. The degree of hyperkalemia can be affected by the intravascular volume status, the amount of dietary potassium intake, medications, and presence of kidney failure.

A. Intravascular Volume Status

Older adults are at risk for decreased intravascular volume for several reasons. First, older adults commonly experience dehydration secondary to hypodipsia. Decreased fluid intake leads to increased sodium and water reabsorption (hypernatremia) and decreased potassium secretion with subsequent hyperkalemia. Older adults are also subject to intravascular volume depletion as a result of volume overload states, such as congestive heart failure or other edematous states where there is third spacing of fluid. Persons with hypoaldosteronism (primary adrenal failure caused by autoimmune disease, hemorrhage, or tumor infiltration), hyporeninemic hypoaldosteronism (commonly caused by diabetes), or tubular unresponsiveness to aldosterone (interstitial renal disease) are most vulnerable to the effects of decreased intravascular volume.

B. Potassium Intake

Increased potassium consumption is also a cause of hyperkalemia. This may result from increased dietary potassium or potassium supplements. Older adults have higher rates of potassium supplement use as these are commonly prescribed concurrently with loop or thiazide diuretics to prevent hypokalemia. In addition, older adults may use nonprescription supplements that contain potassium either out of concern about potassium deficiency or inadvertently, not realizing that such supplements contain potassium as one of the ingredients. Similarly, older adults may be using salt substitutes in their diets to control hypertension or edema. Many of these salt substitutes use potassium rather than sodium and can result in a potentially dangerous potassium load to predisposed individuals.

C. Medication-Induced Hyperkalemia

The primary etiology of hyperkalemia in older adults is drug-induced. The incidence of hyperkalemia among those patients taking offending medications approaches 10% with older adults at increased risk. Several commonly prescribed classes of medications can cause hyperkalemia (Table 37–5).

D. Kidney Failure

Hyperkalemia occurs in kidney failure because potassium excretion is proportional to glomerular filtration rate (GFR).

Table 37–5. Medications associated with hyperkalemia.

Medication Class	Mechanism of Action
Potassium-sparing diuretics	
Spironolactone	Aldosterone antagonism
Triamterene and amiloride	Blocks sodium channels in principal cells
Nonsteroidal antiinflammatory drugs	Decrease renin and aldosterone
Angiotensin-converting enzyme inhibitors	Decrease aldosterone
	Decrease renal blood flow and glomerular filtration rate
β-Blocking agents	Decrease potassium movement into cells
	Decrease renin and aldosterone
Heparin	Decreases aldosterone synthesis
Digoxin intoxication	Decreases Na-K-ATPase activity
Trimethoprim	Blocks sodium channels in principal cells

As GFR declines, the ability of the kidney to effectively excrete potassium also declines. The degree of hyperkalemia is dependent on potassium intake and is affected by compensatory kidney potassium secretion mechanisms and losses of potassium in the stool. When hyperkalemia occurs in the setting of mild or moderate decreases in GFR (>10% normal), another etiology should be identified.

▶ Clinical Findings

The clinical consequences of hyperkalemia generally occur at severe elevations of serum potassium (>6.5 mEq/L). The clinical manifestations involve neuromuscular signs including weakness, ascending paralysis, and respiratory failure, muscle cramping and cardiac abnormalities including chest pain and progressive ECG changes (peaked T waves → flattened p waves → prolonged PR interval → idioventricular rhythm → widened QRS with deep S waves → ventricular fibrillation → cardiac arrest).

▶ Treatment

Diagnosis of hyperkalemia is made by laboratory evaluation. Elevated potassium levels should be confirmed with a repeated plasma sample as problems with drawing or processing blood samples may result in hemolysis, which releases intracellular potassium, leading to inaccurate serum potassium levels. Once hyperkalemia is confirmed, any exogenous potassium should be discontinued. An ECG should be obtained to determine if there are any changes related to hyperkalemia. The presence of ECG changes determines the urgency of treatment.

A. Acute Hyperkalemia

Emergency treatment of severe hyperkalemia with associated ECG changes may be accomplished using several rapidly acting agents.

1. Calcium infusion—Calcium temporarily antagonizes the cardiac effects of hyperkalemia and allows for the institution of more definitive treatment. The effects of calcium on hyperkalemia are immediate but short-lived, lasting only 30–60 minutes. Calcium may be administered as calcium gluconate or calcium carbonate. Calcium gluconate 1000 mg (10 mL of 10% solution) infused over 3–5 minutes may be administered peripherally. Calcium chloride 500–100 mg (5–10 mL of 10% solution) also can be infused over 3–5 minutes. However, calcium chloride should be delivered via central or deep vein as it can cause vein irritation and extravasation can lead to tissue necrosis.

2. Insulin with glucose—Insulin temporarily translocates potassium into cells by enhancing the activity of the Na-K-ATPase pump in skeletal muscle. Glucose should be administered simultaneously with insulin to avoid hypoglycemia. Several regimens are generally used. Ten units of regular insulin in 10% dextrose solution can be infused over 60 minutes. Alternatively, a bolus of 10 units regular insulin is given followed by 50 mL of 50% dextrose solution (25 g glucose). Serum glucose should be monitored closely because of the risks of hypoglycemia.

3. β_2-Adrenergic agonists—β_2-Adrenergic agonists also enhance the activity of the Na-K-ATPase pump in skeletal muscle and activate the Na-K-2Cl cotransporter to translocate potassium into cells. Albuterol can be administered as a nebulized solution (10–20 mg in 4 mL of saline) over 10 minutes with peak effect at 90 minutes or as an IV infusion (0.5 mg) with peak effect at 30 minutes.

4. Sodium bicarbonate—Sodium bicarbonate raises the systemic pH resulting in release of hydrogen ions with movement of potassium into cells to maintain electroneutrality. Bicarbonate is used to treat hyperkalemia in setting of acidosis and is not recommended as single-agent therapy. In the acute setting, one 50 mL ampule of sodium bicarbonate (50 mEq) IV over 5–10 minutes can be administered.

B. Potassium Removal

The acute treatment of hyperkalemia described above is useful in lowering dangerously high serum potassium levels temporarily but additional therapy is required to remove potassium. There are several modalities available to remove potassium from the body.

1. Loop or thiazide diuretics—Loop and thiazide diuretics increase potassium loss in the urine. These diuretics are particularly effective for patients with normal to moderately impaired kidney function.

2. Sodium polystyrene sulfonate—Sodium polystyrene sulfonate or Kayexalate is a cation exchange resin that binds potassium in the gut and causes an osmotic diuresis when combined with sorbitol. Sodium polystyrene sulfonate is effective at lowering serum potassium levels when given in multiple doses over several days. Sodium polystyrene sulfonate can be used to control hyperkalemia in patients with chronic kidney disease who are not yet on dialysis. This can be delivered orally 15–30 g every 4–6 hours or as a retention enema with 50 g in 150 mL tap water (without sorbitol) for severe hyperkalemia. Lower doses can be used for chronic hyperkalemia. The main concern with use of sodium polystyrene in sorbitol suspension is the potential for intestinal necrosis. Intestinal necrosis is a particular concern for older adults with postoperative ileus, those receiving opiates, and kidney transplant recipients.

3. Dialysis—Dialysis is indicated for the treatment of severe hyperkalemia, hyperkalemia that does not respond to other measures, or conditions where cellular breakdown can release large amounts of potassium such as crush injuries or tumor lysis syndrome. Hemodialysis is the preferred modality because of the faster rate of potassium removal.

NOCTURNAL POLYURIA

▶ General Principles in Older Adults

Nocturnal polyuria is a syndrome in which excessive urine is produced at night. Nocturnal polyuria is highly prevalent in older adults, with estimates suggesting that nearly 90% of adults older than age 80 years are affected. Nocturnal polyuria causes disruptions in sleep, which can lead to daytime somnolence, cognitive impairment, and poorer quality of life.

Nocturnal polyuria is considered to be present when 1 of the following criteria are met: (a) urine production during 8 hours of sleep is >33% of 24-hour urine production; (b) nighttime urine production rate is >0.9 mL/min; and (c) 7 PM to 7 AM urine volume is >50% of total 24-hour volume.

▶ Pathogenesis

The cause of nocturnal polyuria is usually multifactorial. First, there are aging-related changes in the diurnal pattern of ADH secretion that lead to increased urine flow at night, sometimes exceeding that during the day. There are also structural and functional changes in the urinary tract that commonly occur with age, such as decreased functional bladder capacity, bladder outlet obstruction caused by benign prostatic hypertrophy, and detrusor overactivity. These structural and functional changes in the urinary tract can predispose older adults to infections which can cause nocturnal polyuria. Also, many medical conditions that affect older adults, such as diabetes mellitus, DI, congestive heart failure, chronic kidney disease, hypokalemia, and hypercalcemia, may also cause nocturnal polyuria. Finally, many common drugs, such as diuretics, calcium channel blockers, lithium, selective serotonin reuptake inhibitors, caffeine, and alcohol may also contribute to nocturnal polyuria.

▶ Treatment

A careful history and review of medical conditions and medications is important in identifying the etiology and recommending treatment. If urinary tract infection is present, then treatment with antibiotics is indicated and reevaluation is necessary to determine if nocturnal polyuria has resolved. If there is no evidence of infection, then nonpharmacologic treatments, such as reduction of fluid intake and avoidance of diuretics and caffeine before bedtime, should be attempted. In patients with edema, use of compression stockings and elevation of the legs during the day is recommended. In women with urge incontinence, Kegel exercises and scheduled voiding during the day may be helpful. In patients with chronic illnesses contributing to nocturia, treating the underlying disease is the primary treatment.

There are several pharmacologic treatments. Diuretics taken 6–8 hours prior to bedtime may decrease a patient's overall volume status, thus decreasing nocturnal urine production. If benign prostatic hypertrophy is present, α blockers and 5α-reductase inhibitors can be used. In women with detrusor overactivity and urge incontinence, medications such as oxybutynin, propantheline, and solifenacin may be useful. However, caution should be exercised when prescribing anticholinergic medications to older adults because of increased risk of falls. Starting with low doses and slowly escalating to the lowest effective dose is recommended.

Fried LF, Palevsky PM. Hyponatremia and hypernatremia. *Med Clin North Am.* 1997 May;81(3):585-609.

Johanson JF, Sonnenberg A, Koch TR. Clinical epidemiology of chronic constipation. *J Clin Gastroenterol.* 1989;11(5):525-536.

Liamis G, Milionis H, Elisaf M. A review of drug-induced hyponatremia. *Am J Kidney Dis.* 2008 Jul;52(1):144-153.

Miller M. Hyponatremia: age-related risk factors and therapy decisions. *Geriatrics.* 1998;53(7):32-48.

Passare G, Viitanen M, Törring O, Winblad B, Fastbom J. Sodium and potassium disturbances in the elderly: prevalence and association with drug use. *Clin Drug Investig.* 2004;24(9):535-544.

Pilotto A, Franceschi M, Vitale D, et al. The prevalence of diarrhea and its association with drug use in elderly outpatients: a multicenter study. *Am J Gastroenterol.* 2008;103(11):2816-2823.

Whitehead WE, Drinkwater D, Cheskin LJ, Heller BR, Schuster MM. Constipation in the elderly living at home. Definition, prevalence, and relationship to lifestyle and health status. *J Am Geriatr Soc.* 1989;37(5):423-429.

Chronic Kidney Disease

38

C. Barrett Bowling, MD, MSPH
Katrina Booth, MD

ESSENTIALS OF DIAGNOSIS

▶ Evaluation of chronic kidney disease (CKD) includes a thorough medical history, physical exam, and specific laboratory measures.

▶ Symptoms related to CKD may not occur until disease is advanced and include sleep disturbance, decreased attentiveness, nausea, vomiting, weight change, dyspnea, lower extremity edema, fatigue, muscle cramps, peripheral neuropathy and pruritus.

▶ Reduced estimated glomerular filtration rate (eGFR) (<60 mL/min/1.73 m²) should be interpreted in the context of the medical history and other lab abnormalities (eg, history of diabetic retinopathy, rate of eGFR decline, presence of elevated albumin-to-creatinine ratio) before a diagnosis of CKD is made.

▶ General Principles in Older Adults

Chronic kidney disease (CKD) is defined as the presence of reduced glomerular filtration rate (GFR) or evidence of kidney damage for at least 3 months, which becomes increasingly common at older ages. In older populations, GFR should be estimated using a prediction equation. CKD stage should be assigned based on the level of kidney function. The vast majority of older adults with CKD will die without progressing to end-stage renal disease (ESRD); however, even mild-to-moderate CKD is associated with functional decline, cognitive impairment, frailty, and complex comorbidity.

The National Kidney Foundation (NKF) Kidney Disease Outcomes Quality Initiative (KDOQI) disease-specific guidelines have been established to direct the evaluation and management of patients with CKD; however, because of the substantial heterogeneity in life expectancy, functional status and health priorities among older adults with CKD, an individualized, patient-centered approach might be helpful. Special considerations must be made when treating CKD-related comorbidities and complications. Among older adults with advanced CKD, a shared decision-making approach should be used to facilitate decisions about dialysis. Geriatric assessment may be helpful to identify older adults who are vulnerable to functional decline and poor outcomes after initiation of dialysis. Palliative and supportive care should be offered to those who experience a high symptom burden regardless of disease stage and dialysis decision.

▶ Pathogenesis

The NKF/KDOQI Clinical Practice Guidelines provide standardized terminology for the evaluation and stratification of CKD. Based on these guidelines, CKD is defined as the presence of reduced GFR or evidence of kidney damage for at least 3 months. Kidney damage is defined as pathologic abnormalities or markers of damage, most frequently identified by albuminuria. This CKD definition is based on GFR and kidney damage, regardless of the underlying kidney disease etiology.

Among older adults, serum creatinine is a poor marker of kidney function. However, because measuring GFR is not clinically feasible, GFR should be estimated using prediction equations based on the serum creatinine and other factors affecting creatinine production including age, race and gender. Multiple estimating formulas are available (see www.kidney.org/professionals/kdoqi/gfr_calculator.cfm) including the Modification of Diet in Renal Disease (MDRD) and Chronic Kidney Disease Epidemiology Collaboration (CKD-EPI) equations. Although there is no consensus on which formula should be used for older adults, the CKD-EPI equation may be superior, especially among patients with normal GFR.

After estimating GFR, CKD stage should be assigned based on the level of kidney function. The stages range

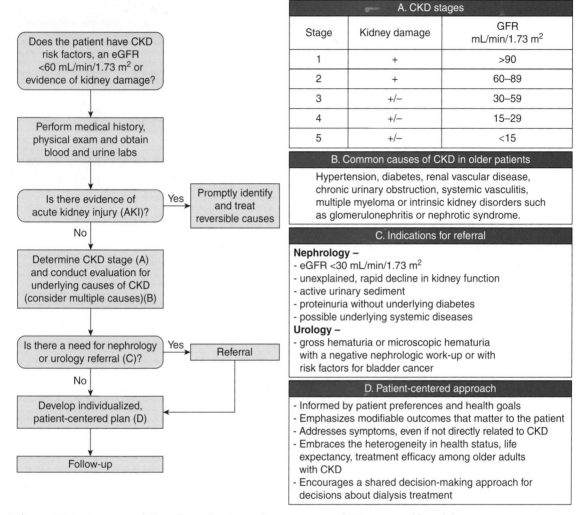

▲ Figure 38-1. Recommendations for evaluation and management of CKD among older adults.

from 1 to 5, with a higher stage indicating more severe CKD (Figure 38–1). The guidelines include a clinical action plan based on the CKD stage. In early stages, the focus is on diagnosis of CKD, treatment of comorbid conditions, and slowing CKD progression. In later stages, guidelines recommend preparation and initiation of renal replacement therapy.

Although age-specific cutpoints for CKD staging have been proposed, current recommendations do not support age-specific cutpoints. A revised staging system that incorporates level of GFR and urinary albumin-to-creatinine ratio (ACR: normal <30, high 30–300, and very high >300 mg/g) has also been proposed.

The prevalence and incidence of CKD increases markedly with age. In a large analysis of data from a U.S.

population-based study of more than 30,000 participants, the prevalence of CKD defined as an eGFR <60 mL/min/1.73 m^2 was 1%, 10%, 27%, and 51% among those <60, 60–69, 70–79, and ≥80 years old, respectively. The prevalence of albuminuria defined as an ACR ≥30 mg/g was 7%, 14%, 21%, and 33% among those <60, 60–69, 70–79 and ≥80 years old, respectively.

Among older adults, CKD is associated with adverse health outcomes, including mortality, cardiovascular disease (CVD), and ESRD. The natural history of CKD has traditionally been described as a progressive decline in kidney function with an expectation that a significant proportion of these patients will develop ESRD and require renal replacement therapy. Accordingly, a priority of CKD management is to identify and treat patients with early stage CKD to slow disease progression. However, more than 95% of older adults with CKD die without progressing to ESRD. Although the risk of ESRD may decrease with age, even mild-to-moderate CKD is associated with functional decline, cognitive impairment, and frailty.

Clinical Findings

A. Common Risk Factors

Risk factors for new-onset CKD include older age, obesity, smoking history, diabetes, and hypertension. Other important risk factors include history of CVD, family history of CKD or ESRD, history of urinary tract infection or urinary obstruction, and systemic illnesses that may affect the kidney (eg, systemic lupus erythematosus, multiple myeloma).

B. Screening for Chronic Kidney Disease

Because of the age-related decline in kidney function, poor correlation between eGFR and pathologic findings on kidney biopsy, and concerns about the validity of GFR estimating equations in older populations, using eGFR to screen all older adults for CKD is not recommended. For an older patient, reduced eGFR (<60 mL/min/1.73 m^2) should be interpreted in the context of the medical history and other lab abnormalities (eg, history of diabetic retinopathy, rate of eGFR decline, presence of elevated ACR) before a diagnosis of CKD is made.

C. Medical History and Physical Exam

Evaluation of CKD includes a thorough medical history, physical exam, and specific laboratory measures. The goal of this evaluation is to identify the underlying cause or causes, as multifactorial disease is common among older adults. A further goal is to identify CKD-related complications.

The medical history should include information on diabetes, hypertension, CVD, lower urinary tract disease and an evaluation for symptoms suggestive of vasculitis. Patients should be asked if they have a family history of CKD or ESRD. Typically, symptoms related to CKD do not occur until disease is advanced (eGFR <15 mL/min/1.73 m^2) and include sleep disturbance, decreased attentiveness, nausea, vomiting, weight change, dyspnea, lower-extremity edema, fatigue, muscle cramps, peripheral neuropathy, and pruritus. A review of medications should also be performed to assess for medications that may be exacerbating kidney injury, such as nonsteroidal antiinflammatory drugs (NSAIDs), or medications that may be contraindicated or require dose reductions in CKD, such as hypoglycemic agents, oral and intravenous antimicrobials, antihypertensive agents, and opioids. Several resources are available to further assist in medication dosing and management for patients with CKD.

Because of the disproportionately higher rates of geriatric syndromes among older adults with CKD, comprehensive geriatric assessment for functional status, cognition, depression, and impaired mobility should be considered in this population.

The physical exam should include vital signs, orthostatic blood pressure and pulse, evaluation of volume status, and evaluation of skin and extremities.

D. Lab Evaluation

Diagnostic testing should include urinalysis and random ACR. Twenty-four-hour urine collections for protein and creatinine clearance can be considered, but may be difficult for older adults. Blood work includes sodium, potassium, chloride, bicarbonate, blood urea nitrogen, creatinine, glucose, calcium, phosphorus, albumin, total protein, lipid profile, and complete blood count with differential. Additional tests may be indicated if the differential diagnosis includes causes other than diabetes or hypertension.

E. Evaluation for Underlying Causes

Prior to attributing reduced eGFR to CKD, an evaluation for reversible conditions causing acute kidney injury (AKI) should be considered. In addition, a rapid reduction in eGFR in a patient with known CKD should be considered AKI and evaluated promptly (see Figure 38–1).

Hypertension and diabetes are the 2 most common causes of CKD. However, multiple factors may contribute to the risk for CKD in the older population, including renal vascular disease, chronic urinary obstruction, systemic vasculitis, multiple myeloma, or intrinsic kidney disorders such as glomerulonephritis or nephrotic syndrome. High levels of proteinuria, abnormal urinary sediment with red or white blood cells, or rapidly progressive loss of kidney function should prompt work-up for causes other than diabetes or hypertension.

Complications

CKD-related complications include fluid and electrolyte abnormalities, bone and mineral disease, anemia and poor nutrition. Many of these complications can be treated by a primary care physician, but as kidney disease progresses and complications become more complex, referral to a nephrologist may be helpful. There are also special considerations for treating CKD-related complications among older adults (Table 38–1).

Treatment

A. In the Primary Care Setting

Because of the large number of older adults with mild-to-moderate CKD, care for these patients is often provided by

Table 38-1. Recommendations and special considerations for the treatment of CKD-related comorbidities and complications in geriatric patients.

Comorbidities	Treatment Recommendations	Special Considerations for Geriatric Patients
Hypertension	• Goal ≤140/90 mm Hg (among those with ACR <30 mg/g) and ≤130/80 mm Hg (among those with ACR ≥30 mg/g) • ACEIs or ARBs are first-line treatment in patients with proteinuria with goal urine protein-to-creatinine ratio of <0.2 or a ACR <30 mg/g	• Lower treatment targets may be harmful in frail older adults • There is limited evidence for BP goals for older CKD patients • Older adults underrepresented in clinical trials of ACEIs and ARBs in CKD
Diabetes	• Goal HgbA1c ~7% • Oral hypoglycemic agents and insulin may need to be dose reduced or are contraindicated	• In frail older adults, hypoglycemia may be dangerous (avoid glyburide) • Patients with limited life expectancy are unlikely to benefit from tight glucose control • Consider higher HgbA1c target
Cardiovascular disease	• Goal LDL <100 mg/dL • Low-dose aspirin unless contraindicated • Smoking cessation	• No change in goals, but must weigh risk-to-benefit of polypharmacy
Complications		
Fluid and electrolyte abnormalities	• Use loop diuretics and dietary restriction to maintain euvolemia and normal electrolyte ranges	• Burden of treatment (ie worsening urinary incontinence) vs. benefit must be considered • Elderly patients often decrease dietary intake; restrictions may not be necessary
Bone and mineral disease (BMD)	• Check levels of 25-hydroxyvitamin D, calcium, phosphorus, intact PTH, alkaline phosphatase • Maintain 25-hydroxyvitamin D in normal range with repletion • Maintain normal calcium and phosphorus with dietary restriction or phosphate binders • Check labs every 3-12 months depending on stage of CKD	• Burden of frequent serologic assessment, dietary restriction and polypharmacy should be considered with patient input • Older adults are at risk for concurrent osteoporosis • Bone densitometry may be less accurate in advanced CKD • Bisphosphonates are contraindicated if GFR <30 mL/min/1.73 m²
Anemia	• Check CBC with differential, iron saturation, ferritin, folate, B₁₂, and rule out other causes • Consider ESA in patients with adequate iron stores and symptomatic anemia with Hgb <10 mg/dL • Treatment with ESA to Hgb >12 mg/dL associated with risk of stroke and cardiovascular mortality	• Anemia in older adults is often multifactorial • ESA use requires self-injections and frequent lab draws and clinic visits • Burden of treatment must be weighed against benefits
Nutrition	• Dietary sodium <2000 mg/day • Limit dietary potassium and phosphorus if serum levels elevated • Consider daily protein restriction in advanced CKD: 0.8-1.0 g/kg body weight	• Elderly patients often decrease oral intake • Encourage adequate nutrition • Hypoalbuminemia is associated with increased risk of death in patients initiating dialysis

ACEIs, Angiotensin-converting enzyme inhibitors; ACR, albumin-to-creatinine ratio; ARBs, angiotensin receptor blockers; CBC, complete blood count; ESA, erythrocyte-stimulating agents; Hgb, hemoglobin; HgbA1c, glycosylated hemoglobin; PTH, parathyroid hormone.

the primary care physician. Routine treatment of CKD in the primary care setting includes monitoring of kidney function, managing CKD-related complications, treating CVD risk factors, preventing additional kidney injury, and promoting general health.

Medical optimization of hypertension and diabetes may improve kidney function and prevent progression of kidney disease (see Table 38–1). Preferred medications for blood pressure control in patients with CKD include diuretics, angiotensin-converting enzyme inhibitors (ACEIs) or angiotensin receptor blockers (ARBs), and β blockers. Achieving

blood pressure and hemoglobin A1c goals often requires multiple medications and the benefits of aggressive medical treatments to reach recommended targets should be considered in the context of the patient's health goals and balanced against the risks of treatment, particularly in frail older patients.

Proteinuria is an independent risk factor for progression of kidney disease as well as for mortality. ACEIs or ARBs are recommended as first-line treatment for proteinuria. However, older adults are underrepresented in the clinical trials used to develop CKD guidelines and evidence on the benefits of ACEIs and ARBs in this population is limited. Furthermore many older adults with reduced eGFR do not have proteinuria and the effectiveness of angiotensin blockade in these patients is limited. Finally, older adults are at risk for adverse drug events, therefore after initiation or dose increase of an ACEI or ARB, the serum creatinine and potassium should be measured.

In addition to treatment of high blood pressure and hyperglycemia, optimization of other risk factors to prevent CKD progression include smoking cessation and avoidance of nephrotoxins and additional kidney injury. However, there is limited evidence of the effectiveness of these interventions specifically among older adults with CKD.

Intense medical optimization of multiple conditions in geriatric patients often requires polypharmacy and should be considered in the context of the patient's preferences and health care goals. In older adults with CKD, complex comorbidity and geriatric syndromes are common, signs and symptoms often do not reflect a single underlying pathophysiologic process, there can be substantial heterogeneity in life expectancy, functional status and health priorities, and information on the safety and efficacy of interventions is lacking. For all these reasons, an individualized, patient-centered approach to CKD management for geriatric patients may be useful (see Figure 38–1).

B. Referral

The NKF/KDOQI guidelines recommend referral of patients with CKD Stage 4 (eGFR <30 mL/min/1.73 m^2) to a nephrologist for comanagement (see Figure 38–1). Indications for earlier nephrology referral include an unexplained, rapid decline in kidney function, the presence of active urinary sediment, proteinuria without underlying diabetes, or for patients with possible underlying systemic diseases such as multiple myeloma, hepatitis, or HIV. Additionally, patients with significant metabolic derangements may benefit from earlier evaluation and management by a nephrologist. Patients with gross hematuria or microscopic hematuria with a negative nephrologic work-up or with risk factors for bladder cancer should be considered for urologic referral.

C. Dialysis

Older adults represent the fastest growing group with ESRD. Decisions about whether or not to start dialysis can be challenging. While it is ideal to make decisions about dialysis initiation well in advance of a patient's reaching ESRD, because of the difficulty in predicting CKD progression and the competing risk for death this is often not possible. Qualitative research in this area suggests that uncertainty about the expected course of CKD appears to be an important concern among both patients and nephrologists. Because of this uncertainty, nephrologists have also reported avoiding discussions with patients about the future and prognosis.

Overall, progression to ESRD carries a poor prognosis. The benefits of dialysis in geriatric patients are less-well-studied and highly variable, depending on the patient's baseline functional status and other medical conditions. Among patients 80–84 years old initiating dialysis, the average life expectancy was 16 months; however, survival ranged from as short as 5 months to as long as 36 months (interquartile range). Older adults starting dialysis are at increased risk for persistent functional decline, increased hospitalizations and are more likely to die in the hospital than at home. In one study of patients ≥80 years of age, within 6 months of initiating dialysis over 30% had a decline in functional ability and required increased caregiver support or nursing home care. Factors associated with death within one year of initiating dialysis in octogenarian patients were poor nutritional status, late referral to a nephrologist, and functional dependence.

A shared decision-making approach that includes the patient, their family and caregivers along with the nephrologist and primary care physician should be used. It may be helpful to elicit the patient and family's values, preferences and health goals and then use these to guide the decision making discussion. Because of the likelihood of functional decline after dialysis initiation, geriatric assessment before initiation of dialysis that includes measures such as gait speed, functional assessment for basic and instrumental activities of daily living and cognitive testing may be helpful to identify those at highest risk for poor outcomes.

D. Withdrawal of Dialysis

Particularly for older adults with multimorbidity and geriatric syndromes, any early benefit of dialysis may quickly become a burden to the patient and family or may fail to improve symptoms that were attributed to ESRD, such as cognitive deficits. Withdrawal of dialysis is best done with the support of hospice or palliative care, as patients are likely to live for several days after stopping dialysis and have high symptom burden.

E. Kidney Transplant

Transplant is the best option for long-term renal replacement therapy. Advanced age alone should not be a contraindication to consideration for transplantation; several studies have demonstrated comparable outcomes among younger and older transplant patients. However, potential candidates must be selected carefully because of the competing risk of death and high complexity of post-transplant care. Predictive models may help determine which older patients may be appropriate for consideration.

F. Palliative and Supportive Care

Regardless of whether patients decide to pursue or forgo dialysis, patients with advanced CKD experience a high symptom burden and palliative and supportive care that addresses physical, emotional, and social suffering should be considered. For patients not on dialysis, fluid overload can be managed with diuretics if the patient still produces urine. Uremia commonly manifests as nausea, and can be managed with antiemetics. Hyperkalemia can be managed to some extent with diuretics and potassium excreting agents such as Kayexalate (sodium polystyrene sulfonate). The improvement of metabolic parameters achieved with these therapies must be balanced with the burden of treatment (eg, urinary incontinence, diarrhea). Patients with ESRD often report symptom burdens and reductions in quality of life similar to patients with terminal malignancy. Pain is a common symptom and should be treated aggressively; however, caution is needed when using renally cleared opioids such as morphine. Patients nearing the end of life may benefit from hospice or palliative care referral.

Abaterusso C, Lupo A, Ortalda V, et al. Treating elderly people with diabetes and stages 3 and 4 chronic kidney disease. *Clin J Am Soc Nephrol.* 2008;3(4):1185-1194.

Bowling CB, Inker LA, Gutierrez OM, et al. Age-specific associations of reduced estimated glomerular filtration rate with concurrent chronic kidney disease complications. *Clin J Am Soc Nephrol.* 2011;6(12):2822-2828.

Bowling CB, O'Hare AM. Managing older adults with CKD: individualized versus disease-based approaches. *Am J Kidney Dis.* 2012;59(2):293-302.

Coresh J, Selvin E, Stevens LA, et al. Prevalence of chronic kidney disease in the United States. *JAMA.* 2007;298(17):2038-2047.

Eufrasio P, Moreira P, Parada B, et al. Renal transplantation in recipients over 65 years old. *Transplant Proc.* 2011;43(1): 117-119.

Jassal SV, Chiu E, Hladunewich M. Loss of independence in patients starting dialysis at 80 years of age or older. *N Engl J Med.* 2009;361(16):1612-1613.

Kurella M, Covinsky KE, Collins AJ, Chertow GM. Octogenarians and nonagenarians starting dialysis in the United States. *Ann Intern Med.* 2007;146(3):177-183.

National Kidney Foundation. K/DOQI clinical practice guidelines for chronic kidney disease: evaluation, classification, and stratification. *Am J Kidney Dis.* 2002;39(2 Suppl 1):S1-S266.

O'Hare AM, Choi AI, Bertenthal D, et al. Age affects outcomes in chronic kidney disease. *J Am Soc Nephrol.* 2007;18(10): 2758-2765.

Schell JO, Patel UD, Steinhauser KE, et al. Discussions of the kidney disease trajectory by elderly patients and nephrologists: a qualitative study. *Am J Kidney Dis.* 2012;59(4):495-503.

Urinary Incontinence

39

Julie K. Gammack, MD

ESSENTIALS OF DIAGNOSIS

▶ Involuntary loss of urine sufficient to be a problem.

▶ Urinary incontinence is a syndrome, not a single disease, resulting from medical conditions, medications, or lower urinary tract disease. It can herald morbid diseases (eg, cancer and neurologic conditions).

▶ General Principles in Older Adults

Older women and men are more likely to experience urinary incontinence (UI) than younger adults; however, this is not an inevitable condition of aging. Approximately, 15% to 30% of healthy older adults experience some urinary leakage. The prevalence is nearly 50% in frail community dwellers and between 50% and 75% in institutionalized older adults. UI occurs more frequently in women than in men in most age groups, but the prevalence of UI increases with age in both men and women.

UI too often goes unreported because of patient embarrassment or reluctance to discuss the condition. Less than 20% of incontinent adults are assessed for this condition by primary care providers. Underevaluation may be a result of time constraints, underappreciation of the prevalence, or uncertainty about the disease management.

Leading risk factors for incontinence in older adults include increasing age, female gender, cognitive impairment, genitourinary surgery, obesity, and impaired mobility.

The financial impact of incontinence in caregiver time, medication costs, and continence supplies is substantial. An estimated $12 billion is spent annually on incontinence in the United States. This is comparable to the health care costs of other chronic diseases such as osteoporosis and breast cancer.

UI has long been classified as a geriatric syndrome: a symptom complex found more frequently in older adults which is often multifactorial in etiology and which requires a multidimensional approach to risk factor modification and treatment. To understand how to prevent, diagnose and treat the condition accurately, it is important to understand the normal physiology of voiding and how normal voiding can be disrupted.

▶ Normal Voiding

To maintain continence, a person must have intact cognitive, neurologic, muscular, and urologic systems. Consciousness, motivation, comprehension, and attention are needed to properly recognize the need to void and sequence the necessary steps to pass urine in an appropriate time and location. Diseases such as dementia, depression, stroke, and delirium can disrupt the cognitive function needed to exert control over voiding. Muscular dexterity is needed to manipulate clothing and toileting supplies, and to physically reach a toilet or urinal. Arthritis and muscular conditions, which impair ambulation and joint functioning, can result in incontinence episodes.

Neurologically, micturition is a coordinated balance between the spinal cord sympathetic and parasympathetic systems (Figure 39–1) and cerebral signaling. The pontine micturition center coordinates the cognitive inhibition/disinhibition to void and the spinal cord response to urinary tract stimulation. Innervation to the detrusor muscle and distal urethra/pelvic floor comes from the sacral 2–4 nerve roots and the innervations to the proximal urethra comes from the thoracic 11–lumbar 2 nerve roots. The sympathetic system allows urinary storage by contracting the urethral sphincter and relaxing the detrusor muscle. The parasympathetic system allows voiding by contracting the detrusor and relaxing the urethral sphincter. Diseases, such as spinal cord injury and multiple sclerosis, can impede the neurologic balance between the bladder wall and sphincter. The genitourinary organs and tissues can be diseased or damaged to a degree that impairs controlled urination. Prostatic enlargement,

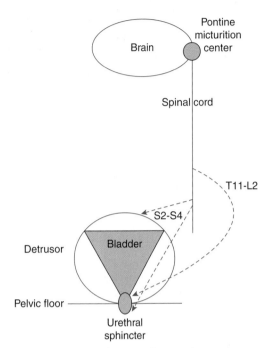

▲ Figure 39–1. Neurologic mechanism for continence control.

bladder prolapse, urethral structuring, bladder stones, and estrogen-deficient tissue atrophy can cause enough anatomic abnormality that incontinence develops.

▶ Prevention

Because UI has many different etiologies, triggers, and risk factors, the timing, frequency and severity of symptoms can be quite variable. Prevention thus focuses on reducing the impact of chronic disease on incontinence-related risk, as well as preventing the development of incontinence itself. It may not be possible to completely prevent UI, but measures to reduce the impact and frequency of the condition may be reasonable goals. Like most geriatric syndromes, prevention of symptoms or events often requires a multifactorial approach, which is designed to eliminate the factors that lead to incontinent episodes.

There are few studies that target primary prevention of UI. Most treatment trials target secondary prevention by attempting to reduce the number of episodes in those who already have some degree of UI. In one primary prevention study of poststroke patients, a multidimensional approach that included dedicated rehabilitation and a continence care team was found to reduce the development of UI. Another study of continent older women who were taught pelvic floor exercises showed a reduction in the later development of incontinence. A small trial of weight loss reduced the development of UI in some obese patients, but increased exercise lead to increased incontinence in others. Diabetes is associated with higher rates of UI. In 1 trial of obese women with prediabetes, a healthy lifestyle that included healthy diet, reduced weight, increased activity levels, and smoking cessation was associated with a lower subsequent development of stress, but not urge, incontinence symptoms. These findings were seen in the younger population, but not in the subgroup of older adults.

Brown JS, Wing R, Barrett-Connor E, et al; Diabetes Prevention Program Research Group. Lifestyle intervention is associated with lower prevalence of urinary incontinence: the Diabetes Prevention Program. *Diabetes Care.* 2006;29(2):385-390.

Diokno AC, Sampselle CM, Herzog AR, et al. Prevention of urinary incontinence by behavioral modification program: a randomized, controlled trial among older women in the community. *J Urol.* 2004;171(3):1165-1171.

Du Moulin MF, Hamers JP, Ambergen AW, Janssen MA, Halfens RJ. Prevalence of urinary incontinence among community-dwelling adults receiving home care. *Res Nurs Health.* 2008;31(6):604-612.

Hu TW, Wagner TH, Bentkover JD, et al. Estimated economic costs of overactive bladder in the United States. *Urology.* 2003; 61(6):1123-1128.

Offermans MP, Du Moulin MF, Hamers JP, Dassen T, Halfens RJ. Prevalence of urinary incontinence and associated risk factors in nursing home residents: a systematic review. *Neurourol Urodyn.* 2009;28(4):288-294.

▶ Clinical Findings

A. Symptoms & Signs

UI is generally classified into 4 different types based on the pathophysiologic cause of the leakage. Many people experience more than 1 type, or "mixed" incontinence. Leakage may be transient (reversible), episodic, or persistent in nature, based on the risk factors contributing to the condition.

1. Functional incontinence

- *Definition*: Loss of urine in the setting of a normal structural and functional urinary system
- *Signs/symptoms*: Impaired awareness/concern, altered cognition, large-volume leakage
- *Potential causes*: Dementia, delirium, depression, immobility, impaired manual dexterity, excessive urine output

2. Stress incontinence

- *Definition*: Loss of urine when abrupt increase in intraabdominal pressure exceeds urethral sphincter closing pressure
- *Signs/symptoms*: Often small volumes, associated with activities such as cough, laugh, sneeze, standing, bending
- *Potential causes*: Genitourinary (GU) atrophy or prolapse, urethral sphincter trauma, pelvic floor weakness

3. Urge incontinence—Also known as overactive bladder (OAB), detrusor hyperactivity, and detrusor instability.

- *Definition*: Loss of urine caused by uninhibited detrusor activity at inappropriately low urinary volumes
- *Signs/symptoms*: Small- or large-volume leakage, abrupt onset, urgency, frequency
- *Potential causes*: Bladder irritants, stones, infection or foreign body, detrusor noncompliance (scarring, fibrosis, and aging)

4. Overflow incontinence

- *Definition*: Loss of urine in the setting of excessive bladder volume as a result of impaired bladder wall contraction or urinary sphincter relaxation
- *Signs/symptoms*: Dribbling, weak urinary stream, intermittency, hesitancy, frequency, nocturia, high postvoid urinary volume
- *Potential causes*: Benign prostatic hyperplasia (BPH), prostate cancer, urethral stricture, GU organ prolapse, anticholinergic medication, neuropathy, spinal cord injury

In men, UI may be associated with other symptoms, which are referred to as lower urinary track symptoms (LUTS). These symptoms include incomplete emptying, frequency, hesitancy, urgency, weak stream, straining, and nocturia. Men with UI should also be asked about erectile dysfunction as previous surgery, cancer treatment, or infections can affect both continence and erectile dysfunction. Both men and women may also have pelvic pain in conjunction with UI. This should prompt a more extensive evaluation for malignant, infectious, or non-GU causes of the symptoms.

Sarma AV, Wei JT. Clinical practice. Benign prostatic hyperplasia and lower urinary tract symptoms. *N Engl J Med*. 2012;367(3):248-257.

B. Clinical Evaluation

The evaluation of UI should include a thorough history of the condition, including duration, frequency, severity, and burden of symptoms. Several tools can be used to evaluate the severity or impact of UI. Some older adults are able to document symptoms using a voiding diary. A 48-hour log of bladder symptoms should include the timing, circumstances, severity, volume, triggers, and frequency of each incontinent episode. The diary should also include timing, volume and frequency of nonincontinent voids. Environmental factors, medication dosing, comorbid illnesses and associated physical symptoms such as pain should also be noted.

The International Prostate Symptom Score (IPSS), which uses the American Urological Association Symptom Score Index (AUA-SI), plus a quality-of-life question, can stratify symptom severity in men with UI associated with LUTS (Table 39–1). Each question is weighted 0 (low) to 5 (high).

Table 39–1. Urinary symptom screening tools.

Tool	Symptoms	Scoring
American Urological Association Symptom Index or Score (AUA-SI)	1. Incomplete Emptying 2. Frequency 3. Hesitancy 4. Urgency 5. Weak Stream 6. Straining 7. Nocturia	• 0–5 points each • 35 points maximum • 0–7 mild • 8–19 moderate • 20–35 severe
International Prostate Symptom Score (IPSS)	Same as AUA-SI plus quality-of-life question	Same as AUA-SI
Overactive Bladder Validated 8 Question Awareness Tool (OAB-V8)	1. Daytime frequency 2. Urinary discomfort 3. Sudden urgency 4. Urinary incontinence 5. Nocturia 6. Sleep disruption 7. Uncontrolled urgency 8. Incontinence with urgency	• 0–5 points each • 40 points maximum • +2 points if male • ≥8 points suggests overactive bladder

The IPSS is helpful to the clinician in gauging the impact of symptoms on the patient and for judging the effectiveness of a symptom-targeted treatment.

The Overactive Bladder Validated 8 Question Awareness Tool (OAB-V8) can be used in both men and women to identify symptoms associated with overactive bladder (see Table 39–1). Each question is weighted 0 (low) to 5 (high) and a score of 8 or more suggests overactive bladder.

Coyne KS et al. Validation of an overactive bladder awareness tool for use in primary care settings. *Adv Ther*. 2005;22(4):381-394.

C. Physical Evaluation

A targeted physical examination should be performed to exclude potential causes of urinary system dysfunction. A cardiovascular exam should document evidence of congestive heart failure or excessive peripheral edema. The abdominal exam should assess for a palpable bladder, pain, or masses. A digital rectal exam is needed to evaluate for an enlarged or tender prostate that would suggest BPH or infection. Rectal or prostate masses would suggest carcinoma, and fecal impaction should be removed as a possible cause of disrupted urinary flow. Rectal tone, perineal sensation, and peripheral motor and sensory exam should be performed to identify spinal cord or neuropathic conditions. The penis should be examined for phimosis, drainage or lesions. An external GU exam in women should identify any organ prolapse or excessive GU tissue atrophy. A bimanual examination should assess for uterine or pelvic masses that may be compromising urinary flow.

D. Laboratory Testing

The evaluation of UI should include a basic laboratory evaluation to exclude metabolic, infectious, and malignant conditions that would affect urinary flow and function: serum electrolytes, glucose, creatinine, calcium, and urinalysis for blood, white cells, protein and culture if indicated. With supporting evidence, a more extensive evaluation for endocrine, neurologic, or malignant conditions may require additional laboratory or radiologic testing.

E. Imaging and Specialized Bladder Testing

It is imperative that bladder overdistention is identified as soon as possible as this may require emergent intervention. The use of an ultrasonic bladder scanner to assess urinary volume after voiding will identify urinary retention. This is performed at the bedside and is available in many hospitals but rarely found in the ambulatory or nursing home setting. Less than 50 mL should be present in the bladder after voiding; more than 200 mL indicates significant bladder dysfunction and requires ongoing evaluation. If unavailable, postvoid urinary catheterization to measure urinary volume will provide necessary information and can relieve urinary obstruction if identified.

Imaging of the kidneys and urinary tract may be helpful in identifying nephrolithiasis, cysts, tumors and obstruction. Renal ultrasound and CT urogram are first-line studies for evaluating the structure and function of the urinary system.

A urinary stress test can be done in women during the external gynecologic examination. The bladder should be full when performing this evaluation. In the lithotomy or standing position, the woman is asked to cough or bear down while observing for evidence of leakage of urine or organ prolapse. Small and immediate leakage of urine suggests stress incontinence; larger volume or delayed leakage suggests detrusor instability.

Urodynamic testing will provide information on bladder storage and voiding pressures but is not routinely indicated unless the initial evaluation and treatment steps are unsuccessful. Urodynamic studies can be helpful in identifying individuals with mixed incontinence and for those considering surgical evaluation for UI. This testing includes measurement of urinary pressure and flow volumes through catheters inserted into the bladder and the rectum or vagina (Figure 39–2). For frail or demented older adults, this testing may not be practical or well tolerated.

Direct observation with cystoscopy may be needed to provide tissue samples, locate and relieve obstruction, and visualize urinary tract structural abnormalities.

Gray M. Traces: making sense of urodynamics testing. Series #1. *Urol Nurs.* 2010;30(5):267-275.

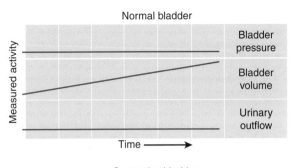

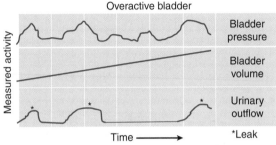

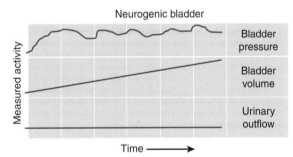

▲ **Figure 39–2.** Urodynamic measures of bladder functioning.

▶ Differential Diagnosis

UI is often the result of a primary GU organ or tissue dysfunction; however, certain diseases or conditions may secondarily cause UI (Table 39–2). In most cases, secondary causes affect the neurologic innervation, structural integrity of the GU tissues, or volume of urine, and thus overwhelm normal bladder functioning. In these cases, treating the secondary cause may alleviate the condition entirely. Malignancies, infections, and obstructing lesions are of highest concern and should be quickly excluded in new or acute onset of UI.

In rare cases, urinary leakage may occur through a fistula between the urinary and genital tract or urinary and gastrointestinal tract. This is generally found in individuals with past surgeries, pelvic radiation therapy, or malignancies of the pelvis.

Table 39–2. Conditions that can exacerbate urinary incontinence.

Condition	Mechanism
Constipation Fecal impaction Cystocele Rectocele Uterine prolapse	Mass effect impeding bladder neck and urethra
Dehydration Recurrent urinary tract infection Nephrolithiasis	Mucosal and bladder wall irritation
Pulmonary edema Peripheral edema Hypercalcemia Hyperglycemia	Increased urinary volume
COPD/asthma Chronic bronchitis	Cough-induced weakening of pelvic musculature
Delirium Dementia Depression	Impaired cognition, consciousness, or motivation to remain dry
Spinal cord injury Multiple sclerosis Parkinson disease Spinal stenosis Cerebrovascular accident	Disrupted neurologic coordination to bladder/sphincter
Tremor Osteoarthritis/rheumatoid arthritis Cerebrovascular accident Frailty	Impaired mobility and dexterity
Urogenital atrophy	Loss of estrogen to tissues

COPD, Chronic obstructive pulmonary disease.

Complications

UI can have significant physical and psychological effects on older adults. Older adults with UI are more likely to self-report an overall poor health status. Studies demonstrated that depressive symptoms are more prevalent in incontinent seniors and the severity of depressive symptoms correlates positively with the severity of incontinence. Men with LUTS have higher rates of anxiety, depression, and sexual dysfunctioning. Women with UI may also report a negative impact on sexual functioning, especially with mixed-type incontinence.

Depending on the type of incontinence, certain complications may be more common in older adults. A systematic review demonstrated that urinary incontinence is associated with an increase in falls for adults with urge but not stress incontinence. Sleep disruption can occur as a result of nocturia with overflow and urge, especially in the setting of excessive nocturnal diuresis. Overflow incontinence, if caused by severe urinary retention, may result in hydronephrosis and renal dysfunction. Urinary retention is also a risk factor for the development of delirium in older adults.

UI can cause embarrassment and social withdrawal. Older adults may avoid leaving home or curtail social activities because of fear of incontinence. If medications, such as diuretics, exacerbate UI, compliance with medications and control of comorbid diseases may be reduced. Many adults will reduce water intake to avoid a full bladder at inopportune times. This increases the risk for urinary tract infection and for dehydration.

Although not recommended for nonobstructive UI, some older adults request a urinary catheter to manage chronic urinary leakage. The use of indwelling and condom-type catheters is associated with an increased risk of urinary tract infections.

Chronic skin wetness from UI may compromise skin integrity. Dermatitis, candidiasis, cellulitis and skin breakdown may occur when the skin is repeatedly moist.

Nicolle LE. Urinary catheter-associated infections. *Infect Dis Clin North Am.* 2012;26(1):13-27.

Treatment

Treatment for UI can include behavioral, pharmacologic, and device or surgical intervention. With all types of incontinence, it is important to maximize treatment for comorbid conditions that can exacerbate urinary symptoms. Medications that contribute to bladder dysfunction and polyuria should be modified if possible (Table 39–3). In some

Table 39–3. Medications that can contribute to urinary incontinence.

Medication/Class	Mechanism
Antihistamines Antimuscarinics Antispasmodics Antipsychotics Antiparkinson Muscle relaxants Tricyclic antidepressants	Anticholinergic effects on bladder wall/sphincter
Diuretics Alcohol	Increased urinary volume and diuresis
Sedative-hypnotics Benzodiazepines	Sedation; impaired cognition
Opioids	Opioid receptor-induced bladder dysfunction
α-Adrenergic agonists	Urethral sphincter constriction

people, reducing dietary diuretics, such as caffeine and alcohol, and bladder irritants, such as spicy foods or acidic fruits, can reduce urinary symptoms. Cautious avoidance of excess liquid intake at certain times of the day may be useful.

A. Behavioral Modifications

Behavioral modification utilizes lifestyle and environmental modifications to reduce episodes of UI.

B. Habit Training

Habit training identifies UI triggers and employs situational bladder emptying to prevent incontinence episodes. Examples include toileting after meals, prior to bedtime, or before vigorous physical exercise if these events are regularly associated with incontinence.

C. Scheduled (Timed) Voiding

Scheduled voiding utilizes regularly timed attempts to void, regardless of urge or sensation to urinate. This approach minimizes large bladder volumes that may result in incontinent episodes. The interval between voids can be increased or decreased based on success in staying dry. This is especially useful in cognitively impaired or nursing home populations where caregivers can plan interval toileting, for example, every 2 hours, to reduce incontinence episodes.

This technique can also be used for bladder retraining in cognitively intact individuals with urge type incontinence. Scheduled voids are first performed at an interval that allows for maximal dryness. The interval is then increased by 30–60 minutes every few days to "train" the bladder to accommodate an increasing volume of urine. With success, time between voiding can reach 3–4 hours without urgency symptoms or leakage.

D. Prompted Voiding

Prompted voiding employs frequent inquiry about the need to pass urine and assistance to the toilet when the response is "yes." This is generally used by caregivers of cognitively impaired adults with functional or urge incontinence.

E. Pelvic Muscle Training

Pelvic muscle training (a.k.a. Kegel exercises) strengthens the urinary sphincter and pelvic floor by exercising the pelvic floor muscles which are under voluntary control. This is most useful in women with stress-type incontinence. The pelvic muscles are contracted for 8–10 repetitions of 6–8 seconds each. To ensure the proper muscles are being used, instruct women to "hold back" the urine flow while voiding on the toilet. Hold these muscles contracted for progressively longer times, up to 10 seconds if possible. Three sets of these contractions should be performed 3–4 times daily to augment the closing pressure of the pelvic floor–urethral

sphincter mechanism. Some women have difficulty localizing the pelvic floor muscles, which are used for continence control. Specially trained gynecologic physical therapists can assist women in isolating and appropriately exercising these muscles. Techniques, such as biofeedback, electrical stimulation, and the insertion of weighted vaginal cones, can be used to improve pelvic floor strength.

Khan IJ, Tariq SH. Urinary incontinence: behavioral modification therapy in older adult. *Clin Geriatr Med.* 2004;20(3):499-509.

Price N. Pelvic floor exercise for urinary incontinence: a systematic literature review. *Maturitas.* 2010;67(4):309-315.

F. Pharmacotherapy

Pharmacotherapy can be effective for all forms of UI, but medication must be carefully selected to target the underlying etiology of the incontinence (Table 39–4). In many cases, medications modulate bladder wall and sphincter function through antimuscarinic or anticholinergic effects on sympathetic or parasympathetic pathways. Because many older adults have mixed type of incontinence, medications must be used cautiously, as improvement in one type of incontinence (eg, urge type) may worsen another form (eg, overflow type).

A meta-analysis has shown that topical estrogen can improve incontinence in women with both stress- and urge-type symptoms. Topical estrogen is usually supplied through vaginal suppositories and creams. For some women, however, ring devices impregnated with estrogen that are placed in the vagina for up to 3 months can be more practical than daily estrogen administration. Systemic (oral) estrogen is not beneficial for control of UI, and, in fact, may worsen urinary symptoms.

Andersson KE, Chapple CR, Cardozo L, et al. Committee 8: pharmacological treatment of urinary incontinence. In: Abrams P, Cardozo L, Khoury S, Wein A, eds. *Incontinence.* 4th ed. Paris, France: Health Publication Ltd 2009:631-700. Available at: http://www.icsoffice.org/Publications/ICI_4/files-book/Comite-8.pdf

Cody JD et al. Oestrogen therapy for urinary incontinence in post-menopausal women. *Cochrane Database Syst Rev.* 2009;(4):CD001405.

1. Anticholinergics—The mainstay of pharmacotherapy for urge incontinence is the use of medications with anticholinergic effects through inhibition of muscarinic postganglionic cholinergic sites on the bladder wall. This reduces bladder wall contraction and thus increases bladder capacity. Numerous medications are now available in this category. These medications may be available in sustained-release oral and transdermal formulations, which are generally better tolerated; however, efficacy is not superior to the immediate-release formulations. Given the heterogeneity in studies and variety of clinical outcomes measured, it is difficult to say with certainty, even with meta-analysis data, that any one medication

Table 39–4. Medications used to treat urinary incontinence.

Medication	Dosing	Type of Incontinence
Estrogen		**Stress; urge**
Estradiol vaginal tablets	10–25 mcg daily to twice weekly	
Estradiol ring	2 mg ring; every 90 days	
Estrogen vaginal cream	0.5–2 g daily to twice weekly	
Antimuscarinics		**Urge**
Darifenacin (IR/ER)	7.5–15 mg daily	
Fesoterodine (IR/ER)	4–8 mg daily	
Oxybutynin IR oral ER oral Patch Topical gel	 2.5–5 mg twice/three times daily 5–30 mg daily 3.9 mg daily 1 g daily	
Solifenacin	5–10 mg daily	
Tolterodine IR oral ER oral	 1–2 mg twice daily 2–4 mg daily	
Trospium IR oral ER oral	 20 mg twice daily 60 mg daily	
α₁-Adrenergic Blockers		**Overflow**
Prazosin	1–10 mg three time daily	
Doxazosin	1–8 mg daily	
Terazosin	1–20 mg daily	
Alfuzosin	10 mg daily	
Silodosin	8 mg daily	
Tamsulosin	0.4–0.8 mg daily	
5α-Reductase Inhibitors		**Overflow**
Finasteride	5 mg daily	
Dutasteride	0.5 mg daily	
Bethanechol	**10–50 mg 3 times daily**	**Overflow**
Desmopressin	**0.2–0.6 mg daily**	**Urge from nocturia**
Imipramine	**25 mg 3 times daily**	**Stress; urge**

ER, Extended release; IR, immediate release.

is truly superior to another. The anticholinergic side effects of these medications can be troublesome to older adults and include dry eyes and mouth, constipation, headache, dizziness, orthostatic blood pressure changes, and confusion.

Madhuvrata P, Cody JD, Ellis G, Herbison GP, Hay-Smith EJ. Which anticholinergic drug for overactive bladder symptoms in adults. *Cochrane Database Syst Rev.* 2012;1:CD005429.

2. α₁-Adrenergic blockers—The prostate, bladder neck, and urethral tissue contract under the stimulation of α-adrenergic receptors. Alpha blockade allows relaxation of these tissues to improve urine flow and is used most frequently in men with bladder outlet obstruction caused by BPH. The literature clearly demonstrates the benefit of α blockers in reducing urinary retention in this population. A number of α blockers are available. Most of these medications are "nonselective" for urinary tract tissue and also block the α receptors on the vascular system, causing vasodilation and hypotension. Tamsulosin and silodosin are "selective" α₁A blockers, with minimal binding to nonurinary tissues and thus less potential to cause hypotension. These medications are considered preferential for older men because of their more favorable side-effect profile.

Because α blockade allows for urethral relaxation, these medications have potential for use in non-BPH overflow incontinence from neurogenic bladder, urethral obstruction, or urethral noncompliance. Studies show benefit in urinary symptoms and flow rates with use of α-blocker in these conditions. Alpha blockers have also been shown to improve the success in removing an indwelling urinary catheter after placement for urinary retention. Studies suggest that as little as 48 hours of α-blockade treatment may be needed prior to successful catheter removal. There is growing interest in using α blockers for women with bladder outlet obstruction. Recent studies demonstrate improvement in urinary flow and urinary symptoms in women with bladder outlet obstruction or neurogenic bladder, but not with overactive bladder.

3. 5α-Reductase inhibitors—5α-Reductase inhibitors (5αRI) block the conversion of testosterone to the active metabolite, dihydrotestosterone, reduce prostate tissue volume and thus reduce bladder outflow obstruction. Both finasteride and dutasteride have been well studied and demonstrate improvement in overflow incontinence and LUTS in men with BPH (see Chapter 40, "Benign Prostatic Hyperplasia & Prostate Cancer," for more on treatment of benign prostatic hypertrophy).

4. Other bladder agents—Bethanechol is a muscarinic agonist at smooth muscle cholinergic receptors. Although it generally is used to stimulate gastric motility it has the pharmacologic potential to increase detrusor tone and improve bladder emptying in the setting of neurogenic bladder. There is no evidence that bethanechol is clinically efficacious for managing urinary symptoms and the side effects of dizziness, hypotension, nausea, and abdominal cramping make this medication a poor choice for older adults.

5. Tricyclic antidepressants—Because of the anticholinergic properties, tricyclic antidepressants (TCAs) may improve symptoms of detrusor hyperactivity. A few studies have been done to demonstrate efficacy of this class of medication for UI, but most have looked at imipramine. Side effects of TCAs limit use in many older adults.

6. Desmopressin—Nocturia occurs in many older adults as a result of increased nocturnal mobilization of peripheral edema and increased levels of atrial natriuretic peptide. This can lead to nocturnal UI. Studies indicate desmopressin can effectively reduce nocturia and bothersome urinary symptoms; however, significant hyponatremia developed in some older subjects. Routine use of desmopressin for nocturnal UI is not recommended in older adults.

G. Devices and Surgery

Incontinence pads, adult diapers, and incontinence garments are regularly used to manage incontinence episodes. An estimated 4.4 billion dollars are spent annually in United States nursing homes alone for incontinence products, laundry service and continence care.

Urinary collection devices for management of transient or chronic urinary retention include intermittent or indwelling catheters. For the cognitively intact and motivated person (or caregiver), intermittent catheterization is preferable as it is less likely to result in urinary tract infection when compared to other forms of urinary catheterization. External (condom-type) catheters are not appropriate for management of urinary retention but may be desirable for men who want to avoid urinary leakage from other types of UI. These devices also increase the risk of urinary tract infection, and can cause skin irritation or infection, so should be used cautiously.

1. Pessaries—Women with GU organ prolapse can experience overflow urinary incontinence from obstruction or worsening of stress urinary incontinence. Those who do not desire, or are not appropriate surgical candidates, can benefit from placement of a pessary. Pessaries are plastic or silicone devices that are inserted into the vagina to physically prevent the prolapse of surrounding tissues into the vaginal canal. These devices come in a variety of sizes and shapes including ring, cube, and Gellhorn types. Some devices must be removed regularly and require dexterity and motivation for use. Other types can remain in place for several weeks and can be changed for cleaning and inspection by medical providers.

Trowbridge ER, Fenner DE. Practicalities and pitfalls of pessaries in older women. *Clin Obstet Gynecol*. 2007;50(3):709-719.

2. Urethral devices—Temporary urethral blockade may be attained by using internal urethral plugs or external adhesive seals or patches (foam pads). Plugs function like a balloon and must be inserted into the urethra and inflated when continence is desired. These devices are generally used for stress type incontinence. Permanently placed balloon devices can be implanted with adjustable inflation/deflation mechanisms to control continence. These are generally used in men with postprostatectomy destruction of the urethral sphincter. Complete continence is achieved in approximately 30% of men, and complication rates average between 20% and 30%.

Urethral bulking procedures involved the injection of collagen around the bladder neck, external to the urethral sphincter, to increase the urethral impedance to urinary flow. This may be done in women with stress or urge incontinence or in men after prostate surgery. Unfortunately improvement in symptoms is often modest, with low cure rates and deterioration in benefit over time.

An artificial urethral sphincter can be surgically implanted for control of stress-type incontinence. This is usually performed in men after prostate surgery and has been shown to have significant benefit on control of UI. Unfortunately, up to 25% of devices must be revised or replaced within 5 years of implantation because of erosion or mechanical failure of the device.

3. Surgical suspension options—Five major types of surgical suspension procedures are used for management of UI in women and are generally performed for stress-type incontinence: anterior repair, suburethral sling, colposuspension, long-needle suspension, and tension-free vaginal tape (TVT). Anterior repair (colporrhaphy) utilizes sutures or support material to elevate the urethra and/or bladder neck and reconstruct the pubocervical fascia. Cure rates and effectiveness deteriorate substantially with time and this procedure is losing favor for treatment of UI. Needle-suspension procedures are more minimally invasive means of supporting the bladder neck by placing sutures through a transcutaneous approach. This procedure has significantly less success and higher complications than other techniques and is generally not being recommended for the routine treatment of UI. Open colposuspension (also referred to as Burch procedure) uses sutures to elevate the periurethral fascia toward the Cooper ligament. A systematic review of more than 4000 women demonstrated a cure rate of 80% with this procedure, and 60% remained continent at 5 years. Open colposuspension has largely been replaced by the less-invasive suburethral sling or TVT procedures. The sling procedure uses a band of either synthetic or autologous fascial material. The band is guided under the bladder neck and both ends are anchored into the pelvic tissue to approximate normal bladder position. TVT uses a similar suspension technique, but at the midurethra and without anchoring of the material. The evidence suggests that TVT is equally effective as traditional fascial sling operations. TVT is more effective than open colposuspension.

Herschorn S, Bruschini H, Comiter C, Grise P, Hanus T, Kirschner-Hermanns R. Committee 13: surgical treatment of urinary incontinence in men. In: Abrams P, Cardozo L, Khoury S, Wein A, eds. *Incontinence*. 4th ed. Paris, France: Health Publication

Ltd 2009:1121-1190. Available at: http://www.icsoffice.org/Publications/ICI_4/files-book/comite-13.pdf

Smith ARB, Dmochowski R, Hilton P, et al. Committee 14: Surgery for urinary incontinence in women. In: Abrams P, Cardozo L, Khoury S, Wein A, eds. *Incontinence*. 4th ed. Paris, France: Health Publication Ltd 2009:1191-1272. Available at: http://www.icsoffice.org/Publications/ICI_4/files-book/comite-14.pdf

Prognosis

The outcome of treatment for UI is affected by many factors, including the type of UI, severity of symptoms, and underlying comorbidity. In general, with the appropriate treatment significant reduction in symptom burden can be achieved. If an inciting trigger for incontinence can be identified and alleviated, clinical cure may be possible. Surgical interventions for UI are very favorable, but are generally indicated for stress-type incontinence alone. Behavioral interventions can be helpful when applied to the correct type of incontinence but require a motivated and sustained effort on the part of the patient or caregiver. Complete dryness may not be possible but reducing the number and severity of episodes can have substantial benefit on quality of life and caregiver burden. Pharmacologic treatments also can substantially reduce symptom burden are generally not expected to provide a complete clinical cure for all urinary symptoms.

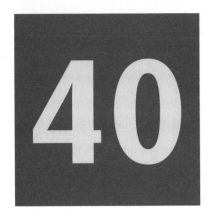

Benign Prostatic Hyperplasia & Prostate Cancer

Serena Chao, MD, MSc
Ryan Chippendale, MD

Disease processes involving the prostate gland are common in older men and can have a significant impact on their quality of life. The diagnostic evaluation and treatment plan of such conditions can be challenging for the primary care clinician, who must align the patients' goals of care with the risks and benefits of the available testing and treatment options. This chapter discusses 2 common prostate issues that frequently occur in older adults: benign prostatic hyperplasia (BPH) and prostate cancer.

BENIGN PROSTATIC HYPERPLASIA

ESSENTIALS OF DIAGNOSIS

▶ Symptoms of obstruction and irritation on voiding.
▶ An elevated American Urologic Association score.
▶ Possible enlargement of prostate on exam.
▶ Absence of other diagnoses that might cause symptoms (such as prostatitis or urinary tract infection [UTI]).

▶ General Principles in Older Adults

BPH remains a common condition in older men that can lead to diminished quality of life. Based on autopsy data, the prevalence of BPH approaches 50% by the sixth decade of life and is close to 90% in men age 80 years and older. However, older men who are symptomatic from BPH underreport their symptoms to their clinicians and, therefore, are less likely to receive medical or surgical treatment for bothersome complaints.

▶ Clinical Findings

A. Symptoms & Signs

When patients develop clinically significant BPH, they complain to clinicians of lower urinary tract symptoms (LUTS) such as increased urinary frequency, nocturia, urinary hesitancy, urine stream weakness, postvoid dribbling, and incomplete bladder emptying. Dysuria and hematuria are not commonly associated with BPH and may be an indication that another disease process is present.

The American Urological Association Symptom Index (AUA-SI) is a 7-item tool that health care providers can use to screen for symptomatic BPH as well as to assess a patient's LUTS severity. Individual item scores are 0 for "not at all" to 5 for "almost always," with a total maximum score of 35 (Table 40–1).

On physical examination, a digital rectal examination (DRE) may reveal a symmetrically enlarged prostate gland with a smooth and rubbery consistency. However, BPH may not be apparent on DRE in up to 52% of cases. Additionally, prostate size on DRE does not correlate with the severity of symptoms related to BPH. If significant urinary retention has resulted from a critically enlarged prostate gland, one may find a distended and tender bladder on palpation of the abdomen.

B. Laboratory Findings

There are no blood tests that confirm the presence of BPH. Though the American Urological Association (AUA) recommends obtaining a serum prostate-specific antigen (PSA) level when patients present with LUTS, it is for the purpose of identifying high PSA levels that might warrant further diagnostic work-up for prostate cancer. Although a PSA level above 2.0 ng/mL is correlated with a prostate volume greater than 40 mL in men older than age 60 years, PSA levels are not universally elevated in all cases of BPH, and other conditions,

Table 40-1. The American Urological Association Symptom Index for BPH.

Patient Name:_____ DOB:_____ ID:_____ Date of assessment:_____

Initial Assessment ( ) Monitor during:_____ Therapy ( ) after:_____ Therapy/surgery ( )_____

		AUA BPH Symptom Score					
	Not at all	Less than 1 time in 5	Less than half the time	About half the time	More than half the time	Almost always	
1. Over the past month, how often have you had a sensation of not emptying your bladder completely after you finished urinating?	0	1	2	3	4	5	
2. Over the past month, how often have you had to urinate again less than two hours after you finished urinating?	0	1	2	3	4	5	
3. Over the past month how often have you found you stopped and started again several times when you urinated?	0	1	2	3	4	5	
4. Over the past month, how often have you found it difficult to postpone urination?	0	1	2	3	4	5	
5. Over the past month, how often have you had a weak urinary stream?	0	1	2	3	4	5	
6. Over the past month, how often have you had to push or strain to begin urination?	0	1	2	3	4	5	
	None	1 time	2 times	3 times	4 times	5 or more times	
7. Over the past month, how many times did you most typically get up to urinate from the time you went to bed at night until the time you got up in the morning?	0	1	2	3	4	5	
						Total Symptom Score	

Reproduced with permission from the American Urological Association Education and Research, Inc. Copyright 2003 by the American Urological Association Education and Research, Inc.

such as recent indwelling bladder catheter placement, prostatitis, and prostate cancer, can cause PSA elevations. In cases where it is necessary to determine prostate volume, ultrasound (either transabdominal or transrectal) of the prostate is the preferred imaging test. However, routine use of ultrasound or other imaging studies to diagnose BPH is currently not recommended.

▶ Differential Diagnosis

When patients complain of LUTS, it is important to obtain additional history to augment information obtained through the AUA-SI. For example, nocturia may be caused by patients' drinking habits prior to bedtime, as well as medications they have been instructed to take at night. Consequently, ask patients to keep a voiding diary, where they record what types of beverages they drink at what time of day, along with

the times they urinate and estimates of urine volume with each void. Consider medications in the differential diagnosis, particularly if the patient is taking diuretics, medications with anticholinergic side effects that might lead to urinary retention (such as diphenhydramine), and nonprescription sympathomimetic decongestants that might exacerbate prostatic smooth muscle contraction (such as pseudoephedrine). Increased urinary frequency, urgency, and nocturia may be presenting symptoms of type 2 diabetes mellitus; if patients have a family history of diabetes and concomitant symptoms of polydipsia, polyphagia, and weight change, this may indicate new-onset diabetes rather than BPH.

If patients complain of dysuria, hematuria, fever, and chills in addition to those symptoms more commonly seen in BPH, obtain a urinalysis and urine culture to rule out UTI. Prostate cancer should be considered if patients present with systemic symptoms (such as anorexia, weight loss, and night sweats) and back pain and/or radiculopathy that might indicate bone metastases with nerve root compression. In addition, DRE may be notable for a nodular prostate, and PSA levels may be more markedly elevated in prostate cancer as compared to BPH. Prostatitis should be considered if patients complain of pain on ejaculation, the prostate is painful and edematous on palpation during DRE, and leukocytosis is seen on urinalysis. Nephrolithiasis should be considered when patients present with concomitant unilateral flank pain and gross or microscopic hematuria.

Certain historical factors, symptoms, signs, and testing results should trigger an immediate referral of the patient with LUTS to urology for further evaluation. These include a history of recurrent UTIs, underlying neurologic disease that could be associated with a primary bladder problem, a palpable bladder on exam, DRE findings that are suspicious for prostate cancer, elevated PSA levels, and hematuria.

▶ Complications

Outlet obstruction from an enlarged prostate may lead to urinary retention, which, in turn, is associated with the development of recurrent UTIs, acute kidney failure, and chronic kidney disease. Acute urinary retention occurs in approximately 20% of cases.

▶ Treatment

Severity of BPH symptoms should guide treatment recommendations.

A. Mild symptoms

If a patient's AUA-SI score indicates symptoms of mild severity (score 0–7), counsel the patient on behavioral modifications, such as minimizing intake of caffeinated and alcoholic beverages, reducing daytime fluid intake if excessive, and eliminating nighttime fluid intake. There is no evidence to support the use of medications in this setting. Patients should also be followed periodically for worsening of symptoms (ie, watchful waiting) that might warrant medical or surgical intervention.

B. Moderate-to-Severe Symptoms

In addition to behavioral modifications, patients with moderately severe symptoms (AUA-SI score 7–35) who are bothered by their symptoms may benefit from medical therapy, which can be initiated by primary clinicians. α-Adrenergic blockers have been found to improve BPH symptoms significantly when compared to placebo, largely through inhibition of prostatic smooth muscle contraction that results in improved urine flow through the urethra. Although doxazosin and terazosin appear on the 2012 Beers Criteria for medications to use with caution in older patients, this warning

applies to their use as primary medical therapy for hypertension and not symptomatic BPH. Orthostatic hypotension and arrhythmias are the most concerning potential adverse effects of these agents. Other side effects of note include dizziness (in up to 19% of cases), headaches, muscle weakness, nausea, and vomiting, dyspepsia, constipation, and diarrhea. When initiating these agents, start with the lowest possible dosages (doxazosin 1 mg or terazosin 1 mg at bedtime) and titrate upwards if needed for better symptom control and as tolerated by the patient. Patients and primary clinicians may prefer these older α blockers because they are inexpensive as compared to tamsulosin and alfuzosin. Tamsulosin should be initiated at 0.4 mg daily, although the dose may need to be increased to 0.8 mg to achieve symptom relief, which might result in increased cost to the patient (it is only available as a 0.4-mg capsule). The recommended and available dosage of alfuzosin is 10 mg daily. Of note, its bioavailability and serum concentrations increase by approximately 50% in the setting of stages II–IV chronic kidney disease (ie, in mild-to-severe renal impairment). Prazosin is no longer recommended for the treatment of BPH-related LUTS because of the associated high risk for adverse events.

Although there is no evidence for a causal relationship between α-blocker use and intraoperative floppy iris syndrome (IFIS), this association has been reported in the literature, with the risk being highest among patients taking tamsulosin as compared to other α blockers. Therefore, initiation of α-blocker therapy should be postponed until after any planned cataract surgeries. It is unknown whether discontinuing α-blocker therapy prior to cataract surgery is effective in preventing IFIS.

5α-Reductase inhibitors (5αRI) may be helpful in delaying progression of BPH, particularly in reducing patients' risk for acute urinary retention and need for prostate surgery. They are most effective in patients with enlarged prostate glands (based on DRE, elevated PSA levels, and/or volume measurement obtained through ultrasound) and should only be used if this circumstance exists. However, some trials suggest that they are not as effective as doxazosin in treating LUTS in the short term. Two medications in this class are currently available: finasteride (dosed at 5 mg daily) and dutasteride (dosed at 0.5 mg daily). Of note, finasteride cannot be crushed and thus can only be given to patients who are able to swallow pills. Dutasteride has a half-life of 5 weeks; therefore, associated adverse side effects of erectile dysfunction and decreased libido may be long lasting in patients on this medication.

Additionally, long-term use (ie, greater than 4 years) of 5αRI and α-blocker combination therapy in patients with documented prostatic enlargement may be more effective than using 5αRI alone in delaying symptom progression, reducing rates of acute urinary retention, and reducing the need for prostate surgery. The 5αRI and α-blocker combinations that have been studied are finasteride with doxazosin and dutasteride with tamsulosin.

Patients may inquire about using complementary and alternative medicines (CAM) to treat BPH symptoms. Several products are currently available for over-the-counter purchase, including supplements containing saw palmetto (*Serenoa repens*), β-sitosterols, and stinging nettle (*Urtica dioica*). To date, there is insufficient high-quality evidence to support the effectiveness of these agents in reducing LUTS related to BPH.

C. Persistent Bothersome Lower Urinary Track Symptoms

In the event that medical therapy does not improve patients' LUTS symptoms, they should be referred to urology for discussion of surgical interventions. Additionally, surgical therapy is indicated when patients have BPH-related renal insufficiency, recurrent UTIs, and bladder stones or gross hematuria caused by BPH. Surgical options include open prostatectomy, transurethral resection of the prostate (TURP), various laser therapies, and transurethral incision of the prostate (TUIP). The choice of which surgical approach to use will depend on the patient's presentation, anatomy, and prostate size; the urologist's experience with the different surgical techniques; the patient's ability to tolerate the procedure based on the patient's preexisting comorbid conditions; and the patient's preferences based on the risk-to-benefit profiles of each individual surgical option. Although there are some minimally invasive therapies now available (specifically transurethral needle ablation of the prostate and transurethral microwave thermotherapy), questions exist about the durability of symptom relief following these procedures.

▶ Prognosis

Increased mortality associated with BPH occurs only when complications arise (such as acute kidney failure or UTI) or in relation to medical or surgical therapies undertaken for the condition. The presence of BPH in itself is not associated with increased mortality.

PROSTATE CANCER

▶ General Principles in Older Adults

Prostate cancer is the most common nonskin malignancy in men. More than 2 million men are currently living with the disease, and a projected 240,000 will be diagnosed in 2012. It is an especially important disease process in the older adult population given that the incidence and mortality rises steadily with age. The Surveillance Epidemiology and End Results (SEER) database estimates that from 2005–2009, 58% of those diagnosed with and 90% of those who died from prostate cancer were 65 years or older.

The prognosis of prostate cancer is largely based on the histologic severity and tumor burden at the time of diagnosis. Current screening modalities, including serum PSA and DRE, are not reliable in predicting associated morbidity and mortality of prostate cancer, thus leading to overdetection. This, coupled with a prostate cancer-specific 5-year survival rate of 99%, has led to mounting controversy among expert panels on general screening recommendations for average-risk men. Even more complex is how to approach the older adult patient with a large burden of competing comorbidities that will likely result in death prior to progression of the prostate cancer itself.

▶ Screening

Both the incidence and prevalence of prostate cancer has increased since 1986 when the FDA approved the use of serum PSA testing, which has allowed diagnosis of prostate cancer in its earliest stages. The SEER estimates a 75% reduction in metastatic presentation of disease and a 42% reduction in prostate cancer-specific mortality associated with the widespread use of PSA screening.

However, an elevated PSA does not always confirm the diagnosis of prostate cancer. Other causes of prostatic cell hypertrophy, such as BPH and prostatitis, can present with elevations of PSA. Thus an elevated PSA may turn out to be a false-positive result, causing anxiety for the patient and the pursuit of unnecessary invasive diagnostic testing, such as prostate biopsy. Diagnostic testing also can lead to considerable adverse side effects (see "Diagnostics" below).

Expert panels disagree on the necessity and frequency of prostate cancer screening in all age groups. The United States Preventative Services Task Force (USPSTF) released guidelines in 2012 recommending against PSA screening in the general U.S. population, stating that the potential harms outweighed the risk of not screening. In contrast, the AUA and American Cancer Society (ACS) urge that providers offer screening to appropriate patients while engaging them in discussions about risks versus benefits of such screening. If there is then an informed decision by the patient to pursue PSA and DRE screening, after careful consideration of the potential risks and benefits of screening and diagnostic work-up for abnormal screening results, it should be offered. The AUA later released the following statement in response to the USPSTF's current recommendation: "it is inappropriate and irresponsible to issue a blanket statement against PSA testing, particularly for at-risk populations, such as African American men."

The majority of expert panels agree that *the overall health status of an individual must be incorporated into the decision to screen.* Those average-risk, asymptomatic patients with a life expectancy of less than 10 years will likely not benefit from routine screening. If the health care provider believes that a patient would not be an appropriate candidate for treatment if prostate cancer is detected, screening should not be offered. Thus, an individualized approach to prostate cancer screening must be adopted by health care providers. One must weigh the risks, benefits, and current uncertainties of scientific evidence, alongside the patient's preferences, estimated life expectancy, and potential effects of treatment on the patient's quality of life. See Chapter 8, "Prevention & Health Promotion," for a comprehensive approach to screening decision making in the older patient.

▶ Prevention

Testosterone plays a significant role in prostate cancer. Knowing this, the National Cancer Institute launched the double-blind, placebo-controlled Prostate Cancer Prevention Trial (PCPT) to study the effects of the 5αRI, finasteride, on the development of prostate cancer. The study was stopped prematurely when significantly fewer men in the treatment arm developed prostate cancer. However, it was later determined that survival was similar for both treatment and control groups, with the predominance of prevented cases found to be of low histologic tumor grade. Of note, high-grade tumors were more common in the treatment group. This result raised questions about whether finasteride could in fact provoke progression of histologic changes. There have been ongoing investigations to further explain this finding.

▶ Clinical Findings

A. Symptoms & Signs

Prostate cancer in its earlier stages is largely asymptomatic. As it becomes more advanced, LUTS can develop, including urinary urgency, frequency, hesitancy, and nocturia. Prostate cancer can also present as new-onset erectile dysfunction, or less frequently with hematuria or hematospermia, which is presence of blood in the urine or semen. A small number of patients may present when the cancer has already metastasized to distant sites. The most common site is bone, presenting with pain or a pathologic fracture.

On physical exam, prostate cancer can be detected through abnormalities on the DRE. These changes include asymmetry, distinct areas of induration, and frank nodules on the prostate gland. However, a negative DRE does not completely rule out prostate cancer, as only the posterior and lateral anatomy of the prostate gland are easily obtained digitally.

B. Laboratory Findings

Elevations in serum PSA can be associated with prostate cancer but also frequently occur in benign conditions such as BPH. A general rule is that the higher the PSA, the higher the likelihood of detecting cancer on subsequent biopsy. Biopsy is

usually recommended if PSA levels are greater than 10 ng/mL. For intermediate levels (PSA between 4 and 10 ng/mL), biopsy will be considered for most older men. However, only 20% of these biopsies will be positive for prostate cancer. Studies that have focused on using age-specific PSA reference ranges, PSA velocity, and free-PSA levels to assist in risk stratifying these intermediate PSA levels have largely failed to show superiority in predicting positive biopsy results. Recommendations for PSA levels less than 4 ng/mL are even less clear. There are a considerable number of patients diagnosed with prostate cancer whose PSA levels fall in the 2–4 ng/mL range. In the PCPT trial, 20% of localized cancers found on biopsy had serum PSAs between 2.6 and 3.9 ng/mL. Men can also experience fluctuations in their serum PSA levels, and thus confirmation of an abnormal PSA is advised prior to biopsy.

C. Diagnostics

A histologic biopsy is required to confirm the diagnosis of prostate cancer after an abnormal PSA or DRE is found. Biopsies are most commonly obtained transrectally, guided with transrectal ultrasonography (TRUS) to increase accuracy. Alternatively, transperineal or transurethral approaches can be used if the transrectal approach is contraindicated. Obtaining a biopsy is a relatively quick and readily available office procedure, but it can have substantial associated morbidities. These include pain, bleeding in the form of hematuria or hematospermia, infection, urinary obstruction, and the potential psychological trauma of a positive result that may not require treatment. Given that approximately 75% of biopsies return negative, candidates must be selected carefully with the assistance of an experienced urologist.

▶ Treatment

Evidence for the most effective prostate cancer treatments in older adults is lacking. This population of patients is largely excluded from current therapeutic trials. Biopsy results, along with TNM (tumor, node, metastasis) and clinical staging, will guide the selection of initial therapy. Equally important to treatment selection is balancing a patient's stated goals and preferences with the risks and benefits of each therapeutic option being considered. Involvement of an interdisciplinary team, including the primary care provider, oncologist, and urologist, will allow formulation of the most comprehensive, patient-centered treatment plan.

A. Localized Prostate Cancer

For localized, organ-confined prostate cancer, the goal of therapy is to balance the risk of death and morbidity with adverse effects that often occur with treatment. The decision on which treatment approach is most appropriate to pursue requires consideration of more than just the patient's chronologic age. It should include the incorporation of the older adult's performance status, comorbidity burden, nutritional status, social supports, and values and preferences.

Definitive treatment options include surgical resection through radical prostatectomy (RP) and radiation via external beam radiation therapy (EBRT) or brachytherapy. With recent advancements in technology, RP and EBRT have resulted in similar disease-specific and overall mortality rates. There are currently no randomized controlled trials comparing brachytherapy to RP or EBRT; therefore, it should be used in carefully selected patients with amenable anatomy.

Because 90% of prostate cancers are clinically localized to the prostate gland and carry a low risk for progression, observation through active surveillance or watchful waiting are also options for the appropriate low-risk patient. The goal of active surveillance is to monitor closely with PSA measurement and biopsy. Curative treatment is only pursued if disease progression is suspected. In contrast, watchful waiting entails close monitoring for the development of symptoms related to the prostate cancer, with palliative treatments offered if these occur. Watchful waiting is most commonly utilized as an option in the older adult patient with a high comorbidity burden. Observation management, in general, is more frequently chosen by men older than 75 years than in younger cohorts.

Androgen deprivation therapy (ADT) alone is not considered standard treatment of localized prostate cancer due to studies suggesting an associated shortened survival and increased mortality. It does still play a role as adjuvant therapy in locally advanced disease.

B. Advanced Prostate Cancer

Treatment of advanced prostate cancer in older adults should largely focus on the promotion of quality of life. Although only approximately 5% of prostate cancers now present initially with metastasis, the symptom burden of these patients can be quite severe. ADT is considered first-line treatment for hormone positive cancers. This involves either surgical castration through bilateral orchiectomy or chemical castration often with gonadotropin-releasing hormone (GnRH) agonists and antiandrogens.

Castrate-resistant prostate cancer in a man with optimal health and functional status is generally treated with the first-line chemotherapeutic regimen of docetaxel and prednisone. The frequency and dosing of this regimen can be altered based on the patient's response to therapy, including how well the patient tolerates associated side effects. For those patients who have severe symptom burden and are castrate-resistant, palliative options are also available. Use of analgesics, local radiation therapy, and bisphosphonates are helpful in treating symptoms associated with bone metastases. Radiation therapy has also been shown to be beneficial for relieving the symptom burden associated with pelvic disease.

Complications

Older men have higher surgical complication rates with RP. Urinary incontinence and erectile dysfunction are quite common and result from urinary sphincter and penile nerve damage, respectively. Nerve-sparing procedures have improved impotence rates, which have been as high as 90% in patients who underwent traditional RP. Urinary leakage has been shown to be more common with RP than other methods of treatment, affecting up to 35% of patients.

Gastrointestinal and genitourinary symptoms are the most common adverse effects of localized radiation therapy (RT). Some studies suggest that older patients may develop side effects earlier in treatment, although comorbidity burden is also thought to play an important role. Bowel urgency is more common with RT than in other treatments, but still only affects 3% of recipients long-term.

ADT therapy for the treatment of advanced prostate cancer also has several potential complications, including osteoporosis and fractures, metabolic syndrome, diabetes, and cardiovascular disease. Men also report experiencing vasomotor symptoms, gynecomastia, testicular atrophy, fatigue, and depression as a result of treatment. With such an extensive side-effect profile, the prescribing provider must consider the potential interactions with already present underlying comorbidities, as these may be exacerbated during treatment.

Sexual dysfunction is a common adverse effect that can result from all treatment options, with incidence rates between <5% and 60%. This potential adverse outcome should be discussed with patients prior to initiation of therapy as quality of life can be significantly compromised when it occurs.

Prognosis

A larger number of men who are diagnosed in or after their seventh decade of life die of prostate cancer than younger populations. This is especially true if a more advanced, higher grade cancer is present at the time of diagnosis. Still, in observational studies, prostate cancer-specific and overall survival rates remain quite high in older adults, with competing comorbidities more commonly the cause of mortality.

American Cancer Society guideline for the early detection of prostate cancer: update 2010. *CA Cancer J Clin.* 2010;60(2):70-98.

American Geriatrics Society 2012 Beers Criteria Update Expert Panel. American Geriatrics Society updated Beers criteria for potentially inappropriate medication use in older adults. *J Am Geriatr Soc.* 2012;60:616-631.

American Urological Association (AUA). *Prostate Specific Antigen Best Practice Statement: 2009 Update.* Linthicum, MD: American Urological Association Education and Research, Inc.; 2009.

American Urological Association Information Sheet: Prostate-Specific Antigen (PSA) Testing for the Early Detection of

Prostate Cancer. Accessed June 2, 2012. Available at: http://www. auanet.org/content/media/USPSTF_information_sheet.pdf.

Basch EM, Somerfield MR, Beer TM, et al. American Society of Clinical Oncology endorsement of the Cancer Care Ontario practice guideline of nonhormonal therapy for men with metastatic hormone-refractory (castration-resistant) prostate cancer. *J Clin Oncol.* 2007;25(33):5313-5318.

Berry SJ, Coffey DS, Walsh PC, Ewing LL. The development of human benign prostatic hyperplasia with age. *J Urol.* 1984;132(3):474-479.

Caroll P, Albertsen PE, Greene K, et al. Prostate-specific antigen best practice statement: 2009 update. Accessed June 2, 2012. Available at: http://www.auanet.org/content/guidelines-and-quality-care/clinical-guidelines/main-reports/psa09.pdf.

Din OS, Thanvi N, Ferguson CJ, Kirkbride P. Palliative prostate radiotherapy for symptomatic advanced prostate cancer. *Radiother Oncol.* 2009;93(2):192-196.

Droz JP, Balducci L, Bolla M, et al. Management of prostate cancer in older men: recommendations of a working group of the International Society of Geriatric Oncology. *BJU Int.* 2010;106(4):462-469.

Farwell WR, Linder JA, Jha AK. Trends in prostate-specific antigen testing from 1995 through 2004. *Arch Intern Med.* 2007;167(22):2497-2502.

Fleshner N, Zlotta AR. Prostate cancer prevention: past, present, and future. *Cancer.* 2007;110(9):1889-1899.

Garnick MB. Prostate cancer: screening, diagnosis and management. *Ann Intern Med.* 1993;118(10):804-818.

Konety BR, Cowan JE, Carroll PR; CaPSURE Investigators. Patterns of primary and secondary therapy for prostate cancer in elderly men: analysis of data from caPSURE. *J Urol.* 2008;179(5):1797-1803.

Lin K, Lipsitz R, Miller T, Janakiraman S; U.S. Preventive Services Task Force. Benefits and harms of prostate-specific antigen screening for prostate cancer: an evidence update for the U.S. Preventative Services Task Force. *Ann Intern Med.* 2008;149(3):192-199.

Loblaw DA, Virgo KS, Nam R, et al; American Society of Clinical Oncology. Initial hormonal management of androgen-sensitive metastatic, recurrent, or progressive prostate cancer: 2006 update of an American Society of Clinical Oncology practice guideline. *J Clin Oncol.* 2007;25(12):1596-1605.

McConnell JD, Roehrborn CG, Bautista OM, et al; Medical Therapy of Prostatic Symptoms (MTOPS) Research Group. The long-term effect of doxazosin, finasteride, and combination therapy on the clinical progression of benign prostatic hyperplasia. *N Engl J Med.* 2003;349(25):2387-2398.

McVary KT, Roehrborn CG, Avins AL, et al. *American Urological Association Guideline: Management of Benign Prostatic Hyperplasia (BPH) Revised, 2010.* Linthicum, MD: American Urological Association Education and Research, Inc.; 2010.

Miller DC, Hafez KS, Stewart A, Montie JE, Wei JT. Prostate carcinoma presentation, diagnosis and staging: and update from the National Cancer Database. *Cancer.* 2003;98(6):1169-1178.

Moyer VA; U.S. Preventative Services Task Force. Screening for prostate cancer: U.S. Preventative Services Task Force recommendation statement. *Ann Intern Med.* 2012;157(2):120-134.

Naslund MJ, Gilsenan AW, Midkiff KD, Bown A, Wolford ET, Wang J. Prevalence of lower urinary tract symptoms and prostate enlargement in the primary care setting. *Int J Clin Pract.* 2007;61(9):1437-1445.

Pal SK, Katheria V, Hurria A. Evaluating the older patient with cancer: understanding frailty and the geriatric assessment. *CA Cancer J Clin.* 2010;60(2):120-132.

Pettaway CA, Lamerato LE, Eaddy MT, Edwards JK, Hogue SL, Crane MM. Benign prostatic hyperplasia: racial differences in treatment patterns and prostate cancer prevalence. *BJU Int.* 2011;108(8):1302-1308.

Pierorazio PM, Humphreys E, Walsh PC, Partin AW, Han M. Radical prostatectomy in older men: survival outcomes in septuagenarians and octogenarians. *BJU Int.* 2010;106(6):791-795.

Roehrborn C, Siami P, Barkin J, et al; CombAT Study Group. The effects of dutasteride, tamsulosin, and combination therapy on lower urinary tract symptoms in men with benign prostatic hyperplasia and prostatic enlargement: 2-year results from the CombAT study. *J Urol.* 2008;179(2):616-621.

Tacklind J, Fink HA, MacDonald R, Rutks I, Wilt TJ. Finasteride for benign prostatic hyperplasia. *Cochrane Database Syst Rev.* 2010;(10):CD006015.

Tacklind J, MacDonald R, Rutks I, Stanke JU, Wilt TJ. Serenoa repens for benign prostatic hyperplasia. *Cochrane Database Syst Rev.* 2009;12:CD001423.

Terakawa T, Miyake H, Kanomata N, Kumano M, Takenaka A, Fujisawao M. Inverse association between histologic inflammation in needle biopsy specimens and prostate cancer in men with serum PSA of 10-50 ng/ml. *Urology.* 2008;72(6):1194-1197.

Thompson IM, Goodman PJ, Tangen CM, et al. The influence of finasteride on the development of prostate cancer. *N Engl J Med.* 2003;349(3):215-224.

Thompson I, Thrasher JB, Aus G, et al; AUA Prostate Cancer Clinical Guideline Update Panel. Guideline for the management of clinically localized prostate cancer: 2007 update. *J Urol.* 2007;177(6):2106-2131.

Wilt T, Ishani A, MacDonald R, Stark G, Mulrow C, Lau J. Beta-sitosterols for benign prostatic hyperplasia. *Cochrane Database Syst Rev.* 2000;(2):CD001043.

Wilt TJ, MacDonald R, Rutks I, Shamliyan TA, Taylor BC, Kane RL. Systematic review: comparative effectiveness and harms of treatments for clinically localized prostate cancer. *Ann Intern Med.* 2008;148(6):435-448.

Thyroid, Parathyroid, & Adrenal Gland Disorders

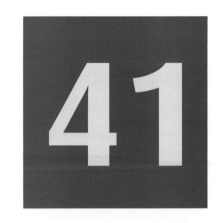

Steven R. Gambert, MD

Ravi Kant, MD

Myron Miller, MD

▼ DISEASES OF THE THYROID GLAND

SUBCLINICAL HYPOTHYROIDISM

▶ General Principles in Older Adults

Subclinical hypothyroidism affects a relatively large number of older persons. Although a small percentage of these cases will progress to overt clinical hypothyroidism each year, individuals with high levels of antimicrosomal antibodies are at greater risk of decline in thyroid function. Several studies have observed beneficial effects of thyroxine (T_4) therapy in patients with subclinical hypothyroidism; no studies have specifically addressed this question in older patients.

▶ Clinical Findings

Older patients with subclinical hypothyroidism may present with few or no complaints. Studies have demonstrated increased intestinal transit time, increased intraocular pressure, higher low-density lipoprotein-cholesterol levels, an increased risk for atherosclerosis, reduced cognitive function, and changes in cardiac performance and congestive heart failure. Older women with atherosclerosis, and an even higher percentage of those with a history of myocardial infarction, have a higher incidence of subclinical hypothyroidism. Treatment with L-thyroxine compared with placebo results in an overall improvement in general well-being. In addition, noninvasive indexes of myocardial contractility also improved, as did memory, psychomotor speed, and serum cholesterol levels. Subclinical hypothyroidism progresses to frank hypothyroidism in 5% to 8% of affected persons each year, with higher rates in those with high levels of antimicrosomal antibodies.

▶ Treatment

Although some physicians advocate replacement therapy for all persons with subclinical hypothyroidism, many believe that treatment is best reserved for those individuals with thyroid-stimulating hormone (TSH) levels >10 mU/L or for those with serum TSH levels between 5 and 10 mU/L with coexisting high levels of antimicrosomal antibodies. If treatment is not initiated, careful follow-up is essential because a percentage of these individuals will develop hypothyroidism each year. The goal of treatment, when initiated, is to normalize serum TSH values as long as the dose of thyroid hormone that is required produces no unwanted clinical effects. Most experts recommend targeting a normal TSH range in older patients, although it should be noted that serum TSH concentrations increase with age and 1 study examining individuals with "extreme longevity" noted serum TSH to be significantly higher in centenarians, with 7.5 mU/L considered to be the true upper limit of normal for those age 80 years and older.

Atzmon G, Barzilai N, Hollowell JG, Surks MI, Gabriely I. Extreme longevity is associated with increased serum thyrotropin. *J Clin Endocrinol Metab.* 2009;94(4):1251-1254.

Bremner A, Feddema P, Leedman PJ, et al. Age-related changes in thyroid function: a longitudinal study of a community-based cohort. *J Clin Endocrinol Metab.* 2012;97(5):1554-1562.

Canaris GJ, Manowitz NR, Mayor G, Ridgway EC. The Colorado thyroid disease prevalence study. *Arch Intern Med.* 2000;160(4):526-534.

Cooper DS. Clinical practice. Subclinical hypothyroidism. *N Engl J Med.* 2001;345(4):260-265.

Ladenson PW, Singer PA, Ain KB, et al. American Thyroid Association guidelines for detection of thyroid dysfunction. *Arch Intern Med.* 2000;160(11):1573-1575.

Ochs N, Auer R, Bauer DC, et al. Meta-analysis: subclinical thyroid dysfunction and the risk of coronary heart disease and mortality. *Ann Intern Med.* 2008;148(11):832-845.

SUBCLINICAL HYPERTHYROIDISM

▶ General Principles in Older Adults

Subclinical hyperthyroidism is a term used to identify individuals with suppressed levels of serum TSH with normal levels of circulating thyroid hormones.

▶ Clinical Findings

Subclinical hyperthyroidism may occur as a consequence of thyroid hormone replacement for hypothyroidism. Although still maintaining circulating levels of T_4 within normal range, these individuals are taking higher doses than necessary to normalize serum TSH. Shorter systolic time intervals, atrial fibrillation, and osteopenia are associated with this entity. Epidemiologic data also suggest that this problem affects 1% to 4% of persons older than age 60 years who are not on thyroid hormone therapy. Unfortunately, there is little in the literature to help determine whether treatment is indicated. Most agree that treatment should be initiated if there are clearly associated symptoms, such as a worsening of cardiovascular function or cardiac arrhythmias, excessive wasting of muscle, anorexia, depression, or significant osteoporosis. Atrial fibrillation has been described in 10% of these patients. As with subclinical hypothyroidism, subclinical hyperthyroidism is also associated with an increased incidence of congestive heart failure in older persons. Patients with subclinical hyperthyroidism are at increased risk of both cardiovascular and all-cause mortality.

▶ Treatment

While all agree that individuals receiving excessive thyroid hormone replacement therapy that suppresses TSH should have their dose of thyroid hormone reduced, it is less clear what to do for individuals with subclinical hyperthyroidism who are not on thyroid hormone. Varied outcomes are reported for affected individuals. Of affected individuals, 47% to 61% have normal serum TSH levels on retesting within 1 year without any intervention, while 1.5% to 13% develop hyperthyroidism. It remains unclear exactly when to treat subclinical hyperthyroidism because therapy has the potential for toxicity and expense, and in some patients the problem may resolve on its own. Treatment is best considered on an individual basis with careful follow-up because hyperthyroidism in older adults often presents in a non-specific manner, and may lead to a decline in functional capacity before or without more classic signs or symptoms of hyperthyroidism. Treatment of subclinical hyperthyroidism may improve bone mineral density and atrial fibrillation if identified. If treatment is selected, ablation therapy with iodine-131 is the preferred modality.

Nanchen D, Gussekloo J, Westendorp RG, et al. PROSPER Group. Subclinical thyroid dysfunction and the risk of heart failure in older persons at high cardiovascular risk. *J Clin Endocrinol Metab.* 2012;97(3):852-861.

Parle JV, Maisonneuve P, Sheppard MC, Boyle P, Franklyn JA. Prediction of all-cause and cardiovascular mortality in elderly people from one low serum thyrotropin result: a 10-year cohort study. *Lancet.* 2001;358(9285):861-865.

Sawin CT, Geller A, Wolf PA, et al. Low serum thyrotropin concentrations as a risk factor for atrial fibrillation in older persons. *N Engl J Med.* 1994;331(19):1249-1252.

Toft AD. Clinical practice. Subclinical hyperthyroidism. *N Engl J Med.* 2001;345(7):512-516.

HYPOTHYROIDISM

▶ General Principles in Older Adults

Hypothyroidism is a common disease of older adults, with a reported prevalence of 0.9% to 17.5%. Hypothyroidism in older adults most commonly results from an autoimmune thyroiditis. Prior radioiodine treatment and subtotal thyroidectomy are also potential causes. The risk of hypothyroidism is >50% after the first year of radioiodine treatment, with an additional annual incidence of 2% to 4% each year thereafter. Hypothyroidism may also be the natural end point to previous Graves disease. Medications may also lead to hypothyroidism, particularly in persons with autoimmune thyroiditis. The most common medications associated with hypothyroidism include iodine-containing radiographic contrast agents, lithium, amiodarone, and iodine-containing cough medicines. Hypothyroidism may also result from a secondary cause: either a pituitary or hypothalamic abnormality.

▶ Clinical Findings

Many of the presenting complaints are confused with other age-prevalent disorders. This problem is further compounded by the often insidious onset of illness. Fatigue and weakness are common. Whereas younger patients commonly present with weight gain, cold intolerance, paresthesia, and muscle cramps, older patients may not, or they may have these or other classic symptoms such as constipation without a thyroid disorder. Many persons who are later discovered to be hypothyroid are unable to identify exactly when the symptoms actually began. Neurologic findings may include dementia, ataxia, and carpal tunnel syndrome, and a delay in the relaxation of deep tendon reflexes may not be easily apparent in a person of advancing age. Hypercholesterolemia may be more common in both circumstances as well. For these reasons, the examining physician should maintain a high index of suspicion of hypothyroidism when evaluating any older person, especially women and those with a personal or family history of some form of thyroid disease.

Primary hypothyroidism is associated with an elevated serum TSH concentration. Changes in protein binding may reduce the level of total T_4; triiodothyronine (T_3) may be reduced in persons with significant medical illness or malnutrition. Even measures of free T_4 may be misleading; T_4 may be suppressed in individuals with T_3 toxicosis. For these reasons, an increase in serum TSH remains the best way to detect primary failure of the thyroid gland regardless of age. During the recovery phase after an acute nonthyroidal illness, however, an elevation of serum TSH level may not represent true clinical hypothyroidism; in this case, the serum TSH returns to the range of normal within 4–6 weeks. Although uncommon in older adults, hypothyroidism can be secondary to pituitary or hypothalamic failure, with low serum TSH and T_4 levels. TSH >10, female sex, and positive antithyroid antibody are associated with an increased risk of progression to overt hypothyroidism. In patients with TSH <10, testing for antithyroid antibodies can be helpful and favors the treatment with levothyroxine. TSH screening is indicated in those older patients with cognitive problems, goiter or history of thyroid abnormality, hypercholesterolemia, or family history of thyroid illness.

Differential Diagnosis

Many of the presenting signs and symptoms of hypothyroidism in persons of any age resemble findings common to many other age-prevalent disorders, notably congestive heart failure and unexplained ascites resulting from cardiac or hepatic abnormalities. A thick tongue may result from primary amyloidosis. Anemia may result from vitamin B_{12}, folate, or iron deficiency or volume expansion. Depression may be present, and other alterations in cognition may be caused by medication toxicity or dementia.

Treatment

L-Thyroxine is the preferred medication to treat hypothyroidism. In general, consistent use of one of the brand name preparations is suggested to minimize variability that may occur with generic preparations. It is also easier for the older person to identify medication with a consistent color and shape. Older patients generally require a smaller amount of L-thyroxine to normalize their thyroid status, on average, 110 µg/day. Because of the age-related increase in T_4 half-life, approximately 9 days in persons 80 years of age and older, it will take longer to reach a steady state. A longer time between dose increases is necessary to reduce unwanted side effects.

The commonly used adage of "start low and go slow" should be followed when starting any older patient on thyroid hormone replacement therapy. Because many older patients with hypothyroidism may have underlying cardiovascular disease, therapy should start with 25 µg/day, with gradually increasing increments of 25 µg every 4–6 weeks. Individuals with significant cardiac disease may require dose changes as low as 12.5 µg and should even be started at that dose. Once a dosage of 75 µg/day is achieved without side effects, increments of 12.5 µg are advised. The final dose required is the amount of L-thyroxine that reduces the serum TSH into the range of normal and does not have associated side effects.

A euthyroid state may exacerbate cardiac symptoms in patients with significant coronary artery disease. In this circumstance, the use of a β-adrenergic blocking agent may allow a clinically euthyroid state to be reached without induction of symptoms of myocardial ischemia. Monitoring of TSH is necessary to avoid inducing iatrogenic subclinical hyperthyroidism from excessive doses of replacement thyroid hormone.

Prognosis

With early treatment, return to a normal state of health is expected. Complete response to thyroid treatment, however, may take months, and patients will require replacement therapy with thyroid hormone and periodic monitoring with thyroid function tests for life.

MYXEDEMA COMA

General Principles in Older Adults

Myxedema coma is a serious consequence of untreated or inadequately treated hypothyroidism. Although rare, it almost exclusively occurs in older patients. Coma is seen in the most severe cases; more common features include alteration in cognition, lethargy, seizures, psychotic symptoms, and confusion and disorientation. In most cases, the affected individual has had a precipitating event such as a severe infection, cold exposure, alcoholism, or the use of psychoactive medications, sedatives, or narcotics. Early treatment is essential.

Clinical Findings

A history of increased fatigue and somnolence is common, as is a history of treatment of a thyroid disorder or use of narcotic, sedative, or antipsychotic medication. Infections, particularly pneumonia and urosepsis, are common. Physical examination may demonstrate classic signs and symptoms of hypothyroidism, including dry, scaly skin, bradycardia, and edema. Profound hypothermia, as well as hypoventilation and hypotension, may exist. Headaches, ataxia, nystagmus, psychotic behavior, muscle spasms, and sinus bradycardia may precede the coma. There may also be a pericardial effusion, ileus, megacolon, and easy bruising.

Laboratory findings classically include a markedly elevated serum TSH and reduced total and free serum T_4. Hypoglycemia and hyponatremia are common. Autoimmune deficiency states, including diabetes mellitus and adrenal insufficiency, are sometimes associated with hypothyroidism and other autoimmune disorders. Creatine phosphokinase of muscle origin is often elevated as a result of muscle breakdown. Myocardial infarction can occur in the presence of myxedema coma or even be the precipitating event, and may complicate the initiation of thyroid hormone therapy. In rare circumstances, myoglobinuria and rhabdomyolysis may occur. Arterial blood gases usually demonstrate a decrease in partial pressure of oxygen and an increase in partial pressure of carbon dioxide, indicating acute or impending respiratory failure. Anemia is also a common finding and is often normochromic, normocytic, or macrocytic. Cardiomegaly is often seen on chest x-ray film. Evoked potentials may have abnormal amplitude or latency, and electroencephalogram may demonstrate triphasic waves that disappear with thyroid replacement.

▶ Differential Diagnosis

Included in the differential diagnosis are dementia, sepsis, intracranial bleed or tumor, hepatic encephalopathy, congestive heart failure, and hypothyroidism.

▶ Treatment

In most cases, patients with severe illness and coma are started on thyroid hormone replacement based on clinical suspicion before obtaining confirming laboratory data. When deciding on therapy, the following principles should be considered:

1. Myxedema coma has a very high mortality rate if treatment is delayed or is inadequate.

2. The uncertainty of diagnosis before receiving laboratory results must be balanced with empiric therapy, especially if the patient is later found not to be hypothyroid.

3. Supportive therapy must be provided and includes ventilatory support for respiratory failure, antibiotics for infection as indicated, and management of hypothermia by external rewarming. Hypotension may be treated with fluid replacement, although dopamine infusion might be required. Hyponatremia must be treated, although thyroid hormone replacement in itself will result in a decrease in antidiuretic hormone (ADH) and produce a brisk diuresis. Hypoglycemia and anemia will need to be monitored carefully and treated on the basis of individual needs. Care must be taken to prevent aspiration, fecal impaction, pressure sores, and urinary retention.

4. Prompt initiation of thyroid hormone replacement is essential. The initial dose for treatment of myxedema coma is between 300 and 500 µg of L-thyroxine given intravenously. This high dose is necessary to occupy hormone-binding sites that have been left free as a result of significant and prolonged hormone deficiency. In addition, precipitating factors, such as infection, may increase the turnover of T_4, and thus warrant a higher initial replacement dose. High doses can increase myocardial oxygen consumption and the potential for myocardial infarction. Once there is evidence of a clinical response, usually noted by a diuresis and increase in body temperature and heart rate, the daily dose of L-thyroxine should be reduced to 50–100 µg and can be given orally and adjusted as necessary. The use of T_3 or a combination of T_4 and T_3 has been suggested by some clinicians because of the shorter onset of action of T_3 and reduced ability to deiodinate T_4 to the more active T_3 in persons with significant illness and/or malnutrition. Data are not available upon which to make a more definitive recommendation.

5. Because adrenal insufficiency may coexist with myxedema coma, suspicion of cortisol deficiency should be high. A suggestive history, physical examination, or electrolyte abnormalities calls for administration of intravenous glucocorticoids. Initiating glucocorticoid therapy for all patients with myxedema coma is controversial. In life-threatening situations, blood for measurement of plasma cortisol should be drawn, and intravenous stress doses of corticosteroids should be administered and continued until there is laboratory confirmation of adrenal status and a decision can be made to continue, taper, or stop the corticosteroids.

▶ Prognosis

Myxedema coma is a serious condition that occurs largely in older hypothyroid persons. Aggressive supportive therapy and thyroid hormone therapy are essential while possible contributing factors are evaluated and treated as necessary. Close monitoring is required when treatment is initiated to avoid toxicity from the relatively large starting doses of thyroid hormone. Even under the best of circumstances, there is considerable mortality related to delay in diagnosis and presence of coexisting morbidities.

Dutta P, Bhansali A, Masoodi SR, Bhadada S, Sharma N, Rajput R. Predictors of outcome in myxoedema coma: a study from a tertiary care centre. *Crit Care.* 2008;12(1):R1.

Kwaku MP, Burman KD. Myxedema coma. *J Intensive Care Med.* 2007;22(4):224-231.

Yamamoto T, Fukuyama J, Fujiyoshi A. Factors associated with mortality of myxedema coma: report of eight cases and literature survey. *Thyroid.* 1999;9(12):1167-1174.

HYPERTHYROIDISM

▶ General Principles in Older Adults

Hyperthyroidism is the result of an excessive amount of circulating thyroid hormone either from endogenous production or iatrogenic sources. Clinically, this disorder is accompanied by a broad spectrum of signs and symptoms that vary among individuals and can differ markedly between young and old persons. A greater percentage of affected individuals is older than age 60 years. Several studies of prevalence indicate the presence of hyperthyroidism in 1% to 3% of community-residing older persons. Hyperthyroidism is far more common in women than in men, with estimates ranging from 4:1 to 10:1.

Graves disease remains the most common cause of hyperthyroidism in young persons, and may still be present in older patients. With increasing age, however, more cases of hyperthyroidism result from multinodular toxic goiter. Although multinodular goiters are commonly found in older persons and are not usually associated with clinical disease, they may evolve into toxic multinodular thyroid goiters. A toxic adenoma may cause hyperthyroidism and is usually identified on thyroid scan as a solitary hyperfunctioning nodule with suppression of activity in the remaining portion of the thyroid gland.

Rarely, hyperthyroidism may result from ingestion of iodide or iodine-containing substances. Iodine may be introduced from seafood, although this problem is more common after exposure to iodinated radiocontrast agents and to amiodarone. Up to 40% of patients taking amiodarone will have serum T_4 levels above the normal range as a result of the drug's effect on T_4 metabolism; far fewer (5%) will develop clinically apparent thyrotoxicosis. The hyperthyroidism can be of rapid onset and severe in magnitude.

Hyperthyroidism must always be considered in the older person who is already receiving thyroid hormone therapy. This is particularly important if the dose is >0.15 mg of L-thyroxine daily, although even smaller doses may be excessive, especially in small individuals of advanced age. Persons taking the same dose of thyroid hormone for many years may become hyperthyroid simply because of an age-associated decline in the body's ability to degrade T_4.

Although extremely rare, a TSH-producing pituitary tumor may be the cause of hyperthyroidism. Nonsuppressed levels of serum TSH in the presence of increased amounts of circulating thyroid hormone are seen with these tumors. Hyperthyroidism may also rarely result with overproduction of thyroid hormone from a widespread metastatic follicular carcinoma.

Transient hyperthyroidism may occur in patients with silent or subacute thyroiditis as a result of increased release of thyroid hormone into the circulation during the inflammatory phase of the illness. Radiation injury, which may be caused by radioactive iodine therapy for hyperthyroidism, may also result in an outpouring of thyroid hormone.

Hyperthyroidism is usually accompanied by elevated levels of both T_4 and T_3. However, a subgroup of older hyperthyroid individuals have isolated elevations of T_3 alone. T_4 is either within the normal range or may, in fact, be suppressed. This circumstance is referred to as T_3 toxicosis. Although it can occur with any type of hyperthyroidism, it is most commonly seen in older patients with toxic multinodular goiter or solitary toxic adenomas. The diagnosis is made on clinical grounds and measurements demonstrating an elevated level of serum T_3 and a suppressed level of serum TSH. T_4 toxicosis, or an isolated increase in serum T_4 without an elevation in serum T_3, most commonly occurs in a sick older person with hyperthyroidism. Disease or malnutrition interferes in the normal removal of iodine from the 5′ position of T_4 and thus a decreased ability to convert T_4 to T_3.

► Clinical Findings

A. Symptoms & Signs

Clinical findings associated with hyperthyroidism in the older adult vary greatly. In general, the clinical presentation of hyperthyroidism at this time of life differs from the more classic findings noted earlier in life (Table 41–1). The presenting feature may be a decline in functional capacity. There may be increased fatigue, muscle weakness, cognitive changes, loss of appetite, weight loss, cardiac arrhythmias, and congestive heart failure. Eye findings associated with the hyperthyroidism are less commonly noted in older adults. Rather than frequent bowel movements, more commonly there is a resolution of preexisting constipation. Anemia and hyponatremia are often noted and thought to be caused by other coexisting illnesses. Although this relative lack of the classic findings of hyperthyroidism does not occur in every older person with hyperthyroidism, a subgroup develops an apathetic hyperthyroid state. In this circumstance, the patient lacks the hyperactivity, irritability, and restlessness common to young patients who are hyperthyroid and presents instead with severe weakness, lethargy, listlessness, depression, and the appearance of a chronic wasting illness. Often the person is incorrectly diagnosed as having a malignancy or severe depression.

Table 41–1. Frequency of signs and symptoms of hyperthyroidism in young versus elderly patients.

Symptom/Sign	Young (%)	Elderly (%)[a]
Palpitation	100	61.5
Goiter	98	61.0
Tremor	96	63.0
Excessive perspiration	92	52.0
Weight loss	73	77.0
Eye signs	71	42.0
Arrhythmias	4.6	39.0

[a]Data represent a compilation of several studies.

Symptoms less common in older patients include nervousness, increased diaphoresis, increased appetite, and increased frequency of bowel movements. More common symptoms include marked weight loss, present in >80% of older patients, poor appetite, worsening angina, agitation, confusion, and edema.

Similarly, physical findings differ in older patients. Hyperreflexia, palpable goiter, and exophthalmos are usually absent, although lid lag and lid retraction may be present. The pulse rate tends to be slower. Cardiac manifestations are particularly important in the older person who may have coexisting heart disease. An increased heart rate with a related increase in myocardial oxygen demand, stroke volume, cardiac output, and shortened left ventricular ejection time underlie the clinical consequences of palpitations. There is also an increased risk of atrial fibrillation (often with slow ventricular response), exacerbation of angina in patients with preexisting coronary artery disease, and precipitation of congestive heart failure that responds less readily to conventional therapy.

Gastrointestinal problems may occasionally include abdominal pain, nausea, and vomiting. Diarrhea and increased frequency of bowel movements resulting from the effect of the thyroid hormone on intestinal motility can occur, but these symptoms are often absent and constipation is still common. There may be an alteration in liver enzymes, including elevation of alkaline phosphatase and γ-glutamyltranspeptidase levels, which become normal after a return to the euthyroid state. Weakness, especially of proximal muscles, is a major feature of hyperthyroidism in older persons and is often accompanied by muscle wasting and functional decline. Disorders of gait, postural instability, and falling may be noted. Tremor is noted in >70% of older persons with hyperthyroidism. The tremor is usually more coarse than in other common tremors. A rapid relaxation phase of the deep tendon reflex is difficult to identify in the older thyrotoxic individual. Central nervous system (CNS) manifestations may be prominent and include confusion, depression, changes in short-term memory, agitation and anxiety, and a decreased attention span. Other findings associated with hyperthyroidism include worsening of glucose tolerance, mild increases in serum calcium, and osteoporosis resulting from increased bone turnover.

B. Laboratory Tests

The altered and often atypical presentation of hyperthyroidism in the older patient warrants a high degree of suspicion among clinicians and the initiation of appropriate laboratory studies. Serum free T_4 and a measurement of serum TSH are the preferred tests for diagnosing thyroid dysfunction. The findings of a normal or low serum free T_4 with a suppressed serum TSH raises the possibility of T_3 toxicosis and warrants a measurement of serum T_3 by radioimmunoassay. Although the finding of anti-TSH receptor antibodies confirms the diagnosis of Graves disease, it is rarely necessary to obtain this test.

C. Special Tests

Thyroid scanning with technetium and measurement of 24-hour ^{131}I uptake can be useful in distinguishing Graves disease from toxic multinodular goiter. Scanning may also demonstrate the presence of a small, diffusely active goiter that could not be detected on physical examination. Very low ^{131}I uptake in a patient with elevated circulating thyroid hormone levels suggests exogenous thyroid hormone ingestion, the hyperthyroid phase of painless or subacute thyroiditis, or iodine-induced hyperthyroidism.

▶ Differential Diagnosis

Patients with hyperthyroidism in later life commonly have coexisting illness, and it is important not to attribute all presenting signs and symptoms to the hyperthyroid state itself. The most common differential diagnoses to consider include anxiety, malignancy, depression, diabetes mellitus, menopause, and pheochromocytoma.

▶ Treatment

Therapy should be directed at the specific cause of the hyperthyroid state. Therefore, the underlying cause must be determined to exclude the possibility of one of the transient forms of illness, such as excessive hormone ingestion, iodine exposure, or subacute thyroiditis. The majority of older patients with either Graves disease or multinodular toxic goiter can be treated with antithyroid medications, radioactive iodine, or surgery. The preferred treatment, however, is radioactive iodine.

A useful initial step in treating suspected hyperthyroidism is to administer a β-adrenergic blocking agent such as long-acting propranolol, metoprolol, nadolol, or atenolol. These agents quickly control associated palpitations, angina, tachycardia, and agitation. Caution is advised, however, in persons with congestive heart failure, chronic obstructive pulmonary disease, or diabetes mellitus being treated with insulin.

Once a diagnosis of Graves disease or toxic nodular goiter is confirmed, treatment should be initiated with one of the antithyroid drugs: propylthiouracil or methimazole. These agents impair biosynthesis of thyroid hormone, thus depleting intrathyroidal hormone stores and ultimately leading to decreased hormone secretion. A decline in serum T_4 concentration is usually seen within 2–4 weeks after initiation of antithyroid drug therapy, and the dose should be tapered once thyroid hormone levels reach the normal range to avoid hypothyroidism. In 1% to 5% of patients, the antithyroid medications may result in fever, rash, and arthralgias. A drug-induced agranulocytosis may be more common in older patients and will most likely occur within the first 3 months of treatment, especially in those who receive >30 mg/day of methimazole. Periodic white blood cell count monitoring should be considered, with discontinuation of the antithyroid medication if there is evidence of neutropenia.

Long-term antithyroid medication use can be effective in patients older than age 60 years with Graves disease, who appear to respond fairly quickly and have a greater likelihood of a long-lasting remission. Because these medications rarely will provide a long-lasting effect for those with a toxic multinodular goiter, more definitive therapy is needed once the patient returns to an euthyroid state on medication. The recommended treatment in most older persons with hyperthyroidism is thyroid gland ablation with [131]I. Once the patient achieves a euthyroid status on antithyroid medication, these agents should be stopped for 3–5 days, after which ^{131}I is given orally. Therapy with β blockers can be maintained and antithyroid agents restarted 5 days after radiotherapy and should be continued for 1–3 months until the major effect of radioiodine is achieved. Although some physicians attempt to calculate a specific dose that will render the patient euthyroid without subsequently developing hypothyroidism, many patients will still develop permanent hypothyroidism. For this reason, most clinicians advocate treating the older person with hyperthyroidism with a relatively large dose of ^{131}I to ensure ablation of thyroid tissue and thus avoid the possibility of hyperthyroidism recurrence.

After treatment, the patient is closely monitored in order to start replacement doses of thyroid hormone, because hypothyroidism may develop in as few as 4 weeks after treatment. Regardless of dosing regimen used, 40% to 50% of patients will be hypothyroid within 12 months of ^{131}I administration, with 2% to 5% developing hypothyroidism each year thereafter.

Prior treatment with antithyroid medication prevents the possibility of radiation-induced thyroiditis after ^{131}I therapy. However, in some circumstances, when clinical and laboratory features suggest a mild case of hyperthyroidism and no cardiac problems are noted, it may be appropriate to treat the hyperthyroid patient with ^{131}I without antithyroid medication pretreatment. When this option is chosen, the patients should be started on a β-blocker and continue with it until thyroid hormone levels return to normal.

Surgery is not recommended as a primary treatment for hyperthyroidism in older patients. Coexisting illness, particularly cardiac, increases operative risk. In addition, postoperative complications of hypoparathyroidism and recurrent laryngeal nerve damage are significant risks. Surgery may be indicated in the rare patient with tracheal compression secondary to a large goiter.

Atrial fibrillation occurs in 10% to 15% of hyperthyroid patients. Treatment of the underlying disease is essential; cardioversion and anticoagulation are considered on an individual basis. The longer the hyperthyroid period, the less likely is the return to normal sinus rhythm; most benefit is found in those who become euthyroid within 3 weeks. Cardioversion is usually reserved for those patients who still remain in atrial fibrillation after 16 weeks of euthyroidism. Many older individuals with hyperthyroidism who develop atrial fibrillation are at greater risk of thromboembolic events, especially those with a history of thromboembolism, hypertension, or congestive heart failure and those with evidence of left atrial enlargement or left ventricular dysfunction. In the absence of contraindications, anticoagulant therapy should be given with warfarin in a dose that will increase the international normalization ratio to 2.0–3.0. Warfarin should be continued until the patient is euthyroid and normal sinus rhythm has been restored.

Allahabadia A, Daykin J, Holder RL, Sheppard MC, Gough SC, Franklyn JA. Age and gender predict the outcome of treatment for Graves' hyperthyroidism. *J Clin Endocrinol Metab.* 2000;85(3):1038-1042.

Trivalle C, Doucet J, Chassagne P, et al. Differences in the signs and symptoms of hyperthyroidism in older and younger patients. *J Am Geriatr Soc.* 1996;44(1):50-53.

NODULAR THYROID DISEASE & NEOPLASIA

▶ General Principles in Older Adults

Multinodular thyroid glands occur more commonly in individuals who have lived in areas of iodine deficiency. Often there is a history of goiter dating to childhood or young adulthood. Very large multinodular goiters, particularly those with a significant substernal component, may compress the trachea and lead to problems of dyspnea and wheezing, or problems with swallowing. All patients with thyroid nodules should be questioned regarding prior exposure to external radiation of the head, neck, and upper thorax. Radiation to these areas markedly increases the risk of thyroid malignancy. Radiation increases the risk of thyroid malignancy as well as benign nodules and parathyroid adenomas. Approximately 16% to 29% of persons who received low-dose radiation to the head and neck as children will develop palpable thyroid nodules; approximately 33% become malignant and clinically detected only after 10–20 years, reaching a peak incidence 20–30 years after radiation exposure.

▶ Clinical Findings

A. Symptoms & Signs

Thyroid nodules usually remain asymptomatic, being discovered by the patient inadvertently or by the physician during a routine physical examination. On occasion, a thyroid nodule may result in an acute onset of neck pain and neck tenderness. This may be an acute or subacute thyroiditis or hemorrhage into a preexisting nodule. Although a single thyroid nodule is more commonly associated with malignancy than is a multinodular thyroid gland, only 5% of clinically apparent solitary nodules will be malignant. The vast majority of thyroid nodules are benign, and include follicular and colloid adenomas, Hashimoto thyroiditis, and thyroid cysts.

Malignant thyroid neoplasms may be papillary, follicular, medullary, or anaplastic carcinomas; lymphoma; or, in rare cases, metastatic disease to the thyroid. Nonthyroid lesions may appear as nodules on physical examination; these include lymph nodes, aneurysms, parathyroid cysts and adenomas, and thyroglossal duct cysts. The risk that a solitary thyroid nodule will prove to be malignant is increased by a history of radiation exposure, age >60 years, rapid increase in size, hoarseness of the voice suggesting an impingement of the recurrent laryngeal nerve, and hardness on palpation. Age is also a factor in predicting the histologic type of malignancy. The overall histologic distribution of all thyroid cancer is 79% papillary, 13% follicular, 3% Hürthle cell, 3.5% medullary, and 1.7% anaplastic. In patients older than 60 years, papillary carcinoma accounts for 67% of thyroid cancers. Follicular carcinoma peaks in frequency between the fourth and sixth decades of life (mean age at diagnosis: 44 years). Together with Hürthle cell carcinoma, these cancers account for 20% of thyroid malignancies in the older-than-age-60-years population. Medullary carcinoma has a peak incidence during the fifth and sixth decades of life and represents approximately 5% of thyroid cancers in the older adult (Table 41–2). Anaplastic carcinomas occur almost exclusively in older populations and account for approximately 6% of thyroid cancers in older patients. Anaplastic carcinoma is characterized by rapid growth, rock-hard consistency, and local invasiveness. Involvement of the recurrent laryngeal nerve and compression of the trachea are common. Lymphoma and metastatic cancers occur infrequently in the older patient. Lymphoma usually presents with a rapidly enlarging painless neck mass that may cause compressive symptoms. Coexisting Hashimoto thyroiditis is common.

B. Laboratory Tests

The major objective in evaluating an older person with a thyroid nodule is to rule out the presence of a malignancy. Blood tests of thyroid function will usually be normal unless there is a hyperfunctioning adenoma or toxic multinodular goiter. An elevated serum TSH may be noted in persons with subclinical hypothyroidism and nodular disease, as may result from longstanding Hashimoto thyroiditis. Serum thyroglobulin is often elevated in the setting of thyroid cancer but cannot differentiate malignancy from benign nodules or thyroiditis with any degree of certainty. It is, therefore, more commonly used as a marker for recurrence or metastasis in patients with papillary or follicular carcinoma who have undergone total thyroidectomy. An elevation of serum calcitonin concentration is indicative of a medullary carcinoma, but is not part of the initial evaluation, unless there is a family history of multiple endocrine neoplasia.

C. Special Tests

Fine-needle aspiration (FNA) of the thyroid remains the best way to obtain tissue for cytologic or histologic examination. FNA is indicated in any patient with a solitary nodule and when there is suspicion of thyroid malignancy based on clinical evaluation, ultrasonography, or thyroid scan. This procedure, when performed by a skilled clinician, has proven to be safe, inexpensive, and capable of determining the presence or absence of malignancy with an accuracy of close to 95%, and even greater accuracy with sonographic guidance. In general, cytopathologic findings from FNA are divided into 4 categories: positive for malignancy, suspicious for malignancy, negative for malignancy, and nondiagnostic. A repeat FNA is indicated for a nondiagnostic but clinically suspicious nodule. Malignant cells found on FNA indicate the need for surgery. The combination of suspicious cytology by FNA and a cold-appearing nodule on thyroid scan also indicates the need for surgical excision of the suspicious nodule. Benign cytology in either a solid or cystic nodule warrants observation. If the FNA is suggestive of a lymphoma, a repeat biopsy using a large-needle or even a surgical biopsy is indicated.

Isotopic scanning is no longer considered the initial diagnostic test in evaluating a suspicious nodule because of its relatively high false-positive and false-negative rates and high cost. Isotope imaging is best used when evaluating a patient with a thyroid nodule who has had a nondiagnostic result from FNA. Because malignant tissue is more likely unable to take up iodine, the identification of a nodule as hot on ^{123}I or technetium scanning makes malignancy in the nodule less likely, although clearly still possible. Scanning may also reveal an apparent single nodule that is, in fact, part of a multinodular thyroid gland, again decreasing the risk of malignancy. The presence of a nonfunctioning or a cold nodule is not proof of a malignancy because 95% of thyroid nodules will prove to be cold; the frequency of malignancy in cold nodules is 5%. Hot nodules associated with normal circulating levels of thyroid hormone and no compressive symptoms should be observed with repeat examinations performed at 6- to 12-month intervals. These nodules may eventually result in hyperthyroidism; thus, clinical correlation is also warranted. High-resolution ultrasonography can detect thyroid lesions as small as 2 mm and can also permit classification

Table 41–2. Thyroid malignancy in the older patient.

Cancer Type	Patients Affected (%)		10-Year Survival
	> Age 40	> Age 60	> Age 60
Papillary/mixed	79	64	<65
Follicular	13	20	<57
Medullary	3	5	<63
Anaplastic	2	6	0
Lymphoma	3	5	99+

of a nodule as solid, cystic, or mixed solid-cystic. It will often identify multinodularity in a gland even when a single nodule is palpated clinically. This technique cannot be used to distinguish with any degree of certainty malignant from benign nodules because there is a great deal of overlap in the characteristics identified using ultrasonography. Ultrasonography is best used to detect recurrent or residual thyroid cancer, as well as to screen persons with a history of radiation exposure earlier in life.

Computed tomography (CT) and magnetic resonance imaging (MRI) are expensive and add little to the initial assessment of malignancy. They may be useful in evaluating the extent of disease in patients found to have anaplastic carcinoma or lymphoma and may provide useful information regarding compression of neck structures and the size and substernal extent of nodules and goiters.

Medullary carcinoma of the thyroid gland can be monitored using blood calcitonin measurements, both in the basal state and after stimulation. Blood levels of carcinoembryonic antigen may also be elevated in patients with residual or recurrent medullary carcinoma.

Differential Diagnosis

The differential diagnosis includes thyroid duct cysts, benign adenomas, toxic thyroid nodule, thyroid malignancy, hemorrhage, and multinodular thyroid gland.

Treatment

Although the basic principles for treating thyroid cancer do not differ significantly between the young and old, older individuals need to be more carefully evaluated for comorbid conditions and risk of surgery. Surgery for thyroid cancer should be performed only by an experienced surgeon. Papillary or follicular carcinoma is usually treated with near-total thyroidectomy because of the high frequency of multicentricity of malignancy and the need to remove functional thyroid tissue to monitor the patient with total-body radioiodine scanning. Thyroid remnants detected postoperatively are ablated with [131]I. At 6 months, and subsequently at yearly intervals, scanning should be obtained and serum thyroglobulin measured to determine whether residual functional tissue exists. If active tissue is found, large ablative doses of ^{131}I should be administered. This approach has reduced the recurrence rate of both papillary and follicular carcinomas and prolonged survival.

Patients treated for malignancy are treated judiciously with suppressive doses of L-thyroxine as tolerated with the desired objective of reducing serum TSH to below normal as measured by third-generation TSH assays. The administration of suppressive doses of L-thyroxine carries a substantial risk of precipitating or aggravating ischemic heart disease and arrhythmias as well as accelerating bone turnover. The

older patient will need to be monitored closely and the dose of thyroid hormone reduced if cardiac symptoms develop. An acceleration of bone loss will occur and necessitate treatment with antibone resorption agents in some circumstances (eg, in osteopenic women). Medullary carcinoma of the thyroid gland is best treated with a total thyroidectomy because the disease is often multicentric. The majority of medullary carcinomas do not respond to ^{131}I treatment; therefore, palliative therapy is recommended using external irradiation if residual thyroid tissue or recurrent disease is detected. Thyroid lymphoma should be clinically staged using CT or MRI. External irradiation in combination with chemotherapy has been associated with a survival rate close to 100%.

Prognosis

Age at diagnosis is an important factor in predicting cancer aggressiveness and mortality from differentiated thyroid cancer. Individuals diagnosed after age 50 years have a higher rate of recurrence and death (see Table 41–2). The 10-year survival for patients with papillary carcinoma is approximately 97% in those younger than 45 years and <65% for those older than 60 years at diagnosis. The 10-year survival rate for persons with follicular carcinoma is 98% for those younger than 45 years and <57% for those older than 60 years at diagnosis. The older the person is when a follicular carcinoma is diagnosed, the greater the risk of recurrence and death.

The 10-year survival rate for persons with medullary carcinoma is 84% for individuals younger than 45 years and decreases with advancing age. Persons in the seventh decade of life have a high rate of persistent disease even after surgery. Anaplastic carcinoma of the thyroid gland is rarely associated with more than a 1-year survival after diagnosis because of its rapid progression and high propensity to metastasize. Palliative treatment of compressive symptoms may be achieved by surgery followed by high-dose external radiation. Chemotherapy with doxorubicin or cisplatin, or a combination, may be beneficial in combination with surgery and external irradiation.

Cooper DS, Doherty GM, Haugen BR, et al. American Thyroid Association Guidelines Taskforce. Management guidelines for patients with thyroid nodules and differentiated thyroid cancer. *Thyroid.* 2006;16(2):109-142.

Mazzaferri EL. An overview of the management of papillary and follicular thyroid carcinoma. *Thyroid.* 1999;9(5):421-427.

DISEASES OF THE ADRENAL CORTEX

Advancing age is associated with a reduced metabolic clearance rate of cortisol, but with a compensatory decrease in secretion rate. Consequently, basal levels of serum cortisol are unaffected over the life span. Basal adrenocorticotropic hormone (ACTH) levels are unchanged or slightly increased with age in healthy individuals. Diurnal cortisol rhythm is reported to show a significant age-related phase advance (earlier peak and nadir level) similar to that observed in depressed patients. This is thought to be related to changes in sleep patterns.

The adrenal androgen precursor dehydroepiandrosterone (DHEA) reaches peak blood levels in both men and women by age 20–30 years, and then declines steadily, so that, after age 70 years, levels are <20% of the peak. Although early reports and popular lay literature have attributed a number of antiaging properties to DHEA, more recent studies in which DHEA has been administered for 6–12 months have shown little or no effect on objective measures of physiologic function. Some studies, however, suggest a beneficial effect on mood and sense of general well-being.

The hypothalamic–pituitary–adrenal axis response to known major stimuli remains intact with increasing age. Stimulation tests of this axis using insulin-induced hypoglycemia or metyrapone administration, result in a normal or slightly longer period of cortisol and ACTH secretory response in older persons. Peak cortisol response to stress is also greater, and both cortisol and ACTH levels remain elevated for a longer period in older compared with younger persons. Moreover, dexamethasone causes less inhibition of cortisol in older patients. It is unknown whether this age-related hyperresponsiveness of the pituitary–adrenal axis to stressful situations contributes to age-prevalent illness, including osteoporosis, glucose intolerance, muscle atrophy, and immunosuppression. Adrenal cortical response to exogenous ACTH, measured by circulating cortisol levels, is unaffected by aging.

ACUTE ADRENAL INSUFFICIENCY

▶ General Principles in Older Adults

Acute adrenal insufficiency results from a deficiency in cortisol secretion and, in older people, occurs most often as a result of failure of the adrenal gland rather than a pituitary gland disorder. The adrenal gland may be unable to produce an adequate amount of corticosteroids and mineralocorticoids because of an autoimmune process involving the entire adrenal gland or from a replacement of healthy adrenal tissue with tumor or infection, such as in tuberculosis. Adrenal crisis may also result from an increased demand for glucocorticoids in an individual unable to increase output sufficiently. This occurs most commonly as a result of chronic adrenal suppression from exogenous corticoid use and less often from stress from trauma, surgery, hemorrhage, or infection. Rarely, this may result from a sudden increase in the metabolic turnover of corticosteroids, as can occur when a patient with both adrenal insufficiency and hypothyroidism is treated with thyroid hormone. Corticosteroid-induced adrenal suppression can occur after as few as 3–4 weeks of exogenous steroid

treatment with doses >15 mg of prednisone or the equivalent dose of other glucocorticoids. In general, individuals on long-term glucocorticoid therapy who have stopped treatment before the return of function of the suppressed adrenal glands or who need a higher dose will have a less clear picture because of the ability of renin and angiotensin to maintain aldosterone function despite suppression of glucocorticoid activity in the adrenal gland.

▶ Clinical Findings

A. Symptoms & Signs

Patients with adrenal insufficiency often have nausea and vomiting and abdominal pain, and may have an altered mental state and fever. In general, blood pressure is low. Signs of primary adrenal insufficiency may include hyperpigmentation and evidence of dehydration. Older persons commonly have sparse or absent pubic and axillary hair; therefore, this is less commonly noted as a presenting sign in older patients.

B. Laboratory Tests

Laboratory findings may include hyponatremia or hyperkalemia. Hypoglycemia and elevation of blood urea nitrogen (BUN) and creatinine are common. Eosinophilia may be noted as well. Cultures may be positive if there is an underlying infection. The cosyntropin (ACTH 1–24) stimulation test is abnormal, and plasma ACTH is usually elevated in persons with primary failure of the adrenal gland. With this test, patients are given 0.25 mg of cosyntropin intravenously over 2–3 minutes, and serum cortisol is measured immediately before and 30 and 60 minutes after administration. Under normal circumstances, serum cortisol rises by at least 7 µg/dL to at least 20 µg/dL. Hydrocortisone administration will interfere with the test results, but other glucocorticoids, such as dexamethasone or prednisone, do not interfere with the specific assay for cortisol.

▶ Differential Diagnosis

Although adrenal insufficiency should be considered in any patient who presents with hyperkalemia and hypotension, other possible causes for these findings should be considered.

Other causes of hypotension in particular include sepsis, hemorrhage, and cardiogenic diseases. Renal insufficiency may cause hyperkalemia as may gastrointestinal bleeding, rhabdomyolysis, and medications such as spironolactone and angiotensin-converting enzyme inhibitors. Hyponatremia may occur in hypothyroidism, with diuretic use, in drug and disease states associated with inappropriate ADH secretion, and with malnutrition, cirrhosis, and vomiting. Eosinophilia may be associated with blood dyscrasias, allergies, medication reactions, and parasitic infections. The associated gastrointestinal findings of nausea, vomiting, and abdominal pain may, in fact, be caused by other gastrointestinal tract disorders common during later life. Hyperpigmentation may not be noted in older persons of dark complexion or who have sun-induced skin damage.

Treatment

Replacement of both glucocorticoids and mineralocorticoids is needed in severe cases of adrenal insufficiency. Because hydrocortisone has some mineralocorticoid activity, it is the corticosteroid of choice for patients with mild cases and is effective in doses of 25–37.5 mg orally; two-thirds of the dose is given in the morning and one-third in the late afternoon or evening. If salt-retaining effects from this therapy are insufficient, fludrocortisone is added to the daily regimen in dosages of 0.05–0.3 mg orally each day or every other day. The exact dose required varies with the individual and, therefore, should be clinically adjusted in relation to postural blood pressure changes, level of potassium, and body weight. The dose is reduced if hypokalemia, hypertension, or edema occurs, especially when fluid and electrolyte management is complicated by cardiac disease or renal insufficiency. Underlying factors that may have contributed to the onset of adrenal insufficiency, particularly infections, should be sought. The dosage of hydrocortisone may need to be adjusted upward to a stress dosage as high as 300 mg/day, although usually 50 mg intravenously or intramuscularly every 6 hours will be sufficient, even for the most stressful situations.

Prognosis

With adequate replacement therapy, adrenal insufficiency is a treatable illness. When accompanied by other illnesses, the risk mortality is increased. If the underlying cause is an autoimmune disease, other endocrine problems, such as diabetes mellitus and hypothyroidism, as well as pernicious anemia, may be present.

Parker CR Jr, Slayden SM, Azziz R, et al. Effects of aging on adrenal function in the human: responsiveness and sensitivity of adrenal androgens and cortisol to adrenocorticotropin in premenopausal and postmenopausal women. *J Clin Endocrinol Metab.* 2000;85(1):48-54.

CUSHING SYNDROME

General Principles in Older Adults

Cushing syndrome is caused by an excessive amount of circulating corticosteroids. In older patients, it most commonly results from exogenous exposure to corticosteroids given for a variety of medical disorders. The most frequent endogenous cause is ectopic production of ACTH by neoplasms, especially small cell carcinoma of the lung and carcinoid tumor.

Cushing disease (ie, oversecretion of ACTH by a pituitary tumor) is less common in older than in younger patients, is usually associated with a small benign adenoma, and occurs more often in women than in men. Approximately 15% of cases of endogenous Cushing syndrome are non-ACTH dependent and result from an adrenal adenoma, carcinoma, or bilateral nodular adrenal hyperplasia. Although adrenal adenomas are generally small and produce mostly glucocorticoids, carcinomas tend to be larger on presentation and more commonly produce excessive amounts of both glucocorticoids and androgens, often resulting in virilization and hirsutism.

Clinical Findings

A. Symptoms & Signs

Although central obesity, thin arms and legs, and a round "moon face" are classic findings, these may be harder to detect in older patients. For example, the "buffalo hump" deposition of fat at the back of the neck may, in older women, be confused with kyphosis resulting from osteoporosis. Thin, transparent skin, bruising, muscle atrophy and weakness, diabetes mellitus, and hypertension are other common findings easily confused with many other age-prevalent disorders. Thirst is less often reported by older adults compared with younger patients. Polyuria may result from increases in blood sugar from glucocorticoid-induced diabetes. Blood glucose is often elevated, and glycosuria may be present. Occasionally, there is a leukocytosis and hypokalemia. Wound healing may be impaired, and changes in mental function, including anxiety, psychosis, and depression, may occur.

B. Laboratory Tests

A 1-mg overnight dexamethasone suppression test, urine free cortisol, late-night salivary cortisol (2 measurements), or longer low-dose dexamethasone suppression test (2 mg/day for 48 hours) can be used to screen for hypercortisolism, based on its suitability for a given patient. In a 1-mg overnight dexamethasone suppression test, dexamethasone 1 mg is given orally at 11 PM, and serum is collected at 8 AM the next morning for cortisol. A cortisol level <1.8 µg/dL is considered normal and excludes a diagnosis of Cushing syndrome. If there is failure of suppression, further evaluation should include a 24-hour urine collection for free cortisol and creatinine, and late-night salivary cortisol (2 measurements). A 2-mg dexamethasone suppression test using 0.5 mg of dexamethasone administered orally every 6 hours for 48 hours can also be used as a screening test. Serum cortisol is measured 6 hours after the last dose of dexamethasone and cortisol level <1.8 µg/dL is considered normal suppression. Longer low-dose dexamethasone suppression test excludes hypercortisolism with improved specificity compared to 1-mg dexamethasone suppression test.

Once hypercortisolism is confirmed, plasma ACTH should be determined. A level of ACTH below the normal range indicates a probable adrenal tumor; an elevated level indicates overproduction by either the pituitary or an ectopic ACTH-secreting tumor. MRI of the pituitary can identify a pituitary adenoma with considerable accuracy. Selective inferior petrosal venous sampling for ACTH can be done to confirm a pituitary source of ACTH and to help distinguish its origin from other sites. A CT or MRI scan of the chest and abdomen to look for ectopic sources of ACTH is indicated and can localize a tumor of the adrenal glands.

Differential Diagnosis

Hypercortisolism can result from iatrogenic use of steroid medications. Alcoholic patients and those with depression may also have increased levels of cortisol. Abnormal dexamethasone suppression tests have been described in patients with morbid obesity, depression, and a variety of CNS disorders. In these patients, urine free cortisol should be measured and an attempt made to assess diurnal variation in cortisol secretion because these tests are usually within normal limits in the setting of obesity. Hypertension resulting from other causes is common in the older adults, and estrogen replacement therapy may alter normal dexamethasone suppressibility.

Treatment

Cushing disease is best treated by removing the pituitary adenoma responsible for the increase in ACTH secretion. After its removal, the adrenal gland remains unable to respond to normal stimulation for a prolonged time, and there is an altered ability to respond under conditions of stress. Hydrocortisone replacement therapy is necessary until normal pituitary–adrenal axis function returns, often taking as long as 6–24 months. Radiation therapy has also been used to treat Cushing disease, with an approximate cure rate of 25%. For patients who are not surgical candidates, inhibition of adrenal steroid biosynthesis can be useful in controlling symptoms and has been achieved with metyrapone, 500 mg every 6 hours, in combination with aminoglutethimide, 250–500 mg every 6 hours, and ketoconazole, 200 mg every 6 hours. Physiologic replacement doses of a glucocorticoid may be necessary to avoid drug-induced adrenal insufficiency.

Adrenal neoplasms secreting cortisol should be resected when possible and often can be removed laparoscopically. Because the nonaffected adrenal gland is usually suppressed, once again hydrocortisone replacement is indicated until the gland returns to normal function. Metastatic adrenal carcinoma can be managed with the medications just mentioned or with mitotane, 2–10 mg daily in divided doses. Ectopic ACTH-secreting tumors should be surgically resected. If this is not possible, once again, medications may be used to suppress the high levels of cortisol. The somatostatin analogue octreotide has been used to suppress ACTH secretion successfully in as many as 33% of cases in which it has been attempted.

Prognosis

Patients who have hypercortisolism as a result of iatrogenic use of corticosteroids can usually expect a return to normal after discontinuation of the steroid therapy. In hypercortisolism, the best prognosis for total recovery is seen when a benign adrenal adenoma is easily removed. Pituitary adenomas are more difficult to treat and, even in the best of hands, have a failure rate of 10% to 20%. Even those who respond have a 15% to 20% recurrence rate over the next decade. The prognosis of patients with ectopic ACTH-producing tumors depends on the underlying type and degree of tumor involvement.

Papanicolaou DA, Yanovski JA, Cutler GB Jr, Chrousos GP, Nieman LK. A single midnight serum cortisol measurement distinguishes Cushing's syndrome from pseudo-Cushing states. *J Clin Endocrinol Metab*. 1998;83(4):1163-1167.

HYPERPARATHYROIDISM

General Principles In Older Adults

Hyperparathyroidism is a common disorder that affects predominantly postmenopausal women, with an incidence of approximately 2 per 1000 women. At least 50% of patients have no or minimal nonspecific symptoms or signs. Although a primary abnormality in 1 or all of the parathyroid glands may be responsible (primary hyperparathyroidism), suboptimal levels of vitamin D are associated with elevated parathyroid hormone (PTH) levels, although usually with normal or low levels of calcium. PTH concentrations are also influenced by a number of other factors and are higher in older individuals, especially older women; in blacks relative to whites; in those with low calcium; and in obese individuals.

Primary hyperparathyroidism (PHPT) is caused by the inappropriate secretion of PTH, which results in hypercalcemia. The most frequent underlying disease is a single benign parathyroid adenoma. Less commonly, multiple gland involvement or 4-gland hyperplasia may be present. With the availability and more widespread usage of PTH assays, normocalcemic hyperparathyroidism is being increasingly identified. In making the diagnosis of normocalcemic hyperparathyroidism, it is critical to exclude other causes of elevated PTH and normal serum calcium (secondary hyperparathyroidism). These individuals may have isolated hypercalciuria and are predisposed to renal calculi.

Secondary hyperparathyroidism (SHPT) is the result of the parathyroid's response to hypocalcemia in an attempt to maintain calcium homeostasis. The common causes of

SHPT are chronic renal failure, vitamin D insufficiency, malabsorption syndromes, drugs (bisphosphonates, furosemide, anticonvulsants, phosphorus), hypercalciuria caused by renal leak, and pseudohypoparathyroidism type1b. Tertiary hyperparathyroidism (THPT) occurs because of prolonged hypocalcemia leading to parathyroid gland hyperplasia and autonomous oversecretion of PTH resulting in hypercalcemia.

▶ Clinical Findings

A. Symptoms and Signs

The most common clinical circumstance is an unanticipated finding of hypercalcemia during a routine blood test. Mild nonspecific complaints may include fatigue and generalized weakness. CNS symptoms of depression or mild cognitive impairment may be present. Questioning may disclose increased thirst and polyuria thought to be caused by the antagonistic effect of hypercalcemia on the renal action of ADH. A history of renal calculi, fracture, loss of height, and/or disproportionately low-for-age bone mineral density on dual energy x-ray absorptiometry scan calls for measurement of serum calcium. In SHPT and THPT, patients may have symptoms from the primary disease process. Even if asymptomatic, PHPT patients with calcium stones and or nephrocalcinosis are categorized as having symptomatic disease.

B. Laboratory Findings

When serum calcium is minimally or only intermittently increased, measurement of ionized calcium can establish the presence of hypercalcemia. Vitamin D deficiency and insufficiency in patients with PHPT may mask hypercalcemia and calcium levels will become increased in most cases after repletion of vitamin D. It is recommended that 1,25-dihydroxyvitamin D_3 (1,25[OH]2) levels be measured in all patients with PHPT. The diagnosis is confirmed by measuring serum intact PTH and correlating to levels of serum calcium. Levels of PTH are almost always elevated above the upper limit of normal or within the normal range but inappropriately high for the level of hypercalcemia. Renal imaging by ultrasound is recommended if kidney stones are suspected. Serum BUN and creatinine should be measured because SHPT is often found in the presence of renal insufficiency. PTH levels tend to rise steadily with the progression of renal disease. A rise of PTH up to the 3-fold normal range is generally accepted as a "physiologic" mechanism of compensating for low 1,25(OH)2, but reverts to normal when vitamin D is repleted.

Once the diagnosis of PHPT is confirmed biochemically, bone mineral density should be measured. Parathyroid adenomas can be localized with a high degree of sensitivity and specificity by means of isotopic scanning with technetium-99m sestamibi. Imaging studies are not appropriate for confirming the diagnosis of PHPT or for screening patients for surgical referral. Selective sampling of veins draining the parathyroid glands for step-up in PTH levels can be done in patients who have had previous parathyroid surgery with failure to identify abnormal parathyroid tissue or if the sestamibi scan is nondiagnostic.

▶ Differential Diagnosis

The finding of hypercalcemia along with low-normal or low serum phosphorus levels suggests the diagnosis of PHPT. Other causes of hypercalcemia are usually associated with a lowered level of PTH and include a number of malignancies with or without bone metastases (squamous cell carcinoma of the lung, breast cancer, renal cell carcinoma, multiple myeloma, lymphoma). Hypercalcemia in many of these malignancies may be mediated by tumor-secreted PTH-related protein. Other causes of hypercalcemia include thiazide diuretics, vitamin D toxicity, sarcoidosis, hyperthyroidism, and familial hypocalciuric hypercalcemia (FHH). FHH has traditionally been diagnosed in families by the presence of hypercalcemia and relative hypocalciuria. The calcium-to-creatinine clearance ratio is of particular value, and is usually below 0.01 in FHH; this ratio is usually above 0.01 in typical PHPT. It is important to ensure that other causes of hypercalcemia and relative hypocalciuria are excluded, including concurrent treatment with thiazide diuretics or lithium.

▶ Treatment

Parathyroidectomy should be offered to patients who meet the criteria for surgery established by the 2008 National Institutes of Health consensus panel (Table 41–3) or who are symptomatic. Older patients are at risk for sudden elevation of serum calcium if they become dehydrated or immobile for whatever reason. The increased risk of fracture in the older woman with significant osteoporosis can be reduced by correction of the hyperparathyroidism. Calcimimetic cinacalcet may be used as a therapeutic trial to determine the effect of lowering serum calcium and the potential benefits of parathyroidectomy in complex cases with significant

Table 41–3. Indications for surgical treatment of primary hyperparathyroidism.

Symptomatic primary hyperparathyroidism
Asymptomatic primary hyperparathyroidism
a. Serum calcium level >1.0 mg/dL (0.25 mmol/L) above the upper limits of normal
b. Creatinine clearance (calculated) reduced to <60 mL/min
c. Bone mineral density with T-score less than –2.5 at any site and/or previous fragility fracture
d. Patient age <50 years
e. Medical surveillance not desirable or possible

comorbidity. In the case of parathyroid adenoma, identification and removal of the adenoma will be curative. If parathyroid hyperplasia is found, 3.5 of 4 identified glands must be removed. Intraoperative rapid PTH assay, if available, can confirm that the surgeon has successfully removed the abnormal tissue.

When surgery is not recommended medical monitoring is critical. Recommended surveillance includes annual measurement of serum calcium and creatinine levels, and annual or biannual bone density testing. Vitamin D replacement in patients with suboptimal vitamin D is associated with reductions in serum PTH, and has not resulted in further increases in serum calcium. It would be appropriate to consider vitamin D supplementation in all individuals with PHPT if serum levels are below 50 nmol/L (20 ng/mL) before making any medical or surgical management decisions. Guidelines for calcium intake should be the same as for patients without PHPT.

Medical options for patients unable to undergo parathyroidectomy include antiresorptive treatments, such as bisphosphonates; raloxifene; and calcimimetic cinacalcet. Several randomized control trials have reported that bisphosphonate therapy and estrogen replacement therapy in PHPT decrease bone turnover and increase bone mineral density (BMD), but fracture outcomes have not been evaluated. Very limited data are available in regard to the biochemical and skeletal effects of raloxifene in postmenopausal women with PHPT. If skeletal protection is the primary reason for intervention, bisphosphonates are the drug of choice. If present, vitamin D deficiency should be corrected first, as it increases the risk of hypocalcemia with bisphosphonate therapy. Bisphosphonates should be used cautiously in the presence of renal insufficiency. Only calcimimetic cinacalcet effectively lowers serum calcium and PTH levels during long-term therapy in PHPT, but has not been shown to alter bone turnover or increase BMD. At present, use of this agent in PHPT is limited to management of symptomatic hypercalcemia in patients who are unable to undergo corrective surgery and in whom bisphosphonates are ineffective or are contraindicated.

Goals of medical management in SHPT are the normalization of calcium and skeletal protection. Medical therapy starts with prevention of the development of severe SHPT with close monitoring of serum calcium, phosphate, PTH and vitamin D_3. Principles of managing SHPT in end-stage renal disease include normalization of hyperphosphatemia, regulation of serum calcium, and lowering PTH secretion (calcitriol and calcimimetic administration). Whenever possible, the underlying cause of SHPT should be treated. THPT should be managed by parathyroidectomy especially in the presence of severe metabolic bone disease.

Marx SJ. Hyperparathyroid and hypoparathyroid disorders. *N Engl J Med*. 2000;343(25):1863-1875.

Silverberg SJ, Shane E, Jacobs TP, Siris E, Bilezikian JP. A 10-year prospective study of primary hyperparathyroidism with or without parathyroid surgery. *N Engl J Med*. 1999;341(17):1249-1255.

Diabetes

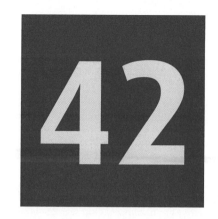

42

Josette A. Rivera, MD
Jessamyn Conell-Price, MS
Sei Lee, MD, MAS

ESSENTIALS OF DIAGNOSIS

- ▶ Hemoglobin A1c ≥6.5, *or*
- ▶ Fasting (no caloric intake for ≥8 hours) plasma glucose ≥126 mg/dL (7.0 mmol/L), *or*
- ▶ Symptoms of hyperglycemia plus random plasma glucose ≥200 mg/dL (11.1 mmol/L), *or*
- ▶ 2-hour plasma glucose ≥200 mg/dL (11.1 mmol/L) during a 75-g oral glucose tolerance test.

▶ General Principles in Older Adults

Diabetes mellitus (DM) is a common condition in older adults and is associated with increased risk of morbidity and mortality. The prevalence of DM (diagnosed and undiagnosed) in the U.S. population of older adults has been estimated at 10.9 million, or 27% of people older than age 65 years. If current trends continue, 16.8 million adults older than age 65 will have diabetes by 2050. There are many reasons for the increasing prevalence of diabetes in older adults, including declining beta cell function, relative insulinopenia, and insulin resistance. Furthermore, the risk of developing DM type 2 increases with obesity, lack of physical activity, and loss of muscle mass, all of which commonly occur with aging. Compared to younger people with diabetes, people older than age 65 years tend to have longer duration of diabetes, with a median duration of 10 years, higher rates of diabetic complications and comorbid disease, and more functional dependence.

The population of older adults with diabetes is incredibly diverse. Some older adults have had type 1 diabetes for many decades and reach old age with significant end-organ complications. Others develop insulin resistance and diabetes in their 70s or 80s, and have no clear evidence of related complications. Some are able to effectively self-manage their disease, whereas others cannot because of cognitive, visual, or functional impairments. Thus, the management of an older patient with diabetes must account for this tremendous heterogeneity and decision making should be individualized, focusing on patient factors such as the duration of diabetes, presence of complications, comorbid conditions, life expectancy, patient goals and preferences, and functional abilities.

Boyle JP, Honeycutt AA, Narayan KM, et al. Projection of diabetes burden through 2050: impact of changing demography and disease prevalence in the U.S. *Diabetes Care.* 2001;24(11): 1936-1940.

Centers for Disease Control and Prevention (CDC). *National Diabetes Fact Sheet: National Estimates and General Information on Diabetes and Prediabetes in the United States, 2011.* Atlanta, GA: Centers for Disease Control and Prevention US Department of Health and Human Services, 2011.

▶ Pathogenesis

Most patients older than 65 years with diagnosed DM have type 2 DM and a small minority has type 1 DM. Type 1 DM is an autoimmune disease in which pancreatic beta cells are destroyed, resulting in absolute insulinopenia, subsequent hyperglycemia, and risk for ketoacidosis. Exogenous insulin is required for survival and glucose control.

In contrast, type 2 DM results from insulin resistance, increased insulin requirements to maintain euglycemia and ultimately, relative insulin deficiency when the pancreatic beta cells are unable to meet the higher insulin requirements. In older patients, decreased insulin production (rather than insulin resistance) can be the predominant factor in the pathogenesis of type 2 DM. Treatment for type 2 DM includes exercise, carbohydrate control, and oral glucose-lowering agents with or without insulin.

Stumvoll M, Goldstein BJ, van Haeften TW. Type 2 diabetes: principles of pathogenesis and therapy. *Lancet.* 2005;365(9467):1333-1346.

▶ Prevention

Numerous studies show that, for obese adults with impaired glucose tolerance who are at high risk for developing type 2 DM, lifestyle modification that focuses on diet, exercise, and weight loss can delay or prevent progression to diabetes. The largest of these trials was the Diabetes Prevention Program (DPP), a nationwide multicenter trial that examined whether metformin or lifestyle modification decreases progression to diabetes in high-risk adults. In older adults (>60 years), lifestyle modification was especially powerful, decreasing the incidence of diabetes 71% compared to usual care in the 2.8 years of follow-up. Metformin, however, decreased the incidence of diabetes by only 11% in older adults, compared with 44% in younger adults (age 25–44 years). Thus, for obese older adults at high risk for diabetes, the focus of diabetes prevention should be on lifestyle modification (diet, exercise, and weight loss) rather than metformin.

Knowler WC, Barrett-Connor E, Fowler SE, et al. Diabetes Prevention Program Research Group. Reduction in the incidence of type 2 diabetes with lifestyle intervention or metformin. *N Engl J Med.* 2002;346(6):393-403.

Li G, Zhang P, Wang J, et al. The long-term effect of lifestyle interventions to prevent diabetes in the China Da Qing Diabetes Prevention Study: a 20-year follow-up study. *Lancet.* 2008;371(9626):1783-1789.

Saito T, Watanabe M, Nishida J, et al. Zensharen Study for Prevention of Lifestyle Diseases Group. Lifestyle modification and prevention of type 2 diabetes in overweight Japanese with impaired fasting glucose levels: a randomized controlled trial. *Arch Intern Med.* 2011;171(15):1352-1360.

Tuomilehto J, Lindström J, Eriksson JG, et al. Finnish Diabetes Prevention Study Group. Prevention of type 2 diabetes mellitus by changes in lifestyle among subjects with impaired glucose tolerance. *N Engl J Med.* 2001;344(18):1343-1350.

▶ Complications

A. Acute Complications

Acute complications of DM are primarily metabolic and infectious.

Diabetic ketoacidosis (DKA) is characteristic of type 1 DM, but can also occur in type 2 DM, particularly among Hispanic and African American individuals. Insulin deficiency, most commonly a result of inadequate insulin therapy in type 1 DM, leads to decreased glucose metabolism, resulting in increased lipolysis, free fatty acid metabolism, and subsequent ketoacidosis. Common precipitating factors for DKA include pneumonia, myocardial infarction, and stroke, and are thought to lead to DKA by invoking a systemic stress response with increased cortisol, glucagon, and catecholamines that counteracts some of the effects of insulin. Typically, patients present with symptoms of dyspnea, acidosis, dehydration, abdominal pain, nausea, and vomiting. Mental status alteration and coma may be present. Effective

management focuses on identifying and treating the precipitating factors as well as treating the metabolic derangements with insulin and volume repletion.

Hyperglycemic hyperosmolar state occurs predominantly in older patients with type 2 DM and results in marked hyperglycemia (often glucose >600 mg/dL), hyperosmolarity, severe volume depletion, and associated acute kidney injury. Patients typically have a several-week history of hyperglycemia and osmotic diuresis, leading to dehydration and altered mental status. As with DKA, precipitating factors include serious infection, stroke, and myocardial infarction. Besides identifying and treating the precipitating condition, volume resuscitation with fluids can lead to rapid, dramatic improvements in hyperglycemia and hyperosmolarity. Mental status alterations often take longer to normalize.

Older patients with diabetes are at increased risk of infections. Hyperglycemia is associated with worse outcomes in common infections such as pneumonia, and diabetes is a potent risk factor for unusual infections such as malignant otitis externa that are uncommon in patients without diabetes. A number of causes for increased infection risk have been proposed, including impaired immune function caused by decreased neutrophil chemotaxis, phagocytosis, and opsonization. Lower-extremity soft tissue and bone infections are common, because of vascular insufficiency and repeated trauma that is unrecognized by the patient as a result of neuropathy. Urinary tract infections are more common in patients with diabetes because of glucosuria and urinary retention from autonomic neuropathy.

Kitabchi AE, Umpierrez GE, Miles JM, Fisher JN. Hyperglycemic crises in adult patients with diabetes. *Diabetes Care.* 2009;32(7):1335-1343.

Rajagopalan S. Serious infections in elderly patients with diabetes mellitus. *Clin Infect Dis.* 2005;40(7):990-996.

B. Chronic Complications

Older adults are at high risk for all of the chronic complications of diabetes seen in younger adults including microvascular (retinopathy, neuropathy and nephropathy) and macrovascular disease (coronary artery disease, stroke and peripheral vascular disease). Because vascular pathology plays a central role in diabetes-related complications, prevention and treatment should focus on vascular risk factors, such as smoking cessation, and blood pressure, lipid, and glycemic control.

1. Macrovascular complications (myocardial infarction, stroke and peripheral vascular disease)—Cardiovascular disease (CVD) is the major cause of morbidity and mortality for older adults with diabetes. Diabetes imparts a 2-fold risk in coronary heart disease and stroke, and increases the risk of amputation 10-fold. Diabetes often co-occurs with other CVD risk factors, such as hypertension and hyperlipidemia, and studies suggest a multifaceted approach addressing multiple risk factors is most effective in decreasing cardiovascular risk. Currently, the American Diabetes Association (ADA) recommends aspirin for patients with diabetes and known CVD. Furthermore, the ADA also recommends blood pressure control to 130/80 mm Hg and lipid control to low-density lipoprotein <100 mg/dL. For frail older adults at higher risk for complications of treatment such as orthostatic hypotension, less-aggressive goals may be more appropriate.

American Diabetes Association. Standards of medical care in diabetes—2012. *Diabetes Care*. 2012;35 Suppl 1:S11-S63.

2. Microvascular complications: retinopathy—Diabetes is a leading cause of blindness in the United States. Early detection and treatment of proliferative retinopathy with laser photocoagulation has been shown to decrease the risk of visual loss by more than 50% at 6 years. Further, because visual compromise is insidious, most patients do not recognize declining visual acuity, increasing the importance of regular screening to detect retinopathy at an early, treatable stage. The ADA currently recommends a dilated eye exam by an ophthalmologist at diagnosis, with regular follow-up exams every 1–3 years, depending on the individual patients' risk factors and initial exam results. In addition to retinopathy, older patients with diabetes also have a 2-fold risk of cataracts and a 3-fold risk of glaucoma compared to older patients without diabetes.

Mohamed Q, Gillies MC, Wong TY. Management of diabetic retinopathy: a systematic review. *JAMA*. 2007;298(8):902-916.

3. Microvascular complications: neuropathy—Diabetic neuropathy is generally classified by the types of nerves that are affected. The most common type of neuropathy is the sensory distal symmetric polyneuropathy, or "glove-and-stocking" neuropathy. Common symptoms include numbness and burning pain of the hands and feet. Because sensory neuropathy predisposes patients to unrecognized lower-extremity trauma, which can ultimately progress to infection and amputation, annual screening with a 10-g monofilament at the plantar aspect of the hallux and metatarsal joint is recommended. Autonomic diabetic neuropathies include diabetic gastroparesis, which can cause nausea and vomiting after eating as a result of impaired gastric emptying, as well as erectile dysfunction and neurogenic bladder. Unlike many other microvascular complications, diabetic gastroparesis can improve quickly and dramatically with improved glycemic control.

Boulton AJ, Vinik AI, Arezzo JC, et al; American Diabetes Association. Diabetic neuropathies: a statement by the American Diabetes Association. *Diabetes Care*. 2005;28(4):956-962.

4. Microvascular complications: nephropathy—Diabetic nephropathy is the most common cause of end-stage renal disease and is strongly associated with cardiovascular

mortality. Diabetic nephropathy is also more common in older diabetic patients than younger patients; however, the association between severity of nephropathy and mortality appears to be weaker in older adults. Compared to other common causes of kidney disease, diabetic nephropathy leads to more albuminuria and less early declines in glomerular filtration rate. This is reflected in the diagnostic criteria for diabetic nephropathy, which is albuminuria >300 g/day in a patient with known diabetes without other potential causes of albuminuria. Many studies have shown that treatment with angiotensin-converting enzyme inhibitors or angiotensin receptor blockers slow the progression of diabetic nephropathy and decrease the risk of cardiovascular events. Thus, the ADA recommends annual screening for microalbuminuria, which can be accomplished by measuring the urinary albumin-to-creatinine ratio on a spot urine specimen.

Bakris GL, Williams M, Dworkin L, et al. Preserving renal function in adults with hypertension and diabetes: a consensus approach. National Kidney Foundation Hypertension and Diabetes Executive Committees Working Group. *Am J Kidney Dis*. 2000;36(3):646-661.

C. Geriatric Syndromes

Geriatric syndromes are common, serious conditions in older adults that often present similarly in different patients despite disparate causes. For example, delirium may present as an acute confusional state with a fluctuating level of consciousness in patients with urinary tract infections as well as a myocardial infarction. DM appears to increase the risk of many geriatric syndromes, including cognitive impairment, depression, urinary incontinence, falls, and functional decline.

Araki A, Ito H. Diabetes mellitus and geriatric syndromes. *Geriatr Gerontol Int*. 2009;9:105-114.

Brown AF, Mangione CM, Saliba D, Sarkisian CA. California Healthcare Foundation/American Geriatrics Society Panel on Improving Care for Elders with Diabetes. Guidelines for improving the care of the older person with diabetes mellitus. *J Am Geriatr Soc*. 2003;51(5 Suppl Guidelines):S265-S280.

Inouye SK, Studenski S, Tinetti ME, Kuchel GA. Geriatric syndromes: clinical, research, and policy implications of a core geriatric concept. *J Am Geriatr Soc*. 2007;55(5):780-791.

Vischer UM, Bauduceau B, Bourdel-Marchasson I, et al. Alfediam/SFGG French-speaking group for study of diabetes in the elderly. A call to incorporate the prevention and treatment of geriatric disorders in the management of diabetes in the elderly. *Diabetes Metab*. 2009;35(3):168-177.

1. Cognitive impairment—In epidemiologic studies, DM appears to increase the subsequent risk of Alzheimer dementia by 50% to 100% and vascular dementia by 100% to 200%. Although some studies suggest that poor glycemic control and hyperglycemia may lead to elevated risk of dementia, there is also evidence that hypoglycemia may increase the risk of subsequent dementia.

Cognitive impairment is an especially important comorbidity in patients with diabetes, because patient activation and self-management is a cornerstone of effective diabetes treatment. Patients with even mild cognitive impairment may be less able to manage their diet, exercise, and medication regimen, and less able to identify symptoms of early hypoglycemia. Thus, the American Geriatrics Society recommends screening for cognitive impairment during the initial evaluation of the older adult with diabetes, and repeating the screening if increased difficulty with self-care or self-management is suspected.

Biessels GJ, Staekenborg S, Brunner E, Brayne C, Scheltens P. Risk of dementia in diabetes mellitus: a systematic review. *Lancet Neurol.* 2006;5(1):64-74.

Whitmer RA, Karter AJ, Yaffe K, Quesenberry CP Jr, Selby JV. Hypoglycemic episodes and risk of dementia in older patients with type 2 diabetes mellitus. *JAMA.* 2009;301(15):1565-1572.

2. Depression—Depression is a common condition in older adults and is associated with adverse outcomes, including poor health-related quality of life, functional decline, and death. Diabetes and depression commonly co-occur, with 30% of older adults with diabetes reporting depressive symptoms and 5% to 10% of older adults with diabetes meeting criteria for major depressive disorder. Like cognitive impairment, depression may interfere with an older adult's ability to self-manage their diabetes care, leading to worse diabetes control. Thus, the American Geriatrics Society (AGS) recommends screening for depressive symptoms with a validated instrument. Repeat screening may be warranted if an older patient with diabetes has new difficulty with self-management.

Egede LE. Diabetes, major depression, and functional disability among U.S. adults. *Diabetes Care.* 2004;27(2):421-428.

Maraldi C, Volpato S, Penninx BW, et al. Diabetes mellitus, glycemic control, and incident depressive symptoms among 70- to 79-year-old persons: the health, aging, and body composition study. *Arch Intern Med.* 2007;167(11):1137-1144.

3. Urinary incontinence—Urinary incontinence is very common in older women with diabetes, with studies reporting a prevalence of >50%. Studies suggest a strong relationship between DM and urinary incontinence, with diabetes associated with a 3-fold increased prevalence of urge incontinence and a 2-fold increased prevalence of stress incontinence. Body mass index appears to be an important risk factor for incontinence, and weight loss reduces the incidence of new incontinence. Although many have suggested poor glycemic control may lead to worse incontinence through glycosuria, studies to date have not confirmed this hypothesis. Very little data exists for incontinence in older men with diabetes.

Brown JS, Wing R, Barrett-Connor E, et al; Diabetes Prevention Program Research Group. Lifestyle intervention is associated with lower prevalence of urinary incontinence: the Diabetes Prevention Program. *Diabetes Care.* 2006;29(2):385-90.

Jackson SL, Scholes D, Boyko EJ, Abraham L, Fihn SD. Urinary incontinence and diabetes in postmenopausal women. *Diabetes Care.* 2005;28(7):1730-1738.

4. Falls and fractures—Falls are common in older adults and associated with increased morbidity and mortality. Overweight patients are more likely to have a higher bone mass and diabetes, leading some to initially hypothesize that patients with diabetes may be less susceptible to injurious falls. However, subsequent studies have shown nearly a 2-fold increased risk of injurious falls in older adults with diabetes compared to older adults without diabetes. Insulin use, poor vision, and peripheral neuropathy appear to further increase the risk of falls. The AGS recommends screening for falls risk in older adults with diabetes to identify potentially modifiable risk factors for falls and fractures.

Schwartz AV, Hillier TA, Sellmeyer DE, et al. Older women with diabetes have a higher risk of falls: a prospective study. *Diabetes Care.* 2002;25(10):1749-1754.

5. Functional decline—Functional limitations are strongly associated with quality of life, as well as mortality and nursing home admission. Diabetes increases the risk of functional limitations, with increased rates of difficulty with activities of daily living (bathing, transferring, toileting, dressing and eating), as well as walking and shopping. The association between diabetes and functional limitations persisted even after accounting for other chronic conditions (such as coronary artery disease, peripheral vascular disease, and depression) as well as age, gender, and duration of diabetes. One observational study in frail, nursing home-eligible, older adults suggests that a hemoglobin A1c level between 8% and 9% is associated with best functional outcomes over 2 years.

Gregg EW, Mangione CM, Cauley JA, et al. Study of Osteoporotic Fractures Research Group. Diabetes and incidence of functional disability in older women. *Diabetes Care.* 2002;25(1):61-67.

Yau CK, Eng C, Cenzer IS, Boscardin WJ, Rice-Trumble K, Lee SJ. Glycosylated hemoglobin and functional decline in community-dwelling nursing home-eligible elderly adults with diabetes mellitus. *J Am Geriatr Soc.* 2012;60(7):1215-1221.

▶ **Treatment**

A. Glycemic Treatment

Hyperglycemia is the core pathologic finding in DM and control of hyperglycemia is a cornerstone of diabetes treatment. However, it is important to recognize that blood pressure control and lipid control appear to be as important (if not more important) in preventing and minimizing most end-organ complications of diabetes. Thus, when prioritizing

Table 42–1. Change in average glucose level by HbA1c.

Hemoglobin A1c (%)	Average Glucose in mg/dL (95% CI)
5	97 (76–120)
6	126 (100–152)
7	154 (123–185)
8	183 (147–217)
9	212 (170–249)
10	240 (193–282)
11	269 (217–314)
12	298 (240–347)

Table 42–2. Guideline recommendations for hemoglobin A1c targets for older patients with limited life expectancy.

	Year	A1c Target
American Diabetes Association (ADA) and the European Association for the Study of Diabetes (EASD)	2012	7.5–8.0 or even slightly higher
American Geriatrics Society (AGS)	2013	8.0–9.0
Veterans Affairs and Department of Defense (VA/DoD)	2010	8–9.0

interventions in medically complex older adults with diabetes, focusing first on blood pressure is a reasonable approach in most patients.

1. Glycemic control targets—Hemoglobin A1c (HbA1c) has been shown to correlate closely with average glucose levels and are strongly predictive of microvascular complications. A reasonable rule of thumb is that each 1% increase or decrease in HbA1c is equivalent to a corresponding approximately 30 mg/dL change in average glucose levels, as shown in Table 42–1.

The goals of glycemic treatment differ in healthy and frail older patients, resulting in different recommended glycemic targets. Studies suggest that tight glycemic control to HbA1c ≤7% decreases the rates of microvascular complications over 8 years. Thus, the ADA recommends HbA1c <7% for healthy older adults with an extended life expectancy.

However, tighter glycemic control has also been associated with increased rates of hypoglycemia and mortality. For older patients with limited life expectancy, tight glycemic control exposes them to a higher risk of adverse events with little chance that they would survive to benefit from decreases in microvascular complications. Because very poor glycemic control can lead to immediate symptoms such as fatigue, older patients with limited life expectancy should receive glycemic treatment that is aimed at avoiding symptomatic hyperglycemia while minimizing the risk of hypoglycemia. A recent guideline from the AGS suggests an HbA1c target of 8% for older adults. For older adults who are healthy, with few comorbidities, few functional limitations and extended life expectancy, HbA1c target of 7% to 8% is appropriate. Conversely, for older adults with extensive comorbidities, functional limitations and limited life expectancy, HbA1c target of 8% to 9% is appropriate (Table 42–2).

Brown AF, Mangione CM, Saliba D, Sarkisian CA. California Healthcare Foundation/American Geriatrics Society Panel on Improving Care for Elders with Diabetes. Guidelines for improving the care of the older person with diabetes mellitus. *J Am Geriatr Soc.* 2003;51(5 Suppl Guidelines):S265–S280.

Inzucchi SE, Bergenstal RM, Buse JB, et al. American Diabetes Association (ADA); European Association for the Study of Diabetes (EASD). Management of hyperglycemia in type 2 diabetes: a patient-centered approach: position statement of the American Diabetes Association (ADA) and the European Association for the Study of Diabetes (EASD). *Diabetes Care.* 2012;35(6):1364-1379.

Lee SJ, Eng C. Goals of glycemic control in frail older patients with diabetes. *JAMA.* 2011;305(13):1350-1351.

Management of Diabetes Mellitus Update Working Group. *VA/DoD Clinical Practice Guideline for the Management of Diabetes Mellitus. Version 4.0.* Washington, DC: Veterans Health Administration and Department of Defense; 2010.

Nathan DM, Kuenen J, Borg R, Zheng H, Schoenfeld D, Heine RJ; A1c-Derived Average Glucose Study Group. Translating the A1C assay into estimated average glucose values. *Diabetes Care.* 2008;31(8):1473-1478.

Ray KK, Seshasai SR, Wijesuriya S, et al. Effect of intensive control of glucose on cardiovascular outcomes and death in patients with diabetes mellitus: a meta-analysis of randomised controlled trials. *Lancet.* 2009;373(9677):1765-1772.

2. Glycemic control targets in hospitalized patients—Many older patients with diabetes are admitted to the hospital, most often for conditions other than diabetes. The goals for glycemic control in older hospitalized patients are to maintain euglycemia, avoid adverse events, and return to a stable outpatient regimen as soon as feasible. However, the stress of acute illness and frequent preprocedural fasting can make maintaining euglycemia challenging in hospitalized patients. In noncritically ill patients, the ADA recommends a fasting (premeal) glucose target of 90–140 mg/dL and a random glucose target of <180 mg/dL. The mainstays of glycemic treatment in hospitalized older adults are insulin and volume repletion.

Although initial studies suggested improved outcomes in critically ill surgical patients with tight glycemic control (glucose levels of 80–110 mg/dL), subsequent studies have not shown similar benefits. The ADA recommends glucose levels between 140 and 180 mg/dL in both medical and surgical ICU patients.

Moghissi ES, Korytkowski MT, DiNardo M, et al. American Association of Clinical Endocrinologists; American Diabetes Association. American Association of Clinical Endocrinologists and American Diabetes Association consensus statement on inpatient glycemic control. *Diabetes Care.* 2009;32(6):1119-1131.

Wiener RS, Wiener DC, Larson RJ. Benefits and risks of tight glucose control in critically ill adults: a meta-analysis. *JAMA.* 2008;300(8):933-944.

B. Nonpharmacologic Treatments

1. Diet—Dietary intervention is an integral component of diabetes treatment. For patients with diabetes and a body mass index >30 kg/m², caloric restriction with the goal of weight loss is recommended. There is no role for caloric restriction in patients who are not overweight or obese. A wide variety of diets with varying macronutrient (carbohydrates, proteins, fats) proportions have been studied, but there is little data to suggest one diet is superior to another. Current ADA dietary recommendations mirror the American Heart Association recommendations and suggest (a) limiting saturated fat (<7% of total calories), (b) minimizing trans fats, and (c) limiting cholesterol intake (<200 mg/day). Medical nutritional therapy provided by a registered dietician is a covered Medicare benefit.

It is important to recognize that for some older adults with diabetes, caloric or dietary restriction may be especially difficult or even harmful. First, changes in diet may be especially challenging for older patients who have established dietary habits over a lifetime. Second, older adults with functional difficulties who have difficulty shopping for groceries and preparing food are at risk for undernutrition; recommending a restricted range of foods may lead to weight loss or micronutrient deficiencies. Third, older adults with diabetes are at higher risk for periodontal disease and xerostomia, which may limit their ability to adapt to a new diet. Thus, dietary modifications should be approached with caution in nonobese older patients with diabetes.

Klein S, Sheard NF, Pi-Sunyer X, et al. American Diabetes Association; North American Association for the Study of Obesity; American Society for Clinical Nutrition. Weight management through lifestyle modification for the prevention and management of type 2 diabetes: rationale and strategies: a statement of the American Diabetes Association, the North American Association for the Study of Obesity, and the American Society for Clinical Nutrition. *Diabetes Care.* 2004;27(8):2067-2073.

2. Exercise—Regular exercise has been shown in improve glycemic control, blood pressure, lipids and contribute to weight loss. The ADA recommends that older adults with diabetes should strive to achieve 150 minutes per week of moderate-intensity exercise. For older patients with functional impairments who are unable to accomplish this, the ADA recommends maximizing their physical activity to reap some of the benefits of exercise. Because older patients with diabetes are at high risk for CVD, exercise regimens should start with low-intensity physical activity and gradually increase in intensity and duration.

Colberg SR, Sigal RJ, Fernhall B, et al. American College of Sports Medicine; American Diabetes Association. Exercise and type 2 diabetes: the American College of Sports Medicine and the American Diabetes Association: joint position statement executive summary. *Diabetes Care.* 2010;33(12):2692-2696.

C. Pharmacologic Therapy (Table 42–3)

1. Biguanides—Most guidelines recommend metformin as first-line oral therapy for type 2 DM because it is efficacious (decreasing HbA1c approximately 1.5%), is not associated with weight gain or hypoglycemia, and appears to be associated with decreased cardiovascular complications compared to sulfonylureas. Large registry-based observational data suggests that patients taking metformin were at 15% to 21% decreased hazard of cardiovascular complications compared to patients taking glyburide or glipizide. Furthermore a 5-year randomized trial showed 46% decreased risk of cardiovascular outcomes in patients treated with metformin versus glipizide.

Mild renal insufficiency (serum creatinine >1.5 mg/dL or creatinine clearance <30 mL/min) has been a relative contraindication to metformin because of the concern for lactic acidosis. However, lactic acidosis appears to be exceedingly rare with metformin, with an incidence of less than 1 per 10,000 person-years of treatment. A recent Cochrane review of 347 studies representing 126,000 patients found that metformin was not associated with an increased risk of lactic acidosis compared to other anti-hyperglycemic medications.

Hong J, Zhang Y, Lai S, et al. SPREAD-DIMCAD Investigators. Effects of metformin versus glipizide on cardiovascular outcomes in patients with type 2 diabetes and coronary artery disease. *Diabetes Care.* 2013;36(5):1304-1311.

Nathan DM, Buse JB, Davidson MB, et al. American Diabetes Association; European Association for Study of Diabetes. Medical management of hyperglycemia in type 2 diabetes: a consensus algorithm for the initiation and adjustment of therapy: a consensus statement of the American Diabetes Association and the European Association for the Study of Diabetes. *Diabetes Care.* 2009;32(1):193-203.

Qaseem A, Humphrey LL, Sweet DE, Starkey M, Shekelle P. Clinical Guidelines Committee of the American College of Physicians. Oral pharmacologic treatment of type 2 diabetes mellitus: a clinical practice guideline from the American College of Physicians. *Ann Intern Med.* 2012;156(3):218-231.

Roumie CL, Hung AM, Greevy RA, et al. Comparative effectiveness of sulfonylurea and metformin monotherapy on cardiovascular events in type 2 diabetes mellitus: a cohort study. *Ann Intern Med.* 2012;157(9):601-610.

Salpeter SR, Greyber E, Pasternak GA, Salpeter EE. Risk of fatal and nonfatal lactic acidosis with metformin use in type 2 diabetes mellitus. *Cochrane Database Syst Rev.* 2010;(4):CD002967.

Table 42–3. Noninsulin therapies for hyperglycemia.

Class	Drug	Action	Expected Decrease in A1c (%)	Advantages	Disadvantages	Cost
Biguanides	Metformin	Decrease hepatic glucose production	1–2	No weight gain No hypoglycemia Decreased cardiovascular mortality (UKPDS)	Nausea, diarrhea Lactic acidosis (rare)	$
Sulfonylureas	Glipizide Glyburide	Stimulate insulin secretion	1–2	Generally well tolerated	Hypoglycemia (especially with glyburide) Weight gain	$
Meglitinides	Repaglinide Nateglinide	Stimulate insulin secretion	1–2	Decrease postprandial hyperglycemia	Hypoglycemia Weight gain Frequent preprandial dosing	$$
α-Glucosidase inhibitors	Acarbose Miglitol	Decrease intestinal carbohydrate absorption	0.5–1	Not absorbed, limiting possibility of drug–drug interactions	Gastrointestinal side effects	$$
Thiazolidinediones	Pioglitazone Rosiglitazone	Increase peripheral insulin sensitivity	1–2	Little hypoglycemia	Weight gain Heart failure exacerbation Increased cardiovascular events (especially with rosiglitazone)	$$$
GLP-1 agonists	Exenatide Liraglutide	Increase glucose-dependent insulin secretion Delay gastric emptying	1–2	Weight loss	Nausea, vomiting, diarrhea Acute pancreatitis	$$$
DPP-4 inhibitors	Sitagliptin Saxagliptin Linagliptin	Accentuates GLP-1 activity Decrease glucagon	0.5–1	No weight gain No hypoglycemia	Acute pancreatitis Modest potency	$$$
Amylin mimetics	Pramlintide	Delays gastric emptying Promotes satiety Decreases postprandial glucagon secretion	0.5	Generally well tolerated	Frequent injections Cannot be mixed with insulin	$$$

UKPDS, United Kingdom Prospective Diabetes Study.

Schramm TK, Gislason GH, Vaag A, et al. Mortality and cardiovascular risk associated with different insulin secretagogues compared with metformin in type 2 diabetes, with or without a previous myocardial infarction: a nationwide study. *Eur Heart J.* 2011;32(15):1900-1908.

2. Sulfonylureas—The sulfonylureas in common use include glipizide and glyburide. Because sulfonylureas act predominantly by increasing pancreatic insulin secretion, weight gain is common and hypoglycemia may occur. Studies suggest that the risk of hypoglycemia is 1.5–2 times higher with glyburide than glipizide, possibly as a result of active metabolites; thus, glyburide should be avoided in older adults. Generally, most of the therapeutic effect occurs with half of the maximum recommended dose, and a decrease in HbA1c of 1% to 2% can be expected. Starting doses should be low, perhaps half that used for younger patients, and education regarding hypoglycemia provided. Sulfonylureas

should be used with caution in patients with kidney disease since active metabolites are excreted slowly.

Gangji AS, Cukierman T, Gerstein HC, Goldsmith CH, Clase CM. A systematic review and meta-analysis of hypoglycemia and cardiovascular events: a comparison of glyburide with other secretagogues and with insulin. *Diabetes Care.* 2007;30(2): 389-394.

3. α-Glucosidase inhibitors—The α-glucosidase inhibitors acarbose (Precose) and miglitol (Glyset) inhibit the absorption of carbohydrates in the gut and decrease postprandial hyperglycemia. Consequently, they do not cause hypoglycemia or weight gain. Because α-glucosidase inhibitors are not systemically absorbed at usual doses (especially acarbose), they generally can be safely used in older adults and with either renal or hepatic insufficiency. The primary drawbacks of α-glucosidase inhibitors are gastrointestinal discomfort including flatulence and diarrhea, and low potency with HbA1c decreasing by approximately 0.5%.

Johnston PS, Lebovitz HE, Coniff RF, Simonson DC, Raskin P, Munera CL. Advantages of alpha-glucosidase inhibition as monotherapy in elderly type 2 diabetic patients. *J Clin Endocrinol Metab.* 1998;83(5):1515-1522.

4. Thiazolidinediones—The thiazolidinediones rosiglitazone (Avandia) and pioglitazone (Actos) act as insulin sensitizers. Thiazolidinediones have fallen out of favor as mounting evidence suggests increased cardiovascular risk, heart failure, and hepatotoxicity, especially with rosiglitazone.

Lincoff AM, Wolski K, Nicholls SJ, Nissen SE. Pioglitazone and risk of cardiovascular events in patients with type 2 diabetes mellitus: a meta-analysis of randomized trials. *JAMA.* 2007;298(10):1180-1188.

Nissen SE, Wolski K. Rosiglitazone revisited: an updated meta-analysis of risk for myocardial infarction and cardiovascular mortality. *Arch Intern Med.* 2010;170(14):1191-1201.

5. Meglitinides—Meglitinides are short-acting insulin secretagogues that can decrease postprandial hyperglycemia. Repaglinide and nateglinide are the meglitinides available in the United States. Nateglinide appears to have a faster onset and shorter duration of action than repaglinide. There is limited experience with either drug in older adults, but they may be effective for patients with fasting euglycemia and postprandial hyperglycemia. Both medications should be taken before each meal, which may make medication adherence more difficult.

Black C, Donnelly P, McIntyre L, Royle PL, Shepherd JP, Thomas S. Meglitinide analogues for type 2 diabetes mellitus. *Cochrane Database Syst Rev.* 2007;(2):CD004654.

6. Incretin modulators: glucagon-like peptide-1 (GLP-1) analog and dipeptidyl peptidase-4 (DPP-4) inhibitors—Incretins, such as GLP-1 and DPP-4, are gastrointestinal hormones that modulate postprandial glucose homeostasis. Incretin modulators can decrease postprandial hyperglycemia by increasing glucose-dependent insulin secretion and slowing gastric emptying. Although these medications do not cause hypoglycemia when used alone, they may aggravate hypoglycemia when used with insulin or sulfonylureas.

Exenatide and liraglutide are the GLP-1 analogs available in the United States. Exenatide is a synthetic analog of exendin-4, a component of Gila Monster saliva. Exendin-4 is structurally similar to GLP-1 (which decreases postprandial hyperglycemia) but is resistant to DPP-4 degradation, leading to more prolonged action. Both GLP-1 analogs appear to decrease HbA1c by approximately 1%. Because of delayed gastric emptying, nausea and weight loss are common. Acute pancreatitis is a rare but serious complication.

Sitagliptin, saxagliptin, and linagliptin are the DPP-4 inhibitors available in the United States. They lead to HbA1c decreases of approximately 0.5%. They are generally well tolerated with less nausea and weight loss than GLP-1 analogs. As with GLP-1 analogs, acute pancreatitis has also been observed with DPP-4 inhibitors.

There is little clinical experience with these medications in older adults. Given their cost and uncertainty regarding long-term safety, they should not be considered first-line agents for older adults.

Amori RE, Lau J, Pittas AG. Efficacy and safety of incretin therapy in type 2 diabetes: systematic review and meta-analysis. *JAMA.* 2007;298(2):194-206.

Shyangdan DS, Royle P, Clar C, Sharma P, Waugh N, Snaith A. Glucagon-like peptide analogues for type 2 diabetes mellitus. *Cochrane Database Syst Rev.* 2011;(10):CD006423.

7. Insulin—Insulin is required in all patients with type 1 diabetes, and in many patients with moderate or severe type 2 diabetes. There is more than 75 years of clinical experience with insulin. With proper dosing, it can be used safely in cases of renal or hepatic insufficiency, as well as in the hospital, nursing home, or as an outpatient. Disadvantages of insulin include the risk of hypoglycemia, weight gain, and patient psychological barriers to injection.

Many different types of insulin have been developed to provide flexible treatment options for different patterns of hyperglycemia (Table 42–4). Commonly used longer-acting insulins include glargine and neutral protamine Hagedorn (NPH), which are used once or twice daily, respectively, to provide basal insulin for control of fasting glucose levels. Commonly used shorter-acting insulins include lispro and regular before meals to provide bolus insulin to control postprandial glucose levels. Insulin mixtures such as 70/30 (70% NPH and 30% regular) may help simplify insulin regimens for many patients. For many older patients with type 2 diabetes, once-daily long-acting insulin at nighttime, often in addition to metformin, may be a reasonable starting regimen.

Holman RR, Farmer AJ, Davies MJ, et al. 4-T Study Group. Three-year efficacy of complex insulin regimens in type 2 diabetes. *N Engl J Med.* 2009;361(18):1736-1747.

Table 42–4. Commonly used insulin products in the United States.

Type	Onset of Action	Peak Action	Duration	Cost
Lispro	15 min	30–90 min	2–4 h	$$
Aspart	15 min	30–90 min		$$
Regular	30–60 min	2–3 h	4–6 h	$
NPH	2–4 h	6–10 h	10–16 h	$
Glargine	—	—	22–24 h	$$

Horvath K, Jeitler K, Berghold A, et al. Long-acting insulin analogues versus NPH insulin (human isophane insulin) for type 2 diabetes mellitus. *Cochrane Database Syst Rev.* 2007;(2):CD005613.

Qayyum R, Bolen S, Maruthur N, et al. Systematic review: comparative effectiveness and safety of premixed insulin analogues in type 2 diabetes. *Ann Intern Med.* 2008;149(8): 549-559.

Singh SR, Ahmad F, Lal A, Yu C, Bai Z, Bennett H. Efficacy and safety of insulin analogues for the management of diabetes mellitus: a meta-analysis. *CMAJ.* 2009;180(4):385-397.

8. Amylin mimetic—Amylin is a peptide that is cosecreted with insulin and modulates glucose homeostasis by delaying gastric emptying, promoting satiety, and decreasing postprandial glucagon secretion. Pramlintide is the only amylin mimetic available in the United States; it is approved for subcutaneous use for patients with type 1 or 2 diabetes taking insulin. Although generally well-tolerated, its effect is modest, decreasing HbA1c approximately 0.5%. Pramlintide must be injected separately from insulin, complicating medication adherence.

Riddle M, Pencek R, Charenkavanich S, Lutz K, Wilhelm K, Porter L. Randomized comparison of pramlintide or mealtime insulin added to basal insulin treatment for patients with type 2 diabetes. *Diabetes Care.* 2009;32(9):1577-1582.

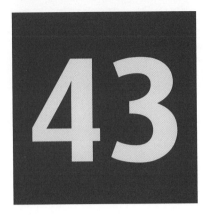

43

Anemia

Gary J. Vanasse, MD

► General Principles in Older Adults

Anemia is a common condition in older adults and is an increasingly recognized contributor to increased morbidity and mortality. Similar to the younger adult anemic patient, anemia in older adults is most commonly defined according to the 1968 World Health Organization (WHO) criteria of a hemoglobin (Hgb) <13 g/dL in men and <12 g/dL in women. Although anemia has often been considered a normal consequence of aging, its association with adverse clinical outcomes merits a thorough evaluation into the underlying pathophysiology. Recent studies suggest that anemia may arise as a result of accumulated effects of age-related comorbidities acting in concert with poorly understood age-specific changes in early hematopoietic progenitors, that combine to influence erythrocyte production. A greater understanding of the pathogenesis of anemia in older adults will likely have important implications for the prevention, diagnosis, and therapy of this common problem.

► Pathogenesis

It is estimated that more than 3 million Americans age 65 years and older are anemic, with anemia being highly prevalent in noninstitutionalized, ambulatory older adult populations. The Third National Health and Nutrition Examination Survey (NHANES III) study revealed that the prevalence of anemia in men and women older than age 65 years was 11% and 10.2%, respectively, and rose rapidly after age 50 years, approaching a rate greater than 20% in those individuals age 85 years or older. This finding has been validated in other population-based studies, most of which have shown that the degree of anemia in older adults is relatively mild, with most patients presenting with Hgb >10 g/dL.

Race appears to significantly influence Hgb levels. In NHANES III, the prevalence of anemia using WHO criteria was found to be 3 times higher in non-Hispanic blacks compared with non-Hispanic whites. Examination of Hgb,

hematocrit (Hct), and mean corpuscular volume (MCV) in 1491 black individuals as compared with more than 31,000 white subjects in the Kaiser Permanente database revealed that all 3 parameters were lower in blacks than in age-matched whites, whereas the serum ferritin was higher. Although racial genetic variation may influence an individual's ability to respond to anemic triggers, it is likely that additional factors besides race significantly contribute to the risk of anemia across various populations.

A. Etiology and Risk Factors

There are presently no studies specifically designed to address causality in older individuals with anemia. The high frequency of comorbid conditions in older populations has also confounded our ability to identify which mechanisms, if any, independently predispose to age-associated reductions in Hgb. Although there appears to be a component of age-related anemia even in healthy individuals, the incidence is much higher in patients with comorbid disease. NHANES III revealed that anemia in older adults is comprised of 3 broad categories: one-third have anemia as a result of nutritional deficiencies (iron, folic acid, or vitamin B_{12}); one-third have anemia of inflammation (AI) on the basis of iron studies; and one-third have unexplained anemia (UA). It is important to remember that these definitions of anemia in NHANES III were based solely on laboratory parameters without the benefit of clinical examination or bone marrow biopsies, making it difficult to evaluate the full clinical impact of anemia in this population. Furthermore, a "hierarchical" categorization of parameters was used to define anemia subtypes, making it difficult to address the independent contributions of factors in subjects with anemia caused by multiple etiologies.

A Stanford University study examining the etiology of anemia defined by WHO criteria in 190 community-dwelling people age 65 or older also found a high prevalence of UA, comprising 35% of participants, a proportion of whom demonstrated mild increases in inflammatory markers and lower-than-expected erythropoietin (EPO) levels compared to nonanemic controls. In contrast to the NHANES III study, participants in the Stanford study underwent a comprehensive evaluation of their anemia, including a complete history and physical examination, laboratory evaluation, and peripheral blood smear review.

1. Anemia of inflammation—AI has historically been termed the "anemia of chronic disease" and is most commonly seen in chronic illnesses, including infection, rheumatologic disorders, and malignancy. It is classically characterized biochemically by the presence of low serum iron and low iron-binding capacity in the setting of an elevated serum ferritin. Although the etiology of classical AI has been attributed to decreased red cell survival, disordered iron-limited erythropoiesis, and progressive EPO resistance of erythroid progenitors, the relative role and interplay of these three mechanisms in the development of anemia remain unknown, as are the potential common pathways that may link them.

Our understanding of AI has been transformed by the discovery of the antimicrobial peptide hepcidin, which is synthesized in the liver and is a key regulator of iron metabolism. In humans, increased hepcidin production has been found in patients with inflammatory disease, infections, and malignancy. NHANES III preceded the identification of hepcidin, and the contribution of hepcidin to anemia was not assessed. Regulation of hepcidin synthesis is complex and involves several inflammatory-mediated cellular pathways, including interleukin 6 (IL-6), which is the primary inflammatory mediator of hepcidin synthesis and is thought to mediate iron-limited erythropoiesis in patients with both acute and chronic inflammatory states. However, recent studies have failed to correlate hepcidin and stimulatory cytokines like IL-6 or inflammatory markers like C-reactive protein, raising questions about the relative contributions of hepcidin-dependent and -independent pathways to the pathogenesis of AI. Future mechanistic studies will be necessary to fully characterize the contribution of increased hepcidin levels in cohorts of older patients with AI and to determine its utility as a clinical diagnostic biomarker of inflammatory anemia.

2. Unexplained anemia in older adults—UA typically presents as a mild anemia characterized predominantly as hypoproliferative, with a low reticulocyte count and low reticulocyte index, suggesting absence of the bone marrow's normal compensatory response to a low red cell mass environment. The pathophysiology of UA in the older adults is poorly understood, and it remains primarily a diagnosis of exclusion.

The role of a chronic proinflammatory state in the pathogenesis of UA in older adults has stirred much debate. There is strong evidence that many markers of inflammation, including tumor necrosis factor-α and IL-6, are increased in the older population regardless of health status. However, studies detailing evidence for chronic inflammation contributing to UA have been few in number and limited by small sample sizes and diverse study designs. Presently, the available data would argue against a role for chronic inflammation in the etiology of UA in older adults.

As anemia is the most common hematologic abnormality in patients with myelodysplastic syndromes (MDS), a heterogenous group of disorders that primarily affects older adults, it is appealing to surmise that MDS may be an important contributor to the pathogenesis of UA. On the contrary, evidence from small studies suggests that MDS may play only a limited role in the etiology of UA, with prevalence of MDS in older adults with UA thought to be in the range of 5% to 16%. These data are limited by small sample sizes, heterogeneity of MDS, and reflect present diagnostic limitations in identifying subjects with low-grade, subclinical MDS.

3. Erythropoietin resistance and aging—EPO is the major cytokine influencing red cell development and is induced in the setting of anemia through an oxygen sensing mechanism in the kidney. Impaired EPO responsiveness of hematopoietic stem cells has been implicated in the pathophysiology of anemia in older adults, with some, but not all, studies showing increased EPO levels with age, even in healthy adults. The Baltimore Longitudinal Study on Aging demonstrated that EPO levels rose with age in healthy, nonanemic individuals, and that the slope of the rise was greater for individuals without diabetes or hypertension. Those with anemia also had a lower slope of rise, suggesting that anemia reflected a failure of a normal age-related compensatory rise in EPO levels. Reduced EPO levels have been preferentially associated with UA in older adults, but the mechanism for this inadequate EPO response remains to be determined and the findings of these studies need to be confirmed in larger cohorts of older patients.

This progressive EPO resistance may reflect a cell intrinsic feature of aging hematopoietic stem cells and/or the combined effects of age-associated comorbidities that promote inflammatory-mediated impairment of normal EPO-dependent cellular pathways, decreased EPO production, and/or decreased EPO-sensitivity of bone marrow erythroid progenitors. We surmise that in some aging patients with chronic inflammation, sufficient hepcidin expression may induce the classic biochemical iron profile of AI, whereas in others hepcidin-independent proinflammatory pathways promote either EPO insufficiency or EPO resistance of committed erythroid progenitors and development of UA. Supporting this hypothesis is the observation that concomitant administration of EPO and intravenous iron can ameliorate anemia in some patients with AI.

B. Associated Conditions

1. Frailty—Anemia and inflammation are strongly associated with and may contribute to the development of "frailty," a poorly defined syndrome of older adults associated with weight loss, impaired mobility, generalized weakness, and poor balance. A systematic review of the literature suggests that elevated proinflammatory markers are associated with development of frailty. A pilot study examining 11 frail and 19 nonfrail individuals age 74 years or older found that frail subjects had significantly higher serum IL-6 levels and lower Hgb and Hct than did nonfrail subjects. In addition, an inverse correlation between serum IL-6 level and Hgb was noted only in frail subjects, suggesting that IL-6-mediated pathways and possibly increased hepcidin may provide a common pathway for anemia development in the setting of frailty.

2. Vitamin D deficiency—Our group examined the association of vitamin D deficiency with anemia in adults age 60 years or older in NHANES III. Anemia was defined according to WHO criteria and subdivided into the following subtypes (nutritional, AI, UA, chronic renal disease). Reviewing data on 5100 participants, we found that vitamin D deficiency was associated with anemia independent of age, sex, and race/ethnicity, with the odds for anemia being increased approximately 60% in the presence of vitamin D deficiency. Furthermore, among those with anemia, vitamin D deficiency was most prevalent among those with AI, with the risk of AI significantly increased in vitamin D deficient versus nondeficient participants. Although this population based study demonstrates an association between vitamin D deficiency and anemia in older adults, there are no data to suggest a causal role for vitamin D deficiency in the pathogenesis of elderly anemia.

3. Other nutrients—A recent analysis of 1036 subjects age 65 years or older in the InChianti Study found an association between elevated carboxymethyl-lysine and decreased plasma selenium and anemia. Of 472 participants who were nonanemic at enrollment, 15.3% developed anemia over a 6-year follow-up period, with incident anemia being significantly associated with the highest quartile elevation in plasma carboxymethyl-lysine and the lowest quartile of plasma selenium levels. Although this study raises the intriguing possibility that anemia may be associated with parameters of oxidative stress, no causal relationship has been shown to date.

4. HIV disease—Anemia is the most common hematologic complication of HIV infection and is associated with decreased survival, increased progression of disease, and decreased quality of life. As the population of those infected with HIV continues to age, individuals are at risk for anemia related to HIV as well as the anemia of aging. The etiology of anemia in the setting of HIV infection is multifactorial and includes opportunistic infections, decreased EPO levels, effects on the kinetics of hematopoietic cell differentiation, nutritional deficiency, and associated malignancy and

medications. Our group has found that a high-expressing single nucleotide polymorphism in the leptin gene was independently associated with anemia in HIV+ but not HIV– subjects. Although our study provides novel insight into the association between genetic variability in the leptin gene and anemia in HIV+ individuals, future studies are required to determine whether aberrant leptin signaling plays a causal role in anemia development or alters EPO responsiveness.

▶ Prevention

There are presently no recommended or agreed upon strategies for the prevention of anemia in older populations.

▶ Clinical Findings

It has become increasingly recognized that even mild forms of anemia are associated with increased morbidity, mortality, and frailty in older adults. The relationship between anemia subtypes and mortality was examined in the Women's Health and Aging Study I, where investigators found that mortality was significantly increased in those with anemia caused by renal disease or AI. Although anemia has been shown to impact physical performance, cognitive function, and mood in older populations, it remains controversial whether the impact of anemia on performance measures is truly independent of concomitant disease co-morbidities.

A. Symptoms & Signs

Because anemia in older adults is commonly mild in severity, patients will often be asymptomatic. When symptomatic, the clinical presentation of anemia in the older adult is similar to that of younger adult populations. However, because of the increased presence of comorbid disease, it is often difficult to determine whether symptomatic complaints in older adults are directly related to anemia, the underlying cause of anemia, or the presence of comorbidities. Additionally, age-related increases in comorbid disease often make older adults more susceptible to multifactorial anemia.

Clinical symptoms of anemia are dependent on the severity of anemia, on the rate with which anemia develops, and on the patient's oxygen demand. In older adults, symptomatic anemia typically reflects impaired oxygen delivery to tissues as a consequence of decreased Hgb concentrations, which may lead to increased cardiac output states and increased tissue hypoxia and a progressive decline in organ function. In general, anemia that develops slowly over time tends to present with fewer symptoms than rapid onset anemia, regardless of the underlying etiology. As in younger adults, rapidly developing anemia may additionally cause symptoms because of the effects of hypovolemia. Such symptomatic illness may be more profound and less-well tolerated in older adults, however, because of increased frailty and decreased performance status often related to the presence of multiple chronic comorbidities. The primary symptoms of anemia may include any or all of the following:

1. Varying degrees of fatigue
2. Dyspnea on exertion or dyspnea at rest
3. Some combination of tachycardia, palpitations, sensation of bounding pulses reflecting a hyperdynamic cardiac state

More severe anemia may additionally present with:

1. Lethargy and loss of drive
2. Confusion
3. Severe cardiac symptoms, including congestive heart failure, arrhythmias, angina, or myocardial infarction

Anemia as a result of acute blood loss or severe acute hemolysis may initially present with the following symptoms that reflect physiologic hypovolemia:

1. Lightheadedness
2. Orthostatic hypotension
3. Syncope
4. Symptoms associated with hypovolemic shock, including coma and death

B. Laboratory Findings

In general, the laboratory evaluation of anemia in older adults is similar to that performed in younger adult populations with a few exceptions. All anemic individuals should receive a complete history and physical examination. Review of the complete blood count and peripheral blood smear is mandatory, as this will help focus on red cell abnormalities, such as unexplained macrocytosis, leucopenia, or leukocytosis, or dysplastic features of white cells or platelets that may provide morphologic evidence suggesting underlying MDS or other diseases. Examining the MCV and red cell indices will help classify anemia as microcytic, normocytic, or macrocytic, and review of the absolute reticulocyte count or reticulocyte index will help determine whether anemia is hyper- or hypoproliferative. Given the increased prevalence of monoclonal gammopathy in older adults, serum and urine protein electrophoresis with immunofixation is warranted in patients with normocytic anemia to evaluate for the presence of an underlying plasma cell dyscrasia.

1. Nutritional anemia—Although the diagnostic approach to nutritional anemia is similar to that in younger adults, there are some special circumstances to consider in older adults. For example, iron deficiency typically presents with microcytic and hypochromic red cells. However, when found in combination with macrocytic causes of anemia, such as MDS or vitamin B_{12} deficiency, the MCV may be in the normocytic range. Such multifactorial anemia common in older adults may be further elucidated by the presence of an increased red cell distribution width. The diagnostic evaluation of vitamin B_{12} and folate deficiencies in older adults is similar to that in younger adults.

Iron-deficiency anemia is commonly diagnosed by the presence of low serum iron, increased total iron-binding capacity, and decreased serum ferritin, with serum ferritin <12 µg/L being the most sensitive peripheral blood laboratory measure of reduced iron stores. However, ferritin also functions as an acute phase reactant, and serum levels may be falsely elevated in the presence of chronic inflammatory conditions, making it difficult to identify iron deficiency in the backdrop of underlying AI. Ferritin levels may also increase with age, but it remains to be determined whether this occurs in healthy older adults or whether it reflects increases in age-related inflammatory comorbidities.

In an attempt to better delineate iron deficiency in the setting of chronic inflammation, some have examined the utility of measuring the soluble transferrin receptor (sTfR)/log ferritin index, which is calculated by dividing sTfR by the log ferritin. In a prospective analysis of 145 anemic patients diagnosed with iron deficiency and AI, the sTfR index more than doubled the detection of iron-deficiency anemia (92%) compared with ferritin alone (41%). A second prospective controlled study of 49 patients age 80 years or older compared the sTfR index to bone marrow examination for the detection of marrow iron stores and found that the sTfR index diagnosed iron deficiency in 43 of 49 subjects (88%), nearly approaching the sensitivity of bone marrow examination (100%). However, because of a lack of standardization of sTfR/log ferritin testing, data interpretation may prove challenging, and ferritin remains the most important first-line measure of total-body iron stores, with the sTfR/log ferritin index serving as an adjunctive test. Bone marrow examination to evaluate the presence or absence of iron in erythroid progenitors remains the gold standard for measuring total-body iron stores.

A thorough diagnostic evaluation of iron deficiency in older adults is warranted to determine the source of iron deficiency. As it is highly uncommon in the industrialized world for iron deficiency to be caused by inadequate dietary intake of iron, gastrointestinal (GI) blood loss remains the most likely cause for iron deficiency in older adults. Because of the increased incidence of GI malignancies in older adults, a thorough upper and lower GI evaluation in patients diagnosed with iron-deficiency anemia is recommended in patients deemed clinically well enough to tolerate diagnostic evaluation and who may be candidates for therapeutic interventions.

2. Anemia of chronic renal disease—Renal disease leads to a blunted EPO response, with lower serum EPO levels seen in patients with declining renal function. The body's oxygen sensing mechanism in the kidney responds to increased hypoxia associated with decreased Hgb concentrations and results in a logarithmic increase in EPO levels that corresponds to anemia severity.

As aging is associated with a decline in renal function, anemia associated with chronic renal disease is an important consideration in older adults. However, the required degree of renal disease to promote the development of anemia remains in question. In the InCHIANTI Study, a creatinine clearance (CrCl) of <30 mL/min was significantly associated with an increased risk of anemia, as well as age- and Hgb-adjusted serum EPO levels in 1005 participants age 65 years or older. In contrast, a cross-sectional study involving 3222 subjects with a mean age of 65 years found that estimated CrCl levels of <50 mL/min were associated with 3-fold and 5-fold increased risks of anemia in women and men, respectively. These differences highlight the fact that the overall impact of moderate degrees of renal disease on the risk of anemia and decline in EPO synthesis requires more rigorous determination. Furthermore, measurement of serum EPO levels is often unhelpful in diagnosing anemia in older adults because serum EPO levels typically increase significantly only at Hgb levels <10 g/dL, a more severe degree of anemia than typically seen in the majority of older adults regardless of the degree of severity of renal dysfunction.

3. Unexplained anemia—During the evaluation of UA in the older adult, a diagnostic work-up of MDS may be justified. Formal diagnosis of MDS typically requires a bone marrow biopsy with morphologic and cytogenetic analyses. However, given the limited treatment options for patients with mild MDS, the necessity of a bone marrow evaluation should be judged in the context of whether information garnered will help inform therapeutic decisions.

▶ Complications

Complications may arise as a result of the chronic impact of anemia or may be associated with specific therapeutic interventions. Chronic anemia may predispose to symptoms associated with high-output congestive heart failure. Common complications of therapy include the following:

1. Adverse effects of oral iron therapy include abdominal pain, constipation, diarrhea, nausea, and vomiting.
2. Adverse effects of parenteral iron administration include allergic reactions, back pain, generalized muscle aches, dizziness, skin rash or erythema, fever, dizziness, headache, hypotension, or anaphylaxis. Anaphylaxis is rare, especially with newer iron formulations, and typically occurs within several minutes of administration.

3. Folic acid therapy may mask coexisting vitamin B_{12} deficiency, allowing for progression of unrecognized neurologic symptoms of vitamin B_{12} deficiency.
4. Erythropoiesis-stimulating agents (ESAs) may worsen underlying hypertension.

▶ Treatment

In general, effective management of anemia in older adults should be based on identification of treatable causes of anemia, with therapy following similar guidelines as for younger adults. Monitoring of treatment in the older adult with anemia should also follow similar guidelines as established for younger patients and should focus on the individual's response to therapy and the impact of anemia on clinical status, with therapeutic adjustments made as clinically indicated. Treatable causes of anemia in older adults include the following:

1. Nutritional deficiencies of iron, vitamin B_{12}, and folic acid
2. Underlying disorders related to the development of a chronic proinflammatory state, including infection, rheumatologic disease, and malignancy
3. MDS
4. Hypothyroidism
5. Renal disease
6. Acute blood loss

A. Nutritional Anemia and AI

Management of anemia caused by nutritional deficiencies in older adults follows the same recommendations as those in younger adults. Similar to younger adults, the use of oral iron therapy is as effective as administration of parenteral iron, provided there is normal enteric iron absorption. As there are no currently proven therapies that directly target inflammatory pathways in patients with AI, management of AI should be targeted to the underlying disorder.

B. Anemia of Chronic Renal Disease

For treatment of anemia caused by chronic renal disease, the United States Food and Drug Administration (FDA) has approved the use of ESA therapy. Guidelines for use of ESAs in older adults with both hemodialysis-dependent and -independent renal disease are similar to those in younger adults. However, recent studies have highlighted the potential for adverse cardiovascular outcomes, such as thrombosis and stroke, with the use of ESAs in anemic patients with renal disease. The Trial to Reduce Cardiovascular Events with Aranesp Therapy (TREAT) evaluated the effect of darbepoetin alfa in 1872 patients with anemia, diabetes and nondialysis dependent chronic kidney disease and found that the risk of stroke was double in those patients receiving darbepoetin alfa compared with placebo. The etiology of these adverse cardiovascular outcomes is unclear but may involve attempts to normalize Hgb levels in resistant subpopulations of patients. For this reason, the FDA recently placed a black-box warning on the use of ESAs in patients with anemia caused by renal disease, with recommendations targeting Hgb levels between 10 g/dL and 12 g/dL.

C. Unexplained Anemia

The majority of older adults with UA present with mild anemia that does not require initiation of therapy. For those symptomatic patients, currently available therapies are limited to red cell transfusions and ESAs. It should be noted that there is no absolute Hgb level that requires the initiation of therapy, and therapeutic intervention should be based on the individual patient, with consideration placed on the following factors: performance status, clinical impact of disease comorbidities, and quality of life assessment. The benefits of red cell transfusions must be weighed against the associated risks of iron overload, infectious complications, anaphylaxis, and red cell alloimmunization.

The use of ESAs in older adults with UA is not currently FDA-approved and there are few studies that have evaluated their use in this population. In one exploratory, randomized trial examining the impact of epoetin alpha in a cohort of 62 predominantly black older women with AI or UA, 69% receiving epoetin alpha achieved a greater than 2 g/dL increase in Hgb compared with those taking placebo ($P <0.001$) and demonstrated improvement in their assessment of fatigue. However, the target Hgb in this study was 13.0–13.9 g/dL, which represents a level above current FDA guidelines and one associated with adverse effects in numerous studies. Future randomized, controlled studies are needed to effectively determine the safety and efficacy of ESA therapy in older patients with UA and to determine whether there exists appropriate and safe target Hgb levels.

Agnihotri P, Telfer M, Butt Z, et al. Chronic anemia and fatigue in elderly patients: results of a randomized, double-blind, placebo-controlled, crossover exploratory study with epoetin alfa. *J Am Geriatr Soc.* 2007;55(10):1557-1565.

Adamson JW. Renal disease and anemia in the elderly. *Semin Hematol.* 2008;45(4):235-241.

Berenson JR, Anderson KC, Audell RA, et al. Monoclonal gammopathy of undetermined significance: a consensus statement. *Br J Haematol.* 2010;150(1):28-38.

Beutler E, West C. Hematologic differences between African-Americans and whites: the roles of iron deficiency and alpha-thalassemia on hemoglobin levels and mean corpuscular volume. *Blood.* 2005;106(2):740-745.

Carmel R. Nutritional anemias and the elderly. *Semin Hematol.* 2008;45(4):225-234.

den Elzen WP, Willems JM, Westendorp RG, de Craen AJ, Assendelft WJ, Gussekloo J. Effect of anemia and comorbidity on functional status and mortality in old age: results from the Leiden 85-plus Study. *CMAJ.* 2009;181(3-4):151-157.

Erslev AJ, Besarab A. Erythropoietin in the pathogenesis and treatment of the anemia of chronic renal failure. *Kidney Int.* 1997;51(3):622-630.

Ferrucci L, Guralnik JM, Bandinelli S, et al. Unexplained anaemia in older persons is characterised by low erythropoietin and low levels of pro-inflammatory markers. *Br J Haematol.* 2007;136(6):849-855.

Ferrucci L, Semba RD, Guralnik JM, et al. Proinflammatory state, hepcidin, and anemia in older persons. *Blood.* 2010;115(18):3810-3816.

Guralnik JM, Eisenstaedt RS, Ferrucci L, Klein HG, Woodman RC. Prevalence of anemia in persons 65 years and older in the United States: evidence for a high rate of unexplained anemia. *Blood.* 2004;104(8):2263-2268.

Hyjek E, Vardiman JW. Myelodysplastic/myeloproliferative neoplasms. *Semin Diagn Pathol.* 2011;28(4):283-297.

Liu K, Kaffes AJ. Iron deficiency anaemia: a review of diagnosis, investigation and management. *Eur J Gastroenterol Hepatol.* 2012;24(2):109-116.

Lucca U, Tettamanti M, Mosconi P, et al. Association of mild anemia with cognitive, functional, mood and quality of life outcomes in the elderly: the "Health and Anemia" study. *PLoS One.* 2008;3(4):e1920.

Nahon S, Lahmek P, Aras N, et al. Management and predictors of early mortality in elderly patients with iron deficiency anemia: a prospective study of 111 patients. *Gastroenterol Clin Biol.* 2007;31(2):169-174.

Penninx BW, Guralnik JM, Onder G, Ferrucci L, Wallace RB, Pahor M. Anemia and decline in physical performance among older persons. *Am J Med.* 2003;115(2):104-110.

Perlstein TS, Pande R, Berliner N, Vanasse GJ. Prevalence of 25-hydroxyvitamin D deficiency in subgroups of elderly persons with anemia: association with anemia of inflammation. *Blood.* 2011;117(10):2800-2806.

Price EA, Mehra R, Holmes TH, Schrier SL. Anemia in older persons: etiology and evaluation. *Blood Cells Mol Dis.* 2011;46(2):159-165.

Roy CN, Andrews NC. Anemia of inflammation: the hepcidin link. *Curr Opin Hematol.* 2005;12(2):107-111.

Roy CN, Semba RD, Sun K, et al. Circulating selenium and carboxymethyl-lysine, an advanced glycation end product, are independent predictors of anemia in older community-dwelling adults. *Nutrition.* 2012;28(7-8):762-766.

Semba RD, Ricks MO, Ferrucci L, et al. Types of anemia and mortality among older disabled women living in the community: the Women's Health and Aging Study I. *Aging Clin Exp Res.* 2007;19(4):259-264.

Skikne BS, Punnonen K, Caldron PH, et al. Improved differential diagnosis of anemia of chronic disease and iron deficiency anemia: a prospective multicenter evaluation of soluble transferrin receptor and the sTfR/log ferritin index. *Am J Hematol.* 2011;86(11):923-927.

Solomon SD, Uno H, Lewis EF, et al. Erythropoietic response and outcomes in kidney disease and type 2 diabetes. *N Engl J Med.* 2010;363(12):1146-1155.

Sullivan PS, Hanson DL, Chu SY, Jones JL, Ward JW. Epidemiology of anemia in human immunodeficiency virus (HIV)-infected persons: results from the multistate adult and adolescent spectrum of HIV disease surveillance project. *Blood.* 1998;91(1): 301-308.

Szczech LA, Barnhart HX, Inrig JK, et al. Secondary analysis of the CHOIR trial epoetin-alpha dose and achieved hemoglobin outcomes. *Kidney Int.* 2008;74(6):791-798.

Tettamanti M, Lucca U, Gandini F, et al. Prevalence, incidence and types of mild anemia in the elderly: the "Health and Anemia" population-based study. *Haematologica.* 2010;95(11): 1849-1856.

Vanasse GJ, Berliner N. Anemia in elderly patients: an emerging problem for the 21st century. *Hematology Am Soc Hematol Educ Program.* 2010:271-275.

Vanasse GJ, Jeong JY, Tate J, et al. A polymorphism in the leptin gene promoter is associated with anemia in patients with HIV disease. *Blood.* 2011;118(20):5401-5408.

Weiss G, Goodnough LT. Anemia of chronic disease. *N Engl J Med.* 2005;352(10):1011-1023.

Woodman R, Ferrucci L, Guralnik J. Anemia in older adults. *Curr Opin Hematol.* 2005;12(2):123-128.

Common Cancers

44

Joanne E. Mortimer, MD, FACP

Janet E. McElhaney, MD

▶ General Principles in Older Adults

Older patients with cancer provide a unique challenge to the oncologist, whether the intent is cure or palliation of symptoms. Curative therapy may require aggressive and potentially morbid operations, radiation therapy, or chemotherapy. Such aggressive approaches are often more toxic in older patients, who tend to be less resilient.

Cancers in older patients may demonstrate a distinct natural history that differs from that of younger patients. For example, breast cancers tend to have a more favorable prognosis in older populations, whereas acute leukemias have a worse prognosis. In addition, because toxicities from therapeutic intervention may be more frequent in older patients, more severe modifications in therapy may be required. Although radiation therapy is generally well tolerated, alterations in the radiation fields and doses may be necessary to decrease toxicity without significantly compromising efficacy.

Most of the antineoplastic agents are cytotoxic to rapidly dividing cells and are not specific for cancer cells. This lack of specificity results in myelosuppression, mucositis, and hair loss. In general, older patients experience more frequent and more severe normal tissue toxicities. Both the peripheral neuropathy from vincristine and the cardiotoxicity from doxorubicin develop at lower cumulative doses than is typically seen in younger patients. Similarly, mucositis from the combination of 5-fluorouracil (5-FU) and leucovorin is also more common and more severe in older patients. Alterations in renal and, to a lesser extent, hepatic function occur with age and should be considered in the selection and dosing of chemotherapy. Agents such as methotrexate, cisplatin, and bleomycin are normally excreted by the kidney and may produce excessive toxicity in older adults if administered in conventional doses. With an awareness of the normal aging physiology and knowledge of the pharmacology of antineoplastic agents, chemotherapy may be safely administered. Because most clinical trials have enrolled mostly younger individuals, evidence-based data that addresses the challenges of cancer treatment in the older population, is often lacking. Thus, in the addition to current age-based recommendations, life expectancy, functional status, and the patient's preferences and goals of care should be taken into consideration when making decisions regarding cancer screening and treatment in the older population.

▶ Treatment

Diagnosis-specific therapies are described in the sections below. If it has been determined that the cancer is not curable or that the patient is unable to tolerate aggressive therapy, the goal becomes palliation of cancer-related symptoms, which may include, but are not limited to, nausea, dyspnea, and pain. Cancer pain management should be tailored to the individual patient's pain needs and may require nonpharmacologic interventions such as radiation therapy. Attention should be paid to the effective management of potential complications of pain management such as constipation and delirium (see Chapter 11, "Geriatrics & Palliative Care," and Chapter 54, "Managing Persistent Pain in Older Adults").

BREAST CANCER

▶ General Principles in Older Adults

The median age for the development of breast cancer is 61 years. The incidence of breast cancer increases with age and plateaus in the seventh decade. In 1973, 37% of breast cancer were diagnosed in women older than 65 years. Between 1996 and 2000 that number increased to 44.2% with 22.5% ≥75 years. The natural history of breast cancer in older populations is unique. When prognostic factors such as estrogen receptor (ER), histologic grade, ploidy, p5p3, epithelial growth factor receptor (EGFR), and human epidermal growth receptor 2 (HER2) status are assessed, it appears that tumors become less aggressive with advancing age. Despite this, 60% of breast cancer-related deaths involve women 65 years of age and older. The high mortality rate may be explained by several factors. First, breast cancer is a common disease in this age group, and patients often have life-threatening comorbid conditions. Second, physicians tend to treat older patients less aggressively than younger individuals.

1. Primary Breast Cancer

▶ Treatment

Treatment recommendations should be made on an individual basis, taking into consideration comorbid conditions and expectations of therapy. Whenever possible, patients should be encouraged to participate in clinical trials designed to assess how cancers can best be managed.

A. Breast Conservation Therapy

Although modified radical mastectomy and breast conservation therapy with lumpectomy and radiation share similar survival rates, older women are less likely to undergo breast conservation therapy. Possibly some women choose mastectomy because they find the 6–7 weeks of daily radiation treatments for breast conservation cumbersome. It has also been shown that physicians are less likely to offer breast conservation therapy to older women.

Data suggest that, after surgical removal of the primary cancer, tamoxifen without radiation therapy may be adequate in select patients. However, by eliminating breast irradiation, ipsilateral breast cancer recurrences are more common and are generally treated by mastectomy for local control of the primary cancer. Despite the higher rate of "in-breast" recurrences, the survival for women treated with this less-aggressive approach is identical to that among women treated with conventional surgery and radiation therapy. Resection of the primary tumor and administration of tamoxifen may be appropriate for select women with small, ER+ breast cancers, and a finite life expectancy. Older women with a favorable long-term outlook should be treated as aggressively as younger women.

B. Adjuvant Therapy

For women with localized ER+ breast cancers, 5 years of adjuvant endocrine therapy decreases the recurrence rate and incidence of contralateral breast cancers. In older women on tamoxifen, the incidence of venous thromboemboli and uterine cancer is higher than in younger women; however, the benefits of adjuvant tamoxifen outweigh the risks. Adjuvant aromatase inhibitors (anastrozole, letrozole, and exemestane) are generally prescribed in postmenopausal women. When chemotherapy is indicated, the reduction in recurrence and survival advantage is identical to that observed in younger women. Less-toxic chemotherapy regimens are less effective than conventional chemotherapy.

Although one must weigh comorbid conditions when making treatment recommendations, appropriately administered adjuvant therapy is cost-effective. In the absence of severe comorbidities, the guidelines for adjuvant therapy are identical to those used to treat younger women. Women with ER+, node-negative breast cancers should have the primary tumor submitted for the 21-gene, Oncotype Recurrence Score, which is helpful in identifying patients who will benefit from chemotherapy in addition to endocrine therapy. Chemotherapy should be considered for those women whose primary cancers are >1 cm and ER− or HER2-positive, and for those with multiple node involvement. The addition of the humanized monoclonal antibody trastuzumab (Herceptin) to conventional chemotherapy is associated with an improved survival and should be used despite a higher incidence of cardiac toxicity in woman older than age 65 years and in patients with hypertension.

2. Metastatic Disease

▶ Treatment

Because the majority of breast cancers are ER+, endocrine therapy is the mainstay of treatment for advanced breast cancers. The aromatase inhibitors have achieved a higher rate of tumor regression and a longer duration of efficacy and have replaced tamoxifen as first-line therapy for metastatic disease. In ER− disease and cancers that are hormone resistant, chemotherapy may provide effective palliation. Newer, less-toxic single agents such as oral capecitabine are as effective as combination chemotherapy. In women with newly diagnosed HER2-positive breast cancer, anti-HER2 therapy is added either to an aromatase inhibitor in hormone receptor-positive disease or to chemotherapy in hormone receptor-negative of hormone refractory disease. Combined anti-HER2 therapy with trastuzumab and pertuzumab with chemotherapy has been shown to further improve survival compared to trastuzumab and chemotherapy alone.

▶ Screening

A systematic review conducted by the U.S. Preventive Services Task Force (USPSTF) in 2009 led to recommendations for biennial film mammography for women ages 50–74 years; there was insufficient evidence to recommend screening mammography for women age 75 years and older. However, screening mammography decreases breast cancer mortality in women aged 70–79 and identifies early lesions in older women as effectively as in younger women. A single decision analysis and cost-effectiveness study of mammography in women age 70 years and older demonstrated that survival may be favorably affected by screening mammography. Given the heterogeneity of health, particularly in the older-than-75-years population, recommendations should be based on age and health status. For example, the American Geriatrics Society recommends screening mammography in women up to age 85 years, provided that their life expectancy is at least 4 years.

LUNG CANCER

▶ General Principles in Older Adults

Lung cancer is the leading cause of cancer death in both men and women. The majority of patients are older than 65 years. Cancers arising from lung parenchyma are categorized as either small cell or non–small cell (adenocarcinoma, large cell, squamous cell, bronchoalveolar cell, or mixed histologies). A tissue confirmation of cancer and determination of histology provides important diagnostic, prognostic, and therapeutic information. Prognosis is also related to the stage of disease, performance status, gender, and patient's ability to tolerate adequate treatment. Although age is not an independent prognostic factor, older patients do experience more side effects from the chemotherapy used to treat lung cancer. This is especially true of myelosuppression.

▶ Treatment

Treatment is determined by the primary tumor histology (small cell or non–small cell) and disease stage (limited or extensive). Staging work-up should include an fluorodeoxyglucose positron emission tomography (FDG-PET) scan and MRI of the brain.

A. Small Cell Lung Cancer

Small cell lung cancers comprise 15% of all lung cancer histologies and 30% of these patients have disease confined to the hemithorax of origin, the mediastinum or supraclavicular nodes. In this "limited stage" disease, concurrent chemotherapy and radiation prolongs survival. Median survival is 20 months, and 20% of patients remain free of disease after 5 years. Because anthracycline-based chemotherapy regimens appear to be more toxic and are probably less effective, etoposide with cisplatin or carboplatin is administered every 21 days for 4–6 cycles. Overall survival and local control of the primary tumor are greater when radiation is initiated with the first cycle of chemotherapy. It has been shown that older patients are more likely to require delays in chemotherapy or dose reductions as a result of toxicity. Yet, despite the need to modify chemotherapy, the likelihood of response to treatment and overall survival are similar to that for younger patients treated with higher doses of chemotherapy. The efficacy of treatment does not appear to be compromised by these alterations in therapy.

For patients with extensive-stage disease, chemotherapy prolongs the median survival from 6–8 weeks to 8–10 months. Patients who are able to receive ≥4 cycles of chemotherapy appear to have a better survival than those who receive fewer cycles. Such data should be viewed with caution because it is possible that the patients who were able to tolerate "more" chemotherapy had a better prognosis. New regimens that are less dose intensive and toxic are being tested in older populations. The survival rates reported with these regimens appear comparable to those for younger patients using more toxic regimens.

B. Non–Small Cell Lung Cancer

The majority of lung cancers are of non–small cell histology and 10% are identified in patients who are nonsmokers. With the development of newer targeted agents, systemic therapy is further individualized based on the presence or absence of target markers such as EGFR and anaplastic lymphoma kinase (ALK) mutations. Rarely, patients have a solitary nodule that may be removed surgically for cure. Appropriate staging includes a mediastinoscopy with nodal sampling before removal of the primary tumor. If nodal metastases are identified, the patient is diagnosed with limited-stage disease and treated accordingly. Adjuvant chemotherapy and radiation therapy may be indicated in patients with selected tumors following definitive resection. Fit older patients with locally advanced disease that is not amenable to surgical resection will benefit from concurrent chemotherapy and radiation therapy, although they experience more myelosuppression. In older patients, chemotherapy doses are often attenuated because of declining performance status or because of an increased incidence of mucositis or myelosuppression.

In metastatic non–small cell lung cancer, chemotherapy has been shown to palliate symptoms and improve quality of life in the Elderly Lung Cancer Vinorelbine Italian Study (ELVIS trial). In patients >70 years of age, the combination of carboplatin with paclitaxel was compared to either single agent vinorelbine or gemcitabine. Although the combination was associated with more side effects, survival was significantly prolonged. Chemotherapy should be offered to patients with extensive-stage non–small cell lung cancer, especially those who have not lost weight and have a good performance status. Although lung cancer is most often fatal, meaningful improvement in survival and quality of life can be achieved. By modifying chemotherapy doses and schedule, toxicity can be minimized without compromising efficacy. In contrast to younger patients, the addition of bevacizumab to carboplatin and paclitaxel in advanced non–squamous cell cancers had no impact on progression free or overall survival in patients age >65 years. In treating cancers with the EGFR mutations, the single agent erlotinib appears to be as effective as other first-line single agents and is associated with increased side effects when used as second- and third-line therapy. Studies of the newer targeted agents are being tested in older populations.

▶ Screening

Although still controversial, in 2012, the American Cancer Society and the American College of Chest Physicians recommended that adults between the ages of 55 and 74 with at least a 30 pack-year history of current or prior cigarette use receive annual low-dose CT scans of the chest to screen for lung cancer. The USPSTF has not updated its 2004 recommendation that there is "insufficient evidence for or against screening asymptomatic persons for lung cancer."

COLORECTAL CANCER

1. Rectal Cancer

The natural history of rectal cancer differs from colon cancer. Because the rectum lies in close proximity to the sacral plexus, uterus, bladder, and prostate, a wide radial margin is often difficult to obtain with surgery, and local recurrences are common. To prevent local disease recurrence, 5-FU in conjunction with radiation therapy is administered either before or after surgical resection. In the Medicare population, the advantages of combined-modality treatment of rectal cancer are similar to those observed in younger patients.

2. Metastatic Colorectal Cancer

Although most large bowel cancers metastasize to the liver, the pattern of disease recurrence differs somewhat depending on whether the primary tumor arises from the colon or rectum. The drainage of the colon is via the portal vein, and the liver is the most common site, and possibly the only site, of metastasis. Because the inferior mesenteric vein receives drainage from the rectum, systemic metastasis to sites in addition to the liver may develop.

Metastatic colorectal cancer is generally incurable. However, resection of liver metastases may provide long-term disease-free survival for select patients. 5-FU–based regimens may provide both improved quality of life and prolongation in survival. The oral agent capecitabine is better tolerated than 5-FU, and is equally effective in this population. The addition of irinotecan to 5-FU and leucovorin produces improvement with a greater likelihood of tumor regression and possibly a longer survival than is achievable with 5-FU and leucovorin alone. Bevacizumab is a component of first-line chemotherapy, but has not been specifically studied in older patients who tend to experience more thrombotic and thromboembolic events with this agent.

▶ Complications

If the primary tumor is not removed, perforation, bleeding, and obstruction may develop, requiring emergency surgical intervention. Emergency operations performed in patients age 70 years and older are associated with higher-than-expected morbidity and mortality.

▶ Treatment

The treatment of colorectal cancers in older patients does not differ from that for younger individuals. Surgical resection of the primary tumor has been the mainstay of treatment, even in patients with metastatic disease. For patients with newly diagnosed cancers, the resection specimen provides important staging information.

When the regional nodes are involved, 32 weeks of adjuvant 5-FU and leucovorin is recommended. In this setting, the leucovorin is administered not to "rescue" the patient from chemotherapy toxicity (as with methotrexate), but to potentiate the antitumor effect of 5-FU. In the Medicare population, a regimen of adjuvant 5-FU and leucovorin has been shown to reduce the risk of death by 27%, an advantage equivalent to that demonstrated in younger patients. The addition of oxaliplatin to 5-FU+leucovorin was not found to improve survival in patients older than 70 years, although it is superior to 5-FU+leucovorin in younger patients (Adjuvant Colon Cancer Endpoints [ACCENT] trial). Possibly because this regimen is relatively nontoxic, adjuvant chemotherapy can be appropriately administered to older patients.

▶ Screening

Colonoscopy has been established as a cost-effective screening tool. The initial screening should begin at age 50 years and is repeated every 10 years until age 85 years. If polyps are identified, the procedure should be repeated every 3–5 years. As with any screening test, the decision to screen should weigh life expectancy and goals of care with the potential risks and benefits of screening. For a more detailed approach to decision making regarding screening see Chapter 3, "Goals of Care & Consideration of Prognosis," and Chapter 8, "Prevention & Health Promotion."

▶ Prognosis

Prognosis is related to the depth of invasion of the primary tumor, involvement of regional structures (eg, bladder or uterus), and nodal involvement.

PANCREATIC CANCER

▶ General Principles in Older Adults

More than 66% of pancreatic cancers develop in individuals 65 years of age and older. Even when it appears that the disease is confined to the organ, few patients survive 5 years.

▶ Treatment

Pancreaticoduodenectomy may provide long-term survival for a small percentage of patients. However, the complications of the procedure are significantly higher in patients 70 years of age and older.

Pain is a common and debilitating problem in patients with pancreatic cancer. Even if the patient is found to have unresectable disease at the time of surgical exploration, palliation of pain and prevention of future pain may be achieved by neurolysis of the celiac ganglion.

If the disease is localized to the pancreas but not resectable, combined chemotherapy and radiation therapy may provide both palliation and a slight survival advantage. Candidates for such an approach should be carefully selected because this therapy is toxic. Once the disease has metastasized, palliation is the goal of any intervention. Single-agent gemcitabine has been shown to improve quality of life, with superior pain control and a modest survival advantage.

OVARIAN CANCER

▶ General Principles in Older Adults

The incidence of ovarian cancer increases with age, peaking at 80–84 years. There are no widely accepted screening modalities, and in 2012, the USPSTF recommended against routine screening for ovarian cancer.

▶ Treatment

Most women present with advanced stages of the disease and are treated with surgery and chemotherapy. Ideally, patients should undergo surgery for both staging and treatment. A total abdominal hysterectomy with bilateral salpingo-oophorectomy and surgical debulking of visible tumor should be performed. Staging also includes nodal sampling, and cytologic examination of smears obtained from the cul-de-sac and diaphragms bilaterally.

The most effective initial chemotherapy combines paclitaxel with cisplatin or carboplatin. Although chemotherapy is effective and relatively nontoxic, older women are less likely to receive treatment. The serum marker CA-125 is an excellent indicator of disease and is of value in monitoring the efficacy of chemotherapy.

LEUKEMIA

1. Chronic Lymphocytic Leukemia

Chronic lymphocytic leukemia (CLL) is the most common form of leukemia and its incidence rises with age. As many as 50% of patients are asymptomatic at the time of diagnosis. The clinical course may be indolent, and chemotherapy or radiation may be reserved until the patient becomes symptomatic. The natural history of CLL is defined by the initial stage at diagnosis, cytogenetics, and tumor markers. Although CLL is not curable, chemotherapy may delay the course of the disease and improve quality of life. Treatment should be initiated only when symptoms are manifested: either B-symptoms (fever, night sweats, 10% weight loss over 6 months) or symptoms from enlarged nodes. Symptoms referable to nodal enlargement may also be palliated with chemotherapy or localized radiation therapy. A number of combination chemotherapy regimens are effective in controlling the disease. In frail older patients, the oral alkylating agent, chlorambucil, was found to be as effective as intravenous fludarabine.

2. Acute Nonlymphocytic Leukemia

The incidence of acute nonlymphocytic leukemia (ANL) increases with age and the prognosis is inversely related.

▶ Treatment

Of all patients treated, 70% of individuals go into remission and these are durable for 15–20% of those who achieve a complete remission. ANL in patients older than 40 years is more aggressive and less amenable to therapy. In older people, ANL frequently develops after a history of myelodysplasia and adverse cytogenetic abnormalities, which predict a poor outcome. Leukemic cells from older patients are also more likely to express genes that confer drug resistance. These factors predict resistance to conventional induction regimens. The treatment-related mortality during induction is as high as 25% and complete remissions are achieved in only 45% of older patients; long-term remissions are rare. When lower doses of chemotherapy are used to minimize treatment-related complications, the remission rate is significantly less as well.

Patients and their families should understand that the treatment for ANL is toxic and relatively ineffective. Whenever possible, patients should be referred to oncologists who enter patients in clinical studies that address improved methods of supportive care and innovative regimens. For frail and elderly patients with significant comorbidities, it is reasonable to provide only palliative care.

LYMPHOMA

1. Indolent Histologies

Lymphomas are classified as Indolent, Aggressive and Highly Aggressive based on the WHO *Classifications of Tumours of Haematopoietic and Lymphoid Tissues*. As with CLL, treatment of low-grade lymphomas does not appear to alter the natural history of the disease, even though the disease is sensitive to treatment.

▶ Treatment

Chemotherapy and radiation therapy are reserved for the treatment of symptoms produced by the disease.

2. Aggressive Histologies

More than 50% of the aggressive histologic subtypes develop in individuals older than 60 years, and age >60 years has been identified as a poor prognostic factor by the International Prognostic Factors Project.

▶ Treatment

Patients with stage I and stage II disease are treated with chemotherapy and radiation therapy, and, regardless of age, have a favorable prognosis. Patients with more advanced-stage disease (stage III and stage IV) are treated with chemotherapy with or without the anti-CD20 antibody, rituximab.

For more than 2 decades, the combination of cyclophosphamide, doxorubicin, vincristine, and prednisone (CHOP) has been the standard chemotherapy. Patients older than 60 years are more likely to experience neutropenia and fever than are younger patients. However, when doxorubicin has been deleted from the regimen or the dose has been attenuated, the efficacy has been significantly compromised. After the first cycle of chemotherapy, the use of colony-stimulating factors will decrease the incidence of neutropenia.

It is expected that chemotherapy will produce complete remission of disease in the majority of patients, with 30% to 40% remaining disease free after 5 years. The benefits of chemotherapy are somewhat less for patients who are older than 60 years or who have 1 or more comorbid medical conditions. The addition of rituximab to CHOP has been shown to further improve disease outcome and survival and is the new standard of care in this population.

For Prostate Cancer, see Chapter 40, "Benign Prostatic Hyperplasia & Prostate Cancer."

AGS Panel on Persistent Pain in Older Persons. The management of persistent pain in older persons. *J Am Geriatr Soc.* 2002; 50(6 Suppl);S205-S224.

Baum M, Budzar AU, Cuzick J, et al; ATAC Trialists' Group. Anastrozole alone or in combination with tamoxifen versus tamoxifen alone for adjuvant treatment of postmenopausal women with early breast cancer: the first results of the ATAC randomised trial. *Lancet.* 2002;359(9324):2131-2139.

Bernabai R, Gambassi G, Lapane K, et al. Management of pain in elderly patients with cancer. SAGE Study Group. Systematic Assessment of Geriatric Drug Use via Epidemiology. *JAMA.* 1998;279(23):1877-1882.

Breast cancer screening in older women. American Geriatrics Society Clinical Practice Committee. *J Am Geriatr Soc.* 2000;48(7):842-844.

Chan JK. The new World Health Organization classification of lymphomas: the past, the present and the future. *Hematol Oncol.* 2001;19(4):129-150.

Cleeland CS. Undertreatment of cancer pain in elderly patients. *JAMA.* 1998;279(23):1914-1915.

Coiffier B, Lepage E, Briere J. CHOP chemotherapy plus rituximab compared with CHOP alone in elderly patients with diffuse large-B-cell lymphoma. *N Engl J Med.* 2002;346(4): 235-242.

Diab SG, Elledge RM, Clark GM. Tumor characteristics and clinical outcome of elderly women with breast cancer. *J Natl Cancer Inst.* 2000;92(7):550-556.

Dighiero G, Maloum K, Desablens B, et al. Chlorambucil in indolent chronic lymphocytic leukemia. French Cooperative Group on Chronic Lymphocytic Leukemia. *N Engl J Med.* 1998;338(21):1506-1514.

Early Breast Cancer Trialists Collaborative Group. Tamoxifen for early breast cancer: an overview of the randomised trials. *Lancet.* 1998;351(9114):1451-1467.

Effects of vinorelbine on quality of life and survival of elderly patient with advanced non-small-cell lung cancer. Elderly Lung Cancer Vinorelbine Italian Study Group. *J Natl Cancer Inst.* 1999;91(1):66-72.

Extermann M, Balducci L, Lyman GH. What threshold for adjuvant therapy in older breast cancer patients? *J Clin Oncol.* 2000;18(8):1709-1717.

Frasci G, Lorusso V, Panza N, et al. Gemcitabine plus vinorelbine versus vinorelbine alone in elderly patients with advanced non-small-cell lung cancer. *J Clin Oncol.* 2000;18(13):2529-2536.

Frazier AL, Colditz GA, Fuchs CS, Kuntz KM. Cost-effectiveness of screening for colorectal cancer in the general population. *JAMA.* 2000;284(15):1954-1961.

Fyles A et al. Preliminary results of a randomized study of tamoxifen ± breast radiation in T1/2 N0 disease in women over 50 years of age. *Proc Am Soc Clin Oncol.* 2001;21:92.

Hughes KS et al. Comparison of lumpectomy plus tamoxifen with and without radiotherapy in women 70 years of age or older who have clinical stage I estrogen receptor positive breast cancer. *Proc Am Soc Clin Oncol.* 2001;21:93.

Ires L et al. SEER cancer statistics review, 1973–1999. National Cancer Institute; 2002.

Iwashyna TJ, Lamont EB. Effectiveness of adjuvant fluorouracil in clinical practice: a population-based cohort study of elderly patients with stage III colon cancer. *J Clin Oncol.* 2002; 20(19):3992-3998.

Kaufmann M, Bajetta E, Dirix LY, et al. Exemestane is superior to megestrol acetate after tamoxifen failure in postmenopausal women with advanced breast cancer: results of phase III randomized double-blind trial. The Exemestane Study Group. *J Clin Oncol.* 2000;18(7):1399-1411.

Kerlikowske K, Salzmann P, Phillips KA, Cauley JA, Cummings SR. Continued screening mammography in women aged 70 to 79 years: impact on life expectancy and cost-effectiveness. *JAMA.* 1999;282(22):2156-2163.

Kouroukis CT, Browman GP, Esmail R, Meyer RM. Chemotherapy for older patients with newly diagnosed, advanced-stage, aggressive-histology non-Hodgkin lymphoma: a systematic review. *Ann Intern Med.* 2002;136(2):144-152.

Miller TP, Dahlberg S, Cassady JR, et al. Chemotherapy alone compared with chemotherapy plus radiotherapy for localized intermediate- and high-grade non-Hodgkin's lymphoma. *N Engl J Med.* 1998;339(1):21-26.

Mouridsen H, Gershanovich M, Sun Y, et al. Superior efficacy of letrozole versus tamoxifen as first-line therapy for postmenopausal women with advanced breast cancer: results of a phase III study of the international letrozole breast cancer group. *J Clin Oncol.* 2001;19(10):2596-2606.

National Cancer Institute: Surveillance and end results program (Public use CD-Rom 1973–1995). Washington, DC: Cancer Statistics Branch, National Cancer Institute; 1998.

Neugut AI, Fleischauer AT, Sundararajan V, et al. Use of adjuvant chemotherapy and radiation therapy for rectal cancer among the elderly: a population-based study. *J Clin Oncol.* 2002;20(11):2643-2650.

O'Mahony S, Coyle N, Payne R. Current management of opioid-related side effects. *Oncology (Williston Park).* 2001;15(1):61-73,77.

Poen JC, Ford JM, Niederhuber JE. Chemoradiotherapy in the management of localized tumors of the pancreas. *Ann Surg Oncol.* 1999;6(1):117-122.

Ries LAG, Eisner MP, Kosary CL, et al. *SEER Cancer Statistics Review, 1975-2000.* Bethesda, MD: National Cancer Institute; 2003.

Sargent DJ, Goldberg RM, Jacobson SD, et al. A pooled analysis of adjuvant chemotherapy for resected colon cancer in the elderly. *N Engl J Med.* 2001;345(15):1091-1097.

Slamon DJ, Leyland-Jones B, Shak S, et al. Use of chemotherapy plus a monoclonal antibody against HER2 for metastatic breast cancer that overexpressed HER2. *N Engl J Med.* 2001;344(11):783-792.

Sonnenberg A, Delcò F, Inadomi JM. Cost-effectiveness of colonoscopy in screening for colorectal cancer. *Ann Intern Med.* 2000;133(8):573-584.

Sundararajan V, Hershman D, Grann VR, Jacobson JS, Neugut AI. Variations in the use of chemotherapy for elderly patients with advanced ovarian cancer: a population-based study. *J Clin Oncol.* 2001;20(1):173-178.

US Preventive Services Task Force. Screening for breast cancer: U.S. Preventive Services Task Force recommendation statement. *Ann Intern Med.* 2009;151(10):716-726, W-236.

Warren JL, Brown ML, Fay MP, Schussler N, Potosky AL, Riley GF. Costs of treatment for elderly women with early-stage breast cancer in fee-for-service settings. *J Clin Oncol.* 2001;20(1): 307-316.

Westeel V, Murray N, Gelmon K, et al. New combination of old drugs for elderly patients with small cell lung cancer: a phase II study of the PAVE regimen. *J Clin Oncol.* 1998;16(5): 1940-1947.

USEFUL WEBSITES

National Cancer Institute's Surveillance Epidemiology and End Results database. http://seer.cancer.gov/index.html

U.S. Preventive Services Task Force. http://www.uspreventive servicestaskforce.org/adultrec.htm

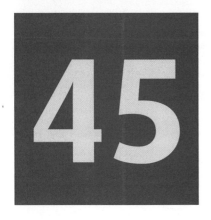

Depression & Other Mental Health Issues

David Liu, MD, MS

Mary A. Norman, MD

Bobby Singh, MD

Kewchang Lee, MD

DEPRESSION

ESSENTIALS OF DIAGNOSIS

▶ Depressed mood.

▶ Loss of interest or pleasure in almost all activities.

▶ Unintentional weight change, lack of energy, change in sleep pattern, psychomotor retardation or agitation, excessive guilt, or poor concentration.

▶ Suicidal ideation or recurrent thoughts of death.

▶ Somatic rather than mood complaints in the elderly.

▶ General Principles in Older Adults

By 2020, depression will rank second only to cardiovascular disease as a cause of global disability and a major public health problem in older people. The prevalence of major depression is estimated at 1% to 2% for elders in the community and 10% to 12% for those in primary care settings. However, even in the absence of major depression as defined by *Diagnostic and Statistical Manual of Mental Disorders* (5th ed.; *DSM-5*) criteria, up to 27% of elders experience substantial depressive symptoms that may be relieved with intervention. For institutionalized elders, the rates of major depression are much higher: 12% for hospitalized elders and 43% for permanently institutionalized elders.

The World Health Organization Primary Care Study reported that 60% of primary care clinic patients treated with antidepressant medication still met criteria for depression 1 year later, with similar efficacy rates for antidepressants reported in older adults and those younger than the age of 60 years. However, depression is often missed or inadequately managed in older adults, sometimes because of the belief that depression is an inevitable process of aging or because

treatment may be risky or ineffective. Indeed, there are several reasons why optimal treatment of depression in the geriatric population may differ from that for younger populations. Higher rates of physical and cognitive comorbidity in older adults, different social circumstances, greater potential for polypharmacy, and age-related pharmacodynamic and pharmacokinetic susceptibility all suggest that this population should be considered separately.

Women are twice as likely to experience major depression as men. Other risk factors include prior episodes or a personal family history of depression, lack of social support, use of alcohol or other substances, and a recent loss of a loved one. Several medical conditions are also associated with an increased risk of depression, including Parkinson disease, recent myocardial infarction, and stroke. These conditions share common threads of loss of control of body or mind, increasing dependence on others, and increased social isolation.

Depression is associated with poorer self-care and slower recovery after acute medical illnesses. It can accelerate cognitive and physical decline and leads to an increased use and cost of health care services. Among depressed older adults who have had a stroke, rehabilitation efforts are less effective and mortality rates are significantly higher.

▶ Clinical Findings

A. Symptoms & Signs

Major depression is defined as depressed mood or loss of interest in nearly all activities (anhedonia) or both for at least 2 weeks, accompanied by a minimum of 3 or 4 of the following symptoms (for a total of at least 5 symptoms): insomnia or hypersomnia, feelings of worthlessness or excessive guilt, fatigue or loss of energy, diminished ability to think or concentrate, substantial change in appetite or weight, psychomotor agitation or retardation, and recurrent thoughts of death or suicide. Severity of depression varies and is important in determining optimal treatment and prognosis. Mild depression is marked by few, if any, symptoms in excess of the minimum number required to meet the diagnostic criteria defined above, and it is accompanied by minimal impairment in functioning. Moderate depression includes a greater number and intensity of depressive symptoms and moderate impairment in functioning. Patients with severe depression experience marked intensity and pervasiveness of depressive symptoms with substantial impairment in functioning. Patients with less-severe depressive symptoms who do not meet criteria for major depression may also benefit from psychotherapy and pharmacotherapy.

B. Screening Tools

Older patients can have fewer mood and more somatic complaints, which are often difficult to differentiate from underlying medical conditions. Special screening tools that consider this difference have been developed for the older population. The Geriatric Depression Scale is widely used and validated in many different languages. Its shortened 15-item scale (Table 45–1) is often used for ease of administration. A separate 2-item scale consisting of 2 questions about depressed mood and anhedonia has also been shown effective in detecting depression in older adults (see Table 45–1). Screening alone has not been found to benefit patients with unrecognized depression, but in combination with patient support programs, such as frequent nursing follow-up and close monitoring of adherence to medication, it improves outcomes.

▶ Differential Diagnosis

Diagnosing depression in older adults can be challenging because of the presence of multiple comorbid conditions. Many patients with mild cognitive impairment may have predominantly depressive symptoms. With effective treatment of depression, their cognitive performance frequently improves; however, their risk for developing dementia in their lifetime is roughly double the risk of nondepressed seniors. Bereavement often manifests with depressed mood, which may be appropriate given a patient's recent loss. However, if depressive symptoms persist, further evaluation may be warranted.

Older patients who experience delirium caused by an underlying medical illness may have mood changes. Other comorbid psychiatric illnesses must also be considered, such as anxiety disorder, substance abuse disorder, or personality disorders. Patients with bipolar disorder or psychotic disorders may have depressed mood; thus, it is important to ask patients about prior manic episodes, hallucinations, or delusions.

Depression can also be confused with other medical conditions. Fatigue and weight loss, for example, may be

Table 45–1. Geriatric depression scale (short form).[a]

Depression Scale	
1. Are you basically satisfied with your life?	Yes/**No**
2. Have you dropped many of your activities and interests?	**Yes**/No
3. Do you feel that your life is empty?	**Yes**/No
4. Do you often get bored?	**Yes**/No
5. Are you in good spirits most of the time?	Yes/**No**
6. Are you afraid that something bad is going to happen to you?	**Yes**/No
7. Do you feel happy most of the time?	Yes/**No**
8. Do you often feel helpless?	**Yes**/No
9. Do you prefer to stay at home rather than going out and doing new things?	**Yes**/No
10. Do you feel that you have more problems with memory than most?	**Yes**/No
11. Do you think it is wonderful to be alive now?	Yes/**No**
12. Do you feel pretty worthless the way you are now?	**Yes**/No
13. Do you feel full of energy?	Yes/**No**
14. Do you feel that your situation is hopeless?	**Yes**/No
15. Do you think that most people are better off than you are?	**Yes**/No
SCORE:	_____
Directions: Score 1 point for each bolded answer. A score of 5 or more is a positive screen for depression.	
Two-Question Case-Finding Instrument[b]	
1. During the last month, have you often been bothered by feeling down, depressed, or hopeless?	**Yes**/No
2. During the last month, have you often been bothered by having little interest or pleasure in doing things?	**Yes**/No
Directions: Yes to either question is a positive screen for depression.	

[a]Reproduced with permission from Yesavage JA, Brink TL, Rose TL, et al. Development and validation of a geriatric depression screening scale: a preliminary report. *J Psychiatr Res.* 1982-1983;17(1):37-49.
[b]Reproduced with permission from Whooley MA, Avins AL, Miranda J, Browner WS, et al. Case-finding instrument for depression. Two questions are as good as many. *J Gen Intern Med.* 1997;12(7):439-445.

associated with diabetes mellitus, thyroid disease, underlying malignancy, or anemia. Patients who have Parkinson disease may first present with depressed mood or flat affect. Sleep disturbances as a result of pain, nocturia, or sleep apnea may also lead to daytime fatigue and depressed mood.

A complete history and physical examination, including assessment of cognitive status, is critical in the evaluation of depression in older adults. Because depression is a clinical diagnosis, no routine laboratory tests are indicated. Testing may be tailored to each patient based on their underlying comorbidities and presenting symptoms. A complete review of medications, both prescription and nonprescription, is essential. Medications, such as benzodiazepines, opioid analgesics, glucocorticoids, interferon, and reserpine, may cause depressive symptoms. Contrary to earlier beliefs, β blockers have not been proven to cause depression. Screening for alcohol and other substance use or addiction is another important part of the medical history. Substance use can interfere with compliance and contribute to high relapse rates, although active substance abuse should not preclude treatment for depression. For patients who struggle with addiction, "dual diagnosis" programs (alcohol or other substance dependence and psychiatric disorder) may be optimal.

▶ Treatment

A. Patient & Family Education/Supportive Care

Educating patients and families about depression is the cornerstone of successful treatment. Depression continues to carry a stigma in many communities and cultures. Appropriate education can help patients understand that their condition results from a combination of inherited factors and personal and environmental stressors. Providers should also emphasize that physical symptoms and sleep disturbances are characteristic of depression; thus, relief of depression could make other physical symptoms more bearable. Encouraging physical activity with a family member or friend can be a simple, effective step toward improving social support and overall well-being.

Involving families in the care of older patients is crucial for both diagnosing depression and developing an effective treatment plan. However, caregivers of older patients, especially if impaired physically or cognitively, may experience considerable stress and depression as well. Referred to as caregiver burden, this is an all-encompassing term used to describe the physical, emotional, and financial toll of providing care. In particular, when patients with dementia have depression, their caregivers report higher levels of burden. Many programs are available that may alleviate stress and promote positive social interactions for patients. Adult day programs, senior centers, and senior support groups can be helpful resources for patients and their families, and geriatric social workers can assist with finding appropriate programs for each patient. Caregiver support groups and formal respite programs are also available in many communities.

B. Pharmacotherapy

1. Antidepressants

a. Selection—Overall, antidepressants, including tricyclic antidepressants (TCAs), selective serotonin reuptake inhibitors (SSRIs), and selective serotonin-norepinephrine reuptake inhibitors (SNRIs), are equally effective in the treatment of geriatric depression. However, because of side-effect profiles and propensity for drug interactions, monoamine oxidase inhibitors (eg, phenelzine and tranylcypromine) and tertiary amine TCAs (eg, amitriptyline, imipramine, and doxepin) are rarely used in older adults. The SSRI class includes citalopram, escitalopram, fluoxetine, paroxetine, and sertraline; examples of SNRIs are venlafaxine, desvenlafaxine, and duloxetine. Fluoxetine is generally avoided in older adults because of its long half-life and inhibition of the P450 system. Choice of therapy among the remaining drugs is generally determined by side-effect profile and the patient's comorbid symptoms such as anxiety, insomnia, pain, and weight loss, although anxiety and insomnia do not necessarily predict a better response to more sedating medications. Renal and hepatic functions are also important considerations in older adults and should be assessed before initiation of therapy.

SSRIs are relatively safe in overdose. Thus, they are a reasonable first choice in treating older patients with depression. However, the Food and Drug Administration has recently posted a warning of cardiac arrhythmias associated with high doses of the SSRI citalopram hydrobromide (Celexa). Citing increased risk of QT interval prolongation and torsade de pointes through postmarketing reports of citalopram, the FDA announced a maximum daily dose of 20 mg for all patients older than age 60 years. The warnings do not apply to its racemic drug, escitalopram (Lexapro), which is the S-enantiomer of the citalopram molecule.

Other agents offer unique advantages: Mirtazapine stimulates appetite and can help with insomnia, and bupropion can reduce craving in smoking cessation. Secondary amine TCAs (eg, nortriptyline, desipramine) can offer beneficial effects for patients with neuropathic pain, detrusor instability, or insomnia. SNRIs, which have serotonergic and noradrenergic activity, are other effective alternatives that may also be useful in treating anxiety and neuropathic pain.

b. Dosage—In general, older patients should begin an antidepressant by taking half of the manufacturer-recommended starting dose (to minimize side effects), but the medication should be titrated to the recommended target dose in weekly increments. Older patients are frequently undertreated because the provider fails to adequately titrate the dose to a therapeutic level. If minimal or no benefit occurs by 4–6 weeks and side effects are tolerable, the dose should be increased. The full effect may not be seen for 8–12 weeks in older patients. If a therapeutic dose has been reached and maintained for 6 weeks and the patient has not adequately responded, one should consider switching to a different agent or augmenting with an additional agent. Although serum drug levels are not useful for SSRIs, levels of TCAs can be measured to assess adherence.

c. Side effects—Side effects differ depending on the type of antidepressant. Most side effects lessen within 1–4 weeks from the start of therapy, but weight gain and sexual dysfunction may last longer. For the SSRIs, the most common side effects include nausea and sexual dysfunction. Sexual dysfunction may respond to treatment with sildenafil, but switching antidepressant medication or lowering the dose of SSRI and augmenting with an additional agent may be necessary. The TCAs have more anticholinergic properties and may lead to dry mouth, orthostasis, and urinary retention.

d. Cautions & interactions

1. Cardiovascular disease—TCAs can be associated with orthostatic hypotension and cardiac conduction abnormalities, leading to arrhythmias. Recently, citalopram has been implicated in potentially dangerous arrhythmias. Therefore, electrolyte and/or electrocardiographic monitoring is recommended for patients at risk for arrhythmias if these agents are considered.

2. Hypertension—Venlafaxine and desvenlafaxine may increase systolic and diastolic blood pressure.

3. Electrolyte abnormalities—Serotonin-reuptake inhibitors may induce hyponatremia.

4. Hepatic disease—Most antidepressants are hepatically cleared and should be used with caution in patients with liver disease. Nefazodone in particular should not be used in patients with liver disease or elevated transaminases because it has been associated with an increased risk of hepatic failure and interacts with other hepatically cleared medications, including simvastatin and lovastatin.

5. Falls—Serotonin-reuptake inhibitors have been associated with an increased risk in falls particularly in older patients with dementia. Fall risk assessment should be included in part of overall medical evaluation.

6. Bleeding risk—Serotonin-reuptake inhibitors may increase bleeding risk and interact with anticoagulant medications such as warfarin. International normalized ratio levels should be closely monitored with initiation of treatment with SSRI's.

7. Cognitive impairment—TCAs and certain SSRIs, such as paroxetine, have stronger anticholinergic effects and should be avoided in patients with cognitive impairment to avoid increasing confusion.

8. Seizure disorders—Bupropion lowers seizure thresholds.

9. Suicidal ideation—TCAs are lethal in overdose and should be avoided in actively suicidal patients. SSRIs and SNRIs are relatively safe in overdose.

10. Serotonin syndrome—Use of serotonergic antidepressants may lead to serotonin syndrome, a potentially life-threatening condition associated with increased serotonergic activity in the central nervous system. Although classically described as a triad of mental status changes (headache, confusion, agitation), autonomic hyperactivity (diaphoresis, hypertension, tachycardia, nausea, diarrhea), and neuromuscular abnormalities (tremor, myoclonus, hyperreflexia) serotonin syndrome can span a spectrum of clinical findings ranging from benign to lethal. Given the increased use of serotonergic agents in medical practice, and the syndrome's potential for rapid onset, with its clinical course developing over 24 hours, providers are advised to remain vigilant for this condition. The central principles to the management of suspected serotonin syndrome are (a) discontinuation of all serotonergic agents, and (b) supportive care aimed at normalization of vital signs.

2. Psychostimulants—Psychostimulants, such as dextroamphetamine (5–10 mg/day) or methylphenidate (2.5–5 mg/day), are sometimes indicated as either a primary or an adjuvant treatment for depression with predominant vegetative symptoms. A newer stimulant, modafinil (Provigil), which increases monoamines, has also been used as an adjunct to traditional antidepressants. With its additional histaminergic effects, modafinil is considered by some to be a "wakefulness promoting agent," and unlike the classic amphetamine-like stimulants, is considered to have limited abuse potential. At the end of life, patients may not have time to wait 4–6 weeks for the benefits of antidepressant medication, and psychostimulants may offer more immediate relief. In the setting of depression after an acute medical illness, psychostimulants may offer a faster means to enhance recovery and participation in rehabilitation. Typical side effects include insomnia and agitation, but these may be lessened by taking the medication early in the day in divided doses (morning and noon). Another common side effect is tachycardia.

3. Herbal remedies—Many herbal remedies claim to be effective in treating depression, but further evidence is still needed to determine whether these "dietary supplements" (eg, *Hypericum perforatum* [St. John's wort]) have a role in the treatment of depression. *H. perforatum* should not be used in conjunction with SSRIs because the combination may lead to serotonergic syndrome, which is characterized by changes in mental status, tremor, gastrointestinal upset, headache, myalgia, and restlessness. It may lower the concentration of certain drugs, such as warfarin, digoxin, theophylline, cyclosporine, and HIV-1 protease inhibitors. Other common herbal remedies such as kava kava and valerian root have not been proven effective for treating depression. Herbal remedies should not be substituted for proven depression therapies.

C. Psychotherapy

Cognitive–behavioral therapy (CBT), problem-solving therapy, and interpersonal psychotherapy are effective treatments for major depression, either alone or in combination with pharmacotherapy. CBT focuses on identifying negative thoughts and behaviors that contribute to depression and replacing them with positive thoughts and rewarding activities. Problem-solving therapy teaches patients techniques to identify routine problems, generate multiple solutions, and implement the best strategy. Interpersonal psychotherapy focuses on recognizing and attempting to resolve personal stressors and relationship conflicts that lead to depressive symptoms.

Typically, these therapies should be continued once or twice weekly for 6–16 sessions. In patients with severe depression, combination therapy with psychotherapy and pharmacotherapy is superior to either treatment alone. Psychoanalytic and psychodynamic therapies have not proved effective for treatment of major depression.

D. Electroconvulsive Therapy

Electroconvulsive therapy (ECT) is an effective treatment for geriatric depression. Response rates for refractory depression are quite high at 73% for the young-old (age 60–74 years) and 67% for the old-old (age >75 years). Typical side effects include confusion and anterograde memory impairment, which may persist for 6 months. ECT may be first-line therapy for severely melancholic patients, for those at high risk for suicide, and for medically ill patients whose hepatic, renal, or cardiac diseases preclude the use of other antidepressants.

E. Psychiatric Therapy

Psychiatric consultation is recommended for those patients with a history of mania or psychosis, for those who have not responded to a trial of 1 or 2 medicines, and for those who require combination therapy or ECT. Immediate psychiatric evaluation is required for any patients who, after probing, admit to having active plans to harm themselves. Risk factors for suicide in older patients with major depression include older age; male gender; marital status of single, divorced, or separated and without children; personal or family history of a suicide attempt; drug or alcohol abuse; severe anxiety or stress; physical illness; and a specific suicide plan with access to firearms or other lethal means (eg, stockpiled medications). If medications and weapons are present and cannot be removed from the patient's home, consider adding "weapon at home" to the patient's problem list to highlight potential suicide risk.

F. Follow-up

1. Pharmacotherapy—Older patients should be monitored closely during the initial 3 months of treatment. Many medical outpatients who receive a prescription for an antidepressant terminate treatment during the first month, when side effects may be at a maximum and before therapeutic effects are evident. Older patients should be monitored closely in the first 1–2 weeks of therapy to assess side effects and encourage continued therapy. They should have a minimum of 3 visits (in person or by telephone) during the first 12 weeks of antidepressant treatment.

Older patients must be informed that antidepressants usually take 4–6 weeks, but may take 8 weeks or longer, to have a full therapeutic effect and that only approximately 50% of patients respond to the first antidepressant prescribed. Patients who have not responded after an adequate trial of medication or who have had intolerable side effects may switch either to another medication within the same class (different SSRI) or to a different class of medications. When switching among SSRIs or between TCAs and SSRIs, no washout period is required (with the exception of switching from fluoxetine, because of its long half-life). However, abrupt cessation of shorter-acting antidepressants (eg, citalopram, paroxetine, sertraline, or venlafaxine) may result in a discontinuation syndrome with tinnitus, vertigo, or paresthesias. Referral for psychiatric consultation is recommended if a patient fails to respond to 2 different medication trials.

Once remission has been achieved, antidepressants should be continued for at least 6 months to reduce the risk of relapse. Patients who are at high risk of relapse (2 or more episodes of depression in the past or major depression lasting more than 2 years) should be continued on therapy for 2 years or possibly indefinitely. Many recommend lifelong therapy, even if it is the patient's first episode of major depression and especially if depression is severe and related to life changes that are not expected to improve. Follow-up visits should be arranged at 3–6-month intervals. If symptoms return, the medications should be adjusted or changed or the patient referred for psychiatric consultation.

If the patient and physician agree to a trial discontinuation of therapy, medications should be tapered over a 2–3-month period, with at least monthly follow-up by telephone or in person. If symptoms return, the patient should be restarted on medications for at least 3–6 months.

When patients fail to respond to adequate trials of 2 medications for major depression, a diagnosis of treatment-resistant depression is considered. One must review the case and consider that the original diagnosis may be inaccurate. What first appeared as depressive symptoms may be a manifestation of underlying anxiety or cognitive impairment. Apathy may be one of the first symptoms seen in dementia prior to more obvious cognitive symptoms. One must then verify that the patient actually received the medication that was prescribed. A simple investigation may reveal that the patient never filled the prescription or was never given medication by caregivers. Finally, one must ensure that the patient had adequate trials of medications (6–8 weeks) and that this trial was performed at a therapeutic dose.

Any patient who has had an adequate trial of 2 different medications without acceptable response should be referred to a psychiatrist for augmentation therapy. As shown from the federally funded Sequenced Treatment Alternatives to Relieve Depression (STAR*D) trial, the largest real-world study of treatment-resistant depression, patients with persistent depression have the potential to improve after several medication treatment trials; however, the odds of remission diminish as additional treatment strategies are needed. Lithium may be used in low doses in older adults with careful monitoring of side effects. Small doses of liothyronine (T_3) can be used safely in euthyroid patients. In addition, combinations of 2 antidepressant medications may be synergistic, with low doses of 1 antidepressant enhancing response to an antidepressant of another class.

2. Structured psychotherapy—Patients who have been referred to psychotherapy must still be monitored closely by their primary care clinicians because patients tend to discontinue therapy even more frequently than antidepressant treatments. The benefits of psychotherapy are generally evident by 6–8 weeks. The addition of pharmacotherapy should be considered for patients who have not fully responded to psychotherapy alone by 12 weeks. A combination of psychotherapy and pharmacotherapy may be more effective for moderate depression than either treatment alone.

▶ Prognosis

Depression is often a chronic or relapsing and remitting disease. Greater severity of depression, persistence of symptoms, and a higher number of prior episodes are the best predictors of recurrence. The lifetime risk of suicide in patients with major depression is 7% for men and 1% for women.

American Geriatrics Society 2012 Beers Criteria Update Expert Panel. American Geriatrics Society updated Beers Criteria for potentially inappropriate medication use in older adults. *J Am Geriatr Soc.* 2012;60(4):616-631.

American Psychiatric Association. *Diagnostic and Statistical Manual of Mental Disorders,* 4th ed. Washington, DC: American Psychiatric Association, 1994.

Hirschfeld RM, Keller MB, Panico S, et al. The National Depressive and Manic-Depressive Association consensus statement on the undertreatment of depression. *JAMA.* 1997;277(4):333-340.

Sable JA, Dunn LB, Zisook S. Late-life depression, How to identify its symptoms and provide effective treatment. *Geriatrics.* 2002;57(2):18-19, 22-23, 26 passim.

Whooley MA: Diagnosis and treatment of depression in adults with comorbid medical conditions: a 52-year-old man with depression. *JAMA.* 2012;307(17):1848-1857.

Whooley MA, Simon GE. Management depression in medical outpatients. *N Engl J Med.* 2000;343(26):1942-1950.

Wilson K, Mottram P, Sivanranthan A, Nightingale A. Antidepressants versus placebo for the depressed elderly. *Cochrane Database Syst Rev.* 2001;(2):CD000561.

SUICIDE

Many depressed elders contemplate suicide. Primary care providers must recognize the risk factors for suicide in patients with major depression: older age; male gender; being single, divorced, or separated and without children; personal or family history of a suicide attempt; drug or alcohol abuse; severe anxiety or stress; physical illness; and a specific suicide plan with access to firearms or other lethal means. Providers

should ask patients whether they ever think of hurting themselves or taking their life. If the patient responds positively, physicians should ask whether they have a plan and, if so, what it is. Asking patients about stockpiled medications or weapons in their home is also critical in assessing the suicide risk. If medications and weapons are present and cannot be removed from the patient's home, consider adding "weapon at home" to the problem list to highlight potential suicide risk. Actively suicidal patients with intent and plan require emergent psychiatric evaluation either through emergency departments or local psychiatric crisis units.

BIPOLAR DISORDER

 ESSENTIALS OF DIAGNOSIS

▶ History of manic episode: grandiosity, decreased need for sleep, pressured speech, racing thoughts, distractibility, increased activity, excessive spending, hypersexuality.

▶ May be associated with psychosis.

▶ Depressive episodes may alternate with mania.

▶ Mania may present for the first time in elderly patients, usually in those with a history of depressive episodes.

▶ General Principles in Older Adults

Bipolar disorder is a less-common diagnosis in older adults, with an overall low prevalence of <1% in community-dwelling elders, but a 10% rate in some nursing home populations. Many patients with bipolar disease require special considerations as they age because of comorbid conditions and diminished ability to tolerate psychiatric medications. Late-onset mania is often secondary to underlying medical conditions and is frequently associated with neurologic abnormalities such as cerebrovascular accident and cognitive impairment. Older patients with bipolar disorder have an increased 10-year mortality rate compared with those who have depression alone (70% vs. 30%).

▶ Differential Diagnosis

Bipolar disorder is diagnosed when a patient meets criteria for a manic episode. A manic episode is defined as a distinct period of abnormally and persistently elevated, expansive, or irritable mood and abnormally and persistently increased goal-directed activity or energy, lasting at least 1 week and with ≥3 of the following symptoms: inflated self-esteem or grandiosity, decreased need for sleep, pressured speech, racing thoughts, distractibility, increase in goal-directed activity or psychomotor agitation, and excessive involvement in pleasurable activities that have a high potential for painful consequences. Although major depressive episodes are common in bipolar disorder, they are not required for the diagnosis. The presence of mania is key to the differentiation between depressive disorder and bipolar disorder.

A variety of conditions may mimic a manic episode. Patients with dementia, particularly frontotemporal dementia, may be disinhibited and hypersexual. Brain tumors, cerebrovascular accidents, and partial-complex seizures may also lead to bizarre, disinhibited behaviors. Older patients who are prone to delirium can have waxing and waning levels of consciousness with some periods of hyperarousal. In addition, some medications may have unexpected effects in older patients. Glucocorticoids, thyroxine, and methylphenidate may lead to acute mania. Even sedative medications (eg, benzodiazepines) may have a paradoxical effect in older adults and lead to agitation. As in younger populations, substance intoxication or withdrawal from cocaine, alcohol, or amphetamines and endocrine disorders, such as hyperthyroidism or pheochromocytoma, can lead to symptoms consistent with mania.

▶ **Treatment**

Mood stabilizers have been the hallmark of treatment for bipolar disease. Valproic acid and carbamazepine are generally favored over lithium in older adults because of lithium's side effect profile and narrow toxic–therapeutic window (Table 45–2). Antipsychotic medication can be used in acute treatment of manic episodes associated with bipolar, maintenance treatment of bipolar, or when psychotic features are present. In general, the newer antipsychotic agents, such as olanzapine and risperidone, are better tolerated by older adults than the older neuroleptics with their extrapyramidal side effects and high risk of tardive dyskinesia, especially in women. Additionally, recent data have suggested typical antipsychotics, in particular Haldol, may have statistically significantly elevated mortality rates compared to atypical antipsychotics. Among the atypical antipsychotics, olanzapine, risperidone, quetiapine, ziprasidone, and asenapine are approved for acute treatment of mania and as adjunctive treatment with lithium or valproate. Only aripiprazole is approved as monotherapy for the maintenance treatment

of bipolar. Antidepressants are often used as an adjunct to mood stabilizers for patients with depression but should not be used alone because of the risk of transforming a depressive episode into a manic episode.

ANXIETY & STRESS DISORDERS

1. Panic Disorder

ESSENTIALS OF DIAGNOSIS

▶ Sudden, recurrent, unexpected panic attacks, characterized by palpitations, dizziness, sensation of dyspnea or choking.

▶ Attacks may include trembling, chest pain or discomfort, nausea, diaphoresis, paresthesias, and depersonalization.

▶ Sense of doom, fear of death.

▶ Persistent worry about future attacks.

▶ Can be accompanied by a fear of being in places where attack might occur (agoraphobia).

▶ **General Principles in Older Adults**

The lifetime prevalence rate of panic disorder is 1.5% to 2%, increasing to 4% in the primary care setting. The rate among community-dwelling elders is <1%. Depression is also present in 50% to 65% of patients with panic disorder; the suicide rate for these patients is 20% higher than that for depressed patients without panic disorder. Panic disorder may be associated with agoraphobia, which can be particularly disabling in older adults.

▶ **Differential Diagnosis**

A panic attack is defined as an abrupt surge of intense fear or discomfort with 4 or more of the following symptoms: palpitations; sweating; trembling or shaking; shortness of breath;

Table 45–2. Mood stabilizers.

Generic Name	Trade Name	Initial Dose	Target Dose	Comments
Lithium	Lithobid, Eskalith	300 mg QD or BID	600–1200 mg/day in divided doses BID or TID	Monitor drug levels, renal function, thyroid function; diuretics and ACE inhibitors increase levels; avoid dehydration and many NSAIDs because of toxicity
Carbamazepine	Tegretol	200 mg QD or BID	400–1000 mg/day	Monitor blood count, liver function tests, drug levels
Valproic acid	Depakote	250 mg QD or BID	500–1500 mg/day	Monitor blood count, liver function tests, drug levels

ACE, angiotensin-converting enzyme; NSAIDs, nonsteroidal antiinflammatory drugs.

choking sensation; chest pain or discomfort; nausea or abdominal distress; dizziness or unsteadiness; chills or heat sensations; numbness or tingling; derealization or depersonalization; fear of losing control; and fear of dying. *DSM-5* criteria for panic disorder include recurrent unexpected panic attacks, with at least 1 of the attacks having been followed by 1 month or more of either 1 or both of the following: persistent concern or worry about additional attacks or their consequences, or a significant maladaptive change in behavior related to the attacks.

Because the likelihood of physical disease is much higher than in younger populations, panic disorder is more difficult to distinguish from other life-threatening events in older patients. Acute coronary syndromes, cardiac arrhythmias, acute bronchospasm, and pulmonary embolism may lead to symptoms consistent with panic attacks. Endocrine disorders, particularly hyperthyroidism and pheochromocytoma, can mimic panic disorder. In acutely hospitalized patients, alcohol, caffeine, and tobacco withdrawal may present as agitation, worry, and other physical symptoms. Abrupt discontinuation of a short-acting antidepressant, anxiolytic, or opioid analgesic medication may also trigger panic symptoms. Older patients who suffer from panic disorder often have comorbid psychiatric diagnoses such as posttraumatic stress disorder (PTSD), generalized anxiety disorder, and depression.

Treatment

CBT has been proven effective for the treatment of panic disorder. Patients often go into a complete remission after as few as 12 weekly sessions. CBT is particularly helpful in preventing relapse and treating agoraphobia. Antidepressants, particularly SSRIs and TCAs, are helpful. Benzodiazepines may also be used as a brief adjunctive therapy while awaiting the clinical response to antidepressants or CBT. Whenever possible, long-term therapy with benzodiazepines should be avoided because of the potential risk of falls, cognitive impairment, and dependence.

Perhaps the most important aspect of treatment is education for the patient and family. Understanding the symptoms of panic disorder and developing ways of coping are essential for effective management of the disease.

2. Social & Specific Phobias

ESSENTIALS OF DIAGNOSIS

▶ A phobia is an irrational fear leading to intentional avoidance of a specific feared object, event, or situation.

▶ Exposure to this phobic object may result in symptoms similar to those of a panic attack.

▶ Patient is aware that his or her fear is irrational.

General Principles in Older Adults

The prevalence of phobias is 5% to 6% in older adults. Phobias present with features similar to panic disorder, but are triggered by a specific event. Late-onset phobias are often associated with a recent life event, such as a fall or injury. Social phobias affect 3% of older adults and can lead to increasing isolation. Simple phobias are thought to be more common than social phobias, affecting 5% to 12% of the general population.

Differential Diagnosis

Social phobia, also known as social anxiety disorder, is defined by *DSM-5* criteria as a marked and persistent fear or anxiety about social situations, exposure to which almost always provokes these feelings. The patient fears that the patient's response to the social situation will be negatively evaluated, and either avoids the situation or endures it with great anxiety. The avoidance, fear, or anxiety associated with the situation is disproportionate to any actual posed threat, and interferes with the patient's occupation or relationships. Specific phobia is a fear or anxiety about certain objects or situations that is disproportionate to the actual danger posed by such, and may lead to impairment in a patient's ability to function normally.

In older adults, new phobic symptoms may represent delusions associated with dementia or delirium. Patients with dementia or delirium are not typically aware of the irrational nature of their delusions in contrast to patients with phobia. Less-common causes of phobia include brain tumors or cerebrovascular accidents. The psychiatric differential diagnosis of phobia includes depression, schizophrenia, and schizoid and avoidant personality disorders. Social phobia and alcohol dependence often coexist; therefore, probing for alcohol use is an important part of the assessment. Although both phobic disorders and panic disorder may present with panic attacks, patients with phobias do not experience recurrent unexpected attacks; rather, their anxiety symptoms are always associated with a specific object or situation.

Treatment

The first-line therapy for specific phobias is behavioral therapy. Techniques may include relaxation therapy, cognitive restructuring, and systematic exposure to the feared object or situation. Use of antidepressants, particularly SSRIs, may be beneficial for generalized social phobia. Beta-adrenergic antagonists such as propranolol may also be effective treatments when administered before a foreseeable feared event or situation. Benzodiazepine use may be necessary but in general should be used with caution because of adverse effects on balance and cognition. Most patients are able to adapt or overcome their phobias and can lead relatively normal lives; if not, they should be referred for evaluation by a mental health specialist.

3. Generalized Anxiety Disorder

▶ Unrealistic or excessive worry about 2 or more life circumstances.

▶ Worry is recurrent and difficult to control.

▶ Physiologic symptoms of restlessness, fatigue, irritability, muscle tension, and sleep disturbance.

▶ General Principles in Older Adults

Anxiety symptoms are often a normal reaction to the surrounding environment. Anxiety disorders tend to begin in early adulthood and continue throughout a patient's lifetime with periods of relapses and remissions. The lifetime prevalence of generalized anxiety disorder is 5%; estimates in elders range from 2% to 7%. Anxiety may increase in older adults as a result of isolation, loss of independence, illness, disability, and bereavement.

▶ Differential Diagnosis

The diagnosis of generalized anxiety disorder is characterized by the following according to *DSM-5* criteria:

- Excessive anxiety and worry about a number of events or activities occurring more days than not for at least 6 months.
- Worry is difficult to control.
- Anxiety and worry are associated with at least 3 of the following: restlessness, easy fatigability, difficulty with concentration, irritability, muscle tension, sleep disturbance.

Diagnosing generalized anxiety in elders can be complicated because many underlying illnesses may have similar symptoms. The differential diagnosis for generalized anxiety disorder includes the physical illnesses discussed previously for panic disorder. In addition, chronic medication or substance use and subsequent withdrawal may lead to anxiety symptoms. Caffeine, nicotine, and alcohol are common culprits. Older patients are much more sensitive to commonly used nonprescription medications such as pseudoephedrine, which may cause restlessness, anxiety, and confusion. Up to 54% of patients who suffer from generalized anxiety disorder have comorbid depression. Obsessive–compulsive disorder, somatoform disorder, and personality disorders may also present with symptoms of anxiety. Psychiatric consultation should be initiated if the diagnosis is in question.

▶ Treatment

CBT is one of the most effective treatments for generalized anxiety disorder. Relaxation techniques and biofeedback may also alleviate symptoms. Several antidepressants (paroxetine, extended-release venlafaxine) also have significant anxiolytic properties and may be effective for both anxiety and depression. When depression and anxiety occur together, one should treat the depression first; doing so may improve the symptoms of both disorders. Anxiolytic medications such as buspirone (5–30 mg twice daily) may be effective. Benzodiazepines should be used with caution in older adults because they can cause a paradoxical effect and may also lead to falls and cognitive impairment.

4. Posttraumatic Stress Disorder

▶ History of exposure to a traumatic event.

▶ Intrusive thoughts, nightmares, and flashbacks.

▶ Avoidance of thoughts, feelings, or situations associated with the trauma.

▶ Isolation, detachment from others, emotional numbness.

▶ Symptoms of arousal such as sleep disturbance, irritability, and hypervigilance.

▶ Frequently associated with depression and substance abuse.

▶ General Principles in Older Adults

PTSD is associated with a lifetime prevalence of 1.2% in women and 0.5% in men. Symptoms of PTSD may persist into older age. In addition, symptoms can remain hidden until an older age when patients have new experiences (deaths, medical illness, disability) that trigger memories of former events or lose the capacity to compensate for lifelong symptoms because of cognitive impairment or other medical illness. However, some studies have shown that increased age may actually protect against the development of PTSD. Other protective factors include marriage, social support, and higher socioeconomic status.

▶ Differential Diagnosis

Per *DSM-5* criteria, the patient has been exposed in 1 or more of the following ways to a traumatic event involving actual or threatened death, serious injury, or sexual violence.

Symptoms may be grouped into 3 categories and may persist for >1 month.

1. Intrusive symptoms with ≥1 of the following: recurrent and intrusive recollections, dreams, dissociative reactions (eg, flashbacks), distress at exposure to cues to the event, or marked physiologic reaction to such cues.

2. Avoidant symptoms with 1 or both of the following: avoiding memories, thoughts, or feelings associated with the trauma; avoiding external reminders (eg, people, places, activities) associated with the trauma.

3. Negative alterations in cognition and mood, with >2 of the following: inability to remember aspects of the trauma; exaggerated negative beliefs or expectations about oneself, others, or the world; distorted blaming of oneself or others; persistent negative emotions (eg, fear, anger, guilt, shame); diminished interest or participation in activities; feeling of detachment or estrangement; inability to experience positive emotions.

4. Arousal symptoms indicated by ≥2 of the following: irritability or outbursts of anger, reckless or self-destructive behavior, hypervigilance, exaggerated startle response, difficulty concentrating, or sleep disturbance.

Other anxiety disorders can present with symptoms of hyperarousal similar to those in patients with PTSD. Major depressive disorder and adjustment disorders can also present with numbing or avoidant symptoms. During a period of bereavement, patients can have visions or dreams about the deceased. Other psychotic disorders may be confused with PTSD, but patients with PTSD may also experience psychotic-like symptoms during severe episodes. Substance use or withdrawal may contribute to symptoms. Organic brain syndrome resulting from prior head injury may be associated with symptoms similar to those of PTSD; the presence of visual hallucinations is particularly suggestive of an organic cause. Patients with delirium may also appear hyperaroused or be prone to illusions. There is a high comorbidity of depression and alcohol abuse among patients with PTSD.

▶ Treatment

Antidepressants, particularly SSRIs and TCAs, are indicated for treatment of PTSD. Both individual and group CBTs are also effective in the treatments and may be used alone or in combination with pharmacological therapy. Antiadrenergic agents such as clonidine may be helpful for symptoms of increased arousal, although one must consider related side effects such as orthostasis. However, recent trials have demonstrated the tolerability and effectiveness of prazosin, an α_1-adrenergic receptor antagonist, particularly in managing nightmares associated with PTSD. Benzodiazepines can often worsen symptoms of PTSD and should be avoided. Antipsychotic medications are occasionally necessary for the treatment of associated psychotic symptoms (see Table 45–2); however, recent data put into question the clinical benefits of risperidone (a very widely prescribed second-generation antipsychotic for PTSD), particularly in light of its potential side-effect profile.

SCHIZOPHRENIA & PSYCHOTIC DISORDERS

ESSENTIALS OF DIAGNOSIS

▶ Loss of ego boundaries and gross impairment in reality testing.

▶ Prominent delusions or auditory or visual hallucinations.

▶ Flat or inappropriate affect.

▶ Disorganized speech, thought processes, or behavior.

▶ General Principles in Older Adults

Psychotic symptoms may be attributable to a longstanding psychotic illness that has persisted into older age, or may present for the first time in later life in association with underlying medical conditions, especially dementia. Estimates for schizophrenia in the older population range from 0.1% to 0.5%. The prevalence of other psychotic syndromes, such as paranoid ideation, is higher, estimated at 4% to 6% in the older population, and is frequently associated with dementia. Patients with Alzheimer disease have a particularly high incidence of psychosis; 50% manifest psychotic symptoms within 3 years of diagnosis.

▶ Differential Diagnosis

The diagnostic criteria for schizophrenia include ≥2 of the following characteristic symptoms present for at least 1 month: delusions, hallucinations, disorganized speech, grossly disorganized or catatonic behavior, or negative symptoms such as flattened affect. These symptoms must also be associated with dysfunction in such areas as work, relationships, or self-care. Patients commonly will not volunteer psychotic symptoms unless specifically asked by their provider after a trusting relationship has been established. If psychosis is suspected, it is important to ask patients and family members specifically about auditory and visual hallucinations, delusions, ideas of reference, and paranoid ideation. Visual hallucinations are associated more strongly with underlying organic cause.

Especially in older adults, new psychotic symptoms carry a vast and complicated differential. New-onset psychotic symptoms can be attributed to medications, changes in environment, organic causes, including dementia, or a combination of these factors. Because psychosis may be the presenting sign of dementia, any older patient with new-onset psychosis should have a thorough cognitive screen. Prominent visual hallucinations are one of the hallmarks of Lewy body dementia. Patients with Alzheimer disease frequently have fixed delusions regarding people stealing their possessions or marital infidelity. The dementia associated with Parkinson disease may include negative symptoms of schizophrenia, such as flat affect.

Other central nervous system diseases, such as brain tumors, partial seizures, multiple sclerosis, or cerebral systemic lupus erythematosus, can also cause psychotic symptoms. Patients with major depression or bipolar disorder may experience psychotic features. Infections, endocrinopathies (thyroid, diabetes, adrenal), and nutritional deficiencies (vitamin B_{12}, thiamine) may lead to psychosis. Finally, older patients can be especially sensitive to medications that trigger psychotic symptoms such as steroids or levodopa. Because of the large differential diagnosis, collateral information regarding the patient's baseline mental status, psychiatric history, and onset of symptoms is critical in the evaluation of psychotic symptoms.

▶ Treatment

A. Pharmacotherapy

Atypical antipsychotic agents, such as risperidone, olanzapine, quetiapine, ziprasidone, aripiprazole, are the mainstays of treatment for psychotic symptoms and are approved for use in schizophrenia and bipolar disease (Table 45–3). Because of their lower incidence of extrapyramidal side effects, these agents are much better tolerated than the older antipsychotic agents, such as haloperidol and trifluoperazine. Recent data from multiple studies highlight the increased all-cause mortality rates in seniors with use of antipsychotic medications particularly when used in patients with dementia. Unlike older neuroleptics, which mainly treat positive symptoms (eg, delusions, hallucinations), the newer agents effectively manage both positive and negative psychotic symptoms (eg, flat affect, social withdrawal). The main side effects of newer agents are sedation and dizziness. Patients may experience akathisia and parkinsonism (eg, stiffness and rigidity) and, with longer term use, tardive dyskinesias, although the risk of such side effects is lower than with high-potency traditional antipsychotic drugs. Risperidone has been associated with an increased incidence of strokes in patients with dementia. Unlike other newer agents, ziprasidone does not appear to cause weight gain and is useful in the treatment of obese patients. However, it is associated with QT prolongation and thus should be avoided in patients with underlying conduction disease and QT prolongation at baseline. Clozapine is often the treatment of choice for patients with severe resistant psychosis and those with disabling tardive dyskinesias. Clozapine, however, carries a 1% to 2% risk of agranulocytosis and, therefore, requires weekly blood monitoring. In addition, both clozapine and olanzapine have been associated with glucose dysregulation and thus should be used with caution in patients with diabetes mellitus. Quetiapine

Table 45–3. Commonly used antipsychotics.

Generic Name	Trade Name	Initial Dose (mg)	Target Dosage[a] (mg/day)	Available Routes of Administration
Older agents				
D₂-Antagonists—high potency[b]				
Haloperidol	Haldol	0.5	0.5-1	PO, IV, IM, depot
Newer agents:				
Serotonin dopamine receptor antagonists[c]				
Risperidone	Risperdal	0.5	1-1.5	PO, depot
Olanzapine	Zyprexa	2.5	2.5-5	PO, IM
Quetiapine	Seroquel	25	50-200	PO
Quetiapine XR	Seroquel XR	50	50-200	PO
Ziprasidone	Geodon	20 BID	80 BID	PO (with food), IM
Aripiprazole	Abilify	2.5	15	PO

[a]Target dose is the usually effective dose for organic psychosis or agitation in the elderly. Patients with formal thought disorder may require higher doses in consultation with a psychiatrist.
[b]Typical antipsychotics carry an increased risk, relative to atypical antipsychotics, of extrapyramidal side effects, including akathisia, bradykinesia, rigidity, and tardive dyskinesia.
[c]Atypical antipsychotics may increase glucose and cholesterol levels. Consider monitoring lipids and glucose post initiation of these medications.

is associated with an increase in cholesterol levels; lipid levels should be routinely monitored. Dosages of antipsychotics used in older patients with dementia or acute delirium tend to be lower than those required for management of other psychotic disorders and may be only necessary for short periods of time (see Table 45–3) as these medications now carry a FDA black-box warning for treatment of behavioral symptoms in older patients with dementia. (See Chapter 22, "Cognitive Impairment & Dementia," for further details on dementia and antipsychotics use.)

Neuroleptic malignant syndrome (NMS) is a life-threatening emergency associated with the use of neuroleptic agents. NMS is characterized by a distinctive clinical syndrome of mental status change, rigidity, fever, and autonomic instability, and is associated with elevated plasma creatine phosphokinase. Although NMS is most often seen with the typical high-potency neuroleptic agents (eg, haloperidol, fluphenazine), every class of neuroleptic agents has been implicated, including the low potency (eg, chlorpromazine) and the newer atypical antipsychotic drugs (eg, risperidone, olanzapine), as well as the antiemetic metoclopramide. NMS may even occur when dopaminergic drugs, such as levodopa, are abruptly reduced or discontinued. Developing from over a few days to the first 2 weeks of neuroleptic therapy, this syndrome should be suspected when any 2 of the 4 following cardinal clinical features occur in the setting of neuroleptic use: mental status change, rigidity, fever, or autonomic instability. When there is any suspicion of NMS, neuroleptic agents should be withheld and patients should have close inpatient monitoring of clinical signs and laboratory values.

To decrease inappropriate use of psychotropic medications and improve the quality of care in long-term care facilities, the Health Care Finance Administration's 1987 Omnibus Reconciliation Act (OBRA) outlined indications and prescribing guidelines for psychoactive medications used in the treatment of psychotic disorders and agitated behaviors associated with organic brain disorders. OBRA requires documentation of response in terms of specific target symptoms and careful monitoring of side effects. To avoid long-term side effects such as tardive dyskinesia, OBRA also recommends trial dose reductions of neuroleptics unless clinically contraindicated because of severity of symptoms.

B. Behavioral Therapy

Behavioral therapy may be effective for the management of psychosis and after the acute episode has resolved. Providing a stable living environment is critical to the successful treatment of psychosis. Medical compliance is difficult without close supervision by a family or staff member. Adult day facilities provide structured programs for patients and give critical respite to caregivers, thus allowing patients to remain in the community longer than they would otherwise be able to without nursing home care.

American Psychiatric Association. *Diagnostic and Statistical Manual of Mental Disorders.* 5th ed: DSM-5. Washington, DC: American Psychiatric Association; 2013.

Dada F, Sethi S, Grossberg GT. Generalized anxiety disorder in the elderly. *Psychiatr Clin North Am.* 2001;24(1):155-164.

Howard R, Rabins PV, Seeman MV, Jeste DV. Late-onset schizophrenia and very-late-onset schizophrenia-like psychosis: an international consensus. *Am J Psychiatry.* 2000;157(2):172-178.

Lang AJ, Stein MB. Anxiety disorders: how to recognize and treat the medical symptoms of emotional illness. *Geriatrics.* 2001;56(5):24-27, 31-34.

Targum SD, Abbott JL. Psychoses in the elderly: a spectrum of disorders. *J Clin Psychiatry.* 1999;60 Suppl 8:4-10.

Weintraub D, Ruskin PE. Posttraumatic stress disorder in the elderly: a review. *Harv Rev Psychiatry.* 1999;7(3):144-153.

Whooley MA, Simon GE. Managing depression in medical outpatients. *N Engl J Med.* 2000;343(26):1942-1950.

Young RC. Bipolar mood disorders in the elderly. *Psychiatr Clin North Am.* 1997;20(1):121-136.

USEFUL WEBSITES

Agency for Healthcare Research and Quality. AHCPR supported guidelines" for Diagnosis and Treatment of Depression in Primary Care. http://www.ahrq.gov/professionals/clinicians-providers/guidelines-recommendations/archive.html

American Association for Geriatric Psychiatry. http://www.aagponline.org

American Medical Association. http://www.ama-assn.org/ama/pub/physician-resources/public-health/promoting-healthy-lifestyles/geriatric-health.page?

Depression and Bipolar Support Alliance. http://www.dbsalliance.org/site/PageServer?pagename=home

Depression Awareness, Recognition, and Treatment (DART) program of the National Institute of Mental Health. http://www.nimh.nih.gov/health/topics/depression/index.shtml

Geriatric Mental Health Foundation. http://www.gmhfonline.org/gmhf

International Foundation for Research and Education on Depression (iFred). http://www.ifred.org

National Alliance of Mental Illness. http://www.nami.org/

National Center for PTSD. http://www.ptsd.va.gov/

National Mental Health Association (Campaign on Clinical Depression). http://www.mentalhealthamerica.net/go/depression

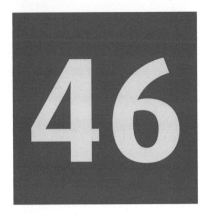

Sexual Health & Dysfunction

Angela Gentili, MD
Michael Godschalk, MD

ESSENTIALS OF DIAGNOSIS

▶ Sexual dysfunction is common among older men and women, and is caused by a combination of physiologic changes, lifestyle choices, psychological factors, and aging-related disease.

▶ In older men, the most common type of sexual dysfunction is erectile dysfunction, and the most common etiology is vascular disease.

▶ In older women, sexual dysfunction is often multifactorial, including lack of estrogen causing vaginal dryness and lack of testosterone decreasing libido.

▶ Evaluation of sexual dysfunction consists of a complete sexual history, review of medications, a targeted physical exam and selected laboratory tests in men.

▶ General Principles in Older Adults

Although older men and women are still interested in sex, sexual activity declines with age. In the Massachusetts Male Aging Study, more than 60% of men age 70 years reported erectile dysfunction and in the Rancho Bernardo Study, 32% of women age 65 years or older reported sexual activity in the previous 4 weeks but only 13% of women age 80 years or older reported being sexually active. This decrease in sexual activity may negatively impact quality of life. Fortunately, there are effective treatments for sexual dysfunction in men and women.

In men, age-related physiologic changes impact sexual function. Alterations in the pituitary–hypothalamic–gonadal axis may result in hypogonadism and decreased libido. Changes in penile innervation make it more difficult to achieve an erection, increase the time it takes to have an orgasm, and prolong the refractory period (the time it takes to have an erection after ejaculation). The increased time to

ejaculate may actually improve sexual function in men who are premature ejaculators.

In women, the 4 phases of sexual response (excitement, plateau, orgasm, and resolution) change with aging. During the excitement phase, there is decreased genital engorgement. Vaginal lubrication is decreased and the woman may need longer foreplay and gentle stimulation to achieve sufficient lubrication for intercourse. During the plateau phase, there is less expansion and vasocongestion of the vagina. During orgasm, there are fewer and weaker contractions, although older women can still achieve multiple orgasms. During the resolution phase, vasocongestion is lost more rapidly. As in younger women, the 4 phases may vary in sequence, overlap, or some may be absent. For example, desire does not always precede arousal. An older woman may engage in sexual activity not out of desire for sex but out of desire for closeness with her partner. If the stimulation is appropriate and she stays focused, her arousal and sexual desire intensifies. A positive experience increases her motivation for future encounters whereas a negative one (eg, from dyspareunia) may decrease her interest in sex.

In addition to the physiologic changes that occur with aging, lifestyle choices, psychological factors, and aging-related diseases and their treatment may affect sexual function in both men and women.

▶ Prevention

A. Men

The most common cause of sexual dysfunction in older men is erectile dysfunction (ED). The National Institutes of Health (NIH) defines ED as the consistent inability to achieve and/or maintain an erection sufficient for satisfactory sexual activity. As noted above, more than 60% of men age 70 years are unable to achieve a rigid erection. ED is the most common chronic disease in men, and vascular disease is the most common cause of ED.

Risk factors for vascular disease include lack of exercise, diabetes mellitus, hyperlipidemia, hypertension, and smoking. In many cases, these diseases are preventable by dietary and lifestyle changes. Because of the correlation between ED and vascular disease, ED is a marker for future vascular events, such as myocardial infarction and stroke. However, ED may be a more powerful predictor of cardiovascular disease in men younger than 60 years of age and in patients with diabetes.

Diabetes mellitus (DM) has the greatest impact on sexual function in men. The risk of ED in DM is directly related to the duration of diabetes, the A1c level, and increasing age. Early aggressive control of DM may prevent ED or delay its onset.

The second most common causes of ED are neurogenic. The autonomic dysfunction seen in DM and Parkinson disease prevents penile vasodilatation and erection. DM may cause both vascular and neurogenic ED. Neurogenic ED is frequently seen after prostatectomy or radiation therapy for prostate cancer. Nerve sparing surgery reduces this risk.

Another common cause of ED is medications. Anticholinergics, such as antipsychotics and oxybutynin, block parasympathetic-mediated vasodilatation. Antihypertensives, including beta blockers and thiazides, also increase the risk of ED. Angiotensin-converting enzyme inhibitors and calcium channel blockers do not have an adverse impact on erections.

Psychogenic ED is the least-common etiology. Patients with psychogenic ED usually describe the sudden onset of ED related to an event in their lives (argument with their partner, losing a job, etc). Of note, patients with ED caused by a nonpsychogenic etiology may have anxiety and/or depression because of the ED.

Testosterone's role in ED is controversial. Low testosterone is associated with decreased libido, but hypogonadal men can still achieve an erection and most men with ED have normal testosterone levels. Studies in animals suggest that testosterone is needed for a rigid erection. Studies also show that testosterone replacement in hypogonadal men improves their response to phosphodiesterase type 5 inhibitors.

Premature ejaculation (PE) occurs in approximately 30% of men. These patients are also referred to as "rapid ejaculators." PE is defined as orgasm with minimal stimulation. The most common cause is neurophysiologic. PE may also be psychogenic. Most PE is chronic. Patients with acute onset of PE may have a prostate infection (prostatitis). As men age, PE becomes less of a problem because of changes in penile innervation resulting in decreased penile sensation.

Retrograde ejaculation is a common complaint in men who have DM or have undergone transurethral prostatic resection. In both cases, the proximal sphincter does not close during ejaculation and semen goes into the bladder.

Orgasmic failure is uncommon in men. When it does occur, it may be a result of nerve damage (prostate cancer, radical prostatectomy, or DM) or may be medication-induced (gabapentin). With the exception of stopping gabapentin, treatment is usually unsuccessful.

B. Women

A decrease in estrogen levels with menopause can have a negative effect on sexuality by causing vaginal dryness. The normal vaginal pH is 3.5–4.5; after menopause it increases up to 7.0–7.39. A pH higher than 5 increases the risk of urogenital atrophy and bladder infections.

Women with poor self-reported physical health and women with diabetes are less likely to be sexually active than healthy older women.

These sexual difficulties constitute a "dysfunction" only if they cause significant distress to the woman, so if lack of interest in sex does not bother the woman, she cannot be diagnosed as having sexual dysfunction. Female sexual dysfunction is classified depending on whether the main problem is in one of these 4 areas: arousal, orgasm, desire, or pain.

Like in men, libido in women is thought to be dependent on testosterone. Estrogen replacement can improve vulvovaginal atrophy symptoms, but it has little effect on libido or sexual satisfaction. The ovaries and adrenals are the main sources of androgens in women. The effects of lack of testosterone in women were originally identified in women treated for advanced breast cancer with oophorectomy and adrenalectomy. When deprived of androgens, these women reported loss of libido. As there are no normative data on plasma total and free testosterone in women and there is no well-defined clinical syndrome of androgen deficiency, the Endocrine Society does not recommend making a diagnosis of androgen deficiency in women.

In older women, the etiology of sexual dysfunction depends on whether the patient presents with decreased desire, decreased lubrication, delayed or absent orgasm, or pain with intercourse (Table 46–1), but often the cause is multifactorial. For example, the patient may have decreased desire because of poor health and medication side effects and at the same time have painful intercourse.

Painful intercourse or "dyspareunia" can be caused by psychological or organic factors or a combination thereof. The most common cause of dyspareunia is vaginal atrophy caused by postmenopausal estrogen deficiency. The fear of experiencing pain may perpetuate the dyspareunia as it limits the woman's ability to become aroused and have adequate lubrication. Other causes of dyspareunia include lack of lubrication, vaginismus, localized vaginal infections, cystitis, Bartholin cyst, or even poor male technique. Pain can occur from pelvic thrusting and can be attributable to the woman's position during intercourse, retroverted uterus, postoperative adhesions, pelvic tumors, endometriosis, pelvic inflammatory disease, ovarian cysts, or urinary tract infections.

▶ Clinical Findings

A. Symptoms & Signs

1. Men—The evaluation of sexual dysfunction in men includes taking a good sexual history, physical exam, and a

Table 46–1. Treatment options for sexual dysfunction in older women.

Symptom	Common Causes	Therapy
Decreased desire	Low testosterone from natural or surgical menopause Chronic illness Depression Relationship problems Medications	Testosterone patch[OL] is not FDA approved in women Treatment of underlying illness Antidepressant medication Marital therapy Review of drugs ingested
Decreased lubrication	Vaginal dryness or atrophy from postmenopausal status Anticholinergic medications	Longer foreplay, regular intercourse, lubricants, topical estrogens Review of medications, including OTC drugs
Delayed or absent orgasm	Neurologic disorders, diabetes Psychologic problems	Treatment of underlying illness Cognitive-behavioral therapy, masturbation, Kegel exercises
Pain with intercourse	Organic cause Vaginal dryness, atrophy Vaginismus (involuntary vaginal contractions)	Treatment of underlying physical condition Longer foreplay, regular intercourse, lubricants, topical estrogens Psychotherapy, cognitive-behavioral therapy

OL, Off Label; OTC, over-the-counter.

Reproduced with permission from *Geriatrics Review Syllabus: A Core Curriculum in Geriatric Medicine*, 7th ed., American Geriatrics Society, 2010.

few lab tests. Patients may be reluctant to talk about their sexual function and the International Index of Erectile Dysfunction (IIEF-5) can be used to start this discussion. The IIEF-5 is self-administered and consists of 5 questions about sexual function during the past month. The IIEF-5 can be given to male patients to complete before the visit.

Obtaining a thorough history is the most important part of the evaluation of sexual dysfunction. The first step is to determine the specific nature of the problem. Does the patient have decreased libido, difficulty obtaining and/or maintaining an erection, PE, retrograde ejaculation, or anorgasmia?

The patient should be then asked about the onset (gradual vs. sudden) of the problem, the presence or absence of sleep-associated erections, and about any treatments that he has tried (both prescription and nonprescription). In men with ED, the onset and presence or absence of sleep-associated erections (SAEs) can help distinguish between psychogenic, medication-induced, and organic ED. Patients with psychogenic ED will describe a sudden onset but will still have SAEs. Men with medication-induced ED will also report a sudden onset, but will deny having SAEs. Finally, patients with organic ED will have a gradual onset and absent SAEs.

The physical exam targets signs of hypogonadism, vascular, and neurologic disease. Signs of hypogonadism include gynecomastia, decreased body hair, scant pubic hair or a female escutcheon. The vascular exam involves checking for bruits and palpating pedal pulses. The neurologic exam includes rectal sphincter tone, bulbocavernosus reflex and deep tendon reflexes. During the rectal exam the prostate should be checked for nodules. Finally, the penis should be examined for plaques (Peyronie's disease).

2. Women—As for men, the most important part of the evaluation is a careful history but the older woman might be reluctant to talk about her sexual function. There are several

self-reported and interview-based screening tools, a simple screen comprises just 3 questions:

1. Are you sexually active?

2. Are there any problems?

3. Do you have pain with intercourse?

If the woman is not satisfied with her sexual life, further questioning is necessary to understand whether the problem is mainly with arousal, desire, orgasm, or pain or a combination of these areas. The woman should be asked about duration and consistency of the problem, quality of relationship and sexual communication between the couple, thoughts during sexual activity, amount and adequacy of vaginal lubrication, symptoms of depression and history of negative experiences, like rape, child abuse, or domestic violence.

The medical history is important as several chronic illnesses can cause sexual dysfunction: diabetes and other conditions that cause debility and poor function like rheumatic diseases, conditions that cause poor self-image like mastectomy, the presence of stoma, advanced pelvic organ prolapse, or incontinence. In 1 study, 22% of women with urinary incontinence feared that intercourse would cause urine loss.

The clinician should elicit a complete drug history as several drugs can contribute to sexual dysfunction, including selective serotonin-reuptake inhibitors, antipsychotics, antihypertensives, antiestrogens, antiandrogens, alcohol, and illicit/recreational drugs. Chronic use of opioids can affect sexual function by causing opioid-induced androgen deficiency. Anticholinergic drugs decrease normal vaginal lubrication.

In the older woman, the physical exam is directed by symptoms elicited during the history and is particularly important in older women who have not received regular medical care. A pelvic examination should be done if the patient complains of vaginal dryness and/or dyspareunia. The exam should also include blood pressure and peripheral pulses as vascular disease affects arousal, a musculoskeletal exam as rheumatologic disorders can cause pain and difficulty with sexual activity, thyroid exam as hypothyroidism can cause decreased desire or arousal, and screening for neuropathy as neurological disorders can cause decreased desire, arousal or anorgasmy.

B. Laboratory Findings

1. Men—The laboratory evaluation of men with sexual dysfunction should include a hemoglobin A1c, a lipid panel and total testosterone. Because of its diurnal secretory pattern, testosterone should be obtained between 8 AM and 10 AM. If the testosterone is low, it should be repeated and luteinizing hormone (LH) level obtained. If the testosterone is low and the LH is high, the problem is at the level of the testes. If the testosterone is low and LH is low or normal, the patient has a hypothalamic or pituitary disorder and will need further testing.

2. Women—Routine laboratory testing is not necessary to evaluate female sexual dysfunction. Testosterone levels do not correlate with sexual function. Prolactin and thyroid-stimulating hormone levels should be done only if the history or physical exam suggest possible abnormalities.

▶ Treatment

1. Men—The choice of treatment in men depends on the etiology of the sexual dysfunction. In men with psychogenic ED, discussion and reassurance are frequently effective. If the patient continues to have ED, referral to a sex therapist may be necessary.

In men with decreased libido who are hypogonadal, testosterone replacement therapy may improve their sex drive. Contraindications to testosterone treatment include a history of prostate or breast cancer, polycythemia, severe lower urinary tract symptoms, or obstructive sleep apnea.

Neurophysiologic PE is treated with medications that delay ejaculation. These include the serotonin reuptake inhibitors, alpha blockers, and topical anesthetics. If a patient has prostatitis, an antibiotic usually cures the PE. In men with psychogenic PE, psychotherapy may help.

Retrograde ejaculation is a benign condition. Reassurance is the main treatment. The patient should be reminded that even without visible ejaculate, impregnation is still possible (if his partner is fertile).

The most common cause of sexual dysfunction in men is ED. However, before treating ED clinicians need to determine if it is safe for the patient to engage in sexual intercourse. The person on top during intercourse expends the equivalent of the energy needed to climb 2 flights of stairs. If a patient is sedentary and has cardiac risk factors (hypertension, DM, hyperlipidemia, or tobacco use) and/or known cardiovascular disease, a cardiac evaluation including a stress test may be needed before starting treatment for ED.

In patients with drug-induced ED, if possible the offending drug should be discontinued or changed to another agent/ different drug class. For example, replace a beta-blocker with an erection-sparing agent, such as a calcium channel blocker. Of note, patients with drug-induced ED frequently have underlying vascular disease, now unmasked by the drug. If the ED is longstanding, patients may not see improvement in their erectile function with the change in agents.

However, in the majority of cases, ED is caused by vascular and/or neurologic disease. The only Food and Drug Administration (FDA)-approved treatments for ED are vacuum devices, phosphodiesterase type 5 inhibitors, intraurethral suppositories, and intracavernosal injection of a vasodilator (Table 46–2).

a. Vacuum constrictive device—The vacuum constrictive device (VCD) was patented in 1917! It works by having the patient insert his penis in a plastic tube that is connected to a pump. He then pumps the air out of the tube and the resultant vacuum pulls blood into the penis and makes it erect. A rubber ring is slipped off the tube onto the base of the penis. The ring traps the blood in the penis and thereby maintains the erection. Patients or their partners may be reluctant to try VCDs because they are mechanical and take the spontaneity out of sex. However, VCDs are successful in 70% to 80% of patients who try them. Men should be warned not to leave the ring on for more than 30 minutes because the rings act like a tourniquet. VCDs with a battery powered pump are available for patients who have arthritis or another condition that limits their ability to use a manual pump.

b. Phosphodiesterase type 5 inhibitors—When a man becomes aroused, there is stimulation of the penile nerve that results in the activation of nitric oxide synthase. Nitric oxide synthase catalyzes the production of nitric oxide from L-arginine. Nitric oxide diffuses into penile smooth muscle cells and activates guanyl cyclase which produces cyclic guanosine monophosphate (cGMP). cGMP relaxes smooth muscle resulting in vasodilatation and erection. cGMP is metabolized by phosphodiesterase type 5 (PDE5). PDE5 inhibitors prevent the breakdown of cGMP thereby increasing vasodilation and erection.

There are 4 FDA-approved PDE5 inhibitors in the United States: avanafil (Stendra®), sildenafil (Viagra®), tadalafil (Cialis®), and vardenafil (Levitra®). Avanafil, sildenafil and vardenafil are taken "on demand." Tadalafil has both "on demand" and daily dosing. With the exception of the daily tadalafil, these medications are taken at least 30 minutes before initiation of sexual activity. The starting doses are 100 mg for avanafil, 25 mg for sildenafil, 10 mg for tadalafil, and 5 mg for vardenafil. The starting daily dose of tadalafil is 2.5 mg.

Table 46–2. Nonsurgical treatment for ED.

Treatment	Route	Dosage	Cost/Dose	Common Adverse Effects	Serious Adverse Effects
Vacuum Devices	EXT	—	$100	Penis cool to touch Ring may cause vaginal irritation	Ring left on for >30 minutes may cause penile ischemia Do not use in patients with sickle cell anemia
Sildenafil	PO	25–100 mg	$21	Erythema, flushing, indigestion, headache, insomnia, visual disturbance, epistaxis, nasal congestion, rhinitis	MI, sickle cell anemia with vasoocclusive crisis, nonarteritic ischemic optic neuropathy, sudden hearing loss, priapism
Vardenafil	PO	5–20 mg	$16–$19	Flushing, dizziness, headache, rhinitis	Chest pain, MI, prolonged QT interval, seizure, nonarteritic ischemic optic neuropathy, sudden hearing loss, priapism
Tadalafil	PO	5–20 mg	$5–$22	Flushing, indigestion, nausea, backache, myalgia, headache, nasopharyngitis	Angina, Stevens-Johnson syndrome, CVA, seizure, nonarteritic ischemic optic neuropathy, sudden hearing loss
Avanafil	PO	50–200 mg	Unavailable	Flushing, backache, headache, nasal congestion, nasopharyngitis	Priapism, nonarteritic ischemic optic neuropathy, sudden hearing loss
Alprostadil	TU	125–1000 mcg	$52–$60	Urethral discomfort, pain in penis, pain in testicle	Priapism
Alprostadil	ICI	1.25–60 mcg	$50–$65	Pain in penis, pain in testicle, fibrosis of penis	Priapism

CVA, cardiovascular accident; EXT, external; ICI, intracavernosal; MI, myocardial infarction; PO, oral; TU, transurethral.

Cost data for medications from Epocrates®; cost data for vacuum devices from Internet; drug adverse events from MicroMedex®.

Side effects are usually mild and related to smooth muscle relaxation. They include headache, flushing, esophageal reflux and rhinitis. Sildenafil may cause "blue haze," a transient disturbance in color vision, because of its effect on retinal PDE6. Tadalafil may cause muscle aches and back pain from its effect on PDE11. Vision loss, from nonarteritic anterior ischemic optic neuropathy, and sudden hearing loss have been reported in a small number of men taking PDE5 inhibitors. The relationship between these events and PDE5 inhibitors is unclear. However, patients should be warned to stop taking PDE5 inhibitors and seek immediate medical attention for sudden decreases or loss of vision or hearing.

Because of their mechanism of action, PDE5 inhibitors potentiate the effects of nitrates and may cause profound hypotension and death. Use of PDE5 inhibitors with any form of nitrates is contraindicated. Also, because PDE5 inhibitors are vasodilators, they may augment the hypotensive effects of antihypertensives. Patients should be warned about possible orthostatic symptoms. Doses of PDE5 inhibitors should be decreased in patients with significant liver or kidney disease, or in men taking P450 inhibitors.

There are many oral, nonprescription, non-FDA approved treatments for ED. Yohimbine is one of the most commonly used nonprescription treatments for ED. It blocks presynaptic α_2 receptors and may improve libido and increase blood flow into the penis. Based on reports from the authors' patients, yohimbine is not an effective treatment of ED.

If patients fail VCDs and PDE5 inhibitors, the next step may be transurethral alprostadil (Medicated Urethral System for Erection or MUSE®). Alprostadil (prostaglandin E$_1$) increases cyclic adenosine monophosphate, resulting in vasodilatation and erection. Alprostadil can be given as an intraurethral pellet or by penile injection. The pellet is inserted into the urethra using a plastic applicator. It dissolves and is absorbed into the surrounding tissue producing an erection. It works in approximately 50% of older patients. Side effects include urethral burning, prolonged erections (priapism), and hypotension.

Alprostadil (Caverject® or Edex®) given as an intracavernosal injection (ICI) is a very effective treatment for ED. Unfortunately, it is the least-popular treatment because it requires an injection into the penis each time the patient wants to have intercourse. Penile pain, priapism, and penile fibrosis (Peyronie disease) are some of the side effects seen with ICI.

2. Women—The first step is to assess goals and establish reasonable expectations. Medical conditions that contribute to sexual dysfunction should be addressed and medications reviewed to minimize sexual side effects.

Dyspareunia from atrophic vaginitis and decreased lubrication responds well to low-dose topical estrogen therapy (Table 46–3). The absorption of vaginal estrogen creams depends on the dose. In 2008, the FDA approved a low-dose

Table 46–3. Low-dose topical estrogens with minimal systemic absorption.

Estrogen	Dose	Comment
Cream: Conjugated estrogen (Premarin® cream)	Continuous regimen: 0.5 g or ⅛ applicator (0.3 mg conjugated estrogen) twice weekly	Low dose approved by the FDA in 2008 for moderate-to-severe dyspareunia
Tablet: Estradiol tablet 10 mcg (Vagifem®)	10 mcg daily × 2 weeks then twice weekly	10 mcg tablet replaced the 25-mcg tablet in 2010
Ring: Estradiol ring 2 g (Estring®)	7.5 mcg/24 h over 90 days	Often preferred by women for ease of use and comfort

conjugated estrogen cream regimen (0.3 mg twice weekly) as it does not cause significant proliferation of the endometrial lining. Vaginal estradiol rings or tablets deliver low-dose estrogen locally with low systemic absorption. In a Cochrane review, women favored the vaginal ring because of ease of use and comfort. According to the 2012 American Geriatrics Society Beers Criteria, low-dose vaginal estrogens are safe even in women with breast cancer, especially at dosages of estradiol <25 mcg twice weekly. Nonhormonal vaginal moisturizers with additional lubricants during intercourse are helpful for vaginal dryness, but they do not reverse the atrophic changes. Additionally, local stimulation through regular intercourse helps maintain a healthy vaginal mucosa. Longer foreplay allows more time for vaginal lubrication, just as older men often need longer and more direct stimulation to achieve an adequate erection.

Hypoactive sexual desire disorder with decreased libido may respond to a low-dose testosterone patch. Several randomized trials have demonstrated that low-dose testosterone patch improves sexual desire in women with decreased libido, taking systemic estrogen with or without progestin and either surgically induced or natural menopause. Androgenic side effects such as acne and hirsutism were uncommon and there was no decrease in high-density lipoprotein-cholesterol as seen in studies using oral methyltestosterone. More recently, it was demonstrated that the testosterone patch is also effective in women with natural or surgically induced menopause who have decreased libido and are not concurrent users of estrogens/progestin. The side-effect profile (hair growth) was acceptable to the women and did not make them discontinue the medication. Although testosterone patch seems effective, there is limited data on its long-term safety: 1 follow-up study demonstrated a good safety profile after 4 years of use in women taking estrogens (Nachtigall et al, 2011). A 300-mcg testosterone patch (Intrinsa®, Procter & Gamble Pharmaceutical) for postmenopausal women is available in Europe. In the United States, no testosterone formulation is FDA approved for women, pending more long-term safety data.

Treatment of urinary incontinence can improve sexual functioning, especially in patients with coital incontinence. If the coital incontinence is caused by detrusor overactivity, it

can be cured in approximately 60% of patients with an antimuscarinic agent.

As the cause of sexual dysfunction in the older woman is often multifactorial, a team approach may be the most helpful. The primary care provider addresses medical issues and medication review. Physical/occupational therapists can improve function in the older woman with limited mobility. A gynecologic referral may be needed if dyspareunia is not caused by genital atrophy or does not respond to topical estrogens. A sex therapist can educate the older couple about sexuality and changes with aging. A couples therapist can address conflicts or poor communication between the couple and if there is underlying depression, anxiety or substance abuse other mental health referrals may be appropriate.

American Geriatrics Society 2012 Beers Criteria Update Expert Panel. American Geriatrics Society updated Beers Criteria for potentially inappropriate medication use in older adults. *J Am Geriatr Soc.* 2012;60(4):616-631.

Bacon CG, Hu FB, Giovannucci E, Glasser DB, Mittleman MA, Rimm EB. Association of type and duration of diabetes with erectile dysfunction in a large cohort of men. *Diabetes Care.* 2002;25(8):1458-1463.

Bachmann G, Lobo RA, Gut R, Nachtigall L, Notelovitz M. Efficacy of low-dose estradiol vaginal tablets in the treatment of atrophic vaginitis: a randomized controlled trial. *Obstet Gynecol.* 2008;111(1):67-76.

Basson R. Women's sexual dysfunction: revised and expanded definitions. *CMAJ.* 2005;172(10):1327-1333.

Basson R. Clinical practice. Sexual desire and arousal disorders in women. *N Engl J Med.* 2006;354(14):1497-1506.

Carey JC. Pharmacological effects on sexual function. *Obstet Gynecol Clin North Am.* 2006;33(4):599-620.

Daniell HW. Opioid endocrinopathy in women consuming prescribed sustained-action opioids for control of nonmalignant pain. *J Pain.* 2008;9(1):28-36.

Davis SR, Davison SL, Donath S, Bell RJ. Circulating androgen levels and self-reported sexual function in women. *JAMA.* 2005;294(1):91-96.

Davis SR, Moreau M, Kroll R, et al; APHRODITE Study Team. Testosterone for low libido in postmenopausal women not taking estrogen. *N Engl J Med.* 2008;359(19):2005-2017.

Davis SR, Braunstein GD. Efficacy and safety of testosterone in the management of hypoactive sexual desire disorder in postmenopausal women. *J Sex Med.* 2012;9(4):1134-1148.

Feldman HA, Goldstein I, Hatzichristou DG, Krane RJ, McKinlay JB. Impotence and its medical and psychosocial correlates: Results of the Massachusetts Male Aging Study. *J Urol.* 1994;151(1):54-61.

Frank J, Mistretta P, Will J. Diagnosis and treatment of female sexual dysfunction. *Am Fam Physician.* 2008;77(5):635-642.

Gorkin L, Hvidsten K, Sobel RE, Siegel R. Sildenafil citrate use and the incidence of nonarteritic anterior ischemic optic neuropathy. *Int J Clin Pract.* 2006;60(4):500-503.

Graziottin A. The aging woman. *J Mens Health Gend.* 2006;3(4):326.

Guay AT. Testosterone and erectile physiology. *Aging Male.* 2006;9(4):201-206.

Impotence. *NIH Consensus Statement.* 1992;10(4):1-33.

Kaiser FE. Sexuality in the elderly. *Urol Clin North Am.* 1996;23(1):99-109.

Kammer-Doak D, Rogers RG. Female sexual function and dysfunction. *Obstet Gynecol Clin North Am.* 2008;35(2):169-183, vii.

Kaplan HS, Owett T. The female androgen deficiency syndrome. *J Sex Marital Ther.* 1993;19(1):3-24.

Krychman ML. Vaginal estrogens for the treatment of dyspareunia. *J Sex Med.* 2011;8(3):666-674.

Maggi M, Filippi S, Ledda, F. Erectile dysfunction: from biochemical pharmacology to advances in medical therapy. *Eur J Endocrinol.* 2000;143(2):143-154.

Masters WH, Johnson VE. Sex and the aging process. *J Am Geriatr Soc.* 1981;29(9):385-390.

Miner M, Seftel AD, Nehra A, et al. Prognostic utility of erectile dysfunction for cardiovascular disease in younger men and those with diabetes. *Am Heart J.* 2012;164(1):21-28.

Nachtigall L, Casson P, Lucas J, et al. Safety and tolerability of testosterone patch therapy for up to 4 years in surgically menopausal women receiving oral or transdermal oestrogen. *Gynecol Endocrinol.* 2011;27(1):39-48.

Penay N, Al-Azzawi F, Bouchard C, et al. Testosterone treatment of hypoactive sexual desire disorder (HSDD) in naturally menopausal women: the ADORE study. *Climateric.* 2010;13(2):121-131.

Plouffe L Jr. Screening for sexual problems through a simple questionnaire. *Am J Obstet Gynecol.* 1985;151(2):166-169.

Ratner ES, Erekson EA, Minkin MJ, Foran-Tuller KA. A special focus on women with gynecologic pathology. Sexual satisfaction in the elderly female population. *Maturitas.* 2011;70(3):210-215.

Rhoden EL, Ribeiro EP, Riedner CE, Teloken C, Souto CA. Glycosylated haemoglobin levels and the severity of erectile function in diabetic men. *BJU Int.* 2005;95(4):615-617.

Rosen RC, Barsky JL. Normal sexual response in women. *Obstet Gynecol Clin North Am.* 2006;33(4):515-526.

Rosen RC, Cappelleri JC, Smith MD, Lipsky J, Peña BM. Development and evaluation of an abridged 5-item version of the International Index of Erectile dysfunction (IIEF-5) as a diagnostic tool for erectile dysfunction. *Int J Impot Res.* 1999;11(6):319-326.

Sainz I, Amaya J, Garcia M. Erectile dysfunction in heart disease patients. *Int J Impot Res.* 2004;16(Suppl 2):S13-S17.

Serati M, Salvatore S, Uccella S, Nappi RE, Bolis P. Female urinary incontinence during intercourse: a review on an understudied problem for women's sexuality. *J Sex Med.* 2009;6(1):40-48.

Suckling J, Lethaby A, Kennedy R. Local estrogen for vaginal atrophy in postmenopausal women. *Cochrane Database Syst Rev.* 2006;4:CD001500.

Thompson IM, Tangen CM, Goodman PJ, Probstfield JL, Moinpour CM, Coltman CA. Erectile dysfunction and subsequent cardiovascular disease. *JAMA.* 2005;294(23):2996-3002.

Trompeter SE, Bettencourt R, Barrett-Connor E. Sexual activity and satisfaction in healthy community-dwelling older women. *Am J Med.* 2012;125(1):37-43.e1.

Weismiller DG. Menopause. *Prim Care.* 2009;36(1):199-226, x.

Wierman ME, Basson R, Davis SR, et al. Androgen therapy in women: an Endocrine Society Clinical Practice guideline. *J Clin Endocrinol Metab.* 2006;91(10):3697-3710.

Common Infections

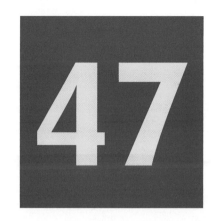

Lona Mody, MD, MSc
James Riddell IV, MD
Keith S. Kaye, MD, MPH
Teena Chopra, MD, MPH

ESSENTIALS OF DIAGNOSIS

► Diagnosing infections in older adults may be challenging because of atypical presentations and the frequent presence of cognitive impairment.

► Delirium, falls, or functional decline may be the presenting and, sometimes, only sign of an infection. Fever may be absent.

► Hospitalization and deaths as a consequence of pneumonia, influenza, and other respiratory tract infections are common.

► Urinary tract infection remains the most common overdiagnosed bacterial infection. Asymptomatic bacteriuria is common in older adults and requires no treatment.

► Optimal management of chronic disease, immunizations, prevention of pressure ulcers, attention to infection prevention practices, such as hand hygiene compliance, appropriate gown and glove use, oral hygiene and judicious antibiotic usage, are key preventive measures to reduce infections and enhance quality of care in older adults in skilled nursing facilities.

▷ General Principles in Older Adults

Infections remain a major cause of mortality and morbidity in older adults. With significant progress made in cancer management and cardiovascular diseases, deaths caused by infectious diseases appear to be rising. Pneumonia, influenza, and bacteremia are among the top 10 causes of death in older adults. Approximately 1.5–2.0 million infections occur in skilled nursing facilities per year, making their prevalence a major quality-of-care concern. Infections can lead to increased hospitalizations for this population, exposing them to nosocomial pathogens and resultant complications, such as functional disability, delirium, pressure ulcers, and adverse events. Common infections in older adults include urinary tract infections, upper and lower respiratory tract infections, gastroenteritis including *Clostridium difficile* diarrhea, skin and soft-tissue infections, including surgical site infections, and osteomyelitis. HIV/AIDS in aging populations will also be an emerging concern as those infected as younger adults now have an increasing life expectancy because of the effectiveness of antiretroviral therapy, and because the number of new infections in older adults is also on the rise.

▷ Pathogenesis

The risks of developing an infection, its severity, and the outcome from that infection depend on the relationship between the virulence of the pathogen, its inoculum, and the host's defense system. The ability of a pathogen to attach and replicate in a host environment determines its virulence. In aging adults, macrophage function is altered, mucocutaneous defenses are compromised, cytokine production is diminished, and T-cell function is suboptimal. Comorbid conditions, such as renal failure, diabetes, congestive heart failure, chronic lung diseases, and malnutrition, further exacerbate defense mechanisms. A paucity of presenting signs and symptoms leads to delayed recognition of infection, which can result in poor outcomes. Subtle changes in functional and cognitive decline are often early warning signs. Other presenting atypical symptoms include falls, loss of appetite, fatigue, and failure to thrive. Febrile response is often blunted, especially in frail older adults residing in long-term care facilities. As a result, the Practice Guidelines Committee of the Infectious Diseases of America recommends a clinical evaluation for residents in skilled nursing facilities with single oral temperature over 100°F (37.8°C), or persistent oral temperature of over 99°F (37.2°C). Two or

Table 47–1. Definition of fever.

Fever, defined as either:
1. A single oral temperature >100°F (37.8°C)
2. Repeated oral temperatures >99°F (37.2°C) or rectal temperatures >99.5°F (37.5°C)
3. An increase in temperature of >2°F (1.1°C) over the baseline temperature

more readings of greater than 2°F (1.1°C) over the baseline temperature should also prompt an evaluation by a physician (Table 47–1).

Principles of Antimicrobial Therapy

Similar to younger populations, the general principles of antimicrobial use in older adults include early and accurate diagnosis of infection, prompt decision to initiate broad-spectrum antibiotics, with equal attention to narrowing or discontinuation of antibiotics based on clinical progress, and identification of the implicating pathogens. In institutionalized older adults, infectious diseases often become a diagnosis of exclusion, leading to inappropriate antibiotic use. A paucity of clinical findings can pose a challenge to prompt initiation of an appropriate antibiotic regimen. Recent literature identifies the minimum criteria to initiate antibiotics, as well as surveillance definitions of infections in older long-term care residents (Table 47–2). Selection of a specific antimicrobial agent depends on the identification of the pathogen, known local susceptibility patterns, and pharmacokinetics and pharmacodynamics of antibiotics in older adults. Several physiologic changes, such as increased gastric emptying time, reduced gastric acidity, reduced lean body mass, increased fat, reduced albumin, reduced glomerular filtration, and/or reduced hepatic blood flow, can impact antibiotic dosing and response.

Prevention

Like cardiovascular disease and cancer, in infection, prevention is key. Administration of influenza vaccine to older adults as well as health care workers lowers infection rates, saves lives, and reduces complications. Recommended vaccinations in older adults include yearly influenza vaccine, pneumococcal vaccine once after age 65 years, zoster vaccine, and Tdap if there is anticipated contact with a child less than 12 months of age. Tdap can be replaced by Td if there is no anticipated contact. Optimal management of chronic diseases, prevention of pressure ulcers, attention to infection prevention practices, such as hand hygiene compliance, appropriate gown and glove use, and judicious antibiotic usage, are all additional preventive measures to reduce infections and enhance quality of care in older adults in skilled nursing facilities.

URINARY TRACT INFECTIONS

General Principles in Older Adults

Urinary tract infection (UTI) remains the most common and the most overdiagnosed bacterial infection in older adults. Asymptomatic bacteriuria is frequent in older adults, both in the community and in health care institutions. Prevalence of asymptomatic bacteriuria ranges from 2% to 10% in the community and can be as high as 40% to 50% in skilled nursing facilities. Bacteriuria is nearly universal after 30 days of urinary catheterization. Asymptomatic bacteriuria with a paucity of typical infectious symptoms creates a challenging diagnostic dilemma for clinicians and frequently leads to overprescription of antimicrobials, particularly among patients who have a fever and an indwelling urinary catheter.

The risk factors for UTIs include prostatic hypertrophy with retention, prior history of recurrent UTIs, loss of the protective effect of estrogen on bladder mucosa, functional disability, cognitive impairment, and presence of a urinary catheter. Approximately 5% to 10% of skilled nursing facility residents have a urinary catheter. It is estimated that 50% of these people will have symptomatic catheter-associated UTI. UTI is a frequent cause of bacteremia in both community-dwelling and institutionalized older adults.

Prevention

Indwelling urinary catheter removal when appropriate, adequate nutrition and hydration, and reducing functional disability can reduce the frequency and adverse consequences from UTIs. Whenever possible, indwelling urinary catheters should be discontinued. If absolutely indicated, indwelling urinary catheters can be replaced with a condom catheter or intermittent straight catheterization when appropriate. Chronic indwelling urinary catheters require diligent health care worker attention to maintain a closed drainage system, and to keep the drainage bag positioned below the level of the bladder. Hand hygiene compliance, as well as glove use during any catheter manipulation, are important components of infection prevention. Routine urinalysis, bladder irrigations or catheter changes are not useful in UTI prevention.

Independence in ambulation reduces the risk of hospitalization from a UTI in skilled nursing facility residents. Low-dose prophylactic antibiotics can be considered in women with more than 3 symptomatic UTIs a year and no other urologic abnormalities. The role of prophylactic antibiotics in institutionalized older adults remains unclear; however, there is no indication that prophylactic antibiotics are effective. Although oral estrogens have not been shown to be effective in reducing UTIs, vaginal estrogens may be effective in community-dwelling older adults with recurrent UTIs. Anecdotal evidence suggests that cranberry juice may be effective in reducing asymptomatic bacteriuria, but its effectiveness in reducing symptomatic UTIs needs to be established.

Table 47–2. McGeer's surveillance definitions and minimum criteria to initiate antibiotics.

	McGeer's Surveillance Criteria	Minimum Criteria
Urinary Tract Infections (UTI)		

A. For residents without an indwelling urinary catheter	A. Both criteria 1 and 2 must be present
	  1. At least 1 of the following sign or symptom subcriteria
	    a. Acute dysuria or acute pain, swelling, or tenderness of the testes, epididymis, or prostate
	    b. Fever or leukocytosis
	      i. Fever
	        1. Single oral temperature >37.8°C (100°F) *or*
	        2. Repeated oral temperatures >37.2°C (99°F) or rectal temperatures >37.5°C (99.5°F) *or*
	        3. Single temperature >1.1°C (2°F) over baseline from any site (oral, tympanic, axillary)
	      ii. Leukocytosis
	        1. Neutrophilia (>14,000 leukocytes/mm³) *or*
	        2. Left shift (>6% bands or ≥1,500 bands/mm³) *and*
	      iii. At least 1 of the following localizing urinary tract subcriteria
	        1. Acute costovertebral angle pain or tenderness
	        2. Suprapubic pain
	        3. Gross hematuria
	        4. New or marked increase in incontinence
	        5. New or marked increase in urgency
	        6. New or marked increase in frequency
	    c. In the absence of fever or leukocytosis, then 2 or more of the following localizing urinary tract subcriteria
	      i. Suprapubic pain
	      ii. Gross hematuria
	      iii. New or marked increase in incontinence
	      iv. New or marked increase in urgency
	      v. New or marked increase in frequency
	  2. One of the following microbiologic subcriteria
	    a. At least 105 cfu/mL of no more than 2 species of microorganisms in a voided urine sample
	    b. At least 102 cfu/mL of any number of organisms in a specimen collected by in-and-out catheter
		A. Must have:
		  1. Acute dysuria alone *or*
		  2. Fever (>37.9°C [100°F] (or a 1.5°C [2.4°F] increase over baseline temp) or chills
		  And at least one of the following:
		    a. New/increased urgency
		    b. Frequency
		    c. Suprapubic pain
		    d. Urinary incontinence

(continued)

Table 47–2. McGeer's surveillance definitions and minimum criteria to initiate antibiotics. (*continued*)

	McGeer's Surveillance Criteria	Minimum Criteria
B. For residents with indwelling urinary catheter	B. Both criteria 1 and 2 must be present 1. At least 1 of the following sign or symptom subcriteria 　a. Fever, rigors, or new-onset hypotension, with no alternate site of infection 　b. Either acute change in mental status or acute functional decline, with no alternate diagnosis and leukocytosis 　c. New-onset suprapubic pain or costovertebral angle pain or tenderness 　d. Purulent discharge from around the catheter or acute pain, swelling, or tenderness of the testes, epididymis, or prostate 2. Urinary catheter specimen culture with at least 10^5 cfu/mL of any organism(s)	B. Must have at least one of the following: 1. Fever (>37.9°C [100°F] or 1.5°C [2.4°F] increase above baseline 2. New costovertebral tenderness 3. Rigors (shaking chills) with or without an identified cause 4. New onset of delirium

Pneumonia (PNA)

	All 3 criteria must be present 1. Interpretation of a chest radiograph as demonstrating pneumonia or the presence of a new infiltrate 2. At least 1 of the following respiratory subcriteria 　a. New or increased cough 　b. New or increased sputum production 　c. O_2 saturation <94% on room air or a reduction in O_2 saturation of >3% from baseline 　d. New or changed lung examination abnormalities 　e. Pleuritic chest pain 　f. Respiratory rate of ≥25 breaths/min 3. At least 1 of the constitutional criteria 　a. Fever 　　i. Single oral temperature >37.8°C (100°F) *or* 　　ii. Repeated oral temperatures >37.2°C (99°F) or rectal temperatures >37.5°C (99.5°F) *or* 　　iii. Single temperature >1.1°C (2°F) over baseline from any site (oral, tympanic, axillary) 　b. Leukocytosis 　　i. Neutrophilia (>14,000 leukocytes/mm³) *or* 　　ii. Left shift (>6% bands or ≥1,500 bands/mm³) 　c. Acute change in mental status from baseline (all criteria must be present) 　　i. Acute onset 　　ii. Fluctuating course 　　iii. Inattention 　　iv. Either disorganized thinking or altered level of consciousness 　d. Acute functional decline: A new 3-point increase in total activities of daily living (ADL) score (range, 0–28) from baseline, based on the following 7 ADL items, each scored from 0 (independent) to 4 (total dependence) 　　i. Bed mobility 　　ii. Transfer 　　iii. Locomotion within LTCF 　　iv. Dressing 　　v. Toilet use 　　vi. Personal hygiene 　　vii. Eating	A. Febrile resident If resident has temp >38.9°C [102°F], must have at least one of the following: 1. Respiratory rate >25 breaths per minute 2. Productive cough If resident has temp >37.9°C [100°F] (or a 1.5°C [2.4°F] increase over baseline temp) but ≤38.9°C, must include presence of cough and at least one of the following: 1. Pulse >100 beats per minute 2. Delirium 3. Rigors (shaking chills) 4. Respiratory rate >25 breaths per minute B. Afebrile resident If afebrile resident has COPD, must include: 1. New/increased cough with purulent sputum production If afebrile resident does not have COPD, must have presence of new cough with purulent sputum production and at least one of the following: 1. Respiratory rate >25 breaths per minute 2. Delirium C. In the setting of new infiltrate on chest radiograph though to represent PNA, any one of the following constitute appropriate minimum criteria: 1. Respiratory rate >25 breaths per minute 2. Productive cough 3. Fever (>37.9°C [100°F] or 1.5°C [2.4°F] increase above baseline

(*continued*)

Table 47–2. McGeer's surveillance definitions and minimum criteria to initiate antibiotics. (*continued*)

	McGeer's Surveillance Criteria	Minimum Criteria
Skin and Soft Tissue Infections (SSTI)		

	At least 1 of the following criteria must be present
	1. Pus present at a wound, skin, or soft tissue site
	2. New or increasing presence of at least 4 of the following sign or symptom subcriteria
	  a. Heat at the affected site
	  b. Redness at the affected site
	  c. Swelling at the affected site
	  d. Tenderness or pain at the affected site
	  e. Serous drainage at the affected site
	  f. One constitutional criterion
	    i. Fever
	      1. Single oral temperature >37.8°C (>100°F) *or*
	      2. Repeated oral temperatures >37.2°C (99°F) or rectal temperatures >37.5°C (99.5°F) *or*
	      3. Single temperature >1.1°C (2°F) over baseline from any site (oral, tympanic, axillary)
	    ii. Leukocytosis
	      1. Neutrophilia (>14,000 leukocytes/mm³) *or*
	      2. Left shift (>6% bands or ≥1,500 bands/mm³)
	    iii. Acute change in mental status from baseline (all criteria must be present)
	      1. Acute onset
	      2. Fluctuating course
	      3. Inattention
	      4. Either disorganized thinking or altered level of consciousness
	    iv. Acute functional decline: A new 3-point increase in total activities of daily living (ADL) score (range, 0-28) from baseline, based on the following 7 ADL items, each scored from 0 (independent) to 4 (total dependence)
	      1. Bed mobility
	      2. Transfer
	      3. Locomotion within LTCF
	      4. Dressing
	      5. Toilet use
	      6. Personal hygiene
	      7. Eating
		Must have one of the following:
		1. New or increasing purulent drainage at a wound, skin or soft tissue site
		2. At least two of the following:
		  a. Fever (37.9°C [100°F] or 1.5°C [2.4°F] increase above baseline
		  Or new or increased at the affected site:
		  b. redness
		  c. tenderness
		  d. warmth
		  e. swelling

▶ Clinical Findings

Presenting findings of symptomatic UTIs among community-dwelling older adults include dysuria, increased urgency and frequency of urination, worsening of incontinence, hematuria, changed character of urine, and suprapubic discomfort. Pyelonephritis can present as fever, vomiting, and abdominal pain. A paucity of these signs and symptoms in older, frail, cognitively impaired skilled nursing facility residents is relatively common and poses a substantial and frequent clinical challenge. A change in the character of urine can be caused by either an infection or dehydration. Residents with cognitive impairment may not be able to communicate their symptoms. Fever can be infrequent. Despite these challenges, a careful history, physical examination, discussion with nursing and other ancillary staff, and rehydration can lead to reduced inappropriate antimicrobial usage in institutionalized older adults. Recent studies show that the triad of dysuria, change in character of urine, and recent mental status change is most predictive of a symptomatic UTI. Pyuria is usually present in the setting of both symptomatic and asymptomatic bacteriuria, hence pyuria alone cannot be diagnostic of UTI. A positive urine culture is usually required to accurately diagnose a symptomatic UTI. Although a positive culture alone is not adequate to define a symptomatic UTI, a negative culture in the setting of nonspecific findings can help to rule out UTI and reduce inappropriate antimicrobial use.

▶ Treatment

Treatment of asymptomatic bacteriuria is not recommended and may even be harmful. Asymptomatic bacteriuria should only be treated with antibiotics prior to genitourinary procedures or surgery so as to prevent sepsis and bacteremia. Treatment of symptomatic UTI requires appropriate antimicrobial therapy, attention to hydration, and efforts to reduce dysuria. Choice of antimicrobial agent usually depends on the organism isolated from urine cultures and local susceptibility patterns. Broad-spectrum antibiotics targeting Gram-negative organisms and enterococci may be required if the patient appears significantly ill. Oral empiric therapy with trimethoprim/sulfamethoxazole is appropriate for most community-dwelling older adults. Fluoroquinolones can be used in the setting of known or likely trimethoprim-sulfamethoxazole resistance, or if a patient is allergic to sulfa. A combination of beta-lactam/beta-lactamase inhibitors, third-generation cephalosporins, or quinolones is appropriate initial choices if sepsis is suspected. Skilled nursing facility residents with urinary catheters may require a broader spectrum antibiotic regimen to incorporate coverage for resistant Gram-positive organisms such as methicillin-resistant *Staphylococcus aureus* (MRSA). Once identification and susceptibility test results are available, appropriate antibiotics can be selected and the treatment period determined.

The duration of antimicrobial therapy usually depends on the risk group. Older community-dwelling women with uncomplicated UTIs can usually be effectively treated with a 3-day regimen of trimethoprim-sulfamethoxazole or a quinolone. Ten to 14 days of treatment is usually required for men with a UTI, and for women with more severe symptoms, such as fever or pyelonephritis. For a catheter-associated UTI, a prompt response may indicate that 7 days of therapy is adequate.

RESPIRATORY TRACT INFECTIONS

▶ General Principles in Older Adults

Hospitalization and deaths as a consequence of pneumonia, influenza, and other respiratory tract infections are common in older adults. Pneumonia in older adults can be community acquired, hospital acquired, or skilled nursing facility acquired. Rates of community-acquired pneumonia increase from 18.2 cases per 1000 person-years in those 65–69 years of age to 52.3 cases per 1000 person-years in those older than 85 years of age. Adults older than age 65 years bear a disproportionately higher brunt of influenza-associated deaths. Deaths among this age group also account for 90% of overall estimated average annual influenza-associated deaths with underlying respiratory and circulatory causes. Outbreaks of seasonal influenza are reported frequently, particularly in the skilled nursing facility setting.

Recent data suggest that pneumonia and respiratory tract infections surpass symptomatic UTIs as the most common infection among skilled nursing facility residents. These residents constitute 10% to 18% of all people hospitalized with pneumonia, corresponding to an average hospital cost of about $10,000 per admission. Aspiration pneumonia is common among this population and is often associated with oropharyngeal dysphagia and regurgitation of gastric contents. Dental plaque contains as many as 25,000 species of bacteria, many of which are likely capable of causing infections under the right conditions.

The risk factors for pneumonia include older age, male gender, history of aspiration, functional disability, history of smoking, chronic bronchitis or emphysema, heart disease, malignancy, neurologic conditions such as cerebrovascular diseases, recent surgery or intensive care unit stay, and presence of a feeding tube. With age, lung parenchyma loses its elastic recoil, there is reduced chest wall compliance, along with a loss of alveoli and alveolar ducts, all of which can increase the risk of pneumonia in the setting of functional disability and acute illness.

▶ Prevention

The prevention strategies for respiratory tract infections are largely driven by risk factors. Yearly influenza vaccination by older adults and health care workers, along with pneumococcal vaccination of older adults can reduce the incidence and complications related to respiratory tract infections in the older population. Daily oral hygiene measures in combination with regular dental care have been shown to reduce the risk associated with aspiration. A systematic review of randomized controlled studies shows that appropriate oral hygiene can prevent respiratory infections in both older hospitalized and skilled nursing facility residents. Smoking cessation can also reduce bronchitis and respiratory infections.

▶ Clinical Findings

Like most other infections, pneumonia in older adults manifests with atypical symptoms and signs such as fatigue, loss of appetite, functional decline, and new confusion. A quarter of this population with pneumonia may not mount a fever and is less likely to present with chills or pleuritic chest pain. Despite these limitations, an increased respiratory rate of greater than 25 breaths/min and hypoxia do portend poor prognosis and are useful tools for risk assessments. Clinical presentation should be confirmed rapidly with diagnostic testing, including chest radiographs, white cell count, and blood cultures. The yield from blood cultures may not be high, but if positive, may help drive appropriate antibiotic choice. Sputum studies are often not helpful or feasible in older adults.

The clinical presentation of influenza in older adults differs from younger adults with the older population having fewer respiratory symptoms. Cough, fever, and altered mental status predominate as presenting findings in older adults hospitalized with documented influenza. Older adults with influenza may have more gastrointestinal symptoms when compared with other respiratory viruses. Clinical presentation can be confirmed with diagnostic tests such as rapid antigen testing, viral cultures and serology, reverse-transcriptase polymerase chain reaction (PCR) testing, and immunologic assays. Rapid tests that can detect either influenza A or B or both are available and can detect influenza viruses within 30 minutes. The sensitivity and specificity of these tests increase when they are performed close to the illness onset.

▶ Treatment

Several risk indices can predict outcomes and particularly mortality in older adults. These include the pneumonia severity index (a 20-item 2-step system more applicable to younger adults), CURB (4 items: confusion, urea, respiratory rate, and blood pressure), and modified CURB65 (confusion, urea, respiratory rate, blood pressure, and age ≥65 years) from the British Thoracic Society (Table 47–3), and SOAR (systolic blood pressure, age ≥65 years, oxygenation, and respiratory rate). These scoring systems can assist in making treatment recommendations, particularly toward the end of life. These scoring systems can also help identify older adults who can potentially be treated as outpatients.

Table 47–3. CURB65: risk index to predict mortality from community-acquired pneumonia.

Symptom	Points
Confusion	1
Urea >7 mmol/L	1
Respiratory rate >30 breaths/min	1
Systolic blood pressure <90 mm Hg, diastolic blood pressure <60 mm Hg	1
Age ≥65 years	1
Total (30-day mortality risk)	0 (0.6%), 1 (3.2%), 2 (13%), 3 (17%), 4 (41.5%), 5 (57.5%)

Empiric therapy varies and depends on several host and environmental factors. For a community-dwelling older adult with no comorbidities, empiric treatment for community-acquired pneumonia includes a macrolide or doxycycline. For older adults with comorbidities such as chronic lung disease, chronic renal failure, diabetes, or immunosuppression, a respiratory quinolone or beta-lactum plus macrolide might be prudent. Older adults with skilled nursing facility-acquired pneumonia or nosocomial hospital-acquired pneumonia may require an initial parental antibiotic regimen such as pipercillin-tazobactam and vancomycin to cover for *Pseudomonas*, MRSA, and/or other nosocomial Gram-negative organisms. In choosing empiric antimicrobial therapy, local antimicrobial susceptibilities should be considered. Empiric therapy can be narrowed to target a specific pathogen once it has been identified.

GASTROINTESTINAL INFECTIONS

▶ General Principles in Older Adults

Gastrointestinal infections are fairly common in older adults. Deaths attributable to diarrheal diseases, like other infections, affect older adults disproportionately. Infection is generally by fecal–oral spread. Hypochlorhydria and achlorhydria, impaired gastric motility, inappropriate use of antibiotics, and waning immunity increase the predisposition to diarrheal illnesses in older adults. Viral gastroenteritis (caused by rotavirus, enteroviruses including Norwalk virus), bacterial gastroenteritis (caused by *C. difficile*, *Bacillus cereus*, *Escherichia coli*, *Campylobacter*, *Clostridium perfringens*, or *Salmonella*) and parasites are well-known causes of diarrhea in skilled nursing facilities.

▶ Prevention

Compliance with hand hygiene guidelines remains key in preventing diarrheal illnesses particularly *C. difficile*-associated diarrhea and viral gastroenteritis such as norovirus. Yet, hand hygiene compliance rates remain poor in all settings. The use of alcohol-based hand rub has increased hand hygiene rates; however, its effectiveness may be diminished in certain diarrheal illnesses, particularly *C. difficile* diarrhea. Inappropriate antibiotic use should be reduced whenever possible and may be considered as a quality improvement process measure.

▶ Clinical Findings

Patient history is often an initial guide to appropriate diagnostic evaluation. Information on food history and exposure, travel history, antimicrobial usage, use of immunosuppressive medications, frequency of diarrhea, tenesmus, and presence of blood and mucus in the stool should be obtained at the initial evaluation. History of exposure and symptoms in other family members or close contacts should be obtained as well. The physical exam should initially focus on the severity of the diarrheal illness including symptoms of dehydration, such as dry mucous membranes, fatigue, loss of appetite, change in mentation, reduced blood pressure, and tachycardia. An abdominal exam may be useful, although it can often be misleading because of a paucity of positive findings.

Treatment

Initial laboratory tests should include electrolytes and complete blood count. Stool studies for blood cells, stool culture, assessment for ova and parasites, and *C. difficile* toxin tests are clinically appropriate. Initial treatment should address dehydration and electrolyte disorders. If indicated, antimicrobials should be started promptly as well. In severe cases, vital signs should be closely monitored. Antimotility agents (loperamide, diphenoxylate) are frequently abused in older adults, and their use should be generally restricted.

Travelers' diarrhea is generally self-limited. Adequate hydration and rest are often sufficient. Using prophylactic quinolones early is sometimes advocated to enhance quality of life during travel. Norovirus can present with nausea, vomiting, and diarrhea. Supportive treatment is key to early recovery. Antibiotic-associated diarrhea is common and is usually self-limited. However, *C. difficile*-associated diarrhea can often be severe and can lead to increased hospitalization, morbidity, and mortality. Diagnoses of *C. difficile* diarrhea should be prompt and treatment should include rehydration and removal of any implicating antibiotics, as well as treatment with either metronidazole or oral vancomycin. Use of oral vancomycin might increase the risk of vancomycin-resistant enterococci, but this risk should be balanced against the risk of poor outcomes from suboptimally treated *C. difficile* diarrhea.

SKIN AND SOFT-TISSUE INFECTIONS

General Principles in Older Adults

Older adults are at greater risk for skin and soft-tissue infections (SSTIs) owing to immunosenescence, multiple comorbid conditions (specifically diabetes, peripheral vascular disease, underlying skin conditions [eg, eczema, venous stasis, and edema]), and/or frequent trauma. Defective cutaneous immunity with aging increases the susceptibility of older adults to SSTIs. Additionally, older adults have a greater likelihood of being bed-bound and hence at an increased risk for pressure ulcers.

Common types of SSTIs in older adults include cellulitis, necrotizing fasciitis, frunculosis, carbunculosis, pressure ulcers, and surgical site infections (SSIs). The incidence of each of these SSTIs varies; 1% to 9% for cellulitis and 2% to 24% for pressure ulcers in long-term care facility residents. Older adults with SSTIs have a higher mortality, morbidity, and attributable hospital costs compared to younger adults with SSTIs. For example, older adults with SSIs are 3 times more likely to die as compared to younger adults with SSIs.

Prevention

The prevention of SSTIs varies by type. Cellulitis can be prevented by elevating the limb to aid adequate fluid drainage and prevent edema, using medical stockings, and treating macerated skin with topical antifungals to prevent recurrences. Similarly, furuncles and carbuncles can be prevented by practicing good hand hygiene, using antibacterial soap baths, and not sharing personal items, which will target infections by community-acquired methicillin-resistant *S. aureus* (CA-MRSA). Prevention strategies for pressure ulcers include frequent turning of bed-bound patients, good nutrition, and maintaining moist sacral skin. The principles of preventing of SSIs are very similar in older and younger adults including rigorous glucose control, preventing hypothermia, smoking cessation, and appropriate timing and dosing of prophylactic antibiotics.

Clinical Findings

Similar to other infections, SSTIs may manifest atypically in older adults with absence of fever and declining mental status as compared to SSTIs in younger adults. Infected pressure ulcers may go unnoticed in chronically bed-bound older adults.

Cellulitis presents with limb swelling, redness, and tenderness, whereas erysipelas involves the dermis causing a raised rash with sharp borders. Both cellulitis and erysipelas are usually caused by *Streptococci* species and *S. aureus*. Necrotizing fasciitis (type 1 and type 2) is a more severe form of SSTI that involves deeper subcutaneous tissue destroying the fascial planes. Type 1 is polymicrobial (*E. coli, Klebsiella pneumoniae, Pseudomonas aeruginosa*, and anaerobic bacteria), which commonly follows surgical procedures or patients with pressure ulcers, whereas type 2 is monomicrobial (usually *Streptococcus pyogenes*) and relatively common in older adults with diabetes. In both types of disease, the area is extremely tender and red, often with an exudate. A Gram stain of cells from the edge of the lesion can aid in diagnosis; however, a strong index of clinical suspicion is needed. Pressure ulcers are often polymicrobial and most commonly affect the sacrum, heels, elbows, and lower extremities. Diagnosis is clinical and treatment is dependent on the Gram stain results and culture of the ulcerative matter.

Scabies is a commonly missed diagnosis in older adults and hence responsible for outbreaks in skilled nursing facility residents. It is caused by a mite (*Sarcoptes scabiei*), which can cause normal scabies or crusted scabies, both of which can be difficult to diagnose in older adults. Normal scabies presents as raised, red, itchy lesions called burrows, typically in interdigital areas and ankles. Crusted scabies, on the other hand, presents more atypically (itching being present in only 50% of patients) in older adults owing to their lack of ability to scratch and mount an immune response. The burden of mites on the skin is much higher in crusted scabies than in normal scabies, hence there are more opportunities for outbreaks. Skin scraping and testing helps to confirm the diagnosis for crusted scabies as it is often confused with psoriasis or eczema.

▶ Treatment

Both cellulitis and erysipelas are usually caused by *Streptococci* species or *S. aureus* and hence antimicrobial therapy targeting these organisms should be used. Antimicrobial choices include first-generation cephalosporins, vancomycin, and clindamycin. In cases where CA-MRSA is suspected (eg, a purulent SSTI), therapy with vancomycin, daptomycin, clindamycin, or linezolid should be considered. The decision between oral versus intravenous therapy generally depends on the severity at presentation and comorbidities. Necrotizing fasciitis can be especially severe in older adults. Surgical intervention is the gold standard diagnostic and treatment modality. In addition to antimicrobial therapy, it is important in infection management. For severe streptococcal or clostridial necrotizing fasciitis infections, clindamycin and penicillin are the antimicrobials of choice, whereas for mixed polymicrobial infections, a broad coverage for Gram-positive and Gram-negative bacteria and anaerobes is warranted. Because all pressure ulcers, like the skin, are colonized with bacteria, antibiotic therapy is not appropriate for a positive surface-swab culture without the signs and symptoms of infection. True infection of a pressure ulcer (cellulitis, osteomyelitis, or sepsis) is a serious condition, generally requiring broad-spectrum parenteral antibiotics, sometimes leading to surgical debridement in an acute-care facility.

Therapy for rashes without confirming the diagnosis of scabies unnecessarily exposes residents to the toxic effects of the topical agents. Because scabies can be transmitted by linen and clothing, the environment should be cleaned thoroughly. This includes cleaning inanimate surfaces, hot-cycle washing of washable items (clothing, sheets, towels, etc), and carpet cleaning. Topical permethrin cream with a repeat application after a week is the recommended treatment of choice for both kinds of scabies. Oral treatment with Ivermectin may be considered in patients with erosive skin from crusted scabies. Prevention is the key to avoiding outbreaks. Major preventive strategies include cleaning of fomites, adequate hand hygiene and personal protective equipment use by staff, retreatment of patients after a week to prevent reinfestation, and avoiding overcrowding in skilled nursing facilities.

PROSTHETIC JOINT INFECTIONS AND OSTEOMYELITIS

▶ General Principles in Older Adults

With the increasing number of total joint arthroplasties in older adults, the rate of prosthetic joint infections is expected to increase. Prosthetic joint infections in older adults are classified into early onset (within 3 months of surgery; usually caused by more virulent organisms like *S. aureus* and Gram-negative organisms) and late onset (3–24 months after surgery; caused by coagulase-negative *Staphylococcus* or *Pseudomonas* organism). Osteomyelitis (OM) is the second most common musculoskeletal infection after SSTIs in older adults, and manifests in a very similar way as in younger adults. Given the increasing frequency of falls (hence bone trauma) and underlying risk factors including peripheral vascular disease, diabetes, dental procedures, frequent surgeries, and prosthetic joint replacements, the incidence of OM is increasing in older adults. Age is also a very common risk factor for septic arthritis and is often associated with poor outcomes; a recent study showed a mortality of 9.5% in adults older than 80 years of age with septic arthritis. The risk factors for septic arthritis in adults 60 years of age and older include diabetes, neoplasm, and prosthetic joint and underlying joint disease. *S. aureus* is the most commonly isolated organism; however, group B streptococcus is very common in adults older than age 80. Of note, *E. coli* should be considered as a possible pathogen in older adults with UTIs and a prosthesis, because of the risk of urosepsis leading to seeding of the prosthesis. Similar to other infections, septic arthritis in older adults might manifest atypically with poor inflammatory response and is often mistaken as preexisting joint disease.

▶ Clinical Findings

Prosthetic joint infections are difficult to diagnose because of the lack of an inflammatory response, especially in patients with delayed onset infections. A Gram stain and culture of joint fluid can be diagnostic. Additionally, the organism can be identified via biopsy of periprosthetic tissue (which might be performed when removing the prosthesis). Older adults with total joint arthroplasty can also present with OM, which usually manifests with loosening of the prosthesis. Elevated erythrocyte sedimentation rate (ESR) in OM differentiates mechanical loosening of a prosthesis from loosening of a prosthesis caused by OM. Similar to younger adults, OM in older adults can be acute, subacute, or chronic. Acute OM is most commonly caused by *S. aureus*. In older adults, it can occur after an injury, which can cause a closed or open trauma to the bone. Pain is a common presenting finding. Fever and chills may or may not be present.

Subacute OM in older adults is most commonly vertebral, which can be either pyogenic or tuberculous. *S. aureus* is the most common pathogen in cases of hematogenous spread; however, aerobic Gram-negative organisms are commonly found in men with UTIs and vertebral OM. Computer-guided tomography biopsy helps in definitive diagnosis and treatment based on the underlying organism. Chronic OM is considered if it persists for more than 6 weeks or recurs after initial treatment. In older adults, the 2 main types of chronic OM include mandibular (caused by periodontal disease or poor dentition) and sternal (manifesting weeks to months after an open heart surgery). Among the most common organisms in the mandibular OM are oropharyngeal flora; in sternal OM, *S. aureus* is the most commonly identified organism. Other causes of chronic OM in older adults include OM complicating pressure ulcers, diabetic foot, and ulcers from peripheral vascular disease.

▶ Treatment

Treatment includes both antimicrobial therapy and surgical debridement. Whether the prosthesis is removed or not depends on the host's factors, type of prosthesis, and the surgeon. Prevention is similar to preventing SSIs in general, as described previously. ESR is often elevated in OM. Therapy for OM involves extensive surgical debridement and removal of the prosthesis. Therapy for septic arthritis is notably delayed in older adults given their poor inflammatory response and presence of underlying joint disease (rheumatoid arthritis, gout, etc). The therapy for OM is very similar to younger adults and depends on the underlying organism(s). A bone scan is diagnostic in acute OM. Therapy is empiric parenteral antimicrobials directed against *S. aureus*, followed by specific antimicrobials based on cultures from bone in patients with open fracture or blood in closed trauma patients. These patients often need extensive surgical debridement and even amputations besides antimicrobial therapy.

HIV/AIDS

▶ General Principles in Older Adults

According to the most recent statistics available, there are now more than 1 million adults in the United States infected with HIV which causes AIDS. There are approximately 50,000 people who become newly infected with HIV each year in this country. Of those new infections, more than 4000 occurred in patients older than age 55 years, including 853 people 65 years of age or older. Most new infections occur in men who have sex with men as a risk factor; however, approximately 25% of new cases happen as a result of unprotected heterosexual contact, and therefore women are also at risk. Cumulatively, there are more than 80,000 people older than age 55 years who carry an AIDS diagnosis. Based on this epidemiologic data, it is clear that the HIV epidemic is

having a significant effect on the aged population. As patients with established HIV infection age, there are several unique considerations and complications that can emerge, such as increased risk of cardiovascular disease and abnormalities of bone metabolism, as well as overall accelerated aging.

▶ Prevention

It is thought that older patients are now more than ever at risk for contracting HIV as a result of increased sexual activity related to the availability of erectile dysfunction treatments and the overall lack of awareness of HIV risk factors. Furthermore, there is a dearth of HIV education geared toward older demographics. In general, older adults do not consider themselves to be a high-risk group for sexually transmitted diseases, and because women are not concerned about the risk of pregnancy, condom use is often limited. Therefore, taking a sexual history in older adults and educating patients regarding the risk of HIV transmission is important. Discussing the importance of condom use in older patients is critical not only for the prevention of HIV, but also to prevent other sexually transmitted infections such as syphilis, gonorrhea, and chlamydia.

▶ Clinical Findings

The Centers for Disease Control and Prevention (CDC) now recommends that HIV screening tests be performed as part of routine health care up to the age of 64 years unless the prevalence of HIV in a particular community is documented to be less than 1 per 1000. A thorough sexual history is imperative with all older adults because patients who have high-risk behaviors should be screened on a yearly basis. Approximately 80% of patients who contract HIV will develop the acute retroviral syndrome, which consists of symptoms of fever, lymphadenopathy, pharyngitis, transient rash, myalgias, and, occasionally, aseptic meningitis. These symptoms tend to develop 2–4 weeks after an exposure. The screening test for HIV is a serology that detects antibodies that develop to antigens on the surface of the HIV structure, as well as capsid antigens. These antibodies tend to only fully develop over the course of 4–5 weeks. Therefore, if acute infection is considered, nucleic acid testing in the form of quantitative PCR for HIV is indicated. False-positive and false-negative tests can occur with any testing modality. Thus, HIV infection is only able to be confirmed with both a positive HIV enzyme-linked immunosorbent assay and Western blot test that demonstrates at least 2 bands, including p24, gp41, or gp120/160.

Occasionally patients may present with immune dysfunction related to AIDS if infection is of long standing and undiagnosed. Therefore, HIV screening should be performed in older patients with unexplained thrush, recurrent bacterial pneumonia or any opportunistic infection, such as *Pneumocystis* pneumonia. The development of opportunistic neoplasms, such as B-cell lymphoma, may also indicate the presence of HIV infection.

Complications

The development of AIDS-associated opportunistic infections and neoplasms are the most well-known complications of HIV infection. However, with effective antiretroviral therapy and earlier diagnosis and treatment, many patients are now leading healthy active lives with close-to-normal immune function. Many of the health problems faced by patients infected with HIV are now related to adverse events related to therapy or the long-term effects of HIV infection independent of immune dysfunction. The D:A:D study demonstrated that there is an excessive risk of myocardial infarction in patients with HIV receiving antiretroviral therapy. Others have shown that patients with HIV infection have a much higher risk of osteoporosis, which is likely related to the effects of certain antiretroviral agents on bone metabolism. There also is an increased risk of non–AIDS-defining cancers in patients with HIV infection. When colon cancer screening is performed, adenomas were found more commonly in HIV-infected patients compared to controls in one study. Human papillomavirus-related rectal cancer is the most common non–AIDS-related neoplasm found in patients with HIV infection. Therefore, routine health care maintenance screening in an aging population with HIV infection remains of paramount importance.

Treatment

Since the advent of the common use of highly active antiretroviral therapy (HAART), the mortality associated with HIV and AIDS has decreased dramatically. However, there are about 15,000 patients per year who die with HIV infection in the United States. When stratifying for survival by age group, those older than age 55 years have a significantly worse prognosis than younger patients, according to epidemiologic data collected by the CDC. This excess mortality has been confirmed in other studies that have shown that the risk of death related to comorbidities is as high as 72% in those older than the age of 50 years compared with 36% for patients up to age 30 years. Because retrospective studies and some prospective trials have demonstrated that patients who initiate HAART early in the course of their infection have fewer non–AIDS-related comorbid complications, the most recent treatment guidelines suggest initiating antiretroviral therapy for all patients with HIV infection regardless of CD4 cell count. Preferred initial combination therapy consists of 2 nucleoside reverse transcriptase inhibitors combined with either a non-nucleoside reverse transcriptase inhibitor, protease inhibitor, or integrase inhibitor. Adherence to antiretroviral is critical

because of the risk for the development of resistant virus if exposed to subtherapeutic levels of drug. One study demonstrated significantly better adherence among patients who were older than age 50 years (87.5%) compared with younger patients who took 78.3% of their medication dosages. Older patients who adhered poorly to their regimen were found to have abnormalities on neuropsychological testing. Because older patients are at higher risk for drug interactions and complications of therapy, including toxicity related to bone loss, kidney disease, and cardiovascular disease, intensified monitoring in this group of patients is important.

Anderson DJ, KS Kaye. Skin and soft tissue infections in older adults. *Clin Geriatr Med.* 2007;23(3):595-613, vii.

Atmar RL, Estes MK. The epidemiologic and clinical importance of norovirus infection. *Gastroenterol Clin North Am.* 2006;35(2):275-290, viii.

Bini EJ, Green B, Poles MA. Screening colonoscopy for the detection of neoplastic lesions in asymptomatic HIV-infected subjects. *Gut.* 2009;58(8):1129-1134.

Braithwaite RS, Justice AC, Chang CH, et al. Estimating the proportion of patients infected with HIV who will die of comorbid diseases. *Am J Med.* 2005;118(8):890-898.

Branson BM, Handsfield HH, Lampe MA, Janssen RS, Taylor AW, Lyss SB, Clark JE. Revised recommendations for the HIV testing of adults, adolescents, and pregnant women in health-care settings. *MMWR Recomm Rep.* 2006;55(RR-14);1-17.

Brown TT, Qaqish RB. Antiretroviral therapy and the prevalence of osteopenia and osteoporosis: a meta-analytic review. *AIDS.* 2006;20(17):2165-2174.

Castle SC. Clinical relevance of age-related immune dysfunction. *Clin Infect Dis.* 2000;31(2):578-585.

Centers for Disease Control and Prevention (CDC). Monitoring selected national HIV prevention and care objectives by using HIV surveillance data—United States and 6 U.S. dependent areas—2010. HIV Surveillance Supplemental Report 2012; 17(No. 3, part A). Published June 2012.

Cunha BA. Osteomyelitis in elderly patients. *Clin Infect Dis.* 2002;35(3):287-293.

Fry AM, Shay DK, Holman RC, Curns AT, Anderson LJ. Trends in hospitalizations for pneumonia among persons aged 65 years or older in the United States, 1988–2002. *JAMA.* 2005;294(21):2712-2719.

Gavet F, Tournadre A, Sourbrier M, Ristori JM, Dubost JJ. Septic arthritis in patients aged 80 and older: a comparison with younger adults. *J Am Geriatr Soc.* 2005;53(7):1210-1213.

High KP, Bradley SF, Gravenstein S, et al. Clinical practice guideline for the evaluation of fever and infection in older adult residents of long-term care facilities: 2008 update by the Infectious Disease Society of America. *Clin Infect Dis.* 2009;48(2): 149-171.

Hinkin CH, Hardy DJ, Mason KI, et al. Medication adherence in HIB-infected adults: effect of patient age, cognitive status, and substance abuse. *AIDS.* 2004;18 Suppl 1:S19-S25.

Juthani-Mehta M, Quagliarello VJ. Prognostic scoring systems for infectious diseases: their applicability to the care of older adults. *Clin Infect Dis.* 2004;38(5):692-696.

Juthani-Mehta M, Quagliarello V, Perrelli E, Towle V, Van Ness PH, Tinetti M. Clinical features to identify urinary tract infection in nursing home residents: a cohort study. *J Am Geriatr Soc.* 2009;57(6):963-970.

Lim WS, van der Eerden MM, Laing R, et al. Defining community acquired pneumonia severity on presentation to hospital: an international derivation and validation study. *Thorax.* 2003;58(5):377-382.

Loeb M, Bentley DW, Bradley S, et al. Development of minimum criteria for the initiation of antibiotics in residents of long-term care facilities: results of a consensus conference. *Infect Control Hosp Epidemiol.* 2001;22(2):120-124.

McGeer A, Campbell B, Emori EG, et al. Definitions of infection for surveillance in long-term care facilities. *Am J Infect Control.* 1991;19(1):1-7.

Nicolle LE. Infection control in long-term care facilities. *Clin Infect Dis.* 2000;31(3):752-756.

Nicolle LE. Urinary catheter-associated infections. *Infect Dis Clin North Am.* 2012;26(1):13-27.

Nicolle LE. Urinary tract infections in the elderly. *Clin Geriatr Med.* 2009;25(3):423-436.

Norman DC. Factors predisposing to infection. In: Yoshikawa TT, Norman DC, eds. *Infectious Disease in the Aging.* 2nd ed. New York, NY: Humana Press; 2009:11-18.

Panel on Antiretroviral Guidelines for Adults and Adolescents. *Guidelines for the Use of Antiretroviral Agents in HIV-1-Infected Adults and Adolescents.* Department of Health and Human Services. Accessed September 26, 2012. Available at http://www.aidsinfo.nih.gov/contentfiles/lvguidelines/adultandadolescentgl.pdf.

Prejean J, Song R, Hernandez A, et al. Estimated HIV incidence in the United States, 2006–2009. *PLoS One.* 2011;6(8):e17502.

Reddy M, Gill SS, Rochon PA. Preventing pressure ulcers: a systematic review. *JAMA.* 2006;296(8):974-984.

Shuman EK, Malani PN. Prevention and management of prosthetic joint infection in older adults. *Drugs Aging.* 2011;28(1):13-26.

Simor AE. Diagnosis, management, and prevention of *Clostridium difficile* infection in long-term care facilities: a review. *J Am Geriatr Soc.* 2010;58(8):1556-1564.

Smith PW, Bennett G, Bradley S, et al. SHEA/APIC guideline: infection prevention and control in the long-term care facility. *Infect Control Hosp Epidemiol.* 2008;29(9):785-814.

Stevens DL, Bisno AL, Chambers HF, et al. Practice guidelines for the diagnosis and management of skin and soft-tissue infections. *Clin Infect Dis.* 2005;41(10):1373-1406.

Stone ND, Ashraf MS, Calder J, et al. Surveillance definitions of infections in long-term care facilities: Revisiting the McGeer Criteria. Shea/CDC Position Paper. *Infection Control and Hospital Epidemiology.* 2012;33(10):965-977.

The Strategies for Management of Antiretroviral Therapy (SMART) Study Group, El-Sadr WM, Lundgren J, Neaton JD, et al. CD4+ count-guided interruption of antiretroviral treatment. *N Engl J Med.* 2006;355(22):2283-2296.

Thompson MA, Aberg JA, Hoy JF, et al. Antiretroviral treatment of adult HIV infection: 2012 recommendations of the International Antiviral Society–USA panel. *JAMA.* 2012;308(4):387-402.

Tjioe M, Vissers WH. Scabies outbreaks in nursing homes for the elderly: recognition, treatment options and control of reinfestation. *Drugs Aging.* 2008;25(4):299-306.

Vukmanovic-Stejic M, Rustin MH, Nikolich-Zugich J, Akbar AN. Immune responses in the skin in old age. *Curr Opin Immunol.* 2011;25(4):525-531.

Pressure Ulcers

48

David R. Thomas, MD, FACP, AGSF, GSAF

ESSENTIALS OF DIAGNOSIS

▶ Pressure ulcers are caused by pressure applied to susceptible tissues. Tissue susceptibility may be increased in the presence of maceration and by friction and shear forces.

▶ Comorbid conditions, especially immobility and decreased tissue perfusion, increase the risk of pressure ulcers.

▶ Most pressure ulcers develop over bony prominences, most commonly the sacrum, heels, and trochanteric areas.

▶ Most pressure ulcers develop in acute hospitals; the risk is greatest in orthopedic and intensive care unit patients.

▶ Pressure ulcers can be stage I (blanchable hyperemia), stage II (extension of the ulcer through the epidermis), stage III (full-thickness skin loss with damage or necrosis of subcutaneous tissue), or stage IV (full-thickness wounds with extensive destruction, tissue necrosis, or damage to muscle, bone, or supporting structures).

▶ Pressure ulcers do not necessarily progress from stage I through stage IV.

▶ General Principles in Older Adults

A. Causes

Pressure ulcers are the visible evidence of pathologic changes in the blood supply to dermal tissues. The chief cause is attributed to pressure, or force per unit area, applied to susceptible tissues. However, external pressure or shear force is increasingly viewed as a necessary but insufficient cause for pressure ulcers. In patients exposed to the same pressure load and duration of surgery, individual intrinsic factors appear to play a larger role in development of a pressure ulcer than the tissue interface pressure. Intrinsic factors leading to

derangement in tissue perfusion may account for the development of a pressure ulcer, despite the provision of common prevention measures that include pressure reduction. These factors are beginning to be identified but more research is needed.

Thomas DR. Does pressure cause pressure ulcers? An inquiry into the etiology of pressure ulcers. *J Am Med Dir Assoc.* 2010;11(6):397-405.

B. Management

Therapy for pressure ulcers is generally empiric, based on anecdotal experience, or borrowed from the treatment of patients with acute wounds. It is problematic because of multiple comorbidities, chronic duration of pressure ulcers, and, frequently, the physician's relative unfamiliarity with options.

Recognition of risk, relief of pressure, and optimizing nutritional status are components of both prevention and management guidelines. For persons with identified pressure ulcers, assessing the wound and implementing strategies for local wound care are paramount.

Thomas DR. Issues and dilemmas in the prevention and treatment of pressure ulcers: a review. *J Gerontol A Biol Sci Med Sci.* 2001;56(6):M328-M340.

Thomas DR. Prevention and management of pressure ulcers. *Rev Clin Gerontol.* 2008;17:1-17.

Thomas DR. Prevention and treatment of pressure ulcers: what works? What doesn't? *Cleve Clin J Med.* 2001;68(8):704-707, 710-714, 717-722.

C. Incidence

The primary source of pressure ulcers appears to be the acute hospital. Among patients who experience pressure ulcers, 57% to 60% do so in the acute hospital. Incidence in hospitalized patients ranges from 3% to 30%; common estimates range from 9% to 13%. A randomized national sample of

Medicare beneficiaries estimated a 4.5% incidence of a new hospital-acquired pressure ulcer from 2006 thru 2007. The incidence differs by hospital location; ICU patients and orthopedic patients are at greatest risk. In patients with a hip fracture, 15% develop a pressure ulcer during hospital admission, and one-third develop a pressure ulcer in 1 month. Pressure ulcers develop early in the course of hospitalization, usually within the first week. The incidence of pressure ulcers in nursing homes is difficult to quantitate.

After discharge from the hospital, pressure ulcers remain a major problem in community care settings. Characteristics associated with pressure ulcers include recent institutional discharge, functional impairment, incontinence, and having had a previous ulcer.

D. Risk Assessment & Risk Factors

In theory, persons who are at high risk for pressure ulcers can be identified, and an increased effort can be directed to preventing ulcers. The classical risk assessment scale is the Norton Score, developed in 1962 and still widely used. Patients are classified using 5 risk factors graded from 1–4. Scores range from 5–20; higher scores indicate lower risk. The generally accepted at-risk score is ≤14; patients with scores <12 are at particularly high risk.

A commonly used risk assessment instrument in the United States is the Braden Scale. This instrument assesses 6 items: sensory perception, moisture exposure, physical activity, mobility, nutrition, and friction/shear force. Each item is ranked from 1 (least favorable) to 3 or 4 (most favorable), with a maximal total score of 23. A score of ≤16 indicates a high risk.

Both the Norton Score and the Braden Scale have good sensitivity (73% to 92% and 83% to 100%, respectively) and specificity (61% to 94% and 64% to 77%, respectively), but poor positive predictive value (approximately 37% at a pressure ulcer incidence of 20%). In populations with a lower incidence of pressure ulcers, such as those in nursing homes, the same sensitivity and specificity produce a positive predictive value of 2%. The net effect of poor positive predictive value means that many patients who will not develop pressure ulcers will receive expensive and unnecessary treatment.

In clinical practice, risk assessment is problematic. A systematic review of 33 clinical trials of risk assessment found no decrease in pressure ulcer incidence that could be attributed to the use of an assessment scale. In long-term care settings, a Braden score had no predictive value for the development of a pressure ulcer.

Because most pressure ulcers develop in the acute hospital, risk assessment in this setting is particularly important. In an ICU, 5 factors contribute to the risk of pressure ulcer after adjusting for 18 univariately significant risk factors: norepinephrine infusion, Acute Physiology and Chronic Health Evaluation (APACHE) II score, fecal incontinence, anemia, and length of stay in the ICU. Independent risk factors for the development of a pressure ulcer after admission to a surgical service include emergency admission (which increased the risk 36-fold), age, days in bed, and days without nutrition.

Risk factors for the prevalence of pressure ulcers at admission include the presence of a fracture (increasing the risk 5-fold), fecal incontinence (increasing the risk 3-fold), and decreased serum albumin level (increasing the risk 3-fold). Applied prospectively to at-risk patients without pressure ulcers, these factors were associated with development of a pressure ulcer.

In functionally limited (bed- or chair-confined) hospitalized patients, 9 factors were associated with the development of pressure ulcers, including nonblanchable erythema (increasing the risk 7-fold), lymphopenia (increasing the risk almost 5-fold), and immobility, dry skin, and decreased body weight (each of which increase the risk 2-fold).

Not surprisingly, risk factors in long-term care populations differ. In this population, the factors associated with development of pressure ulcers are facility dependent. In low-risk nursing homes, difficulty in ambulation, difficulty feeding oneself, and male gender were associated with a 2- to 4-fold risk of pressure ulcer. In high-risk nursing homes, difficulty with ambulation, fecal incontinence, difficulty feeding oneself, and diabetes mellitus predicted pressure ulcer development.

The risk of pressure ulcer may include a history of cerebrovascular accident (5-fold increase), bed or chair confinement (3.8-fold increase), and impaired nutritional intake (2.8-fold increase). In data derived from the Minimal Data Set, logistic regression analysis determined that dependence in transfer or mobility, confinement to bed, history of diabetes mellitus, and a history of pressure ulcer were significantly associated with an existing stages II–IV pressure ulcer.

In community-dwelling persons age 55–75 years, the presence of a pressure ulcer was predicted by self-assessed poor health, current smoking, dry or scaly skin on examination, and decreased activity level.

The importance of these epidemiologic risk predictors lies in understanding which factors are amenable to correction. Risk factor predictors from various sites suggest that immobility, dry skin, and nutritional factors are potentially modifiable. Efforts have centered on correction of these problems.

▶ Prevention

A. Quality of Care

Pressure ulcers are increasingly used as indicators of quality of care. Whether or not pressure ulcers are preventable remains controversial. When aggressive measures for prevention of pressure ulcers have been applied, a "floor effect" for incidence has been noted. Pressure ulcers often occur in terminally ill patients, for whom the goals of care may not include prevention of pressure ulcers. Pressure ulcers also occur in severely ill patients, such as orthopedic patients or ICU patients, for whom the necessity for immobilization may preclude turning or the use of pressure-relieving devices.

Systematic efforts at education, heightened awareness, and specific interventions by interdisciplinary wound teams suggest that a high incidence of pressure ulcers can be reduced. Over time, reductions of 25% to 30% have been reported. The reduction may be transient, unstable over time, vary with changes in personnel, or occur as a result of random variation. Development of pressure ulcers can be, but is not always, a measure of quality of care.

B. Pressure Relief

The first efforts toward prevention should be to improve mobility and reduce the effects of pressure, friction, and shear forces. The theoretical goal is to reduce tissue pressure below capillary closing pressure of 32 mm Hg. If the target pressure reduction is unachievable, then pressure must be intermittently relieved to allow time for tissue recovery.

The most expedient method for reducing pressure is frequent turning and positioning. A 2-hour turning schedule for spinal injury patients was deduced empirically in 1946. However, turning the patient to relieve pressure may be difficult to achieve despite best nursing efforts and is very costly in terms of staffing. The exact interval for optimal turning in prevention is unknown. The interval may be shortened or lengthened by host factors. Despite commonsense approaches to turning, positioning, and improving passive activity, no published data support the view that pressure ulcers can be prevented by passive positioning.

Because of the limitations and cost of turning schedules, a number of devices have been developed to prevent pressure injury. Devices can be defined as pressure relieving (consistently reducing interface pressure <32 mm Hg) or pressure reducing (less than standard support surfaces but not <32 mm Hg). The majority of devices are pressure reducing. Pressure-reducing devices can be further classified as static or dynamic. Static surfaces attempt to distribute local pressure over a larger body surface. Examples include foam mattresses and devices filled with water, gel, or air. Dynamic devices use a power source to alternate air currents and promote uniform pressure distribution over body surfaces. Examples include alternating pressure pads, air suspension devices, and air–fluid surfaces.

Some pressure-reducing devices have been proven more effective than "standard" hospital foam mattresses in moderate- to high-risk patients. Pressure-relieving mattresses in the operating theater have reduced the incidence of pressure sores postoperatively. Limited evidence suggests that low-air-loss beds reduce the incidence of pressure sores in ICUs. The differences among devices are unclear and do not demonstrate a superior device compared with other devices. There is some evidence that air–fluid beds and low-air-loss beds improve healing rates.

Krapfl LA, Gray M. Does regular repositioning prevent pressure ulcers? *J Wound Ostomy Continence Nurs.* 2008;35(6):571-577.

McInnes E, Dumville JC, Jammali-Blasi A, Bell-Syer SE. Support surfaces for pressure ulcer prevention. *Cochrane Database Syst Rev.* 2011;(12):CD009490.

C. Nutritional Interventions

One of the most important reversible factors contributing to wound healing is nutritional status. Of newly hospitalized patients with stage III or stage IV pressure ulcers, most were below their usual body weight, had a low prealbumin level, and were not taking in enough nutrition to meet their needs.

The results of trials to increase improve pressure ulcer healing have been disappointing. Only 1 of 5 trials has shown a small effect of nutritional supplements on prevention of pressure ulcers. In addition, overnight supplemental enteral feeding has not been shown to affect development of pressure ulcers and severity.

Basal metabolic rate appears to be similar or slightly increased in persons with a pressure ulcer. Clinical judgement and prediction equations suggest an caloric intake of 30 kcal/kg per day. An optimum dietary protein intake in patients with pressure ulcers is unknown but may be much higher than current adult recommendations of 0.8 g/kg per day. Half of chronically ill older persons are unable to maintain nitrogen balance at this level. Increasing protein intake beyond 1.5 g/kg per day may not increase protein synthesis and may cause dehydration. A reasonable protein requirement is, therefore, between 1.2–1.5 g/kg per day.

The deficiency of several vitamins has significant effects on wound healing. However, supplementation of vitamins to accelerate wound healing is controversial. There is no substantial evidence to support use of a daily vitamin C supplement for healing pressure sores.

Zinc supplementation has not been shown to accelerate healing except in zinc-deficient patients. High serum zinc levels interfere with healing, and supplementation >150 mg/day may interfere with copper metabolism.

Immune function declines with age, which increases risk for infection, and is thought to delay wound healing. Specific amino acids such as arginine and branched-chain amino acids have not demonstrated an effect on pressure ulcer healing.

Houston S, Haggard J, Williford J Jr, Meserve L, Shewokis P. Adverse effects of large-dose zinc supplementation in an institutionalized older population with pressure ulcers. *J Am Geriatr Soc.* 2001;9(8):1130-1132.

Thomas DR. Improving outcome of pressure ulcers with nutritional interventions: a review of the evidence. *Nutrition.* 2001;17(2):121-125.

Thomas DR. The role of nutrition in prevention and healing of pressure ulcers. *Clin Geriatr Med.* 1997;13(3):497-511.

▶ Clinical Findings

Several differing scales have been proposed for assessing the severity of pressure ulcers. The most common staging, recommended by the National Pressure Ulcer Task Force, is derived from a modification of the Shea Scale. Under this schematic, pressure ulcers are divided into 6 clinical stages.

The first response of the epidermis to pressure is hyperemia. Blanchable erythema occurs when capillary refilling occurs after gentle pressure is applied to the area. Nonblanchable erythema exists when pressure of a finger in the reddened area does not produce a blanching or capillary refilling. A stage I pressure ulcer is defined by nonblanchable erythema of intact skin. Nonblanchable erythema is believed to indicate extravasation of blood from the capillaries. A stage I pressure ulcer always understates the underlying damage because the epidermis is the last tissue to show ischemic injury. Diagnosing stage I pressure ulcers in darkly pigmented skin is problematic.

Stage II ulcers extend through the epidermis or dermis. The ulcer is superficial and presents clinically as an abrasion, blister, or shallow crater. With stage III pressure ulcers, there is full-thickness skin loss involving damage or necroses of subcutaneous tissue that may extend down to, but not through, underlying fascia. The ulcer presents clinically as a deep crater with or without undermining of adjacent tissue.

Stage IV pressure ulcers are full-thickness wounds with extensive destruction, tissue necrosis, or damage to muscle, bone, or supporting structures. Undermining and sinus tracts are frequently associated with stage IV pressure ulcers. Stage I pressure ulcers occur most frequently, accounting for 47% of pressure ulcers, followed by stage II ulcers (33%). Stages III and IV ulcers comprise the remaining 20%.

This staging system for pressure ulcers has several limitations. The primary difficulty lies in the inability to distinguish progression between stages. Pressure ulcers do not progress absolutely through stage I to stage IV, but may appear to develop from the inside out as a result of the initial injury. Healing from stage IV does not progress through stage III to stage I; rather, the ulcer heals by contraction and scar tissue formation. Second, clinical staging is inaccurate unless all eschar is removed, because the staging system reflects only depth of the ulcer.

Because the staging system is based only on the depth of an ulcer, an ulcer that is covered by eschar, or when the depth is unable to be assessed, is designated as "unstageable."

Muscle tissue, subcutaneous fat, and dermal tissue are differentially susceptible to injury, in that order. The differential effect of pressure on the tissue layers suggests that injury occurs first in muscle tissue before changes are observed in the skin. This is the basis for the so-called deep tissue injury. In many cases, the changes visible at the surface of the tissue are minor compared to the damage seen at the deepest layers of tissue. The surface discoloration is often classified as a stage I pressure ulcer, which rapidly evolves into a deep stage IV ulcer. This differential tissue susceptibility suggests that a number of factors are involved in the development of pressure ulcers, including the type of pressure load and biochemical changes in the tissue because of reperfusion injury or tissue compression.

Because pressure ulcers heal by contraction and scar formation, reverse staging is inaccurate in assessing healing. No single measure of wound characteristics has been useful in measuring healing. Several indexes of ulcer healing have been proposed but lack validation studies. The Pressure Ulcer Status for Healing (PUSH) tool (Figure 48–1) was developed and validated by the National Pressure Ulcer Advisory Panel to measure healing of pressure ulcers. The tool measures 3 components—size, exudate amount, and tissue type—to arrive at a numerical score for ulcer status. The PUSH tool adequately assesses ulcer status and is sensitive to change over time.

Stotts NA, Rodeheaver GT, Thomas DR, et al. An instrument to measure healing in pressure ulcers: development and validation of the pressure ulcer scale for healing (PUSH). *J Gerontol A Biol Sci Med Sci.* 2001;56(12):M795-M799.

Thomas DR. Does pressure cause pressure ulcers? An inquiry into the etiology of pressure ulcers. *J Am Med Dir Assoc.* 2010;11(6):397-405.

▶ Differential Diagnosis

Acute wounds proceed through an orderly and well-described process to produce healing with structural and functional integrity. Chronic wounds fail to proceed through this process and result in poorly healing wounds of long duration. There are 4 types of chronic wounds: peripheral arterial ulcers, diabetic ulcers, venous stasis ulcers, and pressure ulcers. Each of these wounds differ in their underlying pathophysiology, and, more importantly, differ with respect to local wound treatment.

Arterial ulcers tend to occur over the distal part of the leg, especially the lateral malleoli, dorsum of the feet, and the toes. The clinical appearance is that of gangrene, which can be wet or dry. Arterial ulcers tend to be painful, and pain control features prominently in their management. Peripheral arterial disease results from atherosclerosis of aorta, iliac and lower extremity arteries. Ischemic vascular ulcers are difficult to heal, and therapy is aimed at improving blood flow. A careful examination for arterial pulses may be useful, but is dependent on the examiner's skill and may be misleading. An ankle-brachial pressure index is an inexpensive and accurate diagnostic test for peripheral arterial disease.

The etiology of diabetic ulcers is multifactorial. Among these, the presence of neuropathy is the most important factor in the development of a diabetic ulcer, while inadequate vascular supply is the most important factor in healing. Diabetic ulcers typically occur in areas of repetitive trauma, producing a callus formation. Microvascular changes in

Patient name: _____ Patient ID#: _____

Ulcer location: _____ Date: _____

Directions: Observe and measure the pressure ulcer. Categorize the ulcer with respect to surface area, exudate, and type of wound tissue. Record a subscore for each of these ulcer characteristics. Add the subscore to obtain the total score. A comparison of total scores measured over time provides an indication of the improvement or deterioration in pressure ulcer healing.

	0	1	2	3	4	5	
Length	0 cm^2	<0.3 cm^2	0.3–0.6 cm^2	0.7–1.0 cm^2	1.1–2.0 cm^2	2.1–3.0 cm^2	
x Width		6 3.1–4.0 cm^2	7 4.1–8.0 cm^2	8 8.1–12.0 cm^2	9 12.1–24.0 cm^2	10 >24.0 cm^2	**Subscore**
Exudate amount	0 None	1 Light	2 Moderate	3 Heavy			**Subscore**
Tissue type^a	0 Closed	1 Epithelial tissue	2 Granulation tissue	3 Slough	4 Necrotic tissue		**Subscore**
							Total score

Length × Width: Measure the greatest length (head to toe) and the greatest width (side to side) using a centimeter ruler. Multiply these two measurements (length × width) to obtain an estimate of surface area in square centimeters (cm^2). Caveat: Do not guess! Always use a centimeter ruler and always use the same method each time the ulcer is measured.

Exudate amount: Estimate the amount of exudate (drainage) present after removal of the dressing and before applying any topical agent to the ulcer. Estimate the exudate (drainage) as none, light, moderate, or heavy.

Tissue type: This refers to the types of tissue that are present in the wound (ulcer) bed. Score as a "4" if there is any necrotic tissue present. Score as a "3" if there is any amount of slough present and necrotic tissue is absent. Score as a "2" if the wound is clean and contains granulation tissue. A superficial wound that is reepitheliazing is scored as a "1". When the wound is closed, score as a "0".

^{a}**Necrotic tissue (eschar):** black, brown, or tan tissue that adheres firmly to the wound bed or ulcer edges and may be either firmer or softer than surrounding skin. **Slough:** yellow or white tissue that adheres to the ulcer bed in strings or thick clumps or is mucinous. **Granulation tissue:** pink or beefy red tissue with a shiny, moist, granular appearance. **Epithelial tissue:** for superficial ulcers. New pink or shiny tissue (skin) that grows in from the edges or as islands on the ulcer surface. **Closed/resurfaced:** wound is completely covered with epithelium (new skin).

▲ **Figure 48–1.** Pressure Ulcer Status for Healing (PUSH) tool version 3.0. (Reproduced with permission from National Pressure Ulcer Advisory Panel.)

blood flow lead to a deep crater-like appearance, especially in areas of foot deformity.

The underlying pathophysiology of venous leg ulcers includes reflux, obstruction, or insufficiency of the calf muscle pump, involving the superficial venous system (greater and smaller saphenous vein), the deep venous system, or the veins that perforate between those systems. The etiology of chronic deep venous disease results from primary (often idiopathic) or secondary causes (postthrombotic obstruction), but most commonly represents a combination of both. The skin in chronic venous stasis disease demonstrates hyper- or hypopigmentation, lipodermatosclerosis, weeping

of the skin, and ulceration. Edema is often present but not necessary for the diagnosis. A venous leg ulcer is irregularly shaped and shallow, but with well-defined borders. Location is usually from the malleolar area upwards to the knee (the "gaiter" area, so-called because this area is covered by leggings known as gaiters). The ulcer bed is often exudative, and bacterial and fungal overgrowth on the wound and surrounding skin surface is common.

Pressure ulcers are the visible evidence of pathologic changes in the blood supply to dermal tissues. Pressure ulcers usually occur over bony prominences, when the tissue is compressed to pressures above capillary closing pressure.

However, patient-specific intrinsic factors may lessen the time or pressure amounts required to produce tissue damage. The most common site for the development of a pressure ulcers is the sacrococcygeal area, followed by the heels.

All of the 4 types of chronic wounds have in common some relationship to pressure. However, the classification of these wounds should be related to the underlying pathophysiology in respect to treatment.

▶ **Complications**

Colonization of chronic wounds with bacteria is common and unavoidable. All chronic wounds become colonized, usually with skin organisms followed in 48 hours by Gram-negative bacteria. The presence of microorganisms alone (colonization) does not indicate an infection in pressure ulcers. The primary source of bacterial infections in chronic wounds appears to be the result of suprainfection resulting from contamination. Therefore, protection of the wound from secondary contamination is an important goal of treatment.

Evidence suggests that occlusive dressings protect against clinical infection, although the wound may be colonized with bacteria. Occlusive dressings very rarely cause a clinical infection.

It is often difficult to determine the presence of an infection in chronic pressure ulcers. The diagnosis of infection in chronic wounds must be based on clinical signs: advancing erythema, edema, odor, fever, or purulent exudate. When there is evidence of clinical infection, topical or systemic antimicrobials are required. Topical treatment may be useful when the wound is failing to progress toward healing. Systemic antibiotics are indicated when the clinical condition suggests spread of the infection to the bloodstream or bone.

Wounds with extensive undermining create pockets for infection with an increased likelihood for infection with anaerobic organisms. Obliteration of dead space reduces the possibility of infection.

Thomas DR. When is a chronic wound infected? *J Am Med Dir Assoc.* 2012;13(1):5-7.

▶ **Treatment**

Maintaining a moist wound environment increases the rate of healing. Moist wound healing allows experimentally induced wounds to resurface up to 40% faster than air-exposed wounds. Any therapy that dehydrates the wound such as dry gauze, heat lamps, air exposure, or liquid antacids is detrimental to chronic wound healing.

Dressings allow moisture to escape from the wound at a fixed rate measured by the moisture vapor transmission rate (MVTR). An MVTR of <35 g of water vapor/m^2/h is required to maintain a moist wound environment. Woven gauze has an MVTR of 68 g/m^2/h, and impregnated gauze has an MVTR of 57 g/m^2/h. In comparison, hydrocolloid dressings have an MVTR of 8 g/m^2/h.

Dressings that maintain a moist wound environment are occlusive, describing the propensity of a dressing to transmit moisture vapor from the wound to the external atmosphere. The available dressings differ in their properties of permeability to water vapor and in wound protection.

A. Topical Dressings

Occlusive dressings can be divided into broad categories of polymer films, polymer foams, hydrogels, hydrocolloids, alginates, and biomembranes. Each has several advantages and disadvantages. The choice of a particular agent depends on the clinical circumstances. The agents differ in the ease of application. This difference is important in pressure ulcers in unusual locations or when considering their use for home care. Dressings should be left in place until wound fluid is leaking from the sides, a period of days to 3 weeks.

1. Polymer films—Polymer films are impermeable to liquid but permeable to both gas and moisture vapor. Because of low permeability to water vapor, these dressings are not dehydrating to the wound. Nonpermeable polymers such as polyvinylidene and polyethylene can be macerating to normal skin. Polymer films are not absorptive and may leak, particularly when the wound is highly exudative. Most films have an adhesive backing that may remove epithelial cells when the dressing is changed. Polymer films do not eliminate dead space and do not absorb exudate.

2. Hydrogels—Hydrogels are 3-layer hydrophilic polymers that are insoluble in water but absorb aqueous solutions. They are poor bacterial barriers and do not adhere to the wound. Because of their high specific heat, these dressings are cooling to the skin, aiding in pain control and reducing inflammation. Most of these dressings require a secondary dressing to secure them to the wound.

3. Hydrocolloid dressings—Hydrocolloid dressings are complex dressings similar to ostomy barrier products. They are impermeable to moisture vapor and gases (their impermeability to oxygen is theoretically a disadvantage) and are highly adherent to the skin. In addition, they offer bacterial resistance. Their adhesiveness to surrounding skin is higher than some surgical tapes, but they do not adhere to wound tissue and do not damage epithelialization of the wound. The adhesive barrier is frequently overcome in highly exudative wounds. Hydrocolloid dressings cannot be used over tendons or on wounds with eschar formation. Several of these dressings include a foam padding layer that may reduce pressure to the wound.

4. Alginates—Alginates are complex polysaccharide dressings that are highly absorbent in exudative wounds. This high absorbency is particularly suited to exudative wounds. Alginates do not adhere to the wound; however, if the wound is allowed to dry, damage to the epithelial tissue may occur with removal.

Table 48–1. Comparison of occlusive wound dressings.

Variables	Moist Saline Gauze	Polymer Films	Polymer Foams	Hydrogels	Hydrocolloids	Alginates, Granules	Biomembranes
Pain relief	+	+	+	+	+	±	+
Maceration of surrounding skin	±	±	–	–	–	–	–
O₂ permeable	+	+	+	+	–	+	+
H₂O permeable	+	+	+	+	–	+	+
Absorbent	+	–	+	+	±	+	–
Damage to epithelial cells	±	+	–	–	–	–	–
Transparent	–	+	–	–	–	–	–
Resistant to bacteria	–	–	–	–	+	–	+
Ease of application	+	–	+	+	+	+	–

Adapted and reproduced with permission from Helfman T, Ovington L, Falanga V. Occlusive dressings and wound healing. *Clin Dermatol.* 1994;12(1):121-127, and Witkowski JA, Parish LC. Cutaneous ulcer therapy. *Int J Dermatol.* 1986;25(7):420-426.

5. Biomembranes—Biomembranes offer bacterial resistance but are very expensive and not readily available. These dressings could be problematic in wounds contaminated by anaerobes, but this effect has not been demonstrated clinically.

6. Saline-soaked gauze—Saline-soaked gauze that is not allowed to dry is an effective wound dressing. Moist saline gauze and occlusive-type dressings have similar pressure ulcer-healing abilities. The use of occlusive-type dressings has been shown to be more cost-effective than traditional dressings primarily because of a decrease in nursing time for dressing changes. Table 48–1 provides a comparison of dressing types. Table 48–2 presents general guidelines.

B. Growth Factors

Acute wound healing proceeds in a carefully regulated fashion that is reproducible from wound to wound. A number of growth factors have been demonstrated to mediate the healing process, including transforming growth factor-α and -β, epidermal growth factor, platelet-derived growth factor, fibroblast growth factor, interleukin-1 and -2, and tumor necrosis factor-α. Accelerating healing in chronic wounds using these acute wound factors is attractive. Several of these factors have been favorable in animal models; however, they have not been as successful in human trials.

In pressure ulcers, recombinant platelet-derived growth factor (rhPDGF-BB) failed to improve the rate of complete healing, although a 15% difference in percentage of initial volume of ulcers has been shown with PDGF-BB. One report showed that more subjects had >70% wound closure with basic fibroblast growth factor. Sequential application of growth factors to mimic wound-healing progression has not been effective in pressure ulcers.

C. Adjunctive Therapies

Alternative or adjunctive therapies include electrical therapy, electromagnetic therapy, ultrasound therapy, low-level light therapy/laser therapy, and vacuum-assisted closure. None of these interventions has been clearly proven effective despite widespread clinical use.

Table 48–2. Therapeutic recommendations for treatment of pressure ulcers.

Stage	Needs	Dressing Options
I and II	Clean, moist surface Protection from environment	Wet-to-moist saline gauze Thin-film polymer Hydrocolloid dressing
III and IV		
With dead space, exudate	Clean, moist surface Protection from environment Adsorption of exudate Elimination of dead space	Wet-to-moist saline gauze Hydrocolloid dressing Synthetic adsorption dressing Hydrogel
With necrosis	Clean, moist surface Protection from environment Debridement	Surgical Mechanical Enzymatic Autolytic
Heel pressure ulcers	Protection from environment	Pressure reduction

Cullum N, Nelson EA, Flemming K, Sheldon T. Systematic reviews of wound care management: (5) beds; (6) compression; (7) laser therapy, therapeutic ultrasound, electrotherapy and electromagnetic therapy. *Health Technol Assess.* 2001;5(9):1-221.

D. Debridement

Necrotic debris increases the possibility of bacterial infection and delays wound healing. The preferred method of debriding pressure ulcers remains controversial. Options include mechanical debridement with dry gauze dressings, autolytic debridement with occlusive dressings, application of exogenous enzymes, or sharp surgical debridement.

Surgical sharp debridement produces the most rapid removal of necrotic debris and is required in the presence of infection. Mechanical debridement can be easily accomplished by allowing a saline gauze dressing to dry before removal. Remoistening of gauze dressings in an attempt to reduce pain can defeat the debridement effect.

Both surgical and mechanical debridement can damage healthy tissue or fail to clean the wound completely. Debridement with a dry gauze should be stopped as soon as a clean wound bed is obtained because dry dressings have been associated with delayed healing.

Thin portions of eschar can be removed by occlusion under a semipermeable dressing. Both autolytic and enzymatic debridement require periods of several days to several weeks to achieve results. Enzymatic debridement can dissolve necrotic debris, but whether it harms healthy tissue is debated. Penetration of enzymatic agents is limited in eschar and requires either softening by autolysis or cross-hatching by sharp incision before application.

Only 1 enzyme preparation is available in the United States for débridement. Topical collagenase reduced necrosis, pus, and odor compared with inactivated control ointment and produced debridement in 82% of pressure ulcers at 4 weeks compared with petrolatum. Papain produced measurable debridement in 4 days compared with a control ointment. The issues of when to debride and which method to use remain controversial. Whether debridement improves the rate of healing remains undetermined.

A total of 5 trials have not shown that the use of enzymatic agents increased the rate of complete healing in chronic wounds compared with control treatment.

E. Surgical Therapy

Surgical closure of pressure ulcers results in a more rapid resolution of the wound. The chief problems are frequent recurrence of ulcers and inability of frail patients to tolerate the procedure.

The efficacy of surgical repair of pressure ulcers is high in the short-term; however, its long-term efficacy has been questioned. Problems with surgical repair include suture line dehiscence, nonhealing, and recurrence.

The proportion of pressure ulcers suitable for operation depends on the patient population, but normally only a low percentage are candidates for surgery. However, among selected groups of patients, such as those with spinal cord injury and deep stage III or IV pressure ulcers, surgery may be indicated for the majority. If the factors contributing to the development of the pressure ulcer cannot be corrected, the chance of recurrence after surgery is very high.

▶ Prognosis

Pressure ulcers have been associated with increased mortality rates in both acute and long-term care settings. Death has been reported during acute hospitalization in 67% of patients who develop a pressure ulcer compared with 15% of at-risk patients without pressure ulcers. Patients who develop a new hospital-acquired pressure ulcer are 2.8 times as likely to die in the hospital compared to persons without a pressure ulcer. The odds ratio for mortality in 30 days is 1.7 times as high, and readmission within 30 days is 1.3 times as high. In long-term care settings, development of a pressure ulcer within 3 months among newly admitted patients was associated with a 92% mortality rate compared with 4% among residents who did not subsequently develop a pressure ulcer. Residents in a skilled nursing facility who had pressure ulcers experienced a 6-month mortality rate of 77.3% compared with 18.3% in those without pressure ulcers. Patients whose pressure ulcers healed within 6 months had a significantly lower mortality rate (11% vs. 64%) than those whose pressure ulcers did not heal.

Despite this association with death rates, it is not clear how pressure ulcers contribute to increased mortality. Patients with stage II pressure ulcers have been equally as likely to die as those with stage IV pressure ulcers. In the absence of complications, it is difficult to imagine how stage I or II pressure ulcers contribute to death. Pressure ulcers may be associated with mortality because of their occurrence in otherwise frail, sick patients.

Thomas DR. Are all pressure ulcers avoidable? *J Am Med Dir Assoc.* 2001;2:297.

Common Skin Disorders

Christine O. Urman, MD
Daniel S. Loo, MD

49

► General Principles in Older Adults

Aging skin is subject to both intrinsic aging processes, as well as many years of environmental assault. With increasing age, skin's barrier function declines, making it much more difficult to maintain moisture. Thus, dry skin in older adults is almost inevitable. This has multiple consequences, the most common being pruritus. Dry skin is also more susceptible to environmental insults, which can cause eczematous dermatitis because of an irritant or an allergen.

After many years of being subject to oxidative damage from environmental pollution and radiation, skin cells have accumulated many mutations. Thus skin cancers are prevalent in the older population.

Aberrant responses of the immune system increase with age; consequently, autoimmune skin diseases as well as allergic contact dermatitis become more common. As normal function of the immune system declines, certain infectious diseases are also more common, such as herpes zoster and onychomycosis.

Certain benign tumors are extremely common in older adults. These include acrochordons, seborrheic keratoses, and cherry angiomas. Although a frequent cause of alarm in a patient, they only require reassurance. On the other hand, benign nevi are extremely uncommon in this age group, and any new mole should raise a suspicion of melanoma.

SEBORRHEIC KERATOSIS

ESSENTIALS OF DIAGNOSIS

► Seborrheic keratosis is the most common benign epithelial tumor of adulthood.
► The trunk is affected more than the extremities, head, and neck.
► Primary lesions are 5–20-mm light brown to dark brown–black papules and plaques with a rough, warty surface (Figure 49–1).
► Differential diagnosis includes: solar lentigo, melanocytic nevus, verruca vulgaris, and lentigo maligna melanoma.

► Complications

Friction, pressure, and trauma to these lesions may cause irritation or inflammation.

► Treatment

Irritated or inflamed lesions can be treated with cryotherapy (Box 49–1), curettage, or shave removal. Lesions on cosmetically sensitive areas are best treated with light electrodessication to minimize scarring and dyspigmentation.

EPIDERMAL INCLUSION CYST

ESSENTIALS OF DIAGNOSIS

► This cutaneous cyst is an epithelium-lined sac filled with keratin and located within the dermis.
► Distribution is more common on the trunk than the face and extremities.
► Primary lesions are 0.5–4-cm flesh-colored to yellow dermal to subcutaneous nodules (Figure 49–2).
► Cysts are freely mobile on palpation. With pressure, cheese-like keratin can often be expressed through a central punctum.
► Differential diagnosis includes lipoma.

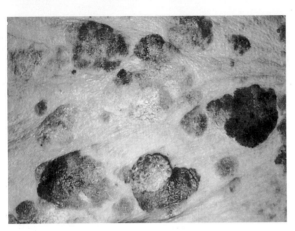

▲ **Figure 49–1.** Seborrheic keratoses. Waxy, stuck-on papules and plaques, with varying shades of brown and a verrucous surface. (Reproduced with permission from Neill Peters, MD.)

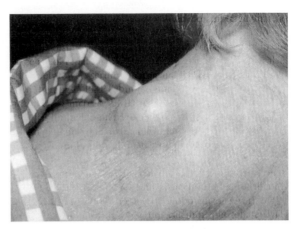

▲ **Figure 49–2.** Epidermal inclusion cyst. This large 4 × 5-cm cyst on the left shoulder is tense but freely mobile over underlying tissues.

Box 49–1. Cryotherapy

A. Indications
   Liquid nitrogen can be used to treat
   Actinic keratosis
   Seborrheic keratosis (irritated)
   Warts

B. Dipstick technique
   1. Roll extra cotton over the tip of the cotton applicator.
   2. Dip tip into liquid nitrogen.
   3. Apply tip of applicator to lesion until 1-2 mm of normal surrounding skin turns white.
   4. Wait until lesion completely thaws back to normal color.
   5. Repeat (number of freeze-thaw cycles depends on the lesion being treated).

C. Open-spray technique
   (Requires hand-held nitrogen unit and C-tip aperture.)
   1. Nozzle should be 1-2 cm from target lesion and perpendicular to it.
   2. Squeeze trigger to emit continuous burst of spray.
   3. The lesion and not more than 1 mm of surrounding normal skin should be frosted.
   4. Wait until lesion completely thaws back to normal color.
   5. Repeat (number of freeze-thaw cycles depends on the lesion being treated).

D. Adverse effects
   Patients must be informed that
   1. During application treated area will sting or burn followed by throbbing.
   2. Treated area will become erythematous and edematous and will vesiculate or blister within hours.
   3. Hypopigmentation is common in darkly pigmented individuals.

▶ Complications

Rupture of the cyst wall leads to extrusion of keratin debris into the dermis and a foreign-body inflammatory response. The area becomes tense, tender, and painful.

▶ Treatment

These cysts do not resolve spontaneously. Permanent removal can be achieved only by excising the entire cyst wall. Incision and drainage may temporarily relieve pressure, but is not curative. In the case of a ruptured cyst, the use of antibiotics is controversial because this is not a true infection (abscess), but rather an inflammatory reaction to foreign material. However, minocycline or doxycycline have an antiinflammatory effect, and a dosage of 100 mg twice daily may be helpful. If there is no improvement within 1 week, incision and drainage followed by infiltration of the area with triamcinolone acetonide, 10 mg/mL, will provide relief. Surgery of inflamed tissue is not recommended. If any portion of the cyst wall remains after treatment, recurrence is likely.

WARTS (VERRUCA VULGARIS & VERRUCA PLANTARIS)

 ESSENTIALS OF DIAGNOSIS

▶ These human papillomavirus-induced growths are found most frequently on the hands and feet, followed by arms, legs, and the trunk.

▶ Primary lesions are 5–15-mm flesh-colored papules and plaques with a verrucous or filiform surface. Reddish-brown punctate dots (thrombosed capillary loops) are diagnostic (Figure 49–3). The lesion may require paring with a no. 15 blade to visualize the capillary loops.

▶ Differential diagnosis includes flat warts, seborrheic keratosis, and squamous cell carcinoma.

▶ Treatment

Multiple plantar warts are often stubborn regardless of the treatment modality. Several treatments may be needed before significant improvement occurs. Immunocompromised patients may have widespread involvement and are refractory to standard treatment modalities.

A. Cryotherapy (see Box 49–1)

Two to 3 freeze–thaw cycles are recommended to induce blistering. Treatment is repeated every 3–4 weeks. Plantar warts are thicker and often require paring with a no. 15 blade before freezing.

B. Cantharidin

Cantharidin 0.7% (Cantharone) is a chemical agent that induces blistering. It must be applied in the office setting because of potential side effects, including blistering, dyspigmentation, and scarring. It is applied to the wart using the wood end of a cotton-tipped applicator, allowed to dry, covered for 8–12 hours, and then washed off with soap and water. A blister develops within 1–2 days. Treatment is repeated every 3–4 weeks. Cantharidin may be used alone or in combination with podophyllin and salicylic acid. Patients are asked to avoid removing the blister roof; however, if the blister is tense and causing discomfort, they may puncture it with a clean needle to relieve some of the pressure.

C. Salicylic Acid

Salicylic acid 40% plasters can be used at home. The plaster is cut to fit over the wart and left in place for 24 hours. This is repeated daily. Between treatments, the superficial macerated debris can be removed with a pumice stone or emery board.

ONYCHOMYCOSIS

ESSENTIALS OF DIAGNOSIS

▶ Characteristic features include distal thickening of the nail plate, yellow discoloration, and subungual debris (Figure 49–4).

▶ Because visual appearance is insufficient to make a diagnosis, microscopy is necessary.

▶ Differential diagnosis includes pincer nails, onychogryphosis, psoriasis, lichen planus, and repeated trauma.

▶ General Principles in Older Adults

Yeast or dermatophyte infection of the nail plate requires laboratory confirmation. Nail dystrophy alone is not sensitive or specific for onychomycosis. There are 3 diagnostic tests:

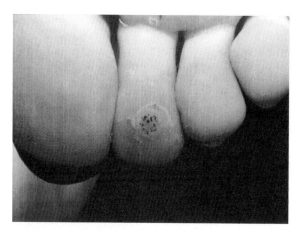

▲ **Figure 49–3.** Plantar wart. The 2–3-mm punctate brown papules are thrombosed capillary loops.

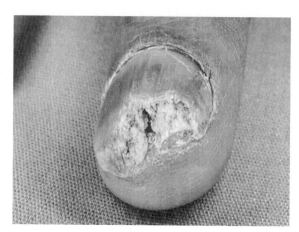

▲ **Figure 49–4.** Onychomycosis. This fingernail demonstrates the characteristic thick subungual hyperkeratosis and debris.

A. Direct Microscopy

Trim back the distal edge of the involved nail. Use a small 1-mm curette or No. 15 blade to scrape the undersurface of the nail plate and nail bed. Place the sample on a glass slide and add 1 drop of potassium hydroxide (KOH) 20% with dimethylsulfoxide (DMSO). Demonstration of hyphae after a few minutes confirms the diagnosis. Sensitivity is highly variable and dependent on experience.

B. Culture

Obtain sample as just described and place on Sabouraud dextrose agar containing chloramphenicol and cycloheximide (Mycosel or mycobiotic agar). Nail clippings are poor specimens for culture. If there is no growth within 3 weeks, the test is negative. Sensitivity is 50% to 60%.

C. Pathology

Send a nail clipping in a formalin container for periodic acid-Schiff (PAS) stain. Sensitivity is >90%.

▶ Pathogenesis

Public exercise facilities and pools are common sites for transmission of dermatophytes, usually via the feet. Tinea pedis can spread to the adjacent nail and often precedes onychomycosis. Toenails are affected more often than fingernails.

▶ Prevention

Treatment of tinea pedis with topical antifungals can prevent onychomycosis and decrease risk of recurrence.

▶ Treatment

Before initiating therapy, patients should be informed that toenails grow very slowly, approximately 1 mm per month. Thus, if half of the nail is involved, it will take 6–9 months to clear. If the entire nail is involved, it will take 12–15 months to clear. Systemic antifungals maintain an effective concentration in the nail matrix for 6–9 months after therapy is discontinued.

A. Systemic Antifungals

Table 49–1 compares dosing regimens and mycologic cure rates.

1. Terbinafine—This is the treatment of choice for dermatophyte onychomycosis, providing superior long-term clinical efficacy and lower rates of relapse compared with pulse itraconazole. Terbinafine may increase levels of theophylline, nortriptyline, and caffeine, and decrease the level of cyclosporine. Rifampin, cimetidine, and terfenadine may

Table 49–1. Systemic antifungal treatment of toenails.

Drug	Dosing Regimen	Mycological Cure (18 months)
Terbinafine	Continuous: 250 mg/day × 3 months	76%
Itraconazole	Continuous: 200 mg/day × 3 months	59%
	Pulse: 400 mg/day × 1 week/month × 3 months	63%
Fluconazole	150 mg × 1 day/week × 9 months	48%

alter serum levels of terbinafine. Terbinafine is best avoided in patients with active hepatitis B or C, cirrhosis, or other chronic hepatic disorders. In healthy individuals, baseline liver function tests are optional.

2. Itraconazole—This is the treatment of choice for onychomycosis caused by yeast (*Candida*) or molds. Itraconazole is contraindicated in patients taking astemizole, terfenadine, triazolam, midazolam, cisapride, lovastatin, or simvastatin. Itraconazole may increase drug levels of oral hypoglycemic agents, immunosuppressants, HIV-1 protease inhibitors, and anticoagulants. Anticonvulsants, antituberculosis agents, nevirapine, H_2 antihistamines, proton pump inhibitors, and didanosine may alter serum levels of itraconazole. Itraconazole is best avoided in patients with active hepatitis B or C, cirrhosis, or other chronic hepatic disorders. In healthy individuals, baseline liver function tests are optional.

B. Ciclopirox Nail Lacquer Solution

Nail lacquers are generally ineffective, with the exception of patients with only 1–2 nails affected and minimal involvement of the distal nail plate. It is brushed onto affected nails daily for 6 months. Nails should be trimmed, with regular removal of the unattached infected nail.

▶ Prognosis

With the use of systemic antifungals, relapse rates range from 20% to 50%. Prophylactic weekend application of topical antifungals may prevent recurrences.

DRY SKIN, PRURITUS, & ASTEATOTIC DERMATITIS

ESSENTIALS OF DIAGNOSIS

▶ Dry skin is a common problem and manifests itself predominantly as pruritus.

▶ More than 80% of older persons have symptoms related to skin problems; the most frequent complaint is pruritus from dry skin.

▶ Symptoms are more common in the winter.

▶ Indoor heat and low humidity combined with hot showers and overuse of soaps result in dryness and cracking of the skin.

▶ Dry skin may lead to asteatotic dermatitis, with erythematous patches and slightly raised plaques on the anterior shins and extensor surfaces of the arms and less involvement of the trunk. Cracking and dry scaling may also be seen.

▶ Differential diagnosis includes atopic dermatitis, contact dermatitis, and irritant dermatitis.

General Principles in Older Adults

Pruritus in older adults can be caused by a variety of dermatologic and systemic conditions, but the most common cause is dry skin and asteatotic dermatitis (Figure 49–5).

Prevention

A humidifier in the bedroom is helpful. Daily use of moisturizers, especially those containing lactic acid or urea, is recommended to heal dry skin. Moisturizers should be used after bathing, while the skin is still slightly moist. Use of bath oils should be avoided because of the risk of slipping.

Treatment

Patient education about preventing dry skin includes:

• Shower or bathe with warm, not hot water

• Reducing use of soaps and rinsing well.

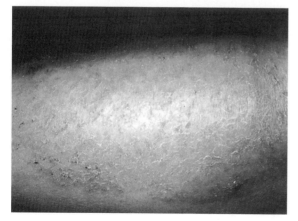

▲ **Figure 49–5.** Asteatotic dermatitis. This plaque on the left lateral shin demonstrates fine crackling or fissuring.

• Application of hydrophilic petrolatum or urea 10% cream to moist skin immediately after bath or shower.

• Reducing vigorous rubbing of the skin with towels, which may exacerbate pruritus.

• In asteatotic dermatitis, application of a class 4 topical steroid ointment to eczematous patches twice daily for 2–3 weeks may be required to break the itch–scratch cycle. (Table 49–2 provides topical steroid potency ratings.)

Table 49–2. Steroid cream potency rating.

Class	Trade Name	Generic
1	Temovate 0.05%	Clobetasol propionate
	Diprolene 0.05%	Betamethasone dipropionate
2	Lidex 0.05%	Fluocinonide
	Psorcon 0.05%	Diflorasone diacetate
3	Aristocort A 0.5%	Triamcinolone acetonide
	Topicort LP 0.05%	Desoximetasone
4	Elocon 0.1%	Mometasone furoate
	Kenalog 0.1%	Triamcinolone acetonide
5	Westcort 0.2%	Hydrocortisone valerate
	Dermatop 0.1%	Prednicarbate
6	Desowen 0.05%	Desonide
	Aristocort A 0.025%	Triamcinolone acetonide
7	Hytone 1%	Hydrocortisone
	Hytone 2.5%	Hydrocortisone

A. Steroid ranking from
   Class 1 (strongest) → class 7 (weakest)
   1. Most steroids come in both a cream and ointment. For the same concentration, the ointment is slightly more potent than the cream (fluocinonide .05% ointment is stronger than fluocinonide .05% cream).
   2. Most topical steroids are applied twice daily.
   3. Class 1 steroids should be used in severe inflammatory or pruritic skin conditions (psoriasis, contact dermatitis, scabies).

B. Adverse effects
   1. Atrophy, telangiectasia, and striae may occur with prolonged use of potent topical steroids (classes 1 and 2). For instance, clobetasol cream applied twice daily for >1 month may result in atrophy. The FDA limits the duration of use of all class 1 steroids to 2 weeks.
   2. The face, genitals, intertriginous areas, and mucosal surfaces absorb steroids more readily and are more prone to these side effects. Potent topical steroids should not be used >2 weeks on the face, genitals, intertriginous areas, and mucosal surfaces.
   3. Potent topical steroids applied to >50% total body surface area may have systemic effects.

SEBORRHEIC DERMATITIS

ESSENTIALS OF DIAGNOSIS

▶ The face (especially between the eyebrows and nasolabial folds), scalp, and chest are affected (Figure 49–6).

▶ Primary lesions are erythematous patches and plaques with secondary changes of greasy scales.

▶ Rosacea, eczema, lupus, and photosensitivity disorders must be considered in the differential diagnosis.

▶ General Principles in Older Adults

Overgrowth of commensal yeast, *Malassezia globosa*, results in this common dermatitis.

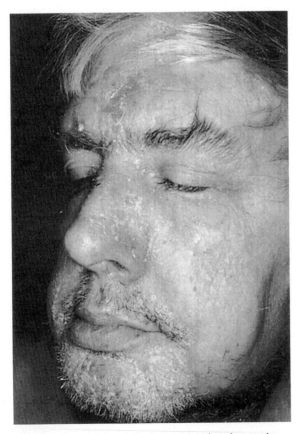

▲ **Figure 49–6.** Seborrheic dermatitis. Abundant scale distributed over the medial eyebrows, nasolabial folds, mustache, and beard.

▶ Treatment

A. Antidandruff Shampoos

Nonprescription zinc pyrithione 1%, selenium sulfide 1%, or ketoconazole 1% shampoo can be applied to the scalp every day for 1 week and then tapered to once or twice weekly to prevent recurrence. The lather should be massaged into the skin for a few minutes before rinsing. Ketoconazole 2% shampoo may be more effective.

B. Topical Treatment

Topical treatment may be needed for patients unresponsive to shampoos alone.

1. Facial involvement—Apply ketoconazole 2% cream twice daily for 2–3 weeks or class 6 steroid cream twice daily for 2–3 weeks. Sodium sulfacetamide 10%/sulfur 5% cream or wash are also effective when used once or twice daily.

2. Scalp pruritus—A class 5 steroid solution can be applied daily as needed.

STASIS DERMATITIS

ESSENTIALS OF DIAGNOSIS

▶ Chronic venous insufficiency results from pooling of venous blood in the lower extremities and increased capillary pressure.

▶ Chronic venous insufficiency is most commonly associated with varicose veins.

▶ Anterior shins are affected most, followed by calves, dorsal feet, and ankles.

▶ Primary lesions are red-brown to brown hyperpigmented macules and patches (Figure 49–7), often with pedal edema.

▶ Erythematous patches with fine crackling and scales can be seen as secondary changes.

▶ Ulceration may occur in up to 30% of patients.

▶ Pigmented purpuric dermatosis, minocycline hyperpigmentation, and contact dermatitis are included in the differential diagnosis.

▶ Prevention

Compression stockings and leg elevation in patients with varicose veins may help prevent stasis changes.

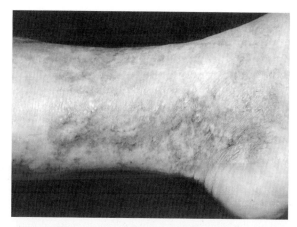

▲ **Figure 49-7.** Stasis dermatitis. Hyperpigmented macules and patches involving the left medial malleolus. (Reproduced with permission from Neill Peters, MD.)

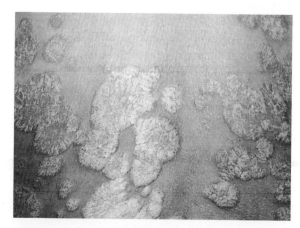

▲ **Figure 49-8.** Psoriasis. Plaques with thick micaceous scale on the lower back.

▶ Treatment

Compression stockings at 20–30 mm Hg can be applied. Elevation of the legs above the level of the heart whenever sitting or lying down will reduce venous pooling. Class 5 steroid ointment applied twice daily will relieve any eczematous patches or plaques.

PSORIASIS

ESSENTIALS OF DIAGNOSIS

▶ This is a heritable T-cell–mediated inflammatory dermatosis; 33% of those affected have a positive family history.

▶ Psoriasis may be precipitated by streptococcal pharyngitis (guttate psoriasis).

▶ There is symmetric involvement of extensor surfaces (elbows, knees, lumbosacral) and scalp. The flexures and genitals may also be involved (inverse psoriasis).

▶ Primary lesions are erythematous papules and plaques with secondary changes of thick micaceous scale (Figure 49-8).

▶ Nails may demonstrate yellow-brown oil spots, pitting (Figure 49-9), and onycholysis.

▶ The prevalence of psoriatic arthritis in patients with psoriasis is approximately 10%.

▶ Differential diagnosis includes eczema, seborrheic dermatitis, and lichen planus.

▶ Complications

Arthritis of the small and large joints may accompany psoriasis. Generalized pustular psoriasis and erythrodermic psoriasis may be life threatening and require hospitalization. There is an increased prevalence of the metabolic syndrome in patients with moderate to severe psoriasis, a known risk factor for cardiovascular disease.

▶ Treatment

Choice of therapy is dependent on disease severity. For individuals with <10% total-body surface area affected, topical therapies are generally effective.

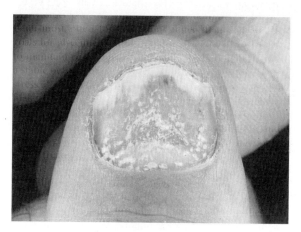

▲ **Figure 49-9.** Nail psoriasis. This thumbnail demonstrates pitting and distal onycholysis.

A. Topical Corticosteroids

1. Trunk & extremities—Class 1 steroid ointment is applied to plaques twice daily for 2–3 weeks or until flattening of lesional skin occurs.

2. Face, intertriginous sites—Class 5 steroid cream is applied to plaques twice daily for 2–3 weeks or until flattening of lesional skin occurs.

B. Calcipotriene

Calcipotriene, 0.005% ointment applied twice daily, has a slower onset of action compared with topical steroids and is somewhat effective for mild plaque psoriasis. Irritation is the most common side effect.

C. Natural Sunlight

Natural sunlight, when practical, is often very helpful. Before 10 AM and after 2 PM, the patient should lie flat for 15–20 minutes on each side 2–3 times a week. For those patients with >10% total body surface area affected, referral to a dermatologist for phototherapy or systemic immunosuppressive agents should be considered.

D. Acitretin

Acitretin is an oral retinoid that is used when the palms and the soles are affected, or if the lesions are covered with very thick scale. It is frequently used in combination with topicals or with phototherapy; however, acitretin can be effective as monotherapy for palmoplantar psoriasis. It is given at doses 10–50 mg daily. At higher doses, severe dryness of the skin is the main side effect. Acitretin is contraindicated in women who are pregnant or plan to become pregnant, as females cannot become pregnant for 3 years after discontinuing the drug. Tetracyclines have to be avoided during treatment because of a drug interaction that may increase the risk of pseudotumor cerebri. Hyperlipidemia may occur in up to one-third of patients. Thus, triglycerides and cholesterol should be monitored closely.

▶ Prognosis

Psoriasis is a chronic disease characterized by exacerbations and remissions. A positive family history, early onset, and extensive involvement are poor prognostic factors.

ROSACEA

 ESSENTIALS OF DIAGNOSIS

▶ Sometimes referred to as adult acne, rosacea is most common in women age 40–50 years and is characterized by flushing.

▶ Lesions affect the central face (nose, cheeks, forehead, and chin).

▶ Primary lesions are erythematous papules and pustules (Figure 49–10).

▶ Secondary changes include confluent telangiectasias with erythema.

▶ Differential diagnosis includes acne, perioral dermatitis, and systemic lupus erythematosus.

▶ Pathogenesis

Although the cause of rosacea is unknown, any stimulus that increases skin temperature of the head and neck can trigger flushing, including sunlight, hot showers, exercise, alcohol, hot beverages, and spicy foods. Frequent flushing, in turn, can cause inflammatory and microvascular changes leading to the development of rosacea.

▶ Complications

Ocular involvement (blepharitis, conjunctivitis) may occur in up to 50% of patients. Some cases can progress to rhinophyma (enlarged bulbous nose).

▶ Treatment

A. Sunscreen

Patients may be able to reduce symptoms by avoiding triggers and applying sunscreen with a sun protection factor of ≥30 daily. Broad spectrum sunscreens that protect from both UVA and UVB should be recommended.

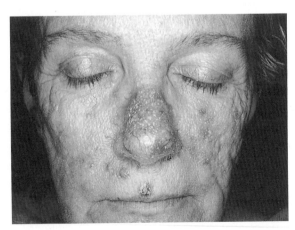

▲ **Figure 49–10.** Rosacea. Papules and pustules of the central face with enlarged nose and telangiectasias.

B. Topical Antibiotics

Topical antibiotics include metronidazole, 0.75% cream or gel applied twice daily, and sodium sulfacetamide 10%/sulfur 5% lotion applied twice daily.

C. Systemic Antibiotics

Systemic antibiotics are effective for treatment of inflammatory papules or pustules. Minocycline 100 mg orally twice daily, or doxycycline 100 mg orally twice daily are most commonly prescribed. Maintenance dose of doxycycline 20 mg twice daily is also effective in those who do not respond to topical alone. This dose has antiinflammatory effects only, and thus a reduced side-effect profile.

D. Laser Treatment

For telangiectasia, the patient can be referred to a dermatologist for pulsed-dye laser treatment. This is most effective, although it does not prevent development of new telangiectasias.

CONTACT DERMATITIS

ESSENTIALS OF DIAGNOSIS

▶ Contact dermatitis is a delayed-type hypersensitivity reaction to an antigen (allergen) that contacts the skin and causes severe pruritus.

▶ Symptoms can be acute or chronic:

• Acute contact dermatitis can be localized or generalized and has linear or artificial patterns (Figure 49–11). Primary lesions include vesicles and erythematous, edematous plaques. Secondary changes include erosions, exudates, and crusts.

• Chronic contact dermatitis can be localized or generalized and occurs in linear or artificial patterns (indicative of external contact). Primary lesions appear as lichenified plaques. Secondary changes include hyperpigmentation.

▶ Differential diagnosis: atopic dermatitis, scabies, and irritant dermatitis.

▶ Prevention

Patients should be advised to avoid sources of known allergens. Table 49–3 lists the most frequent contact allergens and their sources.

▶ Complications

Left untreated, dermatitis may spread, causing debilitating pruritus.

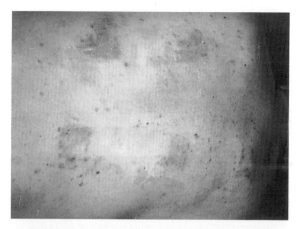

▲ **Figure 49–11.** Contact dermatitis. These square-shaped, itchy plaques resulted from electrode adhesive pads from a transcutaneous electrical nerve stimulation unit.

▶ Treatment

If <10% of the surface area is involved, a class 1 steroid ointment can be applied 3 times a day for 2–3 weeks or until the dermatitis and pruritus resolves. If >10% of body surface area is affected, a prednisone taper is appropriate (Box 49–2). For chronic and extensive dermatitis, the patient should be referred to dermatology for patch testing and possibly chronic systemic immunosuppressive therapy.

Table 49–3. Most frequent contact allergens & their sources.

Contact Allergens	Common Sources
Nickel	Jewelry
Gold	Jewelry
Fragrance mix	Skin or hair care products
Thimerosal	Vaccines, eye and nasal medications
Quaternium-15	Cosmetics (preservative)
Neomycin	Antibiotic ointment
Formaldehyde	Nail polish, cosmetics (preservative)
Methylchloroisothiazolinone/ methylisothiazolinone	Cosmetics (preservative)
Bacitracin	Antibiotic ointment
Thiuram	Latex gloves, shoes (rubber products)
Balsam of Peru	Fragrance in cosmetics
Cobalt	Metal-plated objects (buckles, button, zippers)
P-paraphenylenediamine	Hair dye
Carba mix	Rubber elastic of undergarment

Box 49-2. Prednisone Taper

A. Indications
   (severe pruritus from a variety of conditions)
   1. Contact dermatitis >10% surface area
   2. Severe eczema
   3. Drug eruption

B. Dosing
   Start with 1 mg/kg (maximum 60 mg/day) and then taper by 5 mg each consecutive day.
   1. For 130-lb patient, start with 60 mg and taper by 5 mg each day for 12-day course.
   2. Severe cases may require a prolonged taper over 2–3 weeks.
   3. Medrol dosepaks are inadequate for most adults.

C. Side effects
   (Review patient's history for hypertension, diabetes, glaucoma.)
   1. Water retention
   2. Weight gain
   3. Increased appetite
   4. Mood swings
   5. Restlessness
   6. Avascular necrosis of the hip

DRUG ERUPTION (MORBILLIFORM)

ESSENTIALS OF DIAGNOSIS

▶ Maculopapular eruptions, the most common type of drug eruption, usually occur during the first 2 weeks of a new medication.

▶ The most common drugs implicated in drug eruptions are penicillins (ampicillin, amoxicillin), sulfonamides (trimethoprim-sulfamethoxazole), nonsteroidal antiinflammatory drugs (naproxen, piroxicam), anticonvulsants (carbamazepine, phenytoin), and antihypertensives (captopril, diltiazem).

▶ Distribution of drug eruptions is bilateral and symmetric, usually beginning on the head and neck or upper trunk and progressing down the limbs.

▶ Primary lesions are erythematous macules and/or papules with areas of confluence (Figure 49–12).

▶ Pruritus is occasionally present.

▶ Differential diagnosis includes viral exanthem, bacterial infection, and collagen vascular disease.

▶ Complications

Drug hypersensitivity syndrome is potentially life threatening and presents as a triad of fever, skin eruption (80% morbilliform), and internal organ involvement (hepatitis, nephritis, lymphadenopathy). This occurs on first exposure

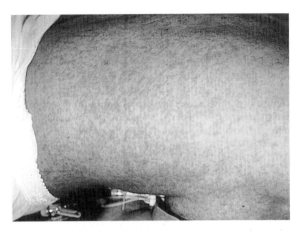

▲ **Figure 49–12.** Morbilliform drug eruption. Macules and papules of the right flank and back with areas of confluence. (Reproduced with permission from Melvin Lu, MD.)

to the drug, with symptoms starting 1–6 weeks after exposure. Laboratory tests to evaluate potential asymptomatic internal organ involvement include transaminases, complete blood cell count, urinalysis, and serum creatinine.

Stevens-Johnson syndrome is a severe form of a bullous drug reaction that involves 2 or more mucosal sites; cutaneous blisters quickly peel off to reveal denuded skin. Hospitalization, close monitoring, and supportive care are required early in the course of the disease.

▶ Treatment

The drug most likely to have caused the eruption should be stopped along with any unnecessary medications.

Topical and oral steroids provide symptomatic relief. Regimens include class 1 steroid cream twice daily for 2–3 weeks or prednisone taper (see Box 49–2) if creams are ineffective. Resolution usually occurs within several weeks.

HERPES ZOSTER

ESSENTIALS OF DIAGNOSIS

▶ Herpes zoster is caused by reactivation of varicella-zoster virus in the dorsal root ganglion.

▶ Distribution of grouped vesicular lesions is unilateral (Figure 49–13) and within 1–2 adjacent dermatomes (ophthalmic branch of trigeminal nerve, thoracic, and cervical are most commonly affected).

▶ Primary lesions are vesicles (Figure 49–14) on an erythematous base. Secondary changes consist of pustules and crusts.

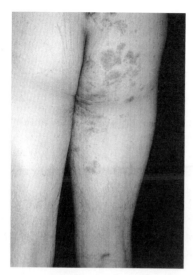

▲ **Figure 49–13.** Herpes zoster. Unilateral S1 and S2 distribution.

► Immunosuppression, especially hematologic malignancy, and HIV infection, substantially increase the risk for herpes zoster as well as dissemination.

► Differential diagnosis includes herpes simplex, eczema herpeticum, varicella, and acute contact dermatitis.

General Principles in Older Adults

Pain precedes the eruption in >90% of cases. Rarely, the eruption does not develop, and neuralgia is the only manifestation of zoster (zoster sine herpete). In most cases, grouped

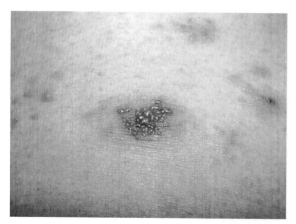

▲ **Figure 49–14.** Herpes zoster. The same patient as in Figure 49–13 has grouped vesicles on an erythematous base.

vesicles in a dermatomal distribution are enough to establish the diagnosis. A positive Tzanck smear cannot distinguish between herpes simplex and varicella-zoster virus. Viral cultures identify herpes simplex within 2–3 days; however, varicella-zoster culture can take 1–2 weeks with frequent false-negative results.

► Complications

Patients with cutaneous involvement of the V_1 branch of the trigeminal nerve may experience ocular complications (keratitis, acute retinal necrosis) and need to undergo immediate slit-lamp examination by an ophthalmologist, particularly if skin lesions involve the side and tip of the nose (Hutchinson sign). Immunocompromised patients are at risk for dissemination, defined as >20 vesicles outside the primary and immediately adjacent dermatomes. Cutaneous dissemination may be followed by visceral involvement (lung, liver, brain) in 10% of these high-risk patients.

Postherpetic neuralgia is pain that persists after resolution of the cutaneous eruption. This most common complication is age dependent, affecting at least 50% of patients older than age 60 years, and most frequently involves the face.

► Treatment

The systemic antiviral drugs (acyclovir, famciclovir, valacyclovir) are effective in the acute phase of zoster and should be used within 48–72 hours of rash onset. These drugs reduce acute pain, accelerate healing, prevent scarring, and reduce the incidence of postherpetic neuralgia. Systemic corticosteroids (prednisone) may help to reduce acute pain but have no effect on incidence or severity of postherpetic neuralgia. Although the safety profile for the antiviral drugs is excellent, headache, nausea, diarrhea, and central nervous system, renal, and hepatic dysfunction can occur. In more severe cases, especially in disseminated zoster, initial intravenous acyclovir should be considered. Studies indicate that oral therapy is as effective as intravenous therapy in ophthalmic zoster.

► Prevention

Herpes zoster vaccine (Zostavax) can be used in patients 60 years of age and older to boost their waning immunity to the varicella virus so as to prevent herpes zoster reactivation and decrease the risk of postherpetic neuralgia.

► Prognosis

The affected dermatome usually heals within 3–4 weeks, and occasionally may scar. Postherpetic neuralgia is the major cause of morbidity.

SCABIES

ESSENTIALS OF DIAGNOSIS

▶ The *Sarcoptes scabiei* mite inhabits the human stratum corneum. Characteristic initial lesions are 3–8-mm linear or serpiginous ridges (burrows; Figure 49–15), often with a gray dot at one end (mite).

▶ The interdigital web spaces of the hands, volar wrists, penis, and areolas are commonly involved.

▶ Secondary changes include papules and nodules (nodular scabies), diffuse eczematous dermatitis, thick hyperkeratotic crusted plaques (crusted or Norwegian scabies), and vesicles or bullae (bullous scabies).

▶ Pruritus is intractable and debilitating.

▶ Differential diagnosis includes atopic dermatitis, contact dermatitis, drug eruption, and urticarial bullous pemphigoid.

▶ General Principles in Older Adults

Close body contact is the most common mode of transmission. Fomite transmission is rare because the female mite cannot survive away from the host for >24–36 hours. Risk factors include nursing home residence, HIV and AIDS, and crowded living conditions.

▶ Microscopic Findings

Diagnosis is confirmed (finding mites, eggs [Figure 49–16], or feces) using direct microscopy in a simple bedside test.

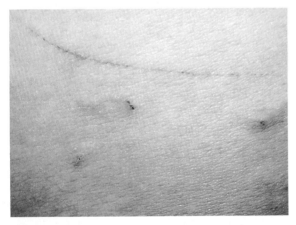

▲ **Figure 49–15.** Scabies. Serpiginous 3–8-mm burrows above a linear excoriation.

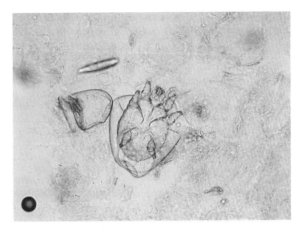

▲ **Figure 49–16.** Direct microscopy. Scabies mite hatched from an egg. (Reproduced with permission from Neill Peters, MD.)

A. Specimen Collection

Place a drop of mineral oil on the center of a glass slide. Touch the sharp part of a No. 15 blade to the drop (so that the specimen will adhere to the blade). Holding the blade perpendicular to the skin, scrape an epidermal burrow to remove the stratum corneum. Pinpoint bleeding indicates the correct depth. Wipe contents onto the center of the glass slide. Choose 2 other burrows, and repeat steps 2–4 to increase the yield. Place coverslip over specimen and gently press down.

B. Microscope Settings

Use ×4 objective to scan the slide.

▶ Complications

Nodular scabies is a pruritic hypersensitivity reaction to remnants of the mite. The lesions are firm erythematous to red-brown nodules occurring on the genitals and the axillae. Patients who are immunocompromised may develop crusted or Norwegian scabies with extensive yellow crusting. Norwegian scabies is extremely contagious because each crust contains hundreds of mites. Epidemics of scabies in nursing homes are relatively common and often go undetected for long periods.

▶ Treatment

Goals of therapy include mite eradication, alleviation of pruritus, and prevention of transmission.

A. Scabicide

The patient and all close contacts should be treated simultaneously, including those who are asymptomatic.

1. Permethrin—Permethrin 5% cream is the most effective topical treatment. A 60-g tube is prescribed for whole-body application. Patients can be instructed to take a bath or shower and completely dry before application. Cream should be applied to the entire skin surface (from the neck down), with particular attention to finger web spaces, feet, genitals, and intertriginous sites. The cream should be washed off in 8 hours. This regimen is repeated in 1 week. Compliance will result in >90% cure rate.

2. Ivermectin—Ivermectin, 0.2 mg/kg as an oral dose and repeated at 10–14 days, is a safe and efficacious alternative to topical treatment. However, two doses two weeks apart must be used, as the drug only kills the mite and not the eggs.

B. Pruritus

Even after successful mite eradication, severe pruritus can persist for 3–4 weeks. This often debilitating symptom is frequently overlooked and leads to unnecessary discomfort and suffering. Patients may receive repeated treatment for scabies in the mistaken belief that infestation persists.

Class 1 steroid ointment can be applied 2–3 times daily for 2–4 weeks or until complete resolution of pruritus. Prednisone taper (see Box 49–2) may be required to manage patients with debilitating pruritus.

C. Transmission Prevention

All clothes worn within 2 days of treatment, towels, and bedsheets should be machine washed in hot water or dry cleaned. Management of nursing home outbreaks requires clinical and epidemiologic expertise and possibly involvement of public health experts.

▶ Prognosis

Immunocompetent individuals do well with standard therapy. Crusted scabies, usually in the immunosuppressed, may require >2 applications of topical scabicides or ivermectin or a combination.

BULLOUS PEMPHIGOID

ESSENTIALS OF DIAGNOSIS

▶ Bullous pemphigoid is an autoimmune disease in which antibodies target components of skin's basement membrane.

▶ Distribution of lesions may be localized or generalized on the extremities or trunk.

▶ Primary lesions are tense vesicles or bullae filled with serous or serosanguineous fluid (Figure 49–17). Primary lesions in urticarial bullous pemphigoid are wheals and edematous erythematous plaques. The latter presentation is less common (Figure 49–18).

▶ Secondary changes are erosions, ulcers and crusts.

▶ Pruritus can be debilitating.

▶ Differential diagnosis includes bullous drug reactions, pemphigus, contact dermatitis, scabies, and arthropod bites.

▶ General Principles in Older Adults

Bullous pemphigoid (BP) is a chronic disease that occurs primarily in older adults and may be associated with significant morbidity. Occasionally BP can be caused by drugs. Diuretics, antibiotics, and angiotensin-converting enzyme inhibitors have been implicated. Diagnosis of BP requires

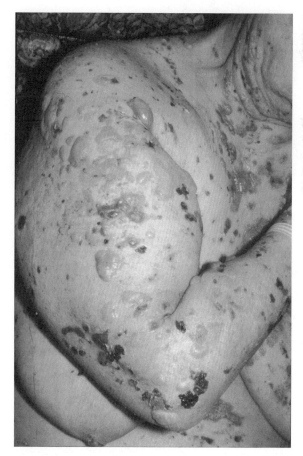

▲ **Figure 49–17.** Bullous pemphigoid. One- to 3-cm tense blisters with secondary erosions and hemorrhagic crusts. (Reproduced with permission from Dana Sachs, MD.)

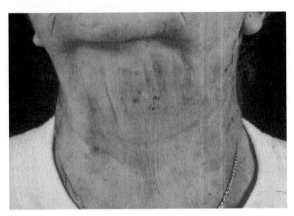

▲ **Figure 49–18.** Urticarial bullous pemphigoid. Erythematous slightly edematous plaques with pinpoint hemorrhagic crusts and excoriations.

2 biopsies to confirm the diagnosis. A 4-mm punch biopsy of the edge of a blister demonstrates a subepidermal split with eosinophils and lymphocytes. A perilesional biopsy for direct immunofluorescence demonstrates binding of immunoglobulin G and C3 in a linear pattern along the basement membrane zone.

▶ Complications

Complications are usually caused by extensive scratching, which causes erosions and ulcers that may become secondarily infected and eventually scar.

▶ Treatment

Superpotent topical corticosteroids can be used successfully in localized disease (less than 5% total body surface area) with significantly lower risks than oral corticosteroids.

Nicotinamide (1.5 g/day) in combination with minocycline (100 mg twice a day) or tetracycline (2 g/day) can be tried in patients with contraindications to oral corticosteroids that did not adequately respond to topical therapy alone.

Oral corticosteroid therapy has been widely used and is very effective when used in high doses and tapered over a long period of time (eg, prednisone 0.5–1 mg/kg tapered slowly over 6–12 months); however, in older adults, the side effects can be substantial, including osteoporosis, diabetes, and hypertension. For patients taking >5 mg/day for more than 3 months, prophylaxis against osteoporosis includes initiation of a bisphosphonate and daily calcium (1500 mg/day) and vitamin D (800 IU/day) supplementation.

Difficult-to-treat cases should be referred to a dermatologist for treatment with a steroid-sparing immunosuppressive agent, such as methotrexate, cyclosporine, azathioprine, or mycophenolate mofetil.

▶ Prognosis

BP is a chronic disease with multiple remissions and exacerbations. Morbidity and mortality are increased in patients with BP, but can be reduced with adequate and prompt treatment.

ACTINIC KERATOSIS

 ESSENTIALS OF DIAGNOSIS

▶ Actinic keratosis is a precursor lesion to squamous cell carcinoma.
▶ Distribution of lesions includes the face, lips, ears, dorsal hands, and forearms (photodistribution).
▶ Primary lesions are 3–10-mm rough, adherent, scaly white papules and plaques (Figure 49–19), often on an erythematous base.
▶ Palpation reveals a gritty, sandpaper-like texture. Lesions are often more readily palpated than visualized.
▶ Differential diagnosis includes dry seborrheic keratosis and retention hyperkeratosis.

▶ General Principles in Older Adults

Actinic keratoses are more common in whites and are directly related to cumulative lifetime sun exposure. Immunosuppressed patients, particularly transplant

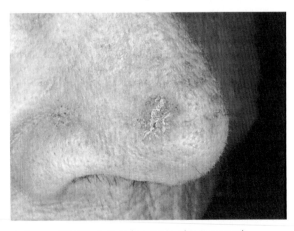

▲ **Figure 49–19.** Actinic keratosis. This is a rough, adherent, scaly papule on the right nasal bridge.

recipients, are at higher risk for actinic keratoses. Daily sunscreen, long-sleeve shirts, broad-brimmed hats, and avoidance of sun can prevent these lesions.

Complications

Conversion rates of actinic keratoses to nonmelanoma skin cancers are estimated to range from 6% to 10% over a 10-year period.

Treatment

Cryotherapy (see Box 49–1) with 2 freeze–thaw cycles is recommended for actinic keratoses. For extensive actinic damage field therapy using a topical treatment is recommended. Imiquimod 5% cream and 5-fluorouracil 5% cream are 2 FDA-approved medications for topical treatment of actinic keratoses.

5-Fluorouracil 5% cream is applied twice a day for 3–4 weeks until the end point of erythema and crusting is attained. The application is then discontinued and the skin is allowed to heal. Application of topical corticosteroids may be needed if the reaction is exuberant or the patient experiences extensive pruritus. Cure rate is approximately 50% (ie, 50% of patients have complete clearance of all lesions).

Imiquimod 5% cream is applied twice a week for 16 weeks. Reactions to imiquimod are less predictable that those with 5-fluorouracil as the molecule is an immunomodulator and its action depends on the host's immune status. Cure rate is around 50%.

The main drawbacks of topical treatment are severe inflammatory reactions that may be uncomfortable and possibly lead to scarring. Imiquimod may also cause a systemic inflammatory response with flu-like symptoms, fevers, chills, and malaise. The added benefit of topical therapy is treatment of subclinical lesions.

Patients with actinic keratoses should be examined annually and are also at risk for basal cell carcinoma, squamous cell carcinoma, and melanoma.

BASAL CELL CARCINOMA

ESSENTIALS OF DIAGNOSIS

▶ Basal cell carcinoma is the most common skin cancer (~75%) and is related to chronic ultraviolet light exposure.

▶ Basal cell carcinoma is derived from stem cells in the basal layer of the epidermis.

▶ The head and neck are most frequently involved; the nose is the most common site.

▶ Primary lesions are translucent or pearly papules or nodules (Figure 49–20), often with visible telangiectasias. Secondary changes include central ulceration or crusting.

▶ Chief complaint is that the lesion "breaks down, bleeds, or does not heal".

▶ Biopsy (rolled shave or punch technique) is required to confirm the diagnosis.

▶ Squamous cell carcinoma, keratoacanthoma, and sebaceous hyperplasia are included in the differential diagnosis.

Complications

Although basal cell carcinoma (BCC) rarely metastasizes, if left untreated, it may become locally invasive and extend to underlying cartilage, fascia, muscle, and bone.

Treatment

Electrodesiccation and curettage (ED&C) and excision have comparable cure rates of 90% for low-risk tumors.

Mohs surgery is the most effective technique (98% to 100% cure rate) and is indicated for high-risk tumors.

Topical therapy for biopsy-proven superficial BCC may be performed with either 5-fluorouracil 5% cream or imiquimod 5% cream on small lesions (less than 2 cm) located on the trunk and proximal extremities. Cure rates are around 90% for 5-fluorouracil and 80% for imiquimod 5% cream. Patient adherence to the manufacturers' treatment regimen is required to achieve these cure rates.

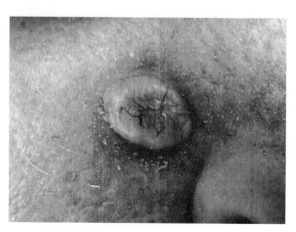

▲ **Figure 49–20.** Basal cell carcinoma. A 1.5-cm shiny nodule with telangiectasias adjacent to the right nasal ala.

▶ Prognosis

BCC patients determined to be at high risk for recurrence and metastasis have 1 or more of the following: recurrent tumor; tumor on the trunk and extremities >2 cm; tumor on the head and neck >1 cm; tumor with poorly defined borders; tumor with immunosuppressed host; and tumor occurring at a site of prior radiation. Recurrence rate with standard modalities (ED&C or excision) for these high risk tumors is >10%.

For patients with a prior BCC, the 3-year cumulative risk for BCC recurrence is approximately 44%. For most patients, an annual skin exam is sufficient for detecting new BCCs. Because the number of previous skin cancers is a strong risk factor for subsequent skin cancers, patients with multiple BCCs should be seen more frequently.

SQUAMOUS CELL CARCINOMA

ESSENTIALS OF DIAGNOSIS

▶ Squamous cell carcinoma is derived from keratinocytes above the basal layer of the epidermis, often with actinic keratoses as precursor lesions.

▶ The head, neck, dorsal hands, and forearms are affected.

▶ Primary lesions are firm indurated papules, plaques, or nodules (Figure 49–21). Secondary changes include rough adherent scale, central erosion, or ulceration with crust.

▶ The lesion does not heal and breaks down or bleeds.

▶ Biopsy with rolled shave or punch technique is required to confirm the diagnosis.

▶ Differential diagnosis includes basal cell carcinoma and keratoacanthoma.

▶ General Principles in Older Adults

Squamous cell carcinoma (SCC) comprises approximately 20% of all skin cancers and has the capacity to metastasize. If SCC is suspected, palpation of regional lymph nodes is recommended. SCC should be suspected in any persistent nodule, plaque, or ulcer, especially when occurring in sun-damaged skin, on the lower lip, in areas of prior radiation, in old burn scars, or on the genitals. Immunosuppressed patients (eg, transplant recipients) are at higher risk for SCC because of impaired cell-mediated immunity.

▶ Complications

SCC on the lips or ears has a 10% to 15% risk of spread to cervical nodes. The overall rate of metastasis from all skin sites ranges from <1% to 5%.

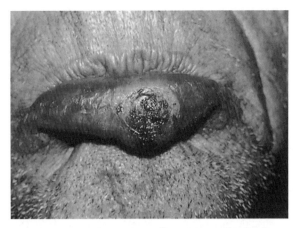

▲ **Figure 49–21.** Squamous cell carcinoma. This hard 2.5 × 2.5-cm nodule with overlying dry hemorrhagic crust is at risk for spread to cervical nodes. (Reproduced with permission from Melvin Lu, MD.)

▶ Treatment

ED&C and excision have comparable cure rates of 90% for low-risk tumors. Mohs surgery is the most effective technique (98% to 100% cure rate) and is indicated for high-risk tumors.

▶ Prognosis

SCC patients considered to be at high risk for recurrence and metastasis have 1 or more of the following: recurrent tumor; tumor on the trunk and extremities >2 cm; tumor on the head and neck >1 cm; tumor occurring on the genitals, lips, ears, site of prior radiation, or scar; tumor with poorly defined borders; and tumor with immunosuppressed host. Recurrence rate with standard modalities (ED&C or excision) is greater than 10%.

For patients with a prior SCC, the 3-year cumulative risk for another SCC is approximately 18%. Annual follow-up examinations for at least 3 years is recommended. Because the number of previous skin cancers is a strong risk factor for subsequent skin cancers, patients with multiple SCCs should be seen more frequently.

MELANOMA

ESSENTIALS OF DIAGNOSIS

▶ Melanoma, derived from melanocytes, has the greatest potential for metastasis.

▶ The trunk and legs are affected more than the face and neck, although the face and neck are more likely to be affected in older adults.

▶ The primary lesion is a brown–black macule, papule, plaque, or nodule with ≥1 of the following features (Figure 49–22): asymmetry, border irregularity, color variegation, diameter >6 mm.

▶ Patients may notice an increase in size (diameter) of a pigmented lesion and bleeding.

▶ Lesions should be excised with a margin of clinically normal skin down to subcutaneous fat.

▶ Differential diagnosis includes seborrheic keratosis, solar lentigo, dysplastic nevus, and pigmented BCC.

General Principles in Older Adults

The incidence of melanoma is increasing faster than any other cancer. The lifetime probability of developing melanoma in an individual in the United States born in 2012 is estimated at 1 in 36 for a man, and 1 in 55 for a woman. Melanoma is the fifth most common cancer in men and the sixth most common cancer in women.

Older men have the highest incidence of melanoma and the highest mortality rates from melanoma. In the United States, the incidence of thick tumors (>4 mm) has continued to increase in men 60 years of age and older. Nearly 50% of all melanoma deaths involve white men 50 years of age and older.

Risk factors include light complexion (red–blond hair), blistering sunburns during childhood, tendency to tan poorly and sunburn easily, and a positive family history. Additional risk factors in the middle-aged population include age >50 years, male sex, and a history of actinic keratoses or nonmelanoma skin cancers.

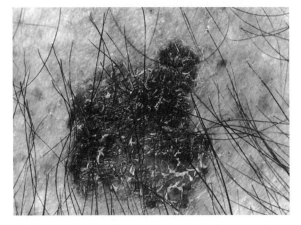

▲ **Figure 49–22.** Melanoma. A 2 × 2-cm plaque on the chest with varying shades of brown to black, asymmetry, and irregular borders.

Complications

Untreated melanoma has a high risk of metastasis to lymph nodes, liver, lungs, and brain.

Treatment

Melanoma is treated by surgical excision with margins determined by histologic tumor thickness (Breslow depth). Evaluation of nodal involvement with sentinel lymph node biopsy is recommended for primary melanomas deeper than 1 mm and for tumors ≤1 mm when histologic ulceration or mitoses are present. Frequency of follow-up, laboratory tests, and imaging studies depends on stage of disease.

Prognosis

Tumor thickness and presence or absence of histologic ulceration are the most important prognostic factors. Patients with thin melanomas (<1 mm) have the best prognosis (>90% 5-year survival rate), whereas those with thick tumors (>4 mm) have a 49% 5-year survival rate. For patients with nodal involvement, the number of affected nodes determines the overall prognosis.

Balch CM, Gershenwald JE, Soong SJ, et al. Final version of 2009 AJCC melanoma staging and classification. *J Clin Oncol.* 2009;27(36):6199-6206.

Currie BJ, McCarthy JS. Permethrin and Ivermectin for scabies. *N Engl J Med.* 2010;362(8):717-725.

Draelos ZD. The multifunctionality of 10% sodium sulfacetamide, 5% sulfur emollient foam in the treatment of inflammatory facial dermatoses. *J Drugs Dermatol.* 2010;9(3):234-236.

Giesse JK, Rich P, Pandya A, et al. Imiquimod 5% cream for the treatment of superficial basal cell carcinoma: A double-blind, randomized, vehicle-controlled study. *J Am Acad Dermatol.* 2002;47(3):390-398.

Marcil I, Stern RS. Risk of developing a subsequent nonmelanoma skin cancer in patients with a history of nonmelanoma skin cancer. *Arch Dermatol.* 2000;136(12):1524-1530.

National Comprehensive Cancer Network (NCCN) clinical practice guidelines in oncology. Basal cell and squamous cell skin cancers. Version 2.2013. http://www.nccn.org/professionals/physician_gls/pdf/nmsc.pdf

National Comprehensive Cancer Network (NCCN) clinical practice guidelines in oncology. Melanoma. Version 3.2014. http://www.nccn.org/professionals/physician_gls/pdf/melanoma.pdf

Sigurgeirsson B Olafsson JH, Steinsson JB, Paul C, Billstein S, Evans EG. Long-term effectiveness of treatment with terbinafine vs itraconazole in onychomycosis: a 5-year blinded prospective follow-up study. *Arch Dermatol.* 2002;138(3):353-357.

Sullivan JR, Shear NH. Drug eruptions and other adverse drug effects in aged skin. *Clin Geriatr Med.* 2002;18(1):21-42.

Walker GJ, Johnstone PW. Interventions for treating scabies. *Cochrane Database Syst Rev.* 2000;(2):CD000320.

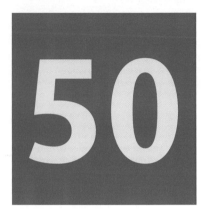

Sleep Disorders

Diana V. Jao, MD
Cathy A. Alessi, MD

▶ Patients with insomnia may have complaints of poor sleep quality, daytime fatigue, irritability, or problems with concentration.

▶ Nighttime symptoms of sleep apnea may include snoring, choking, and altered breathing.

▶ Some sleep disorders are common with neurologic disorders, such as dementia and Parkinson disease.

▶ Depending on the particular sleep disorder, diagnoses are made clinically or using polysomnography.

▶ General Principles in Older Adults

The Institute of Medicine's report, "Sleep Disorders and Sleep Deprivation: An Unmet Public Health Problem," highlighted the prevalence and associated deleterious health consequences of these issues. Sleep difficulties and several primary sleep disorders increase in prevalence with age. However, in older adults, insomnia is most often associated with other conditions, rather than presenting as a primary insomnia. This "comorbid insomnia" often coexists with and can exacerbate or lead to additional medical and psychosocial conditions. For this reason, sleep disorders in older adults should often be approached as a geriatric syndrome as the causes are generally multifactorial.

The prevalence of sleep difficulties varies based on how these problems are identified and defined, but studies suggest that more than 50% of community-dwelling older persons and >65% of long-term care facility residents experience sleeping difficulties. Many community-dwelling older persons use nonprescription or prescribed sleeping medications.

Sleep architecture can be described based on findings of polysomnography, which involves multiple channels (eg, electroencephalogram, electrooculogram, electromyogram) of physiologic recording during sleep. Based on polysomnography, sleep can be categorized into 2 states: nonrapid eye movement (NREM) and rapid eye movement (REM) sleep. NREM sleep is further divided into 3 stages, where N1 is the lightest sleep, N2 is where the majority of sleep time is spent, and N3 is deep sleep. N1 and N2 sleep increase with age, whereas N3 sleep decreases. Altered sleep patterns include decreased sleep efficiency (time asleep as percentage of time in bed), decreased total sleep time, increased sleep latency (time to fall asleep), more arousals during the night, more daytime napping, and other changes.

Patients may not report sleep complaints unless specifically asked. Presenting symptoms overlap significantly among common sleep disorders (Figure 50–1).

INSOMNIA

▶ Clinical Findings

A. Symptoms & Signs

Occasional difficulty falling asleep or staying asleep is common. To diagnose insomnia, the *International Classification of Sleep Disorders*—2nd edition (ICSD2), requires that the individual must have a sleep complaint (ie, difficulty initiating sleep, difficulty maintaining sleep, waking up too early, or sleep that is nonrestorative or of poor quality), the sleep complaint must occur despite adequate opportunity and circumstances for sleep, and there must be daytime impairment related to the nighttime sleeping difficulty (eg, fatigue or malaise, mood disturbance or irritability, daytime sleepiness). Insomnia can be classified based on symptom duration, but definitions based on duration vary. Generally, insomnia must be present for at least a month to be considered a chronic insomnia.

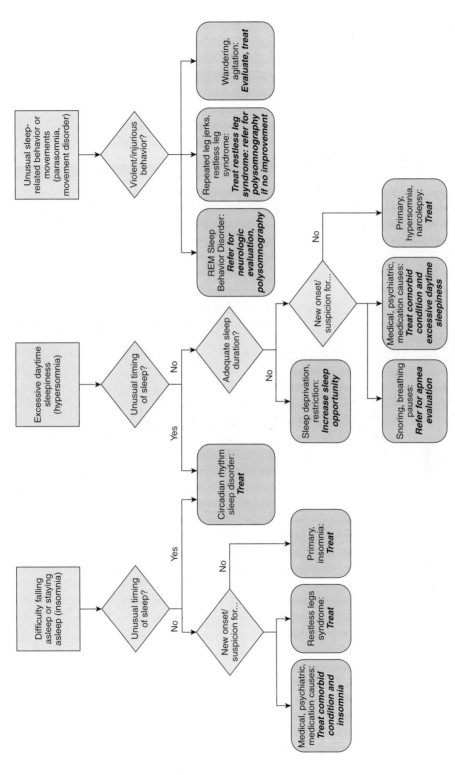

▲ **Figure 50-1.** Evidence-based recommendations for the assessment and management of sleep disorders in older persons. (Reproduced with permission from Bloom HG, Ahmed I, Alessi CA, et al. Evidence-based recommendations for the assessment of sleep disorders in older persons. *J Am Geriatr Soc.* 2009;57(5):761-789.)

B. Patient History

A detailed history is essential in determining the causes of insomnia. Key factors include recent stressors, and symptoms of depression, anxiety, or other psychiatric disorders.

C. Special Tests

Instruments that can be helpful in the evaluation of insomnia include sleep questionnaires, sleep logs, symptom checklists, psychological screening tests, and interviews of bed partners. Examples of self-administered questionnaires are the Insomnia Severity Index (specific to insomnia) and the Pittsburgh Sleep Quality Index (a general questionnaire of sleep problems). Polysomnography and/or wrist actigraphy (which estimates sleep and wakefulness based on wrist movements) are not indicated for the routine evaluation of insomnia unless suggested by signs and symptoms of comorbid sleep disorders. Laboratory tests should be similarly guided based on signs or symptoms of comorbid conditions that appear associated with the insomnia.

▶ Differential Diagnosis

In older adults, psychological problems, symptoms related to underlying medical illnesses, and the effects of medications are common causes of insomnia. Often, multiple factors may contribute to insomnia in the older patient.

Many medical conditions can interfere with sleep, including chronic pain, dyspnea, gastroesophageal reflux disease, and nocturia. Medications reportedly account for 10% to 15% of cases of insomnia. Table 50–1 lists common offending agents. Many other agents can disrupt sleep, including caffeine and nicotine. Caffeine is an ingredient in many nonprescription medications and foods, and many people are unaware that they are ingesting caffeine-containing products. Nighttime alcohol use, while causing initial drowsiness, can interfere with sleep architecture later in the night and worsen sleep. Withdrawal from sedative–hypnotic agents can also lead to worsening insomnia.

▶ Treatment

A. Behavioral

Most published guidelines recommend psychological and behavioral treatments as first-line therapy for the management of chronic insomnia. Cognitive–behavioral therapy for insomnia generally combines several treatments, including stimulus control, sleep restriction and cognitive therapy. Stimulus control promotes behaviors such as establishing regular morning rising and bedtimes, using the bedroom only for sleep and sexual activity, going to bed only when sleepy and getting out of bed if unable to fall asleep, and avoiding or limiting naps. Sleep restriction therapy seeks to

Table 50–1. Agents that can cause insomnia.

Cardiovascular Medications
Furosemide
Beta blockers
Respiratory Medications
Pseudoephedrine
Beta agonists
Theophylline
Phenylpropanolamine[a]
Antidepressants
Bupropion
Fluoxetine
Paroxetine
Sertraline
Venlafaxine
Others
Corticosteroids
Cimetidine
Phenytoin
Caffeine and caffeine-containing drugs
Nicotine
Alcohol

[a]Removed from the U.S. market, but still available in Europe.

improve sleep efficiency by causing modest sleep deprivation (by limiting time in bed) and then gradually increasing time in bed as sleep efficiency improves. Cognitive therapy focuses on correcting inaccurate ideas and thoughts about sleep. Cognitive–behavioral therapy for insomnia is generally provided by a psychologist with expertise in behavioral sleep medicine, but simpler approaches have been developed and tested for use by other personnel, such as nurses.

Sleep hygiene is often a component of more comprehensive behavioral interventions for insomnia. Sleep hygiene addresses lifestyle and environmental factors (Table 50–2). However, simple sleep hygiene alone is rarely effective in the patient with a longstanding, severe chronic insomnia. Other behavioral interventions may include meditation and relaxation techniques to guide patients in recognizing and relieving tension and anxiety.

B. Pharmacologic

1. Prescription medications—Pharmacologic agents (Table 50–3) can be considered if behavioral interventions

Table 50–2. Examples of measures to improve sleep hygiene.

1. Regular morning rising time.
2. Avoid daytime napping or limit to <1 hour in the morning or early afternoon.
3. Exercise during the day but not in the evening and before bedtime.
4. Avoid caffeine, nicotine, and alcohol in the evening.
5. Avoid excessive fluid intake at night to reduce nighttime urination.
6. Avoid large meals before bedtime, but a light snack may promote sleep.
7. Follow a nighttime routine of preparation for bedtime and wear comfortable bedclothes.
8. Ensure a comfortable nighttime environment, minimizing noise and light and keeping room temperature comfortable.

are not fully successful, or the patient has an acute problem with insomnia and the benefits appear to outweigh the risks of these medications. Thoughtful selection of agents to minimize adverse side effects and drug interactions is reached by evaluating symptom types (eg, problem with sleep onset vs. awakening during the night), agent characteristics, comorbid conditions, and cost. In older adults, the starting dose should be the lowest available. Patient dosage self-adjustment should be discouraged.

Benzodiazepines and related drugs are commonly prescribed for sleep. Long-acting benzodiazepines (eg, flurazepam) should not be used in older patients because of the risk of daytime carryover (sedation), falls, and fractures. Short- and intermediate-acting benzodiazepines can be used in older people; however, caution is warranted because of the risk of tolerance to the hypnotic effects of the medication and

the potential for rebound insomnia on withdrawal. These agents also result in an increased risk of falls, and their half-life can be longer in older people.

Nonbenzodiazepine hypnotics may have fewer side effects, and less daytime carryover, compared with benzodiazepines. Although structurally different from benzodiazepines, these agents also act at the gamma-aminobutyric acid (GABA) benzodiazepine receptor, but perhaps with greater specificity for sedative effects. In the United States, currently available nonbenzodiazepine agents include zolpidem, zaleplon, and eszopiclone (see Table 50–3). Caution is also warranted in the use of these newer sleeping medications for the management of chronic insomnia in older adults.

The melatonin receptor agonist ramelteon is approved for sleep-onset insomnia. It is not a scheduled agent. With a half-life of 2.6 hours, it has been shown to reduce sleep latency and to increase total sleep time without rebound or withdrawal effects.

There is some evidence for using a low-dose sedating antidepressant at night (with a more stimulating antidepressant during the day) for depressed patients who also report insomnia. Most published guidelines discourage use of a sedating antidepressant for insomnia unless the patient has failed other agents, or has an indication for an antidepressant. Low-dose doxepin is the only antidepressant that has been FDA approved for insomnia. However, like other sedating tricyclic antidepressants (eg, amitriptyline), it is not recommended for use in older patients because of its strong anticholinergic side effects.

2. Nonprescription medications—Nonprescription sleeping aids often contain a sedating antihistamine (eg, diphenhydramine) alone or in combination with an analgesic. Diphenhydramine and similar compounds are not recommended for older people because of potent anticholinergic

Table 50–3. Examples of commonly used prescription sleeping medications in older people.

Generic Name (Trade Names)	Class	Usual Dose Range in Older People	Half-Life
Temazepam (Restoril)	Intermediate-acting benzodiazepine	7.5–15 mg	3.5–18.4 h
Zolpidem (Ambien)	Benzodiazepine receptor agonist	5 mg	1.5–4.5 h (10 h in cirrhosis)
Zolpidem extended-release (Ambien CR)	Benzodiazepine receptor agonist	6.25 mg	?
Zolpidem sublingual (Edluar)	Benzodiazepine receptor agonist	5 mg	2.4 h
Zolpidem low dose sublingual (Intermezzo)	Benzodiazepine receptor agonist	1.75 mg	2.4 h
Zolpidem oral spray (Zolpimist)	Benzodiazepine receptor agonist	5 mg	2.5 h (?)
Zaleplon (Sonata)	Benzodiazepine receptor agonist	5 mg	1 h
Eszopiclone (Lunesta)	Benzodiazepine receptor agonist	1–2 mg	6 h
Low-dose doxepin (Silenor)	Sedating antidepressant	3–6 mg	15 h
Trazodone (Desyrel) (off-label)	Sedating antidepressant	25–150 mg	2–4 h

effects and the development of tolerance to sedating effects over time. A bedtime dose of an analgesic agent alone (eg, acetaminophen) may be safe and helpful if pain disrupts sleep. The herbal product valerian does not have sufficient evidence to support routine use. However, there is some evidence for use of prolonged-release melatonin.

SLEEP APNEA

▶ General Principles in Older Adults

Sleep apnea is the repetitive cessation (or marked decrease) of airflow during sleep. In obstructive sleep apnea (OSA), the cessation or decrease in breathing is associated with continued ventilatory effort.

▶ Clinical Findings

A. Symptoms & Signs

Increased body mass index is an important predictor of sleep apnea, although the relationship between obesity and OSA is not as strong in older adults, and many older adults with OSA are not obese. The prevalence of OSA is higher in men than women, and in older age groups. Prevalence rates of OSA of up to 40% are reported in people age 65 years and older. There is also a higher prevalence of OSA among older adults with dementia. OSA is common among patients presenting with insomnia, although excessive daytime sleepiness is the most frequent complaint. Other associated signs or symptoms include poorly controlled hypertension and morning headache. The bed partner may be very helpful in reporting loud snoring, choking and gasping sounds, or apneic periods.

The clinical consequences of sleep apnea are related to sleep fragmentation, hypoxia, and hypercapnia. Sleep apnea, especially if untreated, is associated with cardiovascular diseases such as hypertension and coronary artery disease, and increased mortality rates. Other adverse consequences include cognitive impairment and a higher rate of motor vehicle accidents.

B. Screening Methods

Polysomnography in an overnight sleep laboratory remains the gold standard in diagnosing OSA. If unavailable, an ambulatory (home-based, outpatient) approach is an alternative. The optimal patients for home testing are those with high suspicion for OSA with no comorbidities (eg, chronic obstructive pulmonary disease and congestive heart failure) that may require medical attention during the study period. Limitations may include the need for a repeat or formal laboratory study to confirm negative results or resolve technical issues (such as monitoring leads slipping off during sleep). In addition, most ambulatory sleep monitoring systems do not screen for other sleep disorders, such as parasomnias (eg, abnormal nocturnal movements and REM behavior disorder).

▶ Treatment

Positive airway pressure (PAP) is the treatment standard for moderate-to-severe OSA as defined by the apnea-hypopnea index (AHI), the sum of apneas and hypopneas per hour of sleep. One classification suggests that AHI >30 per hour denotes severe OSA, 16–30 per hour that of moderate OSA, and 5–15 per hour for mild OSA. Consistent PAP use improves hypertension and congestive heart failure treatment responses and may also rectify some metabolic problems such as lipid abnormalities. The primary challenge with PAP usage is adherence. Initial experience with PAP is predictive of use as adherence is often established as early as the first week. Initial close follow-up to resolve issues interfering with regular use may promote long-term adherence.

Auto-adjusting positive airway pressure (APAP) is gaining more interest for use in uncomplicated moderate-to-severe OSA. Instead of supplying a continuous fixed pressure (as in continuous PAP), APAP titrates to the minimum pressure that will sustain airway patency. Effective pressure can vary with body position and weight fluctuation.

Alternatively, some patients may respond better to bi-level PAP. A sleep specialist will use polysomnography results to determine the most appropriate treatment.

Patients should be advised to avoid alcohol and sedative use, and to lose weight if obese. For those who fail or are unable to tolerate PAP treatment, other approaches may be considered. Oral–dental devices that reposition the jaw or tongue can be tried. Surgical procedures (eg, laser-assisted uvuloplasty, mandibular-maxillary advancement) offer mixed results, with little evidence for use in older adults. Although rarely performed for this indication, tracheostomy may be appropriate for those with severe life-threatening OSA who do not respond to other therapies.

PERIODIC LIMB MOVEMENT DURING SLEEP & RESTLESS LEGS SYNDROME

▶ General Principles in Older Adults

Among older adults, the prevalence of periodic limb movements during sleep (PLMS) ranges from 20% to 60% and for restless leg syndrome (RLS) from 2% to 15%. RLS may cause insomnia and nighttime restlessness and discomfort. RLS and PLMS often coexist; the latter are present in 80% of patients with RLS. Prevalence of PLMS increases with age and appears to be higher in those of Northern and Western European descent and lower in Asians. The cause of both conditions is unknown, but increased age, family history, uremia, and low iron stores have been suggested as risk factors.

Clinical Findings

A. Symptoms & Signs

PLMS is characterized by recurring episodes of stereotypic rhythmic movements during sleep, generally involving the legs. The diagnosis of PLMS is reserved for individuals with PLMS that causes a sleep disturbance that is not explained by the presence of another disorder. Many patients who exhibit PLMS-like movements are asymptomatic or may have another sleep disorder (eg, OSA).

RLS has 4 features: (a) an uncontrollable urge to move the legs, usually accompanied or caused by uncomfortable and unpleasant sensations in the legs, (b) symptoms begin or worsen during periods of rest or inactivity, (c) symptoms are partially or entirely relieved with movement, and (d) symptoms are worse in the evening or night.

B. Special Tests

The diagnosis of PLMS, but not RLS, requires polysomnography. RLS is diagnosed clinically based on history. Subjective scales such as the International RLS Rating Scale may help evaluate RLS severity and assess treatment outcomes. Patients with RLS should be screened for iron deficiency with a serum ferritin test.

Treatment

The treatment of PLMS depends on the severity of symptoms and their impact on the patient's general well-being. If another sleep disorder is present (eg, OSA), that disorder should be treated first, as PLMS-like movements may improve with treatment of that disorder.

RLS may improve with leg stretching, and avoidance of caffeine, alcohol, and medications that precipitate symptoms, such as antihistamines, antidepressants, and promotility agents. A low ferritin should prompt iron replacement (and appropriate evaluation of iron deficiency) as RLS symptoms may resolve after iron replacement.

Pharmacotherapy should be considered for RLS when these maneuvers are ineffective or when symptoms are severe. Medication choice should depend on evidence of effectiveness and comorbid conditions. Dopaminergic agents are the best studied agents for both RLS and PLMS and are considered to be the treatment of choice in older patients. Treatment near bedtime with a dopamine agonist (eg, pramipexole 0.125 mg, ropinirole 0.25 mg or higher) may be effective for both RLS and PLMS. Adverse effects of dopamine agonists include excessive daytime sleepiness, hallucinations and compulsive behaviors (eg, uncontrolled shopping, gambling, eating, and sexual urges). Carbidopa-levodopa (one-half to 1 full tablet of 25/100-mg tablets, or higher) has also been suggested. Rebound symptoms (which occur as the medication wears off) or augmentation (shift of symptoms to early in the day) can occur with treatment. Augmentation is more common

with carbidopa-levodopa than with the dopamine agonists. Both rebound and augmentation resolve with medication discontinuation. There is also some evidence for use of gabapentin in RLS. Opioids such as oxycodone and hydrocodone may help patients with severe symptoms unresponsive to other therapies, but the side effects of these agents may limit their usefulness for RLS in the older patient.

NARCOLEPSY

General Principles in Older Adults

Narcolepsy is a disorder of recurrent, uncontrollable, brief episodes of sleep that interfere with wakefulness, and which are often associated with hypnagogic hallucinations (which occur near the onset of sleep or awakening), cataplexy, and sleep paralysis. This disorder generally presents in adolescence or young adulthood, and only rarely presents for the first time in old age.

Clinical Findings

A. Symptoms & Signs

The key clinical features of narcolepsy are excessive daytime sleepiness and cataplexy (a sudden and transient loss of muscle tone triggered by emotions). Other common symptoms include sleep paralysis (a transient inability to move or speak during the transition between sleep and wakefulness) and hypnagogic hallucinations (ie, vivid perceptions at the onset of sleep).

B. Special Tests

Polysomnography typically reveals a shortened sleep latency and sleep-onset REM (ie, REM sleep present soon after sleep onset). A structured daytime sleep study, the Multiple Sleep Latency Test (MSLT), is performed to determine the extent of daytime sleepiness and to identify sleep episodes with early onset of REM. In patients without typical cataplexy, the diagnosis of narcolepsy requires performance of nighttime polysomnography and MSLT.

Differential Diagnosis

Narcolepsy can be complicated by other sleep disorders, including sleep apnea, periodic limb movements, and REM behavior disorder. These other disorders would generally be identified during polysomnography.

Treatment

Nonpharmacologic interventions involve maximizing nighttime sleep, supplemented by scheduled daytime naps, and avoiding emotional situations that precipitate attacks.

Various medications are available including stimulants such as modafinil, selective serotonin reuptake inhibitors (SSRIs), serotonin–norepinephrine reuptake inhibitors, tricyclic antidepressants, and sodium oxybate for severe cataplexy. Treatment of narcolepsy typically requires input from a sleep specialist.

CIRCADIAN RHYTHM SLEEP DISORDERS

▶ General Principles in Older Adults

Circadian rhythm sleep disorders (CRSDs) may be primarily intrinsic (eg, advanced sleep phase, delayed sleep phase) or situational, as in time zone change (jet lag) syndrome or shiftwork disorders. Correlations have been made between changes in circadian rhythms and advancing age.

▶ Clinical Findings

A. Symptoms & Signs

Commonly, older people experience an advanced sleep phase, which leads to a pattern of an early bedtime and early morning awakening. The alteration in circadian rhythm can be marked in people who are bed-bound. When the internal clock is completely desynchronized, as may occur in severe neurodegenerative disorders, the sleep–wake cycles become irregular, with sleep occurring during the day and wakefulness at night or alternating periods of sleep and wakefulness throughout the 24-hour period. This irregular pattern is particularly common among nursing home residents.

B. Special Tests

Wrist actigraphy and/or sleep logs can be used for making a diagnosis and for monitoring treatment response. Polysomnography is indicated when the diagnosis is unclear or another sleep disorder is suspected.

▶ Treatment

Depending on the specific CRSD, treatments may include appropriately timed bright light exposure, appropriately timed melatonin use, prescribed sleep scheduling, and other measures. Special expertise is generally needed in the management of severe, chronic CRSDs.

REM BEHAVIOR DISORDER

▶ General Principles in Older Adults

Although rare in the general population, REM behavior disorder (RBD) usually presents in late life, more commonly in men than women.

▶ Clinical Findings

A. Symptoms & Signs

RBD presents with symptoms of dream enactment behavior along with a lack of the normal muscle atonia present during REM sleep. Patients act out dreams with forceful movements and behaviors during sleep. They usually present for medical care as a result of injury to themselves or their bed partners; these injuries can be quite severe. Medications such as SSRIs or other antidepressants can precipitate RBD. It has also has been associated with brain disorders, including dementia and stroke. It is particularly common among the neurodegenerative disorders termed *synucleinopathies*, including Parkinson disease, Lewy body dementia, and multiple system atrophy.

B. Special Tests

Polysomnography is required to confirm the diagnosis and to rule out other conditions.

▶ Treatment

Environmental measures should be taken to make the sleeping environment safe for the patient and the bed partner. Evidence-based guidelines suggest the use of nighttime clonazepam for RBD. However, caution is warranted in using clonazepam in older adults, especially if there is comorbid OSA, dementia, or gait disorders. There is some evidence for using melatonin in older adults and acetylcholinesterase inhibitors (eg, donepezil) to treat RBD in older patients with neurodegenerative disorders.

SLEEP PROBLEMS IN SPECIAL POPULATIONS

A. Sleep Patterns In Dementia

Most research on sleep problems with dementia has focused on Alzheimer disease. Compared with older people without dementia, those with dementia have more sleep disruption, more arousals and lower sleep efficiency. Sundowning, a worsening of confusion or agitated behaviors at night, is present in 12% to 20% of patients with dementia. Their inability to voice their symptoms or actively participate in their care may also compound sleep difficulties. Antipsychotic and sedative hypnotic agents have not been consistently effective. Sensory interventions (aromatherapy, thermal bath and calming music with hand massage) may be beneficial. Polysomnography does not appear to be clinically useful in diagnosing sleep changes with dementia, but may be useful in select cases where primary sleep disorders (eg, OSA) are suspected and if treatment would be warranted.

B. Sleep Disturbance in Long-Term Care Facility Residents

Superimposed on the multifactorial etiologies leading to sleep problems in older adults, long-term care residents have other factors that may contribute to sleep disturbance. The common pattern of sleep disturbance among these residents involves frequent nighttime arousals and daytime sleeping. Many factors seem to affect quality of sleep, including multiple physical illnesses and medications that can interfere with sleep, debility and inactivity, increased prevalence of primary sleep disorders, minimal sunlight exposure, and environmental factors, including frequent nighttime noise and light and disruptive nighttime nursing care activities.

An increase in daytime activity levels to enhance wakefulness may lead to improved nighttime sleep in nursing home residents. Socialization and exercise programs are modestly helpful. Bright light therapy may also improve total nighttime sleep and decrease daytime sleeping. Reduction of nighttime noise and consistent sleep hygiene practices are also recommended. Application of multicomponent nonpharmacological interventions to improve sleep/wake patterns in nursing home residents may have some modest effect but results are mixed.

Bloom HG, Ahmed I, Alessi CA, et al. Evidence-based recommendations for the assessment and management of sleep disorders in older persons. *J Am Geriatr Soc.* 2009;57(5):761-789.

Vaz Fragoso CA, Gill TM. Sleep complaints in community-living older persons: a multifactorial geriatric syndrome. *J Am Geriatr Soc.* 2007;55(11):1853-1866.

USEFUL WEBSITES

American Academy of Sleep Medicine. http://www.aasmnet.org

National Institutes of Health National Center on Sleep Disorders Research. http://www.nhlbi.nih.gov/sleep

National Sleep Foundation. http://www.sleepfoundation.org

Sleep Research Society. http://www.sleepresearchsociety.org

▶ Sleep Questionnaires

Insomnia Severity Index. http://www.journalsleep.org/ViewAbstract.aspx?pid=28127

Pittsburg Sleep Quality Index. http://www.sleep.pitt.edu/content.asp?id=1484

International Restless Leg Rating Scale. http://www.medicine.ox.ac.uk/bandolier/booth/RLS/RLSratingscale.pdf

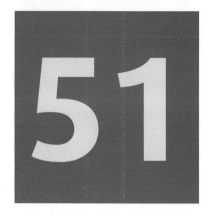

Oral Diseases & Disorders

Dick Gregory, DDS, FASGD

Bonnie Lederman, DDS, BSDH

Susan Hyde, DDS, MPH, PhD, FACD

ESSENTIALS OF DIAGNOSIS

▶ The physical examination for oral health and diseases includes lymph nodes, lips, tongue, mucosa lining cheeks, floor and roof of the mouth, gingiva (gums), saliva, natural teeth, artificial teeth, and observation of oral cleanliness.

▶ Xerostomia (dry mouth) resulting from decreased salivary flow, hypofunction of salivary glands, or changed salivary composition affects 10% to 40% of older adults, seriously impairs oral function (lubrication, cleansing, chewing, swallowing), promotes dental caries (tooth decay), exacerbates periodontal disease (gum disease), and compromises nutritional intake.

▶ Periodontal disease is marked by the loss of alveolar bone and supporting tissues around teeth; advanced periodontitis (severe bone loss) leads to increasing tooth mobility and loss of teeth, and has been found to be associated with many systemic diseases.

- Periodontal disease (gum disease) is the sixth leading complication of diabetes and threatens glycemic control. Poor glycemic control is associated with a 3-fold increase in the risk of periodontal disease. Treatment of periodontal disease results in a 10% to 20% improvement in glycemic control.

- Xerostomia (dry mouth) seriously impairs oral function, promotes dental caries (tooth decay), and exacerbates periodontal disease. Decreased salivary flow is a side effect of 500+ medications, including tricyclic antidepressants, antihistamines, antihypertensives, and diuretics.

- Oral cancer is the eighth most common cancer in men and is 7 times more likely to occur in older adults.

- Aspiration pneumonia is the major reason for hospital admission from nursing homes and has a mortality rate of 20% to 50%. Effective daily oral hygiene lowers the incidence of aspiration pneumonia among patients in nursing facilities and hospitals.

By addressing oral health needs, health care professionals play a critical role in improving the health and quality of life of older adults. Clinicians should be familiar with normal and pathologic oral morphology. Clinicians have a positive impact by counseling patients on effective preventive measures, including regular dental visits.

A. Oral Disease & Access to Care

Although changes in oral health are not inevitable consequences of aging, profound, yet often asymptomatic, untreated oral disease is frequently present in older adults. Twenty-three percent of older adults have untreated dental caries, and 70% have periodontal disease. Almost a third of older adults are fully edentulous (missing all natural teeth). Seniors older than age 65 years average 19 remaining teeth. The World Health Organization recognizes that of the original 32 teeth, 20 constitute the minimum adequate functional

▶ General Principles in Older Adults

Oral health is essential to general health and quality of life for older adults. Chronic disease increases the burden of oral disease, predisposing older adults to oral microbial infections, pain, altered taste, difficulty chewing and speaking, and dysphagia. Clinical research demonstrates the benefits of maintaining oral health and the deleterious consequences of oral neglect.

- Weight loss and failure to thrive are common in patients with poor oral health. Concomitant psychosocial consequences undermine self-esteem, compromise social interaction, and contribute to chronic stress and depression.

dentition. Seventeen percent of older adults experience oro-facial pain, including jaw joint, facial, oral sores, burning mouth, and toothache. Chronic orofacial pain can be associated with increased frailty, social withdrawal, decreased activities of daily living, and diminished quality of life.

Only about half of older adults have had a dental visit during the past year, with lower access to care for minority, impoverished, or institutionalized elders. Medicare and most state Medicaid programs do not cover preventive or restorative dental treatment for older adults. Dental insurance is typically not a retirement benefit. As a result, older adults pay a significant portion of their dental expenses out-of-pocket, limiting their treatment choices and ability to receive care.

B. Periodontal Disease

Gingivitis, the earliest and most common form of periodontitis, is limited to the gingiva. It is associated with plaque, hormonal changes, or a foreign-body response. Gingivitis normally reverses with no lasting damage upon effective plaque removal. It often progresses to periodontitis, resulting in inflammatory destruction of periodontal ligament and bone attached to the tooth root.

Periodontal disease and associated pathogens have been linked with diabetes, peripheral vascular disease, cerebrovascular disease, and coronary vascular disease. Causation has not been established. However, inflammatory cytokines produced in periodontitis are implicated in atherogenesis. Periodontal disease can progress rapidly in those with impaired immune systems. Smoking and poor oral hygiene are the most common risk factors for periodontitis. Periodontal disease is marked by the loss of alveolar bone around teeth. Advanced periodontitis leads to increasing tooth mobility and loss. Treatment with oral antibiotics and chlorhexidine mouth rinse can slow progression, however, a dental referral for root surface debridement may be necessary.

C. Teeth & Dental Caries

Fifty-nine percent of those age 60–69 years and 72% of those age 70+ years have fewer than 20 remaining teeth. Having fewer than 20 teeth compromises masticatory function and nutritional status. It is associated with smoking, low socioeconomic status, low physical and social activity, frailty, living alone or in a nursing home, poor access to care, and higher mortality rates. Even with dentures, fewer than 20 teeth leads to decreased blood levels of vitamins and minerals; decreased consumption of vegetables, fruits and fiber; overprepared and overcooked foods; and increased caloric intake as a result of preferential consumption of fats and sugars.

Dental caries is an infection. Oral bacteria colonize exposed tooth surfaces, metabolize carbohydrates and release acids that demineralize tooth surfaces, potentially leading to a cavitated lesion. Twenty-three percent of older adults have untreated dental caries, a rate similar to children. Root caries is the major cause of tooth loss in older adults, and tooth loss is the most significant oral health-related negative variable of quality of life for older adults. Recurrent caries constitute new infection around existing fillings and crowns. Caries can destroy the structural integrity of a tooth before the patient experiences pain. Metastatic bacterial infections of dental origin have been reported in virtually every organ system. Those with active or recurrent dental caries benefit from fluoride varnish applications and high-fluoride toothpaste, available by prescription.

D. Artificial Teeth

Restorative dentistry offers patients several tooth replacement options:

- A complete denture replaces all the teeth in the maxilla and/or mandible.
- A removable partial denture replaces some teeth and is connected by clasps to remaining natural teeth.
- Fixed bridges replace 1 or more missing teeth and are connected by crowns to the adjacent teeth.
- Dental implants are surgically placed into the jaw and can be used to support individual crowns, fixed bridges and removable dentures.

Properly made, well-fitting complete dentures restore only 10% to 15% of masticatory function. Patients with complete dentures commonly have difficulty eating and may be dissatisfied with their facial appearance. Over time, as the alveolar bone remodels, the ridges upon which the dentures rest resorb and change shape. Unless dentures are periodically relined, the vertical dimension of the lower face is lost and dentures can become ill fitting, impairing speech, compromising self-image, and further reducing masticatory function. Poorly fitting dentures can disrupt the normal flora and result in oral candidiasis infection. Angular cheilitis is a common consequence of the loss of vertical dimension.

E. Oral Candidiasis

Oral candidiasis is the most common fungal infection in humans, and is underdiagnosed among older adults. Up to 65% of denture-wearers experience oral candidiasis. Dentures that are worn for excessive periods of time with improper removal and cleaning can result in an overgrowth of fungus and cause burning sensation and irritation to the roof of the mouth, denture stomatitis or papillary hyperplasia (pebbly appearance). To reduce the likelihood of denture stomatitis, a candidiasis infection, and accelerated bone resorption, dentures should not be worn overnight. Individuals with dentures should be instructed to remove the denture for at least 8 hours daily to allow tissue bearing areas to heal and recover. To treat oral candidiasis, topical anti-fungal agents are applied to both the oral tissues and denture, typically for several weeks.

F. Oral Cancer

Oral cancer is the eighth most common cancer in men and is seven times more likely to occur in older adults. Squamous cell carcinoma comprises 96% of oral and pharyngeal malignancies. Age is the primary risk factor, along with the use of tobacco and alcohol. Both leukoplakia (white patch) and erythroplakia (red patch) persisting for more than 2 weeks, particularly those that progress to raised plaques of mixed appearance and ulceration, should be referred for biopsy. A persistent erythroplakia is an early manifestation of oropharyngeal squamous cell cancer.

G. Aspiration Pneumonia

Aspiration pneumonia is the major reason for hospital admission from nursing homes and has a mortality rate of 20% to 50%. Risk of aspirating increases when frail patients are dependent for assistance with feeding and oral hygiene. Patients with poor oral health have an increased risk for aspiration pneumonia. Improving oral hygiene decreases the bacterial load and results in a 40% reduction in aspiration pneumonia. Postural adjustment, allowing extra time for feeding assistance, feeding smaller quantities per bite, and instructing patients to chew longer prior to swallowing reduces the risk for aspiration.

H. Xerostomia

Saliva should be free flowing and watery. It lubricates the intraoral tissues and the lips facilitating speech, taste, mastication, and swallowing. It decreases the risk of dental caries and periodontal disease. Saliva contains antimicrobial elements that modulate plaque formation, buffer intraoral pH against bacterial acid production, and promote re-mineralization of tooth surfaces with calcium and phosphate salts to repair incipient caries. In normal aging, the amount of saliva remains stable. However, saliva becomes thicker as a result of a reduction in serous flow relative to mucous, resulting in decreased lubrication.

Xerostomia resulting from decreased salivary flow or changed salivary composition affects 10% to 40% of older adults, seriously impairs oral function, promotes dental caries and exacerbates periodontal disease. Xerostomia is associated with autoimmune diseases such as rheumatic disease, Sjögren syndrome; and after chemo-/radiation therapy. In addition, decreased salivary flow is a side effect of 500+ medications, including tricyclic antidepressants, antihistamines, antihypertensives, and diuretics. Oral lubricants and salivary substitutes may be used as needed. However, relief is temporary, and they provide none of the protective properties of saliva. Any of several nonprescription oral lubricants and salivary substitutes are readily available.

I. Osteonecrosis of the Jaw

Bone antiresorptive agents currently include IV and oral bisphosphonates and the recently approved denosumab. All are associated with osteonecrosis of the alveolar bone (ONJ). Cancer patients receiving IV bisphosphonates or denosumab minimize the risk of developing ONJ by receiving a thorough dental evaluation and completion of all dental treatment prior to initiating therapy. During bone antiresorptive therapy, excellent daily oral care, no smoking, limited alcohol consumption, no invasive dental procedures, and dental hygiene maintenance appointments every 3 months are recommended. Evidence of ONJ requires an immediate referral to an oral surgeon for therapeutic and palliative care. Denosumab-related ONJ may resolve more rapidly with a drug holiday than bisphosphonate-related ONJ because the pharmacodynamics and pharmacokinetics of the 2 classes of bone antiresorptive agents differ.

▶ Treatment

A. Patients Requiring Assistance

Older adults suffering from stroke, arthritis, and dementia are likely to have problems maintaining their own oral hygiene. Compromised dexterity, dementia, and depression can have a negative impact on patients' ability or willingness to practice prevention, and correlate with increased periodontitis. Patients with dementia and other disabilities may not be able to communicate their oral pain or problem. Instead, they resort to behavioral signs such as pulling at their face or mouth, exhibiting aggression or agitation, chewing on their lip, tongue, or hand, and not eating. Specialized hygiene aides can facilitate plaque removal for patients with impaired dexterity as well as for the caregivers assisting with the task. Table 51–1 offers suggestions to maintain oral health for older adults requiring assistance.

B. Oral Health Assessment for Nondentists

There is no gold-standard oral health assessment tool for non-dentist clinicians. The Kayser-Jones Brief Oral Health Status Examination (BOHSE) is an instrument developed for nurses in long-term care, and has been validated in a variety of older adult populations, including individuals with cognitive impairment. The 10-item BOHSE reflects oral health, with a higher score indicating more problems. The cumulative score is important, and individuals who score on items with an asterisk should be referred for an immediate dental examination. The BOHSE (available at: http://consultgerirn.org/) does not replace clinical oral examinations and dental radiographs for diagnosis.

Performing the BOHSE

The BOHSE assessment begins with extraoral observation and palpation of lymph nodes in the head and neck and ends with an evaluation of the oral cavity. Using a penlight, tongue depressor, and gauze, the clinician examines and grades on a three point scale the conditions of the oral cavity, surrounding tissues, and natural/artificial teeth. Comprehensive oral assessment should be performed with dentures removed.

Step 1: Lymph Nodes
Infection from the teeth and associated oral tissues usually remains localized and forms an abscess with a fistula to skin, oral mucosa or bone, allowing natural drainage. Occasionally, infection can spread through the lymphatics and vasculature to tissues and organs.

Observe and palpate the lymph nodes of the head and neck for firm, tender, enlarged, or warm lymph nodes indicating an infection.

- **Anterior cervical nodes** (superficial and deep to the sternocleidomastoid muscles from the angle of the jaw to the clavicle) drain the third molars, internal structures of the throat, posterior pharynx, tonsils, and thyroid.
- **Submandibular nodes** (inferior border of the mandible) drain the floor of the mouth, and all the teeth except mandibular incisors and third molars.
- **Submental nodes** (below the chin) drain the mandibular incisors and associated tissues.

Step 2: Lips
Examine the lips at rest to identify facial deformities or extraoral lesions.

Normal:
- The lips should appear smooth, pink and moist, not dry or chapped.

Abnormal:
- *Angular cheilitis, a Candidiasis and Staphylococcal infection,* appears as red cracking at the corners of the mouth and is common in patients with extensive tooth loss.
- *Squamous cell carcinoma* of the lip appears as a dry, scaly or ulcerated lesion of more than two weeks' duration. Lip cancer is strongly correlated with smoking and sun exposure.

Step 3: Tongue
Gently grasp the tip of the tongue with gauze to inspect it along its length (lateral borders).

Normal:
- Normal appearance is rough on the dorsum, pink and moist. Surfaces of the tongue should not appear coated, smooth, patchy, or severely fissured.
- Age-related changes include fissuring on the dorsal surface and sub-lingual varicosities.

Abnormal:
- Pathology is most often found on the lateral borders and the ventral surface of the tongue.

Step 4: Cheeks, Floor and Roof of Mouth
Normal:
- The mucosa of the cheeks, roof and floor of the mouth, and pharynx should appear pink and moist.

- The anterior portion of the roof of the mouth has normal surface irregularities called *rugae.*
- Bony exostoses or tori are histologically normal osseous overgrowth thought to be secondary to excessive functional jaw loading during bruxing (clenching and grinding the teeth). They may be found in the mid-palate, bilaterally on the lingual aspect of the mandible, and on the buccal aspect of both dental arches. While not pathological, large maxillary and mandibular tori may be prone to superficial injury while eating and can interfere with dentures.

Abnormal:
- Dry mucosa interferes with denture retention and oral function.
- Note any dry, shiny, rough or swollen mucosa, white or red patches, bleeding, or ulcerations.

Step 5: Gingiva
Normal:
- The gingival tissue should appear firm, smooth and pink.
- When examining the gingiva, include the area between teeth and/or under artificial teeth.

Abnormal:
- Swollen or bleeding gingiva, generalized redness or tenderness around the teeth indicates a periodontal infection.

Step 6: Saliva
Normal:
- Saliva should be free flowing and watery.

Abnormal:
- Dry, sticky, parched and reddened tissues and/or a patient's perception of dry mouth indicate a problem of reduced salivary flow.

Step 7: Natural Teeth
- Observe and count natural teeth.

Normal:
- No decayed or broken teeth or tooth roots.

Abnormal:
- Decayed, broken teeth.

Step 8: Artificial Teeth
Normal:
- Intact dentures should fit comfortably and be worn most of the day.

Problematic:
- Missing or broken denture teeth, loose or unstable dentures.
- Dentures worn only for eating or cosmetic purposes indicate the need for a dental referral.

Step 9: Oral Cleanliness
- Observe the appearance of teeth and dentures. They should appear clean and free of food particles, plaque, and tartar (calculus). Check for food pocketing in the vestibules and under dentures and bridges.

Table 51–1. Maintaining oral health for older adults requiring assistance.

Activity/Condition	Intervention
Plaque control	• Effective daily plaque removal and regular dental visits. • Floss daily. • Flexibility of soft-bristled toothbrushes, manual or powered, is most effective at plaque removal and prevent damage to the gingiva. • Brush for 2 minutes at least twice a day with a soft brush using fluoridated toothpaste. • Foam or rubber handles can be slipped over manual toothbrushes to improve ease of use. • Electric toothbrushes are more efficient in removing plaque and typically have a larger diameter handle making them easier to grip. • Use of mouth props and behind-the-patient positioning make the job of brushing another person's teeth easier. • Additional Hygiene Aides: floss holders, tongue scrapers, Collis Curve™ and Surround™ toothbrushes. Proxabrushes for wider gaps between teeth, dental floss with prestrung heads and extended handles for people with dexterity issues and for caregivers. • Allow toothbrush bristles to dry between uses to reduce bacterial transmission. • Replace tooth brush every 3-4 months or after an illness. • **In long-term care facilities:** Label all dental supplies; separate individual patient's dental supplies; don't store dental supplies near toilets.
Caries risk reduction	• Use 0.5% sodium fluoride mouth rinse for those with xerostomia and at high risk for decay. • Control of the amount and frequency of food and drinks with high sugar content. • Fluoride varnish applications and high-fluoride toothpaste, available by prescription.
Oral lesions	• Refer for immediate dental evaluation any red or white patch or ulceration persisting longer than 2 weeks.
Denture care	• Label dentures with patient's name. • Keep dentures clean. • Denture acrylic should remain hydrated; store in a plastic container, covered by water when not in use. • Dentures can be soaked with commercial denture cleansers or prescription chlorhexidine, but not bleach. • To prevent bacterial plaque accumulation, dentures should be brushed on all surfaces using a soft toothbrush with nonabrasive liquid soap, and rinsed thoroughly. • Toothpaste abrades the acrylic surface, predisposing it to plaque formation, and should not be used to clean dentures. • Denture adhesives and home-reline kits should be avoided; if needed, use adhesive sparingly. • Dentures should not be worn overnight.
Xerostomia	• Keep the mouth moist and clean with frequent sips of water and rinsing with alcohol-free chlorhexidine. • Avoid alcohol, caffeine, and smoking. • Salivary flow may be stimulated by pilocarpine (5–10 mg q8h), chewing sugarless gum, sucking on sugarless candy, or Salene lozenges (online). • Lanolin keeps the lips moist and protected better than petroleum jelly. • Prescribe medications with minimal oral side effects.

C. Pharmacologic Considerations

Many medications prescribed for older adults have oral side effects. In addition to xerostomia,

- More than 200 medications can alter taste and lead to weight loss, depression, and compensation with sugary foods that promote dental caries.

- Phenytoin, methotrexate and calcium channel blockers cause gingival hyperplasia. Periodontal disease is exacerbated in type 2 diabetics taking nifedipine.

- Gastric reflux caused by progesterone, nitrates, beta blockers, and calcium channel blockers erodes the surfaces of teeth.

- Drug preparations and nutritional supplements containing sugar promote dental caries.

- Chemotherapy and radiation therapy cause oral mucositis and stomatitis.

- Patients taking steroids are more susceptible to candidiasis infections.

- The 2007 American Heart Association guidelines require antibiotic prophylaxis only for patients with a history of previous endocarditis, posttransplant valvulopathy, unrepaired congenital heart disease, indwelling vascular catheters, arteriovenous hemodialysis shunts, and prosthetic heart valves.

- The 2012 guidelines from the American Academy of Orthopedic Surgeons discontinued the routine prescribing of prophylactic antibiotics for all total joint replacement patients undergoing dental procedures, and instead recommended a shared decision-making tool for patients and their health care providers.

- Noninvasive procedures such as cleanings, fillings, crown preparation, and simple extractions may be performed without interrupting anticoagulation or antiplatelet therapy.

- Most dental procedures may be performed with an international normalized ratio between 1.8 and 2.5.

▶ Prognosis

Collaboration among physicians, nurses, therapists, pharmacists and dentists is critical to individualized oral health planning. Older adults who are medically complex and have functional limitations are in particular need of care coordination. Oral daily care is important to lifelong oral health. Health professionals who care for older adults have an important role in promoting oral hygiene practices and identifying the need for referral.

By addressing oral health needs, health care professionals play a critical role in improving the health and quality of life of older adults. Clinicians should be familiar with normal and pathologic oral morphology. Clinicians have a positive impact by counseling patients on effective preventive measures, including regular dental visits.

American Academy of Orthopaedic Surgeons and the American Dental Association. *Prevention of Orthopaedic Implant Infection in Patients Undergoing Dental Procedures Guideline.* Rosemont, IL: American Academy of Orthopaedic Surgeons; 2012. Available from: http://www.aaos.org/Research/guidelines/PUDP/PUDP_guideline.pdf

Budtz-Jørgensen E, Chung JP, Mojon P. Successful aging—the case for prosthetic therapy. *J Public Health Dent.* 2000;60(4):308-312.

Ettinger R. The role of the dentist in geriatric palliative care. *J Am Geriatr Soc.* 2012;60(2):367-368.

Griffin SO. New coronal caries in older adults: implications for prevention. *J Dent Res.* 2005;84(8):715-720.

Kayser-Jones J. An instrument to assess the oral health status of nursing home residents. *Gerontologist.* 1995;35(6):814-824.

Langmore SE, Terpenning MS, Schork A, et al. Predictors of aspiration pneumonia: how important is dysphagia? *Dysphagia.* 1998;13(2):69-81.

Mashberg A, Samit A. Early diagnosis of asymptomatic oral and oropharyngeal squamous cancers. *CA Cancer J Clin.* 1995;45(6):328-351.

Ruggiero SL, Dodson TB, Assael LA, Landesberg R, Marx RE, Mehrotra B; Task Force on Bisphosphonate-Related Osteonecrosis of the Jaws, American Association of Oral and Maxillofacial Surgeons. American Association of Oral and Maxillofacial Surgeons position paper on bisphosphonate-related osteonecrosis of the jaw–2009 update. *Aust Endod J.* 2009;35(3):119-130.

Smith BJ, Shay K. What predicts oral health stability in a long-term care population? *Spec Care Dentist.* 2005;25(3):150-157.

Shimazaki Y. Influence of dentition status on physical disability, mental impairment, and mortality in institutionalized elderly people. *J Dent Res.* 2001;80(1):340-345.

Terpenning MS, Taylor GW, Lopatin DE, Kerr CK, Dominguez BL, Loesche WJ. Aspiration pneumonia: dental and oral risk factors in an older veteran population. *J Am Geriatr Soc.* 2001;49(5):557-563.

USEFUL WEBSITES

Academy of General Dentistry. *Know Your Teeth.* http://www.knowyourteeth.com/

American Dental Association. http://www.ada.org/public.aspx

Apple Tree Dental (an innovative nonprofit community collaborative clinic model for oral health assessment and care delivery). http://www.appletreedental.org

Center for Disease Control Division of Oral Health. http://www.cdc.gov/oralhealth/

HIV Dent. http://www.hivdent.org/ (provides extensive pictorial and print resources on the oral health care of patients with HIV/AIDS).

Kayser-Jones Brief Oral Health Status Examination (BOHSE) tool. http://consultgerirn.org/uploads/File/trythis/try_this_18.pdf

National Institute of Dental and Craniofacial Research (links to numerous oral topics across the life span, including special-needs patients, handouts in Spanish, and links to low cost care). http://www.nidcr.nih.gov/oralhealth/

Smiles for Life (excellent online resource, developed by The Society of Teachers of Family Medicine Group on Oral Health). http://www.smilesforlifeoralhealth.org

Smiles for Life. Adult oral health pocket card and acute dental problems pocket card. http://smilesforlifeoralhealth.talariainc.com/buildcontent.aspx?pagekey=62954&lastpagekey=62948&userkey=11190072&sessionkey=2071443&tut=555&customerkey=84&custsitegroupkey=0

Evaluating Confusion in Older Adults

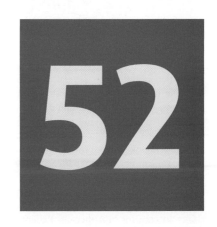

Caroline Stephens, PhD, MSN

▶ General Principles in Older Adults

Confusion is a common presenting problem in many older patients, but it is not a normal part of aging. Most adults experience some cognitive changes as they age, such as decreases in the speed of processing information, lessened spontaneous recall, and small decreases in executive skills. Confusion, however, is not normal aging. When an older patient presents with confusion, it is important to determine whether the confusion is acute or chronic in nature. For example, is it a recent change (days to weeks) or has the change been more chronic and progressive in nature (months to years)? Sometimes the change will be manifested as an acute or sudden change in behavior, such as increased agitation, aggression, wandering, or falls, or a change in function. Understanding the nature and time line of the events will give you an indication regarding the potential underlying diagnosis.

Knowledge of baseline cognitive and physical functional status are key assessment parameters when evaluating confusion. Gathering baseline cognitive and functional status information from patients as well as caregivers, family, and friends will help you determine if the patient's confusion represents an acute change as a result of delirium or if the confusion is more chronic and insidious, such as that related to dementia. It is important to note that while confusion is most commonly a symptom of delirium or dementia, it can also be associated with psychoses and affective disorders, specifically major depression.

▶ Differential Diagnoses

A. Delirium

Delirium, often presenting as acute confusion, is a highly prevalent, preventable, life-threatening clinical syndrome in acutely ill older adults. It is characterized by an acute change in cognition and attention, with disturbances in

consciousness, orientation, memory, thought, perception and/or behavior. In contrast to dementia, which is a chronic confusional state, delirium typically develops over a short period of time (hours to days), fluctuates over the course of the day (often worsening at night) with varying inability to concentrate, maintain attention, and sustain purposeful behavior. Anxiety, irritability, and psychomotor restlessness with insomnia are common. These patients may pick at their intravenous lines, take off their oxygen, disconnect monitoring equipment, exhibit poor safety awareness, and/or talk to people who are not present. Other perceptual disturbances (often visual hallucinations) are also commonly accompanied by paranoid delusional thinking exacerbating the patient's behavioral and emotional manifestations. Agitated behaviors commonly associated with delirium often lead to use of physical and chemical restraints, further compounding the risk of functional loss and serious complications.

Family and caregivers may report the patient was "fine" during the day, but became confused, restless, and agitated during the middle of the night. The change, however, may be even more subtle: "She isn't acting quite right." When family and caregivers can pinpoint such a subtle change over the course of a day or week, that should be taken seriously, and delirium should be ruled out. Delirium is considered a medical emergency and should always be ruled out prior to assuming the patient only has dementia or another psychiatric disorder.

B. Dementia

Unlike delirium, dementia is more chronic in nature and develops insidiously over months to years. Specifically, dementia is a clinical syndrome characterized by a cluster of signs and symptoms including difficulties in memory, disturbances in language, psychological and psychiatric changes, and impairments in activities of daily living. Although there are many different types of dementia (see Chapter 22, "Cognitive Impairment & Dementia"), Alzheimer disease is the most common cause, occurring in an estimated 50% to 80% of all cases.

Such a dementia typically first appears as forgetfulness of recent events or conversations. Family and loved ones may report that over the past several months or year the patient has been increasingly getting lost in familiar areas; misplacing items; having language difficulties (eg, finding the name of familiar objects); having problems performing tasks that require some thought, but that used to come easily (eg, balancing a checkbook, playing card games, learning new information or routines); and/or experiencing personality changes or a loss of social skills leading to inappropriate behaviors. As the dementia slowly progresses, these symptoms become much more apparent and severe, and interfere with the patient's ability to care for him-/herself. Patients may also begin to exhibit psychosis, mood and behavioral difficulties (eg, paranoid delusions, hallucinations, depression, physical and/or verbal aggression; social withdrawal), or sleep disturbances (eg, often waking at night), with increasingly poor insight and judgment. Many of these behaviors often present significant caregiving challenges and burden, frequently resulting in institutionalization. In the severe stages, patients are unable to perform basic activities of daily living, recognize family members, understand language, speak, or ambulate independently.

It is important to note that confusion or a decline in cognitive functioning that is abnormal for age and education but does not meet criteria for dementia should *not* be attributed to normal aging. Mild cognitive impairment (MCI) is the intermediate-stage neurocognitive disorder between normal cognitive aging and dementia. MCI is associated with an increased lifetime risk for developing dementia. A person with MCI will have problems with memory, language, or another mental function severe enough to be noticeable to others and show up on testing, but not serious enough to interfere with daily life. Understanding the degree of functional incapacitation is a key component to determining whether the person has MCI or early dementia.

C. Depression

Depression is the most common psychiatric disorder in the older adult population, primarily affecting those with chronic medical illnesses, cognitive impairment, and disability. It is clinically defined as a syndrome of either depressed mood or loss of interest or pleasure in most activities of the day and these symptoms must represent a change from the person's usual functioning and be present for at least 2 weeks. Personality changes (eg, social withdrawal, apathy, irritability), forgetfulness, and mood changes (eg, complaints of decreased ability to think, feelings of hopelessness/helplessness, changes in sleep or appetite, psychomotor slowing/agitation) may be signs of depression, dementia, or both. Patients with depression may recognize their feelings of sadness, experience somatic complaints or simply exhibit decreased engagement

Table 52–1. The 8 major diagnostic neurovegetative symptoms of depression (SIGECAPS).

Sleep disturbance* (increased during day or decreased at night)
Interest reduced (loss of interest in previously enjoyable activities)
Guilt (worthlessness*, hopelessness*, regret, self-blame)
Energy loss or fatigue*
Concentration impairment*
Appetite change* (usually decreased; occasionally increased)
Psychomotor change (retardation/lethargy or agitation/anxiety)
Suicidal thoughts/preoccupation with death

Note: To meet the diagnosis of major depression, a patient must have 4 of the symptoms plus depressed mood or anhedonia, for at least 2 weeks. To meet the diagnosis of dysthymic disorder, a patient must have 2 of the 6 symptoms marked with an asterisk (*), plus depression, for at least 2 years.

Adapted and reprinted with permission from The psychiatric review of symptoms: a screening tool for family physicians. *Am Fam Phys.* 1998;58(7). Copyright © 1998 American Academy of Family Physicians. All Rights Reserved.

in activities of daily living. The mnemonic "SIGECAPS" (Table 52–1) can help you remember the 8 major diagnostic symptoms of depression.

Unlike dementia, confusion in a patient with depression is more specific than global. For example, the patient may have difficulties with certain activities, like paying bills, but remains capable of completing equally difficult tasks, such as doing a crossword puzzle. Similarly, the patient may not initiate or engage in conversation, but retains the ability to speak. A person with depression is also more likely to relate many themes of loss, as well as detail their cognitive complaints, whereas someone with dementia may be unaware of their cognitive difficulties and/or try to mask their deficits.

▶ Diagnostic Approach

My patient appears confused. What should I know? What should I be looking for? And what are my next steps once I have determined what's going on?

When a patient presents with confusion, it is critical to perform a detailed history and in-depth physical exam, including a mental status exam, as well as laboratory and diagnostic tests. Interviewing the family/caregiver, as well as the patient, is also critical to better understanding the nature and course of the patient's confusion.

A. History and Physical Exam

A thorough history should focus on the specific cognitive, functional and behavioral changes, how these symptoms have evolved over time, and symptoms that may link them to medical, neurologic or psychiatric conditions. Table 52–2 details key

Table 52–2. Key history domains when evaluating confusion.

- Vascular risk factors
- Neurologic diseases, including Parkinson disease, seizures, or known cerebrovascular disease
- Prior episodes of delirium
- Head trauma or falls
- Psychiatric history
- Recent stressors and losses
- Past or current alcohol or drug use
- History of surgery and response to anesthesia
- Functional status
- Safety concerns
- Behavioral disturbances, such as problems with impulse control, physical or verbal aggression, wandering or disrobing inappropriately
- Family history of neurologic or psychiatric disorders, esp. dementia & depression
- Vision and hearing impairment
- New onset urinary incontinence
- Falls

Table 52–3. The Confusion Assessment Method (CAM) diagnostic algorithm.

The diagnosis of delirium using the CAM requires the presence of #1 and #2 and either #3 or #4:

Evidence	
#1: Acute onset and fluctuating course	Positive responses (usually obtained from a family member or nurse) to the following questions: "Is there evidence of acute change in mental status from the patient's baseline? Did the abnormal behavior fluctuate during the day, that is, tend to come and go or increase and decrease in severity?"
#2: Inattention	Positive response to the question: "Did the patient have difficulty focusing attention, for example, being easily distractible, or having difficulty keeping track of what was being said?"
#3: Disorganized thinking	Positive response to the question: "Was the patient's thinking disorganized or incoherent, such as rambling or irrelevant conversation, unclear or illogical flows of ideas, or unpredictable switching from subject to subject?"
#4: Altered level of consciousness	An answer other than "alert" to the question: "Overall, how would you rate this patient's level of consciousness?" (Alert [normal], Vigilant [hyperalert], Lethargic [drowsy, easily aroused], Stupor [difficult to arouse], or Coma [unarousable])

Data from Inouye SK, van Dyck CH, Alessi CA, Balkin S, Siegal AP, Horwitz RI. Clarifying confusion: the confusion assessment method: a new method for detection of delirium. *Ann Intern Med.* 1990;113(12):905-948.

additional past history domains to assess. The medical evaluation should incorporate data from the psychosocial assessment, review of medications (including nonprescription/complementary alternative therapies), and include a complete physical examination with laboratory and diagnostic studies. The general physical exam should focus on the cardiovascular, neurologic and psychiatric systems, unless otherwise indicated by the patient's history.

B. Mental Status Exam

Mental status should be assessed in the domains of memory, abstract thinking, judgment, mood/affect, orientation, attention or concentration, level of consciousness (wakefulness or sleepiness), communication or language abilities, and personality changes (eg, suspiciousness or loss of impulse control). Standardized mental status questionnaires, diagnostic rating scales and symptom inventories can also assist in this assessment process. Together with the history and physical examination, instruments such as the Montreal Cognitive Assessment (MOCA), Confusion Assessment Method (CAM; Table 52–3) and Geriatric Depression Scale (GDS), can aid the clinician in differentiating among dementia, delirium and depression. Recognize, however, that the results of these tools cannot be interpreted in isolation. Assessment findings must be interpreted within the context of an individual's socioeconomic status, cultural background, education and literacy level, current/previous occupation, and other psychosocial factors.

In addition, the way patients respond to these standardized assessment instruments is just as critical as the score they achieve. For example, a patient with depression may perform poorly on the MOCA as a result of poor effort, apathy, and frequent answers of "I don't know," whereas someone with dementia may put forth great effort, attempt to rationalize mistakes, and/or feel bad if they are unable to answer questions appropriately. Alternatively, someone with delirium may exhibit poor attention and concentration by being easily distracted and/or falling asleep during the assessment process. Table 52–4 presents a comparison of the key diagnostic features to help differentiate delirium, dementia, and depression.

▶ Further Diagnostic Studies

Initial laboratory tests should include blood chemistry panel, complete blood count, thyroid panel, liver function, vitamin B_{12}, and serum drug levels (eg, digoxin). Structural

Table 52–4. Comparison of the clinical features of delirium, dementia, and depression.

Clinical Feature	Delirium	Dementia	Depression
Onset/course	Abrupt/acute; precise identifiable onset within hours/days with diurnal fluctuations in symptoms (worse at night, in darkness and on awakening)	Chronic; generally insidious/gradual onset; symptoms progressive yet relatively stable over time (depends on cause)	Fairly abrupt; coincides with major life changes; diurnal effects typically worse in morning
Duration	Hours/days to weeks (or longer)	Months to years	At least 6 weeks, can be months to years
Awareness/alertness	Reduced; fluctuates; lethargic or hypervigilant	Generally clear/normal until more advanced stages	Generally clear/normal
Attention/concentration	Impaired; very short attention span; fluctuates	Generally normal, until more advanced	Minimal impairment but may have difficulty concentrating
Orientation	Disorientation early; severity varies	Disorientation later in the disease (usually after months to years)	Usually normal, but may have selective disorientation
Memory	Recent and immediate impairment	First recent and then later remote impairment	Selective or "patchy" impairment; "islands" of intact memory
Thinking	Disorganized; inattentive; fragmented, incoherent speech, either slow or accelerated; changes in consciousness	Word finding difficulties; difficulty with abstraction, calculation, agnosia; thoughts impoverished later in disease	Some difficulty with concentration; may have slowed processing/speech; themes of loss, hopelessness or self-deprecation
Perception	Distorted; illusions, delusions and hallucinations; difficulty distinguishing between reality and misperceptions	Variable depending on type of dementia; paranoid delusions (people stealing items) and visual hallucinations most common	Generally intact; may have paranoid ideation and/or hallucinations in severe cases
Psychomotor behavior	Marked changes (hyperactive, hypoactive or mixed)	Generally normal until late stage; may have apraxia	Variable, psychomotor retardation or agitation
Sleep/wake cycle	Disturbed; cycle reversed; hour-to-hour variation	Fragmented with day/night reversal but not hour-to-hour variation	Insomnia common—may have difficulty with sleep onset and/or early morning awakening; also hypersomnia
Associated features	Variable affective changes; symptoms of autonomic hyperarousal; exaggeration of personality type; associated with acute physical illness	Affect tends to be superficial, inappropriate and/or labile; attempts to conceal deficits in intellect; personality changes, aphasia, agnosia may be present; lacks insight	Affect depressed; dysphoric mood; exaggerated/detailed complaints, often many themes of loss; preoccupied with personal thoughts; insight present
Assessment	Failings highlighted by providers/family; distracted from task; numerous errors	Failings highlighted by family, caregiver, friend; frequent "near miss" answers; struggles with test; puts forth great effort to find an appropriate reply	Failings highlighted by individual; frequently answers "I don't know"; little/poor effort; frequently gives up; indifferent toward test

neuroimaging with CT scanning or MRI is recommended in the assessment of patients with dementia and may be beneficial in the assessment of MCI. An electroencephalogram may be indicated if there is any suggestion of seizure activity or to help differentiate delirium from a psychiatric disorder. Additional lab and diagnostic tests are based on individual presentation, other medical co-morbidity, and findings from the history and physical examination.

Finally, it is important to recognize that when evaluating confusion in an older adult the 3 common clinical syndromes (ie, dementia, delirium, depression) may overlap. For example, between 25% and 75% of patients with delirium have coexisting dementia and the presence of dementia increases the risk of delirium up to 5-fold. Depression also often coexists with dementia in approximately 20% of individuals with Alzheimer disease and is associated with higher levels of functional impairment and reduced enjoyment in activities. In addition, late-life depressive symptoms or syndromes may be an early manifestation of cognitive decline and dementing disorders in older adults. Moreover, there is a syndrome of overlapping depression and delirium that is associated with significant risk of functional decline, institutionalization, and death. Thus, it is critical to be able to recognize and evaluate all 3 syndromes and their complex interplay in order to safely and effectively provide care to older adults presenting with confusion.

Blazer DG. Depression in late life: review and commentary. *Focus: J Lifelong Learning Psychiatry.* 2009;7(1):118-136.

Burns A, Iliffe S. Alzheimer's disease. *BMJ.* 2009;338:b158.

Carlat DJ. The psychiatric review of symptoms: a screening tool for family physicians. *Am Fam Physician.* 1998;58(7):1617-1624.

Fick DM, Agostini JV, Inouye SK. Delirium superimposed on dementia: a systematic review. *J Am Geriatr Soc.* 2002;50(10):1723-1732.

Inouye SK. Delirium in older persons. *N Engl J Med.* 2006;354: 1157-1165.

Inouye S, van Dyck C, Alessi C, Siegal A, Horwtiz R. Clarifying confusion: the confusion assessment method. *Ann Intern Med.* 1990;113(12):941-948.

Panza F, Frisardi V, Capurso C, D'Introno A, et al. Late life depression, mild cognitive impairment and dementia: possible continuum? *Am J Geriatr Psychiatry.* 2010;18(2):98-116.

Peterson RC. Mild cognitive impairment. *N Engl J Med.* 2011;364(23):2227-2234.

Synderman D, Rovner BW. Mental status examination in primary care: a review. *Am Fam Physician.* 2009;80(8):809-814.

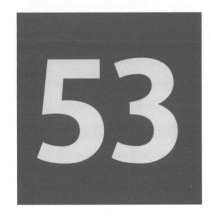

Addressing Polypharmacy & Improving Medication Adherence in Older Adults

David Sengstock, MD, MS
Jonathan Zimmerman, MD, MBA, FACP

▶ General Principles in Older Adults

Older adults are the largest consumers of prescription drugs. A large survey reported that more than one-half of patients 57–85 years old used at least 5 prescription medications, nonprescription medications, and nutritional supplements. Predictably, the number of medications steadily increased with the age of the patient. This survey also reported that 1 in 20 of these patients risked a major drug–drug interaction; half of these interactions included a nonprescription agent. Research demonstrates that polypharmacy is an independent risk factor for adverse outcomes, including hospitalization, nursing home placement, hypoglycemia, falls and fractures, pneumonia, and malnutrition, and death. Older adults are also generally less tolerant to the effects of a medication. This intolerance can manifest as an exaggerated effect of a medication or even a different effect as compared to younger patients, and is described at length in Chapter 9, "Principles of Prescribing for Older Adults."

PROBLEMS CAUSED BY POLYPHARMACY

Table 53–1 lists several major problems caused by polypharmacy. The primary purpose of a medication *also* may be the source of an adverse drug reaction (ADR). A national study of emergency room patients showed that anticoagulants (including both warfarin and antiplatelet drugs) and diabetes drugs (including both insulin and oral medications) were responsible for two-thirds of all medication-related hospitalizations. In contrast, medications considered "inappropriate" by the Beer's criteria accounted for only 7% of hospital admissions. Of these admissions, more than one-half were caused by digoxin alone.

Polypharmacy raises the risk of drug–drug and drug–disease interactions, particularly in older adults. The causes and consequences of such interactions are discussed in Chapter 9. In addition to known interactions, it is likely that clinically important interactions are yet to be discovered. Therefore, physicians should eliminate all unnecessary drugs, regardless of whether they are currently causing an obvious problem.

Similarly, polypharmacy increases the likelihood that patients will not adhere to their medication regimen. Nonadherence to medications contributed to 20% of the ADRs in an ambulatory setting. A number of factors may contribute to nonadherence.

Practice guidelines, for example, are primarily written by specialists for the management of a single condition. Physicians must then combine guidelines in an older patient with multiple conditions. For a hypothetical patient with chronic obstructive pulmonary disease, type 2 diabetes, osteoporosis, hypertension, and osteoarthritis, guidelines require 12 medications with multiple daily dosing regimens. Moreover, prescribing a drug may be easier than more time-consuming interventions such as lifestyle modification or nonpharmacologic treatments. Yet, patients may be less likely to adhere to medications as the regimen grows increasingly complex.

For both patients and the health care system, cost is also an important factor. The hypothetical patient described above would spend $406 each month on medication. It has been estimated that 25% of patients in Medicare part D plans and 40% of patients in employer-based plans are in the Medicare "doughnut hole." When patients reach the doughnut hole, they must cover the cost of all medications until a maximum amount of money is spent in that year. In 2012, the doughnut hole exists between $2930 and $4700. Although the Affordable Care Act slowly eliminates patients' Doughnut hole by 2020, cost remains a problem in health care. Therefore, medication reduction may benefit patient health, improve medication adherence, and reduce costs for patients as well as the overall health care system.

Table 53–1. Problems caused by polypharmacy.

Inherent effects of the medication
Drug-drug interactions
Drug-disease interactions
Nonadherence with the medication regimen
Cost

UNPRESCRIBING: INTERVENING TO REDUCE POLYPHARMACY

Despite clinicians' best intentions to prescribe conservatively, as patients age and medical conditions accumulate, drugs frequently "pile up." The problems listed in Table 53–1 can be ameliorated by decreasing the number and complexity of a patient's medication regimen. At present, no study has demonstrated that trimming a patient's medication list reduces morbidity or mortality. However, studies have demonstrated that pruning a patient's medication list reduces the chance of adverse medication effects, lowers pharmacy cost, and improves patient compliance to their remaining medications. A Cochrane review of multiple systematic approaches to reduce inappropriate medications, for example, found that even with a modest reduction in the number of medications, ADRs could be reduced by 35%. For these reasons alone, *un*prescribing should become as routine a practice as prescribing.

The first step in assessing for inappropriate medications is to determine which medications the patient is taking (including dose and frequency). The traditional way of accomplishing this task is the "brown bag medication review," in which the patient and/or family members collect and bring in *all* medications, including pills and creams, vitamins and supplements, herbal, and nonprescription medications. As each medication is removed from the brown bag, the physician (or office staff) can assess: (a) what the patient is actually taking; (b) what he/she understands about each medication; (c) the medication's effectiveness; and (d) any suspected side effects. Finally, the provider updates the office medication list with the patient's medications. This process may be time-consuming, but much of it can be completed by nonphysician office staff.

Approaches to unprescribing draw on evidence, expert opinion, physician judgment, and patient/caregiver preference. A number of approaches have been described to assist in assessing the appropriateness of a medication, including STOPP (Screening Tool of Older Persons' Potentially Inappropriate Prescriptions), MAI (Medication Appropriateness Index), and ARMOR (Assess, Review, Minimize, Optimize, Reassess). Figure 53–1 illustrates an approach to determine if a medication is a candidate for unprescribing. This approach is built on two published rubrics: the

Good Palliative-Geriatric Practice algorithm and Holmes' Model for Appropriate Prescribing for Patients Late in Life.

After conducting a "brown bag" review, step 2 requires the clinician to reconsider the evidence (or lack thereof) supporting each medication. Older patients are often excluded or underrepresented in trials and geriatric clinical guidelines are often extrapolated from studies of younger patients. Therefore, it is important to remember that what's good for younger patients may not necessarily be good for older patients. Step 2 prompts clinicians to consider unprescribing when a patient is not "comparable" to the population originally examined in a research study. For example, a number of studies support the use of antihypertensive medications in older patients. Similarly, studies support the use of statins in some older populations. However, studies of digoxin for heart failure or atrial fibrillation are limited in older patients. Likewise, analyses of oral hypoglycemic agents or studies supporting specific target A1cs in older patients are scarce. The drugs that lack evidence may be candidates for unprescribing.

Step 3 requires the clinician to personalize the medication that "passed" Step 2. Holmes' "Model for Appropriate Prescribing for Patients Late in Life" is useful. This model suggests that prescribing clinicians should apply 4 considerations to "filter" the medications that passed step 2. These considerations include: (a) the patients' goals of care; (b) individualized treatment targets; (c) life expectancy; and (d) the drug's "time until benefit." Applying this model will result in a personalized set of medications.

To apply the Holmes model, the patient's goals of care may range from curative to solely palliative; treatment targets may range from preventive to symptom management only. A drug's "time until benefit" can vary from minutes (diuretics for congestive heart failure) to years (HMG CoA reductase inhibitors for primary prevention of coronary heart disease). For example, in an older adult with severe emphysema, a long-acting β-agonist inhaler is an evidenced-based, patient-appropriate medication because it improves symptoms in a short timeframe. Statins are also evidenced-based for this patient's hyperlipidemia; however, the patient's limited life expectancy would filter out this preventive medicine.

In step 4, the physician identifies any symptoms of an ADR. It is important to note that symptoms of an ADR may be subtle, such as fatigue or weakness. A good axiom to remember is that all new symptoms are caused by a medication until proven otherwise. The physician should consider unprescribing a medication when a new symptom occurs shortly after that medication was started. This approach will also avoid treating a new symptom by prescribing yet another medication.

In step 5, the physician must decide whether the potential for an adverse effect is likely. The "Beers" listing of potentially inappropriate medications is one helpful resource. Special scrutiny should also be applied to high-risk medications,

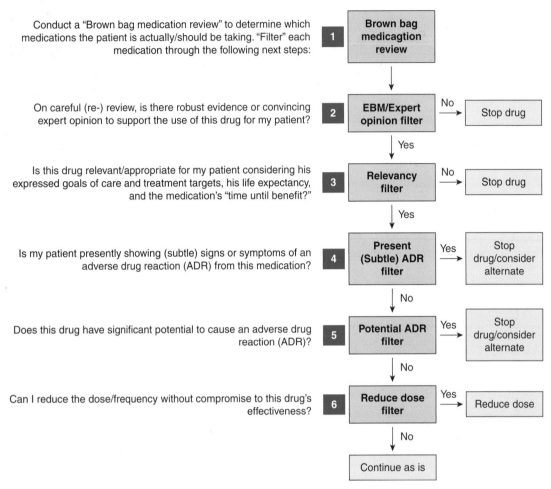

Conduct a "Brown bag medication review" to determine which medications the patient is actually/should be taking. "Filter" each medication through the following next steps:

1 **Brown bag medicagtion review**

On careful (re-) review, is there robust evidence or convincing expert opinion to support the use of this drug for my patient?

2 **EBM/Expert opinion filter** → No → Stop drug

Yes

Is this drug relevant/appropriate for my patient considering his expressed goals of care and treatment targets, his life expectancy, and the medication's "time until benefit?"

3 **Relevancy filter** → No → Stop drug

Yes

Is my patient presently showing (subtle) signs or symptoms of an adverse drug reaction (ADR) from this medication?

4 **Present (Subtle) ADR filter** → Yes → Stop drug/consider alternate

No

Does this drug have significant potential to cause an adverse drug reaction (ADR)?

5 **Potential ADR filter** → Yes → Stop drug/consider alternate

No

Can I reduce the dose/frequency without compromise to this drug's effectiveness?

6 **Reduce dose filter** → Yes → Reduce dose

No

Continue as is

▲ **Figure 53–1.** Filtering algorithm for unprescribing medications.

including hypoglycemic agents, anticoagulation/antiplatelet medications, digoxin, narcotics, antianxiety/sleep aids, antidepressants, and medications with anticholinergic properties. If a drug is the likely cause of an adverse effect, it should be stopped. When unprescribing, clinicians must withdraw drugs carefully. When a medication requires titration up, for example, it will also require titration down. Titrating down is especially important for medications that promote tolerance, such as opiates, sedative-hypnotics, β blockers, clonidine, gabapentin, and selective serotonin reuptake inhibitors. Avoid abrupt, nondiscriminant "drug holidays," and counsel patients to watch for withdrawal symptoms. (Exceptions to titrating down can be made in special circumstances where immediate discontinuation is required.) Finally, step 6 attempts to simply reduce the dose. Reducing dosage and/or frequency may also improve adherence. Further techniques to improve adherence are discussed in the next section.

Interventions beyond physician decision making can also improve prescribing practices. For example, attempts should be made to limit the number of providers who are prescribing medications for a given patient. Studies show that with each additional prescriber there is a 29% increase in ADRs. Likewise, using multiple pharmacies increases this risk. Therefore, clinicians should try to keep a patient's medications with 1 prescriber and 1 pharmacy. Similarly, electronic prescribing (e-prescribing) also holds the potential to decrease the number of inappropriate medications in all patients by instantly reporting drug–drug and drug–disease interactions. E-prescribing programs generate an alert that is sometimes followed by a suggestion of a more appropriate medication. One analysis examined several trials that tested e-prescribing in the ambulatory, hospital, and nursing home settings. The majority of trials showed some decrease in inappropriate prescriptions. However, this decrease was variable, ranging from a decrease of 24% to less than 1%. In addition, excessive (and often irrelevant) alerts were not helpful, leading to "alert fatigue" for physicians. Although e-prescribing holds much promise, the magnitude of the effect on polypharmacy remains uncertain.

ADHERENCE

▶ Improving Immediate Medication Adherence

In addition to prescribing only essential medications, prescribing clinicians must ensure that patients take the medicines that are prescribed. Centuries ago, Hippocrates noted that patients did not consistently take prescribed medicines. Today, multiple medications and frequent dosing regimens decrease adherence. Other factors that have been shown to influence medication adherence include inadequate education about the purpose, importance, and side effects of each medication, excessive cost, and limited physician knowledge of the indicators for a medication. Older adults also have additional medical and social challenges that may affect adherence. These challenges include difficulties in hearing and comprehending physician instructions, remembering discussions because of cognitive impairment, managing multiple medications with complex dosing regimens, accessing medications as a result of reduced social support, purchasing medications because of limited financial and transportation resources, and taking medications as a consequence of poor manual dexterity and vision. Patients may also take their medications intermittently, such as omitting diuretics before bedtime or social events. Together, these factors make nonadherence to medical treatments a serious and common concern in this age group. There may be good reasons that patients cannot adhere to their medicines. Clinicians should ask about barriers to adherence in a nonjudgmental way.

Physicians are often unable to identify which patients are not adhering to their medications; patients are also often reluctant to admit to nonadherence. However, physicians can directly improve many factors that affect medication adherence. Counting pills and asking patients and families about refill history, for example, can be helpful in identifying patients with adherence problems. Table 53–2 lists some simple, evidence-based interventions to improve adherence.

First and foremost, clinicians should always consider improving their relationship and communication with their patients as a means of improving medication adherence. Ultimately, the patient is responsible for taking medications, so a shared decision-making model is more likely to be successful in achieving adherence. A poor patient–provider relationship is likely to frustrate any attempt to improve medication adherence. Clinicians often are trained to believe that many medical problems are lifelong. However, patients may believe that medical problems can be "cured." This

Table 53–2. Interventions to improve medication adherence.

Educate the patient that the disease process requires long-term treatment.
Discuss the purpose of each medication and expected side effects.
Prescribe lower-cost generic medications.
Use combination pills.
Prescribe medications once daily if possible.
Provide simple, clear instructions.

belief is often reinforced by "high-tech" procedures that "fix the blockage" or "stop the bleeding." To adhere to a medication, a patient must understand that an illness continues despite undergoing a medical procedure. The patient may believe that a medication is ineffective, unneeded, or simply not worth the expense. Even when the medication list is reduced, a patient may believe that he/she is taking too many medications, the side effects are too onerous, or a medication is frankly dangerous.

These misconceptions can be addressed only by effective patient–provider communication, including a discussion that emphasizes the chronic nature of a disease. A discussion of the long-term need for the appropriate medication should follow. Research suggests that poor communication commonly leads to medication nonadherence. Older adults report that they must understand the rationale for a medication before they will take it faithfully. Research also shows that many older adults are quite capable of understanding the purpose of a medication, despite the stereotypes to the contrary. The patient should receive education on the purpose, side effects, and length of time that each medication will be needed. This information is often complex, so a written summary may be needed.

Patients are keenly aware of medication cost. Certainly, patients will be unable to adhere if they cannot afford a medication. There is a clear relationship between the amount of a copayment and whether a patient will pick up a medication. Nonadherence rates triple when the copay reaches $50. Despite this, clinicians generally do not know the cost of most medications. Indeed, research shows that physicians underestimate the cost of expensive medications and overestimate inexpensive ones. This is understandable because drug costs change regularly, as new generics become available. Therefore, a pharmacist's advice is important when choosing appropriate alternative medications. Although cost is certainly an important factor, nonadherence is still problematic in high-risk patients without cost constraints.

Finally, frequent dosing is associated with missed medications. Only 50% of patients adhere to medications that are dosed 4 times daily. Research demonstrates that reducing medication frequency improves adherence. Although combination pills and delayed-release preparations are often available, they are underutilized. Across a wide range of clinical settings, 15 randomized trials have demonstrated that combination pills improve adherence. Although individual dosing (bubble wrapping) also improves medication adherence, it is expensive and only available in special circumstances.

▶ Improving Long-Term Medication Adherence

A considerable amount of research has examined the issue of long-term medication adherence. Research shows that adherence rates are higher when the duration of medication therapy is short, such as in acute illnesses. Adherence is much lower in chronic medications, decreasing dramatically within 6 months. Even in life-threatening conditions, adherence is poor. Only 40% of patients with acute coronary syndromes and 36% of those with stable coronary artery disease remained on statins at the second year of follow-up. Table 53–3 lists several interventions that might improve long-term adherence.

Patients are more likely to adhere to a medication if they believe that they have a medical problem. When a disease has symptoms, for example, adherence to medication is better. Therefore, when possible, clinicians should show patients evidence that demonstrates a medical condition exists and evidence of the beneficial effect of a medication. In general, regular contact between providers and patients is essential to improve and maintain medication adherence. Improved adherence was reported in a study where trained nurses regularly reinforced the need for hypertension medications. Importantly, older patients benefitted the most from this intervention. In a meta-analysis of 41 diabetic management studies, a consistent relationship was identified between frequency of contact and adherence to medication. Face-to-face interaction is critical. Research shows that education programs without a face-to-face visit do not change adherence. Therefore, primary care clinicians must see patients often to reinforce the importance of medications.

Table 53–3. Interventions to improve long-term medication adherence.

Count pills and ask family/pharmacy about refill history to assess compliance.
Provide evidence that medications are working (blood pressure results, heart rate, and cholesterol values).
Consider home-monitoring of blood pressure.
Limit the number and frequency of medications.
Enlist family to help setting up pill boxes.
Ask patients about problems taking their medications.
See patients often to reinforce the need for the medications.

SUMMARY

Awareness of the adverse effects of polypharmacy is quite broad. However, prescribing clinicians often wait for signs of an adverse drug event or reaction to discontinue the culprit medication. The practice of "unprescribing" medications to minimize the potential for adverse effects, to reduce pharmacy cost, and to improve a patient's adherence to their remaining medications has yet to become habit. Several tools and algorithms are available to aid clinicians in unprescribing medications. Once a patient's medication list has been trimmed, clinicians should then turn to techniques to increase medication adherence.

American Geriatrics Society 2012 Beers Criteria Update Expert Panel. American Geriatrics Society updated Beers Criteria for potentially inappropriate medication use in older adults. *J Am Geriatr Soc.* 2012;60(4):616-631.

Acelajado MC, Oparil S. Hypertension in the elderly. *Clin Geriatr Med.* 2009;25(3):391-412.

Allan GM, Lexchin J, Wiebe N. Physician awareness of drug cost: a systematic review. *PLoS Med.* 2007;4(9):e283.

Bain KT, Holmes HM, Beers MH, Maio V, Handler SM, Pauker SG. Discontinuing medications: a novel approach for revising the prescribing stage of the medication-use process. *J Am Geriatr Soc.* 2008;56(10):1946-1952.

Boyd CM, Darer J, Boult C, Fried LP, Boult L, Wu AW. Clinical practice guidelines and quality of care for older patients with multiple comorbid diseases: implications for pay for performance. *JAMA.* 2005;294(6):716-724.

Budnitz DS, Lovegrove MC, Shehab N, Richards CL. Emergency hospitalizations for adverse drug events in older Americans. *N Engl J Med.* 2011;365(21):2002-2012.

Clyne B, Bradley MC, Hughes C, Fahey T, Lapane KL. Electronic prescribing and other forms of technology to reduce inappropriate medication use and polypharmacy in older people: a review of current evidence. *Clin Geriatr Med.* 2012;28(2):301-322.

Garfinkel D, Mangin D. Feasibility study of a systematic approach for discontinuation of multiple medications in older adults: addressing polypharmacy. *Arch Intern Med.* 2010;170(18):1648-1654.

Garfinkel D, Zur-Gil S, Ben-Israel J. The war against polypharmacy: a new cost-effective geriatric-palliative approach for improving drug therapy in disabled elderly people. *Isr Med Assoc J.* 2007;9(6):430-434.

Iskedjian M, Einarson TR, MacKeigan LD, et al. Relationship between daily dose frequency and adherence to antihypertensive pharmacotherapy: evidence from a meta-analysis. *Clin Ther.* 2002;24(2):302-316.

Lee JK, Grace KA, Taylor AJ. Effect of a pharmacy care program on medication adherence and persistence, blood pressure, and low-density lipoprotein cholesterol: a randomized controlled trial. *JAMA.* 2006;296(21):2563-2571.

Osterberg L, Blaschke T. Adherence to medication. *N Engl J Med.* 2005;353(5):487-497.

Patterson SM, Hughes C, Kerse N, Cardwell CR, Bradley MC. Interventions to improve the appropriate use of polypharmacy for older people. *Cochrane Database Syst Rev.* 2012;5:CD008165.

Peikes D, Chen A, Schore J, Brown R. Effects of care coordination on hospitalization, quality of care, and health care expenditures among Medicare beneficiaries: 15 randomized trials. *JAMA.* 2009;301(6):603-618.

Sengstock D, Vaitkevicius P, Salama A, Mentzer RM. Under-prescribing and non-adherence to medications after coronary bypass surgery in older adults: strategies to improve adherence. *Drugs Aging.* 2012;29(2):93-103.

Steinman MA, Hanlon JT. Managing medications in clinically complex elders: "There's got to be a happy medium". *JAMA.* 2010;304(14):1592-1601.

Zeller A, Taegtmeyer A, Martina B, Battegay E, Tschudi P. Physicians' ability to predict patients' adherence to antihypertensive medication in primary care. *Hypertens Res.* 2008;31(9):1765-1771.

Zhang Y, Donohue JM, Newhouse JP, Lave JR. The effects of the coverage gap on drug spending: a closer look at Medicare Part D. *Health Aff.* 2009;28(2):w317-w325.

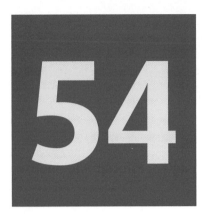

54

Managing Persistent Pain in Older Adults

Vyjeyanthi S. Periyakoil, MD

▶ General Principles in Older Adults

Persistent pain is widely prevalent in older adults and is often underdiagnosed and ineffectively managed. Pain affects more than 50% of older persons living in a community setting and more than 80% of nursing home residents. Pain management disparities are common in older adults for a variety of reasons. Older adults are less likely to report pain owing to (a) a mistaken perception that pain is a normal part of the aging process, (b) not wanting to burden their caregivers, (c) cognitive impairment, and (d) limited health literacy. Even when older adults do report pain, they are less likely to receive opioid analgesics for moderate-to-severe pain and also report lower overall reduction of posttreatment pain scores compared to younger patients. It is also to be noted that any older adults may be reluctant to take opioids as they believe these class of drugs to be too potent, they are concerned about how these drugs may interact with the many other medications they are taking, fear of addiction and dependence, and worries about side effects of feeling "drugged." Data also show that pain is commonly undertreated in cognitively impaired older adults, who receive less analgesic medication than younger cognitively intact persons. Pain limits functional status in older adults and can result in diminished quality of life, sleep disturbances, social isolation, depression, delirium, and increased health care costs and resource utilization (Table 54–1).

Relief of suffering and promotion of patient dignity are primary tenets of geriatric medicine. Timely and effective assessment and management of persistent pain in older adults will help in alleviating their suffering, while maintaining and augmenting quality of life.

A transition from acute to chronic pain in older adults is likely influenced by various factors, including lower socioeconomic status, vivid memory of childhood trauma, obesity, low level of physical fitness, overuse of joints and muscles, chronic illnesses, lack of social support, and elder abuse. The term "persistent pain" is often used interchangeably with the term "chronic pain," and once again denotes pain that persists beyond the expected healing time. Table 54–2 lists other terms commonly used when describing pain.

▶ Screening Tools

A. Assessment

Pain presentation in older adults may be skewed as a result of a variety of factors. In certain acute situations, unlike their younger counterparts, older adults may not report pain. For example, older adults with acute peritonitis or acute myocardial infarction may present with mild or absent pain. A thorough assessment is necessary to formulate a plan to successfully treat persistent pain. The International Association for the Study of Pain (IASP) has developed taxonomy for the classification of pain that identifies five axes as below and these are a helpful framework in assessing pain:

- **Axis I: Anatomic regions**: Ask patient to point out specific areas in the body where the patient has pain.
- **Axis II: Organ systems**: Identify possible organs that may be involved. It is important to remember areas of referred pain, for example, diaphragmatic pain to shoulder.
- **Axis III: Temporal characteristics, pattern of occurrence**: Time the pain occurs, exacerbating and relieving factors are important to assess.
- **Axis IV: Intensity, time since onset of pain**: Some older adults may be able to use numbers (scale of 0 to 10) to describe intensity, whereas other may prefer words (mild, moderate, and severe).
- **Axis V: Etiology**: Underlying etiology of pain should be identified and reversible problems should be corrected.

Persistent pain in older adults is often a result of more than 1 comorbid disease, so thorough assessment should be

Table 54–1. Consequences of poorly treated persistent pain in older adults.

Decreased quality of life
Impaired gait (low-back and lower-limb pain)
Impaired appetite, increased weight loss
Decreased socialization
Impaired sleep
Impaired cognition
Associated depression and anxiety
Agitation in cognitively impaired older adults

performed routinely when the patient is seen in clinic. Pain assessment should include an exploration of effects of pain on functional status, sleep, libido, and emotional and social well-being. Data support the ability of older, cognitively impaired (mild-to-moderate cognitive impairment) patients to rate pain reliably and validly. The choice of scale depends on the presence of language or sensory impairment, level of the patient's health literacy, and numeracy. Scales, such as the McGill Pain Questionnaire and the Pain Disability Scale, measure pain in a variety of domains, including the intensity, location, and affect. Although time-intensive, scales measuring multiple domains can provide a wealth of information about the patient's unique experience of pain. When patients are unable or unwilling to cooperate with time-intensive pain

Table 54–2. Terms commonly used when describing pain.

Nociceptive pain	Nociceptive pain is the perception of nociceptive input, usually as a result of tissue damage (eg, postoperative pain). Nociceptive pain is further subdivided into somatic and visceral pain.
	• Somatic pain: is pain arising from injury to body tissues. It is well localized but variable in description and experience.
	• Visceral pain: is pain arising from the viscera mediated by stretch receptors. It is poorly localized, deep, dull, and cramping (eg, pain associated with appendicitis, hepatic cancer metastasis, bowel ischemia).
Neuropathic pain	Pain initiated or caused by a primary lesion or dysfunction in the nervous system.
Central pain	Pain initiated or caused by a primary lesion or dysfunction in the central nervous system (eg, poststroke pain, phantom limb pain).
Wind-up pain	Slow temporal summation of pain mediated by C fibers. Repetitive noxious stimulation at a rate of <1 stimulus per 3 seconds. It may cause the person to experience a gradual increase in the perceived magnitude of pain.

Table 54–3. Pain Assessment in Advanced Dementia (PAINAD) Scale.

SCORE
Breathing
0 Normal
1 Occasional labored breathing; short period of hyperventilation
2 Noisy labored breathing; long period of hyperventilation; Cheyne-Stokes respirations
Negative vocalization
0 None
1 Occasional moan/groan; low-level speech/negative or disapproving quality
2 Repeated troubled calling out; loud moaning or crying
Facial expression
0 Smiling/inexpressive
1 Sad, frightened, frowning
2 Facial grimacing
Body language
0 Relaxed
1 Tense, distressed, pacing, fidgeting
2 Rigid, fists clenched, knees pulled up, pulling or pushing away, striking out
Consolability
0 No need to console
1 Distracted or reassured by voice or touch
2 Unable to console, distract, or reassure
____ Total

assessments, simple scales, like the Numeric Rating Scale and the Faces Pain Scale, are effective. The patient is asked to rate the patient's pain by assigning a numerical value (with 0 indicating no pain and 10 representing the worst pain imaginable), or a facial expression corresponding to the pain. Older adults, especially those with limited English proficiency or with cognitive impairment, may be unable or unwilling to use numbers to describe their pain (Table 54–3). The Wong-Baker FACES Pain Rating Scale with Foreign Translations is useful for both English and non-English speaking patients.

▶ Treatment

A. Approaches to Persistent Pain Treatment

Cognitively intact patients should be educated about their persistent pain, the underlying causes and how best to track its location and intensity, how to do self-assessment of pain using validated instruments, and how to take medications properly (Box 54–1). They should be encouraged to

Box 54-1. Clinical Pearls for Assessing and Treating Pain

- Pain requires a thorough assessment to determine its source, severity, and impact on the functioning and well-being of the patient.
- Untreated pain can adversely affect the functional and cognitive status of older adults.
- Multiple pain scales are available to help quantify the severity of pain. The selection of a pain scale is based on the cognitive and communication abilities of the patient.
- Local therapies and nonpharmacologic approaches are desirable as they often have limited side effects. Systemic analgesics should be added if needed in the treatment of older adults.
- Nonopioid analgesics should be instituted first and opioid considered only if nonopioid analgesics are ineffective.
- When prescribing opioids, start low and go slow.
- Tolerance to opioids generally develops to the respiratory depression, fatigue, and sedation effects of opioid analgesics but not to the constipating effect.
- "The hand that writes the opioid should write the laxative."
- Given chronic pain's diverse effects, interdisciplinary assessment and treatment may produce the best results for people with the most severe and persistent pain problems.
- Effective management of chronic pain necessitates a collaborative and ongoing partnership between the clinicians, the patient and family.

use nonpharmacologic modalities and exercise regularly. Caregivers of both cognitively impaired and intact patients should be educated as well. The more we are able to empower patients and families to take a central role in their illness management, the better will be their outcomes.

B. Nonpharmacologic Therapy

Recognizing the common overlap of depression, anxiety, and other mood disturbances should prompt early consultation with mental health professionals. Psychological interventions and cognitive–behavioral therapy are also important tools for treatment of persistent pain as they help patients cope with the stresses that accompany persistent pain. In cognitive–behavioral therapy, patients are asked to track their pain and record the thoughts that are associated with the pain experience to identify maladaptive coping strategies. By conscientiously replacing these maladaptive strategies with positive coping strategies, patients can increase control over pain-related experiences and thereby over the pain. When possible, family members and caregivers should be included in the therapy.

Regular physical activity can decrease pain scores, improve mood, boost functional status. For patients with advanced illness who are bedbound, regular repositioning, passive range of motion exercises, and gentle massage are effective interventions. The goals of therapy should include improvements in muscle strength, endurance, and function, and improved quality of life.

An interdisciplinary team approach to treatment may be useful for patients with complex pain or who are poorly responsive to first-line treatments. Incorporating complementary and alternative modalities such as hypnosis, aromatherapy, biofeedback, and music and pet therapy may be effective adjuvant strategies. Suboptimal treatment response should not be viewed as a permanent state, but as an opportunity for input from specialists who have additional expertise in treating these difficult problems (see Chapter 57, "Considering Complementary & Alternative Medicines for Older Adults").

C. Pharmacologic Therapy

1. Nonsystemic therapies—When starting pharmacologic therapy in older adults, the risks and benefits of the treatment should be considered and balanced carefully. If appropriate, nonsystemic therapies should be tried first. For example, patients who primarily have knee pain might respond to intraarticular corticosteroid injections. Topical preparations such as capsaicin or ketorolac gel[OL] or lidocaine patches might be effective as primary or adjunctive therapy for treating neuropathic or myofascial pain syndromes. Patients with myofascial pain may also respond to local treatments such as massage, gentle stretching exercises, ultrasound, and trigger-point injections. If these local therapies are ineffective systemic therapy should be instituted and the patient should be monitored closely to ensure that the treatment is effective and to minimize adverse effects. The pain ladder from the World Health Organization offers an excellent approach towards analgesic management.

2. Acetaminophen—Acetaminophen provides adequate analgesia for many mild-to-moderate pain syndromes, particularly musculoskeletal pain from osteoarthritis, and is recommended as first-line therapy for persistent pain on a regularly scheduled basis. The maximum adult dose is 4 g/day, and in an older adult population, the recommendation is to adhere to a maximum dosage of 3 g/day as older adults may have decreased hepatic phase II metabolism, which increases the risk of hepatotoxicity. In patients at risk of liver dysfunction, particularly those who have a history of alcohol intake, the dosage should be decreased by 50% or acetaminophen should be avoided. Acetaminophen should be administered every 6 hours for patients with creatinine clearance of 10–50 mL/min and every 8 hours for patients with a creatinine clearance of <10 mL/min.

3. Nonsteroidal antiinflammatory drugs—Nonsteroidal antiinflammatories inflammatory drugs (NSAIDs) tend to be more effective than acetaminophen in chronic inflammatory pain and are used after acetaminophen has been tried and proven to be ineffective. Significant adverse effects of NSAIDs include renal dysfunction, gastrointestinal (GI) bleeding, platelet dysfunction, fluid retention, precipitation of heart failure, and precipitation of delirium. As a result of the significant adverse effects profile of NSAIDs, in a recent systematic review of osteoarthritis in older adults, O'Neill et al recommend NSAIDs for short-term use only. According to the 2008 American College of Cardiology Foundation/ American College of Gastroenterology/American Heart Association guidelines, patients are thought to be at high risk for GI toxicity from NSAIDs if they have a history of ulcer disease or complication, are on dual antiplatelet therapy, are on an NSAID with concomitant anticoagulant therapy. Additional risk factors for NSAID GI toxicity include age ≥60 years, corticosteroid use, dyspepsia, or gastroesophageal reflux disease symptoms. Thus in older adults (age >65 years), presence of any of the risk factors listed above should serve as indicators for proton pump inhibitor prophylaxis for NSAID therapy.

The FDA has issued a particular caution against using ibuprofen with aspirin, owing to an interaction that blocks the antiplatelet effect of the aspirin. Ibuprofen (reversible inhibition) and aspirin (irreversible inhibition) occupy nearby sites on cyclooxygenase, such that the presence of ibuprofen interferes with aspirin binding. Thus, ibuprofen interferes with the antiplatelet activity of low-dose aspirin (81 mg, immediate release) when the aspirin is ingested concurrently with ibuprofen. The FDA recommends that patients who use immediate-release aspirin (nonenteric coated) and take a single dose of ibuprofen 400 mg dose the ibuprofen at least 30 minutes after aspirin ingestion, or more than 8 hours before aspirin ingestion to avoid attenuation of aspirin's effect. Misoprostol, a prostaglandin analogue, or a proton-pump inhibitor can be used to reduce the risk of NSAID-induced GI bleeding, but this does not reduce the risks of renal disease, hypertension, fluid retention, or delirium. Topical NSAIDs appear to be safe and effective in the short-term, but longer-term studies are lacking.

4. Opioid medications—Moderate-to-severe pain or pain that requires chronic treatment often requires opioid medications for sufficient relief, although the evidence base supporting the role of long-term opioids in persistent noncancer pain is sparse. A systematic review of existing evidence regarding the efficacy, safety, and abuse/misuse potential of opioids as treatment for chronic noncancer pain in older adults showed that older adults were equally likely to benefit from treatment as compared to their younger counterparts. Common adverse events included constipation (median frequency of occurrence = 30%), nausea (28%), dizziness (22%), and prompted opioid discontinuation in 25% of cases. Abuse/ misuse behaviors were less common with advancing age. Among older adults with chronic noncancer pain and no significant comorbidity, short-term use of opioids was associated with reductions in pain intensity, improved physical functioning, but decreased mental health functioning. The geriatric principle of "start low and go slow" is applicable when starting opioid therapy. Careful and ongoing monitoring for benefits and side effects and tailoring therapy to the

individual patient's response to the therapeutic regimen are keys to successful treatment.

In general, continuous and persistent pain should be treated with long-acting or sustained-release formulations after opioid requirements have been estimated by an initial trial of a short-acting agent (Figure 54–1). Fast-onset medications with short half-lives may be added to cover a transient increase in pain intensity that occurs in patients with persistent pain (breakthrough pain). A typical patient requires approximately 5% to 15% the total daily dose offered every 2–4 hours orally for breakthrough pain. Cost and route of delivery can help guide the choice of medication (Table 54–4).

5. Opioid metabolism—Most opioids are metabolized by the liver and excreted by the kidney. In renal dysfunction, the active metabolites of morphine, including morphine-6-glucuronide and morphine-3-glucuronide, can accumulate, increasing the risk of prolonged sedation and possible neurotoxicity. The dosing intervals should be increased and the dosage decreased to reduce this risk. Limited data suggest that oxycodone may be better tolerated in patients with renal dysfunction because its metabolism results in fewer active metabolites, but this remains controversial.

6. Opioid adverse side effects—Although tolerance develops fairly rapidly to other adverse events of opioids, such as respiratory depression and sedation, constipation usually accompanies opioid use as the opioids bind to the *mu* receptors in the gut and slow down peristalsis. In fact, the most common adverse event of opioid treatment is constipation, and tolerance to constipation does not occur. Experts recommend starting therapy with a stimulant laxative (such as bisacodyl or senna); however, these should be avoided in any patient with signs or symptoms of bowel obstruction. Bulk-forming laxatives, such as fiber and psyllium, should be avoided in patients who are inactive and who have poor oral fluid intake because of the risk of causing fecal impaction and obstruction. For patients who develop opioid-induced constipation despite laxative therapy, treatment with methylnaltrexone, a *mu*-opioid-receptor antagonist, may relieve constipation without precipitating withdrawal symptoms or a pain crisis.

Respiratory depression is the most serious potential adverse effect associated with opioid use, but tolerance to this effect develops quickly. Older adults with a history of lung dysfunction are at particular risk when opioid dosages are increased too rapidly or when a benzodiazepine is prescribed concomitantly. Naloxone, an opioid-receptor antagonist, can reverse opioid-induced respiratory depression. It should be used with caution in patients who have been treated chronically with opioids as it can precipitate a pain crisis and acute withdrawal symptoms. Experts suggest withholding naloxone unless the patient's respiratory rate decreases to <8 breaths per minute or the oxygen saturation drops to <90%. Patients commonly overcome the opioid-induced fatigue and sedation

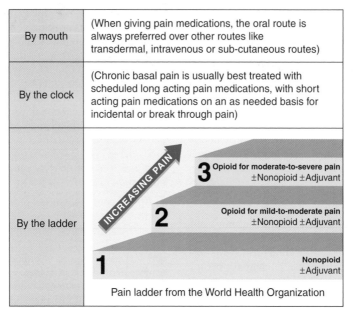

By mouth	(When giving pain medications, the oral route is always preferred over other routes like transdermal, intravenous or sub-cutaneous routes)
By the clock	(Chronic basal pain is usually best treated with scheduled long acting pain medications, with short acting pain medications on an as needed basis for incidental or break through pain)
By the ladder	INCREASING PAIN **3** Opioid for moderate-to-severe pain ±Nonopioid ±Adjuvant **2** Opioid for mild-to-moderate pain ±Nonopioid ±Adjuvant **1** Nonopioid ±Adjuvant Pain ladder from the World Health Organization

▲ **Figure 54–1.** How to institute opioid therapy. Consult this figure for items to remember when dosing opioids for a patient with chronic severe pain. (The pain ladder is reproduced with permission from the World Health Organization.)

over days to weeks as they become tolerant to the medication. It is important to educate patients about the risks of increased falls and instruct them not to drive or operate heavy equipment when opioids are started or the dosage changed.

7. Adjuvant medications—Adjuvant analgesics are medications which aid the primary analgesics in pain management. Adjuvant analgesics include a wide variety of medications, including antidepressants, antiepileptics, medications like clonidine, and others. Adjuvant medications can be used effectively solely or in combination with opioids for treating patients with neuropathic pain or mixed pain syndromes. Tricyclic antidepressants (TCAs) are effective in the treatment of postherpetic neuralgia and diabetic neuropathy. However, they are associated with significant anticholinergic adverse events in older adults, including constipation, urinary retention, dry mouth, cognitive impairment, tachycardia, and blurred vision. Desipramine and nortriptyline may have fewer adverse events. Amitriptyline should be avoided in older adults because of its strong anticholinergic properties.

D. Treatment of Clinical Depression in Patients with Persistent Pain

Clinical depression in patients with persistent pain requires treatment to achieve optimal analgesia and quality of life and selective serotonin reuptake inhibitors are the first-line class

of drugs. Duloxetine, an inhibitor of norepinephrine and serotonin uptake, is approved both as an antidepressant and for the treatment of pain from diabetic neuropathy, and may offer a more favorable adverse-event profile than the TCAs. Anticonvulsant medications such as gabapentin, pregabalin, and clonazepam[OL] are commonly used as treatments for neuropathic pain. Gabapentin and pregabalin have demonstrated clinical efficacy in the treatment of postherpetic neuralgia, and have fewer adverse events than TCAs, although their cost is substantially more. The main adverse side effects of gabapentin and pregabalin include sedation and dizziness. Gabapentin dosage has to be reduced in patients with renal dysfunction. Intravenous bisphosphonates can substantially reduce pain from malignant bone metastases. As bisphosphonates are associated with osteonecrosis of the jaw, a dental consultation is recommended before institution of maintenance bisphosphonates. Meperidine should be avoided in older adults. Meperidine is metabolized to normeperidine, which has no analgesic properties but can accumulate in patients with decreased kidney function and cause tremulousness, myoclonus, and seizures. Tapentadol is a synthetic, oral mu-opioid receptor agonist approved by the FDA in 2009 for the management of moderate-to-severe acute pain and chronic pain in adults. Tapentadol has serotonin norepinephrine reuptake inhibition properties and is structurally and pharmacologically similar to tramadol. Therapy should be initiated at the lowest recommended

Table 54–4. Opioid equivalency table.

Drug	Oral/Rectal Route	Parenteral Route	Conversion Ratio to Oral Morphine	Equianalgesic Dose of Oral Morphine
Morphine sulfate	30 mg oral morphine	10 mg of parenteral morphine	Parenteral morphine is **3 times** as potent as oral morphine	30 mg oral morphine
Oxycodone	20 mg of oral oxycodone	NA	Oral oxycodone is **roughly 1.5 times** more potent than oral morphine	30 mg oral morphine
Hydrocodone	20 mg of oral hydrocodone	NA	Oral hydrocodone is **roughly 1.5 times** more potent than oral morphine	30 mg oral morphine
Hydromorphone	7 mg of oral hydromorphone	1.5 mg of parenteral hydromorphone	Oral hydromorphone is about **4-7 times** as potent as oral morphine. Parenteral hydromorphone is **20 times** as potent as oral morphine	30 mg oral morphine
Fentanyl	NA	15 mcg/h	Transdermal fentanyl is **approximately 80 times** as potent as morphine (This is based on studies converting from morphine to fentanyl. Currently, there are no empirical studies converting fentanyl to morphine.)	30 mg oral morphine
Meperidine. Meperidine is **not** a recommended drug in a palliative care setting and is to be **avoided**. If a patient with chronic pain is on meperidine, convert patient to an equianalgesic dose of one of the other opioids listed in this table.	300 mg of oral meperidine	75 mg of parenteral meperidine	Oral morphine is **about 10 times** more potent than oral meperidine and about twice as potent as parenteral meperidine (mg for mg)	30 mg oral morphine

Created by V.J. Periyakoil, MD, for Stanford eCampus curriculum: http://endoflife.stanford.edu

dosage range in older adults, and the drug should be avoided in severe renal and hepatic impairment. For acute pain, dosage is immediate-release tapentadol at 50 mg q4–6h as needed. For chronic pain, the extended-release formulation can be used at a dosage of 50 mg q12h and titrate to an effective dose in increments of 50 mg and no more frequently than every 3 days. Significant side effects include nausea, vomiting, constipation, dizziness, and somnolence. Also, the extended-release formulation should be titrated off gradually to prevent withdrawal Two other drugs known to cause restlessness and tremulousness in older adults are the mixed agonist–antagonists nalbuphine and butorphanol, and these 2 are best avoided in older adults.

Bhatt DL, Scheiman J, Abraham NS, et al; American College of Cardiology Foundation Task Force on Clinical Expert Consensus Documents. ACCF/ACG/AHA 2008 expert consensus document on reducing the gastrointestinal risks of antiplatelet therapy and NSAID use: a report of the American College of Cardiology Foundation Task Force on Clinical Expert Consensus Documents. *J Am Coll Cardiol.* 2008;52(18):1502-1517.

Chibnall J, Tait R. Pain assessment in cognitively impaired and unimpaired older adults: a comparison of four scales. *Pain.* 2001;92(1-2):173-186.

Feldt KS, Ryden MB, Miles S. Treatment of pain in cognitively impaired compared with cognitively intact older patients with hip fracture. *J Am Geriatr Soc.* 1998;46(9):1079-1085.

Ferrell BA. Pain evaluation and management in the nursing home. *Ann Intern Med.* 1995;123(9):681-695.

Ferrell BA, Ferrell BR, Rivera L. Pain in cognitively impaired nursing home patients. *J Pain Symptom Manage.* 1995;10(8):591-598.

Gibson SJ, Helme RD. Age-related differences in pain perception and report. *Clin Geriatr Med.* 2001;17(3):433-456.

Herr K, Garand L. Assessment and measurement of pain in older adults: pain management in the elderly. *Clin Geriatr Med.* 2001;17(3):457-478, vi.

Hwang U. Richardson LD, Harris B, Morrison RS. The quality of emergency department pain care for older adult patients. *J Am Geriatr Soc.* 2010;58(11):2122-2128.

Kaasalainen S, Middleton J, Knezacek S, et al. Pain and cognitive status in institutionalized elderly: perceptions & interventions. *J Gerontol Nurs.* 1998;24(8):24-31.

Lanza FL, Chan FK, Quigley EM; Practice Parameters Committee of the American College of Gastroenterology. Guidelines for prevention of NSAID-related ulcer complications. *Am J Gastroenterol*. 2009;104(3):728-738.

O'Neil CK, Hanlon JT, Marcum ZA. Adverse effects of analgesics commonly used by older adults with osteoarthritis: focus on non-opioid and opioid analgesics. *Am J Geriatr Pharmacother*. 2012;10(6):331-342.

Papaleontiou M, Henderson CR Jr, Turner BJ, et al. Outcomes associated with opioid use in the treatment of chronic non-cancer pain among older adults: a systematic review and meta-analysis. *J Am Geriatr Soc*. 2010;58(7):1353-1369.

Simsek IE, Simsaek TT, Yumin ET, Sertel M, Ozturk A, Yumin M. The effects of pain on health-related quality of life and satisfaction with life in older adults. *Top Geriatr Rehabil*. 2010;26(4):361-367.

Stolee P, Hillier LM, Esbaugh J, Bol N, McKellar L, Gauthier N. Instruments for the assessment of pain in older persons with cognitive impairment. *J Am Geriatr Soc*. 2005;53(2):319-326.

Warden V, Hurley AC, Volicer L. Development and psychometric evaluation of the Pain Assessment in Advanced Dementia (PAINAD) Scale. *J Am Med Dir Assoc*. 2003;4(1):9-15.

Weiner D, Peterson B, Keefe F. Chronic pain-associated behaviors in the nursing home: resident versus caregiver perceptions. *Pain*. 1999;80(3):577-588.

USEFUL WEBSITES

Stanford School of Medicine. *Successful Aging of Multi-Cultural American Older Adults*. http://geriatrics.stanford.edu

Stanford School of Medicine. *Palliative Care*. http://palliative.stanford.edu

Stanford University Medical School. *Stanford eCampus. End of Life Online Curriculum*. http://endoflife.stanford.edu

Translations of Wong-Baker FACES Pain Rating Scale. http://www.wongbakerfaces.org/

Considering Anticoagulation in Older Adults

55

Anita Rajasekhar, MD, MS

Rebecca J. Beyth, MD, MSc

▶ General Principles in Older Adults

Persons 65 years or older comprise approximately 13% of the U.S. population, yet they are prescribed the greatest proportion of medication; 90% are prescribed at least 1 prescription drug and 65% 3 or more prescription drugs in the last month. They also represent the fastest growing segment of prescription drug users in the United States. Thus, with an increasing number of patients surviving to older age and consuming larger amounts of drugs, it is necessary for clinicians to understand the risk, benefits, and consequences of drug therapy in older patients. This is especially true for anticoagulants, a class of drugs essential for the optimal management of many thromboembolic and vascular disorders that are highly prevalent among older patients. Anticoagulants are unique compared to most pharmacologic agents because even small deviations from "therapeutic levels" place patients at risk for life-threatening complications. While older patients with multimorbidity are particularly susceptible to thrombosis, they also have higher risks of bleeding than the general population. This chapter briefly reviews current anticoagulant therapy and focuses on the newer agents and recommendations for their use in older patients.

Health, United States, 2012, with Special Feature on Emergency Care. United States Department of Health and Human Services, Centers for Disease Control and Prevention, National Center for Health Statistics, May 2013, DHHS Publication No. 2013-1232 Table 1, Page 45, and Table 9, page 282 at http://www.cdc.gov/nchs/data/hus/hus12.pdf#listtables (last accessed December 6, 2013).

AVAILABLE CLASSES OF ANTICOAGULANT THERAPY

Current anticoagulants that are available for use within the United States include unfractionated heparin (UFH), vitamin K antagonists (VKAs), low-molecular weight heparins (LMWHs), indirect selective factor Xa inhibitor, and the direct thrombin (parental and oral) and factor Xa inhibitors. Tables 55–1 and 55–2 summarize the specific pharmacologic characteristics of these agents.

▶ Oral Vitamin K Antagonists

Concerns about the use of anticoagulants in older patients arise from their increased risk for anticoagulant-related bleeding. The major determinants of oral VKA-induced bleeding are the intensity of the anticoagulant effect, as measured by the international normalized ratio (INR), patient characteristics, concomitant use of drugs that interfere with hemostasis or vitamin K metabolism, and the length of therapy. Of these, the INR is the most important risk factor, and this is especially true for the intracranial hemorrhage (ICH), the most feared site of major bleeding. The risk of ICH increases 7-fold with increasing INR levels above 4.0. Patient characteristics, including age and specific comorbid conditions (ischemic stroke diabetes, renal insufficiency, malignancy, hypertension, liver disease or alcoholism), also are associated with increased risk of major bleeding. In general, older patients have approximately a 2-fold increase in major bleeding compared to their younger counterparts. Decision making around the use of anticoagulants is complex because the risk factors that are associated with anticoagulant-related bleeding are similar to those associated with increased risk of thrombosis. The use of anticoagulants medications in older patients is an area where applying the principles of shared decision making is critical. The choice of whether to prescribe anticoagulants and which specific medication to use should be individualized, taking into account not only evidence-based medicine, but also patients' goals and preferences to ensure compliance.

More recently, the genetic polymorphisms of the cytochrome P450 CYP2C9 and the vitamin K epoxide reductase complex subunit 1 (VKORC1) have been found to affect warfarin metabolism and vitamin K reduction. Patients with the CYP2C9*2, CYP2C9*3, and VKORC1 A variants require

Table 55–1. Pharmacologic properties of parental anticoagulants.

Properties	Heparin and Derivatives		Specific Anti-Xa Inhibitor	Parental Direct Thrombin Inhibitors		
	UFH	LMWH	Fondaparinux	Argatroban	Desirudin	Bivalirudin
Subtype		Enoxaparin, Dalteparin, Tinzaparin				
Elimination	Reticuloendothelial system	Renal	Renal	Hepatic	Renal	Enzymatic, 20% renal
Time to peak concentration	IV: immediate SQ: 20–60 minutes	~1.5 hours	~2 hours			
Half-life	~1.5 hours	~2–5 hours	~17–21 hours	~45 minutes	~120 minutes	~25 minutes
Lab monitoring	aPTT, anti-Xa heparin levels	Not required; can measure anti-Xa LMWH levels	Not required; can measure anti-Xa fondaparinux levels	aPTT, ACT	Not required; can monitor aPTT	aPTT, ACT
Prolongation of INR at therapeutic concentrations	No	No	No	Significant	Minor	Minor
Reversible (antidote)	Complete with protamine	Partial with protamine	No	No	No	No
Dose adjustments	None	Renal impairment, extremes of weight: titrate to desired anti-Xa level	Renal impairment: titrate to desired anti-Xa level	Moderate hepatic impairment: 0.5 mcg/kg/min in HIT Severe HF: CI	CrCl <31–60 mL/min: DR unnecessary	CrCl 15–60 mL/min: 15% to 50% DR CrCl <15 mL/min: CI
FDA Indications	• AF with embolization • DIC • Thrombosis prevention in arterial and cardiac surgery • Prophylaxis and treatment of VTE and peripheral arterial embolism • Treatment of unstable angina and NSTEMI	Varies according to subtype of LMWH Includes: • Prophylaxis and treatment of VTE • Prevention of thrombus in hemodialysis circuit • Treatment of unstable angina and NSTEMI	Prophylaxis of DVT in: • Hip fracture surgery • Hip replacement surgery • Knee replacement surgery • Abdominal surgery Treatment of: • Acute VTE when administered with warfarin • Unstable angina and NSTEMI	• Prophylaxis or treatment of thrombosis complicating HIT • HIT with or without thrombosis undergoing PCI	• DVT prevention after THR	• Unstable angina undergoing PTCA • PCI with provisional use of GPI • HIT with or without thrombosis

ACT, activated clotting time; AF, atrial fibrillation; aPTT, activated partial thromboplastin time; CI, contraindicated; CrCl, creatinine clearance; DIC, disseminated intravascular coagulation; DR, dose reduction; DVT, deep vein thrombosis; GPI, glycoprotein inhibitor; HF, heart failure; HIT, heparin-induced thrombocytopenia; IV, intravenous; LMWH, low-molecular-weight heparin; NSTEMI, non-ST elevation myocardial infarction; PCI, percutaneous coronary intervention; PTCA, percutaneous transluminal coronary angioplasty; SQ, subcutaneous; UFH, unfractionated heparin; VTE, venous thromboembolism .

Table 55–2. Pharmacologic properties of oral anticoagulants.

Properties	Vitamin K Antagonist	New Oral Anticoagulants	
Type	Warfarin	Dabigatran	Rivaroxaban
Mechanism of action	Inhibits synthesis of vitamin K-dependent clotting factors	Direct thrombin inhibitor	Direct factor Xa inhibitor
Time to peak concentration	90 minutes (peak anticoagulant effect 5–7 days)	~1.5 hours	~3 hours
Half-life (normal CrCl)	36–42 hours	12–14 hours	4–13 hours
Clearance	Hepatic	80% Renal	60% Renal
Dose reductions	Avoid in hepatic insufficiency	CrCl 15–30: 75 mg BID; CrCl <15, severe hepatic disease: contra-indicated	CrCl 15–50: caution; CrCl <15: contraindicated
Lab monitoring	INR	Not required; TT/TCT or aPTT	Not required; anti-Xa assay
Reversible (antidote)	Vitamin K, fresh-frozen plasma, prothrombin complex concentrates, rFVIIa	No	No

aPTT, activated partial thromboplastin time; BID, twice daily; CrCl, creatinine clearance; INR, international normalized ratio; rFVIIa, recombinant activated factor VII; TT/TCT, thrombin time/thrombin clotting time.

lower maintenance doses of warfarin and are at increased risk of over-anticoagulation and major bleeding. Thus, on average, dosage reductions of approximately 19% to 33% are needed to avoid over-anticoagulation. The International Warfarin Pharmacogenetics Consortium found that an algorithm based on clinical plus pharmacogenetic data performed better compared to either pure clinical algorithm or fixed dose approach in predicting the appropriate warfarin dose. Subsequently, the Food and Drug Administration revised the labeling for warfarin in 2010 to reflect that CYP2C9 and VKORC1 genotyping could assist in warfarin dosing. Yet, the clinical utility of pharmacogenetic-based warfarin dosing in older patients is not clear. Schwartz et al noted in a cohort of patients ≥65 years (mean age: 81 years) that included nursing home and senior care community residents on warfarin with stable therapeutic INRs that the addition of genotype information helped to explain a greater proportion of the INR variability when compared to those without genotype information (50% vs. 12%; P <0.0001). However, when comparing estimated warfarin doses to actual warfarin doses in patients requiring <2 mg per day of warfarin, dosing was overestimated despite the use of pharmacogenetic information; that is, the addition of genotype information did not improve the dosing management. Because earlier studies observed increasing age is associated with increasing response to the effects of warfarin as manifested by lower daily doses, the applicability of pharmacogenetic dosing algorithms to older patients requiring lower warfarin dosing is somewhat limited. Thus, the adage of "start low and go slow" still remains applicable to warfarin dosing in older patients.

Many drugs are known to interact with anticoagulants, and because the majority of older patients are prescribed more than 1 drug, there is ample opportunity for adverse drug reactions to occur in older patients. Drugs that potentiate the anticoagulant effect (increase the INR) increase the risk of bleeding. Other drugs increase hepatic metabolism resulting in decreasing the anticoagulant effect requiring increased dosage requirements (Table 55–3). When these drugs are discontinued, there can be an increase in INR and bleeding. Thus, additional monitoring with dosage adjustment is required when these drugs are either added to or removed from the medication profile of older patients on warfarin therapy.

Despite its efficacy in treatment and prophylaxis, warfarin has several limitations that make its use cumbersome. These include its slow onset of action, narrow therapeutic window, and the lack of predictability in anticoagulant effect by drug dose, many dietary and drug interactions, and the need for routine INR monitoring. Some of this burden may be lessened with less-frequent INR monitoring (up to every 12 weeks vs. every 4 weeks), which has been shown to be safe in patients with stable INRs. Older patients who are motivated and can demonstrate competency can self-manage and/or self-test. Best practices for ensuring safety include using a coordinated monitoring system with patient education, systematic INR testing, tracking and follow-up, and good communication. (For travel recommendations for older adults on warfarin, see Chapter 20, "The Aging Traveler.")

Aithal GP, Day CP, Kesteven PJ, Daly AK. Association of polymorphisms in the cytochrome P450 CYP2C9 with warfarin dose requirement and risk of bleeding complications. *Lancet.* 1999;353(9154):717-719.

Coumadin (warfarin sodium) tablet and injection. Safety Labeling Changes Approved by FDA Center for Drug Evaluation and Research (CDER)—January 2010. Accessed May 8, 2012. http://www.fda.gov/Safety/MedWatch/SafetyInformation/ucm201100.htm.

Table 55–3. Common warfarin drug interactions.

Drug	Effect on Warfarin	Mechanism
Metronidazole	Potentiates	Inhibition of vitamin K synthesis by intestinal flora and CYP2C9 inhibition
Macrolides	Potentiates	Inhibition of vitamin K synthesis by intestinal flora and CYP2C9 inhibition
Fluoroquinolones	Potentiates	Inhibition of vitamin K synthesis by intestinal flora and CYP2C9 inhibition
Trimethoprim-sulfamethoxazole	Potentiates	CYP2C9 inhibition
Fluconazole	Potentiates	CYP2C9 inhibition
Selective serotonin reuptake inhibitors	Potentiates	CYP2C9 inhibition
Amiodarone	Potentiates	CYP2C9 inhibition
Levothyroxine	Potentiates	Increased vitamin K-dependent clotting factor catabolism
Garlic	Potentiates	Not well understood
Ginger	Potentiates	Not well understood
Gingko-biloba	Potentiates	Not well understood
Ginseng	Potentiates	Not well understood
Carbamazepine	Inhibits	CYP2C9 inducer
Phenytoin	Inhibits	CYP2C9 inducer
Phenobarbital	Inhibits	CYP2C9 inducer
St. John's wort	Inhibits	CYP2C9 inducer

CYP2C9, Cytochrome P450 2C9.

Gurwitz JH, Avorn J, Ross-Degnan D, Choodnovskiy I, Ansell J. Aging and the anticoagulant response to warfarin therapy. *Ann Intern Med.* 1992;116(11):901-904.

Heneghan C, Ward A, Perera R, et al. Self-monitoring of oral anticoagulation: systematic review and meta-analysis of individual patient data. *Lancet.* 2012;379(9813):322-334.

Higashi MK, Veenstra DL, Kondo LM, et al. Association between CYP2C9 genetic variants and anticoagulation-related outcomes during warfarin therapy. *JAMA.* 2002;287(13):1690-1698.

Holbrook A, Schulman S, Witt DM, et al; American College of Chest Physicians. Evidence-based management of anticoagulant therapy: Antithrombotic Therapy and Prevention of Thrombosis, 9th ed: American College of Chest Physicians Evidence-Based Clinical Practice Guideline. *Chest.* 2012; 141(2 Suppl):e152S-e184S.

Hutten BA, Lensing AW, Kraaijenhagen RA, Prins MH. Safety of treatment with oral anticoagulants in the elderly. A systematic review. *Drugs Aging.* 1999;14(4):303-312.

Hylek EM, Singer DE. Risk factors for intracranial hemorrhage in outpatients taking warfarin. *Ann Intern Med.* 1994;120(11): 897-902.

James AH, Britt RP, Raskino CL, Thompson SG. Factors affecting the maintenance dose of warfarin. *J Clin Pathol.* 1992;45(8): 704-706.

Rieder MJ, Reiner AP, Gage BF, et al. Effect of VKORC1 haplotypes on transcriptional regulation and warfarin dose. *N Engl J Med.* 2005;352(22):2285-2293.

Robinson A, Thomson RG; Decision Analysis in Routine Treatments Study (DARTS) team. The potential use of decision analysis to support shared decision making in the face of uncertainty: the example of atrial fibrillation and warfarin anticoagulation. *Qual Health Care.* 2009;9(4):238-244.

Schwartz JB, Kane L, Moore K, Wu AHB. Failure of pharmacogenetic-based dosing algorithms to identify older patients requiring low daily doses of warfarin. *J Am Med Dir Assoc.* 2011;12(9):633-638.

Schulman S, Beyth RJ, Kearon C, Levine M; American College of Chest Physicians. Hemorrhagic complication of anticoagulant and thrombolytic treatment: American College of Chest Physicians Evidence-Based Clinical Practice Guidelines (8th Edition). *Chest.* 2008;133(6 Suppl):257S-298S.

Schulman S, Parpia S, Steward C, Rudd-Scott L, Julian JA, Levine M. Warfarin dose assessment every 4 weeks versus every 12 weeks in patients with stable international normalized ratios: a randomized trial. *Ann Intern Med.* 2011;155(10):653-659.

Takeuchi F, McGinnis R, Bourgeois S, et al. A genome-wide association study confirms VKORC1, CYP2C9, and CYP4F2 as principal genetic determinants of warfarin dose. *PLoS Genet.* 2009;5(3):e1000433.

The International Warfarin Pharmacogenetics Consortium, Klein TE, Altman RB, Eriksson N, et al. Estimation of the warfarin dose with clinical and pharmacological data. *N Engl J Med.* 2009;360(8):753-764.

▶ Injectable Anticoagulants

LMWH and selective indirect anti-Xa inhibitor (fondaparinux) are also used in older patients. The 2 major concerns in older patients are renal impairment and lower body weight. Reduced renal clearance occurs with age and increases the susceptibility to major bleeding, as LMWHs are primarily renally eliminated. The risk of LMWH accumulation and bleeding is dependent on the severity of renal impairment, the dose (prophylactic or therapeutic) and type of LMWH. Among LMWHs, only enoxaparin has approved dose reduction in older patients with renal impairment. Advancing age and renal impairment also reduces clearance of fondaparinux. Reduced-dose fondaparinux appears to have good safety and efficacy in older patients with mild renal impairment, but this has not been validated in those with severe renal impairment. Renal function should not be solely assessed by the serum creatinine as this leads to underestimation of renal failure in older patients, and measurement of the glomerular filtration rate is preferred. Thus, it is prudent to test LMWH or fondaparinux anti-Xa levels in older patients with renal impairment or low body weight to avoid supratherapeutic doses.

Cohen AT, Davidson BL, Gallus AS, et al. Efficacy and safety of fondaparinux for the prevention of venous thromboembolism in older acute medical patients: randomised placebo controlled trial. *BMJ*. 2006;332(7537):325-329.

Lim W. Low-molecular-weight heparin in patients with chronic renal insufficiency. *Intern Emerg Med*. 2008;3(4):319-23.

Turpie AG, Lensing AW, Fuji T, et al. Influence of renal function on the efficacy and safety of fondaparinux 1.5 mg once daily in the prevention of venous thromboembolism in renally impaired patients. *Blood Coagul Fibrinolysis*. 2009;20(2):1141-1121.

New Oral Anticoagulants

For the first time since the introduction of warfarin in 1954, 2 new oral anticoagulants have been FDA approved. Dabigatran is FDA approved for the prevention of stroke and systemic embolism in nonvalvular atrial fibrillation. Rivaroxaban is FDA approved for (a) prophylaxis against venous thromboembolism (VTE) in patients undergoing knee or hip replacement surgery and (b) to reduce the risk of stroke and systemic embolism in patients with nonvalvular atrial fibrillation. Although clinical trials that led to the approval of dabigatran and rivaroxaban included older patients, those with renal and hepatic failure were systematically excluded from these trials. These new oral anticoagulants overcome several of the limitations of warfarin, including slow onset of action, narrow therapeutic window, drug and dietary interactions, and the need for routine laboratory monitoring. As a result of the increased use of these agents in the geriatric population,

clinicians should be aware of the indications, pharmacology, methods for monitoring anticoagulant activity, and recommendations for management of bleeding with these new oral anticoagulants (see Table 55-2 and Tables 55–4, 55–5, and 55–6).

Dabigatran is a novel competitive direct thrombin inhibitor. Dabigatran has a rapid onset of action (peak plasma concentration approximately 1.5 hours following oral ingestion) obviating the need for bridging anticoagulation. The half-life of dabigatran with normal renal function is 12–14 hours, allowing for once or twice-daily dosing. Because the drug is 80% renally cleared, dose reductions (75 mg PO BID) are recommended for creatinine clearance (CrCl) of 15–30 mL/min. Dabigatran is contraindicated in patients with severe renal insufficiency (CrCl <15 mL/min). Consideration should be given to age-related changes in kidney function that lead to a 40% to 60% increase in area under the curve. This increased concentration can lead to greater exposure to the drug and potential bleeding complications. Age-related renal function changes may explain some of this age effect. In the RE-LY study, 2 doses of dabigatran, 110 mg and 150 mg twice daily, were compared to dose-adjusted warfarin in more than 18,000 patients with nonvalvular atrial fibrillation. The mean age in each group was 71 years and the mean weight 82 kg. Patients with CrCl <30 mL/min and clinically significant liver disease were excluded. The trial was therefore neither designed nor powered to detect the safety of dabigatran in older patients with low body weight. A significant proportion of patients in each group were on aspirin concomitantly. Both doses of dabigatran were proven to be as effective as

Table 55–4. Patient characteristics in clinical trials involving dabigatran.

Patient Characteristics	RECOVER	RELY	REMOBILIZE	REMODEL	RENOVATE
Age (years)	55 ± 15.8	71.4 ± 8.6	66.2 ± 9.5	67 ± 9	65 ± 10
	54.4 ± 16.2	71.5 ± 8.8	65.9 ± 9.5	68 ± 9	63 ± 11
		71.6 ± 8.6	66.3 ± 9.6	68 ± 9	64 ± 11
Weight (kg)	85.5 ± 19.2	82.9 ± 19.9	Excluded ≤40 kg	Excluded ≤40 kg	Excluded ≤40 kg
	84.2 ± 18.3	82.5 ± 19.4	88.4 ± 19.1	82 ± 15	79 ± 15
		82.7 ± 19.7	87.6 ± 20	83 ± 15	79 ± 15
			88 ± 19.2	82 ± 15	78 ± 15
CrCl <30 mL/min	Excluded	Excluded	Excluded	Excluded	Excluded
Active liver disease	Excluded	Excluded	Excluded	Excluded	Excluded
CHADS2 Score	NA	2.1	NA	NA	NA
Medications	Excluded if on long-term antiplatelets (<100 mg ASA acceptable)	ASA (40%, 38.7%, 40.6%) ACEI/ARB (66.3%, 66.7%, 65.5%) BB (62.9%, 63.7%, 61.8%)	Excluded in needed long-term antiplatelet agent	Excluded if needed long-term NSAIDs	Excluded if needed long-term NSAIDs

ACEI, angiotensin-converting-enzyme inhibitor; ARB, angiotensin receptor blocker; ASA, aminosalicylic acid; BB, beta blocker; CrCl, creatinine clearance; Kg, kilogram; NA, not applicable; NSAIDs, nonsteroidal antiinflammatory drugs.

Table 55–5. Patient characteristics in clinical trials involving rivaroxaban.

Patient Characteristics	EINSTEIN-DVT	EINSTEIN-PE	RECORD1	RECORD2	RECORD3	RECORD4	ROCKET
Age (years)	57.9	55.8	63.1	61.4	67.6	64.4	Median (IQR)
	57.5	56.4	63.3	61.6	67.6	64.7	73 (65–78)
							73 (65–78)
Weight (kg)	<50 kg	<50 kg	Mean:	Mean:	Mean:	Mean:	Median (IQR)
	1.6%	2.1%	78.1	74.3	80.1	84.7	67 (52–88)
	1.8%	2.9%	78.3	75.2	81.2	84.4	67 (52–86)
CrCl <30 mL/min	Excluded	Excluded	Excluded	Excluded	Excluded	Excluded	Excluded
Active liver disease	Excluded	Excluded	Excluded	Excluded	Excluded	Excluded	Excluded
CHADS2 Score	NA	2.1	NA	NA	NA	NA	3.5

CrCl, creatinine clearance; IQR, interquartile range; Kg, kilogram; NA, not applicable.

warfarin for prevention of stroke or systemic embolism. However, dabigatran 150 mg twice daily was found to be superior to warfarin for stroke prevention (1.11% per year vs. 1.71% per year; p <0.001; RR: 0.65; 95% CI: 0.52–0.81). There was no difference in annual major bleeding rates on dabigatran compared to warfarin (3.32% per year vs. 3.57% per year; p = 0.32; RR: 0.93; CI: 0.81–1.07). However, a subset analysis by age groups revealed that among the 39% of patients older than 75 years old, bleeding was increased in the dabigatran 150 mg arm (HR: 1.18; 95% CI: 0.98–1.43). This effect occurred regardless of renal function. Although not Federal Drug Administration (FDA)-approved for the following indications, dabigatran was also found to be as effective as (a) enoxaparin in the prevention of VTE after total knee arthroplasty and total hip arthroplasty, and (b) warfarin in the prevention of recurrent VTE after acute symptomatic proximal deep venous thrombosis or pulmonary embolism.

Table 55–6. Management of bleeding on anticoagulants.

Anticoagulant	Reversal Agent	Laboratory Monitoring of Reversal	Special Considerations
Warfarin	(1) Vitamin K (2) Fresh-frozen plasma (3) Prothrombin complex concentrates (4) rVIIa	PT/INR	FFP has the potential for volume overload, TRALI, and delays related to preparation and delivery of FFP
LMWHs • Enoxaparin • Dalteparin • Tinzaparin	(1) Protamine (2) rVIIa for life-threatening bleeding	anti-Xa activity	Protamine only partially reverses LMWHs
Factor Xa inhibitor • Fondaparinux • Rivaroxaban	(1) rVIIa for life threatening bleeding	anti-Xa activity	
Parenteral direct thrombin inhibitors • Argatroban • Bivalirudin • Desirudin	(1) DDAVP (2) Cryoprecipitate (3) Antifibrinolytics	aPTT, PT	These anticoagulants have short half-lives
Oral direct thrombin inhibitor • Dabigatran	(1) Oral charcoal (2) rVIIa (3) Prothrombin complex concentrates	aPTT, TT/TCT	Hemodialysis can remove dabigatran

aPTT, activated partial thromboplastin time; DDAVP, desmopressin; HD, hemodialysis; INR, international normalized ratio; PCC, prothrombin complex concentrates; PT, prothrombin time; rFVII, recombinant factor VII; TRALI, transfusion related acute lung injury; TT/TCT, thrombin time/thrombin clotting time.

Rivaroxaban is a reversible direct factor Xa inhibitor with peak plasma concentrations at 3 hours after ingestion. The half-life is 4–9 hours (up to 13 hours in patients age 65 years and older). Rivaroxaban is 60% renally cleared, but no dose reductions are required for mild renal insufficiency. Rivaroxaban is contraindicated with CrCl <30 mL/min. Rivaroxaban was investigated in 4 large phase III trials for prevention of VTE after total hip and knee arthroplasty (RECORD 1–4). All studies included older patients but excluded patients with renal and hepatic insufficiency (see Table 55–5). In all 4 trials, rivaroxaban 10 mg orally daily was superior to enoxaparin for a composite of total VTE and all-cause mortality. There were no significant differences in the rates of major bleeding or hepatic enzyme elevations between the 2 treatments. In the ROCKET study, approximately 14,000 patients with non-valvular atrial fibrillation were randomly assigned to rivaroxaban 20 mg orally daily or dose-adjusted warfarin. Notably, patients with CrCl 30–50 mL/min were included in the trial with a dose reduction to 15 mg orally daily. Rivaroxaban was noninferior to warfarin for the prevention of stroke or systemic embolism (HR: 0.88; 95% CI: 0.74–1.03; P <0.001 for noninferiority). There was no significant between-group difference in the risk of major bleeding, although intracranial (0.5% vs. 0.7%, p = 0.02) and fatal bleeding (0.2% vs. 0.5%, p = 0.003) occurred less frequently in the rivaroxaban group. Rivaroxaban has been shown to be noninferior to warfarin for the treatment of acute VTE, but it has yet to be approved for this indication.

Although the characteristics of a more rapid onset of action, and a more predictable anticoagulant effect make these newer agents an attractive alternative to warfarin, caution is still needed when used in older patients. The convenience of no regular monitoring of coagulation also means there is no mechanism to objectively assess adherence to therapy. This may be more problematic for older patients in whom a fixed-dose regimen may not universally apply because of their variations in renal function and body weight, where the safety and efficacy of these agents is uncertain. Additionally, the lack of monitoring may potentially lead to missed opportunities for early detection of a complication because of lack of regular patient–provider interaction.

Connolly SJ, Ezekowitz MD, Yusuf S, et al. Dabigatran versus warfarin in patients with atrial fibrillation. *N Engl J Med.* 2009;361(12):1139-1151.

EINSTEIN Investigators, Bauersachs R, Berkowitz SD, Brenner B, et al. Oral rivaroxaban for symptomatic venous thromboembolism. *N Engl J Med.* 2010;363(26):2499-2510.

EINSTEIN-PE investigators, Büller HR, Prins MH, Lensin AW, et al. Oral rivaroxaban for the treatment of symptomatic pulmonary embolism. *N Engl J Med.* 2012;366(14):1287-1297.

Eriksson BI, Borris LC, Friedman RJ, et al; RECORD1 Study Group. Rivaroxaban versus enoxaparin for thromboprophylaxis after hip arthroplasty. *N Engl J Med.* 2008;358(26):2765-2775.

Eriksson BI, Dahl OE, Rosencer N, et al. Dabigatran etexilate versus enoxaparin for prevention of venous thromboembolism

after total hip replacement: a randomized, double-blind, noninferiority trial. *Lancet.* 2007;370(9591):949-956.

Eriksson BI, Dahl OE, Rosencher N, et al. Oral dabigatran etexilate vs. subcutaneous enoxaparin for the prevention of venous thromboembolism after total knee replacement: the RE-MODEL randomized trial. *J Thromb Haemost.* 2007;5(11):2178-2185.

Jacobs JM, Stessman J. New anticoagulant drugs among elderly patients is caution necessary?: Comment on "The use of dabigatran in elderly patients". *Arch Intern Med.* 2011;171(14): 1287-1288.

Kakkar AK, Brenner, Dahl OE, et al. Extended duration rivaroxaban versus short-term enoxaparin for the prevention of venous thromboembolism after total hip arthroplasty: a double-blind, randomized controlled trial. *Lancet.* 2008;372(9632):31-39.

Lassen MR, Ageno W, Borris LC, et al; RECORD3 Investigators. Rivaroxaban versus enoxaparin for thromboprophylaxis after total knee arthroplasty. *N Engl J Med.* 2008;358(26):2776-2786.

Patel MR, Mahaffey KW, Garg J, et al. Rivaroxaban versus warfarin in nonvalvular atrial fibrillation. *N Engl J Med.* 2011;365: 883-891.

RE-MOBILIZE Writing Committee, Ginsberg JS, Davidson BL, Comp PC, Francis CW, et al. Oral thrombin inhibitor dabigatran etexilate vs North American enoxaparin regimen for prevention of venous thromboembolism after knee arthroplasty surgery. *J Arthroplasty.* 2009;24(1):1-9.

Schulman S, Kearon C, Kakkar AK, et al; RE-COVER Study Group. Dabigatran versus warfarin in the treatment of acute venous thromboembolism. *N Engl J Med.* 2009;361(24):2342-2352.

Stangier J, Stahle H, Rathgen K. Pharmacokinetics and pharmacodynamics of the direct oral thrombin inhibitor dabigatran in healthy elderly subjects. *Clin Pharmacokinet.* 2008;47(1):47-59.

Turpie AG, Lassen MR, Davidson BL, et al; RECORD4 Investigators. Rivaroxaban versus enoxaparin for Thromboprophylaxis after total knee arthroplasty (RECORD4): a randomized trial. *Lancet.* 2009;373(676):1673-1680.

MANAGEMENT OF BLEEDING IN OLDER PATIENTS ON ANTICOAGULANTS

Bleeding is the primary complication of anticoagulation therapy. Older patients are particularly susceptible to bleeding complications on anticoagulation as a result of their inherent risk for falls; comorbidities such as renal failure, hepatic dysfunction, malnutrition, malignancy, amyloid angiopathy; concomitant use of antiplatelet agents; and noncompliance with drug regimens. Although reversal of older therapeutic agents such as UFH and warfarin is possible, many of the newer anticoagulants, including LMWHs, fondaparinux, parenteral direct thrombin inhibitors, and the novel oral anticoagulants, do not have a complete and specific antidote. Therefore the ideal method to manage bleeding with patients receiving these therapies is not known. Furthermore, accurate and widely available laboratory tests to measure anticoagulant activity may not be available for these newer agents. Although laboratory monitoring is not routinely required for patients on dabigatran or rivaroxaban, special clinical scenarios, such as clinically significant bleeding, may call for measurement of anticoagulant effect. At therapeutic doses, dabigatran prolongs the thrombin time/thrombin clotting time (TT/TCT) and activated partial thromboplastin time (aPTT), and has little effect on the prothrombin time (PT). Even though the TT/TCT and aPTT are the most effective and widely available coagulation assays to determine dabigatran activity, the therapeutic range of these tests is not well defined, and these tests are best used to determine the presence or absence of the drug. Rivaroxaban causes prolongation of both the PT and aPTT but exhibits greater sensitivity for PT. However, PT prolongation is not specific. Anti-factor Xa assays specific for rivaroxaban would be ideal for determining plasma rivaroxaban concentrations. Clinicians should not routinely use these laboratory tests to monitor and adjust dabigatran doses or assess the degree of bleeding risk for surgical procedures. However, in an emergency a normal TT/TCT and aPTT rules out the presence of significant amounts of dabigatran. Similarly, a normal PT and aPTT should indicate negligible amounts of rivaroxaban concentrations. Suggestions for the management of bleeding complications in patients on anticoagulation are described in Table 55–6.

Interruption of anticoagulation before interventions with high-risk of bleeding must be weighed carefully against thrombotic risk. Renal and hepatic impairment, which can prolong clearance of anticoagulants, as well as the long half-life of several of these drugs, need to be considered prior to discontinuation of the drug. Recommendations for interruption of the newer anticoagulants, including LMWHs, fondaparinux, parenteral direct thrombin inhibitors, and the new oral anticoagulants, are available. Restarting anticoagulation in a timely manner postoperatively depends on individualized assessment of risks of bleeding from the procedure and thrombosis for underlying hypercoagulable state. Postoperatively, it is critical to note that, unlike warfarin, the newer anticoagulants have more immediate onsets of action. Therefore, if these drugs are interrupted for surgery, they should not be reintroduced until hemostasis is assured.

Anticoagulants are among the most common drugs used to prevent and treat thrombotic and vascular disorders prevalent in the geriatric population. Special attention must be paid to the unique characteristics of older patients that may affect type, dose, monitoring, and management of bleeding of the anticoagulant chosen. Randomized controlled trials specifically addressing geriatric patients are needed to make evidence-based recommendations on the use of anticoagulants in this population.

Crowther M, Warkentin T. Bleeding risk and the management of bleeding complications in patients undergoing anticoagulant therapy: focus on new anticoagulant agents. *Blood.* 2008;111(10): 4871-4879.

Van Ryn J, Stangier J, Haertter S, et al. Dabigatran etexilate—a novel, reversible, oral direct thrombin inhibitor. *Thromb Haemost.* 2010;103(6):1116-1127.

Warkentin TE, Crowther MA. Reversing anticoagulants both old and new. *Can J Anaesth.* 2002;49(6):S11-S25.

Assessing Antiaging Therapies for Older Adults

56

Milta O. Little, DO

John E. Morley, MB, BCh

General Principles in Older Adults

Most older Americans expect to live longer and more independently than previous generations, and many seek to be involved in their own health through diet, exercise, and participation in health care decision-making. The combination of the desire to be involved in health care, a recent surge in the ready access to information, the wish to promote health and avoid aging, and interest in new ways to approach problems have created tremendous interest in therapies designed to prevent or retard aging.

ANTIAGING THERAPIES

Knowledge about the biologic mechanisms involved in aging and the physiologic changes associated with aging provides a rational basis for the quest for antiaging therapies. An antiaging therapy could act by 1 or more of the following 3 mechanisms:

1. Modifying the biochemical and molecular events that cause aging.
2. Correcting physiologic changes that cause signs or symptoms associated with aging.
3. Lessening the susceptibility of an individual to diseases associated with aging.

Practices that act through the third mechanism (eg, colonoscopy, blood pressure reduction, cholesterol reduction, and other practices that aim to prevent age-associated diseases) are common in medical practice and are dealt with elsewhere in this book.

ETHICAL AND LEGAL ISSUES WITH ANTIAGING THERAPIES

The pursuit of antiaging therapeutics is not without controversy and debate. There are several reasons for this. Most importantly, it has been difficult to come to an agreement on the definition of antiaging, with definitions running the gamut from a simple cosmetic procedure to reduce visible signs of aging to a quest for complete reversal of the body's aging process. Because there are many ways to define antiaging therapeutics, patients and practitioners may have different expectations of therapeutic results. Discussions on definitions and expectations needs to take place before any therapeutic alliance can be successfully built. For our purposes, we exclude aesthetic procedures and focus mainly on treatments aimed at reversing or slowing pathologic aging.

With this in mind, it brings up the second area of controversy. When discussing aging, many cannot agree on what is "normal" aging and what is "pathologic" aging, nor on whether it is ethical to intervene in the aging process at all. Furthermore, extending life may not be a noble goal if the quality of that life is poor. It has been considered "a true failure" of antiaging medicine to significantly prolong a life that is full of functional disability.

Historically, there has been a lack of standardization of therapeutics, no established standard of care, little clinical research, and lack of training or certification of antiaging practitioners. To help with these issues the World Society of Interdisciplinary of Anti-Aging Medicine (WOSIAM) offers international education events and funds research projects to improve the scientific rigor of the antiaging field. In the United States, the American Academy of Anti-Aging Medicine (A4M) offers mini-fellowship and certification opportunities in the categories of regenerative medicine, aesthetics, integrative cancer treatment, and stem cell therapy. Despite these efforts, caution needs to be exercised when using or prescribing antiaging therapies, especially those that are marketed as supplements, which do not undergo rigorous efficacy or safety testing.

A final consideration in the antiaging debate is one of cost. The price of these therapies can be high and is often not covered by insurance. Older patients need to be warned against sacrificing better-proven pharmaceuticals or nonpharmacologic therapies for more expensive, but provocative, antiaging interventions.

Fisher A, Hill R. Ethical and legal issues in antiaging medicine. *Clin Geriatr Med.* 2004;20(2):361-382.

Gammack JK, Morley JE. Anti-aging medicine—the good, the bad, and the ugly. *Clin Geriatr Med.* 2004;20(2):157-177.

▶ TREATMENTS

A. Antioxidants: Vitamin A, Vitamin C, Vitamin E, Beta-Carotene

Aging has long been hypothesized to be partly caused by oxidative stress. Many cellular processes produce reactive oxygen or reactive nitrogen species, which via a free radical mechanism can chemically modify and hence damage proteins, DNA, and lipids. Aged animals show accumulation of oxidative damage, with markers of oxidative damage being elevated 2–3-fold between reproductive maturity and death. Experimental studies in animals have supported a role for oxidative damage in aging.

In humans, oxidative damage may contribute to atherosclerosis, cancer, Parkinson disease, and Alzheimer disease. The antioxidants most commonly used in people are vitamin A and its precursor beta-carotene, vitamin C, and vitamin E. When vitamins are used as antiaging therapies, they are often used in doses that are higher than the replacement doses that are appropriate for vitamin deficiencies. Early epidemiologic data suggested a reduction in mortality and prevention of diseases, such as cardiovascular and cerebrovascular disease, with dietary and nondietary vitamin intake. This caused great excitement among the public and researchers conducted multiple randomized controlled trials to further examine the effects of antioxidant supplementation.

Unfortunately, results of large population-based studies and randomized trials not only fail to show a benefit of antioxidant treatments for most conditions, but give evidence of harm with long-term supplementation with vitamins E, A, beta-carotene, and possibly α-lipoic acid (ALA). How should the largely negative results of randomized studies of the antioxidant vitamins be interpreted? Many theories exist, but the most recent evidence suggests that antioxidants reverse the beneficial effects of oxidation without blocking the harmful effects. Exercise is known to reduce blood pressure, improve insulin sensitivity and enhance nitric oxide availability at the endothelium. In trial subjects who took antioxidants prior to or after exercise, these beneficial effects were ameliorated. Even more alarming are the cumulative data of antioxidant and vitamin supplementation on mortality and longevity in large population studies. The most recent Cochrane review update found that long-term supplementation with vitamin E, beta-carotene, or vitamin A was associated with a significantly increased risk of mortality compared to controls. Vitamin C or selenium was not associated with increased mortality; however, the studies failed to show significant benefit of supplementation with these substances. In conclusion, the aggregated data of antioxidant supplementation indicates limited benefit with evidence of harm for all populations. *Dietary* intake of vitamins and antioxidants as part of an active lifestyle may, however, result in reduced signs and symptoms of aging.

Despite overwhelming evidence against the routine use of antioxidants for prevention or treatment of inflammatory conditions, vitamins A, E, and C have been shown to be beneficial in the treatment of 1 common geriatric condition: age-related macular degeneration. In patients with *preexisting* age-related macular degeneration, a combination of antioxidants decreased progression to advanced macular degeneration in the Age-Related Eye Disease Study. In contrast, 6 years of antioxidant supplementation had no effect on the *incidence* of age-related macular degeneration in smokers in the Alpha-Tocopherol, Beta-Carotene Cancer Prevention (ATBC) trial.

Age-Related Eye Disease Study Research Group. A randomized, placebo-controlled, clinic trial of high-dose supplementation with vitamins C and E, beta carotene, and zinc for age-related macular degeneration and vision loss: AREDS report no. 8. *Arch Ophthalmol.* 2001;119(10):1417-1436.

Bjelakovic G, Gluud LL, Nikolova D, et al. Antioxidant supplements for liver diseases. *Cochrane Database Syst Rev.* 2011;(3):CD007749.

Bjelakovic G, Nikolova D, Gluud LL, Simonetti RG, Gluud C. Antioxidant supplements for prevention of morality in healthy participants and patients with various disease. *Cochrane Database Syst Rev.* 2012;(3):CD007176.

Jeon YJ, Myung SK, Lee EH, et al. Effects of beta-carotene supplements on cancer prevention: meta-analysis of randomized controlled trials. *Nutr Cancer.* 2011;63(8):1196-1207.

Ristow M, Zarse K, Oberback A, et al. Antioxidants prevent health-promoting effects of physical exercise in humans. *Proc Natl Acad Sci U S A.* 2009;106(21):8665-8670.

Roberts CK, Vaziri ND, Barnard RJ. Effect of diet and exercise intervention on blood pressure, insulin, oxidative stress, and nitric oxide availability. *Circulation.* 2002;106(20):2530-2532.

Thomas DR. Vitamins in health and aging. *Clin Geriatr Med.* 2004;20(2):259-274.

Tsiligianni IG, van der Molen T. A systematic review of the role of vitamin insufficiencies and supplementation in COPD. *Respir Res.* 2010;11:171.

Wray DW, Uberoi A, Lawrenson L, Bailey DM, Richardson RS. Oral antioxidants and cardiovascular health in the exercise-trained and untrained elderly: a radically different outcome. *Clin Sci.* 2009;116(5):433-441.

B. α-Lipoic Acid

ALA is considered to be a potent antioxidant because it can oxidize and regenerate other antioxidants, such as vitamin E and glutathione. It has been studied at dosages of 600 mg, 1200 mg, and 1800 mg a day, with the best-tolerated dose being 600 mg. Described side effects include headache, tingling or a "pins and needles" sensation, skin rash, or muscle cramps. In addition, ALA may lower blood glucose and alter thyroid hormone levels so these should be monitored in patients taking this supplement.

Several studies have demonstrated the effectiveness of ALA for the treatment of neuropathy, particularly in diabetics. Early evidence suggests that ALA may have a role in retarding the progression of neurodegenerative diseases, such as multiple sclerosis and Alzheimer dementia. However, the use of ALA for the latter reasons cannot be widely recommended until more rigorous studies can be performed.

Head KA. Peripheral neuropathy: pathogenic mechanisms and alternative therapies. *Altern Med Rev.* 2006;11(4):294-329.

Klugman A, Sauer J, Tabet N, Howard R. Alpha lipoic acid for dementia. *Cochrane Database Syst Rev.* 2004;(1):CD004244.

Vallianou N, Evangelopoulos A, Koutlas P. Alpha-lipoic acid and diabetic neuropathy. *Rev Diabet Stud.* 2009;6(4):230-236.

C. Hormone Replacement (Table 56–1)

1. Growth hormone—Growth hormone (GH) secretion (measured by serum insulin-like growth factor [IGF]-1, levels) reaches its maximum during the growth spurt accompanying puberty before beginning a steady decline with age in both men and women. Much of this decline is a result of a selective reduction in the nocturnal pulsatile secretion of GH. Some of the changes associated with aging are reminiscent of those seen in adult patients with frank GH deficiency, such as reduction in lean body mass, increase in body fat (especially abdominal obesity), decrease in muscular strength, and difficulty with cognitive functioning. As a result, there has been much interest in supplementing GH in older adults.

Most GH studies have titrated the doses to produce IGF levels in the low- to mid-normal range seen in young adults. Treatment with GH increases lean body mass, skin thickness, and vertebral bone mineral density and decreases fat mass, all more pronounced in older men than women. GH-induced increases in muscle mass were not accompanied by increases in physical strength, stamina, or functional status, however. Although widely touted by antiaging practitioners, GH for antiaging therapy is not an approved indication for use, and the effects of exogenous GH on cognition and memory have not been well studied. Side effects of GH include fluid retention, arthralgias, gynecomastia, glucose intolerance, headache, and carpal tunnel syndrome. More seriously is the possible increased risk of cancer related to the cell growth stimulant properties of IGF-1. Additionally, emerging evidence indicates that GH and IGF-1 signaling shorten, rather than prolong, life span. In summary, the limited benefits of GH, its high cost, and potential long-term risks weigh against the use of GH in older adults, and its use should be discouraged.

Table 56–1. Hormone replacement and its actions.

Hormone	Actions	Evidence
Growth hormone	Increase lean body mass	+
	Increase skin thickness	+
	Increase vertebral bone mineral density	+
	Decrease fat mass	+
	Increase physical strength	−
	Increase stamina	−
	Increase functional status	−
	Increase longevity	−
Testosterone		
Males	Increase lean body mass	++
	Decrease fat mass	++
	Increase bone mineral density	++
	Increase sexual functioning	+
Females	Increase libido	+
	Increase bone mineral density	+/−
	Increase muscle mass	+/−
Hormone replacement therapy with estrogen		
Females	Decrease vasomotor symptoms	++
	Prevent osteoporosis	++
	Prevent coronary artery disease	−
	Prevent dementia	+/−
	Prevent colon cancer	+/−
	Improve mental health	−
Dehydroepiandrosterone		
Females	Increase sense of well-being	+
	Increase bone mineral density	+
	Increase sexual interest (those older than 70 years)	+
	Decrease skin pigmentation	+
	Decrease skin sebum production	+
Males	Increase sense of well-being	+
	Increase strength	+
	Increase skin thickness	+
	Increase skin hydration	+
Pregnenolone	Increase memory	−
	Improve sleep	+

Khorram O. Use of growth hormone and growth hormone secretagogues in aging: help or harm. *Clin Obstet Gynecol.* 2001;44(4):893-901.

Liu H, Bravata DM, Olkin I, et al. Systematic review: the safety and efficacy of growth hormone in the healthy elderly. *Ann Intern Med.* 2007;146(2):104-115.

2. Testosterone—In men, testosterone levels peak during late adolescence then decrease by roughly 0.5% to 1% per year. Hypogonadism is present in ≤10% of men age 50–69 years and in ≤30% of men 70 years of age and older. In parallel with the declines in testosterone levels, aging men experience decreases in muscle mass and strength, bone mass, sexual interest and potency, and cognitive function, and increases in fat mass. It is unknown, however, whether these changes can be attributed to declines in testosterone levels. Hypogonadism has also been associated with higher risk of type 2 diabetes mellitus, metabolic syndrome, cardiovascular disease, anemia, and osteoporosis.

Several studies have reported on the supplementation of testosterone in men with low testosterone levels via either injections or a scrotal patch (see Table 56–1). Most studies have shown increases in lean body mass and bone mineral density, and decreases in fat mass. Accompanying the increase in muscle mass has been an increase in either upper- or lower-extremity strength. However, only 1 experimental study has shown an increase in functioning with testosterone replacement. Sexual function has shown mixed results with supplementation, and men with lower initial testosterone levels tend to have the most significant improvements. Three studies suggested small improvements in cognitive function in middle-aged men receiving testosterone, but further data fail to show a benefit of testosterone replacement in improving cognitive impairment.

Concerns have been raised regarding potential effects of prostate disease, cardiovascular risk, and erythrocytosis. Testosterone supplementation does not worsen prostatic hypertrophy, and it is unknown whether it increases risk of prostate cancer. A meta-analysis failed to confirm the risk of adverse cardiovascular events with the use of testosterone for hypogonadism. In fact, testosterone therapy decreases angina, causes coronary artery dilation, and decreases ST depression during exercise stress testing. Administration of testosterone leads to no change or a slight decrease in total cholesterol and low-density lipoprotein cholesterol combined with no change or a slight decrease in high-density lipoprotein cholesterol. Erythrocytosis can be seen in up to 25% of patients receiving treatment. This can be easily managed by either decreasing the dose of testosterone given or using phlebotomy.

Hypogonadism can be detected by the Androgen Deficiency in Aging Males Questionnaire followed by direct measurement of a bioavailable testosterone. This questionnaire also identifies patients with depression, which should be treated before replacement therapy is considered.

Testosterone levels decline from age 20 years to menopause in females. Levels then stay constant through the menopausal transition and then increase after menopause. Estrogen therapy increases sex hormone-binding globulin and, therefore, decreases free testosterone levels. Testosterone replacement therapy in menopausal women improves libido and increases bone mineral density and muscle mass (see Table 56–1). Further studies are required to determine the role of testosterone in women as an anti-aging hormone.

Anawalt BD, Merriam GR. Neuroendocrine aging in men. Andropause and somatopause. *Endocrinol Metab Clin North Am.* 2001;30(3):647-669.

Calof OM, Singh AB, Lee ML, et al. Adverse events associated with testosterone replacement in middle-aged and older men: a meta-analysis of randomized, placebo-controlled trials. *J Gerontol A Biol Sci Med Sci.* 2005;60(11):1451-1457.

Haddad RM, Kennedy CC, Caples SM, et al. Testosterone and cardiovascular risk in men: a systematic review and meta-analysis of randomized placebo-controlled trials. *Mayo Clin Proc.* 2007;82(1):29-39.

Morley JE, Perry HM 3rd. Androgen deficiency in aging men: role of testosterone replacement therapy. *J Lab Clin Med.* 2000;135(5): 370-378.

Morley JE, Unterman TG. Hormonal fountains of youth. *J Lab Clin Med.* 2000;135(5):364-366.

Ottenbacher KJ, Ottenbacher ME, Ottenbacher AJ, Acha AA, Ostir GV. Androgen treatment and muscle strength in elderly men: a meta-analysis. *J Am Geriatr Soc.* 2006;54(11):1666-1673. PMID: 17087692.

3. Dehydroepiandrosterone—Dehydroepiandrosterone (DHEA) and its sulfated derivative, DHEAS, are synthesized by the adrenal cortex and are the most abundant steroid hormones in young adults. After age 30 years, serum levels of DHEA decline approximately 2% per year. As a result, in 80-year-olds, DHEA levels are 10% to 20% of levels in young adults. Low levels of DHEA correlate with an increased risk of breast cancer in premenopausal women, an increase in cardiovascular disease and mortality in older men, a lower bone mineral density in perimenopausal women, a higher likelihood of depressed mood in older women, and a higher likelihood of cognitive decline in both sexes.

Several short-term studies in older persons have supplemented DHEA levels to those seen in young adults with 50–100 mg/day doses (see Table 56–1). In women, DHEA supplementation led to an improved sense of well-being, increased bone mineral density, and, in women older than age 70 years, increased sexual interest and satisfaction. In men, DHEA supplementation has led to improved well-being, increased strength, and decreased fat mass. In both sexes, DHEA supplementation improved skin thickness, hydration, sebum production, and pigmentation. Adverse effects on lipid profile and glycemic control were not seen.

In conclusion, short-term DHEA supplementation appears safe, but the effects have been modest. Routine supplementation is not recommended until long-term studies have demonstrated the safety and benefits of DHEA supplementation.

Gurnell EM, Chatterjee VK. Dehydroepiandrosterone replacement therapy. *Eur J Endocrinol.* 2001;145(2):103-106.

4. Bioidentical hormones—After the many disappointing trials with synthetic hormone replacement, antiaging practitioners began to use individually compounded formulations called *bioidentical hormones.* Compounded bioidentical hormone therapy (CBHT) is the tailoring of plant-derived chemicals identical to the body's natural hormone based on the needs of each individual patient. Typically, this is done by measuring the levels of hormones in a patient's saliva and then compounding the hormones to replete the deficiencies observed. The use of CBHT became widespread after the frightening results of the Women's Health Initiative studies of synthetic estrogen replacement. It is thought to be safer, more efficacious, and better tolerated than the standardized hormones. These formulations are non-FDA approved and therefore not tightly regulated as pharmaceuticals. Furthermore, there is no evidence that levels of hormone in saliva can be correlated to menopausal symptoms and this practice is not recommended for use as monitoring or titrating any hormonal treatments. Finally, wide variations in active ingredients with the paucity of data supporting the beneficial claims of CBHT should cause patients and practitioners to strongly reconsider the use of this form of treatment until more rigorous safety and efficacy data become available.

Bhavnani BR, Stanczyk FZ. Misconception and concerns about bioidentical hormones used for custom-compounded hormone therapy. *J Clin Endocrinol Metab.* 2012;97(3):756-759.

Files JA, Ko MG, Pruthi S. Bioidentical hormone therapy. *Mayo Clin Proc.* 2011;86(7):673-680.

SUMMARY

In conclusion, many antiaging therapies have been developed and used in older patients. Few have resulted in significant advantage and the few benefits are often outweighed by the potential harms. In the end, exercise and a regular diet with plenty of fish and fresh fruits and vegetables are the only proven antiaging measures.

Khaw KT, Wareham N, Bingham S, Welch A, Luben R, Day N. Combined impact of health behaviours and mortality in men and women: the EPIC-Norfolk prospective population study. *PLoS Med.* 2008;5(1):e12.

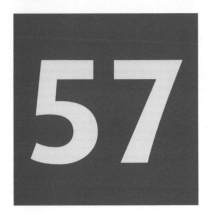

Considering Complementary & Alternative Medicines for Older Adults

Milta O. Little, DO

John E. Morley, MB, BCh

▶ General Principles in Older Adults

Complementary and alternative therapies have been defined as therapies that either fall outside of the conventional thought and approach to a given disease or that are not taught in U.S. medical schools or widely provided by U.S. hospitals. The National Center for Complementary and Alternative Medicine divides these therapies into 5 major domains (Table 57–1).

Among older adults, the most commonly used complementary and alternative therapies are chiropractic therapy, herbal remedies, relaxation techniques, and high-dose or megavitamins.

Patients using complementary and alternative therapies often do not report their use to their physicians. Some therapies, such as herbs, may have side effects or may interact with conventional therapies. Physicians should ask specifically whether older patients are using them or seeing practitioners. Asking about interest in and use of complementary and alternative therapies may also strengthen the physician–patient relationship and facilitate exploration of a patient's needs and expectations.

When an older patient elects to use complementary and alternative treatments, it is important to establish clear goals and endpoints, to apply the same evidence-based medicine principles to the literature, to be knowledgeable and open-minded, and to listen to and hear patient preferences. Practitioners should discuss evidence (or lack thereof) for safety and efficacy of both conventional and alternative options. Do not break the patient's trust by quarreling over placebo effect if you note an improvement, the cost is manageable, there is low toxicity, and the patient is not rejecting other appropriate treatments. Finally, it is recommended that physicians get to know licensed complementary and alternative practitioners and develop a referral base.

Barrett B. Complementary and alternative medicine: what's it all about? *WMJ.* 2001;100(7):20-26.

Eisenberg DM, Davis RB, Ettner SL, et al. Trends in alternative medicine use in the United States, 1990–1997: results of a follow-up national survey. *JAMA.* 1998;280(18):1569-1575.

Eisenberg DM, Kessler RC, Van Rompay MI, et al. Perceptions about complementary therapies relative to conventional therapies among adults who use both: results from a national survey. *Ann Intern Med.* 2001;135(5):344-351.

Foster DF, Phillips RS, Hamel MB, Eisenberg DM. Alternative medicine use in older Americans. *J Am Geriatr Soc.* 2000;48(12):1560-1565.

National Institutes of Health, National Center for Complementary and Alternative Medicine. http://nccam.nih.gov

Pappas S, Perlman A. Complementary and alternative medicine. The importance of doctor-patient communication. *Med Clin North Am.* 2002;86(1):1-10.

Wolsko PM, Eisenberg DM, Davis RB, Ettner SL, Phillips RS. Insurance coverage, medical conditions, and visits to alternative medicine providers: results of a national survey. *Arch Intern Med.* 2002;162(3):281-287.

MASSAGE AND CHIROPRACTIC THERAPY

Massage therapy and chiropractic therapy are the most widely used complementary and alternative therapies in the United States. Swedish massage, the Trager method, and reflexology are the most commonly used types of massage. Studies have consistently found benefit for massage therapy in the treatment of pain, including back pain, fibromyalgia, and headaches. Massage has also been found to be of benefit in the palliative care of patients with HIV, breast cancer, and terminal cancer pain. The improvements include decreases in pain, anxiety, and depression, along with improved sleep.

Chiropractic medicine has spinal manipulation as the core clinical activity. The vast majority of patients seek chiropractic care for back, neck, or head pain. On the basis of history, exam, and x-ray findings, the chiropractic doctor determines whether the patient's condition will be amenable to chiropractic treatment and also plans a treatment regimen. Treatment involves spinal manipulation with or without

Table 57–1. Classifications of complementary and alternative (CAM) treatments.

CAM Domain	Definition	Examples
Alternative medical systems	Complete systems of theory and practice that are completely independent of a biomedical approach	Traditional oriental medicine, homeopathy, naturopathic medicine, and Ayurvedic medicine
Mind–body interventions	Target the potential for the mind to affect the body's basic function and reaction to disease	Meditation, prayer and mental healing, hypnosis
Biologic therapies	The use of herbs, dietary manipulation, supplements, or mixtures prepared from biologic sources to enhance health or treat disease	Herbal remedies, such as ginseng and ginkgo, supplements, such as glucosamine and vitamin E, and mixtures, such as shark cartilage
Manipulative and body-based systems	Therapies use a relationship between form and function to treat disease	Massage, chiropractic manipulation, or osteopathic manipulation
Energy therapies	Modify internal sources or flow of energy or alternately apply external sources of energy to modify body function or health	Use of magnets or electromagnetic fields, which involve external sources of energy, or the practice of Qi Gong or therapeutic touch, which involve manipulating the internal balance or flow of energy

adjunctive treatments such as heat, cold, traction, electricity, and counseling about exercise, fitness, nutrition, weight loss, smoking cessation, and relaxation techniques. Several systematic reviews have found sufficient evidence to support the beneficial use of chiropractic therapy for acute and chronic back pain. Spinal manipulation and mobilization have also shown benefit for mechanical neck pain, migraines, cervicogenic headaches, cervicogenic dizziness, and painful conditions in some extremity joints. Chiropractic treatment has not been shown to be effective treatment of nonmusculoskeletal illnesses, such as hypertension, dysmenorrhea, or asthma. As with most research, older persons make up a small minority of subjects in manipulation research trials.

Common side effects of manipulation and massage are usually mild and transient and include localized pain, headache, and fatigue. More serious side effects are very rare. Cauda equina syndrome from lumbar manipulation or stroke resulting from vertebral artery dissection has been reported. The risk of serious complications from lumbar manipulation has been estimated to be 1 in 100 million manipulations. The risk of stroke from cervical manipulation is also low, estimated at between 1 in 400,000 to 2 million manipulations. The most recent, large, case-control study found no increased risk of vertebrobasilar stroke with cervical manipulation.

Field T. Massage therapy. *Med Clin North Am*. 2002;86(1):163-171.

Gross AR, Goving JL, Haines TA, et al; Cervical Overview Group. A Cochrane review of manipulation and mobilization for mechanical neck disorders. *Spine (Phila Pa 1976)*. 2004;29(4):1541-1548.

Hawk C, Schneider M, Dougherty P, Gleberzon BJ, Killinger LZ. Best practices recommendations for chiropractic care for older adults: results of a consensus process. *J Manipulative Physiol Ther*. 2010;33(6):464-473.

Rubinstein SM, van Middelkoop M, Assendelft WJ, de Boer MR, van Tulder MW. Spinal manipulative therapy for chronic low-back pain. *Cochrane Database Syst Rev*. 2011;(2):CD008112.

HERBS & SUPPLEMENTS

Herbs are the second most common complementary or alternative therapy used by older persons. In contrast to pharmaceuticals, the production, marketing, and sale of herbs and supplements is regulated only by the Dietary Supplement Health and Education Act, which does not regulate the purity, quality, or standardization of preparations. As a result, active ingredients can vary among manufacturers and even from lot to lot for a given manufacturer. Patients and physicians should select products made by larger, more reputable companies, which specify the amounts of ingredients and standardization of the active ingredients to an accepted standard. In addition, most herbs and supplements are not routinely covered by insurance, and as such, may be cost prohibitive for many older individuals on a fixed retirement income. Table 57–2 lists the typical doses and uses of the most common herbs and supplements.

Blumenthal M, Buse WR, Goldberg A, et al, eds. *The Complete German Commission E Monographs: Therapeutic Guide to Herbal Medicines*. Austin, TX: American Botanical Council; 1998. ISBN 096555550X http://nccam.nih.gov/health/herbsataglance.htm

Ernst E, Pittler MH. Herbal medicine. *Med Clin North Am*. 2002; 86(1):149-161.

Massey PB. Dietary supplements. *Med Clin North Am*. 2002;86(1):127-147.

National Centers for Complementary and Alternative Medicine Guide to Herbal Supplements. http://nccam.nih.gov/health/herbsataglance.htm

▶ Ginkgo

Ginkgo is the top-selling herbal medicine in the United States. There are concerns about antiplatelet and warfarin-like effects of gingko, which should be avoided in patients

Table 57-2. Herbal medicines: dose and use.

Herb/Supplement	Dose	Use	Evidence
Gingko	40 mg TID	Dementia	++
		Cerebral/insufficiency	+
		Tinnitus	+
		Claudication	++
St. John's wort	300 mg TID	Depression	−
Glucosamine	1500–2000 mg QD or divided BID	OA	++
Chondroitin	1000–1500 mg QD or divided BID	OA	++
S-adenosyl methionine	1600 mg BID to QID	Depression	+
		OA	++
Saw palmetto	320 mg divided BID to TID	Benign prostatic hypertrophy	+/−
Valerian root	300–900 mg 30–60 min before bedtime	Insomnia	+/−
Ginseng	200–600 mg QD or divided BID	Physical performance	+/−
		Psychomotor performance	+/−
		Immune system function	+/−
Garlic	600–900 mg QD	Hypercholesterolemia	+
		Hypertension	−
		Cancer prevention	+/−
Ginger	0.5–1.0 g QD	Vertigo	+
		Motion sickness	+
		Postoperative nausea	+/−
		OA	+
Omega-3 fatty acid (DHA)	1–3 g/day At least 2 servings of fish in healthy subjects	CV prevention	+/−

CV, cardiovascular; OA, osteoarthritis.

Canter PH, Ernst E. Ginkgo biloba is not a smart drug: an updated systematic review of randomised clinical trials testing the nootropic effects of *G. biloba* extracts in healthy people. *Hum Psychopharmacol.* 2007;22(5):265-278.

Ernst E. The risk-benefit profile of commonly used herbal therapies: ginkgo, St. John's Wort, Ginseng, Echinacea, Saw Palmetto, and Kava. *Ann Intern Med.* 2002;136(1):42-53.

Kurz A, Van Baelen B. Ginkgo biloba compared with cholinesterase inhibitors in the treatment of dementia: a review based on meta-analyses by the Cochrane collaboration. *Dement Geriatr Cogn Disord.* 2004;18(2):217-226.

St. John's Wort

St. John's wort is widely used in Europe to treat depression. St. John's wort is believed to work through selective inhibition of the reuptake of serotonin, dopamine, and norepinephrine in the brain. Several meta-analyses and qualitative systemic reviews have found St. John's wort to be superior to placebo and comparable to tricyclic antidepressants and selective serotonin reuptake inhibitors (SSRIs) with similar side effect rates but fewer withdrawals. St. John's wort may be used cautiously in the treatment of mild depression but is not currently recommended for moderate-to-severe depression, which should be treated with pharmacologic or cognitive–behavioral interventions with more rigorous efficacy data. Patients should not take tricyclic antidepressants, SSRIs, or monoamine oxidase inhibitors while taking St. John's wort. St. John's wort activates P450 enzymes, so care should be used in treating patients who are also taking warfarin, digoxin, or other drugs with hepatic metabolism.

Hypericum Depression Trial Study Group. Effect of *Hypericum perforatum* (St. John's wort) in major depressive disorder: a randomized controlled trial. *JAMA.* 2002;287(14):1807-1814.

Rahimi R, Nikfar S, Abdollahi M. Efficacy and tolerability of *Hypericum perforatum* in major depressive disorder in comparison with selective serotonin reuptake inhibitors: a meta-analysis. *Prog Neuropsychopharmacol Biol Psychiatry.* 2009;33(1):118-127.

Shelton RC, Keller MB, Gelenberg A, et al. Effectiveness of St. John's wort in major depression: a randomized controlled trial. *JAMA.* 2001;285(15):1978-1986.

Glucosamine/Chondroitin

Glucosamine and chondroitin are commonly used for the treatment of osteoarthritis. Both glucosamine and chondroitin are components of proteoglycans found in articular cartilage and synovial fluid. How oral glucosamine or chondroitin work physiologically is not clear, and there is little evidence that patients with osteoarthritis are deficient in these substances or that oral glucosamine or chondroitin is selectively taken to joints. Studies have found these substances to be very safe, with no more side effects than placebo.

taking anticoagulants. Although shown to reduce blood viscosity and clotting factors, gingko does not appear to cause a statistically significant increase in bleeding risk over placebo in patients not on anticoagulants. Ginkgo is clinically used and studied for dementia, memory impairment, cerebral insufficiency, tinnitus, and intermittent claudication. Overall, studies of Ginkgo are weak and the most rigorous trials show benefit for the treatment of tinnitus but speak against the use of ginkgo for treatment of dementia, memory impairment or prevention of cardiovascular events.

Meta-analyses of early clinical trials of glucosamine and chondroitin have shown both to be superior to placebo in improving pain and disability. More recent trials have shown glucosamine, with or without chondroitin, to be as efficacious as nonsteroidal antiinflammatory drugs (NSAIDs) to reduce pain and disability in knee and hip osteoarthritis with fewer side effects. It is unknown whether glucosamine and chondroitin improve symptoms of osteoarthritis at other sites such as the hand or hip.

Ernst E. Complementary and alternative medicine for pain management in rheumatic disease. *Curr Opin Rheumatol.* 2002;14(1):58-62.

Reginster JY, Deroisy R, Rovati LC, et al. Long-term effects of glucosamine sulphate on osteoarthritis progression: a randomised, placebo-controlled clinical trial. *Lancet.* 2001;357(9252): 251-256.

Sawitzke AD, Shi H, Finco MF, et al. Clinical efficacy and safety of glucosamine, chondroitin sulphate, their combination, celecoxib or placebo taken to treat osteoarthritis of the knee: 2-year results from GAIT. *Ann Rheum Dis.* 2010;69(8):1459-1464.

Thie NM, Prasad NG, Major PW. Evaluation of glucosamine sulfate compared to ibuprofen for the treatment of temporomandibular joint osteoarthritis: a randomized double blind controlled 3 month clinical trial. *J Rheumatol.* 2001;28(6):1347-1355.

Towheed T, Maxwell L, Anastassiades TP, et al. Glucosamine therapy for treating osteoarthritis. *Cochrane Database Syst Rev.* 2005;2. Art. No.: CD002946. DOI:10.1002/14651858.CD002946.pub2.

▶ Saw Palmetto

Saw palmetto (also known as *Serenoa repens*) is commonly used to treat symptoms of benign prostatic hypertrophy (BPH) by inhibiting the 5α-reductase enzyme that converts testosterone to 5-dehydrotestosterone, prostaglandin synthesis, and growth factor actions. In Western Europe, saw palmetto is used much more commonly than finasteride or α blockers for BPH. Despite early evidence of benefit, the most recent meta-analysis and several randomized controlled trials found no improvement in urinary symptoms with the use of saw palmetto over placebo. There is also no evidence to support the use of saw palmetto to reduce the size of the prostate. It does not seem to affect prostate-specific antigen levels, but further studies are needed to determine the role of saw palmetto in men with or at risk of prostate cancer. Given the body of evidence speaking against the use of saw palmetto for symptoms of BPH, it should not be recommended for this use.

Barry MJ, Meleth S, Lee JY, et al. Effect of increasing doses of saw palmetto extract on lower urinary tract symptoms: a randomized trial. *JAMA.* 2011;306(12):1344-1351.

Bent S, Kane C, Shinohara K, et al. Saw palmetto for benign prostatic hyperplasia. *N Engl J Med.* 2006;354(6):557-566.

Tacklind J, MacDonald R, Rutks I, et al. *Serenoa repens* for benign prostatic hyperplasia. *Cochrane Database Syst Rev.* 2009;(2):CD001423.

▶ Ginseng

Ginseng is among the best-selling herbal supplements. It is also one of the herbs with the most reported benefits, including central nervous system effects of increased vigilance, increased concentration, increased sense of well-being, and increased relaxation along with systemic anticancer, antidiabetic, and aphrodisiac effects. The incidence of side effects is low but some can be serious, such as vaginal bleeding, Stevens-Johnson syndrome, hypertension, warfarin interactions, and hypoglycemia.

Ginseng is traditionally used as a component of traditional Chinese medicine for overall health and antiaging. Multiple studies have attempted to determine the evidence for the multiple health claims made for ginseng. To date, reviews are limited by significant methodologic issues and possible publication bias. In healthy subjects, ginseng has been shown to improve cognitive performance and may delay onset of dementia. The evidence for benefit in patients with dementia is weaker. Early trials support the use of ginseng for cardiovascular health. Currently, there is moderate and mixed evidence that ginseng improves cardiac function and reduces vascular disease. More rigorous clinical trials are needed to better describe the role and benefit of ginseng as a therapeutic and preventive agent for cardiovascular disease. There is strong evidence that ginseng improves pulmonary function but does not enhance physical performance. Overall, there is limited data to support the widespread recommendation for ginseng.

Ernst E. The risk-benefit profile of commonly used herbal therapies: ginkgo, St. John's Wort, Ginseng, Echinacea, Saw Palmetto, and Kava. *Ann Intern Med.* 2002;136(1):42-53.

Lee NH, Son CG. Systematic review of randomized controlled trials evaluating the efficacy and safety of ginseng. *J Acupunct Meridian Stud.* 2011;4(2):85-97.

Perry E, Howes MJ. Medicinal plants and dementia therapy: herbal hopes for brain aging? *CNS Neurosci Ther.* 2011;17(6):683-698.

▶ Garlic

Garlic is widely advertised and used in the United States with the aims of lowering cholesterol and blood pressure and preventing cancer. The active ingredient is allicin, and most preparations are standardized to contain 0.6% to 1.3% allicin. The most widely studied form is the Kwai powder, which contains 1.3% allicin. Side effects include odor, flatulence, diarrhea, and stomach upset. The most serious, although rare, side effect is increased bleeding, which may be a consequence of reductions in platelet aggregation.

Garlic has been found to be superior to placebo in reducing total cholesterol but not blood pressure. The total reduction in cholesterol is 12–25 mg/dL at 3 months, which is similar to the effect of dietary intervention and less than the effect of statins. None of the underlying studies lasted more than 10 months, and 1 meta-analysis suggested that the benefit of garlic may not last beyond 6 months.

Garlic was associated with reduced rates of stomach and colorectal cancer in cohort and case-control studies, but there are no randomized studies of garlic to support these findings. The effect of garlic on cancer at other sites has not been studied sufficiently to support any conclusions.

Ackermann RT, Mulrow CD, Ramirez G, Gardner CD, Morbidoni L, Lawrence VA. Garlic shows promise for improving some cardiovascular risk factors. *Arch Intern Med.* 2001;161(6):813-824.

Fleischauer AT, Arab L. Garlic and cancer: a critical review of the epidemiologic literature. *J Nutr.* 2001;131(3s):1032S-1040S.

Stevinson C, Pittler MH, Ernst E. Garlic for treating hypercholesterolemia. A meta-analysis of randomized clinical trials. *Ann Intern Med.* 2000;133(6):420-429.

▶ Ginger

Ginger has been used in Chinese and Ayurvedic medicine for more than 2500 years for the treatment of musculoskeletal pain and gastrointestinal illnesses. Ginger has been studied for the prevention of postoperative nausea and motion sickness and the treatment of vertigo and osteoarthritis pain, with mixed but overall slightly positive results.

Altman RD, Marcussen KC. Effects of a ginger extract on knee pain in patients with osteoarthritis. *Arthritis Rheum.* 2001;44(11):2531-2538.

Bliddal H, Rosetzsky A, Schlichting P, et al. A randomized, placebo-controlled, cross-over study of ginger extracts and ibuprofen in osteoarthritis. *Osteoarthritis Cartilage.* 2000;8(1):9-12.

Ernst E, Pittler MH. Efficacy of ginger for nausea and vomiting: a systematic review of randomized clinical trials. *Br J Anaesth.* 2000;84(3):367-371.

▶ Omega-3 Fatty Acids

Omega-3 (n-3) polyunsaturated fatty acids (PUFAs) are the most commonly used supplement in the United States; however, dietary sources appear to be the best way to enrich tissue levels. The richest sources of dietary PUFAs are from oily fish, such as tuna, salmon, sardines, mackerel, and herring. PUFAs can also be found in land meats (beef, pork, and chicken), but in much lower quantities. There is not currently a recommended daily allowance of PUFAs because of the paucity of scientific evidence for adequate intake levels in healthy adults; however, the American Heart Association recommends intake of 8 ounces of fish at least 2 times a week.

Studies suggest 2–3 g/day to lower cholesterol and 1 g/day for secondary cardiovascular prevention. The maximum recommended daily amount is 3 g, although 4 g is often used.

The role of n-3 PUFAs in disease prevention and treatment is still being elucidated, but is most likely a result of antiinflammation and immune modulation. Diseases associated with systemic inflammation increase production of cytokines, which can be modulated by n-3 PUFAs. Studies indicate that those with chronic inflammatory conditions are likely to be more sensitive to the antiinflammatory effects than are healthy people.

The use of PUFAs for prevention of cardiovascular disease remains controversial. Early studies suggested a benefit in mortality and morbidity outcomes for both primary and secondary cardiovascular disease prevention. However, more recent randomized trials fail to reproduce this benefit in secondary prevention. There may still be a role for PUFAs in primary prevention of cardiovascular disease, and they are still recommended as part of a well-balanced, healthy diet. It is also reasonable to recommend PUFAs in people with cardiovascular disease who cannot tolerate HMG-CoA reductase inhibitors. A meta-analysis of 10 randomized controlled trials found a statistically significant reduction in arterial stiffness. Further clinical studies are needed to confirm if this equates to improved cardiovascular fitness and reduced disease and to uncover the role of PUFAs in prevention or treatment of retinal disease, cancer, mental illness, cognitive decline, and autoimmune diseases.

Buhr G, Bales CW. Nutritional supplements for older adults: review and recommendations—part II. *J Nutr Elder.* 2010;29(1):42-71.

Kwak SM, Myung S-K, Lee YJ, Seo HG; Korean Meta-analysis Study Group. Efficacy of omega-3 fatty acid supplements (eicosapentaenoic acid and docosahexaenoic acid) in the secondary prevention of cardiovascular disease: a meta-analysis of randomized, double-blind, placebo-controlled trials. *Arch Intern Med.* 2012;172(9):686-694.

Reidiger ND, Othman RA, Suh M, Moghadasian MH. A systemic review of the roles of n-3 fatty acids in health and disease. *J Am Diet Assoc.* 2009;109(4):668-679.

OTHER FORMS OF ALTERNATIVE OR COMPLEMENTARY MEDICINE

▶ Acupuncture

Acupuncture is a popular alternative therapy that involves the use of sterile, disposable stainless-steel needles to stimulate points on the surface of the body along vital energy meridians. Treatments consist of weekly to biweekly sessions involving the insertion of up to 15 needles at selected points for times ranging from several seconds to 30 minutes. Once inserted, the needles can be stimulated manually or with electricity, heat, or burning herbs. Adverse effects are typically mild and include pain, bleeding, fatigue, nausea, and dizziness. Serious events (pneumothorax or vascular injuries) are rare.

Acupuncture has been shown to be efficacious in the treatment of postoperative and dental pain and for the management of nausea and vomiting resulting from a wide variety of causes. Acupuncture has also been used to treat chronic pain, osteoarthritis, headache, and back pain, but its efficacy in treating these conditions has not been established. A systematic review of the use of acupuncture in the treatment of chronic pain found insufficient evidence of benefit, and one randomized trial found acupuncture to have no benefit in the treatment of chronic back pain. However, acupuncture as a part of traditional Chinese medicine has been shown to be effective for treatment of fibromyalgia. It was shown to be ineffective for functional recovery poststroke or for reducing hot flushes.

Cao H, Liu J, Lewith GT. Traditional Chinese medicine for treatment of fibromyalgia: a systematic review of randomized controlled trials. *J Altern Complement Med.* 2010;16(4): 397-409.

Ernst E, White AR. Prospective studies of the safety of acupuncture: a systematic review. *Am J Med.* 2001;110(6):481-485.

Ezzo J, Berman B, Hadhazy VA, Jadad AR, Lao L, Singh BB. Is acupuncture effective for the treatment of chronic pain? A systematic review. *Pain.* 2000;86(3):217-225.

Kong JC, Lee MS, Shin BC, et al. Acupuncture for functional recovery after stroke: a systematic review of sham-controlled randomized clinical tirals. *CMAJ.* 2010;182(16):1723-1729.

Homeopathy

Homeopathy is an alternative medical system based on the vitalistic theory that illness results from imbalances in the patient's vital force. The goal of homeopathy is to use medications to restore the balance and then to rely on the self-healing potential of the body to lead to a cure. A practitioner selects a remedy, after a thorough history and physical exam, by matching symptoms and findings to remedies.

Homeopathic remedies have been shown to be effective, but are limited by methodologic flaws (eg, small numbers, lack of control groups or randomization, selection bias) and publication bias. Studies of better methodologic quality were more likely to report negative results. Until rigorous studies have validated the use of specific remedies, it would be prudent to approach their use with caution.

Cucherat M, Haugh MC, Gooch M, Boissel JP. Evidence of clinical efficacy of homeopathy. A meta-analysis of clinical trials. HMRAG. Homeopathic Medicines Research Advisory Group. *Eur J Clin Pharmacol.* 2000;56(1):27-33.

Merrel WC, Shalts E. Homeopathy. *Med Clin North Am.* 2002;86(1):47-62.

Teut M, Lüdtke R, Schnabel K, Willich SN, Witt CM. Homeopathic treatment of elderly patients—a prospective observational study with follow-up over a two year period. *BMC Geriatr.* 2010;10:10.

Aromatherapy

The practice of aromatherapy consists of using volatile essential oils extracted from plants for the relief of anxiety and agitation. Essential oils can be topically applied, aerosolized, or used in massage. Side effects are rare and typically mild, making aromatherapy a useful therapeutic adjunct. A systematic review found evidence of a mild anxiolytic effect and improvement in quality of life with essential oils combined with massage in several populations, including terminal cancer patients receiving palliative care and hospitalized dementia patients. Aromatherapy has been safely used in the treatment of behavioral disturbances in people with dementia; however, benefit in clinical dementia trials is short-term and most pronounced when combined with other individualized nonpharmacologic modalities.

Cooke B, Ernst E. Aromatherapy: a systematic review. *Br J Gen Pract.* 2000;50(455):493-496.

O-Connor DV, Ames D, Gardner B, King M. Psychosocial treatments of behavior symptoms in dementia: a systematic review of reports meting quality standards. *Int Psychogeriatr.* 2009;21(2): 225-240.

SUMMARY

When counseling patients regarding complementary and alternative it is most important to maintain a trusting and open therapeutic alliance. Inquire about the use of complementary and alternative and strive to understand the reasons people choose to pursue these therapies. Learning which modalities are supported by the best evidence and which have been shown to not be effective is also important when discussing the pros and cons of using complementary therapies.

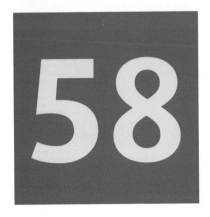

Managing Misuse of Alcohol & Psychoactive Prescription Medications in Older Adults

Frederic C. Blow, PhD

Kristen L. Barry, PhD

▶ General Principles in Older Adults

A growing number of older adults misuse alcohol, psychoactive prescription drugs, and/or other substances, including tobacco. The emerging literature on the baby boom cohort of aging adults (born between 1946 and 1964) indicates that they are continuing to use alcohol and psychoactive prescription medications, in particular, at a higher rate than previous generations, and they are beginning to present larger issues for the health care system and the intervention and treatment communities. The development and refinement of evidence-based practices to address these problems and provide early intervention services is crucial to meeting the needs of this growing population.

Tobacco remains an important concern. A number of programs and medications are available to help individuals stop using tobacco products. Clinicians can guide patients to appropriate programs and/or medications. The important thing to address with older adults is that it is not too late to quit. There are benefits from quitting at any stage in life. (For more on smoking cessation, see Chapter 34, "Chronic Obstructive Pulmonary Disease.")

However, when working with older adults, 2 major categories of substances generate the most concerns for clinicians: (a) alcohol and (b) psychoactive prescription medications (eg, medications for anxiety, medications for sleep, and pain medications). These substances are the focus of this chapter.

The misuse and abuse of alcohol and psychoactive medications in older adults pose challenges for identification of the problem, which interventions will be the most effective, and determinations of the best treatment options, when needed. Problems related to substance use are often unrecognized and, if recognized, generally undertreated in this age group.

There have been a number of community surveys over many years estimating the prevalence of problem drinking among older adults. The prevalence has varied from 1% to 16%, depending on the definitions of "at-risk" and "problem" drinking, and alcohol abuse/dependence.

In 2002, more than 616,000 adults age 55 years and older reported alcohol dependence in the past year: 1.8% of those age 55–59, 1.5% of those age 60–64, and 0.5% of those age 65 or older. Although alcohol and drug/medication dependence are less common in older adults when compared to younger adults, the mental and physical health problems related to higher levels of use can be serious.

HEALTH RISKS ASSOCIATED WITH HAZARDOUS AND HARMFUL USE IN OLDER ADULTS

There are a number of physical health problems that have been related to harmful use of alcohol. Drinking at hazardous levels increases the risk of hypertension and may increase the risk of breast cancer and diabetes, among other medical conditions in both younger and older adults.

However, symptoms of harmful drinking are often not as noticeable in older adults because these symptoms can be masked by social challenges (eg, isolation), medical conditions (eg, gastrointestinal distress), or psychological problems (eg, depressed feelings, confusion). The physiologic aging processes and the presence of health conditions common to old age can reduce a person's tolerance to alcohol. Comparable amounts of alcohol produce higher blood alcohol levels in older adults than in younger persons, and may exacerbate other health problems. Drinking produces higher blood alcohol levels in older adults than in younger persons when comparable amounts of alcohol are drunk, and many problems common among older people, such as chronic illness, poor nutrition, and polypharmacy, may be exacerbated by even small amounts of alcohol.

Although light-to-moderate alcohol use for someone in their 30s may not cause health or social problems, that amount may actually have a number of negative health effects in an older person. Clinicians who treat older patients should assess the amount of alcohol use and should be aware of health implications of any individual's pattern of use.

PSYCHOACTIVE MEDICATIONS

Although older adults, in general, have high rates of medication use compared to younger individuals, there are very few studies that have specifically examined the prevalence of psychoactive medication use, misuse and abuse among older adults. This literature indicates that psychoactive medication misuse affects a small but significant minority of the older adult population.

A relatively recent study found that 25% of older adults use prescription psychoactive medications that have abuse potential. The characteristics of older adults who may be more likely to have problems with psychoactive medications include (a) being female, (b) being socially isolated, and (c) having a history of substance abuse or a mental health disorder. In addition, longer-term use of psychotropic medications, especially benzodiazepines, is associated with cognitive losses and depressed feelings. Also, combining alcohol and psychoactive medications has even more potential for poor health and social outcomes.

DEFINITIONS TO GUIDE SCREENING AND INTERVENTIONS

The National Institute of Alcohol Abuse and Alcoholism (NIAAA) developed drinking limit recommendations for younger and older adults: The following are the drinking limits by age group.

- *Younger than age 65 years:* No more than 7 standard drinks/week for women (no more than 1 drink/day), and no more than 14 standard drinks/week for men (no more than 2 drinks/day).
- *For men and women age 65+:* At risk drinking is no more than 1 drink/day. The limits are the same for both men and women in this age group.

The World Health Organization defines alcohol use in 3 major categories: nonhazardous, hazardous, and harmful use. This categorization allows for variation based on individual differences in metabolism, response, history, and use patterns. It fits particularly well when working with older adults because it avoids stigmatizing terms such as "alcoholic" and "addict."

▶ Nonhazardous or Low-Risk Use

Alcohol use or short-term psychoactive medication use that does not lead to problems is called nonhazardous or low-risk use (see Case 58–1, adapted from Barry and Blow, 2010). People who use alcohol and/or medications at a low risk level can set reasonable limits on alcohol consumption and do not drink when driving a car or boat, operating machinery, or using contraindicated medications. They also do not engage in binge drinking. Among older adults, low-risk use of medications could include short-term use of an antianxiety medication for an acute anxiety state during which the physician's prescription is followed and no alcohol is used, or drinking 1 drink 3 times/week without the use of any contraindicated medications.

Case 58–1

Jenny Martin is a 68-year-old retired social worker who drinks 1 glass of wine when out to dinner or playing bridge with friends, no more than 3 times/week. She does not take any psychoactive medications. She has no family history of alcohol abuse or dependence, and does not take other medications that would interact with alcohol. She receives routine health care from a primary care physician and attends a senior center. A clinician could provide prevention messages regarding her alcohol use in the context of her overall health.

▶ Hazardous Use or At-Risk Use

Hazardous or at-risk use is use that increases the chances that a person will develop problems and complications related to the use of alcohol. These individuals have more than 7 drinks/week or drink in risky situations (see Case 58–2). They do not currently have health problems related to alcohol, but if this drinking pattern continues, problems may result. Misuse of psychoactive medications includes taking more or less medication than prescribed; hoarding or skipping doses of a medication; using medication for purposes other than those prescribed; and using medications in conjunction with alcohol or other contraindicated medications.

Case 58–2

John Fogarty is a 64-year-old marketing executive. He works long hours with few interests outside of work. He drinks 2 drinks/day during the week and 3 or 4 drinks/day on the weekends. His wife has been concerned about his drinking. She would like him to spend more time in activities with her that do not involve drinking. He has gone to a counselor to help him start to plan for retirement. He completed some health and social history questionnaires for the counselor. The message from the counselor included a statement regarding his use of alcohol and concern about potential problems. "You said that, on average, you drink alcohol every day and drink 2 drinks at a time during the week and drink more than that on the weekends. You and I have talked about your stresses at work, your wife's concerns about your use of alcohol, and your own worries about retirement. I am concerned that your pattern of alcohol use could put you at risk for other problems. How do you see this?"

▶ Harmful Use

"Harmful use" includes both "problem use" and "dependence."

A. Problem Use

Problem use refers to a level of use that has already resulted in adverse medical, psychological, or social consequences (see Case 58–3). Although most problem drinkers consume more than the low-risk limits, some older adults who drink smaller amounts may experience alcohol-related problems. As mentioned above, medication misuse can also fit into the problem use category. Assessment is needed by the clinician to determine severity.

Case 58–3

Marina Holbrook is a 70-year-old widow living alone in a small apartment in a medium-size city. Her husband died 3 years ago and she has "felt lost" since then. In a routine visit to her primary care clinic, the nurse practitioner asked some questions about her general health and Mrs. Holbrook said that she is tired all the time and, because she does not sleep well, she is using nonprescription sleeping pills. When asked, she said that she generally drinks 1 glass of wine a day before dinner just as she and her husband did when they were younger, and 1 glass of wine before bed "to help me sleep." She had been taking a prescription medicine for stomach pain for 6 months, but the pain has not improved. Her nurse practitioner discussed with her the potential problems of mixing some medications with alcohol, provided information about the senior center in her neighborhood, suggested she try the center for some activities and that she try to stop the use of alcohol, since it could be starting to cause problems that would get worse with time. "I am concerned about your use of alcohol with the medications for your stomach and the sleeping pills. The stomach medicine you take and the sleeping pills can increase the effect of the alcohol. I'm also concerned that you may not have a lot of opportunities to get together with other people. Would you like me to give you the phone number for the Senior Center in your neighborhood and the name of the person to call at the Center? She is very nice and I know would be happy to hear from you. Ideally, it may be best to discontinue both alcohol and the sleeping pills. You said that you did not want to do that. So do you think that, for the next month, you could stop using the sleeping pills *or* stop the use of alcohol? It is more dangerous to use them both at the same time. We can talk again about what works and what does not work in 1 month and reassess what to do next."

B. Dependence

Dependence is part of the World Health Organization (WHO) "harmful use" category and is a medical disorder characterized by loss of control, preoccupation with alcohol, continued use despite adverse consequences, and, sometimes, physiologic symptoms such as tolerance and withdrawal as in Case 58–4.

A wide range of legal and illegal substances can be abused. Medication abuse involves medication use that results in diminished physical or social functioning, medication use in risky situations, and continued medication use despite adverse social or personal consequences. Dependence includes medication use that results in tolerance or withdrawal symptoms, unsuccessful attempts to stop or control medication use, and preoccupation with attaining or using a medication.

Case 58–4

Leon Culver is a 68-year-old retired electrician. He has had chronic abdominal pain and unresolved hypertension for the past 12 years. He has a history of alcohol problems and had an admission to alcohol treatment 15 years ago. About 4 years ago, after having withdrawal symptoms during a hospital admission for a work-related injury, he again entered an alcohol treatment program. He was abstinent for 2 years and then started drinking again after he retired. He now drinks approximately 5 beers a day plus some additional liquor once a week. His physician and social worker in the primary care clinic are aware that this is a chronic relapsing disorder and continue to work with Mr. Culver to help him stabilize his medical conditions and find longer term help for his primary alcohol dependence. "Mr. Culver, your high blood pressure and stomach pains don't seem to be getting better. The amount you are drinking could interfere with them getting better. I know you've tried hard to deal with your alcohol problems and you really kept those problems in check for a very long time, but now they seem to be getting in the way of your health and well-being again. Would you be willing to talk to someone from the alcohol program here at the medical center to assess whether or not it is time to get some extra help to prevent further problems?"

▶ Screening

Because of the relationship between the amount of alcohol consumed and health problems, questions about consumption (quantity and frequency of use) provide a method to categorize patients into levels of risk for alcohol use. The traditional assumption that all patients who drink have a tendency to underreport their alcohol use is not supported by research. People who are not alcohol dependent often give accurate answers. To assess for misuse of psychoactive medications, key questions include amounts used, other medications taken, and any concomitant use of alcohol.

Clinicians can attain more accurate histories by asking questions about the recent past; embedding the alcohol use and psychoactive medication questions in the context of other health (ie, health history, exercise, nutrition, smoking, medications used, alcohol use). Screening questions can be asked by verbal interview, by paper-and-pencil questionnaire, or by computerized questionnaire. All 3 methods have been shown to have equivalent reliability and validity. To successfully embed alcohol and medication misuse screening into clinical practices, the screening needs to be simple and consistent with other screening procedures already in place.

A. Potential Prescreening Questions

- *Prescreening question:* Do you drink beer, wine, or other alcoholic beverages?
- *Follow-up:* If yes, how many times in the [past year; past 3 months; past 6 months] have you had 4 or more drinks in a day (for older men)/3 or more drinks in a day (for older women)?

- On average, how many days/week do you drink alcoholic beverages? *If weekly or more:* On a day when you drink alcohol, how many drinks do you have?
- *Prescreening questions:* Do you use prescription medicines for pain? Anxiety? Sleep? Do you use any of these prescription drugs in a way that is different from how they were prescribed?
- *Follow-up:* If yes, follow up with additional questions regarding which substances, frequency and quantity of use.

Screening instruments exist that can be used with older adults: the Alcohol Use Disorders Identification Test (AUDIT) developed by the WHO (Table 58–1), the Short Michigan Alcoholism Screening Test–Geriatric Version (SMAST-G) (Table 58–2), and ASSIST, a drug use questionnaire developed by the National Institute on Drug Abuse (NIDA) and modified for older adults to assess misuse of psychoactive prescription medication.

The Substance Abuse and Mental Health Services Administration (SAMHSA), Center for Substance Abuse Treatment (CSAT) developed a series of treatment improvement protocols (TIPs), including TIP #26, "Substance Abuse in Older Adults." The expert panel recommended that all adults age 60+ years should be screened on a yearly basis (generally, embedded with other health-screening questions) and rescreened if there are major life changes that could precipitate increased use and problems (eg, retirement, death of a partner/spouse, etc).

Table 58–1. The alcohol use disorders identification test: AUDIT.

1. How often do you have a drink containing alcohol?
   - ❏ 0 Never
   - ❏ 1 Monthly or less
   - ❏ 2 2 to 4 times a month
   - ❏ 3 2 to 3 times a month
   - ❏ 4 4 or more times a week
2. How many drinks containing alcohol do you have on a typical day when you are drinking?
   - ❏ 0 1 or 2
   - ❏ 1 3 or 4
   - ❏ 2 5 or 6
   - ❏ 3 7 or 9
   - ❏ 4 10 or more
3. How often do you have 6 or more drinks on one occasions?
   - ❏ 0 Never
   - ❏ 1 Less than monthly
   - ❏ 2 Monthly
   - ❏ 3 Weekly
   - ❏ 4 Daily or almost daily
4. How often during the last year have you found that you were not able to stop drinking once you had started?
   - ❏ 0 Never
   - ❏ 1 Less than monthly
   - ❏ 2 Monthly
   - ❏ 3 Weekly
   - ❏ 4 Daily or almost daily
5. How often during the last year have you failed to do what was normally expected from you because of drinking?
   - ❏ 0 Never
   - ❏ 1 Less than monthly
   - ❏ 2 Monthly
   - ❏ 3 Weekly
   - ❏ 4 Daily or almost daily
6. How often during the last year have you needed a first drink in the morning to get yourself going after a heavy drinking session?
   - ❏ 0 Never
   - ❏ 1 Less than monthly
   - ❏ 2 Monthly
   - ❏ 3 Weekly
   - ❏ 4 Daily or almost daily

(continued)

Table 58–1. The alcohol use disorders identification test: AUDIT. (*continued*)

7. How often during the last year have you had a feeling of guilt or remorse after drinking?
   - ❏ 0 Never
   - ❏ 1 Less than monthly
   - ❏ 2 Monthly
   - ❏ 3 Weekly
   - ❏ 4 Daily or almost daily

8. How often during the last year have you been unable to remember what happened the night before because of your drinking?
   - ❏ 0 Never
   - ❏ 1 Less than monthly
   - ❏ 2 Monthly
   - ❏ 3 Weekly
   - ❏ 4 Daily or almost daily

9. Have you or someone else been injured as a result of your drinking?
   - ❏ 0 No
   - ❏ 2 Yes, but not in the last year
   - ❏ 4 Yes, during the last year

10. Has a relative, friend, doctor or other health worker been concerned about your drinking or suggested you cut down?
   - ❏ 0 No
   - ❏ 2 Yes, but not in the last year
   - ❏ 4 Yes, during the last year

Record sum of individual item scores here: ▭

SCORING: The following are standard guidelines for scoring the AUDIT. However, for older adults a score of 3 or more warrants additional assessment of the situation and possible brief counseling; older adults who use contraindicated medications or are experiencing cognitive or health problems should not use alcohol at all.

Standard Scoring: 0–4: Lower risk use; 5–8: At-risk use; 8–10: Alcohol abuse; 11–up: Alcohol dependence.

Reproduced with permission from Babor TF, Higgins-Biddle JC, Saunders JB, Monteiro MG. *AUDIT: The Alcohol Use Disorders Identification Test: Guidelines for Use in Primary Care.* 2nd edition. Department of Mental Health and Substance Dependence, Geneva, Switzerland, World Health Organization, 2001.

Table 58–2. Short Michigan ALCOHOLISM Screening Test-Geriatric Version (SMAST-G).

	YES (1)	NO (0)
1. When talking with others, do you ever underestimate how much you actually drink?	___	___
2. After a few drinks, have you sometimes not eaten or been able to skip a meal because you don't feel hungry?	___	___
3. Does having a few drinks help decrease your shakiness or tremors?	___	___
4. Does alcohol sometimes make it hard for you to remember parts of the day or night?	___	___
5. Do you usually take a drink to relax or calm your nerves?	___	___
6. Do you drink to take your mind off your problems?	___	___
7. Have you ever increased your drinking after experiencing a loss in your life?	___	___
8. Has a doctor or nurse ever said they were worried or concerned about your drinking?	___	___
9. Have you ever made rules to manage your drinking?	___	___
10. When you feel lonely, does having a drink help?	___	___

TOTAL SMAST-G SCORE (0–10) ▭

© The Regents of the University of Michigan, Frederic C. Blow, Ph.D., 1991.

BRIEF INTERVENTIONS

There is a large body of evidence that motivational brief interventions, delivered in a variety of health care and social service settings, can effectively reduce drinking, particularly for at-risk and problem users. Over the past 25+ years, there have been more than 100 preventive intervention trials in a variety of medical and social service care settings that have proven motivational brief interventions to be efficacious in reducing alcohol misuse among younger and older adults. The general form of the interventions in these studies included personalized feedback based on the individual's responses to screening questions, and messages regarding cutting back or stopping use. Results indicate that, across studies, participants reduced their average number of drinks per week by approximately 30% compared to controls. Psychoactive prescription medication misuse has been incorporated into alcohol brief interventions for older adults so as to address these 2 issues in a systematic framework.

▶ Use of a Brief Intervention Workbook

Brief intervention protocols often use a workbook. Using a workbook can make it easier for both the older adult and the clinician to discuss cues to use, reasons for the level of use, reasons to cut down or quit, negotiate an agreement for next steps, and introduce using daily diary cards for self-monitoring. Brief interventions take approximately 20–30 minutes to conduct (Barry, CSAT, 1999).

SUMMARY

Identification of substance-use problems in older adults can take place in many health care-related settings, including primary care clinics, specialty care settings, home health care, elder housing, and senior center programs. Both from a public health standpoint and from a clinical perspective, the aging of the baby boom cohort means that there is a critical need in the health care field to implement effective screening and intervention strategies with older adults who are at-risk for more serious health, social, and emotional problems as a consequence of their use of alcohol, psychoactive prescription medications, and other drugs.

Innovative screening, intervention, and treatment methods have been developed for alcohol and drug misuse among older adults. Successful implementation of these strategies can improve the physical and emotional quality of older adults' lives.

Babor TF, Higgins-Biddle JC. *Brief Intervention for Hazardous and Harmful Drinking: a Manual for Use in Primary Care.* World Health Organization, Department of Mental Health and Substance Dependence. 2001. http://whqlibdoc.who.int/hq/2001/who_msd_msb_01.6b.pdf

Baker SL. Substance abuse disorders in aging veterans. In: Gottheil E, Druley RA, Skiloday TE, Waxman H, eds. *Alcohol, Drug Addiction and Aging.* Springfield, IL: Charles C. Thomas; 1985:303-311.

Barry KL, Fleming MF, Barry KL, Fleming M. Computerized administration of alcoholism screening tests in a primary care setting. *J Am Board Fam Pract.* 1990;3(2):93-98.

Barry KL, Blow FC. Screening, assessing and intervening for alcohol and medication misuse in older adults. In Lichtenberg P, ed. *Handbook of Assessment in Clinical Gerontology.* 2nd ed. New York, NY: Wiley; 2010:310-330.

Barry KL, Center for Substance Abuse Treatment. *Brief Interventions and Brief Therapies for Substance Abuse.* Treatment Improvement Protocol (TIP) Series 34. DHHS Publication No. (SMA) 99-3353. Rockville, MD: Substance Abuse and Mental Health Services Administration; 1999.

Blow FC, Barry KL, Walton MA, et al. The efficacy of two brief intervention strategies among injured, at-risk drinkers in the emergency department: impact of tailored messaging and brief advice. *J Stud Alcohol.* 2006;67(4):568-578.

Blow FC, Center for Substance Abuse Treatment. *Substance Abuse Among Older Adults.* FC Blow, Chair. Treatment Improvement Protocol (TIP) Series 26. DHHS Publication No. (SMA) 98-3179. Rockville, MD: Substance Abuse and Mental Health Services Administration; 1998.

Chermack ST, Blow FC, Hill EM. The relationship between alcohol symptoms and consumption among older drinkers. *Alcohol Clin Exp Res.* 1996;20(7):1153-1158.

Chick J, Lloyd G, Crombie E. Counseling problem drinkers in medical wards: a controlled study. *Br Med J (Clin Res Ed).* 1985;290(6473):965-967.

Culberson J, Ziska M. Prescription drug misuse/abuse in the elderly. *Geriatrics.* 2008;63(9):22-31.

Dealberto MJ, Mcavay GJ, Seeman T, Berkman L. Psychotropic drug use and cognitive decline among older men and women. *Int J Geriatr Psychiatry.* 1997;12(5):567-574.

Fleming MF, Barry KL, Manwell LB, Johnson K, London R. Brief physician advice for problem drinkers: a randomized controlled trial in community-based primary care practices. *Alcohol Alcohol.* 1997;277(13):1039-1045.

Fleming MF, Manwell LB, Barry KL, et al. Brief physician advice for alcohol problems in older adults: a randomized community-based trial. *J Fam Pract.* 1999;48(5):378-384.

Hogan DB, Maxwell CJ, Fung TS, Ebly EM; Canadian Study of Health and Aging. Prevalence and potential consequences of benzodiazepine use in senior citizens: results from the Canadian Study of Health and Aging. *Can J Clin Pharmacol.* 2003;10(2):72-77.

Moore AA, Blow FC, Hoffing M, et al. Primary care-based intervention to reduce at-risk drinking in older adults: a randomized controlled trial. *Addiction.* 2011;106(1):111-120.

National Institute on Alcohol Abuse and Alcoholism. *Helping Patients Who Drink Too Much. A Clinician's Guide, Updated 2005 Edition.* U.S. Department of Health and Human Services, National Institute of Health. NIH Publication No. 07-3769. Rockville, MD: U.S. Department of Health and Human Services; 2005.

Office of Applied Studies. Summary of Findings from the 2002 National Survey on Drug Use and Health. Rockville, MD: Substance Abuse and Mental Health Services Administration, Department of Health & Human Services; 2002.

Rosin AJ, Glatt MM. Alcohol excess in the elderly. *Q J Stud Alcohol.* 1971;32(1):53-59.

Schonfeld L, King-Kallimanis B, Duchene D, et al. Screening and brief intervention for substance misuse among older adults: the Florida BRITE project. *Am J Public Health.* 2010;100(1): 108-114.

Simoni-Wastila L, Yang HK. Psychoactive drug abuse in older adults. *Am J Geriatr Pharmacother.* 2006;4(4):380-394.

Vestal RE, McGuire EA, Tobin JD, Andres R, Norris AH, Mezey E. Aging and ethanol metabolism. *Clin Pharmacol Ther.* 1977;21(3):343-354.

Whitlock EP, Polen MR, Green CA, Orleans T, Klein J; U.S. Preventive Services Task Force. Behavioral counseling interventions in primary care to reduce risky/harmful alcohol use by adults: a summary of the evidence for the U.S. Preventive Services Task Force. *Ann Intern Med.* 2004;140(7):557-568.

Assessing Older Adults for Syncope Following a Fall

59

Natalie A. Sanders, DO, FACP

Mark A. Supiano, MD

"Marked clinical overlap exists between falls, orthostatic hypotension, and dizzy spells, which may all present as syncope. Elderly patients may present with recurrent falls resulting from syncope."

From the *AHA/ACCF Scientific Statement on the Evaluation of Syncope* (2006)

"Given that up to 70% of falls in older persons are not witnessed, these patients may present with a report of a fall rather than syncope."

From the *AGS/BGS Clinical Practice Guideline: Prevention of Falls in Older Persons* (2011)

General Principles in Older Adults

Falls and syncope are commonly encountered syndromes in older adults and both are associated with significant morbidity and mortality. It is often difficult to know when to consider syncope as the primary or a contributing cause to falls in older adults. This chapter provides some guidance for the clinician faced with the question, "Is this patient's fall caused by syncope?"

Most studies estimate that one-third of community-dwelling older adults fall each year. Falls are the leading cause of injury among patients age 65 years and older. Twenty percent to 30% of falls among older adults result in moderate-to-severe injuries. Falls are associated with functional decline, increased risk for nursing home placement, decreased quality of life, and higher health care costs.

Syncope is also common among older adults. Its prevalence in the general population has a bimodal distribution peaking in people age 10–30 years and again in those older than age 65 years. Almost half of emergency room visits for syncope are made by persons 65 years of age or older. Because of underlying multiple comorbidities and increased prevalence of cardiovascular disease in older people, the morbidity

and mortality associated with syncope is higher in older adults compared to younger adults.

GENERAL APPROACH TO THE PATIENT WITH FALLS OR SYNCOPE

Falls

The literature varies widely on the definition of falls, but typically falls are defined as unintentionally coming to rest on the ground or a lower surface. When evaluating a patient with falls, obtaining a detailed history of the fall from the patient and witnesses, if available, is imperative and a good starting point. This history should include the circumstances surrounding the fall, any preceding symptoms, such as dizziness or lightheadedness, whether the fall was witnessed or not, and whether there was loss of consciousness with the fall. A focused physical exam including a cognitive and functional assessment should also be completed. During the evaluation, it is important to remember that falls constitute a geriatric syndrome. As such, the cause of falling in an older patient is rarely the result of a single cause but instead the result of a complex interaction between intrinsic and extrinsic risk factors. In addition to a detailed history and physical exam, identifying and addressing these risk factors is at the core of a falls evaluation. Current guidelines emphasize assessing the following risk factors: (a) history of falls, (b) medications, (c) gait, balance, and mobility, (d) visual acuity, (e) other neurologic impairments, (f) muscle strength, (g) heart rate and rhythm, (h) postural hypotension, (i) feet and footwear, and (j) assessment of environmental hazards (Table 59–1). Medication classes to specifically identify in older adults with falls include anticonvulsants, antipsychotics, benzodiazepines, nonbenzodiazepine hypnotics, tricyclic antidepressants, and selective serotonin reuptake inhibitors. Because of their propensity to worsen postural hypotension, antihypertensive medications should also be evaluated.

Table 59–1. Multifactorial fall risk assessment.

History of previous falls
Medications
Gait, balance, and mobility
Visual acuity
Presence of other neurologic impairments (ie, neuropathy)
Muscle strength
Heart rate and rhythm
Postural hypotension
Feet and footwear
Environmental hazards

Syncope

Fainting is a common problem and encompasses any disorder associated with a real or perceived transient loss of consciousness. Nontraumatic transient loss of consciousness is further classified into syncope, epileptic disorders, psychogenic pseudosyncope, and rare miscellaneous causes, such as cataplexy or drop attacks. Syncope specifically refers to transient loss of consciousness caused by global hypoperfusion. Hallmark features of its presentation are sudden loss of consciousness with associated loss of postural tone and rapid spontaneous recovery. The causes of syncope can be classified into 3 broad categories: reflex-mediated syncope, syncope caused by orthostatic hypotension, and cardiac syncope (Table 59–2).

The initial goal of the evaluation of syncope is risk stratification, that is, to define those patients who warrant urgent cardiac evaluation because of the high short-term risk of recurrence of syncope. Approximately one-third of patients with syncope will have a recurrent event within 3 years. As

Table 59–2. Classification of syncope.

Reflex (neurally mediated) syncope
    Vasovagal
    Situational
    Carotid sinus syndrome
    Atypical forms
Syncope caused by orthostatic hypotension
    Primary autonomic failure
    Secondary autonomic failure
    Drug-induced
    Volume depletion
Cardiac syncope
    Arrhythmia
    Structural

Data from Task Force for the Diagnosis and Management of Syncope; European Society of Cardiology (ESC); European Heart Rhythm Association (EHRA); Heart Failure Association (HFA); Heart Rhythm Society (HRS), Moya A, Sutton R, Ammirati F, et al. Guidelines for the diagnosis and management of syncope (version 2009). *Eur Heart J.* 2009;30(21):2631-2671.

with falls, the evaluation of the patient with syncope should start with obtaining a comprehensive history of the event and physical examination, including checking orthostatic vital signs. An electrocardiogram (ECG) should also be performed. Historical questions should be targeted to try to identify which class of syncope is most likely. A detailed history and physical examination combined with ECG findings can identify the cause of syncope in nearly 25% of patients. Patients in whom the cause of syncope is uncertain may warrant additional tests. These tests include, but are not limited to, echocardiography, stress testing, short-term or long-term ECG monitoring, electrophysiology study, tilt-table testing, and supine and upright carotid sinus massage. Similar to falls, older adults may have more than 1 factor contributing to their syncope. Physiologic changes associated with aging, such as inability to preserve sodium and water, decreased baroreceptor responsiveness and autonomic dysfunction all increase older adults' risk for syncope. The use of multiple medications that affect blood pressure, heart rate, and volume status, such as diuretics and β blockers, also predispose older people to syncope. All of these factors should be kept in mind when evaluating the older adult with syncope.

HOW FALLS AND SYNCOPE OVERLAP

There is increasing evidence of an overlap between nonaccidental falls and syncope. First, because of the lack of a witness account, history provided by the patient may be unreliable. In addition to patients not recalling the circumstances of their fall, several studies indicate patients do not accurately remember the number of falls they have. Individual patient factors that increase the risk of poor fall recall include older age, cognitive impairment, and occurrence of a non-injurious fall. Second, patients may not recall loss of consciousness. Retrograde amnesia for loss of consciousness affects up to 30% of patients with syncope. These data mainly originate from studies evaluating patients with carotid sinus syndrome, although up to two-thirds of patients with orthostatic hypotension may also not report loss of consciousness. Finally, in patients with gait or balance problems, hypotension and bradycardia may be less-well tolerated, resulting in a fall. Both hypotension and bradycardia can decrease cardiac output enough to cause cerebral hypoperfusion and loss of postural tone without causing complete loss of consciousness. These patients may be misclassified as having only suffered a fall and not a syncopal event. Yet, the underlying physiology is the same (decreased global cerebral perfusion) and may be treatable, warranting consideration of syncope in these patients.

WHEN TO CONSIDER SYNCOPE AS A CAUSE OF FALLS

Clinicians should consider evaluating patients for syncope when the following factors are present: (a) history of loss of

Table 59–3. Considering syncope as a cause of falls.

Clinical Situations
History of loss of consciousness
Unexplained nonaccidental fall
Recurrent falls despite adherence to multicomponent treatment program targeting risk factors
Common Diagnostic Categories Associated with Unexplained Falls
Orthostatic hypotension variants
Classical
Delayed
Postprandial
Carotid sinus syndrome
Vasodepressor response
Cardioinhibitory response
Mixed response
Cardiac syncope due to arrhythmia

consciousness with the fall, (b) unexplained non-accidental fall or (c) recurrent falls despite adherence to a multi-factorial targeted treatment program (Table 59–3).

COMMON DIAGNOSTIC CATEGORIES TO CONSIDER

There are 3 diagnostic categories to consider in the differential diagnoses of these patients: orthostatic hypotension and its variants, carotid sinus syndrome, and cardiac syncope due to arrhythmia (see Table 59–3).

▶ Orthostatic Hypotension and Its Variants

A. Classical Orthostatic Hypotension

Classical orthostatic hypotension, defined as a drop in systolic blood pressure of ≥20 mm Hg within 3 minutes of standing, is common in older adults. However, it is often not tested for or may be simply disregarded by patients. In the Cardiovascular Health Study, the prevalence of orthostatic hypotension was 18% in subjects age 65 years or older, yet only 2% of these subjects reported symptoms with standing.

B. Delayed Orthostatic Hypotension

Delayed orthostatic hypotension is characterized by a drop in systolic blood pressure of ≥20 mm Hg after more than 3 minutes of standing. It should be considered in older adults with underlying neurologic disorders, which put them at risk for autonomic dysfunction. These include idiopathic Parkinson disease, multiple system atrophy, and diabetes. Because nearly 40% of patients with this condition will drop their blood pressure only after at least 10 minutes of upright posture, tilt-table testing is typically used to evaluate for delayed orthostatic hypotension.

C. Postprandial Hypotension

Postprandial hypotension is another diagnosis to consider when evaluating patients with falls for the possibility of syncope. Postprandial hypotension is defined as a fall in systolic blood pressure of ≥20 mm Hg within 2 hours of eating a meal. Nearly half of healthy older patients with unexplained syncope have been found to have postprandial hypotension. Patients with classical orthostatic hypotension or autonomic dysfunction are also at higher risk for postprandial hypotension. Obtaining a detailed history of events and their association with meals can help identify patients with possible postprandial hypotension. Some patients may require 24-hour ambulatory blood pressure monitoring to confirm the diagnosis.

▶ Carotid Sinus Syndrome

Carotid sinus hypersensitivity is caused by an exaggerated response to carotid sinus massage. In some studies, up to 70% of patients ≥65 years old with unexplained falls have carotid sinus hypersensitivity during supine and upright tilt-table testing. Carotid sinus syndrome is diagnosed when there is reproduction of a patient's symptoms associated with a systolic blood pressure drop of ≥50 mm Hg (vasodepressor response), an asystolic pause of ≥3 seconds (cardioinhibitory response), or both (mixed response) with carotid sinus massage. Carotid sinus syndrome has been reported to be the cause of unexplained falls in up to 40% of patients. Performing carotid sinus massage in the supine and upright positions increases the sensitivity. Although the evidence is not yet conclusive, permanent cardiac pacing may be helpful in reducing falls in patients with a marked cardioinhibitory response to carotid sinus massage.

▶ Cardiac Syncope Caused by Arrhythmia

Cardiac syncope caused by arrhythmia may be responsible for up to 30% of syncope in older adults. Its high prevalence in older adults is thought to be related to the increased number of underlying cardiovascular comorbidities older adults have as well as the increased prevalence of sinus node dysfunction seen with aging. Atrial fibrillation, one manifestation of sinus node dysfunction, has been found to be an independent risk factor for unexplained non-accidental falls in older adults. Ambulatory ECG monitoring can be used to diagnose syncope caused by arrhythmia. This is often done by using a 30-day event monitor. However, because cardiac syncope caused by arrhythmia may not recur within 30 days, clinical guidelines endorse the use of long-term ECG monitoring with implantable loop recorders for patients with unexplained syncope. Recognizing the overlap between syncope and falls, one may also consider long-term ECG monitoring in a patient with unexplained falls.

SUMMARY

When evaluating an older adult who has fallen or with frequent falls, it is important to: (a) conduct a multifactorial fall risk assessment (see Table 59–1); (b) consider clinical scenarios in which syncope may be the cause of falls (see Table 59–3); and (c) if syncope is the likely cause of the fall, classify syncope to determine next diagnostic and treatment steps (see Table 59–2).

American Geriatrics Society 2012 Beers Criteria Update Expert Panel. American Geriatrics Society updated Beers Criteria for potentially inappropriate medication use in older adults. *J Am Geriatr Soc.* 2012;60(4):616-631.

Anpalahan M. Neurally mediated syncope and unexplained or non-accidental falls in the elderly. *Intern Med J.* 2006;36(3):202-207.

Schatz IJ, Bannister R, Freeman RL, et al. Consensus statement on the definition of orthostatic hypotension, pure autonomic failure, and multiple system atrophy. *J Neurol Sci.* 1996;144(1-2):218-219.

Del Rosso A, Alboni P, Brignole M, Menozzi C, Raviele A. Relation of clinical presentation of syncope to the age of patients. *Am J Cardiol.* 2005;96(10):1431-1435.

Gibbons CH, Freeman R. Delayed orthostatic hypotension: a frequent cause of orthostatic intolerance. *Neurology.* 2006;67(1):28-32.

Narender P, Orshoven V, Jansen P, et al. Postprandial hypotension in clinical geriatric patients and healthy elderly: prevalence related to patient selection and diagnostic criteria. *J Aging Res.* 2010;2010:243752.

Panel on Prevention of Falls in Older Persons, American Geriatrics Society and British Geriatrics Society. Summary of the Updated American Geriatrics Society/British Geriatric Society clinical practice guideline for prevention of falls in older persons. *J Am Geriatr Soc.* 2011;59(1):148-157.

Ryan DJ, Nick S, Colette SM, Roseanne K. Carotid sinus syndrome, should we pace? A multicentre, randomised control trial (Safepace 2). *Heart.* 2010;96(5):347-351.

Sanders NA, Ganguly JA, Jetter TL, et al. Atrial fibrillation: an independent risk factor for non accidental falls in older patients. *Pacing Clin Electrophysiol.* 2012;35(8):973-979.

Strickberger SA, Benson DW, Biaggioni I, et al; American Heart Association Councils on Clinical Cardiology, Cardiovascular Nursing, Cardiovascular Disease in the Young, and Stroke; Quality of Care and Outcomes Research Interdisciplinary Working Group; American College of Cardiology Foundation; Heart Rhythm Society. AHA/ACCF scientific statement on the evaluation of syncope: from the American Heart Association Councils on Clinical Cardiology, Cardiovascular Nursing, Cardiovascular Disease in the Young, and Stroke, and the Quality of Care and Outcomes Research Interdisciplinary Working Group; and the American College of Cardiology Foundation In Collaboration With the Heart Rhythm Society. *J Am Coll Cardiol.* 2006;47(2):473-484.

Tan MP, Kenny RA. Cardiovascular assessment of falls in older people. *Clin Interv Aging.* 2006;1(1):57-66.

Task Force for the Diagnosis and Management of Syncope; European Society of Cardiology (ESC); European Heart Rhythm Association (EHRA); Heart Failure Association (HFA); Heart Rhythm Society (HRS), Moya A, Sutton R, Ammirati F, et al. Guidelines for the diagnosis and management of syncope (version 2009). *Eur Heart J.* 2009;30(21):2631-2671.

Tinetti ME, Kumar C. The patient who falls: "It's always a trade-off". *JAMA.* 2010;303(3):258-266.

Treating Headaches in Older Adults

60

Katherine Anderson, MD

Jana Wold, MD

General Principles in Older Adults

In the headache literature, the term *older adult* usually refers to patients age 50 years and older because of changes in presentation and types of headache that occur in patients older than age 50. Primary headaches tend to abate, whereas secondary headaches, that is, headaches caused by another disease or medical condition, become more common with age. Up to 30% of headache complaints in the older adult are caused by other etiologies, including medical conditions or their associated treatments. Essentials to consider when assessing headaches in older adults include:

- New onset headaches are rare in older adults necessitating evaluation
- Temporal arteritis is an emergency
- Headaches in older adults are frequently due to an underlying medical diagnosis or treatment

General Evaluation

Development of a new headache in an older adult, or a change in pattern of chronic headaches, warrants a thorough medical evaluation. This should include a complete pharmacologic review and comprehensive neurologic examination. Additional work-up may be necessary in the older adult, as new headaches are more often a result of serious conditions or exacerbations of comorbid disorders. Such work-up may include brain imaging with CT and/or MRI; cervical spine radiography to evaluate for facet disease causing cervicogenic headache; arterial imaging in the setting of ischemic headache symptoms; laboratory testing, including a complete blood count, erythrocyte sedimentation rate (ESR), C-reactive protein (CRP), and a complete metabolic panel; overnight oximetry in cases of morning headaches or to evaluate for nonrestorative sleep; and/or referral to ophthalmology to evaluate for vision impairment, glaucoma, or other ocular causes of headache.

Differential Diagnoses

A. Primary Headache

The 3 most common headache types (migraine, tension, and cluster) usually have onset before age 45 years. Generally, the presentation and management of these headaches is similar in younger and older adults; however, some unique features found in headaches in older adults are outlined below.

1. Migraine

a. General considerations—New-onset migraine in adults older than the age of 50 years occurs in approximately 3% of all migraine sufferers. Typically, older adults with a history of migraine experience fewer and milder migraines as they age. Traditional migraine should be differentiated from acephalic migraine (migraine without headache).

Acephalic migraine often begins after the age of 40 years, following a migraine-free period of many years or in the absence of a history of migraine. The overall course is benign, and patients experience predominantly visual symptoms. Other symptoms include migrating paresthesia, speech disturbance, and progression of 1 neurologic symptom to another. Most patients experience 2 or more identical spells, each lasting 15–25 minutes.

b. Clinical findings—Migraine attacks in the older adult are less typical compared with younger individuals. They are more frequently bilateral and have fewer associated symptoms, such as photophobia, phonophobia, nausea, and vomiting; thus they may be misdiagnosed as tension-type headache. Patients may complain of throbbing pain, aura, and traditional triggering and ameliorating factors. Attacks are also more often associated with vegetative symptoms, such as anorexia, dry mouth, and paleness.

Acephalic migraine is more common in people with a history of migraine. Visual symptoms (scintillations, diplopia, oscillopsia, nystagmus) associated with migraine aura tend to evolve slowly. Patients describe bright shimmering lights that tend to enlarge and move across both visual fields before they disappear. These symptoms may raise concern for a transient ischemic attack (TIA). However, in TIA, visual deficits tend to be dark, dim, and static lasting only a few minutes. Paresthesias from migraine usually move up and down the extremities, may be bilateral, and clear in the reverse order. Ischemic paresthesias tend to occur suddenly, clear in the same order as they developed, and 90% last less than 15 minutes.

Menopause has variable effects on migraine. Two-thirds of women with migraine will experience a marked improvement, or complete cessation, once they are completely menopausal. Women who require hormonal therapy may have an increase in headache frequency secondary to therapy. Reducing the dose of estrogen or changing the type of estrogen from a conjugated estrogen to pure estradiol may reduce the number of headaches. The favorable course of migraine postmenopause is primarily attributed to the absence of variations in sex hormone levels.

c. Evaluation—Because of the clinical overlap between acephalic migraine and TIA, stroke imaging, such as brain MRI, is warranted. Vessel imaging, such as a CT or magnetic resonance angiogram, may also be considered to evaluate vascular risk factors.

d. Treatment—Because of their vasoconstrictive effects, abortive agents, such as triptans and ergotamines, should be used cautiously in older adults. They are contraindicated in patients with uncontrolled hypertension or evidence of vascular disease. Effective abortive agents include the limited use of acetaminophen, nonsteroidal antiinflammatory drugs (NSAIDs), and opioid analgesics. Patients on NSAIDs chronically should be monitored for azotemia, hypertension, or worsening cerebral or coronary artery disease. Tricyclic antidepressants (TCAs), such as amitriptyline and nortriptyline, are often used for migraine prevention, however, these are not a first-line choice in older individuals because of their anticholinergic side effects. Calcium channel blockers and β blockers also may be used for prevention, and are often effective at lower doses.

2. Tension headache

a. General considerations—Tension headaches typically begin before age 45 years and are most commonly caused by physical or psychological stress. However, these headaches can develop later in life secondary to age-related musculoskeletal, visual, or dental changes.

b. Clinical findings—Neck spasms, cervical spine and muscle tenderness, or decreased cervical range of motion, all of which can be caused by spinal degenerative changes irritating the cervical muscles, may be present. Additionally, some patients complain of spasms of the temporomandibular joint (TMJ), from teeth-clenching, arthritis in the joint, or an abnormal bite. Cervical nerve root irritation can also occur, resulting in complaints of tenderness over the occipital neurovascular bundle, suggesting occipital nerve involvement.

c. Evaluation—Physical exam should include evaluation for muscle tension in the neck, scalp, and face, and an assessment of the patients posture. Attention to the patients bite and screening for TMJ disorders should be performed. Imaging may be warranted if there are concerns for cervical arthritis.

d. Treatment—Nonpharmacologic therapies include physical therapy for posture, balance, and range of motion in patients with musculoskeletal causes; referral to optometry or ophthalmology in the setting of decreased vision or eye strain; and relaxation therapy when stress is identified as a primary trigger.

Pharmacologic therapies include TCAs, muscle relaxants, and NSAIDs in younger populations, but should be used with caution in older patients because of the adverse side-effect profile. Acetaminophen can be used safely in older patients and should be considered prior to other agents. Nerve blocks may be indicated in settings of nerve root pain.

3. Cluster headache

a. General considerations—Cluster headaches are less of a problem in older individuals, with a decrease in the frequency of attacks. The etiology of these headaches is not completely understood, however, there appears to be genetic links and frequently patients are smokers.

b. Clinical findings—Cluster headaches typically are episodic, severe headaches of the orbital, supraorbital, or temporal area. Associated autonomic symptoms include ptosis, miosis, lacrimation, conjunctival injection, rhinorrhea, and nasal congestion occurring ipsilateral to the side of pain. Characteristically, they are of short duration (15–180 minutes) and unilateral, yet symptoms may switch to the other side during a different cluster attack. Patients may describe feeling restless or the need to pace during an attack.

c. Evaluation—Cranial imaging is recommended with CT or MRI to exclude structural brain lesions, including pituitary abnormalities.

d. Treatment—Abortive therapy with oxygen is usually safe and effective. Oxygen therapy should be used cautiously in patients with severe chronic obstructive pulmonary disease given risk of severe hypercapnia and CO_2 narcosis. Vasoconstrictive drugs, such as triptans, have been shown to be effective, but should be used cautiously in patients with vascular disease because of deleterious side effects. One should consider giving first doses in a monitored setting. Even though often effective, prednisone should be used cautiously as it can worsen other medical conditions, such as osteoporosis and diabetes. Preventative medications, such as verapamil, lithium, and antiepileptic drugs, can usually be safely used in older adults.

4. Hypnic headache

a. General considerations—Hypnic headache syndrome is a rare, benign, recurrent, sleep-related headache disorder that occurs almost exclusively in patients older than 50 years. Painful attacks awaken patients from sleep at a predictable time, often during rapid eye movement stages, and can last from 15 minutes to 2 hours occurring, 1–2 times per night.

b. Clinical findings—Hypnic headaches are not accompanied by autonomic symptoms, differentiating them from cluster headaches. Pain is most often described as bilateral, as opposed to the unilateral location of cluster headaches. Patients describe the pain as a steady discomfort primarily in the frontal area.

c. Evaluation—Diagnosis is based on history and further evaluation is usually not indicated.

d. Treatment—Hypnic headaches are self-limited and may resolve after a few months. In the case in which medication therapy is needed, lithium carbonate has shown a favorable response. TCAs, antiepileptics, or NSAIDs at bedtime may also be effective. The side-effect profile of lithium often precludes use in older patients. At least 1 prospective study has shown that hypnic headaches may be responsive to indomethacin. In the older adult, caffeine and melatonin are often effective, safer options.

B. Secondary Headache

1. Temporal arteritis (Giant cell arteritis)

a. General considerations—Also known as giant cell arteritis (GCA), temporal arteritis is a systemic necrotizing vasculitis occurring primarily in whites and has a female predominance. GCA typically occurs in 70–80-year-olds, but should be considered in patients older than 50 with new-onset headache. It is a medical emergency and may result in permanent visual loss in 15% to 20% of patients.

b. Clinical findings—The first symptom in 70% to 90% of patients is a steady or throbbing headache over the temples. However, pain may involve any portion of the head or scalp and may come in waves, triggered by touching the face, laughing, or chewing. Visual symptoms may include amaurosis fugax, diplopia, and visual loss. Symptoms consistent with polymyalgia rheumatica are present in approximately 66% of patients. Nonspecific symptoms of fatigue, anorexia, low-grade fever, and weight loss may also be present. The temporal artery is often thickened with a diminished or absent pulse, and may be tender to palpation. Jaw claudication is uncommon but is highly specific for temporal arteritis.

c. Evaluation—Temporal artery biopsy is the gold standard for diagnosis. Classic findings consistent with GCA, granulomatous inflammatory infiltrate with giant cells located at the intima-media junction, are only found in 50% of cases.

Ideally, biopsy should be done within 48 hours of initiating treatment. If elevated, CRP and ESR have 97% specificity in diagnosing GCA. Pulses may be diminished and palpation of carotid, brachial, radial, femoral, and pedal pulses is recommended. Funduscopic exam by an ophthalmologist is warranted.

d. Treatment—To prevent blindness, urgent treatment with systemic steroids is the standard of care. Even if temporal artery biopsy is not immediately available, treatment should be initiated because pathologic findings may be present for up to 2 weeks after steroid administration. Usual course includes 1 month of full-dose therapy, followed by a slow taper up to 1–2 years. Intravenous glucocorticoids may be recommended for patients at high risk of blindness.

2. Cerebral vascular disease

a. General considerations—Headache can be the heralding symptom in up to 50% of hemorrhagic strokes and 25% of ischemic strokes. In older adult patients with vascular risk factors and headache, cerebrovascular disease must be considered. See Chapter 23, "Cerebrovascular Disease."

3. Trigeminal neuralgia

a. General considerations—Trigeminal neuralgia (TN) is one of the most common neuralgias seen in older adults, with the incidence increasing with age, and slight female predominance. Classic TN occurs in 80% to 90% of cases, and is thought to be caused by compression of the trigeminal nerve root by an aberrant arterial or venous loop. Secondary TN may be a result of other causes, such as an acoustic neuroma, meningioma, epidermoid cyst, or, rarely, an aneurysm or arteriovenous malformation.

b. Clinical findings—Patients may experience paroxysmal attacks of unilateral sharp, superficial or stabbing pain in the distribution of 1 or more branches of the fifth cranial nerve. Pain is often described as "electric" or "shock-like" and is maximal at onset of an attack. The pain may last only minutes, but often returns in repeated attacks, and usually does not awaken patients from sleep. Episodes may last for weeks to months and may be followed by pain-free intervals. Patients may develop a general dull ache in the distribution of the affected nerve.

c. Evaluation—TN is a clinical diagnosis. Attacks may be triggered during an examination by touching the "trigger zone," usually an area in the distribution of the affected nerve, often near the midline. Actions that may trigger an attack include chewing, talking, brushing one's teeth, cold air against the face, smiling, or grimacing. International Headache Society Diagnostic Criteria for TN are:

1. Paroxysmal attacks of pain lasting from a fraction of a second to 2 minutes, affecting 1 or more divisions of the trigeminal nerve.

2. Pain that has at least 1 of the following characteristics: intense, sharp, superficial, or stabbing; or pain that is precipitated from a trigger area or by trigger factors.

3. Stereotyped attacks in an individual patient.

4. No clinically evident neurologic deficit.

5. No other attributing disorder.

Notably, secondary TN is often indistinguishable from classic TN. Imaging with CT or MRI is warranted to rule out secondary causes. Electrophysiologic tests may be useful in distinguishing classic from secondary causes of TN.

d. Treatment—Pharmacologic therapy is the initial treatment for patients with classic TN. Carbamazepine is the best studied and side effects may be manageable if it is started at low doses with slow titration. Oxcarbazepine is probably effective, along with baclofen, lamotrigine, and pimozide. There is less evidence for the effectiveness of clonazepam, gabapentin, phenytoin, tizanidine, and valproate. Periodic taper or withdrawal trials should be attempted. Secondary TN requires treatment of the underlying condition, however, medications used in treatment of classic TN may provide pain relief. In patients with refractory pain, microvascular decompression or ablative surgical procedures may be considered.

4. Mass lesions

a. General considerations—Older adults have a higher incidence of intracranial tumors than younger adults. Up to 50% of patients presenting with brain tumors complain of headache.

b. Clinical findings—Pain is usually generalized, but may be localized over the tumor. The classic severe morning headache, associated with nausea and vomiting, occurs in approximately 17% of patients. More often, patients complain of symptoms similar to tension or migraine headache.

c. Evaluation—If a mass lesion is suspected, an MRI must be obtained and subspecialty referral pursued.

d. Treatment—Neurosurgical, medical, and/or palliative care options should be considered.

5. Cervicogenic headache

a. General considerations—Cervicogenic headache is referred pain from anatomic structures and soft tissues of the neck. This headache type may be overdiagnosed in the older adult secondary to the large number of geriatric patients with radiographic changes consistent with cervical spondylosis.

b. Clinical findings—Symptoms are elicited by neck movement, certain head positions, or when pressure is applied over cervical musculature. There may be occipital-nuchal pain, limited range of motion of the neck, or spasms of the cervical muscles.

c. Evaluation—Successful anesthetic blockade of the cervical facet joint, nerve root, or occipital nerves is confirmatory.

d. Treatment—Nonpharmacologic therapies include neck massage, physical therapy, and biofeedback. Muscle relaxants and NSAIDs may be necessary but used with caution in the older adult. Procedural treatments include radiofrequency facet joint rhizolysis and occipital nerve cryorhizolysis.

6.   Medication-induced headache—Medications and supplements should be reviewed as a cause of headache. Common offenders include nitrates, calcium channel blockers, estrogens/progestins, histamine blockers, theophylline, and NSAIDs. Overuse, or abrupt discontinuation, of caffeine, analgesics, narcotics, and serotonin antagonists can lead to daily headache. A careful history regarding the timing of headaches in relation to starting or taking a medication is advised.

7. Headache caused by other medical conditions—Older adults often have medical conditions or treatments that may cause or worsen headaches, which should be considered in the differential diagnosis.

Antonaci F, Ghirmai S, Bono G, Sandrini G, Nappi G. Cervicogenic headache: evaluation of the original diagnostic criteria. *Cephalalgia.* 2001;21(5):573-583.

Biondi DM, Saper JR. Geriatric headache: how to make the diagnosis and manage the pain. *Geriatrics.* 2000;55(12):40, 43-45, 48-50.

Bigal ME, Lipton RB. The differential diagnosis of chronic daily headaches: an algorithm-based approach. *J Headache Pain.* 2007;8(5):263-272.

Cantini F, Niccoli L, Nannini C, Bertoni M, Salvarani C. Diagnosis and treatment of giant cell arteritis. *Drugs Aging.* 2008;25(4): 281-297.

Fisher CM. Late life migraine accompaniments—further experience. *Stroke.* 1985;17(5):1033-1042.

Headache Classification Subcommittee of the International Headache Society. The International Classification of Headache Disorders: 2nd edition. *Cephalalgia.* 2004;24 Suppl 1:9-160.

Kunkel R. Headaches in older patients: special problems and concerns. *Cleve Clin J Med.* 2006;73(10):922-928.

Martins KM, Bordini CA, Bigal ME, Speciali JG. Migraine in the elderly: a comparison with migraine in young adults. *Headache.* 2006;46(2):312-316.

Neri I, Granella F, Nappi R, Manzoni GC, Facchinetti F, Genazzani AR. Characteristics of headache at menopause: a clinico-epidemiologic study. *Maturitas.* 1993;17(1):31-37.

Newman LC, Goadsby PJ. Unusual primary headache disorders. In: *Wolff's Headache and Other Head Pain.* New York, NY: Oxford University Press; 2001:310.

Rozen TD, David C, Donald JD, et al. Cranial neuralgias and atypical facial pain. In: *Wolff's Headache and Other Head Pain.* New York, NY: Oxford University Press; 2001:509.

Tanganelli P. Secondary headaches in the elderly. *Neurol Sci.* 2010;31(Suppl 1):S73-S76.

Managing Vision Impairment in Older Adults

61

Meredith Whiteside, OD

▶ General Principles in Older Adults

Vision impairment is relatively rare in people younger than 65 years of age, but its incidence steadily increases to almost 24% of those 80 years and older. Not surprisingly, vision impairment can have a significant impact on a patient's quality of life. It is associated with social isolation, anxiety, depression and a loss of independence. It can affect balance, leading to more frequent falls, and has been shown to negatively affect physical activity.

The following 3 levels are used to categorize the severity of vision loss*:

1. Normal vision: Visual acuity ≥20/40

2. Visual impairment: Visual acuity >20/40 but <20/200

3. Legal blindness: Acuity ≤20/200 in the better eye, or total visual field <20 degrees

NORMAL CHANGES IN THE AGING EYE

Although not meeting the definition of vision impairment, there are still a number of changes in the aging eye leading to diminished vision. In all adults, the crystalline lens gradually becomes less flexible and less able to change its curvature (accommodate) with age. This results in the condition known as presbyopia, in which patients lose the ability to focus their eyes on near objects. The ability to see well in dim light also becomes diminished in older adults as a result of a combination of decreases in pupil size and progressive increases in the light absorption of the lens. This age-related reduction in retinal illumination is substantial. A typical 60-year-old's retina receives only about one-third of the light that a typical 20-year-old receives. As a result of the tendency for opacities to form in the aging lens and cornea, older adults are increasingly sensitive to glare caused by scattered light in the eye. Finally, because of neural changes in the retina, there is an age-related reduction in the ability to adapt to sudden changes in illumination.

▶ Clinical Findings

A. Signs & Symptoms

Starting in the mid-40s, reading glasses may be required to manage presbyopia. Although distance vision remains stable during this time, by the seventh decade and beyond, distance vision also can be reduced because of changes in refractive error. Difficulty with dim lighting and sensitivity to glare may cause problems with driving at night. Dry eye, especially in older women, is also common. Symptoms include a mild foreign-body sensation, burning, small fluctuations in vision, and even (reflexive) tearing because of mild corneal irritation. Table 61–1 includes suggested vision screening tests for older adults.

B. Treatment & Prognosis

Although a number of normal, age-related changes have a negative impact on vision, there are simple ways to compensate for many of them. Because dry eye tends to be chronic and associated with many medications used by older adults, nonprescription artificial tears can help relieve symptoms. In epidemiologic studies, 40% to 60% of older adults have vision worse than 20/40 simply because of problems with their eyeglasses, a problem easily remedied through ensuring regular eye examinations. Finally, other ways to compensate for normal age-related losses of vision include providing bright, but indirect (ie, nonglare) lighting, which significantly improves visual function in most older adults.

---

*It is assumed the patient is wearing the best glasses (or contact lens) correction.

Table 61–1. Suggested vision screening tests for older adults.

Procedure	Description	Causes of Abnormal Findings
Visual acuity	Test left eye (OD), right eye (OS) separately Use habitual glasses to test distance Use bright ambient light	Cataract, uncorrected refractive error, retinal or optic nerve disease, other neurological disease
Visual field by confrontation	Test OD, OS separately Patient fixates examiner's eye opposite of the patient Examiner shows fingers in 4 quadrants of patient's visual field Patient counts fingers	Monocular defect = disorder of retina, optic nerve Binocular defect = chiasm, cortex or bilateral eye disease
Pupils	Check direct and consensual response to light Swinging flashlight test	Asymmetric responses = optic nerve or autonomic nervous system disorder
Extraocular motility	Observe patient with both eyes open for strabismus Test motility of OD, OS separately: patient looks up/down, right/left with head fixed	Deviations or restricted movement = binocular vision disorder, nerve palsy, trauma, or previous ocular surgery
External observation	Observe lids, lashes, conjunctiva, cornea Instill fluorescein, illuminate eye with cobalt blue filter on direct ophthalmoscope	Discharge, crusting of lids or conjunctival injection = infection or allergy Significant corneal staining = abrasion or foreign body
Direct ophthalmoscopy	Darken room illumination Observe red reflex in pupils Examine optic disc, macula, and vasculature	Darkened red reflex often caused by cataract Large cupping = possible glaucoma Disc pallor = optic atrophy or end-stage glaucoma Hemorrhages = possible diabetic or hypertensive retinopathy White spots = macular degeneration or exudate due to diabetes or hypertension

Congdon N, O'Colmain B, Klaver C, et al. Causes and prevalence of visual impairment among adults in the United States. *Arch Ophthalmol*. 2004;122(4):477-485.

Pascolini D, Mariotti SP. Global estimates of visual impairment: 2010. *Br J Ophthalmol*. 2012;96(5):614-618.

Rosenbloom AA, Morgan MM. *Rosenbloom & Morgan's Vision and Aging*. St. Louis, MO: Butterworth-Heinemann; 2007.

▼ ABNORMAL CHANGES IN THE AGING EYE

The leading abnormal ocular changes that cause vision impairment in older adults are cataracts, age related macular degeneration, diabetic retinopathy, and glaucoma.

CATARACTS

▶ General Principles in Older Adults

A cataract is a clouding of the lens and is a leading cause of vision impairment in the United States and globally. Cataracts progress gradually, and may require removal. By age 80 years, more than half of all people in the United States either have a cataract or have had cataract surgery. Risk factors for cataracts include advanced age, diabetes, cumulative exposure to ultraviolet B radiation, smoking, current or previous long-term use of corticosteroids, previous eye surgery, or a history of eye injury.

▶ Prevention

Decreasing UV exposure by wearing sunglasses and hats, encouraging smoking cessation and good glycemic control may delay the onset and progression of cataracts. Currently, there is no evidence that medication or nutritional supplementation prevents, delays the progression of, or cures cataracts.

▶ Clinical Findings

Typical symptoms of cataracts include a gradual onset of blurred vision and increased sensitivity to glare (especially when driving at dusk or night). A common sign of a sight-limiting cataract is an insensitivity to subtle color differences such as those caused by food stains on clothing in an otherwise neatly dressed patient. Observing a white haze in the pupil during pupil testing suggests a moderate or worse cataract. With the pupil dilated, the red eye reflex may exhibit focal or diffuse areas of darkness when viewed with the direct ophthalmoscope or a slit lamp.

Differential Diagnosis

Patients with significant cataracts often present with a history of painless, gradual and progressive deterioration of vision and a normal appearing external eye. Other possibilities include uncorrected refractive error, diseases of the macula or optic nerve, or diabetic eye disease. If vision loss is rapid, consider vitreal or retinal hemorrhage, or other vascular disorders. Associated eye pain and/or conjunctival hyperemia should raise concern for uveitis or angle-closure glaucoma.

Complications

Complications due to cataracts are very rare and include lens-induced glaucoma or uveitis. In the case of glaucoma, the lens pushes the iris forward into the anterior chamber angle, and blocks aqueous drainage. In lens-induced uveitis, disruption of the lens capsule causes an immune-related intraocular inflammation, which can also induce glaucoma by blocking aqueous outflow. In both situations, surgical removal of the lens is curative.

Management & Treatment

Cataracts usually develop slowly, and in the early stages an updated spectacle correction often will improve vision. Environmental modifications, such as avoiding high glare situations (eg, night driving) the use of antiglare sunglasses and providing adequate ambient light, can help patients cope. The only treatment for cataracts is removal. Surgery is usually indicated when visual acuity is approximately 20/40 or when a patient's daily activities are compromised by reduced vision, despite best correction. The decision for surgery should take into account other pathologies, such as macular degeneration or diabetic retinopathy, which may limit postsurgical vision.

A. Pre- and Postoperative Care

Most older adults can tolerate cataract surgery. Patients should be medically stable and ideally be able to lie supine for 30 minutes. Postoperative care typically requires the administration of antibiotic and antiinflammatory eye drops, as well as follow-up office visits. For patients with comorbidities such as chronic obstructive pulmonary disease, poorly controlled blood pressure, coronary artery disease, or diabetes, the ophthalmologist will typically request a medical evaluation by the patient's primary care physician. Although preoperative laboratory testing for any medical problems indicated by the history and physical examination is appropriate, studies show that routine medical testing before cataract surgery does not improve outcomes.

Cataract surgery is usually an outpatient procedure. In patients deemed to have a reasonably healthy cornea, the incision is made through the cornea, which results in minimal or no blood loss and usually requires only topical anesthesia and minimal systemic medications. Because of this, anticoagulant or antiplatelet therapy may be continued, based on the preferences of the eye surgeon and primary care physician.

B. Complications

Serious postoperative complications from cataract surgery are rare (<1.5%). Symptoms of pain or a decrease in vision in the days following surgery suggest intraocular infection (endophthalmitis), and an increase in floaters or flashes of light could signal retinal detachment. Both of these conditions require immediate ophthalmologic consultation. While less vision-threatening, 2 more common complications, cystoid macular edema and the development of opacities on the posterior capsule of the lens, also require consultation because they can reduce visual acuity. Cystoid macular edema occurs at a rate of <3% in the weeks following cataract removal and is typically treated with topical antiinflammatory medications. Posterior capsular opacities (sometimes called secondary cataracts) can develop months to years following lens removal surgery and occur at a rate of 18% to 50%. If the opacity becomes visually significant, a laser is used to ablate the area of membrane that blocks vision.

Prognosis

Age-related cataracts typically progress slowly over time. Through regular evaluations, an optometrist or ophthalmologist can monitor their progress and recommend when the risks of cataract surgery are justified by its potential benefits in terms of ensuring the patient's visual capacities continue to meet the demands of daily living.

Owsley C, McGwin G Jr, Scilley K, et al. Impact of cataract surgery on health-related quality of life in nursing home residents. *Br J Ophthalmol.* 2007;91(10):1359-1363.

West S. Epidemiology of cataract: accomplishments over 25 years and future directions. *Ophthalmic Epidemiol.* 2007;14(4): 173-178.

AGE-RELATED MACULAR DEGENERATION

General Principles in Older Adults

Age-related macular degeneration (AMD) is a disease that progressively destroys the macula, impairing central vision.

It accounts for 54% of all legal blindness and is the leading cause of irreversible vision loss in people older than the age of 65 years. Although the etiology of AMD is unknown, it is likely an inherited disease with environmental factors contributing. Risk factors include advancing age, white race, a family history of AMD, and smoking. There are 2 forms of AMD: nonneovascular (or dry) and neovascular (or wet). Ninety percent of patients have the dry form of AMD, which causes a gradual loss of vision. Even though wet AMD is less common, leakage from the newly growing vessels results in rapid vision loss, and the majority of cases of legal blindness in older adults.

Prevention

Although there are no definitive preventive treatments for either dry or wet AMD, studies suggest that people who eat a diet rich in green, leafy vegetables and fish may have a lower risk of developing AMD. Smoking doubles the risk of AMD. For patients who have been diagnosed with intermediate or advanced dry AMD, taking high doses of antioxidants and zinc may reduce the risk of developing advanced AMD and experiencing severe vision loss. Because severe vision loss is typically associated with the wet form of AMD, the best prevention of blindness is prompt diagnosis and treatment of neovascularization.

Clinical Findings

In its early stages, AMD has no symptoms. As dry AMD progresses, patients note a gradual blurring of central vision, and increased difficulty reading fine print, recognizing faces or seeing street signs. In contrast, wet AMD often presents as a rapid loss of central vision, with metamorphopsia (images that appear distorted) or central scotomas. Even with advanced wet or dry AMD, patients maintain navigational mobility. In dry AMD, drusen—cream colored lesions that represent a build-up of metabolic waste products within the retina—are seen in the macula. Other signs include pigmentary changes or chorioretinal atrophy of the macula. In wet AMD, abnormal blood vessels grow and hemorrhage, causing macular swelling, loss of retinal function and scarring.

Differential Diagnoses

Other conditions causing a reduction in visual acuity with changes in the appearance of the macula include diabetes and hypertension, each of which might cause retinal hemorrhages and/or the deposition of exudates, which may or may not be in the macula.

Complications, Treatment, & Prognosis

Loss of central vision is the main complication of AMD. In wet AMD, the vision loss quickly becomes severe and represents an ocular emergency requiring urgent consultation. Evaluation and treatment for wet AMD frequently involves visualizing the retinal vasculature with fluorescein angiography and then laser photocoagulation of abnormal blood vessels. Unfortunately, while the laser stops leakage and destroys new blood vessels, it also destroys the underlying retina. The development of antivascular endothelial growth factor (anti-VEGF) medications such as bevacizumab that inhibit neovascularization has markedly changed the management of wet AMD. These drugs are injected intravitreally and may be used alone or in conjunction with laser treatment. With prompt recognition and referral to a retinal specialist ophthalmologist, many patients treated with anti-VEGF intravitreal injections will maintain or even have mildly improved vision. Patients who develop unilateral wet AMD have a 30% 6-year risk of neovascularization in the contralateral eye, so frequent follow-up evaluations are recommended.

For patients with dry AMD, vision loss progresses slowly. In mild cases, there is no treatment. For moderate-to-severe dry AMD, vitamin supplements may be recommended to slow progression. According to a 10-year clinical trial, the Age-Related Eye Disease Study (AREDS), a specific formulation of antioxidants and zinc in supplements reduced risk of developing advanced AMD and subsequent severe vision loss. The AREDS formulation is not a cure, nor does it restore vision loss caused by AMD; it simply may delay the onset of advanced AMD and help maintain stable vision.

Chew EY, Lindblad AS, Clemons T; Age-Related Eye Disease Study Research Group. Summary results and recommendations from the age-related eye disease study. *Arch Ophthalmol.* 2009;127(12):1678-1679.

DIABETIC RETINOPATHY

General Principles in Older Adults

Diabetic retinopathy is characterized by a progressive series of abnormal changes in the retinal microvasculature. The early phase of the disease is called nonproliferative (or background) retinopathy. Changes in the microvasculature lead to areas of retinal nonperfusion and to increased vasopermeability, which causes the appearance of microaneurysms and hemorrhages. If the disease progresses, proliferative diabetic retinopathy develops when there is a pathologic propagation of fragile retinal vessels that can break and bleed extensively. Overall, approximately 40% of all diabetics have some stage of diabetic retinopathy. The longer one has diabetes, the more likely retinopathy will develop.

Prevention

Good glycemic and blood pressure control are associated with decreased development and progression of diabetic retinopathy. Although diabetic retinopathy may not be completely avoidable, studies show that severe vision loss can be prevented 90% of the time with timely detection and intervention. Therefore, leading eye care organizations and the American Diabetes Association recommend that all diabetic patients should have an annual dilated, funduscopic examination. In the early stages of nonproliferative retinopathy with no macular edema, management consists of emphasizing the importance of glycemic control and follow-up evaluations. In more advanced cases of retinopathy, laser treatment or other medications may be indicated.

Clinical Findings

Diabetic retinopathy may be asymptomatic in its early more treatable stages. Blurred vision may occur if there is macular edema, but if the contralateral eye is unaffected or the vision loss is subtle, patients may not notice changes. In cases of proliferative retinopathy, new blood vessels can bleed extensively, causing blurred vision, or visual field scotomas. Patients who have had extensive laser photocoagulation for treatment of proliferative disease may have an overall constriction of the visual field. Signs of diabetic retinopathy are best evaluated through dilated funduscopy, and can include hemorrhages, exudates or neovascularization. In areas where there is inadequate access to eye care specialists, fundus photographs reviewed via telemedicine can be a sensitive and effective screening tool for identifying patients with diabetic retinopathy who need to be prioritized for referral to specialty eye care. Specialty diabetic eye examinations typically include retinal examination for subtle signs of macular edema, assessing the location and amount of hemorrhages and assessing the vascular abnormalities that help stage the severity of either nonproliferative or proliferative retinopathy.

Differential Diagnosis

Hypertensive retinopathy, vein occlusions, ischemic disorders, inflammatory or infectious disorders or any other disorder that can cause retinal hemorrhages can be considered in the differential diagnosis of diabetic retinopathy.

Complications

Vision loss caused by diabetic retinopathy is caused mainly by macular edema and proliferative retinopathy, and to a lesser extent, by macular capillary nonperfusion. Macular edema occurs when fluid leaks into the central retina, and may occur with either nonproliferative or proliferative retinopathy.

Treatment

Management of nonproliferative diabetic retinopathy (with no macular edema) typically consists of observation by an optometrist or ophthalmologist who has performed a dilated stereoscopic examination of the fundus. In cases where macular edema or proliferative disease is present or likely to occur (such as in severe nonproliferative retinopathy), referral to an ophthalmologist (preferably one specializing in retina) is indicated. Clinical studies show that treatment of a specific subset of macular edema, clinically significant macular edema (CSME), reduces the risk of moderate vision loss. In proliferative retinopathy, blood vessels can bleed extensively into the vitreous and/or undergo fibrous proliferation, causing vitreoretinal traction and tears in the retina. Treatment for both CSME and proliferative retinopathy can include laser and intravitreal injections of anti-VEGF agents.

Prognosis

Current treatment for diabetic eye disease usually does not restore lost vision. Instead, it is aimed at preventing additional vision loss. Studies show that laser treatment for CSME reduces the risk of moderate vision loss by 50% to 70%, and that panretinal laser photocoagulation for proliferative or severe nonproliferative diabetic retinopathy yields a 50% reduction in the risk for severe vision loss.

Antonetti DA, Klein R, Gardner TW. Diabetic retinopathy. *N Engl J Med.* 2012;366(13):1227-1239.

Mohamed Q, Gillies MC, Wong TY. Management of diabetic retinopathy: a systematic review. *JAMA.* 2007;298(8):902-916.

GLAUCOMA

General Principles in Older Adults

Glaucoma is a progressive, chronic optic neuropathy in which intraocular pressure (IOP) and other currently unknown factors contribute to a characteristic acquired atrophy of the optic nerve that, if left to progress, leads to visual field loss. There are 2 major forms of glaucoma: open angle, in which the intraocular drainage system is open, and closed angle, in which the system is blocked. Primary open-angle glaucoma (POAG) accounts for vast majority of cases of glaucoma. Vision loss caused by glaucoma typically occurs first in peripheral vision, but as the disease advances central vision is lost. Glaucoma is the second leading cause of blindness worldwide, and approximately 50% of those with glaucoma are unaware they have the condition.

In the United States, glaucoma is the leading cause of blindness in African Americans. There is a 3-times-higher prevalence of POAG in African Americans relative to non-Hispanic whites. Studies also suggest that Hispanic/Latinos have a prevalence rate of POAG comparable to African Americans. Besides race, increasing age is also risk factor for glaucoma. POAG occurs in 5.7% of African Americans 73–74 years of age. At age 75 years and older, it increases to 23.2%. Although the prevalence of POAG is much lower in white populations, with older age, it increases from a rate of 3.4% in 73–74-year-olds to 9.4% in those age 75 years and older.

Clinical Findings

Prevention of vision loss from glaucoma is dependent upon early diagnosis and treatment. Unfortunately, because glaucoma is often asymptomatic, most patients fail to notice changes in vision until end-stage disease. Because of this, annual eye examinations are recommended for older adults at higher risk (Table 61–2). For others, an eye examination every 1–2 years is recommended. Clinical examination for glaucoma includes measurement of IOP (tonometry), optic disc assessment, visual field assessment and gonioscopy to assess whether the intraocular drainage system is "open" or "closed." In gonioscopy, a specialized lens is placed on the patient's cornea that allows the examiner to visualize the iridocorneal angle between the cornea and the iris where aqueous humor drains. IOP normally ranges from 10–21 mm Hg; however, IOP outside of this range is not pathognomonic for glaucoma—it is simply a risk factor associated with the development and/or progression of the disease.

Table 61–2. Indications for referral to an optometrist or ophthalmologist for glaucoma screening.

Patients at higher risk for glaucoma	African ancestry, especially older than age 40 years Everyone older than age 60 years, especially Mexican Americans Family history of glaucoma Prolonged corticosteroid use History of eye trauma
Possible indications of glaucoma	Suspicious optic disc cupping with a cup-to-disc ratio >0.5 Asymmetric optic cup, marked interocular asymmetry in disc cupping Elevated IOP

Optic disc examination is one of the most important ways to evaluate for glaucoma. Glaucomatous atrophy causes increased optic nerve cupping. Although most cases of glaucoma are typically bilateral, the presentation can vary between the 2 eyes. Hence, markedly asymmetric cupping between the 2 eyes can indicate glaucoma. In the earliest stage of glaucoma, optic disc findings are usually observed before visual field losses appear. Nonetheless, periodic visual field assessment using standardized perimetry is important for diagnosing, staging, and monitoring disease progression.

Differential Diagnosis

The differential diagnosis of glaucoma encompasses a variety of conditions that affect the optic nerve. In angle-closure glaucoma, narrowing of the intraocular drainage system raises IOP and induces optic atrophy. If the rise in IOP occurs quickly, patients may complain of pain. Gradual rises in IOP may be asymptomatic. In normal tension glaucoma, glaucomatous optic atrophy occurs in the absence of documented elevated IOP. Other possibilities include optic atrophy caused by retinal vascular disease, ischemic disease, or chiasmal tumors. These conditions can be differentiated from glaucomatous atrophy in that they usually cause optic nerve pallor without optic nerve cupping.

Complications & Treatment

Vision loss in glaucoma typically starts in the periphery and extends inward, ultimately destroying central vision until complete blindness. Treatment of POAG consists of lowering IOP, with the goal of preventing progressive visual field loss by slowing optic nerve atrophy. Therapies to lower IOP may include topical or oral medications, laser surgery, such as trabeculoplasty, or incisional surgical procedures, such as a trabeculectomy with or without an iridectomy. Topical medications are often the first line of treatment and work by either decreasing aqueous production or increasing aqueous outflow. As a result of their effectiveness in lowering IOP, simplicity of once-a-day dosing, and few systemic side effects, prostaglandin analogs are among the most frequently prescribed first-line therapies for glaucoma. All medications used for the treatment of glaucoma may have significant local and systemic effects, and should be included in the older patient's chronic medication list (Table 61–3).

Although topical medications are typically first-line therapy, surgery may be an option. If 2 or more topical therapies do not adequately control IOP, or if the topical medications are not tolerated well, surgery will be considered. Other indications for surgical care of glaucoma include poor compliance with medications because of memory impairment

Table 61–3. Commonly used topical glaucoma medications.

Brand Name	Generic Name	Concentration/Dose[a]	Side Effects	Contraindications
β-Blockers				
Betagan, (or generic)	Levobunolol hydrochloride	0.25% BID[b] 0.5%/QD[b]-BID	Bronchospasm Bradycardia Heart block Exacerbation of congestive heart failure Depression Impotence Death	Chronic obstructive pulmonary disease Asthma Bradycardia Hypotension Congestive heart failure (check with cardiologist) >First-degree heart block Diabetes mellitus[c] Myasthenia gravis[c]
Betimol	Timolol hemihydrate	0.25%/QD-BID 0.5%/QD-BID		
Betoptic-S	Betaxolol hydrochloride	0.25% BID		
Istalol	Timolol maleate	0.5% QAM		
Timoptic (or generic)	Timolol maleate	0.25% QD-BID 0.5% QD-BID		
Timoptic XE (or generic)	Timolol maleate	0.25% QD 0.5% QD		
Prostaglandin Analogs				
Lumigan	Bimatoprost	0.01% QPM	Eyelash growth Periocular hyperpigmentation Conjunctival hyperemia Iris color change Cystoid macular edema Uveitis Possible herpes virus activation	Macular edema History of • Herpetic keratitis • Uveitis • Cystoid macular edema
Travatan Z	Travoprost	0.004% QPM		
Xalatan (or generic)	Latanoprost	0.005% QPM		
Zioptan	Tafluprost	0.0015% QPM		
α-Adrenergic Agents				
Alphagan P (or generic)	Brimonidine Tartrate	0.1%, 0.15%, 0.2% TID	Lethargy Dry mouth Allergic reactions Headache	Monoamine oxidase inhibitor therapy
Carbonic Anhydrase Inhibitors				
Azopt	Brinzolamide	1% TID	Altered taste Corneal edema	Corneal endothelium compromise Sulfonamide allergy
Trusopt (or generic)	Dorzolamide hydrochloride	2% TID		
Parasympathomimetic Agents/Miotics				
Generic pilocarpine	Pilocarpine hydrochloride	1%, 2%, 4%, 6% TID-QID	Eye ache Headache Miosis ($\rightarrow$ dim vision) Cataracts	Neovascular, uveitic, or malignant glaucoma Asthma (possibly) History of retinal detachment
Combination Medications				
Combigan	Brimonidine & timolol	0.2% & 0.5% q12h	(See individual medications)	(See individual medications)
Cosopt (or generic)	Dorzolamide & timolol	2% & 0.5% BID		
Simbrinza	Brinzolamide & brimonidine	1% & 0.2% TID		

[a]1 drop, unless otherwise noted.

[b]1 or 2 drops.

[c]Some believe β-blocker use should be avoided in patients with diabetes mellitus because symptoms of hypoglycemia may be masked and those of myasthenia gravis may be exacerbated.

Data from Yanoff M, Duker JS. *Ophthalmology*. London: Mosby Elsevier; 2009; Melton R, Thomas R. Glaucoma review and update. A supplement to Review of Optometry. May 15, 2012; American Academy of Ophthalmology Glaucoma Panel. *Preferred Practice Pattern Guidelines. Primary Open-Angle Glaucoma*. San Francisco, CA: American Academy of Ophthalmology; 2010. Available at: www.aao.org/ppp; American Optometric Association. *Optometric Clinical Practice Guideline. Care of the Patient with Open Angle Glaucoma*. St. Louis, MO: American Optometric Association; 2011. Available at: http://www.aoa.org/documents/optometrists/CPG-9.pdf

and if poor manual dexterity prevents eyedrop application. Finally, when compared to the cost of surgery, the annual cost of medications may become prohibitive for some.

Prognosis

Without treatment, glaucoma causes a progressive loss vision that will eventually lead to complete blindness. Patients who are diagnosed before extensive glaucoma optic nerve atrophy and who are able to achieve good IOP control have a good prognosis for vision.

Deva NC, Insull E, Gamble G, Danesh-Meyer HV. Risk factors for first presentation of glaucoma with significant visual field loss. *Clin Experiment Ophthalmol.* 2008;36(3):217-221.

Leske MC, Heijl A, Hyman L, Bengtsson B, et al. Predictors of long-term progression in the early manifest glaucoma trial. *Ophthalmology.* 2007;114(11):1965-1972.

Quigley HA. Glaucoma. *Lancet.* 2011;377(9774):1367-1377.

▼ VISUALLY IMPAIRED OLDER ADULTS

When working with older patients with or without vision impairment, there are 2 simple ways to maximize their vision: increase contrast and provide adequate lighting. Contrast sensitivity refers to the ability to distinguish an object from its background. Low-contrast objects are harder for older persons to detect, becoming markedly more difficult in those with vision impairment. Patients may demonstrate adequate acuity when tested with a high-contrast, black-on-white eye chart, but their performance drops markedly when reading a low-contrast chart with light gray letters on a white background. This latter test much more closely resembles the everyday situation an older adult faces when trying to step off the curb at the edge of a sidewalk. Providing adequate lighting for these patients means using a light source that brightly illuminates the object of regard without shining directly into the their eyes or producing excessive reflections. This typically involves use of an indirect, high-wattage light source.

In addition to receiving medical eye care, patients with vision impairment will often benefit from referral to a low-vision specialist. These eye doctors specialize in maximizing the patient's remaining functional vision through custom-ized optical devices, such as strong reading glasses, tele-scopes, magnifiers, and electronic devices that enlarge and project reading material onto a video screen. Their efforts often include collaboration with rehabilitation specialists who, in addition to working directly with visually impaired patients, can recommend the use of nonoptical aids, such as large-print books and newspapers, free library services for access to books on tape, and special telephones, clocks, or dials (eg, oven or cooktop) equipped with large, high-contrast numerals.

SYSTEMIC MEDICATIONS AND GLAUCOMA

The use of corticosteroids, such as cortisone and predniso-lone, can increase IOP. Although the majority of patients taking corticosteroids do so without a subsequent elevation in IOP, risk factors for developing increased IOP include a personal or family history of glaucoma, current status as a glaucoma suspect, route of administration and duration of the corticosteroid treatment. Topically or intravitreally applied corticosteroids pose the highest risk. In descend-ing risk are intravenous, parenteral, and inhaled routes of administration. Corticosteroid use for <2 weeks generally does not require special monitoring of IOP. However, any patient taking corticosteroids who uses them chronically or is at risk for glaucoma should have at least an annual eye evaluation.

Most medications that list glaucoma as a contraindica-tion or adverse effect are concerned with the form of glau-coma in which the anterior chamber angle drainage system is narrow. When the patient takes the medication, the drain-age system can narrow even further, sometimes to the point of closure, which causes a rise in IOP. Classes of medications that have the potential to induce angle closure are antispas-molytic agents, antihistamines, antiparkinsonian drugs, antipsychotic medications, tricyclic antidepressants, mono-amine oxidase inhibitors, and topical mydriatics. These warnings do not apply to most glaucoma patients who have the primary open-angle form of the disease. Rather, they are relevant only to those with the relatively uncommon, narrow-angle form. Narrow-angle glaucoma is typically treated surgically, and consultation with an eye specialist may reveal that the above medications can be used safely.

VISUAL SYMPTOMS INDICATING NEED FOR URGENT REFERRAL TO AN EYE-CARE SPECIALIST

Red flags indicating the need for urgent referral include sig-nificant changes in vision and moderate or worse eye pain. Changes in vision may include a sudden onset of decreased visual acuity (even with correction), a report of distorted vision (in metamorphopsia straight lines appear curved or irregular), or the sudden appearance of a scotoma or a visual field defect.

Careful review of the ocular history is important. In the history, the patient should be questioned about, among other things, which eye is affected and the timing and onset of symptoms such as pain, decrease in vision, photophobia, or discharge. If the primary symptom is pain, ask about a his-tory of recent eye surgery, trauma, chemical injury, photo-phobia, or recent use of contact lenses. If there is a reduction in vision, ask about the location of the loss. A reduction in central vision suggests macular involvement and may be a result of macular degeneration, diabetic retinopathy, vascular

Table 61–4. Visual symptoms indicating the need for referral.

Symptom	Possible Etiology	Need for Referral

Decreased central vision
Marked loss
Rapid onset
Monocular (usually)
	Wet age-related macular degeneration
	Macular edema or hemorrhage caused by diabetes
	Vascular occlusion
	Ischemic optic neuropathy
	    Arteritic = patients with temporal arteritis
	    Nonarteritic = patient often has diabetes or hypertension
		ASAP[a]

Decreased central vision Mild loss Slow onset Bilateral (usually)	Dry age-related macular degeneration Cataracts Diabetic retinopathy Refractive error change	Less Urgent
Ocular Pain Monocular Moderate-to-severe photophobia (possibly)	Infection (eg, herpetic keratitis) Corneal abrasion Uveitis Endophthalmitis (usually also reduces vision) Chemical or mechanical trauma Angle-closure glaucoma	ASAP[a]
Loss of peripheral vision Monocular	Retinal detachment[a] Glaucoma (usually bilateral, but asymmetric)	ASAP[a] or Urgent
Loss of peripheral vision Binocular	Lesion in central visual pathway (from chiasm to cortex)	Urgent

[a]ASAP, get telephone consult or refer patient for in-person evaluation by an eye specialist.

occlusive disease, or optic neuropathy. If the vision loss is peripheral, establish whether it is monocular or binocular. If it is monocular, suspect either a retinal or optic neuropathy. In cases of bilateral loss of vision, consider a neurologic cause or, less likely, concomitant bilateral eye disease (Table 61–4).

USEFUL WEBSITE

Lighthouse (provides more information on visual rehabilitation services, education, research, prevention, and advocacy). http://www.lighthouse.org

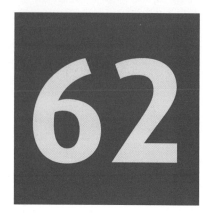

Managing Hearing Impairment in Older Adults

Dane J. Genther, MD
Frank R. Lin, MD, PhD

▶ General Principles in Older Adults

Hearing loss is highly prevalent in older individuals and is often overlooked as a potential contributor to morbidity in this population. In the United States, an estimated 26.7 million adults 50 years of age or older suffer from bilateral hearing loss of 25 dB (decibels) or greater, and up to 79% of adults age 80 years and older may suffer from hearing loss. It is likely that many of these individuals could be adequately treated with current technology; however, evidence suggests that this population is vastly undertreated. For example, in the United States, only 14.2% of adults 50 years of age or older with hearing loss use hearing aids. The rate is similar in England and Wales (17.3%) despite having a health care system that covers the cost of hearing aids.

Hearing loss affects an individual's ability to communicate effectively, but it is often perceived as a normal part of aging, both by patients and health care providers. However, current evidence supports the contrary. Recent studies show that hearing loss is independently associated with incident dementia, accelerated cognitive decline, poorer neurocognitive functioning, and increased falls and gait disturbances. Such significant negative outcomes warrant heightened vigilance by providers in addressing and treating hearing loss in their patients.

▶ Prevention

Age-related hearing loss in older adults represents the sequelae of multiple insults that can progressively damage the cochlea over time. Although many of these factors cannot be modified (eg, intrinsic aging of the cochlea, sex, genetic predisposition), several factors (eg, noise exposure, ototoxic medication use) can be controlled and are discussed below.

▶ Clinical Findings

A. Signs & Symptoms

1. Patient interview—Patients are often unaware of their hearing impairment, especially when it progresses gradually over many years. It is useful to ask a patient if they have difficulty hearing in large groups or in loud, crowded venues, or if they often ask people to repeat what they have said. The interviewee may note that she can hear people but that other people mumble too much or are just speaking too softly. Answers to these questions can provide clues to the provider about the presence of hearing loss. If the patient is aware of the hearing loss, the time course and nature of the progression can give vital information about the etiology. It is important to ask about tinnitus (ringing), ear pain (otalgia), ear drainage (otorrhea), dizziness (vertigo, disequilibrium), other neurologic deficits, and cranial neuropathies. A history of intense and/or prolonged noise exposure, ear trauma, head trauma, ear surgery, or ear infections (even remotely as a child or young adult) are necessary components of any interview.

2. Family member/friend interview—Often, the insightful person or the impetus for the hearing loss-related office visit is a family member or friend. They are often the first to notice that the patient is asking others to repeat themselves or misunderstanding words or entire conversations. They may note that they have to speak louder to interact with the patient, that the patient may not hear them when speaking from a different room, or that the patient turns the radio or television volume to a level that sounds too loud to other listeners. Interviewing people who spend time with the patient is vital to detecting more subtle hearing impairments.

3. Physical exam findings—It is vital that a health care provider inspect the ear with an otoscope. The external auditory canal (EAC) and the tympanic membrane (TM) should be fully

Table 62–1. Interpretation of tuning fork tests.

Results of Weber Test	Results of Rinne Test	Interpretation
Sound does not lateralize	Air conduction greater than bone conduction bilaterally	No hearing loss or equal sensorineural hearing loss bilaterally
Sound does not lateralize	Bone conduction greater than air conduction bilaterally	Equal conductive hearing loss bilaterally
Sound lateralizes to 1 side	Air conduction greater than bone conduction bilaterally	Sensorineural hearing loss on the side opposite of the lateralization
Sound lateralizes to 1 side	Bone conduction greater than air conduction on the side of lateralization	Conductive hearing loss on the side of lateralization
Sound lateralizes to 1 side	Bone conduction greater than air conduction bilaterally	Bilateral conductive hearing loss, greater on the side of lateralization

visualized. Cerumen can accumulate in the EAC and can cause some hearing loss if it fully occludes the EAC. The EAC can also be occluded by other masses, such as tumors, granulation tissue, cysts, polyps, or even a foreign body. The TM should be translucent and grayish in color. Any perforation of the TM, drainage from the TM or middle ear, masses behind the TM (in the middle ear), middle ear effusion, or significant thickening of the TM is abnormal and may cause hearing loss. A tuning fork exam should also be performed, ideally with a 512-Hz tuning fork, using 2 techniques. A Weber test is performed by placing the tuning fork on a bony prominence in the midline, most often on the upper forehead, to identify any lateralization of sound. A normal test is heard equally in both ears. A Rinne test compares bone conduction to air conduction of each ear by, first, placing the tuning fork on the bony prominence at the tip of the mastoid behind the ear (bone conduction) and, then, comparing its sound when held lateral to the patient's ear (air conduction). A normal (positive) Rinne test demonstrates air conduction greater than bone conduction. Table 62–1 demonstrates how to interpret the findings of tuning fork tests.

4. Screening tests—Screening may take the form of direct questioning of the patient as above. Handheld screening instruments, such as the Welch Allyn AudioScope, and survey questionnaires are also available, for example, the Hearing Handicap Inventory for the Elderly (Box 62–1), but offer limited additional utility over careful questioning. The recent U.S. Preventative Task Force report regarding hearing loss screening for adults age 50 years and older serves as a guide. A hearing impairment screen is a required aspect of the initial Medicare annual wellness visit.

5. Referral to audiology and otolaryngology—Any patient with hearing loss should be referred to an audiologist with master's- or doctoral-level training for formal audiometric testing. Referral to a hearing aid dispenser (or hearing

aid specialist) can also be considered. The training for these individuals varies from state to state, with some having only a high school degree. Referral to an otolaryngologist is warranted when a medical concern exists (Table 62–2).

▶ Differential Diagnosis

The classic presentations of various causes of hearing loss are given here, but not all of the associated symptoms or additional symptoms may be present with any given condition. Sensorineural hearing loss (SNHL) constitutes 92% of hearing loss in older adults, with the remainder being conductive or mixed (both sensorineural and conductive components). In the vast majority of cases, hearing loss in older adults is multifactorial, and many etiologies concurrently lead to hearing loss over time. Of note, subjective tinnitus, which is a centrally mediated process, can accompany any type of hearing loss as a result of the alteration of auditory input to the auditory cortex in the temporal lobe.

A. Sensorineural Hearing Loss (Inner Ear Disease)

1. Presbycusis—An audiogram typical of presbycusis (age-related hearing loss) shows a down-sloping SNHL, in which the higher frequencies (toward 8 kHz) are more severely affected than lower frequencies (toward 250 Hz) (Figure 62–1). Patients often are unaware of their degree of hearing impairment because of its gradual progression over years. The patient's friends and family members are often the first to notice and may prompt the patient to seek evaluation and treatment. In some patients, hearing loss may be accelerated due to hereditary factors.

2. Noise damage—Noise-induced hearing loss can result from prolonged exposure to noise, in which case the hearing

Box 62–1. Hearing Handicap Inventory for Elderly Screening

Instructions: The purpose of this scale is to identify the problems your hearing loss may be causing you. Answer *Yes*, *Sometimes*, or *No* for each question. *Do not skip a question if you avoid a situation because of your hearing loss.* It is important that you answer all questions. If you use a hearing aid, please answer the way you hear *without* the hearing aid.

E S

(E1) Does a hearing problem cause you to feel embarrassed when meeting new people?
4_____ Yes
2_____ Sometimes
0_____ No

(E2) Does a hearing problem cause you to feel frustrated when talking to members of your family?
4_____ Yes
2_____ Sometimes
0_____ No

(S3) Do you have difficulty when someone speaks in a whisper?
4_____ Yes
2_____ Sometimes
0_____ No

(E4) Do you feel handicapped by a hearing problem?
4_____ Yes
2_____ Sometimes
0_____ No

(S5) Does a hearing problem cause you difficulty when visiting friends, relatives, or neighbors?
4_____ Yes
2_____ Sometimes
0_____ No

(S6) Does a hearing problem cause you to attend religious services less often than you would like?
4_____ Yes
2_____ Sometimes
0_____ No

(E7) Does a hearing problem cause you to have arguments with family members?
4_____ Yes
2_____ Sometimes
0_____ No

(S8) Does a hearing problem cause you difficulty when listening to a TV or radio?
4_____ Yes
2_____ Sometimes
0_____ No

(E9) Do you feel that any difficulty with your hearing limits or hampers your personal or social life?
4_____ Yes
2_____ Sometimes
0_____ No

(S10) Does a hearing problem cause you difficulty when in a restaurant with relatives or friends?
4_____ Yes
2_____ Sometimes
0_____ No

_____ Emotional Subscale Total
_____ Social Subscale Total
_____ **Total Score**

Remember to answer *all of the questions* and if you wear a hearing aid answer the way you hear *without* the hearing aid.

S, Social Subscale Question; E, Emotional Subscale Question; yes, 4 points; sometimes, 2 points, no, 0 points. Range of results for total score: 0-8, no hearing handicap; 9-24, mild-to-moderate hearing handicap; 25-40, severe hearing handicap.

Reproduced with permission from Ventry I, Weinstein B. The hearing handicap inventory for the elderly: a new tool. *Ear Hear.* 1982;3(3):128-134.

loss would be permanent and occur gradually over months to years, or from brief exposure to intense noise, in which case the hearing loss may be sudden and may be temporary or permanent. The audiogram for these patients typically shows a dip on the audiogram at 3–6 kHz and may be unilateral or bilateral depending upon the nature of the injury. Noise-induced hearing loss is preventable with avoidance and use of ear plugs and other hearing protective devices.

3. Infection—Various infections can cause hearing loss. Viral, bacterial, or fungal labyrinthitis can cause hearing loss that is typically unilateral with associated tinnitus and vertigo. Meningitis, particularly bacterial, can cause partial to complete hearing loss through direct damage to the cochlea. Syphilis and lyme disease are known to cause sudden SNHL. Herpes zoster oticus, known as Ramsay Hunt syndrome, because of reactivation of the zoster virus in the geniculate

Table 62–2. Indications for otolaryngologic referral.

Impacted cerumen that cannot be removed
Mass in the external auditory canal
Significant otorrhea
Persistent otalgia
Persistent perforation of the tympanic membrane
Persistent middle ear effusion
Mass in the middle ear
Severe infection of the external auditory canal or middle ear
Associated vertigo or disequilibrium
Associated cranial neuropathies
Asymmetric hearing loss
Fluctuating hearing loss
Hearing loss for which an audiogram does not provide adequate explanation

ganglion, begins as painful vesicles in and around the external ear followed by any or all of the following: sudden unilateral hearing loss that may be temporary or permanent, tinnitus, nystagmus, disequilibrium or vertigo, and/or facial weakness

that may be temporary or permanent. The diagnosis can be made by isolating the virus from vesicular fluid.

4. Autoimmune inner ear disease—A number of autoimmune diseases are associated with hearing loss that is typically progressive and bilateral in nature, including, but not limited to, systemic lupus erythematosus, polyarteritis nodosum, inflammatory bowel disease, Crohn disease, ulcerative colitis, and granulomatosis with polyangiitis. There are also some patients who experience hearing loss and/or dizziness outside of a known disease process who respond to immunosuppressive therapy. The hearing loss in these conditions is thought to be caused by direct damage to the cochlear and vestibular organs through antibody-mediated attack by the host immune system.

5. Systemic and vascular disease—Multiple systemic diseases can result in hearing loss, primarily through their effects on the vasculature of the cochlea. The blood supply to the cochlea is composed of terminal branches of the intracranial circulation and is subject to vascular insult with subsequent ischemia or even infarction. Diabetes mellitus, small vessel vasculitides, and microthrombotic or embolic events may lead to sudden or gradual hearing loss. Furthermore, hearing

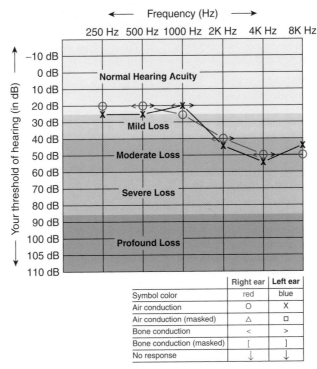

▲ **Figure 62–1.** Audiogram of presbycusis. An audiogram demonstrating moderate SNHL typically seen in presbycusis (age-related hearing loss). Note that the higher frequencies are more affected than the lower frequencies. Physician's Choice Hearing and Dizziness Center. (Available at http://hearinganddizziness.com/. Accessed October 8, 2012. Used with permission.)

Table 62–3. Common ototoxic medications.

Aminoglycoside antibiotics
Gentamicin
Amikacin
Neomycin
Streptomycin
Vancomycin
Erythromycin
Antimalarials
Chloroquine
Quinine
Platinum-based chemotherapy agents
Cisplatin
Carboplatin
Loop diuretics
Furosemide
Torsemide
Nonsteroidal antiinflammatory drugs
Aspirin
Ketorolac

loss, vertigo, and/or nystagmus can be some of the presenting symptoms of a central ischemic or hemorrhagic stroke.

6. Ototoxic medications—Signs and symptoms that a patient may be experiencing ototoxic effects include the development of new tinnitus, vertigo or disequilibrium, and difficulty hearing. If these symptoms develop, the patient should be evaluated and the drug should be stopped immediately if possible. Table 62–3 lists some of the most common ototoxic medications.

7. Acoustic neuroma (Vestibular schwannoma)—These small tumors of cranial nerve VIII typically present with unilateral, slowly progressive, high-frequency SNHL, but may present as sudden SNHL in up to 25% of patients. Commonly associated symptoms included tinnitus in 70% of patients, disequilibrium or vertigo in 50% of patients, cranial nerve (CN) V dysfunction (often subclinical) in 50% of patients, and/or facial weakness or asymmetry in 2% of patients. MRI with gadolinium is the study of choice for diagnosis.

8. Meniere disease—Also known as endolymphatic hydrops, this condition is characterized by episodic rotational vertigo that is typically debilitating and lasts from 20 minutes to 24 hours, but typically 1–2 hours. It is associated with fluctuating low frequency hearing loss, aural fullness, and tinnitus. The symptoms almost always begin unilaterally, but the contralateral ear may become involved in up to 50% of patients over time. The natural history is a relapsing and

remitting course with the disease often "burning out" over time. Recurrent attacks can lead to a permanent SNHL.

9. Trauma—Temporal bone fractures from falls, motor vehicle accidents, assault, or other blunt trauma can cause SNHL if the inner ear is involved. Additionally, patients can suffer facial nerve paresis that can be delayed or immediate and injury to surrounding structures. A temporal bone protocol CT scan without IV contrast will make the diagnosis in these patients.

10. Sudden sensorineural hearing loss—Sudden SNHL is a sudden decrease in hearing thresholds of 30 dB or greater at 3 contiguous audiometric frequencies occurring over 72 hours or less and is an otologic emergency that occurs in an estimated 5–20 per 100,000 people per year. The primary goal in managing these patients is the prevention of permanent SNHL through prompt referral to an otolaryngologist for confirmation and treatment with steroids within 24–48 hours. Distinguishing between sudden SNHL (requiring immediate referral) and an acute conductive loss from an ear infection or middle ear effusion (treated with simple antibiotics or a nasal steroid spray and not requiring urgent referral) can be made using the tuning fork tests described above.

11. Radiation—A history of radiation to the head or neck, for either a neoplastic process or environmental exposure, can lead to SNHL by direct damage to the inner ear and auditory nerve.

B. Conductive Hearing Loss (Middle or External Ear Disease)

Conductive hearing losses are far less common than SNHLs in older adults and can often be diagnosed in the clinic by otoscopic examination or through tuning fork testing. Common causes include EAC obstruction (eg, cerumen), TM perforations, middle-ear effusions, and ossicular chain pathology. Middle-ear effusions caused by eustachian tube dysfunction can often be treated with intranasal steroids and oral antibiotics (if there is a concern for acute otitis media) and followed conservatively for 2 months. Failure of resolution or concern for any other etiology for a conductive hearing loss warrants referral to an otolaryngologist.

► Complications

In addition to impairing verbal communication, hearing loss has been implicated in a number of other negative outcomes. Figure 62–2 models how age-related hearing loss (ARHL) is associated with poorer cognitive and physical functioning through the pathways of cognitive load and social isolation. Poorly encoded auditory signals from an impaired cochlea require greater brain resources for auditory decoding, and this cognitive load results in a smaller pool of resources being available for other cognitive tasks. Concurrently, ARHL has also been associated with poorer social functioning, one of the determinants of morbidity and mortality in older adults.

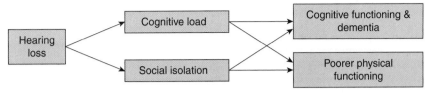

▲ **Figure 62–2.** Working conceptual model of how hearing loss affects domains of health and functioning.

Consistent with this model, epidemiologic evidence demonstrating that ARHL is independently associated with cognitive and physical functioning in older adults is beginning to surface. ARHL has now been found to be independently associated with poorer neurocognitive functioning on both verbal and nonverbal tests of executive function and memory, accelerated cognitive decline, and incident dementia. Compared to individuals with normal hearing, those with a mild, moderate, and severe hearing loss have a 2-, 3-, and 5-fold increased risk of developing dementia, respectively. Cognitive resources are also critical for gait, balance, and other tasks, such as driving. Recent studies demonstrate that ARHL is associated with poorer balance, falls, and impaired driving ability. These relationships may be mediated through the effects of hearing on cognitive load or from reduced awareness of the auditory environment.

▶ Treatment

Most often, the difficulty in treating or attempting to address hearing loss in older adults is convincing them, first, that they have a hearing loss that has potentially significant implications for healthy aging and, second, that current treatment can help them to hear better and improve many aspects of their lives. For a useful review of many aspects of hearing loss in older adults with a substantial section on treatment by Pacala et al, 2012.

A. Adaptive Techniques

Individuals with hearing loss should directly face the person with whom they are speaking. Family members and friends can be encouraged to speak at a normal volume, enunciate clearly, keep hands and other items away from in front of their mouths, and rephrase sentences instead of repeating them when asked. Also, training in speech reading, word recognition, and active listening has shown some benefit in these patients.

B. Environmental Modifications

A person with hearing loss should place herself at the center of the conversation, away from background noise. A setting with minimal background noise should be chosen for

gatherings or conversations if possible. Lighting should be adequate to see the faces of those speaking.

C. Assistive Listening Devices

Multiple devices exist that allow for improved communication through personal amplification without hearing aids. These can be useful in a patient who would like hearing aids but cannot afford or manage them. Assistive listening devices (ALDs) typically use a microphone placed close to the desired sound and transmit this sound to the patient. One device is a "pocket talker," which amplifies nearby sound and sends it to the user through earphones. Many public venues also have listening systems that send sound from the speaker or area of interest to the user through infrared or frequency modulation (FM) signals. Other devices include amplified telephones, telecommunication devices for the deaf (also known as text telephones), closed captioning for television, vibrating alarm clocks, and visual alarm systems (eg, door bells and smoke alarms).

D. Audiologic Evaluation

The goal of the audiologist or hearing aid specialist is not to simply fit a hearing aid, but to ensure that a patient can effectively communicate in all settings. The hearing rehabilitative process therefore entails counseling, proper fitting of hearing aids and amplification devices, rehabilitation, and training in the use of other systems such as ALDs, amplified telephones, and hearing loop induction systems. To identify an audiologist or hearing aid specialist who shares these goals, ask the following: Does she offer regular audiologic rehabilitation sessions for her patients? Does he have an induction loop system installed in his office? Is she a member of the Academy of Rehabilitative Audiology, an organization focused on the comprehensive management of hearing loss? Given the fee-for-service model of audiologic services that are rarely covered by insurance, it is vital to distinguish between audiologists committed to comprehensive rehabilitative care from those who are focused only on hearing aids.

E. Hearing Aids

Fewer than 15% of Americans older than the age of 50 years with hearing loss use hearing aids, despite the evidence for improved speech perception, understanding, and hearing-related quality of life, including social, emotional, and mental wellbeing. This may be a result of hearing aids' cost, appearance, comfort, and performance in different environments. Furthermore, in the United States, most insurance carriers do not cover the cost of hearing aids, which on average cost approximately $1500 each, with premium models costing $3000–$5000 each.

1. Types of hearing aids—Digital hearing aids have become standard over the past decade and offer size and performance advantages over the bulky analog hearing aids commonly used a decade ago. There are 4 main types: behind the ear, in the ear, in the ear canal, and completely in the ear canal.

2. Selection and fitting of hearing aids—Following audiometric testing by a qualified audiologist, hearing aids need to be correctly fitted, customized with appropriate ALDs, and managed over time. The audiologist will help the patient maximize her experience with regard to performance while attending to the patient's preferences for appearance, functionality, and cost. Once the hearing aid is chosen and fitted, the patient should take part in aural rehabilitative training, which a conscientious audiologist should offer to all her patients, during which the patient is educated in proper use of the device, management of the device in different environments, speech perception and communication, and strategies to cope and deal with difficulties that may arise during use. Successful amplification requires an ongoing effort by the audiologist and the patient over multiple visits.

3. Assistive listening devices for use with hearing aids— Although hearing aids perform well when the sound source is within a 6-foot radius, at farther distances they perform less well. Some public venues are equipped with technology that can transmit sound directly to hearing aids through FM, infrared, or induction loop systems. This improves sound quality by reducing the signal-to-noise ratio. Of particular interest, induction loops or "hearing loops" directly transmit sound to the two-thirds of hearing aids currently equipped with a telecoil, dramatically improving sound quality. The system involves a thin wire that is placed around the periphery of a room or area allowing sound to be transmitted to the telecoil through induction. Such systems are installed in concert halls, ticket booths at train stations, houses of worship, and anywhere background noise or proximity to the sound of interest may interfere with communication.

4. Cochlear implants—Cochlear implants are surgically implanted neuroprosthetic devices that are used to treat profound SNHL in patients who do not gain appreciable benefit from optimized hearing aid use. The surgery is typically a 2-hour outpatient operation performed by an otolaryngologist who implants an electrode array into the cochlea by way of a mastoidectomy. Unlike hearing aids, cochlear implants directly stimulate the auditory nerve, functionally replacing the role of the impaired cochlea. Cochlear implantation can substantially improve the ability of older adults to communicate. Many older adults improve from 0% word comprehension preoperatively (without the aid of visual cues) to 100% comprehension several months after surgery. There are no age contraindications to cochlear implant surgery, with many implant centers routinely performing cochlear implantation in adults in their 80s and 90s. Candidates for cochlear implantation are those who have severe-to-profound SNHL even while using optimized bilateral hearing aids. Typically, even while maximally aided, these patients score less than 40% to 50% on word or sentence recognition testing.

▶ Prognosis

In the case of age-related or idiopathic hearing loss, the natural history is that it progresses over time, possibly contributing to social isolation, cognitive load, and morbidity in older adults. There is currently no definitive evidence on whether treating hearing loss could mitigate these negative outcomes. There has only been 1 moderately sized, randomized, clinical trial of hearing aids that has examined effects beyond speech comprehension and quality of life, and it was performed more than 20 years ago. Interestingly, this study demonstrated positive effects of hearing aids on cognition and other functional domains at 4 months posttreatment. A larger trial utilizing more current technology and longer periods of follow-up in a more generalizable study population is currently being planned.

Bisht M, Bist SS. Ototoxicity: the hidden menace. *Indian J Otolaryngol Head Neck Surg.* 2011;63(3):255-259.

Chien W, Lin FR. Prevalence of hearing aid use among older adults in the United States. *Arch Intern Med.* 2012;172(3):292-293.

Chou R, Dana T, Bougatsos C, Fleming C, Beil T. Screening adults aged 50 years or older for hearing loss: a review of the evidence for the U.S. Preventive services task force. *Ann Intern Med.* 2011;154(5):347-355.

Kim HH, Barrs DM. Hearing aids: a review of what's new. *Otolaryngol Head Neck Surg.* 2006;134(6):1043-1050.

Kuhn M, Heman-Ackah SE, Shaikh JA, Roehm PC. Sudden sensorineural hearing loss: a review of diagnosis, treatment, and prognosis. *Trends Amplif.* 2011;15(3):91-105.

Lee CA, Mistry D, Uppal S, Coatesworth AP. Otologic side effects of drugs. *J Laryngol Otol.* 2005;119(4):267-271.

Lin FR. Hearing loss and cognition among older adults in the United States. *J Gerontol A Biol Sci Med Sci.* 2011;66(10):1131-1136.

Lin FR, Ferrucci L, Metter EJ, An Y, Zonderman AB, Resnick SM. Hearing loss and cognition in the Baltimore Longitudinal Study of Aging. *Neuropsychology.* 2011;25(6):763-770.

Lin FR, Metter EJ, O'Brien RJ, Resnick SM, Zonderman AB, Ferrucci L. Hearing loss and incident dementia. *Arch Neurol.* 2011;68(2):214-220.

Lin FR, Yaffe K, Xia J, et al; Health ABC Study Group. Hearing loss and cognitive decline among older adults. *JAMA Intern Med.* 2013;173(4):293-299.

Pacala JT, Yueh B. Hearing deficits in the older patient: "I didn't notice anything". *JAMA.* 2012;307(11):1185-1194.

Mulrow CD, Aguilar C, Endicott JE, et al. Quality-of-life changes and hearing impairment. A randomized trial. *Ann Intern Med.* 1990;113(3):188-194.

Strawbridge WJ, Wallhagen MI, Shema SJ, Kaplan GA. Negative consequences of hearing impairment in old age: a longitudinal analysis. *Gerontologist.* 2000;40(3):320-326.

Ventry I, Weinstein B. The hearing handicap inventory for the elderly: a new tool. *Ear Hear.* 1982;3(3):128-134.

Wallhagen MI, Pettengill E, Whiteside M. Sensory impairment in older adults: part 1: hearing loss. *Am J Nurs.* 2006;106(10):40-48; quiz 48-49.

Wingfield A, Tun PA, McCoy SL. Hearing loss in older adulthood—what it is and how it interacts with cognitive performance. *Curr Dir Psychol Sci.* 2005;14(3):144-148.

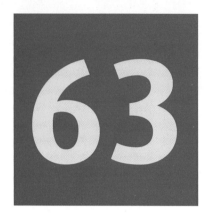

Addressing Chest Pain in Older Adults

Christina Paruthi, MD

Miguel Paniagua, MD, FACP

▶ General Principles in Older Adults

Older patients are more likely than younger patients to have a cardiac event in the absence of chest pain or present to medical care with an atypical clinical presentation of chest pain. Fewer than half of patients whose ultimate diagnosis is acute myocardial infarction (MI) are admitted for acute MI. The National Registry of Myocardial Infarction (NRMI) showed that only 40% of older patients' chief complaints were chest pain, compared to 77% of patients presenting with MI age 65 years or younger. Patients may present with nausea, fatigue, or delirium. The lack of typical symptoms can lead to treatment delay and increased morbidity and mortality in the older patient population (see Chapter 7, "Atypical Presentations of Illness in Older Adults"). For adults age 65 years or older, ischemic heart disease accounts for 81% of mortality, and should therefore be the first diagnosis considered when an older adult presents for medical care with chest pain. However, chest pain in older patients can also be noncardiac in origin or of a cardiac etiology other than coronary artery disease. Noncardiac origins of chest pain include pulmonary and esophageal. Although not all causes of chest pain in the older adult will lead to fatal events, timely diagnosis based on a history of associated factors and a targeted physical exam can improve an older patient's health outcomes in the short-term, as well as longer-term quality of life, functionality, and health outcomes. It is therefore essential that clinicians take a thorough history, perform a targeted physical exam, and have a high level of suspicion to make the correct diagnosis in a timely manner.

▶ Clinical Findings

A. Symptoms & Signs

Typical angina at any age presents as substernal chest pain, often described as "pressure like," with radiation to the jaw, neck, or arm. If a patient has experienced an MI in the past,

asking the patient if this pain is similar to that experienced during a previous MI can be an important clue. Descriptions of chest pain radiating to the back, may be more suggestive of aortic dissection or gastrointestinal pathology such as esophageal reflux. If patients complain that they feel chest pain after eating or when lying flat, one should consider gastroesophageal reflux as a possible diagnosis.

Features suggesting acute coronary syndrome include diaphoresis, cool clammy skin, new or progressive shortness of breath, and/or exertional shortness of breath. Older patients are typically more likely to delay seeking medical care, or be more inclined to attribute their symptoms to "normal aging," which can lead to increased adverse outcomes or death if the etiology of the chest pain is serious in nature. Most older adults with acute coronary syndrome present to medical professionals with dyspnea, diaphoresis, nausea/vomiting, and/or syncope, and not necessarily with chest pain. In addition, given that older adults have a higher prevalence of comorbidities, concurrent disease processes may cloud the presentation of acute coronary syndrome. Moreover, patients with delirium or dementia may have trouble communicating their symptoms accurately to their clinician.

1. Physical examination—Physical examination should begin with vital signs, with special attention to blood pressure, heart rate, and oxygen saturation, to assess the clinical stability of the patient.

Next, the clinician should assess the cardiovascular system. Check blood pressure in both arms, a discrepancy of more than 20 mm Hg systolic between readings, without a history of vascular compromise in either limb should raise suspicion of aortic dissection, especially if the patient describes a "ripping" or "tearing" quality to his chest pain. If heart sounds are muffled on cardiac auscultation, cardiac tamponade should be considered as a cause of distress. Additional signs and symptoms of cardiac tamponade include pulsus paradoxus (a decrease in systolic pressure of >10 mm Hg during inspiration), and hypotension. Cardiac tamponade is more common in the setting of certain chronic illnesses including autoimmune disease, malignancy, or a recent history of acute trauma to the chest. If a cardiac rub is present, a diagnosis of pericarditis should be entertained. A loud new holosystolic murmur, is suggestive of acute coronary pathology and possibly mitral valve papillary dysfunction. Elevated jugular venous pressure and an S_3 gallop suggest congestive heart failure. New congestive heart failure in the setting of chest pain should be considered a medical emergency and prompt swift work up to rule out serious diagnoses such as acute coronary syndrome. In the setting of chest pain that varies with respiration with or without the presence of hemoptysis, pulmonary embolism should be considered. Pain on palpation of the chest wall may indicate musculoskeletal pain or costochondritis and can provide reassurance to the clinician and patient. Lower-extremity edema that is symmetric in both limbs and acute or subacute may be suggestive of right heart failure; however, if there is unilateral swelling, one must suspect venous thromboembolism and consider evaluation for pulmonary thromboembolism as a cause of chest pain. In this scenario, chest pain may also be associated with hypoxia and tachycardia and be exacerbated by respiration.

2. Laboratory findings—The standard cardiac chemistry panel includes creatinine kinase (CK), creatinine kinase–myocardial bound (CK-MB), and troponin I. CK is leaked out of injured muscle cells and is not specific to myocardial injury. CK-MB as an isoenzyme is more specific to myocardial injury; additionally, when a ratio to CK is performed, if >4.5% of the total CK it is suggestive of myocardial injury. Troponin I is more specific and sensitive to myocardial injury; however, it can take up to 8 hours from initial event to abnormal rise in number. In the case of recurrent injury, CK-MB has a shorter half-life and if it were to rise again in a presumed acute setting, would be a more reliable marker of repeat myocardial injury. Other diagnostic tests that may be of use include D-dimer for work up of pulmonary embolism (see Chapter 32, "Peripheral Arterial Disease & Venous Thromboembolism").

3. Diagnostic tests and imaging studies—Electrocardiogram (ECG) is the first step in the chest pain work up of an older patient. It is important to obtain a previous ECG for comparison; in this age group, patients may already have significant cardiac history, thereby further confounding acute findings, particularly without a comparison study. S-T elevations in a specific coronary territory raises concern for acute coronary plaque rupture and ST-segment elevation MI. Diffuse S-T elevations or depressions may be more suggestive of pericarditis in the appropriate clinical context. ECG findings of cardiac tamponade include blunting of the voltage of QRS complexes, in association with dyspnea and the presence of electrical alternans—a beat to beat variation of QRS complexes in an alternating pattern.

On chest radiography, the presence of a widened mediastinum, if clinical history suggests, should raise suspicion of an aortic dissection. Suspicion for pulmonary thromboembolism or aortic dissection should prompt the clinician to order a CT chest with contrast for diagnostic purposes.

4. Special tests—Progressive dyspnea that accompanies chest pain with exertion (angina) should be evaluated with a stress test, either an exercise stress test with an imaging modality such as echocardiogram or nuclear imaging. An imaging modality is absolutely necessary as baseline abnormalities on ECG can confound results during stress testing. Frail older patients may be limited by their functional capacity and unable to complete an exercise stress test. In appropriate patients, using a bicycle instead of a treadmill can sometimes compensate for these functional deficits, for patients who are unable to reach target heart rate with exercise, pharmacologic testing is a viable alternative.

Gastrointestinal causes of chest pain can be mistaken for angina. If the patient notes a correlation of symptoms to food, consider an empiric trial of acid suppression, or if clinically indicated, a barium swallow exam which may show multiple strictures in corkscrew pattern if the patient is suffering from esophageal spasm. Upper endoscopy may be helpful in the diagnosis of esophagitis (see Chapter 35, "Gastrointestinal & Abdominal Complaints," for further discussion of work-up for esophageal and other gastrointestinal disorders).

▶ Differential Diagnosis

The differential diagnosis of chest pain in older patients is as broad as it is in younger adults, with the potential added complication of coexisting medical comorbidity. Initial assessment includes assessment of cardiogenic and pulmonary stability. Once established, chest pain should be assessed for its likelihood of being cardiac or noncardiac, followed by initial assessment for diagnoses associated with the highest mortality or complication rates. Cardiovascular causes of chest pain include acute coronary syndrome, unstable angina, pericarditis, and aortic dissection. The Thrombolysis In Myocardial Infarction (TIMI) risk score is a widely used prognostic scale for risk stratification of chest pain and likelihood for ischemic chest pain. The 7 components include age greater than 65 years, 3 or more risk factors for coronary artery disease, known coronary artery disease, ST-segment deviation on ECG, 2 episodes within 24 hours of presentation, aspirin use in the last 7 days, or elevation of cardiac biomarkers at time of presentation. A higher TIMI risk score reflects an elevated risk of cardiac etiology and is used to guide therapy such as additional anticoagulation and early invasive strategies versus conservative strategies for further testing.

Pulmonary causes of chest pain include acute pulmonary embolism and pleuritis. Pleuritic chest pain, caused by inflammation of the pleural lining of the lung, occurs with inspiration and can lead to chest pain. This inflammation can be caused by any pathologic process causing inflammation or fluid accumulation, including pneumonia or less commonly, a smaller distal pulmonary embolism. A history of chest pain exacerbated by inspiration and associated with fever and/or sputum production would suggest pneumonia. Chest pain can also be the first sign or chief complaint of an older patient who is ultimately found to have lung cancer.

The most common musculoskeletal cause of chest pain is costochondritis or Tietze syndrome (a swelling of the costal cartiladges). Chest pain caused by gastrointestinal diseases is generally related to esophageal reflux, esophagitis or esophageal spasm. Chemical esophagitis (or pill esophagitis) related to medications such as bisphosphonates may be particularly prevalent in older patients, especially those with a high daily pill burden. Suspicion of pill esophagitis should prompt a close examination of the patient's medication list for possible contributors to esophagitis.

▶ Treatment

Treatment is specific to the underlying cause of chest pain. In the case of an ST-elevation MI, rapid diagnosis by ECG and clinical history can lead to prompt activation of the cardiac catheterization team. If no cardiac catheterization is available at location of presentation, and if the patient can be transported to a hospital with cardiac catheterization capabilities within 90 minutes of presentation, then arrangement for transfer should be made immediately. If catheterization is not possible, then pharmacologic thrombolysis can be considered. TIMI risk score can then guide therapy with antiplatelet agents (see Chapter 28, "Coronary Disease").

At presentation, if clinical history of aortic dissection is confirmed by a CT scan, or in some cases, by ECG, this is a surgical emergency, and preparations to take patient to the operating room should be made, after consideration of comorbid disease, functional capacity, life expectancy, patient goals, and advance directives.

Pericarditis requires additional work up after diagnosis to establish the etiology. In addition to treatment of the underlying cause, most cases can be treated with nonsteroidal antiinflammatory agents or aspirin, if there are no contraindications. The antigout medication, colchicine is also very effective in the treatment of pericarditis.

If the diagnosis of pulmonary embolism is definitively made with CT scan or with ventilation perfusion scan, the patient should be started on anticoagulation therapy if no absolute contraindications are present. If the patient experiences recurrent thromboembolic events, consideration can be given to inferior vena cava filter placement.

Pleuritic chest pain is a nonspecific symptom that can have a variety of causes including infectious, autoimmune or other systemic illnesses. Management includes antiinflammatory agents in addition to goal-directed therapy against the underlying cause.

Inflammation and strain of the muscles of the rib cage can lead to chest pain causing significant distress. Once all life-threatening causes of chest pain are effectively ruled out and the physical exam is consistent with costochondritis (such as positional chest pain, and pain reproducible on palpation) the patient can be reassured and pain relief can generally be achieved with an antiinflammatory agent.

Gastrointestinal manifestations of chest pain such as gastroesophageal reflux disease and esophagitis can be managed with antihistamine-1 blockers or with proton pump inhibitors (see Chapter 35, "Gastrointestinal & Abdominal Complaints"). With the diagnosis of esophageal spasm, a calcium channel blocker and avoidance of triggers can effectively manage symptoms.

SUMMARY

Ischemic heart disease is a significant cause of morbidity and mortality in older adults. Age alone puts older adults at higher risk of having cardiac ischemia when chest pain is present. However, in this population, heart disease may not initially present with chest pain, or it may present with atypical chest pain. In addition, when chest pain is present, it may not represent cardiac pathology. It is important for clinicians to differentiate cardiac from noncardiac chest pain and risk stratify patients immediately upon presentation so that proper treatment is not delayed. Tools to accomplish this include physical exam, thorough history, electrocardiography, cardiac biomarkers, and chest rdiography on initial evaluation.

Alexander KP, Newby KL, Cannon CP, et al; American Heart Association Council on Clinical Cardiology; Society of Geriatric Cardiology. Acute coronary care in the elderly part 1: non-ST-segment-elevation acute coronary syndromes: a scientific statement for healthcare professionals from the American Heart Association Council on Clinical Cardiology: in collaboration with the Society of Geriatric Cardiology. *Circulation.* 2007;115(19):2549-2569.

Antman EM, Cohen M, Bernink PM, et al. The TIMI Risk Score for unstable angina/non-ST elevation MI: a method for prognostication and therapeutic decision making. *JAMA.* 2000;284(7):835-842.

Brieger D, Eagle KA, Goodman SG, et al. Acute coronary syndromes without chest pain, an underdiagnosed and undertreated high-risk group: insights from the Global Registry of Acute Coronary Events. *Chest.* 2004;126(2):461-469.

Cannon CP, Weintraub WS, Demopoulos LA, et al; TACTICS (Treat Angina with Aggrastat and Determine Cost of Therapy with an Invasive or Conservative Strategy)—Thrombolysis in Myocardial Infarction 18 Investigators. Comparison of early invasive and conservative strategies in patients with unstable coronary syndromes treated with the glycoprotein IIb/IIIa inhibitor tirofiban. *N Engl J Med.* 2001;344(25):1879-1887.

Chun AA, McGee SR. Bedside diagnosis of coronary artery disease: a systematic review. *Am J Med.* 2004;117(5):335-343.

Chute CG, Greenberg ER, Baron J, Korson R, Baker J, Yates J. Presenting conditions of 1539 population-based lung cancer patients by cell type and stage in New Hampshire and Vermont. *Cancer.* 1985;56(8):2107-2111.

Fuster V, Walsh R, Harrington R, eds. *Hurst's the Heart.* New York, NY: McGraw Hill; 2010.

Gibbons RJ, Balady GJ, Bricker JT, et al. ACC/AHA 2002 guideline update for exercise testing: summary article: a report of the American College of Cardiology/American Heart Association Task Force on Practice Guidelines (Committee to Update the 1997 Exercise Testing Guidelines). *Circulation.* 2002;106(14):1883-1892.

de Groen PC, Lubbe DF, Hirsch, LJ, et al. Esophagitis associated with the use of alendronate. *N Engl J Med.* 1996;335(14): 1016-1021.

Halter JB, Ouslander JG, Tinettie ME, Studenski S, High KP, Asthana S, eds. *Hazzard's Geriatric Medicine and Gerontology.* New York, NY: McGraw-Hill; 2009.

Roger VL, Go, AS, Lloyd-Jones DM, et al; American Heart Association Statistics Committee and Stroke Statistics Subcommittee. Heart disease and stroke statistics—2012 update: a report from the American Heart Association. *Circulation.* 2012;125(1):e2-e220.

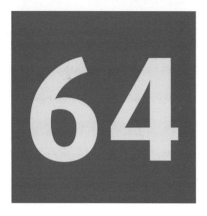

Addressing Dyspnea in Older Adults

Leslie Kernisan, MD, MPH

▶ General Principles in Older Adults

Dyspnea, also known as shortness of breath, is a common symptom affecting the geriatric population. In a 2012 consensus statement, the American Thoracic Society defined dyspnea as follows:

> *"Dyspnea is a term used to characterize a subjective experience of breathing discomfort that is comprised of qualitatively distinct sensations that vary in intensity. The experience derives from interactions among multiple physiological, psychological, social, and environmental factors, and may induce secondary physiological and behavioral responses."*

This chapter discusses special considerations pertaining to the presentation, evaluation, and management of dyspnea in the geriatric patient. This chapter is particularly oriented toward outpatient evaluation in the context of primary care follow-up or the urgent care visit. However, the key principles also can be applied in the acute or long-term care setting.

Dyspnea is often inadequately addressed in the geriatric patient because of factors such as limited appointment time, or a clinician's inappropriate presumption that the dyspnea is caused by a chronic condition and cannot be treated further. In fact, it is common for dyspnea to signal either a new significant medical problem, or a worsening of 1 (or more) of the chronic cardiopulmonary diseases that are prevalent among older adults. Dyspnea is also often a very distressing physical symptom, which, left untreated, can substantially impair physical function and quality of life. For these reasons, dyspnea in the geriatric patient should never be ignored.

Clinicians should consider the following key principles of geriatric care when evaluating and treating the older patient with shortness of breath.

- **Consider soliciting history from caregivers or other knowledgeable informants.**

  Although many geriatric patients are very capable of providing an excellent history, others may be limited by cognitive problems, hearing impairments, or even speech difficulties. Soliciting information from caregivers can uncover additional information of importance, and helps to obtain a more robust and useful history. Clinicians should also bear in mind that other clinicians often fail to recognize or document cognitive impairment. Hence, the absence of a cognitive impairment diagnosis should not preclude a clinician from considering this possibility, and from seeking additional information from a knowledgeable informant, especially if the history is unclear or does not cohere as expected.

- **Consider the possibility of alternative presentations.**

  In some cases, breathing problems in the geriatric patient may manifest as another complaint or symptom, such as fatigue, chest discomfort, or decreased physical activity. Patients with moderate or worse dementia may no longer be able to clearly articulate a breathing complaint. Dyspnea is sometimes identified by the astute clinician after a caregiver simply notes that the patient is not his or her usual self.

- **Pay special attention to medications.**

  Geriatric patients are often prescribed multiple medications for chronic and acute use, and many struggle with medication management (see Chapters 9, "Principles of Prescribing for Older Adults," and 53, "Addressing Polypharmacy & Improving Medication Adherence in Older Adults," for more details on medication management). Careful review of prescriptions and medication use is required, so as to ensure that a breathing complaint is not related to a problem with medication adherence. Special attention should be given to inhalers, which are often difficult to use correctly, as well as to cardiovascular medications. For example, patients sometimes skip diuretics in an attempt to reduce incontinence.

- **Consider multimorbidity.**

  Dyspnea is a symptom associated with many chronic and acute illnesses, which often coexist in the geriatric patient. A thoughtful evaluation is usually required to sort out the underlying etiology of new or worsened shortness of breath, and sometimes a trial of treatment may be required to identify the main cause of the current dyspnea complaint. Patients and families often appreciate clinicians letting them know that more than one condition may be causing the dyspnea, and that a little therapeutic trial-and-error may be required.

- **Consider the benefits and burdens of diagnostic procedures.**

Although an initial office-based assessment for dyspnea can be completed in all geriatric patients, more extensive testing (eg, pulmonary function tests, CT scans, cardiac stress tests, etc) can be burdensome for some frailer patients with limited life expectancy. For these reasons, clinicians should consider benefits and burdens before referring patients for more extensive evaluation, and should attempt to discuss benefits and burdens with patients and families, as part of a shared decision-making process. For more on how to identify older adults with limited life expectancy, see Chapter 3, "Goals of Care & Consideration of Prognosis."

- **Identify key players in medical decision making.**

Many geriatric patients have 1 or more family members or other caregivers involved in their medical decision making. Identifying and involving such caregivers is essential, especially as such caregivers are often integral to implementing any care plan recommended by the clinician.

- **Consider the benefits and burdens of proposed treatment plans.**

Some treatments for dyspnea may be more burdensome or difficult for geriatric patients than others. This is not to say that such treatments should not be proposed; however, it is important to consider the feasibility of implementation for patients and caregivers. Clinicians should attempt to anticipate and minimize the burden that a proposed treatment plan may impose on an older adult and/or caregiver.

- **Consider goals of care.**

Goals of care should be reviewed, especially if more complex diagnostic procedures or treatments are under consideration. As dyspnea can be a very distressing symptom, clinicians should always endeavor to provide at least some degree of symptomatic relief. For further information on how to incorporate goals of care into the clinical care of the geriatric patient, see Chapter 3, "Goals of Care & Consideration of Prognosis."

- **Consider palliative care if advanced chronic cardiopulmonary illness.**

Persisting dyspnea in the geriatric patient is sometimes caused by very advanced cardiopulmonary illness, such as stage IV chronic obstructive pulmonary disease (COPD) or advanced heart failure. In these cases, a palliative care approach, which usually combines a thoughtful discussion of prognosis and goals with an emphasis on symptom control and quality of life, should be considered. Studies have found that patients often progress to very advanced cardiopulmonary illness without any clinician having discussed prognosis with them. Clinicians should consider assessing a patient and family's understanding of prognosis, as treatment preferences may be influenced by this information. For example, a patient and family may be more willing to consider low-dose opiates for treatment of refractory dyspnea in stage IV COPD, if the patient understands his poor prognosis and high likelihood of death in the coming year (see Chapter 3, "Goals of Care & Consideration of Prognosis," and Chapter 11, "Geriatrics & Palliative Care").

▶ Symptoms

To evaluate the symptom of dyspnea in the geriatric patient, the clinician should start with a thorough history and a brief chart review. As noted above, the clinician should consider including a knowledgeable informant, especially if there is any possibility of cognitive impairment. The goals of the history taking are to:

- Determine whether the complaint is a new problem, a worsening of a chronic complaint, or an ongoing complaint that has failed to resolve.

- Obtain more information regarding the dyspnea, such as the duration, severity, frequency, temporal pattern, exacerbating/alleviating factors, and qualitative character.

- Identify the impact on physical and psychological function, by asking about impact on physical activity and on mood.

- Identify other signs and symptoms that may be related and might point toward an underlying etiology.

- Identify chronic conditions or previous conditions associated with dyspnea.

- Check for the presence of environmental or occupational exposures that may provoke or aggravate dyspnea, such as cigarette smoking or urban air pollution.

- Review medication use, with a special focus on adherence to pulmonary and cardiovascular medications.

▶ Quantitative and Qualitative Assessment of Dyspnea

The severity of dyspnea can be quantitatively assessed by asking the patient to report how intense the shortness of breath feels, using either a numerical scale (ie, 1–10) or visual analogue scale. Patients should also be encouraged to describe the character of the dyspnea. Dyspnea can represent a number of qualitatively distinct sensations, some of which have been linked with certain underlying pathophysiologies. For example, research has found that pulmonary edema is often associated with a sensation of "suffocation," whereas acute bronchoconstriction is often described as "chest tightness." Cardiac deconditioning has been linked to the feeling of "heavy breathing." The sensation of increased effort or work of breathing is linked to COPD, asthma, pulmonary fibrosis, and myopathy, whereas air hunger is associated with heart failure and pulmonary embolism, as well as with COPD and asthma.

A. Assessing Functional Impact

Assessing dyspnea's impact on function is important whether the problem is new and acute, or chronic and ongoing. The experience of dyspnea often involves a strong affective component, hence clinicians should inquire about impact on mood and psychological function, as well as on physical function.

Impact on physical function can quickly be assessed by asking the patient and caregiver questions such as, "How far can you walk? How does that compare to before?" or "What activities are you having difficulty with as a result of your shortness of breath?"

Assessing affective impact is especially important in patients suffering from chronic dyspnea, such as those with COPD. This can be briefly assessed by asking questions such as, "How does your breathing difficulty make you feel?" or "How bothersome does your breathing feel to you?" For those patients endorsing feelings of sadness, apathy, or anxiety, more detailed evaluation for depression or anxiety should be considered.

For patients suffering from chronic dyspnea, a variety of assessment tools and questionnaires have been developed; however, these have mainly been used in research settings, and most are too long to be used in common clinical practice. No index is currently widely used in routine clinical practice, although development of a short questionnaire addressing dyspnea severity, functional impact, and distress is underway.

B. Associated Signs & Symptoms

The presence or absence of certain signs and symptoms can help identify the underlying etiology of the dyspnea. In particular, clinicians should ask about:

- Cough and characteristics of sputum, if any
- Fever
- Nasal congestion
- Pain in the chest, pain with deep breaths, or pain elsewhere
- Edema of the legs or elsewhere

C. Relevant Chronic or Past Medical Conditions

Clinicians should note the presence of any chronic medical conditions associated with dyspnea, as these provide an important context in which to consider the current complaint. Past conditions (eg, acute anemia) may have an increased chance of recurrence. The most common chronic conditions associated with dyspnea are:

- Chronic obstructive pulmonary disease
- Heart failure
- Coronary artery disease
- Deconditioning/obesity
- Asthma
- Interstitial lung disease
- Anemia

▶ Findings

All evaluations of dyspnea in the geriatric patient should include, at the very least, a focused physical exam. Additional laboratory and diagnostic testing may be indicated, depending on the history and physical exam findings, and whether the complaint appears to be acute or chronic.

A. Physical Exam

On exam, the clinician should note the following:

- Vital signs including respiratory rate and oxygen saturation; consider ambulatory oxygen saturation if dyspnea on exertion has been reported.
- General appearance, including visible distress and work of breathing.
- Head and neck exam, with attention to signs of upper respiratory infection or obstruction, placement of the trachea, and use of accessory muscles in breathing.
- Lung exam, with special attention to the presence of wheezing, crackles, or other abnormal sounds.
- Cardiovascular exam, with special attention to the cardiac rhythm, jugular venous pressure, and leg edema.

B. Additional Diagnostic Tests

Table 64–1 lists additional tests to consider. The appropriate test depends on the history and acuity of the complaint. For an acute complaint, CT of the chest is generally only indicated for high suspicion of pulmonary embolism. For chronic shortness of breath, CT of the chest is generally only considered for evaluation of interstitial lung disease.

▶ Differential Diagnosis

Table 64–2 details the differential diagnoses to consider for both acute and chronic dyspnea. The differential diagnoses are strongly influenced by whether the dyspnea complaint

Table 64–1. Additional diagnostic tests.

Test	Indication
Electrocardiogram	Suspicion of ongoing or recent cardiac ischemia, or if concern for atrial fibrillation or other symptomatic arrhythmia
Chest radiograph	Suspicion of pneumonia, pleural effusion, or pneumothorax
Laboratory testing	Complete blood count (CBC) if concern for anemia Brain natriuretic peptide (BNP) if concern for heart failure Consider D-dimer if suspicion of deep venous thrombosis (DVT)/pulmonary embolism (PE) (negative predictive value much higher than positive predictive value)
Peak flow	Suspicion of asthma exacerbation
Spirometry and pulmonary function tests	Evaluation of ongoing or chronic dyspnea (not usually performed for acute dyspnea)
Echocardiogram	Consider if concern for heart failure or valve disease
Cardiac stress testing	Consider if concern for coronary artery disease

Table 64–2. Differential diagnoses for dyspnea in the geriatric patient.

Acute Dyspnea	Chronic Dyspnea
Pneumonia	COPD
Acute coronary syndrome	Heart failure
COPD or asthma exacerbation	Deconditioning
Heart failure exacerbation	Interstitial lung disease
Rapid atrial fibrillation or other tachyarrhythmia	Asthma
Aspiration	Anemia
Anemia	
Pulmonary Embolism	
Cardiac tamponade	
Pneumothorax	
Anaphylaxis	
Panic Attack	

appears to be new and acute versus chronic and ongoing. In geriatric patients, it is common to develop acute on chronic dyspnea, either because of an exacerbation of an existing condition, or from the development of a new acute illness in a patient with chronic disease. For subacute presentations (ie, development over days to weeks), both lists in Table 64–2 should be considered.

▶ Next Steps and Treatment

Treatment of dyspnea depends on the underlying illness thought to be causing the symptom. Clinicians should also tailor treatment to fit with the patient's preferences and goals of care, and should assist the patient in considering the expected benefits and burdens when selecting among treatment options.

A. General Recommendations

Clinicians treating a complaint of dyspnea in the geriatric patient should do the following:

- **Provide extremely clear written instructions to patient and caregivers.**

Geriatric patients, especially when feeling unwell, may have difficulty remembering verbal instructions. Furthermore, some caregivers instrumental in managing medications or other aspects of care may not be present during the clinical encounter. Clear, written instructions reduce the chance of misunderstandings and facilitate sharing of the care plan with other caregivers or clinicians involved.

- **Realize that inhalers are often difficult for geriatric patients to use correctly.**

Geriatric patients are at risk of using inhalers incorrectly and of misunderstanding instructions for use (especially if both short-acting and long-acting inhalers are prescribed). Inhalers are also often expensive for patients to obtain, causing many patients to decline to fill the prescription. Clinicians should encourage patients and caregivers to obtain inhaler training, either in clinic or from pharmacists, and should be alert to the possibility of financial strain interfering with adherence. Inhaler regimens should be simplified if possible. Clinicians should also consider ordering a nebulizer for patients; both albuterol and ipratropium, for instance, are much less expensive as generic nebulizer solutions.

- **Arrange prompt follow-up of symptoms and medication adherence.**

Clinicians should arrange prompt follow-up, in order to ensure that a geriatric patient's dyspnea is improving. This is especially important for the more vulnerable geriatric patients, such as those who live alone or with a frail spouse, as well as for those with cognitive impairment.

Patients and caregivers should be asked to bring all medications, including the ones newly prescribed, to the follow-up visit. Difficulty adhering to medication changes or recommendations is a common cause for dyspnea symptoms to persist or even worsen.

B. Special Considerations for Treating Chronic Dyspnea in the Geriatric Patient

Clinicians often encounter geriatric patients with significant chronic dyspnea that is not easily reversible. These cases of chronic dyspnea are most commonly caused by advanced COPD or heart failure. Such patients can be challenging for clinicians, especially when there is no superimposed acute condition to treat, or medication adherence problem to resolve.

Although dyspnea in such patients cannot be cured, it is often possible to make significant gains in symptom relief and psychological well-being. To pursue this, clinicians should begin by confirming that the underlying disease(s) causing dyspnea have been maximally treated. Subsequently (or sometimes concurrently), the following approaches to symptom relief should be considered.

1. Regular and repeated documentation of dyspnea—Clinicians caring for a chronically dyspneic older adult should regularly inquire as to the patient's feeling of dyspnea. In particular, clinicians should document severity, impact on function, and distress. Documenting dyspnea over time allows clinicians reassess the efficacy of the current dyspnea care plan and adjust as needed. Regular inquiry as to chronic dyspnea can also provide much-needed reassurance and support to patient and caregivers, who benefit from feeling a clinician's engagement despite the dyspnea being incurable.

2. Oxygen, medical air, and fans—For patients suffering from chronic hypoxemia, such as stage IV COPD patients, oxygen therapy has been proven to improve dyspnea and quality of life, and is also associated with longer survival. Oxygen also benefits patients with activity-induced hypoxemia; consequently, clinicians should check ambulatory oxygen saturation in patients who do not have resting hypoxemia.

Whether oxygen benefits chronically dyspneic patients who are not hypoxemic remains under study. To address this question, a recent trial randomized patients to oxygen versus medical air. The study found oxygen to be nonsuperior, but interestingly, both groups reported improvements in dyspnea and quality of life, suggesting that in nonhypoxic patients, it may be air flow itself that palliates symptoms, rather than increased oxygen. In another recent randomized trial, nonhypoxic patients suffering from chronic dyspnea experienced symptomatic improvement when a fan was directed to their face.

3. Relaxation, psychosocial support, and cognitive behavioral therapy—Counseling and therapy can help many patients develop better ways to psychologically cope with chronic breathlessness. Such therapy can reduce anxiety and dyspnea-related distress, with resultant improvements in quality of life.

4. Pulmonary rehabilitation and exercise—Pulmonary rehabilitation usually combines supervised exercise training with coaching in breathing technique, dyspnea self-management strategies, and may also include psychosocial support and nutrition support. It has been shown to benefit patients with stages III and IV COPD. Geriatric patients with COPD may benefit from pulmonary rehabilitation, although participation can be limited by cognitive impairment or overall frailty.

Exercise training, both aerobic and resistive, helps reverse deconditioning and can improve well-being. Exercise has been shown to improve exercise tolerance and dyspnea in patients with chronic breathlessness, especially those with COPD.

5. Opiates and other pharmacotherapy—Opiates relieve breathlessness and studies have found that the use of relatively low systemic doses can lead to significant improvements in dyspnea. For example, a recent dose increment study found that 70% of enrolled patients experienced significant symptom improvement with only 10 mg of sustained-morphine daily (approximately half of the 85 participants had COPD). Nebulized opiates, on the other hand, have not shown benefit in placebo-controlled trials. At this time, multiple expert groups recommend clinicians consider systemic opiates to treat refractory dyspnea in patients with very advanced disease.

Although clinicians are often understandably concerned about the potential for respiratory depression from opiates, no study has detected associated decreases in oxygen saturation, or increases in mortality. Still, clinicians prescribing opiates for breathlessness should counsel patients and families regarding the prevention of overdose and of diversion, and should also anticipate common side effects such as drowsiness, constipation, and sometimes nausea (see Chapter 54, "Managing Persistent Pain in Older Adults," on pain management for dosing of opiates and treatment of side effects).

Benzodiazepines are another class of medications often considered for the relief of chronic breathlessness. Evidence in support of this practice is weak: a recent Cochrane review concluded that "there is no evidence for a beneficial effect of benzodiazepines for the relief of breathlessness in patients with advanced cancer and COPD." However, many clinicians have noted anecdotal improvement, especially in patients who are particularly suffering from anxiety related to breathlessness, and 1 small, recent trial of cancer patients did note benefit with midazolam.

Given that benzodiazepines are strongly linked to worsened cognition and balance in the geriatric population, clinicians should use caution in prescribing benzodiazepines to the older patient in the community setting with refractory breathlessness, and should try opiates and other symptom-management techniques first.

SUMMARY

Dyspnea is a common complaint among geriatric patients. Key points to remember in addressing dyspnea in this population include:

- Dyspnea should never be ignored or dismissed. New or worsened dyspnea requires diagnostic evaluation and treatment. Chronic dyspnea can significantly depress function and quality of life, and can often be palliated successfully.

- Clinicians should consider involving a knowledgeable informant when obtaining a history. Difficulty adhering to medications or in properly using inhalers is common among older adults, and clinicians should be alert to these frequent contributors to persisting dyspnea. Caregivers are often instrumental in implementing a treatment plan, and in monitoring symptoms. Treatment instructions should be in writing.

- Goals of care and life expectancy should be considered before engaging in more complicated diagnostic or therapeutic procedures, as the burdens may outweigh the likely benefits in patients who are frail or prefer to have fewer interventions.

- Chronic dyspnea caused by advanced incurable cardiopulmonary disease can often be successfully palliated through techniques such as oxygen or medical air, psychosocial support, pulmonary rehabilitation, or low-dose opiates. Clinicians should consider providing guidance as to prognosis and life expectancy; palliative care referral is also often appropriate for those patients struggling with chronic dyspnea.

Abernethy AP, McDonald CF, Frith PA, et al. Effect of palliative oxygen versus room air in relief of breathlessness in patients with refractory dyspnoea: a double-blind, randomised controlled trial. *Lancet.* 2010;376(9743):784-793.

Casaburi R, ZuWallack R. Pulmonary rehabilitation for management of chronic obstructive pulmonary disease. *N Engl J Med.* 2009;360(13):1329-1335.

Currow DC, McDonald C, Oaten S, et al. Once-daily opioids for chronic dyspnea: a dose increment and pharmacovigilance study. *J Pain Symptom Manage.* 2011;42(3):388-399.

Galbraith S, Fagan P, Perkins P, Lynch A, Booth S. Does the use of a handheld fan improve chronic dyspnea? A randomized, controlled, crossover trial. *J Pain Symptom Manage.* 2010;39(5):831-838.

Kamal AH, Maguire JM, Wheeler JL, Currow DC, Abernethy AP. Dyspnea review for the palliative care professional: assessment, burdens, and etiologies. *J Palliat Med.* 2011;14(10):1167-1172.

Kamal AH, Maguire JM, Wheeler JL, Currow DC, Abernethy AP. Dyspnea review for the palliative care professional: treatment goals and therapeutic options. *J Palliat Med.* 2012;15(1):106-114.

Mahler DA, Fierro-Carrion G, Baird JC. Evaluation of dyspnea in the elderly. *Clin Geriatr Med.* 2003;19(1):19-33, v.

Mahler DA, Selecky PA, Harrod CG, et al. American College of Chest Physicians consensus statement on the management of dyspnea in patients with advanced lung or heart disease. *Chest.* 2010;137(3):674-691.

Navigante AH, Castro MA, Cerchietti LC. Morphine versus midazolam as upfront therapy to control dyspnea perception in cancer patients while its underlying cause is sought or treated. *J Pain Symptom Manage.* 2010;39(5):820-830.

Parshall MB, Schwartzstein RM, Adams L, et al. An official American Thoracic Society statement: update on the mechanisms, assessment, and management of dyspnea. *Am J Respir Crit Care Med.* 2012;185(4):435-452.

Scano G, Stendardi L, Grazzini M. Understanding dyspnoea by its language. *Eur Respir J.* 2005;25(2):380-385.

Simon ST, Higginson IJ, Booth S, Harding R, Bausewein C. Benzodiazepines for the relief of breathlessness in advanced malignant and non-malignant diseases in adults. *Cochrane Database Syst Rev.* 2010;(1):CD007354.

Yorke J, Moosavi SH, Shuldham C, Jones PW. Quantification of dyspnoea using descriptors: development and initial testing of the Dyspnoea-12. *Thorax.* 2010;65(1):21-26.

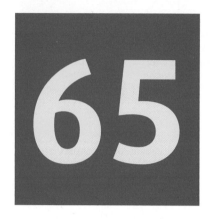

Managing Joint Pain in Older Adults

Lisa Strano-Paul, MD

Gout, calcium pyrophosphate crystal disease (CPPD), and polymyalgia rheumatica are common conditions that can cause joint pain in geriatric patients. These conditions are discussed in this chapter.

GOUT

▶ General Principles in Older Adults

Gout was first described thousands of years ago. Major risks for gout and hyperuricemia include obesity and old age. One study suggests that the incidence of gout is increasing in the geriatric population. The strongest predictor for the development for gout is an elevated uric acid level. Levels between 6 and 8.99 mg/dL predict a 2-fold increase in gout flares and a level >9 predicts a 3-fold rise. Although gout more commonly affects males, male predominance is not seen in patients older than age 60 years, where the incidence of gout in men and women is about equal. Additional risks for gout include high purine diet (red meat, shellfish), alcohol (beer and spirits), high-fructose drinks, renal insufficiency, medications (thiazides), organ transplantation, lead exposure, and genetic factors. Certain diseases that are common in the elderly are also risk factors for gout and include hypertension, diabetes, hyperlipidemia, metabolic syndrome, and hematologic malignancies.

▶ Symptoms

Gout is characterized by episodic self-limited oligoarticular joint pain. The presence of erythema and swelling is characteristic. A history of podagra (first metatarsal joint attack) and or tophi, which are deposits of uric acid crystals around the ear helix or joints, further increases the specificity of diagnosis. Most gout attacks are monoarticular, although recurrent attacks can affect more than 1 joint. Patients may also present with fevers and constitutional symptoms. The ear

and lower extremities are common sites of attacks because lower temperatures favor uric acid deposition. Periarticular structures such as bursa and tendons can also be involved. Gout often develops in previously damaged joints or after a trauma. Gout typically resolves in 3–14 days if untreated; however, crystals remain in affected joints and recurrent attacks are common, ranging from 60% in 1 year to up to 84% in 3 years.

▶ Findings

The gold standard for the diagnosis of gout is the finding of monosodium urate crystals from aspirated fluid from an inflamed joint or tophi. These crystals are needle shaped and seen inside of polymorphonuclear leukocytes from aspirated joint fluid. They are strongly birefringent when viewed under polarized microscopy. Crystals from tophi are seen alone because the tophus material is acellular. Joint fluid in gout is inflammatory, with elevated leukocyte counts, which can result in diagnostic confusion between septic arthritis and gout. Joint aspiration might not always be performed or be successful, and the American College of Rheumatology has developed additional criteria for diagnosis. Six of the following criteria are needed for diagnosis: recurrent acute arthritis; acute inflammation that develops over 1 day; monoarticular arthritis; redness of the joint; unilateral first metatarsal joint pain or swelling; unilateral tarsal joint swelling; suspected tophus; hyperuricemia; asymmetric swelling within a joint on x-ray; subcortical cysts without erosions on x-ray; and negative joint fluid culture during an attack. Additional tests that support the diagnosis of gout are elevated serum uric acid levels, complete blood count and differential, and serum creatinine. Radiography, although not typically helpful in diagnosing acute gout, can show characteristic changes with chronic gout, including subcortical cysts, proliferative bony reaction, and tophi-induced bone destruction away from the joint space.

Differential Diagnoses

Calcium pyrophosphate deposition disease (CPDD) and pseudogout can be confused with gout. The 2 diseases can be distinguished by crystal analysis from joint fluid as calcium pyrophosphate crystals are rhomboid shaped and weakly birefringent on polarized microscopy. CPDD results in cartilage calcification of the knee, symphysis pubis, glenoid and acetabular labrum, and wrist.

Rheumatoid arthritis (RA) presents as a symmetric polyarticular arthritis typically in the hands and feet. Gout, especially recurrent gout, may be polyarticular, but RA is more likely to involve the hands than gout. Rheumatoid synovitis may be confused with gout. Up to 20% of patients with RA will have rheumatoid nodules, but these do not occur in the same locations as gout tophi. Radiographs can distinguish RA from gout as RA results in diffuse joint space narrowing, osteopenia and erosions of small joints.

Septic arthritis also presents as monoarticular or oligoarticular arthritis, associated with pain swelling and redness. Fever can be a common presenting sign with both conditions. The best way to distinguish these 2 conditions is with joint aspiration.

Osteoarthritis doesn't cause joint inflammation but hallus valgus is common and may be confused with podagra.

Psoriatic arthritis affects distal interphalangeal joints of the fingers and nail changes. These are not seen in gout. However, patients with psoriasis can have elevated uric acid levels.

Treatment

Routine treatment of elevated uric acid levels is not recommended. Patients with elevated uric acid levels should be counseled on lifestyle changes, including dietary reduction of purines, weight loss, and reduction of alcohol intake. Also medications known to impair uric acid secretion should be avoided.

Nonsteroidal antiinflammatory drugs (NSAIDs) are usually first-line treatment for acute gout. Patients should be treated with NSAIDs for 2–10 days. Nonprescription drugs, such as ibuprofen or naproxen, are as effective as indomethacin. If a patient is at increased risk for gastrointestinal complications, proton pump inhibitors can reduce the incidence of ulcers related to NSAIDs.

Colchicine is also a first-line agent for acute gout; however, its potential for side effects, especially diarrhea, can limit its effectiveness. The current recommendation is to treat with 0.6 mg 2–3 times a day.

Corticosteroids also can be used for acute gout and are preferred for patients with kidney disease. Intraarticular injections can be useful for monoarticular gout once infection has been ruled out.

Long-term treatment directed at lowering uric acid levels is recommended for a patient who has had more than 2 or 3 acute gout attacks. It should also be given for tophaceous gout, severe attacks of polyarticular gout, joint damage seen on radiographs,

and uric acid nephrolithiasis. Patients with known inborn errors of uric acid metabolism should also be treated. The goal of treatment is to maintain uric acid levels less than 6 mg/dL.

Xanthine oxidase inhibitors include allopurinol and febuxostat. These drugs should be started after the acute gout attack subsides. Concurrent treatment with colchicine reduces gout attacks initially. Dose range for allopurinol is usually 100–800 mg, with the average dose usually in 400–600 mg/day range. The febuxostat dose range is 40–120 mg/day.

Probenecid is the only uricosuric drug available in the United States. To determine if a patient should be treated with probenecid, a 24-hour urine for uric acid and creatinine should be collected while consuming a low purine diet and not during an acute flare. If the uric acid level is less than 600–700 mg/dL, then probenecid can be considered. Probenecid should not be used in patients with known uric acid nephrolithiasis. Probenecid can be combined with allopurinol in resistant patients.

Rasburicase is a recombinant form of urate oxidase that promotes the conversion of uric acid to allantoin. It is used for the prevention of tumor lysis syndrome.

Baker JF, Schumacher HR. Update on gout and hyperuricemia. *Int J Clin Pract.* 2010;64(3):371-377.

Malik A, Schumacher HR, Dinnella JE, Clayburne GM. Clinical diagnostic criteria for gout: comparison with the gold standard of synovial fluid crystal analysis. *J Clin Rheumatol.* 2009;15(1):22-24.

Mandell BF. Clinical manifestations of hyperuricemia and gout. *Cleve Clin J Med.* 2008;75 Suppl 5:S5-S8.

Wallace SL, Robinson H, Masi AT, Decker JL, McCarty DJ, Yü TF. Preliminary criteria for the classification of the acute arthritis of primary gout. *Arthritis Rheum.* 1977;20(3):895-900.

Wallace KL, Riedel AA, Joseph-Ridge N, Wortmann R. Increasing prevalence of gout and hyperuricemia over 10 years among older adults in a managed care population. *J Rheumatol.* 2004;31(8):1582-1587.

Wilson JF. In the clinic. Gout. *Ann Intern Med.* 2010;152(3):ITC21.

CALCIUM PYROPHOSPHATE CRYSTAL DISEASE

General Principles in Older Adults

CPPD is associated with aging. The average age of patients with CPPD is 72 years, with an incidence of greater than 50% in patients older than age 85 years. The sex distribution for disease occurrence is roughly equal for men and women. CPPD may occur in previously traumatized joints or in joints that have required surgery. Some metabolic conditions, including hemochromatosis, hyperparathyroidism, hypophosphatasia, hypomagnesemia, and Gitelman syndrome, should be ruled out when younger patients present with CPPD. The European League Against Rheumatism (EULAR) recently established the following nomenclature for CPPD: Pseudogout for acute attacks of crystal-induced synovitis resembling gout; chondrocalcinosis when calcification is seen in hyaline or fibrocartilage (this finding can also occur with crystal deposition); and pyrophosphate arthropathy describes joint disease or radiographic abnormalities accompanying CPPD crystal disease.

Symptoms and Differential Diagnosis

Clinically, the disease may present in different ways. Asymptomatic disease is common with CPPD crystal deposition seen on radiographs. Pseudogout presents as self-limited acute attacks that resemble gout with acute inflammation and swelling. Fever and elevated leukocyte count can also be seen. These attacks, like gout can be precipitated by trauma, medical illness, but can also be associated with fluctuation in calcium levels that can occur post parathyroidectomy. The joints that are affected by pseudogout differ from gout because the knee is the most commonly affected joint. Urate and CPPD crystal disease can occur together and definitive diagnosis can only be made with joint aspiration. Pseudo-RA (chronic calcium pyrophosphate crystal inflammatory arthritis) should be suspected with more chronic symptoms of inflammatory arthritis in multiple joints associated with CPPD crystal in the joint fluid. The diagnosis can be difficult to distinguish from RA, as patients can experience morning stiffness and synovial thickness. Radiographs can be helpful, as the findings are more suggestive of osteoarthritis than RA. Pseudo-osteoarthritis (OA with CPPD) can occur with or without superimposed acute attacks. Half the patients with symptomatic CPPD will develop joint degeneration. The most common joint affected is the knee, which is often difficult to distinguish from OA. The diagnosis is more straightforward when the joints involved are less typical for OA, such as wrists, metacarpophalangeal, hips, shoulders, elbows, or spine. Pseudoneuropathic joint disease caused by CPPD crystal deposition can lead to joint degeneration and Charcot joint. Spinal involvement can be seen in CPPD and result in spine stiffness resembling ankylosing spondylitis or diffuse idiopathic skeletal hyperostosis.

Findings

Analysis of synovial fluid is the most important diagnostic criterion for CPPD. The presence of positively birefringent rhomboid crystals within leukocytes is pathognomonic for the disease. The synovial leukocyte count will also be elevated. A definitive diagnosis can be made when both weakly positive birefringent crystals are seen in synovial fluid or tissues and cartilage or joint capsule calcification is seen on radiographs.

Treatment

Acute pseudogout is managed in the same way as gout. Pseudogout should be treated with joint aspiration and NSAIDs. Intraarticular steroids can be utilized if infection has been ruled out. Colchicine and oral glucocorticoids are additional options. For patients with recurrent pseudogout attacks who present with 3 or more episodes should be treated with colchicine prophylaxis. The dose is 0.6 mg BID, although in elderly patients or patients unable to tolerate BID dosing, once daily can be considered.

Pseudo-RA can be treated with NSAIDs or colchicine. Second-line agents include low-dose glucocorticoid, methotrexate, and hydroxychloroquine.

For patients with OA with CPPD, treatment is determined by the presence or absence of intermittent episodes of pseudogout. If unaccompanied by acute episodes, then treatment is the same as that for OA.

McCarty DJ. Calcium pyrophosphate dihydrate crystal deposition disease. *Arthritis Rheum.* 1976;19 Suppl 3:275-285.

Zhang W, Doherty M, Bardin T, et al. European League Against Rheumatism recommendations for calcium pyrophosphate deposition. Part I: terminology and diagnosis. *Ann Rheum Dis.* 2011;70(4):563-570.

POLYMYALGIA RHEUMATICA

General Principles in Older Adults

Polymyalgia rheumatica (PMR) is a common condition affecting middle age and older patients. The incidence of PMR increases after the age of 50 years and peaks between 70 and 80 years. It is more common in women than in men. It is related to temporal arteritis or giant cell arteritis in approximately 16% of cases. They may be different phases of the same disease.

Symptoms

PMR should be suspected when a patient older than 50 years presents with typical symptoms, which include at least 1 month of bilateral aching of the shoulders or proximal muscles of the arms and hips or proximal aspects of the thighs. Neck or torso stiffness might also be present. The stiffness is worse in the morning and lasts up to 1 hour. Muscular pain can interfere with activities of daily living. Patients may complain of discomfort with activities that utilize proximal muscles of the arms and legs such as grooming or stair climbing. Shoulder pain is the most typical presenting symptom, with hip and neck less frequently involved.

Findings

On physical examination both passive and active range of motion of the shoulders is reduced because of pain. Joint pain of swelling is not seen with PMR. Systemic symptoms, such as malaise, fever, fatigue, and weight loss, can be seen in up to one-third of patients. Erythrocyte sedimentation rate (ESR) will be greater than 40 mm/h, and other inflammatory markers, such as C-reactive protein, will be elevated. Mild normocytic anemia can also be seen.

Differential Diagnosis

Proximal pain and stiffness can be seen in many rheumatologic diseases that affect older people. Half the cases of PMR have distal symptoms, such as an asymmetric peripheral arthritis, that primarily affect the wrists and knees. Hand swelling with pitting edema of the dorsum of the hand and carpal tunnel syndrome can be seen. When these symptoms are present, it is difficult to differentiate between PMR and RA. A negative rheumatoid factor and absence of joint erosions can distinguish the 2 conditions. The rare condition of remitting seronegative symmetric synovitis with pitting edema also causes pitting edema of the hands and feet and responds to steroids. Rheumatoid factor is negative in this condition, which may be part of the same disease spectrum as PMR.

Systemic lupus erythematosus can present in the elderly with symptoms that mimic PMR. The presence of additional findings such as pericarditis, pleuritis, leukopenia, or thrombocytopenia, and a positive antinuclear antibody will distinguish these conditions.

Late-onset spondyloarthropathy can result in proximal symptoms but the presence of peripheral enthesitis, anterior uveitis, and sacroiliitis differentiate these conditions.

Polymyositis presents with more muscle weakness and causes elevated muscle enzymes. Fibromyalgia patients experience painful trigger points and have a normal ESR.

Primary systemic amyloidosis may share symptoms with PMR, but these patients do not respond to steroids and have a monoclonal band on immunoelectrophoresis.

Treatment

Corticosteroids are the drug of choice for PMR. The dose for prednisone is 10–20 mg, and the response to treatment is rapid. Symptoms typically resolve within days. Treatment with the initial dose should be continued for 2–4 weeks and gradually tapered every 1–2 weeks. Rapid taper can result in recurrent symptoms and caution should be taken to ensure judicious tapering of steroid dose. Even with slow tapering 30% to 50% of patients can have spontaneous recurrence of symptoms requiring increased steroid dose. Monitoring patients by assessment of symptoms and ESR is useful. Steroid dose should not be increased if ESR is increased without recurrent symptoms. Most patients require 1–2 years of treatment.

Methotrexate can be used as a steroid-sparing agent in patients with severe symptoms requiring high doses of steroids.

Dasgupta B, Cimmino MA, Maradit-Kremers H, et al. 2012 provisional classification criteria for polymyalgia rheumatica: a European League Against Rheumatism/American College of Rheumatology collaborative initiative. *Ann Rheum Dis.* 2012;71(4):484-492.

Salvarani C, Cantini F, Boiardi L, Hunder GG. Polymyalgia rheumatica and giant-cell arteritis. *N Engl J Med.* 2002;347(4): 261-271.

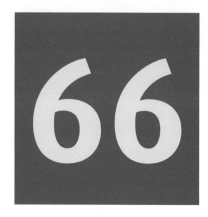

Managing Back Pain in Older Adults

Una E. Makris, MD

Leo M. Cooney Jr, MD

General Principles in Older Adults

Back pain is 1 of the top 3 reasons for physician visits by older adults. Of the 1037 surviving subjects from the original Framingham Heart Study cohort (ages 68–100 years), 22% had back pain on most days. Although back pain in older adults is prevalent, costly, and leads to considerable morbidity, much of the literature has focused on younger populations with this condition.

Back pain is often categorized as acute (lasts less than 4 weeks), subacute (lasts between 4 and 12 weeks), or chronic (lasts longer than 3 months). Although much of the literature evaluates chronic symptoms, a recent article using longitudinal data reported that most back pain in older adults has a recurrent or episodic course. Understanding the various patterns of back pain in older persons is important as prevention and treatment planning may differ. Table 66–1 identifies the terminology used to describe back pain.

In older individuals, there are several specific causes for back pain (eg, lumbar spinal stenosis, osteoporotic vertebral compression fractures, and sacral fractures) that are less common in younger individuals. Systemic conditions, such as malignancy and infections, although rarely the cause of back pain, are more common in older compared to younger age groups. One of the most challenging aspects of assessing and managing back pain is identifying the source(s) of pain in the older adult who often has multiple musculoskeletal comorbidities (eg, trochanteric bursitis, hip osteoarthritis, multilevel lumbar degenerative changes, and lumbar stenosis). These conditions rarely occur in isolation, and pinpointing which one contributes most to the patient's pain is not a trivial endeavor.

A systematic approach to the diagnosis of lower back pain in older adults requires knowledge of the typical presentation of common back conditions of older adults, an understanding of the anatomy of the lumbar spine, the identification of physical findings associated with common abnormalities, and the judicious use of diagnostic imaging studies.

Symptoms

Back pain (with or without radiating symptoms to the buttocks, legs and feet) is the most common symptom that patients will report. The question, "Where is your back pain located?" is most helpful in determining cervical versus thoracic versus lumbar spine pain. Low back pain (lumbar spine) is the most common site of pain. Even though the patient may report low back pain, the pain may originate from the hip and radiate to the spine or legs in a distribution that resembles back disease.

The timing and onset of pain are important to elicit. Back pain is most often characterized by intermittent, positional pain that is worse at onset and that usually improves over time. Pain that is insidious in onset, progressive in its course, nonpositional, associated with night pain and systemic symptoms or signs, and that persists for longer than 1 month should raise concerns about malignancy or infection.

Findings

The physical examination of the back, hips, and legs is essential in the assessment of an older adult with back pain. The finding of subtle, but asymmetric, weakness of the hip, ankle, and foot muscles innervated by the lumbar and sacral nerves can help elucidate the cause of back and leg pain.

The physical exam of an older adult with back pain begins with observation of gait and posture, followed by inspection of the back and palpation of the spine and paraspinal muscles. Patients with lumbar spinal stenosis often bend forward as they walk, while patients with hip disease are more likely to limp. The back exam includes range of motion in 4 planes (forward flexion, extension, side flexion to the left and right) with attention to symmetry. Asymmetric limitation of the range of motion of the lumbar spine, or reproduction of the pain with these maneuvers, often indicates mechanical disease of the lumbar spine. The pain of lumbar spinal stenosis is often reproduced by spinal extension. A straight-leg

Table 66–1. Back pain terminology.

Cauda equina syndrome	Compression of multiple nerve roots resulting in bilateral motor weakness (usually of legs), bowel or bladder incontinence, saddle anesthesia; a surgical emergency.
Kyphosis	Outward curve of the thoracic spine.
Lordosis	Inward curve of the lumbar spine.
Piriformis syndrome	Entrapment resulting in pain, numbness, paresthesia, weakness in the distribution of sciatic nerve. Often after direct trauma to sacroiliac or gluteal region, occasionally caused by repetitive hip or lower-extremity movements or repeat pressure on the piriformis muscle.
Radiculopathy	Impairment of a nerve root usually causing pain, numbness, tingling, or muscle weakness that usually corresponds with the nerve root.
Sciatica	Pain, numbness, tingling in distribution of sciatic nerve. Symptoms radiate down posterior or lateral leg, usually to foot or ankle. Usually caused by mechanical pressure or inflammation of lumbosacral nerve root(s).
Scoliosis	Abnormal, sideways curvature of the spine.
Spinal stenosis	Narrowing of the central spinal canal by bone or soft tissue elements. Pain, numbness often radiate from low back to buttock and/or thigh and often associated with neurogenic claudication.
Spondylolisthesis	Anterior displacement of vertebra on the one beneath. Graded by radiologist base on percentage of slippage on x-rays.
Spondylosis	Arthritis of the spine. Radiographically: disc space narrowing and arthritic changes at facet joints.
Spondylolysis	Fracture in the pars interarticularis where vertebral body and posterior elements, protecting the nerves are joined.

raise test can be informative (indicative of herniated disc, for example) if positive, but a negative test does not exclude any condition.

Each patient with a back complaint should have a complete examination of the hips, focusing on passive range of motion. The examiner should be able to abduct the hip to 40 degrees before the pelvis starts to tilt. The hip should flex beyond 110 degrees, externally rotate 50–60 degrees, and internally rotate 15–20 degrees. The hip is more likely to be the cause of the pain if the individual has pain in the groin, a limp, or limited range of motion of the hip. Back disease is more likely to cause pain when an individual goes from the supine to the sitting position.

For patients who present with leg symptoms, manual examination of the leg muscles can be helpful. Nerve root irritation from a spinal process should affect the muscles innervated by the respective nerve roots. Thus, an individual

with lumbar spine disease at the L4–L5 and the L5–S1 level should have weakness of the hip abductor and hip extensor, as well as of the ankle dorsiflexor, great toe dorsiflexor, and ankle evertor. A patient with a peroneal palsy should have weakness of the great toe extensor, ankle dorsiflexor, and ankle evertors, but no involvement of the hip abductors and hip extensors.

If the older adult presents with persistent pain or a history that strongly suggests systemic disease, a careful evaluation for malignancy (breast, prostate, lymph node exam) and infection is warranted.

Laboratory tests are not specific for back pain, although, if positive in the appropriate clinical setting, may suggest underlying systemic disease. Ordering a complete blood count, erythrocyte sedimentation rate, C-reactive protein, or serum protein electrophoresis may be helpful if the history and physical exam suggest infection or tumor. Keep in mind that older adults may not consistently mount the inflammatory response (indicated by fever, leukocytosis) that we expect to see in younger adults in the face of infection. Other clues, such as altered mental status, may trigger suspicion for infection.

Diagnostic imaging can complicate the evaluation of pain in older adults as the prevalence of anatomic abnormalities unrelated to back pain is high. The lack of specificity of diagnostic imaging heightens the importance of the history and physical examination as an evaluation tool.

Although routine imaging for low back pain in younger populations is not recommended, imaging of the spine may be indicated in older adults with back pain. According to the American College of Radiology, the following criteria should be used to determine who is at higher risk for systemic disease-related back pain and when it may be appropriate to obtain imaging: recent significant trauma or milder trauma (age >50 years); unexplained weight loss or fever; immunosuppression (including diagnoses such as diabetes mellitus); history of cancer; IV drug use; osteoporosis or prolonged use of glucocorticoids; age >70 years; focal neurologic deficits that are progressive or produce disabling symptoms; and, lastly, duration of 6 weeks or more (subacute or chronic). According to these criteria, many older adults who present with new-onset back symptoms will receive an imaging modality.

Initial imaging modalities include lumbar radiographs that evaluate alignment, instability, and scoliosis, as well as postoperative evaluation of instrumentation and fusion. This single diagnostic tool can demonstrate degenerative disc and joint disease, vertebral compression fractures, deformities such as spondylolisthesis and scoliosis, and systemic disorders such as osteoporosis and Paget disease. In certain clinical scenarios, early CT or MRI may be ordered to facilitate diagnosis. For example, CT may be useful in depicting structural bone problems (spondylolisthesis, fracture, or stenosis). MRI short-tau inversion recovery and fat-saturated T2 fast spin-echo sequences may detect facet arthropathy and edema. MRI with contrast can aid in the diagnosis of infection or

Table 66–2. Differential diagnosis for back pain in older persons.

Systemic Causes of Back Pain
Malignancy: Multiple myeloma, metastatic disease, lymphoma, spinal cord tumors, retroperitoneal tumors
Infection: Osteomyelitis, septic discitis, paraspinous abscess, bacterial endocarditis
Inflammatory arthritis: Ankylosing spondylitis, psoriatic arthritis, reactive arthritis, inflammatory bowel disease
Osteochondrosis
Paget disease
Visceral: aortic aneurysm, prostatitis, nephrolithiasis, pyelonephritis, perinephric abscess, pancreatitis, cholecystitis, penetrating ulcer, fat herniation of lumbar space
Nonsystemic/Mechanical Causes of Back Pain
Spinal stenosis
Sciatica
Osteoporotic vertebral or sacral compression fractures
Lumbar strain (muscle)
Herniated disc
Spondylolisthesis
Diffuse idiopathic skeletal hyperostosis (DISH)
Congenital disease: kyphosis, scoliosis
Spondylolysis
Piriformis syndrome
Degenerative disease: spondylosis (discs and facet joints)

malignancy. The first large, randomized, controlled trial to evaluate patient-reported outcome measures in older adults with back pain who receive early imaging compared to no early imaging is currently underway.

▶ Differential Diagnoses

Categorizing back pain into systemic and nonsystemic causes is a helpful way to think about its broad differential diagnosis in older adults (Table 66–2). Nonspecific mechanical back pain (of unclear etiology) and degenerative diseases are the most common diagnoses of back pain in older adults.

The history and physical exam are helpful in distinguishing systemic from nonsystemic/degenerative/mechanical causes of back pain.

A. Systemic Causes of Back Pain

The absence of the typical physical examination findings of motor weakness of the L4 through S1 innervated muscles of the hip and foot may indicate systemic disease. The likelihood

of cancer as a cause of back pain increases in adults ≥50 years old, those with a previous history of cancer, and those with pain that persists longer than 1 month.

Fever, focal vertebral tenderness, and upper lumbar or thoracic nonpositional pain may indicate vertebral infection. Approximately 10% of older adults with endocarditis may present with back pain. Infections leading to back pain are more likely in individuals at risk for endovascular infections.

Visceral disease (abdominal aortic aneurysms, bladder distention caused by urinary retention, large uterine fibroids, intraabdominal infections or tumors) can present with back pain. Referred pain from these conditions is usually suggested by the history, pattern of pain, the absence of positional changes, and a normal physical examination of the lumbosacral spine.

B. Nonsystemic/Mechanical Causes of Back Pain

The pain of mechanical disease is usually intermittent, positional, and often worse at onset. Several of the more common nonsystemic causes of back pain are discussed here.

Lumbar spinal stenosis results from a narrowing of either the central or lateral aspect of the lumbar spine canal. The characteristic symptom of lumbar spinal stenosis is pain in the back or in the legs that worsens with standing or walking. Pain in the calf when walking is called neurogenic or pseudoclaudication and can mimic the symptoms of claudication from arterial insufficiency. Walking can result in paresthesia, numbness, and weakness in 1 or both legs. Positions that flex the spine, such as sitting, bending forward, walking uphill, and lying in a flexed position, relieve symptoms; positions that extend the lumbar spine, such as prolonged standing, walking, and walking downhill, will exacerbate symptoms. Stenosis symptoms are usually progressive and consistent, rather than intermittent. There may be subtle weakness in the muscles innervated by the L4, L5, and S1 nerve roots.

Sciatica, as defined in Table 66–1, may be acute or chronic. Acute sciatica usually occurs spontaneously, with no clear causal event. Although the clinical course of acute sciatica is variable, it usually occurs spontaneously, with no clear precipitating event. The pain may be felt throughout the distribution of the sciatic nerve and is not positional (it does not remit or subside in certain positions). These patients typically have a favorable clinical course, similar to that seen in younger patients.

Lumbar degenerative disc disease is common (but not universal) with the aging spine. The disc space narrowing and arthritis of the facet joints may produce a *relatively* unstable lumbar spine. In addition to the pain in the back, individuals with this condition may also report symptoms of sciatica. The pain usually comes on suddenly after particular movements or activity (eg, carrying or lifting heavy objects, flexing or extending the lumbar spine). The pain may be short-lived (lasting minutes to hours) but often will recur. On physical examination, the patient may exhibit guarded movements of the lumbar spine and pain is exacerbated with moving from flexion to extension. Imaging studies will reveal significant disc space narrowing, vertebral end-plate sclerosis, and osteophytosis at 1 disc space disproportionate to the other spaces.

Diffuse idiopathic skeletal hyperostosis (DISH) occurs most frequently in older, obese men. DISH is characterized by calcification and ossification of spinal ligaments (typically in the thoracic spine) and formation of bridging enthesophytes elsewhere. It is asymptomatic and detected inadvertently on imaging studies. Loss of range of motion and stiffness may be more common than pain.

Osteoporotic vertebral compression fractures are often asymptomatic, although approximately 33% will have severe symptoms. The onset of pain is abrupt. Intense pain is felt at the site of the fracture. The pain is usually worse on standing and walking, and relieved with lying down. Although the pain commonly radiates to the flank, abdomen, and legs, neurologic sequelae usually do not occur in patients with spontaneous osteoporotic fractures. Symptomatic fractures most often affect the lower thoracic and lumbar vertebrae. The pain from an acute vertebral fracture usually lasts at least 3–4 weeks. Patients with these fractures are at high risk for subsequent fractures, are more disabled, and have a higher mortality than those without fractures. Hence, primary and secondary prevention efforts for this condition are paramount.

Osteoporotic sacral fractures are more prevalent among older women than older men and the incidence of associated osteoporotic fractures is high. Sacral fracture often occurs spontaneously and patients will report pain in the lower back, buttock, or hip; sacral tenderness is present on physical examination. On imaging studies, plain films are usually negative, a technetium bone scan may show an H-shaped uptake over the sacrum, and a CT scan shows displacement of the anterior sacrum. These patients have an excellent prognosis and rarely report neurologic deficits or pain beyond 4–6 weeks.

Nonspecific back pain, where there is no particular lesion or etiology identified as the root cause of pain, is a common back pain diagnosis. Keep in mind that most back pain symptoms in older adults will be accompanied by radiographic evidence for degenerative changes, however, it remains questionable if the patient's symptoms correspond to the radiographic changes given what we know about the specificity of these imaging studies. Assessment of back pain in older persons has been limited by a lack of information about the natural history of this condition. A recent study evaluated individuals older than the age of 70 years and found that 80% of episodes in back pain individuals lasted less than 4 weeks. This information is very helpful, as the defined causes of back pain in older persons (tumor, infection, lumbar spinal stenosis, and compression fractures) are not likely to resolve within 4 weeks. Most episodes of back pain in older persons are self-limited, of short duration, likely to recur, and are probably mechanical (noninflammatory) in origin.

▶ Next Steps

Generally, management of back pain in older adults should focus on addressing the structural cause that is the most likely source of pain; identifying this source of pain is usually the most challenging step. The most appropriate therapy for an older patient with back pain must be determined in the context of the individual's comorbid conditions, understanding potential interactions with other medications, and after discussing their preferences and goals of treatment.

Treatment of low back pain usually begins with conservative, nonoperative modalities, including patient education, nonopioid analgesics (acetaminophen or nonsteroidal antiinflammatory drugs, if not contraindicated) and activity modification. Once the acute symptoms subside, a gentle progressive exercise program (initially with supervision from a physical therapist) should be started to strengthen the spinal and abdominal musculature. The goals of therapeutic exercises include increased flexibility by stretching, improved muscle strength by resistive exercise, and improved endurance with repetition. Heat or cold modalities may relieve pain and loosen muscles and may be tried prior to physical therapy exercises. Hot compresses must be used cautiously to avoid skin burns.

Management of chronic mechanical pain is aimed at reducing or eliminating the repetitive movements or activities that result in excessive vertebral motion. Activity modification begins with identifying the activities that result in new or worsening back pain, and, ultimately, avoiding or altering those activities in such a way to reduce pain. Physical therapy and home exercises may help by strengthening the paraspinous and abdominal muscles, essentially providing an internal "brace" for the lumbar spine. These exercises are most helpful if practiced routinely and consistently. In severe cases that have not responded to conservative therapy, surgical options may be considered.

The most important goal of management for vertebral compression fractures is adequate analgesia while avoiding the complications of bed rest and inactivity that result from the acute pain. Because the acute pain is relatively brief, braces and corsets are rarely required. Once the acute pain subsides, gentle spinal extension exercises may be helpful. If conservative measures fail, minimally invasive techniques are available and should be discussed with a surgeon who is experienced in treating the older patient with back pain.

If progressive and resulting in neurologic deficits because of mechanical encroachment on lumbar nerve roots, lumbar spinal stenosis may not respond to conservative therapies. Although epidural corticosteroid injections have been used extensively for the sciatica associated with lumbar spinal stenosis, a review of controlled trials of this therapy did not demonstrate efficacy of injection over controls. Lumbar spinal stenosis is the most common indication for spinal surgery in older adults. In a prospective study of surgery for spinal stenosis, the ideal candidates for surgery were found to be those patients with severe narrowing of the spinal canal, minimal associated back pain, no coexisting conditions that affect walking, and symptom duration of less than 4 years. In 2 randomized, controlled trials and a high-quality observational study, surgery provided earlier and greater pain relief and improvement in functional status.

Indications for referral to a surgeon include cauda equina syndrome, suspected cord compression, and progressive or severe neurologic deficits. Most surgical interventions (decompression, laminectomy, fusion) are nonurgent so it is imperative to work closely with a thoughtful, conservative surgeon who can take time to explain the procedure, risks, and benefits to the older patient.

Atlas SJ. Point of view: in the eye of the beholder: preferences of patients, family physicians, and surgeons for lumbar spinal surgery. *Spine* (Phila Pa 1976). 2010;35(1):116.

Chang Y, Singer DE, Wu YA, Keller RB, Atlas SJ. The effect of surgical and nonsurgical treatment on longitudinal outcomes of lumbar spinal stenosis over 10 years. *J Am Geriatr Soc.* 2005;53(5):785-792.

Chou R, Qaseem A, Snow V, et al. Diagnosis and treatment of low back pain: a joint clinical practice guideline from the American College of Physicians and the American Pain Society. *Ann Intern Med.* 2007;147(7):478-491.

Deyo RA, Mirza SK, Martin BI. Back pain prevalence and visit rates: estimates from U.S. national surveys, 2002. *Spine.* 2006;31(23):2724-2727.

Deyo RA, Weinstein JN. Low back pain. *N Engl J Med.* 2001;344(5):363-370.

Di Iorio A, Abate M, Guralnik JM, et al. From chronic low back pain to disability, a multifactorial mediated pathway: the InCHIANTI study. *Spine.* 2007;32(26):E809-E815.

Edmond SL, Felson DT. Function and back symptoms in older adults. *J Am Geriatr Soc.* 2003;51(12):1702-1709.

Freburger JK, Holmes GM, Agans RP, et al. The rising prevalence of chronic low back pain. *Arch Intern Med.* 2009;169(3):251-258.

Hadjistavropoulos T, Herr K, Turk DC, et al. An interdisciplinary expert consensus statement on assessment of pain in older persons. *Clin J Pain.* 2007;23(1 Suppl):S1-S43.

Hanlon JT, Backonja M, Weiner D, Argoff C. Evolving pharmacological management of persistent pain in older persons. *Pain Med.* 2009;10(6):959-961.

Jacobs JM, Hammerman-Rozenberg R, Cohen A, et al. Chronic back pain among the elderly: prevalence, associations, and predictors. *Spine.* 2006;31:E203-E207.

Katz JN. Lumbar disc disorders and low-back pain: socioeconomic factors and consequences. *J Bone Joint Surg Am.* 2006;88 Suppl 2:21-24.

Lavsky-Shulan M, Wallace RB, Kohout FJ, et al. Prevalence and functional correlates of low back pain in the elderly: the Iowa 65+ Rural Health Study. *J Am Geriatr Soc.* 1985;33:23-28.

Makris UE, Fraenkel L, Han L, Leo-Summers L, Gill TM. Epidemiology of restricting back pain in community-living older persons. *J Am Geriatr Soc.* 2011;59(4):610-614.

Reid MC, Williams CS, Concato J, et al. Depressive symptoms as a risk factor for disabling back pain in community-dwelling older persons. *J Am Geriatr Soc.* 2003;51:1710-1717.

Reid MC, Williams CS, Gill TM. Back pain and decline in lower extremity physical function among community-dwelling older persons. *J Gerontol A Biol Sci Med Sci.* 2005;60(6):793-797.

Rudy TE, Weiner DK, Lieber SJ, Slaboda J, Boston JR. The impact of chronic low back pain on older adults: a comparative study of patients and controls. *Pain.* 2007;131(3):293-301.

Weiner DK, Haggerty CL, Kritchevsky SB, et al. How does low back pain impact physical function in independent, well-functioning older adults? Evidence from the Health ABC Cohort and implications for the future. *Pain Med.* 2003;4(4):311-320.

Determining the Appropriate Use of Exercise for Older Adults

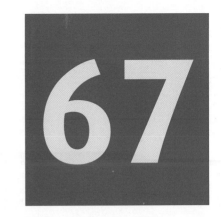

Sara J. Francois, PT, DPT, MS

Jennifer S. Brach, PhD, PT

Stephanie Studenski, MD, MPH

Case Vignette

Ethel, your 75-year-old patient, comes into your office inquiring about starting an exercise program. Some of her friends participate in an exercise group and have been talking about the benefits of exercise. Ethel asks for your advice about starting her own exercise program. She has arthritis and hypertension, for which she takes a β-blocker; otherwise, Ethel is in good health.

▶ General Principles in Older Adults

Physical activity has a profound positive impact on health, chronic disease prevention, function, and fall prevention, especially for older adults; higher levels of physical activity have been linked to reduced morbidity and mortality. New evidence has emerged indicating the positive impact of physical activity on cognition and psychological health. Although physical activity has clear benefits to health and function, most older adults are not physically active or do not engage in activity at high enough intensities to obtain the noted health benefits. In fact, less than 10% of older adults meet the recommended guidelines for physical activity (ie, 30–60 minutes of moderate-to-vigorous physical activity per day, 5 or more days a week), accumulating only 5–10 minutes of moderate-to-vigorous physical activity per day.

Physical activity is not synonymous with exercise. *Physical activity* is "any bodily movement produced by skeletal muscles that results in energy expenditure," whereas *exercise*, a subset of physical activity, is "planned, structured, and repetitive bodily movement done to improve or maintain one or more components of physical fitness." Physical activity may not achieve the increased fitness levels that are often expected with exercise; however, physical activity can reduce the risks and complications of many chronic conditions and increase well-being if it is of sufficient intensity.

Multiple methods exist to identify the level of intensity of an activity. One method compares the energy cost of the activity to the energy cost at rest, assigning metabolic equivalents, or MET values to different activities. Estimates of the MET values are summarized in the *Compendium of Physical Activities*, and the level of intensity of an activity is based on its MET value. However, the *Compendium* was developed based on data from healthy adults. Because energy use may be more inefficient in older adults, the intensity based on the MET value may underestimate the intensity at which the older adult is working. For this reason, the best use of the *Compendium* in the older adult population is to create a hierarchy of activities that can be used to select gradually increasing energy-demanding activities, rather than using it to define the exact intensity of an activity.

Because MET levels may not be the best method to determine the intensity of an activity, other methods should be used to estimate how hard the older adult is working, such as heart rate, rating of perceived exertion (RPE), or the talk test. Using a percentage of the estimated maximum heart rate, traditionally calculated by subtracting the person's age from 220, is a simple way to determine intensity. Moderate intensity is defined as 64% to 76% of estimated maximum, and 77% to 93% of estimated maximum is considered vigorous intensity. Using heart rate methods is not appropriate in the presence of conditions that alter the heart rate response to exercise, such as the use of β blockers, some pacemakers, and many atrial arrhythmias.

Another option is the Borg RPE scale. While participating in an activity, a person rates how hard he is working on a scale from 6–20. Moderate intensity activity would be rated in the 12–13 range.

Another simple, although informal, method for determining intensity level is the talk test. While exercising at moderate intensity, a person should be able to talk, but not sing. If the person can sing, the activity is light intensity; if the person can only respond with a couple of words before needing to take a breath, the activity is vigorous intensity.

Table 67–1. Physical activity/exercise web resources for the patient and the clinician.

Patient Resource	Clinician Resource	Website Information and URL
X	X	Centers for Disease Control and Prevention Physical Activity website. http://www.cdc.gov/physicalactivity/index.html
		Information about many different topics related to physical activity.
X		Exercise: A guide from the National Institute on Aging. http://www.move.va.gov/download/Resources/NIAA_Exercise_Guide.pdf
		PDF about the benefits of exercise, how to exercise safely, and how to keep going with an exercise program; includes descriptions and pictures of exercises.
X		Exercise and Physical Activity: Your Everyday Guide from the National Institute on Aging. http://www.nia.nih.gov/sites/default/files/exercise_guide.pdf
		PDF about the benefits of exercise, how to start and keep going with an exercise program, setting goals and making an activity plan; includes descriptions and pictures of exercises; also includes activity logs and records.
		To order a hard copy of the booklet, go to this website: http://go4life.nia.nih.gov/exercise-guide-video and click "Order Now."
X	X	Exercise is Medicine. http://exerciseismedicine.org/
		Website designed to increase the discussion of physical activity between physicians and patients; includes handouts and fliers for both the clinician and the patient; includes a template for an exercise prescription.
X	X	Go4Life. http://go4life.nia.nih.gov/
		Patients can click on "Get Started" and get information about physical activity. Clinicians can click on "For Health Professionals" and get information and materials from the Go4Life campaign.
X		NIH Senior Health website. http://nihseniorhealth.gov/exerciseforolderadults/healthbenefits/01.html
		Information on the benefits of exercise with links to topics including "How to Get Started," "Exercises to Try," and "How to Stay Active"; also provides links to many other health topics that are important for older adults.
X		President's Council on Fitness, Sports, and Nutrition—Be Active website. http://www.fitness.gov/be-active/
		Information on why physical activity is important, how to be physically active, physical activity guidelines; provides links to other resources, and also provides links to information on eating healthy.

The healthcare provider should assess medical safety for exercise and recommend modifications for different conditions. The provider should also give the older adult key recommendations for safe, unsupervised exercise and be involved in improving patient adherence to exercise programs. Many websites exist for both the patient and the clinician to use as resources (Table 67–1). The challenge for the clinician is to prescribe activity that is appropriate and feasible based on the individual needs of the patient.

▶ Before an Older Adult Begins an Exercise Program

The need to screen an older adult prior to becoming physically active is controversial. Most exercise screening guidelines focus on recognizing conditions that require modifications to activities (Table 67–2) and determining safety during exercise (specifically cardiac screening and contraindications to exercise); however, cardiac screening (ie, exercise stress testing) is difficult to perform for many older adults and uncovers a huge reservoir of silent cardiac disease of unclear clinical significance. Many older adults do not plan to undertake a vigorous activity program, and moderate activity may be associated with negligible accumulated cardiac risk because of the associated cardiac risk reductions. For healthy and asymptomatic older adults, standard recommendations and precautions are appropriate with no need for cardiac screening. Cardiac screening is also not necessary for sedentary older adults beginning a low- to moderate-intensity activity program, especially considering the risks associated with being sedentary are worse than the risks of being physically active. Discussion of the symptoms during exercise that may indicate an inappropriate response to activity (eg, chest/jaw/arm pain, excessive dyspnea, palpitations, etc) is sufficient for these groups. Individuals with known cardiovascular disease are at risk for symptoms during activity and would benefit from cardiac screening prior to beginning an activity program.

The very few contraindications to physical activity include recent myocardial infarction, unstable angina, uncompensated congestive heart failure, severe valvular heart disease, resting systolic blood pressure above 200 mm Hg, resting

Table 67–2. Modifications of exercise prescription for selected conditions.

Condition	Modification
Back pain	Moderate intensity activities, water activities; low resistance, low repetition strength training; flexibility exercises; modified abdominal strengthening activities
Chronic obstructive lung disease	Moderate intensity activities using interval or intermittent approach; low resistance, low repetition strength training; modified flexibility and stretching exercises
Coronary artery disease	Symptom-limited activities: moderate intensity activities (eg, walking, cycling); more vigorous activities at physician's discretion; low resistance, high repetition strength training
Degenerative joint disease	Non-weight-bearing activities: stationary cycling, water exercises, chair exercises; low resistance, low repetition strength training
Diabetes mellitus	Daily, moderate intensity activities; low resistance, high repetition strength training; flexibility exercises
Dizziness, ataxia	Chair exercises; low resistance, low repetition strength training; moderate flexibility activities with minimal movement from supine or prone to standing
Hypertension	Dynamic large-muscle aerobic activities; minimize isometric work and focus on low resistance, high repetition isotonic strength training
Orthostatic hypotension	Minimize movements from standing to supine and supine to standing; sustained moderate intensity activities with short rest intervals
Osteoporosis	Weight-bearing activities with intermittent bouts of activity spaced throughout the day; low resistance, low repetition strength training; chair-level flexibility activities

Data from American College of Sports Medicine, Chodzko-Zajko WJ, Proctor DN, et al. American College of Sports Medicine position stand. Exercise and physical activity for older adults. *Med Sci Sports Exerc.* 2009;41(7):1510-1530; Whaley MH, ed. *ACSM's Guidelines for Exercise Testing and Prescription.* 7th ed. Philadelphia, PA: Lippincott Williams & Wilkins; 2006; and Bryant CX, Green DJ, eds. *Exercise for Older Adults: ACE's Guide for Fitness Professionals.* 2nd ed. San Diego, CA: American Council on Exercise; 2005.

diastolic blood pressure above 100 mm Hg, and significant abdominal aortic aneurysm. Some acute conditions, such as major bone fracture, nonhealing lesion on a weight-bearing extremity, or febrile illness may transiently limit activity.

▶ Exercise Prescription

The exercise prescription is based on the individual's current health and physical activity level. The prescription includes frequency, intensity, duration, and progression, as well as inclusion of warm-up, cool-down, different types of exercise

(eg, aerobic, strength, etc), stretching, and safety precautions. Exercise frequency, intensity, and duration will vary depending on the type of exercise. Moderate intensity is often recommended; however, not all older adults will be able to perform moderate levels of intensity. An activity that is light intensity for one older adult may be vigorous activity for another older adult. The recommended duration of 30 minutes or more for aerobic exercise may be intolerable for more deconditioned older adults. Brief episodes of activity (ie, stopping before fatigued) several times per day can help build toward more sustained activity.

All programs should progress over time so as to induce a level of stress on the body that results in change to the tissues. Duration should be progressed toward bouts of activity that lasts 20–30 minutes before intensity is progressed. It can take weeks or even months to reach this goal in the older adult population. All activity should begin with a warm-up of somewhat easy activities that slightly increase energy demands to prepare the body for exercise. The cool-down after exercise is also important as it is the transition phase for heart rate and oxygen consumption to return to resting levels. Slower walking or biking are examples of appropriate activities for warm-up and cool-down. Stretching should be performed after the warm-up and/or during the cool-down. General safety guidelines (Table 67–3) should also be included in the exercise prescription.

Exercise can be performed in the community, within the healthcare system, or at home, and can be supervised or unsupervised. Advantages and disadvantages exist for each situation, and the best fit for each patient depends on the needs of that patient.

Table 67–3. General patient instructions for exercise.

1. Start slowly and increase gradually.
2. Avoid holding your breath.
3. If you are on a medication or have a heart condition that changes your natural heart rate, do not use your pulse rate to judge how hard you should exercise.
4. Use safety equipment as recommended for the activity.
5. Drink plenty of fluids if performing activities that make you sweat unless your doctor has asked you to limit fluids.
6. Bend from the hips, not the waist, when bending forward.
7. Warm up muscles before stretching.
8. No exercise should be painful.
9. You can find the right amount of effort using the guideline "If you can talk without any trouble at all, your activity is probably too easy. If you cannot talk at all, it is too hard."
10. Always include a warm-up and cool-down that moves your body but doesn't tire you.

Data from Bryant CX, Green DJ, eds. *Exercise for Older Adults: ACE's Guide for Fitness Professionals.* 2nd ed. San Diego, CA: American Council on Exercise; 2005; and the National Institute on Aging at http://www.nia.nih.gov/health/publication/exercise-and-physical-activity-getting-fit-life

Table 67–4. Physical activity prescription by patient type.[a]

Patient Type	Duration (minutes)	Frequency	Examples of Exercise
Overt Disability			
Recently bed bound	5–10	Several times per day	Sitting ADL, passive and active range of motion, progress to standing and walking
Nonambulatory	5–10	Several times per day	Self-propel wheelchair, seated self-care, upper-extremity games and activities individually and in groups
Subclinical Disability			
Very sedentary	5–10	Several times per day	Slow walking program, group recreation
Inactive	20 or more	Most days of the week	Walking, gardening, housework, bicycling
Usual aging	30	Most days of the week	Brisk walking, stair climbing, moderate endurance recreation
Fit	30 or more	Most days	Moderate-to-high intensity: very brisk walks on uneven surfaces and hills, brisk stair climbing, moderate-to-vigorous sports

ADL, activity of daily living.

[a]Prescribing activity: (1) Let the patient select the preferred mode of activity; (2) start with an intensity and duration that is well tolerated; (3) initial exercise sessions should be observed if there has been no recent moderate activity; (4) initial sessions of moderate activity should include assessment of blood pressure and heart rate; (5) increase duration to a target training level (20–30 minutes or a set of 10 reps) before increasing intensity; (6) teach about self-monitoring of effort (eg, percent of maximum heart rate, Rating of Perceived Exertion, talk test, etc).

Most older adults have at least 1 medical condition that requires consideration when prescribing a physical activity program. Activities can be adapted to benefit specific needs or to avoid problems based on the condition (see Table 67–2). Many resources are available that provide specific guidelines and tips on how exercise prescription will differ for various diagnoses. Some older adults may appear independent in activities of daily living but have subclinical disability, demonstrated by reduced physical performance, requiring modifications to the exercise prescription.

Physical Activity

The current public health recommendation for older adults is to accumulate 30 minutes of moderate-intensity physical activity on most days of the week; recommendations for the other types of exercise (strength, flexibility, and balance) are in addition to this recommendation. Physical activity can be easily incorporated into daily life—simple ideas, such as taking the stairs instead of the elevator or parking further from the entrance to a building, can increase physical activity. Cross-training promotes variability in an activity program, reduces boredom, and decreases risk for injury. Activities such as swimming and use of exercise equipment that requires upper extremity effort can complement lower-extremity activities such as walking or bicycling.

Types of Exercise

Exercise is a subset of physical activity. Multiple types of exercise exist, including, but not limited to, aerobic, strength,

flexibility, and balance. The recommendations for aerobic exercise are typically considered to be the physical activity recommendations (ie, 30–60 minutes 5 or more days a week). Strength training to all major muscle groups is recommended 2 or more days per week, but not on consecutive days to allow for muscle recovery. Flexibility exercises should also be performed at least 2 days per week, and can be incorporated into an aerobic or strength program. For those older adults at risk for falls, balance exercises should be performed 3 times per week. Examples of the different types of activities or exercises for each of the categories are provided later in this chapter.

Older adults benefit from a prescription that includes all types of exercise, as all types are important for mobility and function. Major constraints on combined programs are time and fatigue; it is unrealistic for most older adults to undertake a program that demands hours of exercise each day. Some programs combine a mix of aerobic, strength, and balance activities into an hour-long session 3 days a week. The individual's preferences and current level of health should dictate the details of the prescription (Table 67–4).

A. Aerobic

Aging limits peak performance of aerobic exercise, but not the ability to benefit from training. Unsupervised aerobic exercise is appropriate for healthy older adults who are able to walk steadily at a brisk pace. Supervised aerobic exercise is appropriate for persons who have clinical or subclinical disability and cannot exercise continuously at moderate intensity.

Some examples of aerobic activity include walking, jogging/running, biking, and swimming. Other activities can be considered aerobic exercise if done at a high enough intensity; activities such as dancing, golfing, gardening, vacuuming, cleaning windows, and mowing the lawn are just a few examples.

The major risk associated with aerobic exercise is a cardiac event, such as myocardial infarction or death; however, this risk has been described after participation in *vigorous* exercise. Participating in *regular* aerobic exercise improves many cardiac risk factors and subsequently reduces the risk of cardiac events during activity.

B. Strength

Aging is associated with loss of muscle mass and power but both are responsive to strength training in older adults. Strength training can be performed with weight machines, free weights, or using body weight for resistance. Weight machines offer safe ways to lift heavier weights and provide complex systems to control the rate of muscle contraction. Using free weights such as wrist or ankle weights, low-tech items such as elastic bands, or household items like milk jugs or tin cans will work for strength training. Bearing the weight of the whole body in standing, transfers, and walking or performing active range of motion exercises can be a strength training activity for many frail older adults. Examples of body weight exercises include repeated chair stands, wall squats, and step ups.

Strength training should be performed for all major muscle groups, including, but not limited to, the shoulders, arms, hips, legs, ankles, back, and trunk. The lower-extremity muscle groups are larger and more important for functional mobility and independence; however, upper-extremity exercises will induce a higher heart rate response. Initial durations may be much briefer than with lower extremity exercise, as many people tend to have more deconditioned arms than legs.

The major risks with strength training include muscle soreness and musculoskeletal injury. Completing the exercise in good form by moving in a smooth, controlled manner rather than shaking or jerking through the movement will reduce the risk of injury. Starting with a low number of repetitions and a low amount of resistance will also reduce the risk of injury. It is also very important to avoid holding one's breath during strength training as it induces increased blood pressure. Key breathing guidelines are to start by taking a breath before lifting, exhale during lifting, and inhale during controlled release.

C. Flexibility

Flexibility decreases with age and can become significantly restricted with disease or disuse. Loss of range of motion affects mobility and function, and, in the worst case, can result in contractures that limit standing, walking, and reaching. Stretches should last 30–60 seconds and involve all major joints of the upper and lower extremity and trunk. The stretch should cause a sensation of pulling but not acute pain. To prevent injury, light to moderate activity to warm up the muscle before stretching for flexibility is advised. Contraindications to flexibility exercises include acutely inflamed joints, fused joints, and recent fracture.

D. Balance

Balance training is recommended for those older adults at risk for falls. The types of exercises and activities included in "balance training" are rarely defined in the literature, and there is little to no consensus on the frequency, intensity, and duration needed to induce benefits. Healthy older adults can improve balance through recreational activities that require displacement and recovery, such as dancing or tennis. Balance training for the very frail person involves movement practice in a seated position that requires displacement of the trunk and arms. Balance training in water allows patients to explore the margins of their ability to displace and recover without fear of injury, as falls are cushioned by the water.

Balance training requires progression of difficulty, making it inherently more dangerous than other types of exercise due of the increased risk of falling. Therefore, to reduce this risk, an older adult should only begin a balance training program after proper instruction by a health professional.

▶ Gaps in Current Exercise Recommendations

Recommendations exist for physical activity/aerobic exercise, strength, flexibility, and balance; however, these recommendations leave out an important aspect of physical activity in older adults—the timing and coordination of movement. Aging and disease can alter the timing and coordination of walking and subsequently reduce gait efficiency, resulting in older adults working harder to walk than they should be. Performing exercises to improve the timing and coordination of walking (ie, stepping and walking patterns with progression of difficulty) result in improved gait efficiency and subsequently improved walking ability. While the evidence for the benefits of this type of exercise is just emerging, it might be considered as part of an exercise prescription.

Another aspect of physical activity prescription that is often forgotten is that activity should be fun. Common barriers to exercise include the lack of motivation to participate in regular activity and the often boring and repetitive nature of many types of activity (ie, walking, jogging, bicycling, etc). Providing the older adult with examples of ways to make exercise fun, such as listening to music while performing the exercise or doing interactive video-based fitness activities, may be one way to increase participation and adherence.

► Continuing an Exercise Program

Convincing an older person to exercise can be a formidable challenge. Modern civilization has created a living environment that, although immeasurably beneficial, reduces the need for physical activity in daily life. How to begin and adhere to an exercise program is an important aspect of prescribing an activity plan that should be discussed with all patients.

Prior experience, knowledge, and beliefs about exercise will influence attitudes and expectations toward exercise. An older adult is more likely to participate in physical activity if he feels confident in his ability to succeed and that the activity is safe and enjoyable. For many older adults, the opportunity to socialize during exercise is a key motivating factor. Identifying these important contributors to participation and adherence for each older adult will encourage the initiation and maintenance of an exercise program.

A. Progression

All exercise requires a minimum frequency, intensity, and duration to achieve gain by inducing moderate physiological stress; thus, exercise must include a plan for progression over time. Many sedentary older adults are unable to sustain a moderate intensity activity for more than a few minutes. For this reason, the exercise program often must begin with a gradual increase in duration before any effort to increase intensity is considered. A necessary and important part of the exercise prescription includes checking with the older adult as to how the program is going and if the frequency, intensity, or duration of the activities needs to be adjusted.

B. Adherence

Adherence to an activity program improves when an individual commits to personally meaningful and measurable goals, uses a self-monitoring plan such as a calendar to record exercise, receives specific feedback, and has access to support as desired from others. A physician's formal recommendation to exercise, delivered as a prescription based on individualized risks and needs, increases motivation and adherence.

SUMMARY

Physical activity positively impacts multiple aspects of life, and is beneficial to almost all older adults. Very few instances exist in which physical activity is contraindicated. Depending on the needs and preferences of the individual, physical activity programs can be performed in a supervised setting or unsupervised, incorporating all types of exercise. Providing an exercise prescription that is tailored to the individual, sets reasonable and attainable goals, and monitors the individual's maintenance and progression of the activity program are key for initiation and adherence.

Case Vignette (*continued*)

You discuss with Ethel her goals and interests with an activity program. You find that she loves to walk and dance, but she is concerned about falling. You recommend that Ethel start an exercise program in which she performs aerobic exercise 4–5 days a week, starting with walking for as long as she can tolerate before needing a rest break. Given that Ethel is relatively healthy, you would expect her to be able to walk for about 15–20 minutes continuously. However, if Ethel can only tolerate about 5–10 minutes of walking, she should walk for that long, take a short rest break, then walk again, repeating this a few times (for 20–30 minutes of total walking time). You tell her to gradually increase the amount of time she walks until she is able to tolerate 30 minutes continuously. Because of her use of β blockers, you explain the RPE scale and the talk test as ways to measure her level of intensity. You encourage Ethel to find dancing classes that she can attend with her husband, and educate her about swimming or group exercise classes at the local gym. You also advise Ethel about the importance of strength training, giving her a few exercises to perform at home. You schedule a follow-up appointment with Ethel in 3 months to check her progress with her short- and long-term goals and to address any barriers she has noticed, as well as discuss how to progress her current activity program.

Ainsworth BE, Haskell WL, Herrmann SD, et al. 2011 Compendium of Physical Activities: a second update of codes and MET values. *Med Sci Sports Exerc.* 2011;43(8):1575-1581.

American College of Sports Medicine, Chodzko-Zajko WJ, Proctor DN, et al. American College of Sports Medicine position stand. Exercise and physical activity for older adults. *Med Sci Sports Exerc.* 2009;41(7):1510-1530.

American College of Sports Medicine. Physical activity programs and behavior counseling in older adult populations. *Med Sci Sports Exerc.* 2004;36(11):1997-2003.

Bean JF, Vora A, Frontera WR. Benefits of exercise for community-dwelling older adults. *Arch Phys Med Rehabil.* 2004;85(7 Suppl 3): S31-S42.

Borg G. Perceived exertion as an indicator of somatic stress. *Scand J Rehabil Med.* 1970;2(2):92-98.

Brach JS, Wert D, VanSwearingen JM, Studenski SA. The Compendium of Physical Activity underestimates walking intensity in old more so than in young. *J Am Geriatr Soc.* 2009;57:S110.

Bryant CX, Green DJ, eds. *Exercise for Older Adults: ACE's Guide for Fitness Professionals.* 2nd ed. San Diego, CA: American Council on Exercise; 2005.

Capaday C. The special nature of human walking and its neural control. *Trends Neurosci.* 2002;25(7):370-376.

Caspersen CJ, Powell KE, Christenson GM. Physical activity, exercise, and physical fitness: definitions and distinctions for health-related research. *Public Health Rep.* 1985;100(2):126-131.

Centers for Disease Control and Prevention. *Measuring Physical Activity Intensity.* Accessed August 2, 2012. Available at: http://www.cdc.gov/physicalactivity/everyone/measuring/index.html

Centers for Disease Control and Prevention. *Perceived Exertion (Borg Rating of Perceived Exertion Scale).* Accessed August 2, 2012. Available at: http://www.cdc.gov/physicalactivity/everyone/measuring/exertion.html

Centers for Disease Control and Prevention. *Target Heart Rate and Estimated Maximum Heart Rate.* Accessed August 2, 2012. Available at: http://www.cdc.gov/physicalactivity/everyone/measuring/heartrate.html

Costello E, Kafchinski M, Vrazel J, Sullivan P. Motivators, barriers, and beliefs regarding physical activity in an older adult population. *J Geriatr Phys Ther.* 2011;34(3):138-147.

Exercise is Medicine. Your Prescription for Health series. Accessed August 2, 2012. Available at: http://exerciseismedicine.org/YourPrescription.htm

Garber CE, Blissmer B, Deschenes MR, et al. American College of Sports Medicine position stand. Quantity and quality of exercise for developing and maintaining cardiorespiratory, musculoskeletal, and neuromotor fitness in apparently healthy adults: guidance for prescribing exercise. *Med Sci Sports Exerc.* 2011;43(7):1334-1359.

Gill TM, DiPietro L, Krumholz HM. Role of exercise stress testing and safety monitoring for older persons starting an exercise program. *JAMA.* 2000;284(3):342-349.

Grandes G, Sanchez A, Sanchez-Pinilla RO, et al. Effectiveness of physical activity advice and prescription by physicians in routine primary care: a cluster randomized trial. *Arch Intern Med.* 2009;169(7):694-701.

Graves LE, Ridgers ND, Williams K, Stratton G, Atkinson G, Cable NT. The physiological cost and enjoyment of Wii Fit in adolescents, young adults, and older adults. *J Phys Act Health.* 2010;7(3):393-401.

Harris TJ, Owen CG, Victor CR, Adams R, Cook DG. What factors are associated with physical activity in older people, assessed objectively by accelerometry? *Br J Sports Med.* 2009;43(6):442-450.

Howley ET. Type of activity: resistance, aerobic and leisure versus occupational physical activity. *Med Sci Sports Exerc.* 2001;33 (6 Suppl):S364-S369.

Inzitari M, Greenlee A, Hess R, Perera S, Studenski SA. Attitudes of postmenopausal women toward interactive video dance for exercise. *J Womens Health (Larchmt).* 2009;18(8):1239-1243.

Lees FD, Clark PG, Nigg CR, Newman P. Barriers to exercise behavior among older adults: a focus-group study. *J Aging Phys Act.* 2005;13(1):23-33.

Metkus TS Jr, Baughman KL, Thompson PD. Exercise prescription and primary prevention of cardiovascular disease. *Circulation.* 2010;121(23):2601-2604.

National Institute on Aging. *Exercise & Physical Activity: Your Everyday Guide from the National Institute on Aging.* 2011. Accessed August 15, 2012. Available at: http://www.nia.nih.gov/sites/default/files/exercise_guide.pdf

Nelson ME, Rejeski WJ, Blair SN, et al. Physical activity and public health in older adults: recommendation from the American College of Sports Medicine and the American Heart Association. *Circulation.* 2007;116(9):1094-1105.

Physical Activity Guidelines Advisory Committee. *Physical Activity Guidelines Advisory Committee Report, 2008.* Washington, DC: U.S. Department of Health and Human Services; 2008.

Rasinaho M, Hirvensalo M, Leinonen R, Lintunen T, Rantanen T. Motives for and barriers to physical activity among older adults with mobility limitations. *J Aging Phys Act.* 2006;15:90-102.

Studenski S, Perera S, Hile E, Keller V, Spadola-Bogard J, Garcia J. Interactive video dance games for healthy older adults. *J Nutr Health Aging.* 2010;14(10):850-852.

Thompson PD, Franklin BA, Balady GJ, et al. Exercise and acute cardiovascular events. Placing the risks into perspective: a scientific statement from the American Heart Association Council on Nutrition, Physical Activity, and Metabolism and the Council on Clinical Cardiology. *Circulation.* 2007;115(17):2358-2368.

Troiano RP, Berrigan D, Dodd KW, Masse LC, Tilert T, McDowell M. Physical activity in the United States measured by accelerometer. *Med Sci Sports Exerc.* 2008;40(1):181-188.

Tucker JM, Welk GJ, Beyler NK. Physical activity in U.S. adults: compliance with the Physical Activity Guidelines for Americans. *Am J Prev Med.* 2011;40(4):454-461.

Van Norman KA. *Exercise and Wellness for Older Adults: Practical Programming Strategies.* 2nd ed. Champaign, IL: Human Kinetics; 2010.

VanSwearingen JM, Perera S, Brach JS, Cham R, Rosano C, Studenski SA. A randomized trial of two forms of therapeutic activity to improve walking: effect on the energy cost of walking. *J Gerontol A Biol Sci Med Sci.* 2009;64(11):1190-1198.

Wert DM, Brach J, Perera S, VanSwearingen JM. Gait biomechanics, spatial and temporal characteristics, and the energy cost of walking in older adults with impaired mobility. *Phys Ther.* 2010;90(7):977-985.

Whaley MH, ed. *ACSM's Guidelines for Exercise Testing and Prescription.* 7th ed. Philadelphia, PA: Lippincott Williams & Wilkins; 2006.

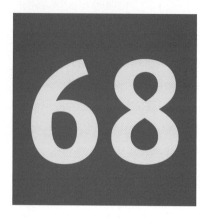

68 Defining Adequate Nutrition for Older Adults

Michi Yukawa, MD, MPH

▶ General Principles in Older Adults

Weight loss and malnutrition are common in older adults. Previous studies have reported that 17% to 65% of hospitalized geriatric patients and up to 59% of geriatric residents in institutions suffered from malnutrition. Over the past 15 years, however, obesity in older adults has increased. Despite an overall weight increase, obese older patients lose lean mass and remain at risk for functional decline and other medical complications much as do older adults with involuntary weight loss. There remains controversy regarding the appropriateness of advocating for weight loss in older adults with body mass index (BMI) greater than 35, which is discussed later in this chapter.

In general, body weight in men tends to increase from age 30–60, plateaus for the next 10–15 years, and then slowly declines. In women, the pattern of weight change is similar, except that changes occur approximately 10 years later in life. Lean body mass (primarily skeletal muscle) begins to decline by middle age as a result of many factors, including decreasing exercise and age-related declines in hormone levels (eg, testosterone, estrogen, and growth factors), metabolism, and muscle protein synthesis. Even during healthy aging, daily energy requirements decline with age. This is a result of decreases in muscle mass and decreases in physical activity. There are many formulas to estimate resting caloric needs (Table 68–1). All of these estimations should take into account activity levels and underlying illness severity.

▶ Recommended Dietary Allowances for Older Adults

Recommended dietary allowances (RDAs) of vitamins and minerals for geriatric patients are not significantly different from those for middle age adults (Table 68–2). Notable differences include recommendations for calcium and vitamin D intake. For men older than age 70 years, recommended

calcium intake increases from 1000 mg/day to 1200 mg/day. For both men and women older than age 70 years, the recommended daily dosage of vitamin D (cholecalciferol) increases from 600 IU to 800 IU. Most nonprescription multivitamins provide adequate vitamins and minerals except for calcium and vitamin D. Supplementation with additional calcium and vitamin D remains warranted.

The RDA of macronutrients for older adults is similar to those for middle age adults (Table 68–3). Protein requirements are influenced by activity level, medications, nonprotein content of the diet, and health status. For example, corticosteroid use, bed rest, injury, infection, and inflammation all increase the risk of negative nitrogen balance, which can lead to rapid loss of lean body mass. Older hospitalized persons who are very ill or recovering from trauma or major surgery may require ≥1.5 g/kg per day of protein to maintain their nitrogen balance. Monitoring protein intake becomes challenging in medical conditions requiring protein restriction, such as liver or renal disease. In these situations, patients and families have to work closely with dietitians to provide adequate protein intake without worsening patients' hepatic or renal failure.

Serum lipid levels remain a strong a predictor of risk for coronary heart disease in older adults as in middle-age adults. Most current recommendations for a healthy diet suggest a diet in which 25% to 30% of total calories come from fat. Some fat in the diet is required for the absorption of fat-soluble vitamins (A, D, E, and K). In addition, essential fatty acids must be consumed because they cannot be synthesized in the body. There are 2 general categories of essential fatty acids, which are omega-6 type and omega-3 type. Omega-6 fatty acids have proinflammatory properties and are the substrate for arachidonic acid, prostaglandins, thromboxanes, and leukotrienes. Omega-3 fatty acids, including eicosapentaenoic acid, docosahexaenoic acid, and prostacyclin, decrease platelet aggregation and vasoconstriction and have antiinflammatory properties. Based on current data, in nonfrail older

Table 68–1. Estimation of daily resting caloric (Kcal) requirements.

Institute of Medicine and National Academies Press
Male: 661.8 − (9.53 × age[y]) = PAC × (15.91 × weight [kg] + 539.6 × height [m])
Female: 354.1 − (6.91 × age [y]) = PAC × (9.36 × weight [kg] = 726 × height [m])

PAC, Physical activity coefficient (sedentary PAC = 1.0; low activity PAC = 1.12; active PAC = 1.27; very active PAC = 1.45); y, age in years.

Data from Institute of Medicine and National Academies Press. Dietary Reference Intakes for Energy, Carbohydrate, Fiber, Fat, Fatty Acids, Cholesterol, Protein, and Amino Acids. 2005. Accessed September 25, 2012. http://www.Nal.usda.gov/fnic/DRI/DRI_Energy/energy_full_report.pdf

adults, fat intake should not exceed 30% of total calories consumed, polyunsaturated and monounsaturated fats should predominate, and saturated fat and partially hydrogenated fat intake should be reduced. However, in those frail older adults who are at high risk for weight loss, fat intake of all types should be encouraged so as to increase total calorie intake.

Carbohydrate requirements are generally calculated after determining total caloric, fat, and protein requirements. Thus, carbohydrates generally make up approximately 55% of total caloric intake. Unrefined, whole-grain products should be emphasized, with decreased intake of simple sugars.

The DASH diet (Dietary Approaches to Stop Hypertension), which is a diet rich in fruits, vegetables, low-fat dairy, and <25% fat, is recommended to reduce blood pressure (http://dashdiet.org). Furthermore increasing whole-grain food intake improves fiber intake. A higher intake of fiber is associated with improved bowel function and is associated epidemiologically with a decreased risk for cardiovascular disease, diverticular disease, and diabetes mellitus type 2. Supplementing the diet with commercially available concentrated fiber sources may be necessary when fiber intake from natural sources is inadequate. Fiber intake should be increased gradually to avoid bloating, excess flatus, and general discomfort. Adequate fluid intake is also needed, particularly with bed-bound or inactive persons, because constipation may actually worsen with fiber alone.

▶ Findings

A. Anthropometrics

1. Adverse effects of unintentional weight loss and malnutrition—Among community-dwelling older adults, significant weight loss is defined as 4% to 5% weight loss over 6–12 months or rapid weight loss of >5% in 1 month. For older adults living in skilled nursing homes, the definition of significant weight loss is either ≥10% weight loss over 180 days or ≥5% weight loss over 1 month. Some of the adverse effects of involuntary weight loss and malnutrition include functional decline, increase in mortality rate (9% to 38% within 1–2.5 years), increased risk for hospitalization, increased risk for developing pressure ulcers, postural hypotension, poor wound healing, cognitive decline, and increased risk for infection as a result of poor immune function. Physical signs of malnutrition besides weight loss include peripheral edema caused by protein malnutrition, alopecia, glossitis, skin desquamation, and dry depigmented hair.

2. Adverse effects of obesity in older adults—In the United States, approximately 42.5% of women 60–79 years old and 19.5% of women older than age 80 years are obese (BMI >30). For men, 38.1% between ages 60 and 79 and 9.6% of men older than age 80 years are obese. Obesity is

Table 68–2. Dietary reference intakes: recommended dietary allowances for older adults.

	Vitamin A (µg/day)	Vitamin B₁ (Thiamine) (mg/day)	Vitamin B₂ (Riboflavin) (mg/day)	Vitamin B₆ (Pyridoxine) (mg/day)	Vitamin B₁₂ (mg/day)	Vitamin C (mg/day)	Vitamin D (IU)	Vitamin K (µg/day)	Niacin (mg/day)	Calcium (mg/day)
Males										
51–70 years	900	1.2	1.3	1.7	2.4	90	600	120	16	1000
>70 years	900	1.2	1.3	1.7	2.4	90	800	120	16	1200
Females										
51–70 years	700	1.1	1.1	1.5	2.4	75	600	90	14	1200
>70 years	700	1.1	1.1	1.5	2.4	75	800	90	14	1200

Adapted from Dietary References Intakes from Food and Nutrition Board, Institute of Medicine, National Academies. Accessed September 3, 2012. http://fnic.nal.usda.gov. Recommended macronutrients are based on the following calories per day: For ages 51–70 years: male 2204 kcal/day and female 1978 kcal/day. For age >70 years: male 2054 kcal/day and female 1873 kcal/day.

Table 68–3. Dietary reference intakes: macronutrients for older adults.

	Carbohydrates (g/day)	Total Fiber (g/day)	n-6 Polyunsaturated Fatty Acids (g/day)	n-3 Polyunsaturated Fatty Acids (g/day)	Protein and Amino Acids (g/day)
Males					
51–70 years	130	30	14	1.6	56
>70 years	130	30	14	1.6	56
Females					
51–70 years	130	21	11	1.1	46
>70 years	130	21	11	1.1	46

Adapted from Dietary References Intakes from Food and Nutrition Board, Institute of Medicine, National Academies. Accessed September 3, 2012. http://fnic.nal.usda.gov. Recommended macronutrients are based on the following calories per day: For ages 51–70 years: male 2204 kcal/day and female 1978 kcal/day. For age >70 years: male 2054 kcal/day and female 1873 kcal/day.

associated with an increase in all-cause mortality rate in community-dwelling older adults. However, for geriatric patients living in skilled nursing homes, increase in mortality was found for BMI ≥35 but not for those with BMI between 30 and 35. Obesity can increase the risk for developing hypertension, dyslipidemia, diabetes mellitus, coronary artery disease, stroke, osteoarthritis, and sleep apnea. Increased risk for breast, prostate and colon cancers have also been associated with obesity. Also, obesity has been associated with increased knee pain from osteoarthritis.

BMI, rather than body weight, is a better measure for determining an individual's nutritional status. BMI adjusts weight in relation to height; however, it does not identify persons who have replaced muscle mass with adipose tissue, nor does it distinguish persons with central obesity. Central obesity is associated with negative health outcomes and thus some researchers believe that waist circumference may be a better measure than BMI for assessment of obesity in older adults.

Skinfold measurement using calipers are prone to many measurement errors and remain primarily a research tool. Bioelectric impedance may prove a better way to assess body composition; however, it is influenced by volume status and also mostly used in research.

B. Laboratory Assessment

The initial laboratory assessment of weight loss should include a complete blood count, glucose, electrolytes, renal and liver function, thyroid-stimulating hormone level, urinalysis, and chest x-ray film. These initial tests should rule out metabolic, endocrine, or infectious causes of weight loss.

Although serum albumin is commonly ordered to assess protein nutrition or status, serum albumin levels have poor sensitivity and specificity as a measure of nutritional health. The half-life of albumin is approximately 3 weeks. Levels respond slowly to adequate nutritional intervention and

may never normalize if inflammation is ongoing. Raising the serum albumin with intravenous albumin replacement does not improve prognosis. However, measurement of serum albumin does have clinical value: A low serum albumin, although not a good indicator of nutritional status, may be a powerful predictor of illness severity and mortality.

Prealbumin (transthyretin) has a short half-life of 2–3 days and is more sensitive than albumin in evaluating acute nutritional change. A low level can be used to confirm the clinical impression of poor nutritional status in the absence of inflammation. A progressively rising prealbumin level may help to confirm improving nutritional status; however, the clinical exam remains the best indicator. Serum cholesterol <160 mg/dL is a marker for increased risk of morbidity and mortality but not a good measure of nutrition.

C. Clinical Assessment

A comprehensive clinical assessment of nutritional status is the most useful way to identify malnutrition, and several assessment instruments exist. The Mini-Nutritional Assessment (Figure 68–1) has become widely used to evaluate nutritional status in geriatric patients. Other screening tools include Seniors in the Community: Risk Evaluation for Eating and Nutrition (SCREEN) (http://www.drheatherkeller.com/index.php/screen/) and the Simplified Nutrition Assessment Questionnaire (SNAQ) (http://www.slu.edu/readstory/newslink/6349).

▶ Differential Diagnosis

A. Potential Causes of Unintentional Weight Loss

As in most geriatric syndromes, unintentional weight loss in older adults is often caused by multiple factors. Possible causes can be categorized into medical, psychosocial,

Mini Nutritional Assessment
MNA®

Nestlé
NutritionInstitute

Last name:		First name:		
Sex:	Age:	Weight, kg:	Height, cm:	Date:

Complete the screen by filling in the boxes with the appropriate numbers. Total the numbers for the final screening score.

Screening

A Has food intake declined over the past 3 months due to loss of appetite, digestive problems, chewing or swallowing difficulties?
0 = severe decrease in food intake
1 = moderate decrease in food intake
2 = no decrease in food intake ☐

B Weight loss during the last 3 months
0 = weight loss greater than 3 kg (6.6 lbs)
1 = does not know
2 = weight loss between 1 and 3 kg (2.2 and 6.6 lbs)
3 = no weight loss ☐

C Mobility
0 = bed or chair bound
1 = able to get out of bed / chair but does not go out
2 = goes out ☐

D Has suffered psychological stress or acute disease in the last 3 months?
0 = yes   2 = no ☐

E Neuropsychological problems
0 = severe dementia or depression
1 = mild dementia
2 = no psychological problems ☐

F1 Body Mass Index (BMI) (weight in kg) / (height in m^2)
0 = BMI less than 19
1 = BMI 19 to less than 21
2 = BMI 21 to less than 23
3 = BMI 23 or greater ☐

IF BMI IS NOT AVAILABLE, REPLACE QUESTION F1 WITH QUESTION F2.
DO NOT ANSWER QUESTION F2 IF QUESTION F1 IS ALREADY COMPLETED.

F2 Calf circumference (CC) in cm
0 = CC less than 31
3 = CC 31 or greater ☐

Screening score (max. 14 points)

12 - 14 points: Normal nutritional status
8 - 11 points: At risk of malnutrition
0 - 7 points: Malnourished ☐☐

References
1. Vellas B, Villars H, Abellan G, et al. Overview of the MNA® - Its History and Challenges. J Nutr Health Aging. 2006;10:456-465.
2. Rubenstein LZ, Harker JO, Salva A, Guigoz Y, Vellas B. Screening for Undernutrition in Geriatric Practice: Developing the Short-Form Mini Nutritional Assessment (MNA-SF). J. Geront. 2001;56A:M366-377.
3. Guigoz Y. The Mini-Nutritional Assessment (MNA®) Review of the Literature - What does it tell us? J Nutr Health Aging. 2006; 10:466-487.
4. Kaiser MJ, Bauer JM, Ramsch C, et al. Validation of the Mini Nutritional Assessment Short-Form (MNA®-SF): A practical tool for identification of nutritional status. J Nutr Health Aging. 2009;13:782-788.
® Société des Produits Nestlé, S.A., Vevey, Switzerland, Trademark Owners © Nestlé, 1994, Revision 2009. N67200 12/99 10M
For more information: www.mna-elderly.com

▲ **Figure 68–1.** The Mini Nutritional Assessment (MNA) short form.

Table 68–4. Potential causes of involuntary weight loss.

Medical factors:	Cancer:	Noncancer:
	GI malignancy (esophageal, pancreatic and gastric cancer) Lung Lymphoma Prostate Ovarian Bladder	GI disorders (motility or swallow dysfunction, mesenteric ischemia, peptic ulcers, gallstones) Congestive heart failure Dementia COPD Endocrine disorder (hyperthyroidism, diabetes mellitus) Stroke End-stage renal failure End-stage liver failure Alcoholism Rheumatoid arthritis Oral or dental problems
Psychosocial factors:	Social:	Psychological:
	Poverty Inability to shop or cook Inability to feed Social isolation Lack of ethnic food variety	Depression Alcoholism Bereavement Paranoia
Medications:	Anorexic: Antibiotic (erythromycin) Digoxin Opiates SSRI (fluoxetine) Amantadine Metformin Benzodiazepines Dry mouth: Anticholinergics Loop diuretics Antihistamines	Nausea/vomiting: Antibiotic (erythromycin) Bisphosphonates Digoxin Dopamine agonist Levodopa Opiates Tricyclic antidepressants SSRI Alter taste or smell: ACE inhibitors Calcium channel blockers Spironolactone Iron Antiparkinsonian medications (levodopa, pergolide, selegiline) Opiates Gold Allopurinol

ACE, Angiotensin converting enzyme; COPD, chronic obstructive pulmonary disease; GI gastrointestinal; SSRI, selective serotonin reuptake inhibitors.

Data from McMinn J, Steel C, Bowman A. Investigation and management of unintentional weight loss in older adults. *BMJ.* 2011;342:d1732 and Chapman IM. Weight loss in older persons. *Med Clin North Am.* 2011;95(3):579-593.

and pharmacologic (Table 68–4). Underlying or previously undiagnosed cancer could be the cause of involuntary weight loss in 16% to 36% of cases according to some studies. Gastrointestinal malignancy such as esophageal, pancreatic, and gastric cancer is more common than other cancers. Other malignancies that are associated with weight loss include lymphomas, and lung, prostate, ovarian, and bladder cancers. Nonmalignant causes of weight loss include chronic illnesses such as dementia, congestive heart failure, chronic obstructive pulmonary disease, endocrine disorders (diabetes mellitus, hyperthyroidism), and end-stage kidney or liver failure. Oral and dental problems, such as ill-fitting dentures or poor dentition, can also lead to weight loss.

Social factors, such as financial constraints, inability to shop or cook, social isolation, and lack of ethnic foods in an institutional facility, can contribute toward unintentional weight loss. Depression and dementia are major causes of weight loss in older adults, and may account for 10% to 20% of weight loss in community-dwelling older adults and in 58% of nursing home residents. People who have dementia lose weight and decrease food intake as a result of dysphagia, the inability to self-feed, and the excess energy expenditure caused by agitation and wandering. Many medications can lead to weight loss from side effects of anorexia, nausea/vomiting, dry mouth, or altered taste or smell (see Table 68–4).

► Next Steps

A. Improve Malnutrition and Weight Loss

Patients often eat better, and more, when fed by family members. One reason for this is the length of time the family member dedicates to unhurriedly feeding and encouraging the patient. Older people also eat more if they are eating with others. Studies have shown that older adults receiving meals-on-wheels eat more if the delivery person stays with them. Successfully motivating undernourished persons to eat requires a multidimensional approach, including treating pain, increasing social supports, and adapting to individual food preferences and meal times. Simple exercise, such as daily walking, may improve appetite in some patients. As stated above, depression is a common cause of anorexia and refusal to eat. Patients should be screened for depression and if needed, referred for evaluation by a psychiatrist or psychologist.

1. Oral supplements—A variety of commercial liquid and powder supplements are used when patients are unable or unwilling to consume enough regular food. Although the most recent Cochrane review on oral nutritional supplements did not show improvement in survival rate, studies using dietary advice with or without oral nutritional supplements have shown improvement in weight and body composition. Nutritional supplements are most effective when consumed at least one hour before meals, so patients do not substitute supplement intake for regular meals. Powder formulations allow the supplement to be masked by mixing it with other food. A major barrier to canned supplements is cost, even with generic brands. For patients with no history of lactose intolerance, instant breakfast powders mixed in milk are a satisfactory and less-expensive alternative.

2. Appetite stimulants—Several medications have been promoted as helping to improve appetite and increase weight; however, none have proven satisfactory in geriatric patients. Megestrol acetate has been shown to increase appetite and weight in AIDS and cancer patients and to increase weight in older adults. Recent studies, however, have shown that megestrol acetate increases adipose tissue rather than lean mass, increases the risk for thromboembolic disease and suppresses the hypothalamic pituitary adrenal axis. Several small clinical trials with dronabinol in older adults showed that they were unable to tolerate the dysphoria associated with dronabinol use. Cyproheptadine has not been shown to be effective in older adults. Anabolic agents such as growth hormone and insulin-like growth factor are expensive and associated with frequent side effects. Ghrelin use in clinical trials has increased body weight and lean body mass in older adults; however, it is currently only available for research purposes. Androgen therapy with testosterone or its analogues also has many side effects, and thus its use for weight gain remains experimental. Antiinflammatory therapies that affect arachidonic acid metabolism and cytokine release, including the omega-3 fatty acids, are also being studied. Persons with persistent anorexia may benefit from a trial of antidepressant therapy such as with mirtazapine.

3. Artificial tube feeding—Before discussing use of artificial tube feeding, patients and their family members should discuss overall goals of care. In certain cases, temporarily use of tube feeding can be beneficial, such as during treatments for head neck cancer or recovery from an acute stroke. Some clinicians initiate artificial feeding as a therapeutic trial for a limited and predetermined duration with the understanding that if certain goals are not achieved (eg, the person will begin to voluntarily consume sufficient calories for survival), the intervention will be discontinued. (For more on the use of feeding tubes, see Chapter 11, "Geriatrics & Palliative Care.")

Previous studies have shown that for patients with end-stage dementia, initiation of artificial tube feeding neither increases survival nor improves function. Furthermore, no method of tube feeding (G-tube or J-tube) will prevent aspiration or pneumonia.

4. Treatment of obesity—Community-dwelling older adults who are obese and have poorly controlled hypertension, diabetes mellitus, functional impairment, or lower-extremity arthritis may benefit from gradual weight reduction. Sustained weight loss generally requires a combination of healthy diet and exercise. Several studies of older obese adults who were placed on a weight loss diet along with

exercise (aerobic exercise and resistance training) demonstrated ability of these subjects to lose weight without losing significant lean body mass. The use of weight loss medication (amphetamines, sibutramine, orlistat) in older adults has not been investigated adequately and thus these medications should not be used or should be used with significant caution. Amphetamines and sibutramine should be avoided in patients with cardiac disease.

Although the effects of obesity have been studied extensively in older adults living in the community, little is known about the effects of obesity in the nursing home. One study showed that nursing home residents with BMI >40 kg/m² were associated with increased mortality compared to those with normal weight (BMI of 19–28). Because of concerns about potential malnutrition and decrease in bone density, weight loss programs for nursing home residents should be initiated with caution. Having a low BMI (<19 kg/m²) is associated with increased mortality rates among nursing home patients, and nursing home residents with a BMI of 30–35 have been shown to have a higher mortality rate.

5. Interaction between medications and food—Certain foods can inhibit or potentiate the effects of commonly prescribed medications for older adults (Table 68–5). Grapefruit juice can inhibit the cytochrome P450 3A4 and thus lead to increased serum levels of statins, calcium channel blockers, and phosphodiesterase inhibitors (sildenafil, vardenafil and tadalafil) (Table 68–5). Dairy products or calcium supplements can diminish the effectiveness of some antibiotics (fluoroquinolones, cefuroxime, tetracyclines) if taken together (Table 68–5). These antibiotics should be taken at least 2 hours before or 6 hours after calcium supplements or calcium-rich foods. For community-dwelling older adults, their local pharmacist is often a good person to consult for how many hours to wait until a food or drink can be consumed after taking a medication. Table 68–5 lists other interactions between food and medications.

SUMMARY

The RDAs of vitamins, minerals and macronutrients for geriatrics patients are not significantly different for younger adults except for increased need for calcium and vitamin D supplements. The DASH diet may serve as a good guideline for healthy older adults to follow. Involuntary weight loss and obesity in older adults can increase morbidity and mortality. Improving malnutrition and weight loss in geriatric patients probably will require multistep approach. Reassessment of social issues, potential psychiatric illness, underlying medical conditions and medications is essential. A combination of healthy diet and exercise should be recommended for obese community dwelling older adults. For obese nursing home residents, weight loss programs should be initiated with caution.

Table 68–5. Food and drug interactions.

Food	Medications	Interaction
Grapefruit juice	Atorvastatin Simvastatin Lovastatin	Decreased metabolism Increased risk for muscle toxicity (myalgia, myopathy, rhabdomyolysis)
	Calcium channel blockers: Amlodipine Nifedipine Nicardipine Verapamil, Felodipine	Decreased metabolism Increased risk for orthostatic hypotension
	Phosphodiesterase inhibitors: Sildenafil Vardenafil Tadalafil	Increased serum concentration Priapism, hypotension, visual disturbances
	Benzodiazepines: Diazepam Temazepam Midazolam	Increased serum concentration Increased central nervous system depressant effect
	Amiodarone	Decreased metabolism Increased risk for bradycardia, CHF, hypotension
Caffeine	Ciprofloxacin	Ciprofloxacin can potentiate the effect of caffeine Increase risk for insomnia
	Cimetidine	Cimetidine can increase caffeine levels
	Theophylline	Caffeine inhibits the metabolism Increase risk for anxiety, insomnia and cardiac arrhythmia
Dairy products or calcium supplements	Fluoroquinolones Ciprofloxacin Levofloxacin Cefuroxime Tetracycline	Decreased absorption
	Bisphosphonates: Alendronate Risedronate Ibandronate	Low bioavailability and drug absorption when taken with dairy products or calcium supplements
Protein-rich foods	Propranolol	Increased bioavailability of propranolol Increased risk for bradycardia, hypotension and bronchoconstriction
	Carbidopa/levodopa	Decreased serum concentration
	Theophylline	Decreased serum concentration
Fiber	Metformin	Decreased serum levels if taken with large amounts of fiber
Tyramine-containing foods (cheese and red wines)	MAOIs: Selegiline Phenelzine Isocarboxazid Tranylcypromine	Potentiate the effect of these medications. Can contribute to serotonin syndrome
	Linezolid	Some MAOI properties
	Isoniazid	MAOI effects
	Tramadol	Weak MAO inhibitor
Green, leafy vegetables	Warfarin	Rich in vitamin K and thus reduce the efficacy of warfarin

CHF, Congestive heart failure; MAO, monoamine oxidase; MAOI, monoamine oxidase inhibitor; SSRI, serotonin selective reuptake inhibitors.

Alibhai SM, Greenwood C, Payette H. An approach to the management of unintentional weight loss in elderly people. *CMAJ.* 2005;172(6):773-780.

Anton SD, Manini TM, Milsom VA, et al. Effects of a weight loss plus exercise program on physical function in overweight, older women: a randomized controlled trial. *Clin Interv Aging.* 2011;6:141-149.

Attar A, Malka D, Sabate JM, et al. Malnutrition is high and underestimated during chemotherapy in gastrointestinal cancer: an AGEO prospective cross-sectional multicenter study. *Nutr Cancer.* 2012;64(4):535-542.

Baldwin C, Weekes CE. Dietary advice with or without oral nutritional supplements for disease-related malnutrition in adults. *Cochrane Database Syst Rev.* 2011;(9):CD002008.

Bradway C, DiResta J, Fleshner I, et al. Obesity in nursing homes: a critical review. *J Am Geriatr Soc.* 2008;56(8):1528-1535.

Chapman IM. Weight loss in older persons. *Med Clin North Am.* 2011;95(3):579-593.

Cullen S. Gastrostomy tube feeding in adults: the risks, benefits and alternatives. *Proc Nutr Soc.* 2011;70(3):293-298.

DiFrancesco V, Fantin F, Omzzolo F, et al. The anorexia of aging. *Dig Dis.* 2007;25(2):129-137.

Flegal KM, Carroll MD, Kit BK, Ogden CL. Prevalence of obesity and trends in the distribution of body mass index among US adults, 1999-2010. *JAMA.* 2012;307(5):491-497.

Gioulbasanis I, Georgoulias P, Vlachostergios PJ, et al. Mini Nutritional Assessment (MNS) and biochemical markers of cachexia in metastatic lung cancer patients: Interrelations and associations with prognosis. *Lung Cancer.* 2011;74(3):516-520.

Grabowski DC, Campbell CM, Ellis JE. Obesity and mortality in elderly nursing home residents. *J Gerontol A Biol Sci Med Sci.* 2005;60(9):1184-1189.

Hulisz D, Jakab J. Food-drug interaction. *US Pharm.* 2007;32:93-98.

Keller HH, Goy RE, Kane SL. Validity and reliability of Screen II (Seniors in the community: risk evaluation for eating and nutrition, Version II). *Eur J Clin Nutr.* 2005;59(10):1149-1157.

Li A, Heber D. Sarcopenic obesity in the elderly and strategies for weight management. *Nutr Rev.* 2011;70(1):57-64.

McMinn J, Steel C, Bowman A. Investigation and management of unintentional weight loss in older adults. *BMJ.* 2011;342:d1732.

Messier SP, Loeser RF, Miller GD, et al. Exercise and dietary weight loss in overweight and obese older adults with knee osteoarthritis: the Arthritis, Diet, and Activity Promotion Trial. *Arthritis Rheum.* 2004;50(5):1501-1510.

Morley JE. Anorexia and weight loss in older persons. *J Gerontol A Biol Sci Med Sci.* 2003;58(2):131-137.

Rutter CE, Yovino S, Taylor R, et al. Impact of early percutaneous endoscopic gastrostomy tube placement on nutritional status and hospitalization in patients with head and neck cancer receiving definitive chemoradiation therapy. *Head Neck.* 2011;33(10):1441-1447.

Saragat B, Buffa R, Mereu E et al. Nutritional and psycho-functional status in elderly patients with Alzheimer's disease. *J Nutr Health Aging.* 2012;16(3):231-236.

Villareal DT, Chode S, Parimi N, et al. Weight loss, exercise, or both and physical function in obese older adults. *N Engl J Med.* 2011;364(13):1218-1229.

Wilson MM, Thomas DR, Rubenstein LZ, et al. Appetite assessment: simple appetite questionnaire predicts weight loss in community-dwelling adults and nursing home residents. *Am J Clin Nutr.* 2005;82(5):1074-1081.

Yaxley A, Miller MD, Fraser RJ, Cobiac L. Pharmacological interventions for geriatric cachexia: a narrative review of the literature. *J Nutr Health Aging.* 2012;16(2):148-154.

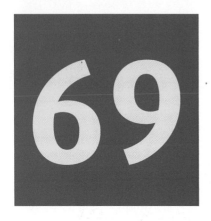

69

Helping Older Adults with Low Health Literacy

Anna H. Chodos, MD, MPH
Rebecca L. Sudore, MD

▶ General Principles in Older Adults

Health literacy is defined as "the degree to which individuals have the capacity to obtain, process, and understand basic health information and services to make appropriate health decisions." The construct of health literacy is complex. It involves reading and writing, listening and verbal communication skills, and computational or numeracy skills required for such tasks as pill counting or insulin dosing. Limited health literacy (LHL) is thought to occur at or below an eighth grade reading level. Language barriers also contribute to LHL, and the number of foreign-born, older adults in the United States who have limited English proficiency is growing. Health literacy is also a function of the health care environment, which places a heavy burden on patients to manage their own complex disease processes and health care benefits.

It is estimated that close to half of U.S. adults have LHL, and up to 90% report difficulty with routine health information. The prevalence of LHL increases among older age groups, with the prevalence reported as high as 60% among older populations. Although the average adult in the United States reads at an eighth-grade level, adults age 65 years or older read at a fifth-grade level. Older adults with LHL have been shown to have significant difficulty weighing the risks and benefits of complex treatment options and to have difficulty reading medical forms. Yet, most health care materials are written at or beyond a college reading level. LHL also results in worse clinical outcomes for older adults including poor functional status, disparities in health care access and the receipt of preventative services, worse chronic disease management, increased hospitalization, and increased mortality. By universally adopting clear health communication techniques outlined in this chapter, clinicians can help ensure informed medical decision making and patient safety for all patients, and especially for older adults with LHL.

UNIQUE HEALTH LITERACY CONSIDERATIONS IN OLDER ADULTS

For all age groups, LHL has been found to be more common among persons of lower socioeconomic status, limited education, and limited English proficiency. However, many unique, patient-related factors contribute to LHL in older populations (Figure 69–1), including a high prevalence of impairments in hearing, vision, and cognition, as well as a high burden of chronic disease and polypharmacy. A caregiver's LHL may also affect a patient's medical care and safety.

▶ Hearing and Vision Impairment

Hearing impairment, a significant contributor to LHL, is common among older adults, with estimates as high as 63% among adults older than age 70 years. Clinicians and patients often miss a diagnosis of hearing loss. Up-to-date audiology evaluations and access to hearing aids is a first step. For patients whose hearing is undercorrected with hearing aids, small portable sound amplifiers (eg, Pocket Talkers) can be worn over hearing aids. Portable amplifiers can be used in the outpatient clinic, inpatient hospital wards, and at home to ensure patient understanding of medical information. Telephone amplifiers, often available through state-supported programs (Table 69–1), can also improve comprehension of medical information relayed by phone.

Visual impairment, which also contributes to LHL, increases with age as a consequence of the high prevalence of macular degeneration, cataracts, and glaucoma. Up-to-date vision evaluations, access to magnifying readers and adequate corrective lenses, and use of prescribed medications for ophthalmic-related conditions can help mitigate visual barriers to adequate health literacy.

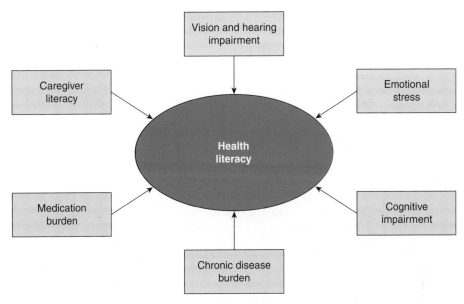

▲ **Figure 69–1.** Unique health literacy considerations in older adults.

▶ Cognitive Impairment

Cognitive impairment contributes significantly to LHL in older adults. Twenty-two percent of U.S. adults 71 years of age or older have mild cognitive impairment and 13.7% have dementia. It is estimated that by 2050 there will be 16 million adults living with Alzheimer disease in the United States.

LHL is highly correlated with cognitive impairment, and therefore, screening for cognitive impairment is crucial. The 3-item Mini Cog is a quick screening test (79% sensitive and 90% specific for cognitive impairment) and the Montreal Cognitive Assessment (MOCA) is a more thorough assessment shown to detect cognitive impairment even in early stages (90% sensitive and 87% specific for mild cognitive impairment). Detecting cognitive impairment early allows the provider to consider pharmacologic interventions, such as acetylcholinesterase inhibitors, and social interventions, such as adult day health care programs that provide cognitive stimulation, to help maintain cognition. The diagnosis of cognitive impairment also signals the need to identify caregivers who can help interpret medical information for the patient.

▶ Multimorbidity and Polypharmacy

Many older adults have multiple chronic conditions resulting in a high volume and burden of medical information, a large number of medications and disease management tasks, and often many doctors and specialists with whom the patient must contend. Conditions or procedures associated with multimorbidity, such as prior strokes, chronic pain, surgery, or acute hospitalization, also impair cognition, impact patients' ability to understand discharge instructions, and impact patients' ability to manage their medical conditions.

Polypharmacy also plays a significant role in LHL, particularly psychoactive medications, such as antidepressants and pain medications. In addition, patients with LHL have difficulty reading and interpreting medication labels and are often nonadherent as a result of poor understanding. The risk of medication nonadherence increases with increased medication burden.

▶ Emotional Stress of Illness

Emotional stress related to multimorbidity can also affect LHL. For example, older adults are more likely to be widowed, to obtain a new diagnosis of cancer, endure new disabilities or chronic pain, and encounter new surroundings during a hospitalization or institutionalization. Stress is associated with impaired memory, poor medication adherence, and poor disease self-management. It is important to inquire about how patients are coping with new diagnoses and cumulative disability and to screen for depression and anxiety. If needed, counseling and/or pharmacologic treatment may improve health information processing.

▶ Caregivers and Limited Health Literacy

Paid and unpaid caregivers are often an important part of older adults' health care. Caregivers may be responsible for

Table 69–1. Health literacy resources.

Informational Websites and General Resources

Center for Disease Control (CDC) health literacy facts and resources:
http://www.cdc.gov/healthliteracy/
Department of Health and Human Resources, Office of Disease
Prevention and Health Promotion, health literacy facts and resources:
http://www.health.gov/communication/literacy/olderadults/
default.htm

Provider Training and Self-Assessment Tools

American Medical Association (AMA) healthy literacy campaign:
http://www.ama-assn.org/ama/pub/about-ama/ama-foundation/
our-programs/public-health/health-literacy-program.page
Harvard School of Public Health, literacy resources and provider/clinic
assessment tools: http://www.hsph.harvard.edu/healthliteracy/
resources/index.html
Health Resources and Services Administration's (HRSA) course in health
literacy training for providers: http://www.hrsa.gov/publichealth/
healthliteracy/index.html

Literacy-Appropriate Written Materials

American College of Physicians Foundation, patient education materials
on COPD, diabetes and heart health: http://www.acpfoundation.org/
materials-and-guides/patient-guides/
Centers for Disease Control and Prevention (CDC) Healthy Literacy guide:
http://www.cdc.gov/healthliteracy/
Health Literacy Missouri: https://www.healthliteracymissouri.org/
our-services/resources
Institute for Healthcare Advancement, Low-literacy Advance Healthcare
Directive (multiple languages): http://www.iha4health.org/default.
aspx/MenuItemID/266/MenuGroup/_Home.htm
Plain Language Action and Information Network, examples of plain
language and health literacy information to customize materials:
http://www.plainlanguage.gov/populartopics/health_literacy/
index.cfm

Resources for Hearing Impairment

Telecommunications Equipment Distribution Program Association
http://www.tedpa.org/StateProgram.aspx

---

health-related tasks, such as medication management, and for obtaining health care instructions from clinicians on behalf of the patient. However, caregivers may themselves have LHL. More than one-third of paid caregivers have LHL and, in 1 study, 60% made medication errors when administering medications in response to written instructions and medication labels. The person responsible for critical health tasks, if not the patient, should be identified and clear health communication techniques should be used for both the patient and the caregiver.

SCREENING

The patient's social history may alert the clinician to potential LHL, such as a history of limited education, limited English proficiency, or lower socioeconomic status; however, providers should have a broad approach to screening and evaluating patients from all backgrounds. Other clues include noncompliance with medical instructions or difficulty completing medical forms. A powerful screening tool for LHL is the medication review. This involves asking patients to bring all medications to a medical visit, including nonprescription medications, to list the name of each medication, to describe what each medication is for, and to describe how the medication is taken. Any confusion likely indicates LHL.

Formal screening tools to identify patients with LHL, such as the Rapid Estimate of Adult Literacy in Medicine (REALM) and Test of Functional Health Literacy in Adults (TOHFLA) are generally used for research purposes. Quick 3-item and 1-item screening questions are also available (eg, "How confident are you filling out medical forms by yourself?"). However, rather than formal screening, we recommend using clear health communication best practices for all older patients universally.

CLEAR HEALTH COMMUNICATION STRATEGIES

Adults with LHL experience shame and feel less empowered in their interactions with health care providers than patients with adequate health literacy, often leading to a breakdown in communication within clinical encounters. Clear health communication techniques are one way to ensure patients are more engaged and empowered.

▶ Clear Verbal Communication

Clear verbal communication techniques are helpful for all patients (Table 69–2). Before offering a recommendation or providing teaching, it is important to tailor communication to the individual. First, assess what patients already know (eg, "What do you already know or believe about…?"). The answer to this question can help clinicians detect misunderstandings and focus their instructions. Next, attempt to learn and then to match instructions to the patient's regular, day-to-day routine. This may help elicit barriers and enhance compliance.

When discussing health-related topics, providers should attempt to slow their speech, use lay language, and avoid jargon, for instance say "high blood pressure" instead of "hypertension." It is also recommended that clinicians limit information to 3 topics or less, and to focus the discussion on concrete instructions about what the patient needs to do when they go home. To improve patient understanding and health outcomes, when possible, every effort should be made to provide information to patients in their native language and to offer interpreters.

Importantly, if a patient is known to be hearing impaired, before beginning a discussion, ensure the patient has working hearing aids or is using an assistive hearing device such as a Pocket Talker. With all patients, the clinician should face the patient to allow for lip reading, which may assist in understanding.

Table 69–2. Clear health communication.

Setting up the discussion:
- Ensure hearing aids and amplification available
- Face the patient
- Involve the caregiver

Tailor communication:
- Ask, *"What do you already know about...?"*
- Ask patients about their day-to-day routine to tailor instructions

Clear communication techniques
- Speak slowly
- Avoid medical jargon; for example, say "not cancer" instead of "benign"
- Keep number of points to ≤3
- Attempt to provide information in patient's native language

Confirm understanding (teach-back)
- Encourage questions by asking,
  - "What questions do you have?"
- Put onus on clinicians by saying:
  - "We have just talked about a lot things. To make sure I did a good job and explained things clearly, can you tell me in your own words/show me...?"

Reinforce instructions
- Offer pictures, graphs, and written information to reinforce verbal communication

Teach-Back

We recommend that all verbal communication be followed by a confirmation of understanding, often called the "teach-back" or "teach-to-goal strategy." Asking, "Do you understand?" or "Do you have any questions?," often conveys to the patient that they should understand. Instead, we recommend clinicians ask, "What questions do you have?" After questions are answered, clinicians can ask patients or caregivers to restate in their own words what was just discussed or to demonstrate what skill was just taught (eg, insulin dosing). We recommend placing the onus of clear communication on the clinician: "We have just talked about a lot things. To make sure I did a good job and explained things clearly, can you tell me in your own words/show me...?" Teach back has been associated with better chronic disease management and informed medical decision making, yet has not been shown to increase the length of a medical visit.

Reinforcing Verbal Communication

Verbal communication can be reinforced with written materials, pictures, or graphs. Using written materials to reinforce verbal instructions has been shown to increase knowledge and improve patient's satisfaction with communication. In addition, literacy appropriate written materials can improve the completion rate of medical forms and can help with chronic disease management (see Table 69–1).

When looking for appropriate written information for older patients, the target grade level should be the fifth grade reading level or lower, and should include clear headings, bright contrasting colors, a font size of 14 points or larger, and a combination of both upper- and lowercase letters (ie, not all capital letters). Because of the high prevalence of ophthalmic-related conditions in older adults, non-serif (sans serif) fonts, such as Arial or Helvetica, and nonglossy, matte materials are recommended because they are easier to see. Sentences should contain 1 topic, be no more than 6–8 words in length, and be written in an active "how to" voice. Written materials should also have a high white-space-to-text ratio and include carefully chosen pictures that explain the text and put written material into context.

When creating health care materials, several resources can be used to ensure the materials are literacy appropriate. The Suitability Assessment of Materials uses criteria standards in 6 categories: content; literacy demand; graphics; layout and typography; learning stimulation/motivation; and cultural appropriateness to help assess if the literacy level is appropriate. The Lexile Framework and the Lexile Analyzer (http://www.lexile.com) can also be used to assess the readability of written materials based on sentence length and word frequency. It is important to include the target population in the design and pilot testing of materials to ensure proper understanding and to improve the material's acceptability.

Strategies for Medically Complex Patients

Patients with multiple medical conditions can benefit from disease-management programs that incorporate strategies for LHL patients. Disease-management programs for heart failure and diabetes that include literacy-appropriate verbal communication, literacy-appropriate written materials with pictures, automated telephone calls, and/or nurse follow-up calls have been shown to improve disease management, decrease hospitalizations, and decrease mortality. New technology, such as tailored, computerized, discharge instructions from virtual nurses also show promise for older adults with LHL. These computer technologies allow patients to repeat the information as often as needed.

Creative use of multidisciplinary teams may improve medical care and patient understanding for all older adults with multimorbidity, and especially for older adults with LHL. Some examples include group medical visits, collaborating with pharmacists to help review medications and fill pill boxes, and asking social workers to help complete advance directive or informed consent forms. The use of health navigators and community health workers may also help patients navigate the health care system and manage their disease processes.

SYSTEMS APPROACHES

The health care environment often places a heavy burden on patients to manage their disease and to navigate the health care system. For health literacy to improve on a public health level, health systems need to be modified. At the clinic and system levels, signs should include large font and pictures. Standard forms, such as intake forms, informed consent forms, and advance directives, should be written at or below a fifth grade reading level. Medication labeling should be consistent and should match written instructions to improve patient safety. In addition, all staff should have training in communication techniques for patients with LHL. Phone triage and menu systems should be carefully designed with no more than 2–3 options at a time. By universally adopting these clear health communication techniques, clinicians can help ensure informed medical decision making and patient safety for all patients, and especially for older adults with LHL.

Alzheimer's Association. 2012 Alzheimer's disease fact and figures. *Alzheimers Dement.* 2012;8(2):131-168.

Baker DW. The meaning and the measure of health literacy. *J Gen Intern Med.* 2006;21(8):878-883.

Baker DW, Gazmararian JA, Sudano J, Patterson M. The association between age and health literacy among elderly persons. *J Gerontol B Psychol Sci Soc Sci.* 2000;55(6):S368-S374.

Baker DW, Wolf MS, Feinglass J, Thompson JA. Health literacy, cognitive abilities, and mortality among elderly persons. *J Gen Intern Med.* 2008;23(6):723-726.

Berkman ND, Sheridan SL, Donahue KE, Halpern DJ, Crotty K. Low health literacy and health outcomes: an updated systematic review. *Ann Intern Med.* 2011;155(2):97-107.

Institute of Medicine. *Health literacy: A Prescription to End Confusion.* Washington, DC: National Academic Press; 2004.

Kripalani S, Weiss BD. Teaching about health literacy and clear communication. *J Gen Intern Med.* 2006;21(8):888-890.

Kutner M, Greenberg E, Baer J. *A First Look at the Literacy of America's Adults in the 21st Century.* Washington, DC: National Center for Education Statistics, U.S. Department of Education; 2005.

Lindquist LA, Jain N, Tam K, Martin GJ, Baker DW. Inadequate health literacy among paid caregivers of seniors. *J Gen Intern Med.* 2010;26(5):474-479.

Paasche-Orlow MK, Parker RM, Gazmararian JA, Nielsen-Bohlman LT, Rudd RR. The prevalence of limited health literacy. *J Gen Intern Med.* 2005;20(2):175-184.

Paasche-Orlow MK, Wolf MS. Evidence does not support clinical screening of literacy. *J Gen Intern Med.* 2008;23(1):100-102.

Pacala JT, Yueh B. Hearing deficits in the older patient: "I didn't notice anything". *JAMA.* 2012;307(11):1185-1194.

Peavy GM, Salmon DP, Jacobson MW, et al. Effects of chronic stress on memory decline in cognitively normal and mildly impaired older adults. *Am J Psychiatry.* 2009;166(12):1384-1391.

Pignone M, DeWalt DA, Sheridan S, Berkman N, Lohr KN. Interventions to improve health outcomes for patients with low literacy. A systematic review. *J Gen Intern Med.* 2005;20(2):185-192.

Schillinger D, Piette J, Grumbach K, et al. Closing the loop: physician communication with diabetic patients who have low health literacy. *Arch Intern Med.* 2003;163(1):83-90.

Sudore RL, Yaffe K, Satterfield S, et al. Limited literacy and mortality in the elderly: the health, aging, and body composition study. *J Gen Intern Med.* 2006;21(8):806-812.

Sudore RL, Schillinger D. Interventions to improve care for patients with limited health literacy. *J Clin Outcomes Manag.* 2009;16(1):20-29.

Sudore RL, Landefeld CS, Perez-Stable EJ, Bibbins-Domingo K, Williams BA, Schillinger D. Unraveling the relationship between literacy, language proficiency, and patient-physician communication. *Patient Educ Couns.* 2009;75(3):398-402.

Wilson RS, Hebert LE, Scherr PA, Dong X, Leurgens SE, Evans DA. Cognitive decline after hospitalization in a community population of older persons. *Neurology.* 2012;78(13):950-956.

Understanding the Effects of Homelessness and Housing Instability on Older Adults

70

Rebecca Brown, MD, MPH
Margot Kushel, MD

General Principles in Older Adults

Homelessness and housing instability are common in the United States, and affect the health and welfare of many older adults. Although definitions of homelessness vary, the most commonly used definition in the United States comes from Congress's 1987 McKinney-Vento Homeless Assistance Act. The McKinney Act defines homeless individuals or families as lacking "a fixed, regular, and adequate nighttime residence," including persons in emergency shelters and places not meant for human habitation. In 2009, Congress expanded the definition of homelessness to include people facing imminent loss of housing (eg, within 14 days after their application for homeless assistance) (Table 70–1).

Most individuals who become homeless have a preceding period of housing instability. *Housing instability* is defined by varying criteria, including difficulty paying a mortgage, rent, or utilities; spending more than 50% of household income on housing; moving frequently; living in overcrowded conditions; and "doubling up" (eg, living temporarily with family or friends).

In the last 2 decades, the proportion of the homeless population in the United States age 50 years or older has increased dramatically. In 1990, only 11% of adults experiencing homelessness in the United States were age 50 years or older; however, by 2003 one-third of these adults were older than age 50 years. This trend has continued over the past decade. In 2003, the median age of adults experiencing homelessness was 46 years, but is now estimated to be 49–50 years. The aging of the homeless population is thought to be the result of a cohort effect: individuals born in the second half of the "baby boom" generation (1954–1964) have an increased risk of homelessness compared to other age groups. As this cohort ages, the median age of the homeless population is expected to continue to increase. In the wake of the foreclosure crisis, the number of adults experiencing housing instability has also increased. To provide appropriate clinical care to older individuals experiencing homelessness and housing instability, clinicians need to understand how housing problems interact with health.

PATHWAYS TO HOMELESSNESS AMONG OLDER ADULTS

Homelessness is not a monolithic experience; it has different manifestations and trajectories, and requires different solutions. A common schema divides homeless people into 3 broad groups: first time/crisis homelessness, episodic homelessness, and chronic homelessness (Table 70–2).

Older adults arrive at homelessness by different paths. Some older adults have experienced a long history of personal challenges, such as severe mental illness, imprisonment, substance use disorders, low educational attainment, and poor job histories. These individuals tend to become homeless as younger adults, then remain chronically homeless for many years as they age. Older adults who have been chronically homeless are likely to benefit from permanent supportive housing.

Other older adults have led lives that are relatively conventional, although economically vulnerable, and become homeless for the first time following a crisis late in life. Crises may include death of a partner, divorce, or disabling illness. Most people who become homeless do so after a period of housing instability; those with fewer social supports are at higher risk of homelessness. These individuals may benefit from rapid rehousing after the initial episode of homelessness, or from efforts to prevent homelessness before it occurs. Interventions to prevent homelessness are critical in this group, because adults who become homeless late in life are at increased risk for becoming chronically homeless and experiencing poor health outcomes.

Clinicians can play an important role in recognizing patients at risk of becoming homeless and working to prevent a first episode of homelessness. If a patient becomes homeless, clinicians can help prevent chronic homelessness by helping patients to regain housing.

Table 70–1. Definition of homelessness, U.S. Department of Housing and Urban Development.

1. An individual or family who lacks a fixed, regular and adequate nighttime residence. Includes persons residing in an emergency shelter, a place not meant for human habitation, or an institution where the person temporarily resided.
2. An individual or family who will imminently lose their housing (eg, within 14 days after the date of their application for homeless assistance).
3. An unaccompanied youth (defined as younger than 25 years of age) and families with children and youth defined as homeless under other federal statutes.
4. An individual or family who is fleeing, or attempting to flee, domestic violence, dating violence, sexual assault, stalking, or other dangerous or life-threatening condition.

Reproduced with permission from the United States Congress. *Homeless Emergency Assistance and Rapid Transition to Housing (HEARTH) Act.* 111th Congress, 1st session. S 896. Washington, DC: U.S. Government Printing Office, 2009. Accessed April 20, 2012. Available at: http://www.hudhre.info/documents/S896_HEARTHAct.pdf

STRATEGIES TO PREVENT HOMELESSNESS AMONG OLDER ADULTS

Though the causes of homelessness are complex, they can be understood in 3 broad categories as defined by Dr. Martha Burt: predisposing personal vulnerabilities (eg, poverty and social isolation); structural factors (eg, availability of low cost housing); and the absence of a safety net (eg, social insurance).

Older adults at risk for homelessness have financial, social, and medical vulnerabilities (Table 70–3). Poverty is nearly universal among older adults at risk for homelessness; financial problems rank first on self-reported causes of homelessness among older adults. One-third of older adults reported that difficulty paying a rent or a mortgage triggered their homelessness, and one-fifth became homeless after losing their housing as a result of external factors (eg, sale by the landlord). Spending more than 50% of household income on rent increases the risk of homelessness, as does not having one's name on a lease.

Social vulnerabilities also increase the risk of homelessness, including social isolation. Older adults who lack

Table 70–2. Categories of homelessness.

1. *Chronic homelessness:* individuals with a disabling condition who have either been continually homeless for a year or more, or who have had at least 4 episodes of homelessness in the last 3 years.
2. *Intermittent homelessness:* individuals who experience 1 or more periods of homelessness of less than a year in total duration.
3. *Crisis homelessness:* individuals who are homeless for the first time, often following a catastrophic life event.

Table 70–3. Risk factors for becoming homeless after age 50 years.

Personal Factors
Death of a relative or close friend
Breakdown of a marital or cohabiting relationship
Disputes with a landlord, cotenant, or neighbor
Domestic or elder abuse
Lack of children, relatives, or friends willing to provide temporary housing
Release from prison

Economic Factors
Job loss
Difficulty paying a mortgage, rent, or utilities
Spending more than 50% of household income on housing
Loss of home (because of foreclosure of one's own home or a home one is renting, sale, conversion, not having one's name on a lease, falling behind on rent, precipitous rise in rent)

Medical Factors
New-onset or increased severity of mental illness
New-onset or increased severity of cognitive impairment

Data from Shinn M, Gottlieb J, Wett JL, Bahl A, Cohen A, Baron Ellis D. Predictors of homelessness among older adults in New York City: Disability, economic, human and social capital and stressful events. *J Health Psychol.* 2007;12(5):696-708; Crane M, Byrne K, Fu R, et al. The causes of homelessness in later life: findings from a 3-nation study. *J Gerontol B Psychol Sci Soc Sci.* 2005;60(3):S152-S159; and Williams BA, McGuire J, Lindsay RG, et al. Coming home: health status and homelessness risk of older pre-release prisoners. *J Gen Intern Med.* 2010;25(10):1038-1044.

children, relatives, or friends willing to house them are at increased risk for homelessness. Breakdown or loss of interpersonal relationships may also precipitate homelessness, such as death of a spouse or relative, divorce or breakdown of a cohabiting relationship, or disputes with landlords, co-tenants, or neighbors. It is not known if elder abuse increases the risk of homelessness, but domestic violence is a well-recognized risk factor. Conditions that are common among older adults at risk of homelessness increase the risk of elder abuse, including shared living situations and social isolation. Imprisonment also contributes to homelessness; older prisoners are at risk for homelessness following release (see Chapter 71, "Understanding the Effects of Criminal Justice Involvement on Older Adults"), and imprisonment of a partner may precipitate homelessness through loss of social or economic support.

Medical vulnerabilities can cause homelessness, including new onset or increasing severity of a chronic illness, mental health condition, or substance use disorder. These problems can lead to significant medical debt, or to job loss and inability to pay rent or a mortgage. The role of cognitive impairment as a risk factor for homelessness is not known, but cognitive impairment could lead to homelessness if impaired cognition causes difficulty holding a job or managing money.

To identify these risk factors for homelessness among older adults, clinicians should perform a detailed social history, including financial resources, ability to manage finances, social supports, substance use, and current housing situation, including if patients are living in market rate versus subsidized housing. If patients are renting, ask if their name is on the lease or sublease. Ask if patients are living temporarily ("doubling up") with friends or relatives, and if so, with whom they are living and how long they will be able to stay. If a patient is doubled-up and the patient's living situation is not stable, help prevent a first episode of homelessness by referring the patient to social work.

Social work referral may also be appropriate to determine eligibility for benefits such as Supplemental Security Income (SSI), Social Security Disability Insurance (SSDI), or the Supplemental Nutrition Assistance Program (SNAP). Although the availability of benefits differs by state, older homeless patients who are indigent and have disabilities that qualify them for SSI are usually eligible for Medicaid. Under the Affordable Care Act, in States that have accepted Medicaid expansion, in 2014, Medicaid benefits will be extended to Americans earning less than 133% of the federal poverty level, with or without disabling conditions. This will extend Medicaid to most homeless individuals.

Individuals facing imminent loss of housing are defined as homeless by Congress, and are therefore eligible for housing relocation and stabilization services, including rental assistance, mediation with property owners, and legal services.

HEALTH STATUS OF OLDER HOMELESS ADULTS

Most older homeless adults are 50–64 years of age; adults age 65 and older currently make up less than 5% of the total homeless population. Homeless adults in their 50s experience chronic illnesses and geriatric syndromes at rates similar to those of housed adults 15–20 years older. Approximately 75% of homeless adults age 50 years and older reported at least 1 chronic medical condition, and half reported 2 or more chronic conditions. The most common chronic illnesses were hypertension, arthritis, and asthma or chronic obstructive pulmonary disease. Because these studies relied on self-report by adults experiencing homelessness, who often have poor access to medical care and may have undiagnosed medical conditions, reported prevalences are likely to be underestimates.

Older homeless adults have high rates of geriatric syndromes. One-third of homeless adults age 50 years and older reported difficulty performing activities of daily living (ADLs), and nearly 60% had difficulty performing instrumental activities of daily living (IADLs). Half of older homeless adults fell in the last year. Cognitive impairment, measured as a Mini Mental State Examination (MMSE) score <24, was present in about one-quarter of older homeless adults. Between one-third and one-half of older homeless adults reported hearing impairment, and approximately 20% had impaired vision, defined as acuity >20/40. Nearly 50% reported urinary incontinence.

Early onset of chronic illnesses and geriatric syndromes in older homeless adults may result from the high prevalence of risk factors for poor health in this population, including poorly controlled chronic illnesses, traumatic brain injury, mental health conditions, and substance use disorders. Several factors contribute to poor control of chronic illnesses, including competing priorities for obtaining health care and lack of health insurance. Nearly three-quarters of older homeless adults experiencing homelessness reported one or more psychiatric conditions, including depression (34% to 60%), anxiety disorder (19%), and posttraumatic stress disorder (12%). Although homeless adults age 50 years and older have lower rates of both lifetime and current substance use disorders compared to their younger homeless counterparts, rates of alcohol and drug use are significantly higher than in the general population.

Because older homeless adults have early onset of chronic illnesses and geriatric syndromes at rates usually found in domiciled adults age 65 years and older, many experts consider homeless adults to be "older" at age 50 years, 15 years earlier than in the general population. This so-called accelerated aging in older homeless adults has important implications for screening and clinical care in this population. Compared to older adults who have housing, older homeless adults have limited ability to modify their environment to match their personal abilities. This mismatch between environmental demands and personal abilities puts older homeless adults at increased risk for adverse outcomes.

INTERACTION BETWEEN HEALTH STATUS AND ENVIRONMENT

Older homeless adults must cope with high rates of chronic conditions in the chaotic setting of homeless shelters or the street. Living in a shelter or on the street is hazardous at any age, but poses special hazards for older adults (see Table 70–3). Most shelters are group living spaces, with bunk beds and shared bathing facilities. These features may increase the risk of falling. Older adults also encounter risks outside of the shelter. Many shelters require occupants to vacate each morning and return in the evening to wait in line for a bed. On the street during the day, homeless adults are exposed to the elements and at risk for victimization. They must navigate a complex web of social services to obtain meals or shelter. Older homeless adults with impaired function, mobility, or cognition may be unable to safely perform these activities, resulting in falls, injuries, or inability to obtain food or shelter. Other hazards include difficulty toileting because of limited public bathroom facilities, and inability to safely store personal items, leading to lost or stolen medications, canes, and glasses.

Although clinicians face many challenges in caring for older homeless adults, several measures may improve care for these vulnerable older patients. These measures include screening for geriatric syndromes, mental health problems, and substance use disorders. As noted above, clinicians should work with other members of the health care team to determine eligibility for benefits and to refer to available community resources.

Most screening tools for geriatric syndromes are not validated in homeless adults, and there are no evidence-based guidelines for when to screen homeless patients for geriatric syndromes. The American Geriatrics Society recommends comprehensive assessment for geriatric syndromes (Chapter 6, "Geriatric Assessment") in frail, older patients who are at risk for functional decline, hospitalization, or nursing home placement. Because older homeless adults have rates of geriatric syndromes and hospitalizations similar to housed adults 15–20 years older, we recommend assessing homeless adults age 50 years and older for geriatric syndromes, as most screening instruments have been validated in these age groups, despite the lack of specific evidence in the homeless population. Based on the pattern of geriatric syndromes among older homeless adults, we recommend screening for functional and mobility impairment, falls, cognitive impairment, and urinary incontinence.

Although the Katz ADL Scale has not been validated in homeless adults, it has been widely used in younger patients with a range of chronic conditions. One-third of older homeless adults have difficulty performing ADLs, yet treatment options are limited because of the difficulty of modifying the environment of the shelter or street. Public or shared bathing facilities may lack modifications like grab bars and raised toilet seats. Informal caregiving by partners or friends is often not possible in the shelter, because shelters are segregated by sex, which may separate individuals from their caregivers. In addition, many adults experiencing homelessness are socially isolated. Furthermore, referrals for formal caregiving services such as home health aides are impractical in a shelter. A physical therapist may be able to recommend portable adaptive equipment for use in the shelter, such as canes, walkers, and dressing aids, but these materials are often stolen or lost.

Standard IADL scales include items that do not apply to homeless adults living in shelters or on the street, such as food preparation and housekeeping. The Brief Instrumental Functioning Scale (BIFS) was developed and validated for homeless adults, and asks about ability to perform the following activities independently or with help: fill out an application for benefits, budget money, use public transportation, set up a job interview, find an attorney to help with a legal problem, and take medications as prescribed by a physician. Homeless patients who are unable to perform these activities independently should be referred to social work and/or case managers.

Taking medications as prescribed poses special challenges in the shelter or on the street, where loss and theft of medications is common. Clinicians should ask if patients have a secure location to store medication, such as a storage locker

Table 70–4. Environmental hazards for older homeless adults.

Environmental Hazard	Associated Risk
Homeless Shelter	
Bunk beds	Falls, injuries
Lack of refrigeration	Inability to properly store medications (eg, insulin)
Lack of secure storage	Stolen/lost medications Stolen/lost adaptive equipment (eg, glasses, hearing aids, canes)
Noisy environment	Disrupted sleep
Group living environment	Victimization, lack of privacy, falls, injuries
Group showers	Victimization, lack of privacy, falls, injuries
Bathing and toileting facilities without adaptive equipment (ie, raised toilet seats, grab bars)	Falls, injuries
Institutional meals, often with high starch and salt content	Limited ability to modify diet to accommodate health conditions
Street	
Lack of public toilet facilities	Urinary incontinence, inability to maintain hygiene
Need to walk long distances between services, requiring higher functional status	Falls, injuries
Need to navigate complex web of social services to obtain food and shelter, requiring intact cognition and executive function	Food insecurity
Exposure to elements	Falls, injuries

at a shelter. If they do not, consider other strategies, such as dispensing medications 1 week at a time. Standard measures that improve medication adherence in older adults may also be helpful (Chapter 53, "Addressing Polypharmacy & Improving Medication Adherence in Older Adults").

The American Geriatrics Society recommends screening for falls beginning at age 65 years. However, homeless adults age 50 years and older fall at rates higher than the general older population and may benefit from earlier screening. A combination of factors may contribute to high rates of falls among older homeless adults, including environmental hazards (Table 70–4), functional and mobility impairment, and substance use disorders. Clinicians may be able to decrease the risk of falls among older homeless patients by ensuring that patients have a pass to sleep on the lower bunk, referring patients with impaired function or mobility to physical therapy, and providing counseling for substance use disorders.

Although screening tests for cognitive impairment have not been validated among homeless adults, most have been widely used in younger patients. Patients who screen positive for cognitive impairment should undergo standard medical assessment for reversible causes (Chapter 22, "Cognitive Impairment & Dementia"). Assess patients with cognitive impairment for decision-making capacity, and refer patients who lack decision-making capacity to social work.

Most screening tests for urinary incontinence have been validated in younger patients, such as the International Consultation on Incontinence Questionnaire (ICIQ). Managing urinary incontinence in shelters and on the street is challenging because of limited access to public toilets and use of shared toileting facilities. Where feasible, consider a trial of standard behavioral interventions, such as bladder training and pelvic muscle exercises.

To screen for depression in older homeless adults, we recommend using a screening tool validated in patients younger than age 65 years, such as the Patient Health Questionnaire 9. Although little is known about the prevalence of other mental health conditions among older homeless adults, consider screening for anxiety and posttraumatic stress disorder, given the high rates of mental health conditions in the general homeless population.

Substance use disorders are often underrecognized in older adults. However, screening for substance use disorders in older adults is particularly important because older adults are at higher risk for adverse effects of substance use as a result of changes in body composition with aging, higher rates of prescription medication use, and impairments in function, gait, and balance, among other factors (Chapter 58, "Managing Misuse of Alcohol & Psychoactive Prescription Medications in Older Adults"). The risk for adverse effects of substance use may be even more acute in older homeless adults, who have higher rates of substance use disorders and geriatric syndromes compared to the general older population.

Clinicians caring for older homeless patients should be aware of several resources for homeless individuals, including rapid rehousing, permanent supportive housing, medical respite, and intensive case management. *Rapid rehousing* provides rental assistance and services, and is most appropriate for individuals who experience barriers to housing but have the potential to sustain housing after the rental subsidy ends. *Permanent supportive housing* is defined as permanent, subsidized housing with onsite or closely linked supportive services (eg, medical, psychiatric, case management, vocational, and substance use services) for chronically homeless individuals. Because permanent supportive housing programs help chronically homeless adults maintain housing and may decrease use of acute health services, the federal government has identified such programs as a priority intervention for people experiencing chronic homelessness. Permanent supportive housing units are available in an increasing number of communities, funded by a combination of resident income, rent subsidies, tax credits, grants, and service-linked funding, such as Department of Mental Health benefits.

Medical respite is also recognized by the federal government as a strategy to decrease the negative impacts of homelessness on health. Medical respite programs provide temporary post-hospitalization care with medically oriented supportive services to homeless people discharged from acute care hospitals, but who are not medically ready to return to a shelter or the street. These services may be less costly compared to longer-term hospitalizations or stays in skilled nursing facilities or nursing homes. Moreover, patients discharged to medical respite instead of directly to shelters or to the street have fewer hospital readmissions. Medical respite services exist in a growing number of cities.

Intensive case management refers to a set of wraparound services delivered by highly trained case managers whose low case load allows for intensive follow-up with clients. Intensive case management programs were originally developed for patients with severe mental illness, and were later adapted to support individuals who used health services frequently, many of whom were homeless. Intensive case management differs from case management, a general term used to describe a range of programs, from peer support to medically oriented services. Many shelters and homeless assistance programs offer case management programs to help individuals experiencing homelessness to identify and access appropriate services.

As in general geriatric medicine, interprofessional teams may help improve care for older homeless adults (Chapter 5, "The Interprofessional Team"). An interprofessional team for an older homeless patient might include a case manager working to obtain permanent supportive housing, clinicians providing medical and psychiatric care, a social worker, and a substance abuse counselor.

CONCLUSIONS & NEXT STEPS

Homelessness and housing instability are associated with poor health. As a result of demographic shifts and the foreclosure crisis, these problems affect a growing proportion of older adults. Although clinicians face challenges in caring for adults experiencing homelessness and housing instability, understanding the unique health problems among homeless adults age 50 years and older and identifying risk factors for homelessness may improve care for these vulnerable groups. Furthermore, a growing number of federal programs provide resources to prevent new homelessness and to end chronic and crisis homelessness.

Brown RT, Kiely DK, Bharel M, Mitchell SL. Geriatric syndromes in older homeless adults. *J Gen Intern Med.* 2012;27(1):16-22.

Burt M, Aron LY, Lee E, Valente J. *Helping America's Homeless: Emergency Shelter or Affordable Housing?* Washington, DC: Urban Institute Press; 2001.

Caton CL, Dominguez B, Schanzer B, et al. Risk factors for long-term homelessness: findings from a longitudinal study of first-time homeless single adults. *Am J Public Health.* 2005;95(10):1753-1759.

Crane M, Byrne K, Fu R, et al. The causes of homelessness in later life: findings from a 3-nation study. *J Gerontol B Psychol Sci Soc Sci.* 2005;60(3):S152-9.

Culhane DP, Metraux S, Bainbridge J. The age structure of contemporary homelessness: risk period or cohort effect? *Penn School of Social Policy and Practice Working Paper.* 2010:1-28.

Garibaldi B, Conde-Martel A, O'Toole TP. Self-reported comorbidities, perceived needs, and sources for usual care for older and younger homeless adults. *J Gen Intern Med.* 2005;20(8):726-730.

Gelberg L, Linn LS, Mayer-Oakes SA. Differences in health status between older and younger homeless adults. *J Am Geriatr Soc.* 1990;38(11):1220-1229.

Hahn JA, Kushel MB, Bangsberg DR, Riley E, Moss AR. Brief report: the aging of the homeless population: fourteen-year trends in San Francisco. *J Gen Intern Med.* 2006;21(7):775-778.

Shinn M, Gottlieb J, Wett JL, Bahl A, Cohen A, Baron Ellis D. Predictors of homelessness among older adults in New York City: disability, economic, human and social capital and stressful events. *J Health Psychol.* 2007;12(5):696-708.

Sullivan G, Dumenci L, Burnam A, Koegel P. Validation of the brief instrumental functioning scale in a homeless population. *Psychiatr Serv.* 2001;52(8):1097-1099.

United States Congress, Homeless Emergency Assistance and Rapid Transition to Housing (HEARTH) Act. 111th congress, 1st session. S 896. Accessed April 20, 2012. Available at http://www.hudhre.info/documents/S896_HEARTHAct.pdf

United States Interagency Council on Homelessness. Opening doors: Federal strategic plan to prevent and end homelessness. Accessed April 20, 2012. Available at http://www.ich.gov/PDF/OpeningDoors_2010_FSPPreventEndHomeless.pdf

Understanding the Effects of Criminal Justice Involvement on Older Adults

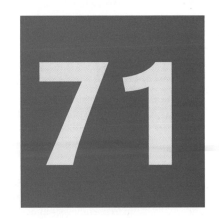

Lisa C. Barry, PhD, MPH

Brie A. Williams, MD, MS

▶ General Principles in Older Adults

Health care providers are increasingly managing the health of older patients who are currently or recently involved in the criminal justice system. These interactions occur in a variety of arenas. Many correctional systems contract with community clinics to provide prisoner-patients with specialty services, such as cardiology, neurology and dialysis. For acute care, prisoners are generally triaged to those hospitals with prison health care contracts, although in urgent or critical situations, a prisoner is brought to the nearest appropriate facility for care. As a result, current and former prisoners are seen daily at community clinics, specialty clinics, hospitals, and emergency departments around the country. Primary care providers are also increasingly taking care of patients who are arrested for the first time, as well as recently released older adults who are reintegrating into the community from prison or jail.

Increased attention from the press, nonprofit advocacy groups, and policymakers has spurred a growing literature in health and criminal justice research aimed at addressing the aging crisis in U.S. correctional systems. Studies suggest that currently and recently incarcerated older adults are a medically vulnerable group and that a history of incarceration is an important life event for health care practitioners to consider when caring for older patients.

EPIDEMIOLOGY

Prisoners age 55 years or older ("older prisoners") are the fastest growing segment of the criminal justice population, both as a result of stricter sentencing policy and an increasing number of older adult arrests. Since 1990, the number of older prisoners in the United States has more than tripled, and it is estimated that older prisoners could comprise up to one-third of the total U.S. prison population by 2030 if current sentencing policies remain unchanged. The percentage of new parolees who are older is also growing. Between 1990 and 1999, the number of state prisoners released to the community on parole nearly doubled and is expected to continue to increase.

▶ Physical Health

In general, older prisoners age prematurely and their physiologic age appears to be about 10–15 years older than their chronologic age. This "accelerated aging" can result from multiple factors—an unhealthy lifestyle prior to prison entry (eg, alcohol abuse, homelessness) and during incarceration (eg, poor diet, minimal exercise), limited lifetime access to preventive health care, and chronic stress during incarceration.

On average, older prisoners tend to have high rates of multimorbidity, geriatric syndromes, and functional impairments. Older prisoners have considerably higher rates of chronic illnesses, such as diabetes, hepatitis C, hypertension, and chronic obstructive pulmonary disease as compared with younger prisoners and age-matched community-living older persons, and they are also likely to take multiple medications. Geriatric syndromes, including vision and hearing impairment, falls, chronic pain, and urinary incontinence are also common in this population and may lead to unique challenges. For example, an older prisoner may be at increased risk for physical confrontation if he fails to respond to another inmate's request as a result of hearing loss or if he aggravates another inmate in close quarters because of incontinence. The prevalence of disability in traditional activities of daily living (eg, bathing, dressing) is higher in older prisoners than in age-matched older adults in the community. Additionally, disability rates in this population increase even more dramatically when considering unique activities that are necessary for independence in prison. These activities of daily living for prison include dropping to the floor for alarms and climbing on and off the top bunk. The inability to keep up with the fast pace of day-to-day prison life because of disability may make older prisoners more vulnerable to victimization by other inmates and at greater risk of disciplinary action from correctional staff.

▶ Mental Health

The prevalence of mental illness is much higher among prisoners as compared with those in the general population, regardless of age. Compared with younger prisoners, older prisoners have a higher likelihood of previous alcohol abuse, lower rates of personality disorders, and higher rates of depression, the most common mental health condition in this population. Similar to older persons living in the community, depression among older prisoners is often undertreated and frequently goes undetected; it may be misdiagnosed as a seemingly appropriate response to a medical illness or medication, or to the process of aging, in general, and it may be difficult to disentangle from conditions such as bereavement, fatigue, or cognitive impairment. High rates of undertreated and undetected depression likely contribute to the high rate of suicide in this population. In addition, although empirical research is lacking, histories of substance abuse, posttraumatic stress disorder, and traumatic brain injury may contribute to high rates of cognitive impairment in older prisoners, with 1 study reporting prevalence of 40%. Yet, early stages of cognitive impairment and dementia may be difficult to detect in the structured prison or jail environment as a consequence of limited opportunities for prisoners to make decisions, make plans, or initiate complex behaviors.

THE CLINICAL ENCOUNTER

With the aging of the population, an increasing number of older adults are coming into contact with the criminal justice system as arrestees, detainees in jail or prison, or as recently released members of the community. Clinicians should consider a recent history of criminal justice contact as a potential warning for underlying cognitive impairment, substance abuse, or psychiatric disease. In addition, given the health risks of incarceration, clinicians should screen those recently released for a history of victimization, depression/suicidality and infectious diseases such as hepatitis B and C and HIV. Recognition of the medical vulnerabilities of older adults involved in the criminal justice system is critical to maintaining the health and safety of this growing population. Table 71–1 details specific

Table 71–1. Considerations for the primary care physician whose patient has come in contact with the criminal justice system.

Clinical Encounter	Consideration	What to Do
Acute care of prisoners (eg, hospital; ER; specialty clinic)	Patients may have untreated or undertreated medical conditions resulting from suboptimal health care during incarceration	Optimize clinical care and evaluate for history of victimization during detainment including rape; screen for depression/suicidality and infectious diseases including tuberculosis (TB), HIV, methicillin-resistant *Staphylococcus aureus* (MRSA), and hepatitis B and C
	Conditions of incarceration (eg, overcrowding) are risk factors for poor health	
Outpatient care of persons who are recently arrested	A first arrest may be indicative of underlying medical condition	Rule out medical conditions (eg, dementia; alcohol or drug abuse/dependence) that may have led to the illegal behavior. Evaluate for common conditions in the criminal justice population including risky sexual encounters; infectious diseases; alcohol or drug abuse/dependence; homelessness
	Poor health may compromise ability to obtain appropriate legal counsel and increase safety risks during jail detainment	If patient is detained, consider contacting the jail Chief Medical Officer (CMO) or patient's legal counsel if there are concerns about patient's ability to participate meaningfully in the legal process or to be safe while in detainment
	Clinicians working in the prison system may have difficulty accessing prisoners' prior medical records and/or reconciling prisoners' medications	Contact physician at the correctional facility to confirm receipt of important clinical records
Outpatient care for persons reintegrating into the community after incarceration	Patients may have untreated or undertreated medical conditions resulting from suboptimal health care during incarceration	Obtain clinical records from correctional facility and optimize clinical care
	Conditions of incarceration (eg, overcrowding) are risk factors for poor health upon community reentry	Evaluate patient for history of victimization during detainment including rape; screen for depression/suicidality and infectious diseases including TB, HIV, MRSA (skin) and hepatitis B and C
	Barriers may hinder appropriate health care management	Evaluate living situation (eg, homelessness; living with adult child); determine availability of social support

considerations to guide the clinical encounter when a criminal justice history is identified. These considerations are further discussed in the following sections.

Care of a Patient Arrested or in Custody

In 2009, more than 530,000 persons age 55 years and older were arrested. These individuals include both first-time arrestees and those who are returning to jail or prison in later life, yet typically have been in the criminal justice system sporadically throughout their lives. The majority of persons who are arrested again in later life have multiple health problems resulting from a lifetime of unhealthy behaviors, including substance abuse, poor diet, risky sexual encounters, and substandard health care both prior to and (sometimes) during incarceration. They are also more likely to have been homeless with few family or community ties. These behavioral and physical health factors can adversely affect an older adult's ability to participate in the legal process or obtain appropriate legal counsel, and can also put them at risk for incarceration and associated decreased safety and worse health. Particularly for those arrested for the first time as an older adult, the event leading to the arrest may be indicative of an underlying medical condition. Clinicians can play a key role in evaluating for diagnoses such as alcohol or drug use, cognitive impairment, dementia, or delirium, which may have contributed to criminal justice involvement or result in implications for sentencing and/or safety during incarceration.

Care of a Patient Returning to the Community from Incarceration

A growing number of persons transitioning from incarceration to the community are older adults. As older prisoners are far less likely to be reincarcerated than younger prisoners, the transition from prison or jail to the community is particularly important. Substantial periods of time away from the community are associated with negative consequences. These include severed relationships with family and friends, and termination of housing and employment. In addition, the reinstatement of cancelled government entitlement programs such as Medicare, Medicaid, Social Security Insurance, and Veterans Health Administration benefits may take several months, thereby causing considerable stress for those returning to the community. Prisonization, or excessive dependence on the institutional routines of prison life, is also common among older inmates who have spent much of their lives in prison and may make it difficult to navigate life outside of prison. Regardless of how long a recently released patient was incarcerated, health problems, which may be exacerbated by the stresses of community reentry, can also lead to additional difficulties with employment, housing, and other important benchmarks of successful reentry. For example, older parolees with dementia could violate parole unintentionally. In general, health care practitioners should know that older adults

who are recently released from a jail or prison are at risk for adverse health outcomes including disproportionately high rates of mortality in the immediate post-release period and an increased risk of suicide after reentry into the community.

SUMMARY

Ideally, clinicians who treat older adults being released from incarceration should be contacted by jail or prison clinicians during the prerelease planning phase to optimize referral to social services such as reinstitution of government benefits including medical insurance and housing support, and continuing medical and mental health care of these individuals. However, this rarely occurs. It is, therefore, critically important to ask new patients about a recent or remote history of arrest, detainment, or incarceration.

Aday RH. Aging prisoners. In: Berkman B, ed. *Handbook of Social Work in Health and Aging*. New York, NY: Oxford University Press; 2006:231-244.

Barry LC, Abou JJ, Simen AA, Gill TM. Under-treatment of depression in older persons. *J Affect Disord*. 2012;136(3):789-796.

Binswanger IA, Stern MF, Deyo RA, et al. Release from prison—a high risk of death for former inmates. *N Engl J Med*. 2007;356(2):157-165.

Enders SR, Paterniti DA, Meyers FJ. An approach to develop effective health care decision making for women in prison. *J Palliat Med*. 2005;8(2):432-439.

Falter RG. Elderly inmates: an emerging correctional population. In: Moore J, ed. Management and Administration of Correctional Health Care. Kingston, NJ: Civic Research Institute; 2003. Chapter 9, p. 1-26.

Fazel S, Hope T, O'Donnell I, Jacoby R. Unmet treatment needs of older prisoners: a primary care survey. *Age Ageing*. 2004;33(4):396-398.

Fazel S, Baillargeon J. The health of prisoners. *Lancet*. 2011;377(9769):956-965.

Fazel S, Hope T, O'Donnell I, Piper M, Jacoby R. Health of elderly male prisoners: worse than the general population, worse than younger prisoners. *Age Ageing*. 2001;30(5):403-407.

Fazel S, Hope T, O'Donnell I, Jacoby R. Hidden psychiatric morbidity in elderly prisoners. *Br J Psychiatry*. 2001;179:535-539.

Hughes T, Wilson D; Bureau of Justice Statistics. Rentry trends in the United States. Available at http://bjs.ojp.usdoj.gov/content/pub/pdf/reentry.pdf

Human Rights Watch. Old Behind Bars: The Aging Prison Population in the United States. New York, NY: Human Rights Watch; 2012.

Kakoullis A, Le Mesurier N, Kingston P. The mental health of older prisoners. *Int Psychogeriatr*. 2010;22(5):693-701.

Kerbs JJ, Jolley JM. A commentary on age segregation for older prisoners: philosophical and pragmatic considerations for correctional systems. *Crim Justice Rev*. 2009;34:119-139.

Kingston P, Le Mesurier N, Yorston G, Wardle S, Heath L. Psychiatric morbidity in older prisoners: unrecognized and undertreated. *Int Psychogeriatr*. 2011;23(8):1354-1360.

Mitchell AJ, Rao S, Vaze A. Do primary care physicians have particular difficulty identifying late-life depression? A meta-analysis stratified by age. *Psychother Psychosom*. 2010;79(5):285-294.

Mitka M. Aging prisoners stressing health care system. *JAMA*. 2004;292(4):423-424.

Murdoch N, Morris P, Holmes C. Depression in elderly life sentence prisoners. *Int J Geriatr Psychiatry*. 2008;23(9):957-962.

Pratt D, Piper M, Appleby L, Webb R, Shaw J. Suicide in recently released prisoners: a population-based cohort study. *Lancet*. 2006;368(9530):119-123.

Williams B, Abraldes R. Growing older: challenges of prison and reentry for the aging population. In: Greifinger RB, ed. *Public Health Behind Bars: From Prisons to Communities*. New York, NY: Springer-Verlag; 2007;56-72.

Williams BA, Baillargeon JG, Lindquist K, et al. Medication prescribing practices for older prisoners in the Texas prison system. *Am J Public Health*. 2010;100(4):756-761.

Williams BA, Lindquist K, Sudore RL, Strupp HM, Willmott DJ, Walter LC. Being old and doing time: functional impairment and adverse experiences of geriatric female prisoners. *J Am Geriatr Soc*. 2006;54(4):702-707.

Williams BA, McGuire J, Lindsay RG, et al. Coming home: health status and homelessness risk of older pre-release prisoners. *J Gen Intern Med*. 2010;25(10):1038-1044.

Yorston GA, Taylor PJ. Commentary: older offenders—no place to go? *J Am Acad Psychiatry Law*. 2006;34(3):333-337.

Detecting, Assessing, & Responding to Elder Mistreatment

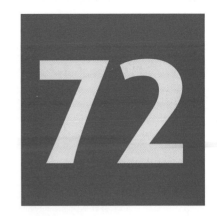

Tessa del Carmen, MD
Mark S. Lachs, MD, MPH

▶ General Principles in Older Adults

Elder mistreatment is a common yet underappreciated health issue affecting an increasing number of older adults each year.

Elder mistreatment can have a detrimental impact on victims' health and well-being and add significant costs to the health care system. Yet barriers to reporting incidences of elder mistreatment are significant. Patients may be unable to report because of cognitive impairment or social isolation. They may feel afraid, embarrassed, or ashamed, and perhaps worry about the repercussions of reporting (ie, retribution from those who are mistreating them, including caregivers or nursing home staff). Health care providers may have concerns about making the situation worse with reporting or intervention, may lack training in recognizing mistreatment, may be uncomfortable confronting the possible abuser, may be afraid of retaliation against the victim, or may not want to be involved in the legal system. That caregivers and family members are themselves most likely to be responsible for mistreatment in the community is a further challenge. As a result, it is estimated that as many as 4 of 5 cases of elder mistreatment remain unreported. By identifying instances of potential elder mistreatment, health care professionals play an important role for victims whose physical and mental health is at risk. The importance of this role is underscored by studies showing that elder mistreatment victims experience a significant increase in mortality. One large longitudinal study found that 9% of victims of elder mistreatment were alive after 13-year follow-up compared to 41% who had not experienced abuse and that victims of elder mistreatment were 3 times more likely to die during one 3-year period. Elder mistreatment victims are also at higher risk for other adverse outcomes including nursing home placement and depression.

According to the National Elder Abuse Incidence Study, 510,000 adults age 60 years and older experience some form of mistreatment each year. Only 21% of cases were reported to and verified by adult protective services (APS) agencies. A growing number of cases are occurring in nursing homes and other long-term care facilities, where some form of abuse is one of the most common complaints among residents. Abuse commonly reported in nursing homes includes physical abuse, neglect, sexual abuse, and financial abuse or misappropriation of property. State long-term care ombudsman programs are now federally mandated to report events of elder mistreatment that occur in institutions, though the majority of complaints to the state programs are filed by residents, family, and others. There were approximately 269,000 complaints of elder mistreatment in long-term care facilities reported to the National Ombudsman Reporting System in 2008, a number that is likely to grow as the population in nursing homes expands to meet the needs of our aging society.

▶ Defining Elder Mistreatment

A. Signs & Symptoms

There are various definitions of elder mistreatment. The American Medical Association describes elder mistreatment as an act of omission or commission that results in harm or threatened harm to the health or welfare of an older adult. As defined by the National Center for Elder Abuse, elder abuse is a term referring to any knowing, intentional, or negligent act by a caregiver or any other person that causes harm, or serious risk of harm, to a vulnerable adult. Elder mistreatment appears in several forms of abuse (Table 72–1): physical, sexual, psychological or emotional, financial, and neglect or self-neglect. The following terms were derived by the NCEA definitions:

1. Physical—Physical abuse is defined as physical contact that may result in any type of pain or injury. Physical abuse also may include unwarranted administration of drugs, physical restraints, force-feeding, or physical punishment.

Table 72–1. Types of elder abuse and associated signs.

Type of Abuse	Signs and Symptoms	Possible Physical Findings	Differential Diagnosis
Physical	Patient's report of abuse	Pattern of bruising or burns Burns in the shape of an object Bruising including bruises that encircle elder person's arms, legs, or torso Broken bones, sprains, dislocations, internal injuries Open wounds, cuts Untreated injuries	Osteoporosis Pathologic fractures Metabolic disorders Frequent falls
Sexual	Patient's report of sexual abuse Unusual sexual behavior Unusual or inappropriate relationship between the patient and possible abuser Patient's report of sexual assault or rape	Bruises on or around the genital area/breasts Unexplained sexually transmitted diseases or genital infections Unexplained vaginal or anal bleeding Torn, stained, or bloody underwear Pain on walking or sitting	Vaginosis, nonsexually transmitted diseases like *Candida* Dementia-related behavior
Psychological/ emotional	Depression Anxiety Agitation Excessive fears Sleep changes Change in appetite	Passive Evasive Fear—possibly in presence of abuser Confusion Agitation Significant weight loss or gain Sudden worsening medical conditions	Psychiatric disorders Cognitive impairment Worsening dementia
Financial	Ambiguity of financial status Inability to pay bills, buy food or medications Sudden changes in legal documents (eg, will, power of attorney, or health care agent) Excessive concern regarding expenses necessary for patient's care by the possible abuser	Living well below the patient's means Discomfort/evasiveness when discussing finances	Psychiatric disorders Cognitive impairment/dementia Neurologic disorders
Neglect	Absence of assisted hearing devices, eyeglasses, dentures or assisted walking devices Sudden changes or decline in health	Malnutrition Dehydration Poor hygiene Inadequate or inappropriate clothing Decubitus ulcers/bedsores	Chronic diseases that can affect nutrition including end stage dementia, dysphagia, Parkinson disease, amyotrophic lateral sclerosis, malabsorption syndromes, malignancy

Physical findings potentially associated with physical abuse include a pattern of bruising or burns, including burns in the shape of an object or bruises that encircle an elder person's arms, legs, or torso, broken bones, sprains, dislocations, internal injuries, open wounds, cuts, and untreated injuries. A patient's report is typically essential in identifying instances of physical abuse.

2. Sexual—Sexual abuse is sexual contact or behavior of any kind with an older adult that is either against their will or with an older adult who lacks capacity to give consent. Physical findings associated with sexual abuse may include bruises or bleeding around the genitals or chest, unexplained sexually transmitted diseases or genital infections, unexplained genital bruising or bleeding, torn, stained, or bloody clothing especially underwear, and new injuries. In addition to the patient's report of sexual abuse, potential signs of sexual abuse include an unusual or inappropriate relationship between the patient and potential abuser.

3. Psychological or emotional—Psychological or emotional abuse is defined as words or actions that spur emotional stress. Physical signs may include functional decline, behavior changes in the patient, significant weight loss or gain, and worsening of medical conditions or new onset medical conditions. Other signs of possible psychological abuse include a passive or evasive affect, fear (possibly in the presence of an abuser), or increased confusion or agitation. Differential diagnosis for depression, cognitive impairment, or worsening dementia is important when evaluating for psychological abuse and is discussed further below. Reporting of psychological abuse is not required in all states (eg, California) and health professionals may wish to seek the outside consultation of a mental health or social worker where psychological abuse is suspected.

4. Financial—Financial abuse the misuse of finances or possessions of an older adult for another's gain. Financial abuse is one of the most common forms and may occur in any context, including among family caregivers, friends, and in nursing homes or long-term care facilities. Financial abuse is often accompanied by social isolation or loneliness when an older adult either agrees to enter into an arrangement where friendship is traded for money or other gain or when the perpetrator isolates older adults to exert undue influence over their finances. Forcing an older adult to the automated teller machine or a check-cashing business to withdraw cash is also common and may be considered both financial abuse and abduction. Older adults who are victims of financial exploitation may have diminished mental capacity to understand their decisions. Potential signs of financial abuse include a findings of a patient living well below the patient's means. Discomfort/evasiveness when discussing finances, ambiguity of the patient's finances, a patient's unexplained inability to pay bills, inability to buy food or medications, unexplained sudden changes to legal documents, and over-eagerness by another in the older patient's assets.

5. Neglect—Neglect is the failure to provide any care or responsibilities that they must provide for the patient. Neglect can be active or passive and can be either intentional or unintentional. Common physical signs of neglect include malnutrition, dehydration, poor hygiene, inadequate or inappropriate clothing, and decubitus ulcers or bedsores. Other signs to look for are sudden or questionable deteriorations of health or the absence of needed assistive devices including assisted hearing devices, eyeglasses, dentures, and walking devices/wheelchairs. Self-neglect occurs when an older adult with cognitive or functional impairment cannot care for themselves nor attain help to get the care needed. Self-neglect may coincide with neglect of family or other caregivers or may occur when an older adult refuses help and/or takes efforts to conceal their inability to meet basic needs.

Differential Diagnosis

A number of chronic illnesses and injuries sustained by older adults may mimic mistreatment. Consequently, it can be challenging for clinicians to make the definitive diagnosis of elder mistreatment or self-neglect. Dramatic injuries such as fractures, burns, contusions and lacerations that are accompanied by a credible patient history pose no diagnostic quandary; however, subtle presentations of medical

Table 72-2. Risk factors for suffering from and committing elder abuse.

Risk factors for suffering from abuse
Living in the same household
Socially isolated
Conditions that increase dependence (advanced age, lack of financial sophistication, disability [physical or mental], and recent personal loss)

Risk factors for committing abuse
Family caregiving
History of mental illness
History of physical abuse in the past
Substance abuse
Elder dependence (ie, emotional, financial)
Single caregiver and perception of stress (ie, caregiver stress)

problems over long periods of time can be difficult to distinguish from elder mistreatment. Therefore, self-neglect or elder mistreatment should be included in differential diagnosis when evaluating older adults. Table 72-1 lists some examples of underlying medical problems that could mimic elder mistreatment.

Risk Factors

Elder abuse affects people of all ethnic backgrounds and social status. It affects both men and women. Similarly, those who commit elder abuse come from all backgrounds and can have close or distant connections to the victim. Table 72-2 lists common risk factors for suffering from and committing elder abuse.

Screening

There are multiple screening and assessment tools for elder mistreatment, but health care professionals may neither have access to them nor have been trained to administer them. To date, there is no widely accepted single screening tool or method of assessment for elder mistreatment. Some tools may be useful to identify those at risk for abuse while others are useful to identify ongoing abuse. Cohen et al have categorized different instruments into 3 categories:

- Direct questioning of the suspected abuse or self-reporting of abuse (eg, Hwalek-Sengstock Elder Abuse Screening Test [H-S/EAST], Vulnerability to Abuse Screening Scale [VASS])

- Tools that look for signs of abuse (eg, Elder Assessment Instruments [EAI] by Fulmer and Wetle)

- Tools that evaluate the risk of abuse (eg, Indicators of Abuse Screen [IOA] by Reis and Namiash)

Table 72–3. Screening for elder mistreatment suggested by the AMA.

Screening Questions for the Patient	Screening Questions for the Possible Abuser
Is someone hurting you? Physically or verbally? Have you been threatened or been called names?	Tell me about the person you give care to and how much care does that person require?
Do you feel you are being cared for properly?	What tasks can the person perform by themselves and what is he/she limited with?
Have you ever been pressured to do something against your will?	What expectations does the person have for you? Can you accomplish what he/she expects?
Do you have any concerns about your finances? Has your money or property ever been used by someone else? Has any of your money or property been taken or signed over to someone else?	Do you have any responsibilities outside of the home?
Does your caregiver rely on you financially?	Elder patient care can be quite difficult; has the patient ever frustrated you?
Are you aware of any behavioral violence, alcoholism, illicit drug abuse, or psychiatric disorders by your caregiver?	Have you ever raised your voice or threatened the patient?
	What kind of support would you need in order to help take care of the patient?

The American Medical Association recommends that all physicians routinely inquire about the physical, sexual, and psychological abuse of an older patient as part of the medical history. Physicians should also consider abuse as a factor in the presentation of medical complaints as abuse may adversely affect patients' health status or ability to adhere to medical recommendations.

A direct approach to a patient who is a possible victim of elder mistreatment is advised. Health care professionals should question the patient and caregiver separately and identify potential red flags. Many health care interactions, such as those that take place in an emergency room, may not allow for a comprehensive elder mistreatment screen. In these cases a single-question or 3-question screen can be used.

- Single question screen: Are you being abused or neglected?
- Three-question screen: Do you feel safe where you live? Who prepares your meals? Who takes care of your checkbook?

Table 72–3 includes additional suggested questions that are commonly used in screening for elder abuse.

▶ **Assessment**

Suspected elder mistreatment victims should undergo comprehensive geriatric assessment in addition to the traditional history and physical exam. This should include an assessment of their psychosocial and functional capabilities or limitations (see Chapter 2, "Consideration of Function & Functional Decline," Chapter 4, "The Social Context of Older Adults,"

and Chapter 6, "Geriatric Assessment"). An interdisciplinary approach to the assessment and plan is highly desirable. The following was adapted from Breckman and Adelman:

A. History Taking

When taking a medical history from an older adult, conduct interviews in a private space and with the patient alone. The patient and examiner should be at eye level, and any assistive devices needed for communication should be provided (ie, hearing devices, amplifiers, glasses, dentures). The health care professional should be cognizant of cultural sensitivity during the history and examination, as cultural differences may contribute to varying perceptions of what constitutes elder mistreatment.

Clinicians must determine the patient's cognitive status (see Chapter 22, "Cognitive Impairment & Dementia"). Assessing the patient's level of cognitive functioning may require further evaluation.

Health care professionals need to differentiate possible signs and symptoms of abuse from medical conditions. It is important to determine the patient's functional status and ability to perform activities of daily living. If the patient needs assistance, then it is essential to find out if the patient has access to help as well as the knowledge of who is to provide assistance.

It is important to explore the patient's living arrangement, as patients and potential abusers may live in the same household. Determining how long the patient has been living with that person(s), as well as who pays the bills and who owns or rents where the patient lives, can provide critical information regarding the potential for mistreatment. Questions about the financial status of the patient can help in assessing potential financial abuse. Identify the person who manages

Table 72–4. Summary of signs and symptoms of elder mistreatment to look for during history taking.

Items from patient history that may signal elder mistreatment
Repeated use of emergency department and admissions; multiple use of different emergency departments
Delays in seeking treatment
Explanation of injuries are inconsistent with medical findings
Inconsistent history of injury
Prior history of similar injuries
Multiple missed medical appointment(s) and/or going to multiple medical providers
Signs from patient demeanor and responses that may signal elder mistreatment
Patient may seem hesitant or afraid to answer questions
Potential abuser answers all questions and prevents examiner from interviewing/examining the patient alone
Patient seems fearful of potential abuser
Potential abuser acts angry or indifferent towards the patient
Potential abuser refuses to provide necessary assistance for patient's care
Potential abuser seems overly concerned at the cost of care for the patient

a patient's finances and whether the patient is dependent on others for living and personal expenses. Social support should be determined as victims of elder mistreatment are often socially isolated. Table 72–4 summarizes the symptoms of elder mistreatment to look for in the medical history.

B. Physical Exam

The physical exam should include full examination of the patient, from head to toe. It should begin with general observation, including appearance, signs of dehydration, weight loss, and hygiene. A complete exam should include visual examination of a patient's body and skin for any evidence of physical abuse, poor hygiene, skin breakdown; a musculoskeletal examination for signs of fractures or previous fractures; a complete neurologic examination to search for possible signs of delirium, cognitive impairment or dementia; and a genitourinary and rectal examination for signs of sexual abuse. If there are any signs of mistreatment, then further laboratory tests and radiologic examinations should be done depending on the findings. Some examples of suggested further testing include diagnostic imaging for fractures, checking electrolytes for dehydration, liver function tests for malnutrition, and/or checking hemoglobin and hematocrit for anemia.

▶ Intervention/Treatment

Elder mistreatment is a complex medical problem that requires a multidisciplinary treatment approach. Each case

of elder abuse or neglect necessitates individualized assessment and treatment planning.

A. Medical Intervention

1. Documentation—Documentation of the abuse or neglect should be completed regardless of the health care setting. The provider should record the chief complaint in the patient's own words if possible. Proper documentation should include a complete medical and social history. If appointments are repeatedly canceled, the name of the caller should be noted. If injuries are present, the type, number, size, location, and color, as well as the patient's overall state of health, the resolution of the problems, and possible causes should be included. The provider should render an opinion on whether injuries were adequately explained by the history. All laboratory or radiologic and imaging studies should be recorded. If it is possible, obtain color photographs. If the police are called, the name of the officer, actions taken, and police incident number should be documented as well as the date and time the report was made to APS and the name of the person taking the report. The diagnosis of elder mistreatment should be included in the medical problem list.

2. Reporting—Health care professionals make up the greatest reporting source of potential elder mistreatment to APS agencies. Legal requirements differ from state to state. Knowing your state's reporting system is crucial. Nearly all states mandate health care providers to report cases of elder abuse. (Colorado, New York, North Dakota, and South Dakota do not currently mandate health care providers to report suspected or identified cases of elder abuse, but have voluntary reporting systems.) In some states, health care providers can be found negligent if they do not report suspected mistreatment. The website for National Center on Elder Abuse, which is part of the Administration on Aging, lists state directory of help lines, hotlines and elder abuse prevention resources (http://www.ncea.aoa.gov).

3. Discharge or ongoing care planning—The provider must ensure that the older adult's medical and safety needs have been met. If the patient does not meet the criteria for admission to the hospital after the provider has documented the findings and filed a report, the provider must be sure that the home environment is safe and that there is assistance at home for functionally and/or cognitively impaired patients. A social work consultation or consultation with an APS specialist may be necessary before discharge in order to develop a safety plan.

Elder mistreatment is often a chronic problem and patient's with history of elder mistreatment should be referred to a physician or medical team with whom the elder can have an ongoing relationship. Elder mistreatment presents special difficulties for the patient in terms of function, decision-making capacity, and health and social support. These inter-related problems are best handled by a team of professionals from medicine, law, and social services. Clinicians should be skilled in the recognition of geriatric syndromes and familiar with local agencies that provide services to a mistreated older patient. Comprehensive geriatric assessment and intervention may be needed for vulnerable abused or neglected elders (see Chapter 6, "Geriatric Assessment"). It is often helpful to discharge the patient to their home with as many appropriate services as possible. Home health agencies can provide in-home assessments by social workers or nurses. Other referral sources include drug and alcohol rehabilitation services, and legal assistance or advocacy groups.

4. Assessment of decision-making capacity—In many instances, the mistreated elder is vulnerable because the elder lacks the capacity to participate fully in decision making. Additionally, acute illness can reduce an older person's ability to make rational and informed decisions. A competent individual has the right to be a fully informed participant in all aspects of decision making and has the right to refuse care. However, patients who lack decision-making capacity and whose expressed choices may lead to harm or even death need protection and assistance. The determination of neglect versus informed personal choices will hinge on an older adult's capacity to participate in the elder's own care. Therefore, it is essential to determine each patient's decision-making capacity whenever assessment for elder abuse or self-neglect is in question (for more on informed decision making, see Chapter 12, "Ethics & Informed Decision Making").

B. Social Services Intervention

APS or similar entities can provide social interventions in almost every jurisdiction in the United States. APS specialists usually receive reports, conduct investigations, and coordinate social interventions. They elicit input from collateral sources such as friends and family members of the patient and consult with other social workers, physicians, and nurses. After the APS specialists complete the investigation and comprehensive in-home assessment of the patient's situation, they develop plans to address mistreatment issues and other problems they have identified. APS works closely with victims, families, and other involved parties. APS's goal is to ensure that the service provided is the least-restrictive alternative, reflects the patient's preferences, and maximizes the older adult's independence. When a patient has the capacity to make informed decisions, the APS specialists advocate for the right to refuse services if the individual does not want intervention. As advocates of a legal jurisdiction, APS specialists are bound by statutory limitation and may not impose services such as medical care if the patient is capable of making decisions.

C. Legal Interventions

Although laws differ from state to state, law enforcement is generally involved in cases in which crimes are committed against older adults, including physical abuse, neglect with malicious intent, financial exploitation and other forms of elder mistreatment. Police officers investigate cases for evidence to help prosecutors pursue perpetrators. Officers of the court and judges participate in guardianship hearings when appropriate. Members of law enforcement and the legal profession help link older persons with agencies and other resources available to victims of crime. Forensic pathologists work closely with law enforcement officers to determine the cause of death in cases of suspected homicide resulting from abuse or neglect.

SUMMARY

Elder mistreatment, particularly abuse, neglect and financial exploitation, can be a common occurrence. Health care providers should screen and assess for potential abuse. Making a diagnosis of elder mistreatment can often be difficult but knowing the signs and symptoms and maintaining a high index of suspicion can help identify potential victims and abusers. Knowledge of your state's reporting system and laws is essential. The goal of treatment for patients who are victims of elder mistreatment is to improve their safety, health, and well-being.

2008 National Ombudsman Reporting System Data Tables, U.S. Administration on Aging Department of Health and Human Services. Accessed May 07, 2010. Available at: www.aoa.gov/AoARoot/AoA_Programs/Elder_Rights/Ombudsman/National_State_Data/2008/Index.aspx

Acierno R, Hernandez MA, Amstadter AB, et al. Prevalence and correlates of emotional, physical, sexual, and financial abuse and potential neglect in the United States: the National Elder Mistreatment Study. *Am J Public Health.* 2010;100(2):292-297.

The Administration on Aging. The National Elder Abuse Incidence Study: final report September, 1998. US Department of Health and Human Services, Administration on Aging (www.aoa.dhhs.gov/abuse/report/default.html).

Ahmad M, Lachs MS. Elder abuse and neglect: what physicians can and should do. *Cleve Clin J Med.* 2002;69(10):801-808.

American Medical Association. Accessed April 28, 2009. Available at: www.ama-assn.org/ama/pub/physician-resources/medical-ethics/code-medical-ethics/opinion202.shtml

American Medical Association Diagnostic Treatment Guidelines on Elder Abuse and Neglect. Chicago, IL: American Medical Association; 1992.

Ansell P, Breckman RS. Assessment of Elder Mistreatment Issues and Considerations. Elder Mistreatment Guidelines for Healthcare Professionals: Detection, Assessment and Intervention. New York: Mt. Sinai/Victim Services Agency Elder Abuse Project; 1988.

Aravanis SC, Adelman RD, Breckman R, et al. Diagnostic and treatment guidelines on elder abuse and neglect. Arch Fam Med. 1993;2:371.

Bass DM, Anetzberger GJ, Ejaz FK, Nagpaul K. Screening tools and referral protocol for stopping abuse against older Ohioans: a guide for service providers. *J Elder Abuse Negl.* 2001;13(2):23-38.

Bonnie RJ, Wallace RB (Eds). Elder Abuse: Abuse, Neglect and Exploitation in an Aging America. Washington, DC: National Academy Press; 2002.

Breckman R, Adelman R. *Strategies for Helping Victims of Elder Mistreatment*. London: Sage Publications; 1988.

Cohen M. Screening tools for the identification of elder abuse. *J Clin Outcomes Manag*. 2011;18(6):261-270.

Cohen M, Halevy-Levin S, Gagin R, et al. Elder abuse: disparities between older people's disclosure of abuse, evident signs of abuse, and high risk of abuse. *J Am Geriatr Soc*. 2007;55(8):1224-1230.

Dyer DB, Heisler CJ, Hill CA, Kim LC. Community approaches to elder abuse. *Clin Geriatr Med*. 2005;21(2):429-447.

Elder Mistreatment: Abuse, Neglect and Exploitation in an Aging America. Washington, DC: National Research Council Panel to Review Risk and Prevalence of Elder Abuse and Neglect; 2003.

Ferguson D, Beck C, Carney MT, Kahan FS, Paris BEC. Elder abuse: is every bruise a sign of abuse? *Mt Sinai J Med*. 2003;70(2):69-74.

Fulmer T, Guadagno L, Bitondo Dyer C, Connolly MT. Progress in elder abuse screening and assessment instruments. *JAGS*. 2004; 52:297.

Fulmer T, Paveza G, Abraham I, Fairchild S. Elder neglect assessment in the emergency department. *J Emerg Nurs*. 2000; 26:436.

Fulmer T, Street S, Carr K. Abuse of the elderly: screening and detection. *J Emerg Nurs*. 1984;10(3):131-140.

Halphen JM, Dyer CB. Elder mistreatment: abuse, neglect, and financial exploitation (Internet); www.uptodate.com; Apr 16, 2012, cited 12/17/13.

Kruger RM, Moon CH. Can you spot the signs of elder mistreatment? *Postgrad Med*. 1999:106;169-183.

Lachs MS. Screening for family violence: what's an evidence-based doctor to do? *Ann Intern Med*. 2004;140:399.

Lachs MS, Pillemer K. Abuse and neglect of elderly persons. *New Engl J Med*. 1995;332:437.

Lachs MS, Pillemer KA. Elder abuse. *Lancet*. 2004;304:1236-1272.

Lachs MS, Williams CS, O'Brien S, et al. The mortality of elder mistreatment. *JAMA*. 1998;280:428.

Lachs MS, Williams CS, O'Brien S, Pillemer KA, Charlson ME. The mortality of elder mistreatment. *JAMA*. 1998;280(5): 428-432.

Mosqueda L, Burnight K, Liao S. The life cycles of bruises in older adults. *J Am Geriatr Soc*. 2005;53(8):1339-1343.

Neale AV, Hwalek MA, Scott RO, et al. Validation of the Hwalek-Sengstock elder abuse screening test. *J Appl Gerontol*. 1991;10:406.

Ploeg J, Fear J, Hutchinson B, et al. A systematic review of interventions for elder abuse. *J Elder Abuse Negl*. 2009;21:187-210.

Pompei P, Murphy JB, eds. Geriatrics Review Syllabus: A Core Curriculum in Geriatric Medicine. 6th ed. New York: American Geriatrics Society; 2006;86-91.

Reis M, Nahmiash D. Validation of the indicators of abuse (IOA) screen. *Gerontologist*. 1998; 38:471.

Schofeld MJ, Mishra GD. Validity of self-report screening scale for elder abuse: Women's Health Australian Study. *Gerontologist*. 2003;43:110-120.

State Ombudsman Data: Nursing Home Complaints. Office of Inspector General, Department of Health and Human Services. Accessed July 01, 2003. Available at: www.oig.hhs.gov/

Swagerty DL, Takahashi P, Evans J. Elder Mmistreatment. *Am Fam Physician*. 1999 May 15;59(10):2804-2808.

Tatara T. The National Elder Abuse Incidence Study. The National Center on Elder Abuse, 1998. Accessed March 09, 2009. Available at: www.ncea.aoa.gov/ncearoot/Main_Site/Library/Statistics_Research/National_Incident.aspx

USEFUL WEBSITES

Administration on Aging. www.aoa.gov

Agency for Healthcare Research and Quality. www.ahrq.gov/

Long-Term Care Ombudsman Resource Center. www.ltcombudsman.org

National Center on Elder Abuse. www.ncea.aoa.gov

National Committee for the Prevention of Elder Abuse. www.preventelderabuse.org

National Council on Child Abuse and Family Violence. www.nccafv.org/elder.htm

WHO: Elder abuse. www.who.int/ageing/projects/elder_abuse/en/

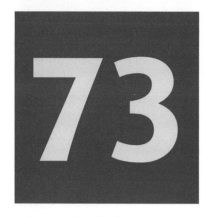

73

Meeting the Unique Needs of LGBT Older Adults

Mark Simone, MD

Manuel Eskildsen, MD, MPH

▶ General Principles in Older Adults

Older adults who are lesbian, gay, bisexual, or transgender (LGBT) are a vulnerable group with specific health care needs that are largely unrecognized. Health care professionals and society in general too often fail to address the sexuality, and sexual orientation, of older adults. However, LGBT older adults are also much more likely than other generations of LGBT adults to hide their sexual orientation, as a result of a lifetime of experiencing discrimination from a society that has only recently evolved to become more accepting of homosexuality.

The general LGBT population is affected by health disparities, and as such, has higher rates of common and life-threatening physical and mental health conditions, and these disparities carry over into older years as well. Older LGBT adults continue to be affected by unequal treatment and ongoing social stigma, which we explore in this chapter. This chapter also describes specific health concerns related to LGBT aging, in addition to psychosocial concerns that are of tremendous importance.

DEFINITIONS

Homosexuality is an orientation toward people of the same gender in sexual behavior, affection, attraction, and/or self-identity. Bisexuals have an orientation toward people of both genders. Transgender includes people whose gender identity and expression do not match, including transsexual, transvestite, androgyne, and intersex individuals; they may or may not also consider themselves homosexual or bisexual.

It is important to note that sexual orientation is much more than just sexual behavior. For instance, some who have same-sex attractions may never engage in same-sex behavior, and those who engage in same-sex behavior may not identify as being homosexual. For some people, sexuality is more fluid, and so sexual orientation may change over time. This may also

be more prevalent in older generations who felt the need to hide their sexual orientation, thus "staying in the closet," by pretending to be heterosexual in order to avoid discrimination and rejection. "Coming out of the closet" refers to the process of disclosing that one identifies as LGBT, and for many, this is a life-long process. As described below, this process has been especially difficult for the older LGBT population.

▶ Demographics

It is difficult to determine the number of LGBT Americans older than age 65 years because of the lack of reliable statistics, and major challenges recording such statistics such as unwillingness to report sexual orientation, but the best estimates are 1–3 million, based on a range of 3% to 8% of the general population being LGBT. By 2030, there will be an estimated 2–6 million older LGBT Americans. U.S. census data from 2000 and 2010 showed that same-sex–headed households existed in >90% of all counties, and that more than 1 in 10 same-sex couples included a partner older than age 65 years.

▶ History of Stigma and Prejudice Linked to Issues of Coming Out and Disclosure

Older LGBT adults came of age during a time in the United States when being LGBT was viewed in an especially negative light. This group of older adults is divided into 2 cohorts, depending on whether they came of age before or after the Stonewall Riots of 1969, which were demonstrations that are considered to be the beginning of the gay civil rights movement in the United States. The current older, pre-Stonewall generation grew up in a society with widespread and accepted discrimination against LGBT persons, and lived most of their lives in a society where the expression of their sexual orientation was criminalized by the government and pathologized by the medical community. For instance, it was not until

1962 that the first state decriminalized private, consensual homosexual acts, and it was not until 1973 that the American Psychiatric Association stopped designating homosexuality a mental disorder that could be treated and cured. Society's views of homosexuality did not begin to change until the late 1960's and 1970's. In contrast to the pre-Stonewall generation, the Stonewall generation of LGBT baby boomers, those currently in their 50s or 60s, came of age during the social unrest of the 1960s and a time of rising social acceptance of LGBT people. And still, a 2006 survey of LGBT baby boomers found that the greatest concern of aging was facing discrimination related to sexual orientation.

The overt discrimination experienced during the pre-Stonewall period severely inhibited the pre-Stonewall generation from coming out as young adults and being out in old age. Thus, they are much more likely to have kept, and continue to keep, their sexual orientation hidden. In contrast, LGBT baby boomers are more likely to be at least partly open about their sexual orientation, with 76% of lesbians and 74% of gay men in 2009 reporting that they were mostly or completely "out of the closet."

Although the climate has changed considerably in the decades since Stonewall, the more persons experienced homophobia as young adults, the less likely they are to be out to their physicians. Studies suggest that discrimination and stigmatization can be associated with lower life satisfaction, lower self-esteem, depression, suicide, substance abuse, and unhealthy and risky behavior. Nondisclosure of sexual orientation may also lead to delay in care, inappropriate care, and prevent the development of a trusting provider–patient relationship.

▶ Patient–Provider Communication

Health care providers should provide culturally competent care that creates the optimal environment for the respectful care of LGBT older adults. All health care providers should ask their older patients about their sexual health, including sexual orientation, while also keeping in mind that LGBT older adults may be unwilling or psychologically unable to disclose their sexual orientation. The intention of asking about sexuality is not to force disclosure of sexual orientation, but rather, to provide an opportunity, and a safe and supportive environment, to come out of the closet if desired. Studies show that poor relationships with providers and mistrust of others in the medical field were some of the reasons why homosexuals, especially lesbians, do not receive appropriate preventive care. This sentiment was also demonstrated in a survey of LGBT baby boomers, where less than half expressed strong confidence that health care professionals would treat them with dignity and respect because of their sexual orientation. Local LGBT centers of the clearinghouse at Services and Advocacy for LGBT Elders (http://www.lgbtagingcenter.org) and the Gay and Lesbian Medical

Table 73–1. Resources for LGBT health and aging.

Name	Website
Services and Advocacy for Gay, Lesbian, Bisexual & Transgender Elders (SAGE)	http://www.sageusa.org
Gay and Lesbian Medical Association (GLMA)	http://www.glma.org
American Society on Aging (ASA)	http://www.asaging.org/lain
National Gay and Lesbian Task Force	http://www.thetaskforce.org/issues/aging
Gay, Lesbian, Bisexual, and Transgender (GLBT) Health Access Project	http://www.glbthealth.org
National Coalition for LGBT Health	http://lgbthealth.webolutionary.com
CenterLink (formerly The National Association of Lesbian, Gay, Bisexual and Transgender Community Centers)	http://www.lgbtcenters.org
Human Rights Campaign	http://www.hrc.org/issues/aging.asp
Vancouver Coastal Health Transgender Health Program	http://www.vch.ca/transhealth
Fenway Health and the Fenway Institute	http://www.fenwayhealth.org

Association website (http://www.glma.org) are good sources of information in finding welcoming providers. Table 73–1 lists additional resources.

HEALTH ISSUES FOR LGBT OLDER ADULTS

Research on health maintenance and medical issues for older LGBT adults is unfortunately limited. There are certain issues that require particular attention in LGBT patients because of health disparities that affect this group (Table 73–2). In addition, older LGBT people may be more susceptible to mental health disorders as a result of the stresses associated with long-term concealment of sexual identity, many years of exposure to discrimination, and greater risk of inadequate support.

▶ Health Issues for Older Gay and Bisexual Men

Sexual health (function, activity, and safer sex methods) should be discussed with older gay and bisexual men so as to assess for and reduce the risk of sexually transmitted diseases. Although the Centers for Disease Control and Prevention (CDC) currently recommends routine HIV testing for all people younger than age 65 years, it is important to consider testing in any sexually active person at any age, especially in the presence of risk factors. Human papillomavirus (HPV)

Table 73–2. Overview of specific health care issues to address in older LGBT adults.

Gay and Bisexual Men	Lesbian and Bisexual Women	Transgender
HIV/AIDs	Prevention/screening	HIV/AIDs
Sexually transmitted diseases/sexual health	Sexually transmitted diseases/sexual health	Sexually transmitted diseases/sexual health
Anal papilloma/anal cancer	Breast cancer/gynecologic cancer	Preventive care/access to health care
Substance abuse	Substance abuse	Substance abuse
Cardiovascular disease	Cardiovascular disease	Hormone therapy
Mental health	Mental health	Mental health
Psychosocial issues	Psychosocial issues	Psychosocial issues

screening should also be offered to men who have sex with men in the form of a routine anal pap smear every 2–3 years, especially in men who have unprotected receptive anal intercourse, or who have HIV, to screen for early signs of precancerous cells caused by certain strains of the HPV virus that can lead to anal cancer.

Younger gay and bisexual men are more likely to smoke cigarettes, and while older gay men appear to have similar rates of smoking compared to heterosexuals, the effects of previously higher rates of smoking in this group may continue to be a risk factor for cardiovascular disease, including stroke and heart attacks. There are also several cancers which may be more common among gay and bisexual men. These include anal cancer, caused by the human papillomavirus; lung cancer caused by smoking; colon cancer, perhaps attributable to reduced rates of screening; liver cancer related to an increase in hepatitides B and C infections.

▶ Older Lesbian and Bisexual Women's Health

There is good evidence that lesbians receive less preventive care, access health care services less often, and enter the health care system later, than heterosexual women. Most of the health disparities experienced by women who have sex with women relate to difficulty in accessing the health care system, which in part is due to prior discrimination or fear of being treated poorly as a result of being lesbian/bisexual. Lesbians have lower rates of Pap screening and mammograms as compared to heterosexuals. In addition, older lesbians and bisexual women should be counseled on safer sex practices and engaged in conversations about sexual health and function. Sexually active lesbians and bisexual women should be screened for cervical cancer, domestic abuse, and sexually transmitted infections. Clinicians should avoid assuming heterosexuality of older patients, and keep in mind that some women are or have been sexually active with both men and women, even if they identify as "straight" or lesbian. Also keep in mind that sexual identity and behavior can change over time, and that many lesbians have had children and grandchildren from heterosexual or homosexual relationships.

Lesbian and bisexual women may be at an increased risk of heart disease because of higher rates of risk factors for cardiovascular disease, such as cigarette smoking and obesity. On average they have a higher body mass index (BMI) than their heterosexual counterparts. They may be at greater risk of cervical and breast cancer as a result of decreased access to screening. Because of increased smoking rates, lesbian and bisexual women may also have greater risk of lung cancer.

▶ Older Transgender Health

Although there has been little research on the health issues of older gay and lesbian patients, there are even fewer studies on transgender health, and the particular challenges of caring for older transgender patients. As transgender adults age, they may encounter health issues that correspond to their biologic sex, leading to additional stress as they cope with a disease or condition associated with the gender they have left behind. Appropriate health screenings for the birth gender is important preventive care for transgender patients. Disease prevention and health education are key for transgender patients, who are often marginalized by society. Prejudice remains a major barrier to appropriate health care for transgender adults. Many lack health insurance or have insurance programs that do not cover health care related to transgender issues, including hormone treatment. The consequence is that many transgender adults use "black market" hormones, lack preventive care, and do not have their mental health needs addressed. Rates of HIV and viral hepatitis infections, as well smoking and substance abuse, are higher in this group compared with the LGB community and heterosexual counterparts. The University of California San Francisco's Center of Excellence for Transgender Health is a rich resource for the care of transgender folks, and provides a primary care protocol, including recommendations for general prevention and screening. For example, they recommend routine mammogram screening in transwomen (MTF: male-to-female transgender persons) older than age 50 years with additional risk factors (estrogen and progestin use >5 years, positive family history, or BMI >35).

Mental Health

There is a link between mental health and health disparities. Communities that suffer health disparities are more likely to have higher rates of mental health issues, particularly depression and anxiety. Older LGBT people who have lived in the closet for much of their lives can have significant stress, loss of self-esteem, and less-fulfilled lives. Trying to manage stigma, marginalization, and self-esteem, can lead to higher rates of depression, suicide, risky sexual behavior, and substance abuse. More research is needed regarding the prevalence of mental health disorders in LGBT older adults. Older LGBT adults appear to have elevated levels of current or lifetime depression, with rates possibly being the highest among transgender people. Very little research has explored mental health problems in transgender adults; what is known is that they have experienced a major life change and many have faced tremendous discrimination. They are more likely to have adjustment disorders, anxiety disorder, posttraumatic stress disorder, depression, and substance abuse.

HIV in Older Adults

Although the topic of HIV is covered in Chapter 47, "Common Infections," it is worth noting that there is not only an increasing prevalence of older adults living longer with HIV, but also an increasing incidence of new HIV infections in older adults. More than 37% of all those infected with HIV in the United States are older than age 50 years, and by 2015, more than half will be older than age 50. More than 17% of new HIV infections occur in older patients, and men who have sex with men remain a large percentage of those infected. Minorities with HIV/AIDS have higher mortality rates: the death rates are 5 times higher among older Hispanics, and 12 times higher in older blacks. Health care providers need to better educate older patients about safer sex, and also need better detect and screen for HIV in older adults. The HIV and Aging Consensus Project is a resource for suggested treatment strategies for caring for older adults with HIV/AIDS.

BIOPSYCHOSOCIAL ASPECTS OF CARE

Social Supports and Family Structure

The social support structures of LGBT older adults tend to be different from those of older adults in the general population. Whereas older adults in the general population tend to rely on spouses and adult children as part of a network of support that is able to meet an older individual's psychosocial and caregiving needs, LGBT older adults are more frequently socially isolated and may rely on informal networks for their social needs.

There are several reasons for this social isolation: LGBT older adults are less likely to be partnered, less likely to have children, and more likely to live alone. Also, lack of societal acceptance can lead to estrangement from biologic family members, like former spouses or adult children. Because of this, LGBT older adults are more likely to rely on informal "families of choice," comprised of extensive networks of friends. Even though these informal networks can be a great asset, they also have some disadvantages. For example, these networks can deteriorate over time as a consequence of the effects of aging and poor health on the stability of the support network, putting the LGBT senior at further risk of isolation. As a result of these informal networks, it is imperative that clinicians carefully document patient choices for surrogate decision makers, who may often be a person that is not the legal default next-of-kin (see "Visitation Rights and Advance Care Planning" below on advanced care planning for LGBT older adults).

Housing and Long-Term Care

Antidiscrimination laws in housing do not extend themselves to LGBT persons. Neither do patterns of spousal inheritance apply for same-sex spouses in most states. If legal provisions are not made through wills and trusts, inheritance of home ownership may bypass a surviving partner and go to the deceased partner's heirs. Legal planning is necessary to secure housing for a surviving partner.

Entering a long-term care facility is a particularly vulnerable and potentially dangerous time for this population. There is a significant amount of real or feared discrimination, from both the staff and the other residents. By 2030, there will be an estimated 120,000–300,000 older LGBT adults living in nursing homes. A 2005 study found that 73% of LGBT adults believed that discrimination exists in retirement settings, 60% believed that they would not have equal access to social and health services, and 34% believed that they would have to hide their orientation upon entry into a retirement facility. Fear of disclosure is a significant and unique concern of LGBT seniors who are entering long-term care facilities, and concealing one's identity and key relationships may prevent them from receiving appropriate care, threaten the ability to make meaning of one's life, and can be very damaging to one's personal identity and emotional, psychological, and physical well-being. Home care agencies and long-term care facilities are making strides in becoming more inclusive of the LGBT community, but more awareness and training is needed. Specific training in these areas is increasingly available, for instance, the LGBT Aging Project (http://www.lgbtagingproject.org/).

▶ Policy Issues Affecting LGBT Older Adults

LGBT elders face many policy challenges to their financial well-being. Some of the challenges derive from their frequent reliance on nontraditional family structures, but many exist because of unequal treatment reflected in laws and regulations. As of this publication, many states and the District of Columbia now recognize same-sex unions; however, the majority of states still do not offer same-sex couples any recognition, thus denying them the scores of protections given to married couples in their jurisdictions. In June 2013, the United States Supreme Court overturned sections of the Defense of Marriage Act (DOMA) that prohibited the federal government from recognizing same-sex marriages performed in the states. With this, same-sex couples that are married in states where there is marriage equality are able to enjoy federal benefits of marriage such as inheritance, tax, social security, and immigration benefits. Notwithstanding, same-sex couples are only able to access those benefits if they marry in jurisdictions were same-sex marriage is legal.

▶ Visitation Rights and Advance Care Planning

Because of the lack of policy recognition for LGBT couples by most states, long-term partners may be seen as "legal strangers" in situations of illness and disease by their health care providers. This often has the practical effect of taking decision-making powers away from "families of choice," and giving them to blood relatives whose relationships with LGBT patients may not be as close, and who may not be as accepting of their relative's homosexuality. Up until 2011, hospital staff in most U.S. states could refuse visitation rights for a sick partner and limit visitation to only family members, choosing to ignore same-sex partners if their relationship were not legally recognized by their state. However, President Obama issued an executive order which took effect January 2011, mandating that all hospitals extend visitation rights to the partners of gay, lesbian, bisexual, and transgender men and women.

Documenting advance health directives is one of the strategies that older LGBT adults can pursue to ensure that their wishes are respected in the health care setting. Through a living will, a person may declare their preferences for their end-of-life care. The main disadvantage of relying solely on this document is that it will not designate a surrogate decision maker, and therefore the desired surrogate decision maker may not be allowed to make decisions for an LGBT patient if not specifically documented. Therefore, drafting a document which specifically designates an alternative decision maker in the case of incapacity is critically important to ensure that LGBT couples can legally safeguard their choice of decision maker (they are named differently in different states, eg, "health care proxy" or "durable power of attorney for health care"; see Chapter 12, "Ethics & Informed Decision Making," for more information on surrogate decision makers and advanced care planning).

CONCLUSION

At least 3% to 8% of older adult patients are LGBT, and these persons have specific medical, psychological, and social needs. Health care providers must be sensitive to the specific challenges faced by this group, and provide the appropriate support and resources that address their needs. For additional resources to aid the provider in caring for older LGBT patients, see Table 73–1. Many older LGBT adults have faced a lifetime of discrimination and health disparities, and health care professionals should consider this when providing appropriate and compassionate care to this vulnerable group. As with all cross-cultural topics, one should not assume that the negative experiences and health disparities described in this chapter are automatically true for every individual LGBT older adult, as there are certainly examples of happy, healthy, and successful individuals who are all the more remarkable for having overcome significant obstacles to live enriched and inspiring lives.

Appelbaum J. Late adulthood and aging: clinical approaches. In: Makadon H, Mayer K, Potter J, Goldhammer H, eds. *The Fenway Guide to Lesbian, Gay, Bisexual and Transgender Health.* Philadelphia, PA: American College of Physicians; 2007: 135-156.

Cahill S, South K, Spade J. *Outing Age: Public Policy Issues Affecting Gay, Lesbian, Bisexual and Transgender Elders.* Washington, DC: The Policy Institute of the National Gay and Lesbian Task Force; 2000.

Dean L, Meyer IH, Robinson K, et al. Lesbian, gay, bisexual, and transgender health: findings and concerns. *J Gay Lesbian Med Assoc.* 2000;4(3):101-150.

HIV and Aging Consensus Project. *Recommended Treatment Strategies for Clinicians Managing Older Patients with HIV.* Accessed April 28, 2012. Available at: http://www.aahivm.org/ Upload_Module/upload/HIV%20and%20Aging/Aging%20 report%20working%20document%20FINAL%2012.1.pdf

LGBT Movement Advancement Progect and SAGE. *Improving the Lives of LGBT Older Adults.* March 2010. Accessed December 2013. Available at: http://www.lgbtmap.org/file/improving-the-lives-of-lgbt-older-adults-large-print.pdf

Simone M, Appelbaum J. Addressing the health needs of older LGBT adults. *Clin Geriatr.* 2011;19(2):38-45.

UCSF Center of Excellence for Transgender Health. Accessed January 2013. Available at: http://www.transhealth.ucsf.edu/ trans?page=home-00-00

Applying Evidence-Based Medicine to Older Patients

74

Kenneth E. Covinsky, MD, MPH

Ideally, the care of older patients should be grounded in the best available evidence about the benefits and harms of treatments. Unfortunately, high-quality evidence rarely exists. Good studies of a clinical condition often exclude older persons. Even when older persons are included, enrollment tends to be limited to healthy robust older persons who may little resemble the patient in front of you.

As a result, one can rarely practice true evidence-based medicine in older patients. Instead, one needs to examine available evidence and then critically assess the extent to which the evidence might apply to the patient being treated. To best make optimal clinical decisions, clinicians need to understand the limitations of applying the clinical research literature to their older patients, and thoughtfully apply existing evidence to the individual patient they are treating.

THE CHALLENGES WITH CURRENT EVIDENCE

Clinicians are generally trained to consider outcomes from clinical trials as the gold standard for how to apply evidence-based medicine to clinical care. Ideally, clinical trials would include any patient who is a logical candidate for the therapy being examined. Unfortunately, most clinical trials include only idealized patients, excluding patients in whom the therapy has a greater risk of side effects, or patients who are at risk for not completing the trial. However, these nonidealized patients who are commonly excluded from clinical research are just the type of patients seen in geriatric practice, and in whom the therapies will often be used and marketed.

Zulman et al have described a framework that outlines the reasons older persons may be excluded from clinical trials. These reasons include explicit age exclusions, implicit age exclusions, and unintentional age exclusions.

▶ Explicit Age Exclusions

Many studies have age-specific cutoffs in which all subjects above a defined age are denied enrollment. Although these

exclusions are common, they can almost never be justified. Most studies with explicit age exclusions present absolutely no rationale to justify the exclusion.

An explicit age exclusion is only justifiable if one clearly would not offer a therapy in clinical practice to persons older than a particular age. In actual practice, most therapies tested in younger patients are eventually offered to older patients. Furthermore explicit age exclusions ignore the vast heterogeneity in health in older persons.

▶ Implicit Age Exclusions

More often, the reasons for excluding older subjects are more subtle. Many studies without an age cutoff have exclusion criteria that differentially restrict the entry of older patients, particularly older patients who are more medically complex. Examples of implicit age exclusions include comorbidity, functional impairments, cognitive impairments, and inability to give informed consent.

A. Comorbidity

Treatment studies often focus on the effect of a specific treatment on health outcomes in persons with a specific condition. But most older people have multiple conditions. Yet many studies of specific conditions exclude patients with additional health conditions other than the condition being studied. For example, a study comparing the effectiveness of bronchodilator and anticholinergic inhalers for chronic obstructive pulmonary disease (COPD) excluded persons with chronic kidney disease or hospitalizations for congestive heart failure (CHF) in the past year. This is very problematic in older persons, as many older persons with COPD have coexisting chronic kidney disease or CHF. In actual practice, comorbidity is the norm, not the exception, and most treatments are still offered to older patients despite this comorbidity. It is difficult to judge the risk and benefits of treatments studied in idealized patients when applied to real patients with complex comorbidity.

B. Functional Impairment

Many studies exclude patients with "poor performance status" or poor functional status. Although there are many simple tools available to define functional status, often studies do not include a definition of poor functional status.

Many older patients have functional limitations and, in practice, these are rarely viewed as contraindications for most therapies. Often, the goal of therapy for older adults may be to prevent further loss of function. However, functional problems, such as falls, can markedly alter the risk and benefits of therapies. The failure to account for functional impairments in most studies makes it difficult to gauge how a patient's functional impairments should affect the decision to offer a treatment.

C. Cognitive Impairment and Inability to Consent

Studies often exclude subjects who have cognitive impairment or are unable to provide informed consent. Often, the studies fail to describe how cognitive impairment or consent capacity was assessed.

Cognitive impairment is extremely common in older patients and older adults with cognitive impairment are usually offered the same therapies as patients without cognitive impairment. Because most studies fail to even describe the cognitive status of their subjects, it is often impossible to know how cognitive impairment might impact the risks and benefits of a treatment. Additionally, in clinical practice, family members are often asked to consent to treatments when the patient is unable to fully understand the risks and benefits. While methods exist for enrolling these patients in studies using similar approaches for surrogate consent, surrogate consent is often not attempted.

D. Nursing Home Patients

Virtually all treatments offered in the community are offered to persons in nursing homes. It is extraordinarily rare to find a study of any therapy that even considers nursing home patients as candidates for enrollment. As a result, there is an extraordinary lack of evidence to guide most therapeutic decisions in nursing home patients.

▶ Unintentional Exclusions

Even when studies have few exclusion criteria, study processes may unintentionally exclude older patients who are potential targets for therapy. For example, many studies have complex procedures for follow-up. Often follow-up procedures require patients to report to a study center for examinations and blood draws. But many older patients no longer drive, making participation difficult. This type of subtle exclusion is important because the same factors that make study follow-up difficult may make the type of monitoring and followup that is needed difficult in the less mobile older patient being considered for treatment. Also, while sensory problems, such as vision and hearing impairment, may not be an explicit study exclusion, sensory impairment may make study enrollment and follow-up difficult for older patients. For example, older adults with hearing impairment may be excluded from studies that screen enrollees over the phone or require answers to phone-based health status questionnaires. Many studies do not budget the extra cost needed for in-person interviews for older participants who are hard of hearing.

APPLYING THE EVIDENCE TO YOUR OLDER PATIENTS

Applying evidence from clinical research to an individual patient can be difficult. However, addressing a series of questions can help a clinician make the best possible inference about how existing evidence might inform the best clinical decision in their patient. In addition to addressing whether patients in existing studies are similar to your patient, one should also think about what outcomes matter to your patient and whether limited life expectancy might affect the risks and benefits of the treatment in question.

▶ How Do the Characteristics of My Patient Differ from Those Patients in the Research Studies?

It is particularly useful to consider the types of aging patients who are excluded in clinical studies. For a relatively healthy older patient, there may be no reason to believe that a treatment that is indicated in a younger patient will not also be useful in the older patient. However, this conclusion might change as one considers the comorbid burden, degree of functional impairment, and cognitive problems in a frailer older patient. In a patient with many comorbid conditions, it is possible that side effects of a treatment may exacerbate one of the comorbid conditions. In a patient with functional impairment, falls may be a particular concern. A medicine that causes slight problems with balance may not be a big concern in a younger patient, but could precipitate a complicated fall in an older patient.

Similarly, if a medicine such as warfarin requires close titration and monitoring to minimize possible complications, the presence of cognitive impairment can markedly impact the risks/benefit titration.

▶ What Outcomes Matter to My Patient?

Many clinical trials focus on outcomes such as mortality, or disease-specific outcomes such as cardiovascular hospitalizations. Even though these outcomes are particularly relevant to older patients, other outcomes, such as preserving mobility, preventing falls, or quality of life, may matter more to many older patients. Because these outcomes are often not included in many studies, clinicians must often make their best inference about how a treatment impacts these outcomes.

Because quality of life is best judged by the patient, a patient's own sense of how a treatment is impacting him or her can be a crucial criterion in assessing the risks and benefits of therapy. This can be especially important for a patient taking multiple medicines. Some patients may not be bothered by taking many medicines, while for others, the addition of another medicine may be sufficiently burdensome and distressing to outweigh a small benefit seen in clinical studies.

How Does My Patient's Life Expectancy Impact the Risks and Benefits of Treatment?

Some treatments confer immediate risks to patients, whereas the benefits accrue over time. Older patients with limited life expectancy may be subject to all of the risks of treatment with few benefits. This concern becomes increasingly important with increasing age, as well as in patients with limited life expectancy as a result of major comorbidity, or severe functional or cognitive impairment. These concerns are addressed in greater depth in Chapter 8, "Prevention & Health Promotion."

Overall, the exclusion of older participants in clinical research can affect the ease with which a clinician applies the evidence base to the clinician's patient. Knowing the important ways that one's patient is similar or different from participants in clinical research, as well as the quality of life factors that are most important to one's patient, should guide all evidence-based medical decisions in geriatric care.

Boyd CM, Darer J, Boult C, Fried LP, Boult L, Wu AW. Clinical practice guidelines and quality of care for older patients with multiple comorbid diseases: implications for pay for performance. *JAMA*. 2005;294(6):716-724.

Covinsky KE. Management of COPD: Let's just pretend older patients don't exist. Accessed August 28, 2012. Available at: http://www.geripal.org/2011/03/management-of-copd-lets-just-pretend.html.

Lee SJ, Eng C. Goals of glycemic control in frail older patients with diabetes. *JAMA*. 2011;305(13):1350-1351.

Zulman DM, Sussman JB, Chen X, Cigolle CT, Blaum CS, Hayward RA. Examining the evidence: a systematic review of the inclusion and analysis of older adults in randomized controlled trials. *J Gen Intern Med*. 2011;26(7):783-790.

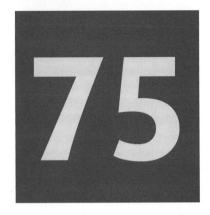

International Perspectives in Geriatric Care

GERIATRIC CARE IN JAPAN

Sandra Y. Moody, MD, BSN, AGSF & Miwako Honda, MD

"Given that the biggest cause of concern among the people at large is being looked after in their old age, it is desirable to enhance the programs for dealing with this."

KEMPOREN, 2011

Japan has the highest life expectancy, at nearly 87 years, and faces the most rapidly aging society in the developed world. This likely has been achieved through a convergence of several factors, but most importantly a decline in infant mortality since the 1920s, an economy that grew rapidly over 2–3 decades beginning in the late 1950s, and the introduction of universal health insurance coverage in 1961, which allowed equal access to health care across the population. Commensurate with the growing proportion of older adults in Japan, the total fertility rate has decreased drastically, and continues to do so, leading to a crossover effect—a rapid growth in the proportion of older adults, with a declining proportion of younger people.

The proportion of adults age 65 years and older has grown substantially from 4.9% in 1950 to 22.7% in 2010. As of March 2012, Japan's total population was estimated to be 127,650,000, with approximately 29,487,150 individuals who were age 65 or older. Furthermore, it is estimated that by 2050, a full 40% of Japan's population will be age 65 years and older. Assuming Japan's total population will decrease during the next 50 years, by 2060, nearly 41 million individuals (40.5% of the population) will be age 65 years or older.

In addition to having the longest life expectancy, Japan also has been noted to have the best healthy life expectancy in the world as of 2007, which is partly attributed to a national health insurance plan that encourages annual health checks and preventative care. For example, on average, Japanese men live in a healthy state for 73 years and women for 78 years. These successes put Japan in a position to serve as a model to other nations as they address similar aging-related issues, including the United States.

▶ Challenges of an Aging Society

Japan faces several challenges given its aging society. These challenges include: (a) how to continue to support and maintain its national health insurance system, and (b) how to prepare a health care workforce that can care for a society that is aging rapidly.

A. Health Care Expenditure in Japan

Japan's national health insurance is a social insurance plan to which all citizens must contribute. Broadly speaking, the health care payment structure consists of insurance premiums and state subsidies. According to the KEMPOREN (the National Federation of Health Insurance Societies), for those who are fully employed, insurance premiums are drawn from their "monthly salary, bonuses, allowances, and all other forms of compensation for work received by the insured person from the employer." This cost, shared by the employee and employer, ranges from 3% to 12% (the proportion employees pay depends on their annual salary). The state pays the administrative costs. Because the payment structure is complex, it is not discussed in detail here.

As of 2008, health care expenditures in Japan were only 8.5% of the gross domestic product compared to approximately 16% for the United States. As fewer younger workers contribute to the coffers of the health care system, Japan will be challenged to keep health care expenditure as low as possible and still pay for its aging society. Many approaches are being considered, but one is to create a social structure that dispenses with forced retirement and encourages older adults to continue to work for as long as possible based on ability and not age.

B. Geriatric Medicine in Japan

The relative underdevelopment of geriatric medicine in Japan poses another challenge to overcome as the society ages. Geriatric medicine was recognized as a subspecialty in 1988 (Japan Geriatrics Society). Currently, there are 6200 members of the Japan Geriatrics Society, which is one of the main organizations that advocates for the care of older adults, but only 1494, as of December 2013 physicians are board certified in geriatrics. This translates into 1 geriatrician for every 34,500 older adults. Not all older adults are in need of a board-certified geriatrician, but because the general population of doctors has not been trained in geriatric medicine, a huge burden rests on those who are.

There are 80 medical schools in Japan and between 30 and 40 university- or hospital-based departments or divisions of geriatrics/gerontology. The care of older persons occurs from 2 perspectives—geriatrics and gerontology. Geriatrics focuses on the care of older persons through research, education, and clinical practice, but the research is the most emphasized. Gerontology focuses on health promotion by way of social welfare, psychology, environmental, and social systems.

Not only is clinical geriatrics underdeveloped, but there is also very little formal geriatrics education in medical school or postgraduate training. Furthermore, medicine in Japan is composed of mostly subspecialists. Primary care in its "purest" form is not widely practiced. For example, general internal medicine and family medicine specialties are in formative stages throughout the country. In general, subspecialists provide both primary and subspecialty care. Nevertheless, geriatrics is gradually being integrated into current practice by on-the-job training ("geriatricizing" currently practicing physicians) through seminars and the availability of an online geriatrics handbook provided by the Japan Geriatrics Society. Additionally, some of the physicians train abroad in geriatrics with the intent of expanding geriatrics practice in Japan. Change is afoot, but there are unmet opportunities to develop the field at a faster rate in response to apparent or projected need.

▶ Innovative Models of Care

One of the most innovative care models in Japan is the *Public Long-term Care Insurance System (LTCI)*, a system that has been updated over the years. Its predecessor, the *Long-term Insurance Act*, was approved by parliament in 1997 and came into effect in April of 2000. The Long-term Insurance Act was created to address the increasing health care needs of the older adult population resulting from a gradual change in societal norms—mainly a breakdown in traditional family supports for older adults. Traditionally, the daughter-in-law of the eldest son became the caregiver for her parents-in-law, but more and more women are working outside the home; fewer people are getting married and when they do, they do

so at an older age; and many women no longer want to be the primary caregivers. As the gap in traditional family supports has increased, the government has stepped in to fill the gap.

According to Tamiya et al, the primary focus of the LTCI is "to help older people lead more independent [lives] and to relieve the burdens of family [caregivers]." They further state that it operates on social insurance principles, in which health care benefits are provided regardless of income or family situation; coverage and benefits are substantial; only services, not cash allowances, are provided; and recipients are free to choose the type of services they will need as well as the entity that will serve as the provider of those services. The providers of care include the local government, semipublic welfare corporations, nonprofit organizations, hospitals, and others. In Japan, the average length of hospital stay is about 2 weeks, but can be prolonged for various reasons if the older person does not have a place that can provide the appropriate level of care upon discharge.

A. The Long-term Care Insurance System

All individuals age 40 years and older are covered under this plan. However, the primary recipients are those who are age 65 years and older. Individuals who are between the ages of 40 and 64 years receive coverage only if they have a "geriatrics-related" illness, such as dementia, stroke, or significant functional disability. To keep costs down, the services are primarily community-based, with the intent of preventing institutionalization—whether acute hospitalization or long-term nursing home care. Fifty percent of the cost derives from public funds and 50% from premiums paid by the recipients. A cap is placed on how much the individual has to pay to prevent financial catastrophe.

The appropriate level of care for each patient is determined by the patient's answers to a 74-item questionnaire that is based on activities of daily living, which are then analyzed to determine 1 of 7 levels of care for which the person is eligible. The levels identify a person is "self-reliant," "needs assistance" (levels 1 and 2), or needs long-term care (levels 1–5). The higher numbers indicate greater needs. Figure 75–1 gives the outline of the LTCI system. According to Tamiya et al, it has been difficult to show the efficacy of LTCI, but there is some evidence that it is effective in reducing caregiver burden.

SUMMARY

Japan faces a rapidly aging society, possesses the oldest society in the developed world, and has the highest healthy life expectancy. It has been successful in creating one of the most innovative long-term care insurance plans worldwide. Yet, it will require a herculean effort for Japan to fully develop the practice of geriatric medicine and to train enough physicians, including more geriatrics specialists, to meet the health care needs of its aging population. Many efforts are currently

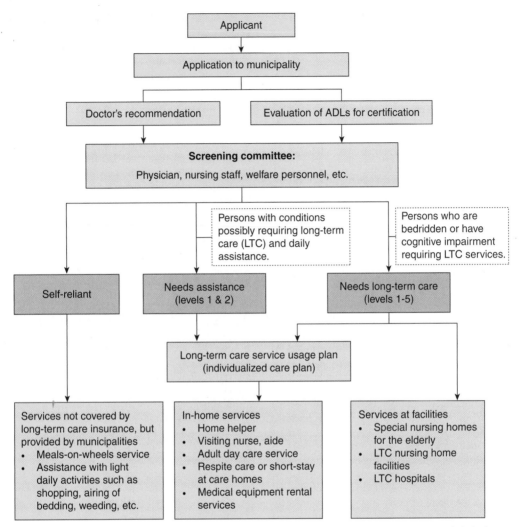

▲ **Figure 75–1.** Organization of the Long-term Care Insurance System in Japan. ADLs, activities of daily living. (Modified from Health Insurance, Long-term Care Insurance and Health Insurance Societies in Japan 2011. Reproduced with permission from KEMPOREN National Federation of Health Insurance Societies, p. 89, June 2011.)

underway, but how successful Japan will be in meeting its goals in a time-sensitive manner is yet to be determined.

Aria H, Ouchi Y, Yokode M, et al; Members of the Subcommittee for Aging. Toward the realization of a better aged society: Messages from gerontology and geriatrics. *Geriatr Gerontol Int.* 2011;12(1):16-22.

Health Insurance, Long-term Care Insurance and Health Insurance Societies in Japan 2011. Published by KEMPOREN National Federation of Health Insurance Societies, pp. 88-101, June 2011.

Ikeda N, Saito E, Kondo N, et al. What has made the population of Japan healthy? *Lancet.* 2011;378(9796):1094-1105.

Reich MR, Ikegami N, Shibuya K, Takemi K. 50 years of pursuing a healthy society in Japan. *Lancet.* 2011;378(9796):1051-1053.

Tamiya N, Noguchi H, Nishi A, et al. Population ageing and wellbeing: lessons from Japan's long-term care insurance policy. *Lancet.* 2011;378(9797):1183-1192.

USEFUL WEBSITES

Japan Geriatrics Society. http://www.jpn-geriat-soc.or.jp

Roster Board Certified Geriatricians Japan Geriatrics. https://www.kktcs.co.jp/jgsmember/secure/senmon/seek.aspx

Ministry of Health, Labour and Welfare; http://www.mhlw.go.jp/english/topics/elderly/care/2.html

National Institute of Population and Social Security Research in Japan. http://www.ipss.go.jp/index-e.asp

GERIATRIC CARE IN ISRAEL

Jochanan Stessman, MD & Jeremy M. Jacobs, MBBS

Comprehensive health care is a universal right of all citizens of Israel. In 1995, the Israeli parliament passed the National Health Insurance law, which guaranteed compulsory membership to 1 of 4 existing health maintenance organizations (HMOs), all of whom are obligated by law to provide a Uniform Benefits Package, locally known as the "health basket." This continually updating umbrella of services includes preventive, ambulatory, emergency, and hospital care of all types, as well as paramedical care. The HMOs compete among themselves for membership, based upon satisfaction of health insureds, quality of care and services provided. Comprehensive coverage is irrespective of age, and older people are of prime importance within the national health care system.

Funding for the health service is derived from health tax (26%), direct government funding (35%), supplementary optional services provided by HMOs and the private sector (38%), and donations (1%). Per capita reimbursement of health taxes to the HMOs is weighted according to certain medical indices and age, with age older than 65 years resulting in a 3.5 factor increase. In 2011, Israel's health expenditure constituted 7.7% of GNP ($2046 per capita), as compared to 17.6% in the United States and 9.4% average in the Organisation for Economic Co-operation and Development (OECD) countries. People age 65+ years account for approximately 35% of HMO expenditure.

Average life expectancy in 2010 for Israeli males and females was 79.7 and 83.5 years, respectively, while life expectancy at age 65 years for males and females was 18.5 and 20.5 years, respectively, ranking high for longevity compared to other countries. Israel is a fairly "young" society in its demographic makeup. In 2009 people age >65 and >75 years formed 9.9% and 4.7%, respectively, of the general population. The number of people age >65 years is expected to increase by 44% from 2009 to 2020 (3.4% annual growth), and by 84% from 2009 to 2030 (3.0% annual growth), as compared to annual growth rates among the general population of 1.4% from 2009 to 2020 and 1.3% and 2009 to 2030.

▶ Geriatric Care

Israel is considered a pioneer in health care technology, with the implementation of electronic medical records for both primary, and general and geriatric hospital care in virtually 100% of the country's health care facilities. The increasingly innovative and efficient use, analyses and sharing of data serve to promote the continuum, quality, as well as efficiency of care. There are 3.36 doctors per 1000 people in Israel.

In 1986, the parliament passed the National Community Long-Term Care Insurance law, which entitled older people living at home to claim state-financed nursing care from the National Insurance Institute (NII), the Israeli equivalent of the U.S. Social Security Administration. According to their dependence in activities of daily living, and financial means testing, older people are entitled to receive between 9.5 and 18 hours per week of home help. In 2011, home help was provided to 16% of older people, of whom about one-fifth received the maximum level of assistance. Aimed at improving quality of life, it is an important step in keeping functionally dependent home bound older people in the community (Table 75-1). Frail older people who are unable to remain at home, mainly for social reasons, are entitled to "sheltered living." These facilities cater to ambulatory, mentally intact, continent older people requiring some degree of assistance in instrumental and certain basic activities of daily living. Unrelated to the health basket, sheltered living is provided by the Ministry of Social Affairs and Welfare Services, and is based upon financial means testing.

Long-term ("nursing home") care in Israel is partially financed by the Ministry of Health, and is not included in the health basket. Most long-term care departments provide a high standard of care, and are under licensing and regulatory control of the Geriatric Division of the Ministry of Health. To be eligible, subjects must be functionally dependent, no longer ambulatory, and/or doubly incontinent. Financial coverage by the Ministry of Health requires financial means testing. Specialized psychogeriatric departments cater to the specific needs of ambulatory dementia patients, who require 24-hour care because of cognitive and affective problems. These departments are also under the auspices of the Ministry of Health, with similar guidelines for licensing and financial assistance.

The continuum of long-term care includes patients with complicated medical needs, whose level of care demands greater medical and nursing supervision than is provided in the regular long-term care. Specialized departments for "complicated long-term care" cater to nursing patients who suffer from major pressure sores, end-stage heart or respiratory lung disease, or hemodialysis, as well as patients receiving end-of-life care for both nononcologic and advanced terminal cancer. Similarly, a growing number of long-term ventilated patients receive care in specialized departments. Complicated long-term care is included in the health basket.

Geriatric rehabilitation plays an important role in the spectrum of geriatric care. In keeping with national guidelines of the Ministry of Health, the health basket provides free geriatric rehabilitation for up to 3 months, either at home or in a geriatric rehabilitation department, according to the patient's

Table 75–1. The spectrum of geriatric services in Israel.

Elderly Service	Financial Responsibility	Place of Care	Within Health Basket
Primary care	HMO	Community	Yes
Home nursing care	NII	Home	No
Comprehensive geriatric assessment	HMO	Community	Yes
Home hospital	HMO	Home	No
General hospitalization	HMO	General hospital	Yes
Subacute hospitalization	HMO	Geriatric hospital	Yes
Complicated LTC	HMO	Geriatric hospital	Yes
Long-term ventilation	HMO	Geriatric hospital	Yes
Rehabilitation	HMO	Community and geriatric/general hospital	Yes
Sheltered living	Ministry of Welfare and Social Services[a]	Sheltered living for frail elderly	No
Long-term nursing care	Ministry of Health[a]	LTC department	No
Long-term psychogeriatric care	Ministry of Health[a]	LTC departments	No

[a]According to financial means testing.

needs. Typically included are common orthopedic and neurologic disorders, as well as deconditioning.

Subacute (postacute) care is a recognized modality included within the health basket, providing an interim period following acute admission and prior to discharge back to the community. Patients transferred to these departments are typically frail older adults with a clear diagnosis and treatment plan and an expected slow recovery. Typically cheaper than treatment in a general hospital, these departments cater to patients requiring close geriatric medical care from a multidisciplinary team, whose emphasis is upon functional gain.

The bulk of community geriatrics exists within primary care practice and is provided by family physicians. Most of the HMOs are working to determine nationwide standards-of-care and quality-of-care indices for geriatric patients. Community-based home-care units provide multidisciplinary care to home-bound older people.

In 1990, the first Home Hospital in Israel was established in Jerusalem by the Clalit HMO, with the explicit goal of providing high-quality physician-led multidisciplinary care at home, as an alternative to in-patient care. The service offers a home-based alternative to a wide spectrum of in-patient geriatric care: acute, subacute, long-term complicated medical care, rehabilitation, and chronic home ventilation, as well as palliative end-of-life care. The model of care has been adopted throughout the country, and in addition to high patient and family satisfaction, has proven itself to be cost-effective.

Comprehensive geriatric assessment is recognized as an important tool, and is thus also included in the health basket. Efforts are being made to introduce routine comprehensive geriatric assessment on a national scale. In addition, social care for older people in Israel is well developed, with formal, informal and volunteer services spanning numerous areas of care.

▶ Challenges

Many challenges face geriatric care in Israel. The growing demand for alternatives to in-patient care is expected to further stimulate the establishment of home care and home hospital units. The contribution of geriatricians is likely to undergo subtle changes, with increased role as educators, planners, and consultants. Family physicians and medical internists will most likely become increasingly empowered as first-line providers of geriatric care. Geriatric medicine is a recognized medical specialty, and geriatric medicine is already a compulsory part of the medical school syllabus. It may also become part of general medical residencies.

The fact that numerous bodies are involved in providing care for the older adult population is often perceived as an obstacle, causing fragmentation rather than continuum of care. An attempt at creating a single unified body responsible for providing the full spectrum of geriatric social, medical, and nursing care has yet to be completed. Recently, it has been suggested that the health basket be widened, to include full financial responsibility of the HMOs for long-term nursing care. Protagonists claim that this step would serve as a stimulus to invest in early identification and treatment of vulnerable older adults, and a far greater interest in preventing functional decline.

Inequalities in health care exist, closely linked to socioeconomic status. The fact that 38% of funding for health care is generated from private or supplementary health packages (outside of the health basket) is cited as a leading cause, and is a subject of public debate.

SUMMARY

Despite numerous challenges, the current state of geriatric care in Israel is both comprehensive and universal. The wide spectrum of available treatment options and care settings ensures that among older people, no one is left behind.

Brodsky J, Shnoor Y, Be'er S. *The Elderly in Israel: Statistical Abstract.* Jerusalem, Israel: Meyers-Joint-Brookdale, Eshel. Center for Aging Research; 2010.

The Central Bureau of Spastics (Israel). 2010. Accessed August 24, 2012. http://www1.cbs.gov.il/publications12/1490/pdf/t02_38.pdf

Jacobs JM, Hammerman-Rozenberg R, Stessman J. Home hospitalization: 15 years of experience. *Ann Intern Med.* 2006;144(6):456.

▼ GERIATRIC CARE IN CHINA*

Shuang Wang, MD & Joseph H. Flaherty, MD

Four societal factors in China are colliding, creating dramatic challenges never before seen in a country's aging population: (a) a previously high fertility rate followed by a rapid decline to a very low fertility rate; (b) migration of young people away from rural areas, where the majority of older Chinese still live; (c) an inordinate burden of family obligations on the adult population (of would be caregivers) that will make traditional filial piety difficult to sustain; and (d) an increase in life expectancy with an associated increase in functional disabilities and chronic diseases.

CHALLENGES FOR THE FUTURE OF CHINA'S AGING POPULATION

Although most discussions about the aging demographics in China point to the 1 child per couple policy as the main cause (instituted in 1979, and strongly enforced in the mid 1980s), the increase that is predicted to occur is the result of a once-high fertility rate (as high as 7.5 in the early 1960s) followed by a rapid decline within 1–2 generations (1.7 in 2003). According to the 2010 national census data, China had more than 119 million older adults (defined as older than 65 years of age), who accounted for 8.87% of the population, with 21 million older than 80 years of age. The annual growth of

the older population in China has been increasing at a rate of 3.3% since 2001, and is expected to reach 437 million by 2051.

An understanding of the changing demographics of the aging population in China requires an understanding of the shifting demographics of the population as a whole. First, the majority of China's population, including older adults, still live in rural areas, where the provision of care to aging residents poses far more challenges than those witnessed in urban areas. Second, migration of the young from rural areas to large cities, which previously included "developed" regions of the country (mostly on the northeast and southern coast), such as Beijing, Shanghai or Guangzhou, is now occurring at a rapid rate in areas considered "underdeveloped," such as Chongqing municipality and Sichuan province (in the southwest). This outmigration from underdeveloped regions might have more negative consequences compared to developed regions.

One of the strongest attributes in Chinese culture that many people are depending on to alleviate some of the challenges of the aging population is the Confucian philosophy and Chinese traditional value of filial piety, a respect for one's parents. Currently, less than 1% of older adults in China live in nursing homes and most older Chinese prefer to stay with families rather than in retirement or nursing facilities. However, the looming question is whether the strong value of filial piety (which is based on having many children) can withstand the pressures of a family structure of 2 working adults in their 40s or 50s taking care of up to 4 aging parents in their 70s and 80s? It is too early to tell how this will turn out, as the first generation of "1-child" children (ie, the future caregivers) will not reach their 40s until around 2025.

With life expectancy in China at 74 years (77.1 for women, 72.8 for men), it is not surprising that functional disabilities and chronic diseases such as atherosclerotic vascular disease, cancer, dementia, depression, fall-related injuries, osteoporosis, and incontinence in the older adult population has increased dramatically. In 2009, there were 9.4 million disabled older persons (1.9 million in urban areas and 7.5 million in rural areas). There were also 18.9 million older persons with partial disability.

▶ Long-term Care in China Today

The next 20 years will be an exciting yet anxious time for all involved in long term care (LTC) in China. The first major challenge is that currently older persons can receive "institutional" LTC under 2 different systems, which have separate funding mechanisms and policies: the social welfare system (run by departments of Civil Affairs at national and regional levels) and the medical care system (run by local Departments of Health).

The social welfare system has traditionally been responsible for institutional LTC in rural areas (but institutions under this system do exist in urban areas). Patients must

---

*The authors would like to thank Dr. Birong Dong, Director of the Geriatrics Department at West China Hospital, Sichuan University, for her insights and review of the manuscript.

Table 75–2. Comparison of aging population demographics and long-term care in China and United States.

	China	United States
Total population	1.3 billion	311 million
Percetnage >65 years of age	8.87%	13.3%
Total population age >65 years of age	119 million	41 million
Percentage >80 years of age	1.6%	3.5%
Total population age >80 years of age	21 million	11 million
Number of nursing home beds	2.66 million	1.7 million
Ratio of nursing home beds to population >65 years of age	1:45	1:24
Occupancy rate	79%	86%
Percent of nursing home residents with dependence in 5 ADLs	17%	51%

ADLs, activities of daily living.

meet certain eligibility requirements for the social welfare system, the most important of which is not having any children or other people with a legal responsibility for support or care. Based on just this system, LTC in China is not as well established as it is in developed parts of the world, such as the United States, Europe, and Japan. A late 2010 report published by the Chinese Ministry of Civil Affairs noted that there were nearly 40,000 National Senior Welfare Agencies in China with approximately 2.66 million beds. Comparing China and the United States, there are far fewer beds per capita for older Chinese (Table 75–2). However, this report may not include private facilities, and does not include "beds" in the medical system (see below).

Although there are reports that claim China needs more LTC facilities now, the need may be overestimated based on current disability rates in the social welfare system. Among residents in social welfare facilities, only 17% are totally disabled (defined as dependence in 5–6 activities of daily living [ADLs]), compared to 51% in the United States.

A limitation of social welfare institutions is the level of medical care. Only approximately 40% of facilities have medical services within the facilities, and most facilities (especially in rural areas) do not have physicians who visit, and physicians who do make visits are not geriatricians.

In most urban areas, the medical care system, in the form of hospitals and rehabilitation wards, has evolved as a major provider of institutional care for older persons. This has happened for 2 reasons. First, hospitals (a typical hospital includes inpatient and outpatient services) have become a common location where many older people go for their routine health care, not just acute care. Thus, as the number of older people with chronic conditions has increased over the past couple of decades, the number of people with chronic conditions who visit hospitals and subsequently are admitted to hospitals, has increased.

Second, because many of these patients are retired military and government officials, they have good health care benefits for acute care but not for LTC. As a result, although social welfare institutions and for-profit LTC institutions exist in urban areas, many older hospitalized patients with chronic diseases, especially dementia, often stay in the medical system (ie, hospitals) for prolonged periods. Transferring patients from acute care to postacute care facilities or LTC facilities has not become common practice.

Third, because the aim of the treatment has traditionally been disease-oriented rather than function-oriented, ADLs are typically done by a privately hired untrained caregiver. This probably perpetuates long stays because patients become more dependent over time and the emphasis in not on functional recovery. However, this situation is changing. One example is West China Hospital, which has more than 200 inpatient beds in the Department of Geriatrics. In the past, almost all inpatients were retired military and government officials for whom comprehensive geriatric assessment (CGA) or interdisciplinary rehabilitation processes were not very useful because they were either younger (young-old) or very disabled. Now, more and more older persons from the general population (nongovernmental workers) are admitted with acute medical problems, which has made geriatric clinical practice (CGA, interdisciplinary teams) as well as geriatric clinical research useful and possible.

The economics of LTC in China is another challenge, not just for the government, but for older individuals and their families. At least in the near future, the quality of a LTC institution one enters will likely depend on personal finances instead of insurance. China first made "old age insurance" available to some rural areas in 1991. Although by 2000, the availability of old age insurance had reached 76% of the nation's towns and townships, only approximately 11% of the rural population had opted to invest in this new program. One reason was the high cost of buying into the insurance plan. Use of retirement insurance for urban residents may be somewhat higher than rural, but still is quite low.

One area of opportunity for innovation and for preventing institutionalization is based on the current architecture and living arrangements of most people in urban areas. Most people (families as well as older persons) still live in apartment-like housing, from short 4–6-story buildings to highrise 20–30-story buildings. This concentration of older populations opens up the possibility of developing community-based programs on a large scale (eg, home care, community-based clinics, preventive health programs, such as falls prevention, and health promotion, such as exercise programs). These types of programs are difficult and costly in places like the United States and Europe, where travel (for patients and health care providers), is often burdensome and not time- or cost-efficient.

Geriatric Education

One of the greatest opportunities to meet the challenges of the aging population in China is in the area of geriatric education. In a cross-sectional survey of 500 physicians who care for older persons in West China (>70% of their patients were older), 77% of the respondents felt that they lacked geriatric knowledge. Only 16% of the respondents had geriatric curriculum before graduation and 26% had received geriatric training after graduation. Most physicians felt that "language barrier" and "insufficient geriatric education in undergraduate medical school and postgraduate education" were the main challenges in practicing geriatric medicine. A government report showed that no more than 30% of nurses who currently work in LTC welfare institutions had geriatric training and only one-third had nursing licenses.

Currently, only a few medical schools in China offer gerontology and geriatrics in their curricula and medical textbooks seldom cover geriatric syndromes and CGA. In Beijing, where the geriatric education resources are relatively sufficient compared to other cities in mainland China, geriatrics was not a part of the interns' rotations at most university-affiliated hospitals, and although postgraduate (research) education has been initiated, it has not been standardized and integrated into the health education system.

Examples of growth and opportunities for large scale impact exist. A collaboration between Peking Union Medical College (PUMC) and John Hopkins University School of Medicine (JHU) has resulted in faculty member exchange between JHU and PUMC, training of physicians and nurses from the Division of Geriatric Medicine and Gerontology of PUMC at JHU, and the establishment of a geriatric inpatient ward at PUMC. Two continuing medical education geriatrics conferences in 2011 occurred as a result of a collaboration between the International Association of Gerontology and Geriatrics (IAGG) with the Sichuan Association of Geriatrics and the IAGG with the Hong Kong Geriatrics Association.

Jackson R, Howe N. *The Graying of the Middle Kingdom: The Demographics and Economics of Retirement Policy in China.* Washington, DC: The Center for Strategic and International Studies; 2004.

Leng SX, Tian XP, Durso S, et al. The aging population and development of geriatrics in China. *J Am Geriatr Soc.* 2008;56(3):571-573.

Leng SX, Tian X, Liu X, et al. An international model for geriatrics program development in China: the Johns Hopkins-Peking Union Medical College experience. *J Am Geriatr Soc.* 2010;58(7):1376-1381.

Li Y, Wang S, Li J, et al. A survey of physicians who care for older persons in southwest China. *J Nutr Health Aging.* 2013;17(2):192-195.

Poston DL, Duan CC. The current and projected distribution of the elderly and eldercare in the People's Republic of China. *J Fam Issues.* 2000;21(6):714-732.

Wu B, Mao Z, Zhong R. Long-term care arrangements in rural China: review of recent developments. *J Am Med Directors Assoc.* 2009;10(7):472-477.

Zhang Y, Goza FW. Who will care for the elderly in China? A review of the problems caused by China's One Child Policy and their potential solutions. *J Aging Stud.* 2006;20(2):151-164.

GERIATRIC CARE IN SWEDEN

Gunnar Akner, MD, PhD

Sweden has a long tradition in geriatrics and gerontology. During the 1970s and 1980s, geriatric medicine in Sweden had a leading international role because of its developing hospital care, nursing home care, day care/night care, home health care, health monitoring, and prevention. Professor Alvar Svanborg (1921–2009) in Göteborg was the architect and international pioneer for this development. He initiated, and for many years headed, the well-known longitudinal population study of aging called H70 (Health for 70 year olds), by including cohorts of 70-year-old people from the Göteborg area and following them prospectively in 5-year intervals. This pioneering work laid the foundation for the approach to geriatrics in Sweden today.

In December 2011, the Swedish total population was 9,482,855, of which 18.8% was age 65 years and older. According to Statistics Sweden, this part of the population will increase by 50% between the years 2011 and 2040, while the age group 90 years and older is estimated to increase by 125%.

Organization of Health Care for the Elderly

In Sweden, health care is socialized and financed by taxes derived principally from 21 county councils and 290 municipalities, and, to a smaller extent, from the state. The public health care system is complemented by a small private sector with a few private hospitals and a small and declining number of private physician clinics.

Two pieces of legislation regulate care of the elderly in Sweden: the Health and Medical Services Act (Hälso-och sjukvårdslagen) of 1982 and the Social Service Act (Socialtjänstlagen) of 2001. Health care for elderly people is divided by these 2 laws into 2 financial and organizational systems: medical health care through the county councils and social and nursing health care through the municipalities. In 1992, a major political reform ("ÄDEL reform") transferred about 40,000 beds and 55,000 staff, including the formal responsibility for long-term care patients, from the county councils to the municipalities. Physicians could also no longer be employed by the municipalities, but would be contracted on commission by the county councils instead. As a result, physicians have no formal role in the organization, team-building work, or staff education in the municipalities, which are responsible for long-term, social, and nursing health care needs of many older Swedes.

A. Hospitals

Since 1992, more than 95% of all geriatric hospital beds in Sweden have been closed and geriatric medicine is now only present in hospitals in larger cities, particularly in the Stockholm area, with a strong focus on acute geriatric medicine. There is also a small number of geriatric rehabilitation centers.

A study of the organization, staffing, and care production in geriatric medicine in Sweden showed, on average, 1 geriatric bed for every 799 individuals age 65 years and older, with a 10-fold variation between the counties. There were 41 independent Departments of Geriatric Medicine with 85 beds per clinic on average, again with a 10-fold variation between the counties. The report concluded that "there is no overall structural plan for the role of geriatric medicine in Swedish health care, with the desired close connection between content and dimensioning of geriatric specialist training and the practical organization of the activities." Since then, the closing of geriatric units has continued, but no current detailed national data on the number of geriatric beds are available. This closing process has been driven by the independent county councils without any strategic national planning or broader discussion about the role of geriatric medicine in Sweden.

This development should be viewed against the fact that 75% of all hospitals open in 1980 in Sweden have since been closed. According to the OECD, Sweden had 2.8 hospital beds per 1000 population in 2009 (compared to the U.S. rate of 3.1 and the OECD average of 4.9), which was the lowest number of hospital beds in Europe. As a consequence, the average inpatient length of stay has been cut in half and many older patients are discharged too early to home care or municipality care.

B. Primary Care

A previous version of the Health and Medical Services Act stated that physicians serving as "stable physician contacts" in primary care must be specialists in general medicine. In the last revision of 2009, this rule was changed to allow patients to choose any specialist working in primary care as their stable physician contact. However, a number of county councils still require that all physicians serving in primary care must be specialists in general medicine. There are only occasional geriatric medicine units in primary care in Sweden, and these focus on "elderly care," not geriatric medicine.

▶ Medical Specialties

The medical specialty in long-term care medicine was instituted in 1969 and renamed geriatric medicine in 1992. In 2006, the Swedish government made geriatric medicine a "basal medical specialty"; that is, it is possible for physicians to specialize only in geriatric medicine. The medical specialties in Sweden were reorganized in 2012. Geriatric medicine in Sweden has no formal subspecialties, but geropsychiatry became an "additional specialty" to both geriatric medicine and psychiatry. However, on the other side of the age spectrum, there are 3 pediatric basal specialties: pediatric surgery, pediatric psychiatry, and pediatric medicine, and the latter has 5 defined additional specialties: allergology, cardiology, neonatology, neurology/habilitation, and oncology.

Physicians' choice of medical specialty is controlled by the local county councils in how they advertise "specialty training positions," and is not regulated by the Swedish National Board of Health and Welfare (Socialstyrelsen). This lack of national planning has led to a longstanding lack of geriatricians, general physicians, and psychiatrists, and a disproportional increase in, for example, cardiologists. According to statistics from the Swedish Medical Association, in October 2012, there were only 628 (63% female) active specialists in geriatric medicine in Sweden, many of whom have other medical specialties as well, and who frequently work part-time in their role as geriatricians (Table 75–3).

Very few geriatricians serve in primary care in Sweden and there are very few care units designated for older adult care in the primary care setting. Thus, geriatricians in Sweden serve almost entirely in hospitals, mostly in acute geriatric medicine wards or in units specializing in certain "geriatric giants," usually falls/fractures/osteoporosis, stroke, and dementia.

Table 75–3. The number of active working medical specialists in 10 medical specialties in Sweden in October 2012.

Medical Specialty	Total Number	Relation to All 22,179 Medical Specialists	Female
Geriatric medicine	628	3%	63%
General medicine	5467	25%	46%
Internal medicine	3000	14%	37%
Cardiology	742	3%	25%
Neurology	400	2%	38%
Obstetrics/gynecology	1213	5%	67%
Oncology	406	2%	54%
Pediatric medicine (including the 5 "additional specialities")	1809	8%	54%
Psychiatry	1595	7%	53%
Surgery	1537	7%	21%

Education

During the 5.5 years of medical school, medical students get 1–2 weeks of formal education and training in geriatric medicine; that is, less than 1% of the total time in medical school. Different aspects of diagnostics, treatment/care, and evaluation of older adults are taught during many other courses, but not presented as a coherent geriatric theme or curriculum during medical school.

Regarding specialist training, only physicians specializing in geriatric medicine are required to train and serve in geriatric medicine. For all other specialists, including primary care specialists (general physicians) and internists, such education is optional and based on individual interest.

For all other health/nursing care staff groups, there is very limited education and training in geriatric medicine during basal educational programs, and what exists is usually not called geriatric medicine, but rather "care of the elderly." A small number of nurses and physiotherapists have 1 year of formal training in geriatrics/gerontology or "care for the elderly." A recent investigation from the Swedish National Board of Health and Welfare found that only 1.6 % of all 12,316 nurses employed in municipality elderly care in Sweden have formal education in "care for the elderly."

In several medical faculties, there are a limited number of shorter courses in geriatric medicine for different health care staff groups, but there are small incentives for employers to allow members of the staff to attend such courses during working hours.

Patients in the Health/Nursing Care System

In Sweden, older patients (age 65+ years), who often have multiple morbidities requiring multiple treatment methods, dominate in all parts of the health care system. In primary care, these patients represent approximately 50% of physician working time. In hospital departments such as internal medicine and its subspecialties, they account for 60% to 70% of all inpatients. In municipality care dedicated to older adults, 100% of all resources is given to older residents. Thus, there is a significant mismatch between the number of older patients with multimorbidities and the competence in geriatric medicine among physicians and health/nursing care staff across all groups.

Research

All medical faculties have university professors in geriatric medicine and there are units for geriatric medicine in all 7 Swedish medical faculties, except for Örebro. The professors in 3 of the faculties are focused on dementia (Stockholm, Uppsala, Linköping) and 1 is focused on osteoporosis (Göteborg). There are about 10 other professors in geriatric medicine in these faculties with different research focuses. Only a few are devoted to the study of multimorbidity in older adults, with a focus on clinical management in primary care/municipality care.

SUMMARY

Sweden is facing a number of future challenges regarding care for the elderly:

1. **Knowledge area**—Geriatric medicine must be widely accepted as the knowledge area that deals with multiple risk factors, multiple manifest health problems and multiple treatments during the whole span of aging.

2. **Focus**—The focus of health care for older persons must switch from the present single-disease management to multiple domain management; from national guidelines and standardized care plans to individual, personalized health analysis and management; and from a reactive to a proactive approach focusing on prevention.

3. **Organization**—The health care organization must be much better suited for and adapted to older persons with multiple morbidities and treatments based on geriatric principles. The present hospital in-patient perspective must be completed by a primary care/municipality perspective.

4. **Medical records**—The most important tool to steer the analysis, evaluation, and management of care for older persons is the medical record. Presently, medical records serve as retroactive diaries and constitute a strong risk factor for multimorbid older people. To enable better care, the electronic medical record should be developed into a prospective "interactive health analysis system" focusing on providing physicians with an overview of the whole health situation, both cross-sectionally and longitudinally. It should stimulate analysis of relations between risk factors, symptoms, manifest diagnoses and various treatments in close cooperation with patients.

5. **Empowerment**—Older patients and their relatives must be empowered to act as codrivers who share responsibility for monitoring their health over time. This includes increased participation in decisions regarding health analysis and treatment towards end of life. In Swedish nursing homes, patient's average 10 medical drug prescriptions per day and it is important that such intensive drug treatment is prescribed in accordance with the patients' wishes and is properly monitored over time.

6. **Education/training**—The basic and continued education and training of physicians and other health care staff groups must have required curricula in geriatric medicine with several separate courses, while also being present in most other courses. There must be incentives to encourage physicians and other health care staff groups to

specialize in geriatric medicine. The designation "care for the elderly" should have a firm base in geriatric medicine.

7. **Living**—There is a strong need to develop a wide range of different types of housing adapted to elderly peoples' needs, particularly intermediate service facilities.

8. **Research**—An extensive study from the Swedish Council on Health Technology Assessment 2003 reported the strong lack of controlled treatment studies in patients age 65 years and older. For patients age 75 years and older, there are only very few such treatment studies, even though this age group, in particular, is prescribed much treatment, usually multiple treatments. This lack of appropriately targeted research has not been addressed in recent years, suggesting the pressing need for treatment trials in older patients, particularly for those with multimorbidity.

The present method of choice for treatment studies, the randomized controlled trial, is not suited to study multiple treatment effect(s) in heterogeneous populations. Thus, a new research methodology for treatment studies must be developed and integrated with routine care for the elderly. Research focusing on primary and secondary prevention for older adults using individual multiple risk factor profiles is also needed.

Further reading for a more complete understanding of problems in the present Swedish system of care for the elderly and related challenges for the future is listed below.

Akner G. Geriatric medicine in Sweden: a study of the organisation, staffing and care production in 2000-2001. *Age Ageing*. 2004;33(4):338-341.

Akner G. *Multimorbidity in Elderly. Analysis, Management and Proposal of a Geriatric Care Center*. VDM Verlag Dr Müller 2011. The book is available from the website: http://dl.dropbox.com/u/78150446/gunnarakner/Gunnar_Akner_homepage/Book_Multimorbidity.html

Akner G. Frailty and multimorbidity in elderly people: a shift in management approach. *Clin Geriatr*. 2013;21: published online 23 Sep 2013. Available at: http://www.clinicalgeriatrics.com/article/frailty-multimorbidity-elderly-shift-management-approach

Swedish National Data Service. *H70: Health for 70-Year-Old Populations. a Prospective Cohort Study on Aging*. Available at: http://snd.gu.se/en/catalogue/study/671.

Swedish Medical Association. *Statistics Regarding Physicians in Sweden 2012*. Available at: http://www.slf.se/upload/Lakarforbundet/Trycksaker/PDFer/Läkarfakta_2012.pdf (in Swedish).

Swedish Society for Geriatric Medicine. *Summary of Geriatric Institutions and Research Units in Sweden*. Available at: http://www.slf.se/Foreningarnas-startsidor/Specialitetsforening/Svensk-Geriatrisk-Forening/Lankar/Geriatriska-institutioner-och-forskningsenheter (in Swedish).

Swedish Council on Health Technology Assessment. *Geriatric Care and Treatment. a Systematic Compilation of Existing Scientific Literature*. 2003. Available at: http://sbu.se/en/Published/Vit/Geriatric-care-and-treatment

Public Policy Intersecting with an Aging Society

76

Gretchen E. Alkema, PhD

Bruce Allen Chernof, MD, FACP

The continuum of care that supports older Americans is at a crossroads. The major policy initiatives framing financing and system design in both the public and private sectors are approximately 50 years old and were designed for a very different time and population. When the Medicare and Medicaid programs became law in 1965, the average life expectancy in the United States was 70 years (Figure 76–1), and most hospitals did not have technologies to significantly prolong life following a life-threatening incident.

Over the course of the twentieth century, particularly in the last 25 years, the United States has experienced a dramatic increase in life expectancy, largely as a result of far more sophisticated medical interventions and treatments. Even though social policy has evolved over this period, the primary focus has been on incremental changes to the policy backbone built decades ago: Social Security, Medicare, and Medicaid. These programs now encompass services, such as dialysis and transplantations, or use delivery system approaches, such as managed care. Yet these programs have not changed substantially to meet the dramatic and different needs of current and future older adults.

THREE SPHERES OF AGING WITH DIGNITY AND INDEPENDENCE

What are the needs that all adults will face as they age? These needs can be categorized into 3 spheres of security: income, health, and functional (Figure 76–2). Public policy has historically focused on 2 of these 3 spheres: (a) health security through Medicare, Medicaid, and other insurance; and (b) income security through Social Security, defined retirement benefits, and savings programs such as 401Ks. Functional security, or those programs that support people in daily living who have functional challenges, is the sphere with the least-developed policy architecture. The increasing need for this type of security is a consequence of individuals

living longer with more chronic illness and functional limitation than in any other previous period.

Most adults are simply not prepared for these substantial needs as they grow older, and often rely on the 2 spheres of income and health security to address them. Seventy percent of Americans who reach the age of 65 years will need some form of long-term services and supports (LTSS) in their lives for an average of 3 years. Most individuals desire to receive these services in their homes and communities rather than in an institution, such as a nursing home. The "oldest old," or those age 85 years and older, have the most substantial need for this type of care, with approximately 30% having moderate-to-severe LTSS needs—three times the proportion among those 75–84 years old. The percentage of those age 85 years and older is expected to increase by more than 25% by 2030. The lack of a comprehensive policy approach to meeting the functional security needs of vulnerable elders remains a critical policy challenge.

The next sections outline the Medicare and Medicaid programs, describe new initiatives aimed at addressing functional security through these 2 programs, and provide a framework for future policy development in this area.

KEY PROGRAMS AND SERVICES FOR OLDER ADULTS

▶ Medicare and Its Role in Supporting Older Americans

Enacted in 1965, Medicare is a federally administered health insurance program that provides coverage for individuals age 65 years and older, individuals younger than age 65 years with permanent disabilities who receive Social Security Disability Insurance payments, and individuals diagnosed with end-stage renal disease or amyotrophic lateral sclerosis. Medicare is funded through payroll taxes,

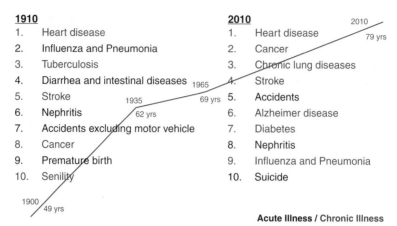

1910		2010	
1.	Heart disease	1.	Heart disease
2.	Influenza and Pneumonia	2.	Cancer
3.	Tuberculosis	3.	Chronic lung diseases
4.	Diarrhea and intestinal diseases	4.	Stroke
5.	Stroke	5.	Accidents
6.	Nephritis	6.	Alzheimer disease
7.	Accidents excluding motor vehicle	7.	Diabetes
8.	Cancer	8.	Nephritis
9.	Premature birth	9.	Influenza and Pneumonia
10.	Senility	10.	Suicide

2010 79 yrs
1965 69 yrs
1935 62 yrs
1900 49 yrs

Acute Illness / Chronic Illness

▲ **Figure 76–1.** Causes of death and life expectancy, 1910–2010. (Adapted from the National Center for Health Statistics, Centers for Disease Control and Prevention. *Leading Causes of Death, 1900–1998.* Available at: http://www.cdc.gov/nchs/data/nvsr/nvsr60/nvsr60_04.pdf; and Murphy S, Xu J, Kochanek K. Deaths: preliminary data for 2010. *Natl Vital Stat Rep.* 2012;60(4):1-52.)

general revenues, and beneficiary premiums and copays. As of 2010, 47 million people rely on Medicare for their health insurance coverage. This includes 39 million people age 65 years and older and 8 million people younger than age 65 with disabilities.

Medicare consists of 4 parts, each covering different benefits.

- **Part A**, also known as the Hospital Insurance program, covers inpatient hospital services, short-term rehabilitative care through a skilled nursing facility or home health agency, and hospice care. Part A is funded by a tax of 2.9% of earnings paid by employers and workers (1.45% each).

- **Part B**, the Supplementary Medical Insurance program, helps pay for physician, outpatient, home health, laboratory, and preventive services. Part B is funded by general revenues and beneficiary premiums ($104.90 per month in 2014). Beneficiaries who have higher annual incomes

Functional security

Public:　ACA opportunities (2010)
　　　　　Medicaid (1965)
　　　　　Older Americans act (1965)

Private:　LTC insurance (1970s)
　　　　　Family / Friends / Neighbors

Income security

Public:　Social security (1935)
　　　　　SSDI/SSI (1956/1972)

Private:　Defined retirement benefit
　　　　　401K–403B
　　　　　Private disability insurance
　　　　　Earned income

Health security

Public:　ACA opportunities (2010)
　　　　　Medicare (1965)
　　　　　Medicaid (1965)
　　　　　VA (1930)

Private:　Medigap/Supp ins. (1965)
　　　　　Retiree health insurance

Pub/Priv:　Medicare managed care (1982)
　　　　　　Medicare + choice (1997)
　　　　　　Medicare advantage/SNP (2003)

▲ **Figure 76–2.** Three spheres of security.

(greater than $85,000/individual, $170,000/couple) pay a higher, income-related monthly Part B premium.

- **Part C**, also known as the Medicare Advantage program, allows beneficiaries to enroll in a private plan, such as a health maintenance organization, preferred provider organization, or private fee-for-service plan, as an alternative to the traditional fee-for-service program. These plans receive payments from Medicare to provide all Medicare-covered benefits. Part C is not separately financed, but instead includes dollars from Parts A, B, and sometimes D if a plan includes prescription drug coverage (see Part D below). Special Needs Plans and the Program of All-inclusive Care for the Elderly (PACE) are included in this statute.

- **Part D**, the outpatient prescription drug benefit, launched in 2006. The benefit is delivered through private plans that contract with Medicare, either as standalone prescription drug plans or Medicare Advantage prescription drug plans. Part D is funded by general revenues, beneficiary premiums, and state payments. Individuals who sign up for a Part D plan generally pay a monthly premium. Those with modest income and assets are eligible for assistance with premiums and cost-sharing amounts.

▶ Medicare Funding for Graduate Medical Training

Medicare has historically provided substantial support to train the next generation of medical professionals, initially funding this on a cost basis. However, when Medicare began paying for inpatient hospital services through the Prospective Payment System in 1983, it recognized that teaching hospitals often serve a vulnerable population and, as a result of the teaching process itself, care in these institutions is more costly than in other hospitals. For this reason, Medicare makes an adjustment to the discharge payment rates in hospitals that train residents called the Indirect Medical Education payment. Also, since 1985, Medicare compensates hospitals for a portion of the costs directly related to training residents through its Direct Graduate Medical Education (DGME) payment. DGME is based on a per-resident amount, which generally includes salaries and fringe benefits for interns and residents, supervisory teaching physician costs, and overhead associated with operating a medical residency training program.

▶ Medicaid and Its Role in Supporting Low-Income Older Americans

Also enacted in 1965, Medicaid is the federal–state jointly funded program that provides medical services and LTSS to millions of low-income Americans across the 50 states, the District of Columbia, and the Territories. Medicaid is the responsibility of both the states and the federal government, with states having primary administrative responsibility. Within national guidelines, each state operates its Medicaid program under a state plan, which describes the populations the state intends to cover, as well as the nature and scope of services it plans to offer. States can establish their own eligibility standards for the program; determine the type, amount, duration, and scope of services that will be provided; and set payment rates for these services. However, Medicaid is an entitlement program, meaning that states must provide certain mandatory services to specified populations in order to receive federal funding. Although participation is voluntary, all states currently participate in the program.

Medicaid financing is a shared responsibility of the federal and state governments. States incur Medicaid costs by making payments to service providers and performing administrative activities and are then reimbursed by the federal government for the "federal share" of these costs. The amount of the federal contribution to Medicaid relative to state dollars is termed the "federal medical assistance percentage" (FMAP) and is determined by a statutory formula set in law that establishes higher FMAPs for states with per capita personal income levels lower than the national average and lower FMAPs for states with per capita personal income levels that are higher than the national average. An FMAP of 50% is the statutory minimum. For fiscal year 2012, state FMAPs ranged from 50% to 74%.

To qualify for Medicaid coverage, an applicant's income and assets must meet program financial requirements. States are required to serve select groups of individuals, also known as "categorically needy" populations, as part of their state plans. At their discretion, states may choose to cover additional "categorically related" groups beyond those required by law. States must also provide certain services through Medicaid, consisting of a basic set of mandatory medical care services (eg, hospital, physician, laboratory services) and institutional LTSS, such as long-stay custodial care in a nursing home. States may choose to offer optional services (eg, dental care, hospice), which vary by state as part of each state's Medicaid plan.

States may also apply to the Centers for Medicare and Medicaid Services to waive certain federal requirements in order to modify their Medicaid programs and implement new approaches in the delivery and payment of services. Medicaid waivers allow states to limit services to special populations (eg, individuals with AIDS) or those with particular needs (eg, care management to older adults with nursing home levels of care) while still being eligible to receive federal matching payments for these services.

▶ Long-Term Services and Supports

As Americans continue to live longer than in previous generations, often with chronic conditions and functional impairment, the number of individuals needing LTSS is expected to increase. LTSS is defined as assistance with activities of daily living (including bathing, dressing, eating, transferring, walking) and instrumental activities of daily living including meal preparation, money management, house cleaning, medication management, transportation) to older people and other adults with disabilities who cannot perform these activities on their own because of a physical, cognitive, or chronic health condition that is expected to continue for an extended period of time, typically 90 days or more. LTSS include such things as human assistance, supervision, assistive technologies, and care and service coordination for people who live in their own home, a residential setting, or an institutional setting, such as a nursing facility. LTSS also include supports provided to family members and other unpaid caregivers.

The cost of LTSS is substantial, impacting family financial resources and their potential to engage in the labor market. Private market costs of LTSS can far exceed most families' resources, particularly for families of older and disabled Americans. In 2011, personal care at home averaged $20 an hour, or about $21,000 annually for part-time help. For people who need extensive assistance through nursing home care, the average annual cost is $78,000 for a semiprivate room.

Many Americans are not prepared for the likelihood of needing these services at some point in their lives. When the need for LTSS arises, individuals and families initially finance this care by utilizing their own resources. Families draw on their income and assets, and family caregivers provide a substantial amount of unpaid care. In 2009, nearly 62 million family caregivers in the United States provided care to an adult with LTSS needs at some time during the year. The estimated economic value of their unpaid contributions was approximately $450 billion in 2009, up from an estimated $375 billion in 2007. Businesses in the United States lose up to $33 billion per year in productivity from full-time caregiving employees. Private long-term care insurance plays a small role in financing LTSS, as about 6–7 million private policies are in force.

When individuals and families have exhausted their resources and can no longer shoulder the costs of LTSS on their own, they reach to Medicaid for help. Individuals who qualify for financial assistance through Medicaid for LTSS generally need this help for the rest of their lives. LTSS services covered by Medicaid include institutional services, such as those provided in a nursing facility or intermediate care facilities for the mentally retarded. LTSS that are provided outside of institutional settings over an extended period of time are referred to collectively as home- and community-based services (HCBS). Noninstitutional LTSS covered by Medicaid include home health, private duty nursing, rehabilitative services, personal care services, PACE, and a variety of HCBS provided through Medicaid waivers.

Nationally, Medicaid is the primary payer of LTSS for millions of Americans. Of the almost $208 billion in total U.S. spending on LTSS in 2010, Medicaid paid for more than 62% ($129.3 billion). These payments represent almost one-third of all Medicaid spending. Individuals age 65 years and older represented approximately 8% of Medicaid enrollees, but approximately 20% of all program expenditures. Of Medicaid LTSS spending for fiscal year 2010, slightly more than half (53%) was for institutional care. This proportion of spending on institutional care relative to HCBS varies across states.

▶ Special Emphasis on Those Eligible for Medicaid and Medicare

There are more than 9 million individuals who are eligible for both Medicaid and Medicare ("dual eligibles"). While dual eligibles account for a smaller percentage of enrollees in both programs, they account for a disproportionate share of the costs. Duals represent 15% of Medicaid enrollees but account for 39% of Medicaid costs. These individuals are universally acknowledged to be a vulnerable and medically fragile group. Thirty-three percent of dual eligibles have 1 or more of the following chronic conditions: diabetes, stroke, dementia, and/or chronic obstructive pulmonary disease. These conditions often result in functional limitations and may require the use of personal care and supportive services. Dual eligibles are more likely to have multiple chronic conditions, use more health services and LTSS, and have higher per capita spending than Medicare-only beneficiaries. For these individuals, the Medicare and Medicaid programs were meant to complement each other, with Medicare covering medical services, while Medicaid provides assistance with Medicare premiums and cost sharing, as well as coverage for LTSS. However, misalignments between the 2 programs often make it challenging for dually eligible individuals to access needed services in a timely and customer-focused manner. Several efforts are currently underway to address these misalignments, including regulatory review and reconciliation at the federal level and development of programs that integrate the delivery of services and financing at the state and local levels.

OPPORTUNITIES IN THE PATIENT PROTECTION AND AFFORDABLE CARE ACT

The passage of the *Patient Protection and Affordable Care Act* (ACA, P.L. 111-148) on March 23, 2010, laid the groundwork for wide-ranging reform of the continuum of care that serves older adults. Although several provisions sought to increase preventative care and reduce cost sharing for key services (eg, prescription drugs), many provisions focused on improving care delivery for individuals with chronic conditions and functional impairment who interact often with the health and long-term care systems. The ACA created new programs to better incentivize providers and organizations to improve service arrangements for vulnerable populations served by the Medicare program. Examples include the creation of Accountable Care Organizations (ACOs), medical homes, and bundled payment programs for acute and postacute services, as well as the Community-Based Care Transitions Program and Independence at Home Demonstration. The ACA also created 2 new offices to enhance the continued pursuit of alternative models for financing services and organizing care through pilot testing: the Center for Medicare and Medicaid Innovation and the Federal Coordinated Health Care Office (now called the Medicare-Medicaid Coordination Office), focusing on bridging the gap between Medicare and Medicaid. The ACA also called for increased efforts to bolster the health care workforce. It established a National Health Care Workforce Commission, provided increased payment incentives for primary care providers, and encouraged states to directly enhance their supply of direct care workers (eg, Certified Nursing Assistants) through workforce development grants.

Specific to Medicaid, the ACA seeks to rebalance LTSS in the states toward increased use of HCBS and away from institutional care by enhancing federal matching for states to implement HCBS and improve the operational efficiency of state LTSS systems. The goal of these initiatives is to encourage a broader range of available services. However, the ACA does not fundamentally recalibrate the financial imbalance that currently favors institutional care services given that they are mandatory.

WHERE DO WE GO FROM HERE?

▶ Focus on Person and Function Versus Patient and Disease

Over the past 2 decades, significant dollars have been spent tackling the assumption that chronic illness alone drives health care use. Even though some tangible improvements have been achieved, there is little evidence that "fixing" the disease will directly result in better care and health outcomes at a lower cost. The reason is that targeting efforts have not been refined enough and have missed a key part of the equation—how chronic disease (and often multiple diseases) impacts a person's daily living, which requires a more robust discussion of functional status.

Our current health care system is built for "patients"—those people who are vessels for illness ideally on the road to wellness under the care of the medical system. This approach works well for a relatively healthy person facing an acute illness where a cure is almost always achievable. This model is fundamentally flawed however for individuals with serious chronic health conditions, as many will never be fully "well" the way a healthy 20-year-old recovers from pneumonia. As a result, people with chronic conditions risk getting stamped as "patients" for life. They get "patient-centered care" for their

list of chronic illnesses as opposed to "person-centered care" focused on their desires to retain choice and independence in their lives inclusive of health conditions and functional status.

Addressing both the patient and the underlying person—the illness and its functional impact—is the key to more effective targeting. About 110 million people in the United States live with chronic illness and nearly 32 million have serious functional limitations. Of key interest is the overlap in these 2 populations, accounting for 27 million people. More than 30% of older Medicare beneficiaries in the top spending quintile have both chronic conditions and functional limitations. On average, Medicare spends almost 3 times more per capita on seniors who live with chronic health conditions and functional impairment compared to seniors with chronic conditions alone. They were nearly twice as likely to have a hospital stay than those with chronic conditions alone. While roughly half of seniors with chronic conditions and functional limitations qualify for Medicaid (dually eligible), more importantly the other half do not. When an older adult with chronic conditions and functional limitations has a daily living crisis, even if not primarily medical in nature, the medical system and particularly hospitals are often the backstop. These data clarify that a chronic disease, "patient-only" perspective to care delivery is simply too broad an assumption for good targeting.

▶ Focus on Quality

Given that older adults have care needs and preferences that are much different from those of a younger population, assessing the performance of providers and organizations should account for the comprehensive set of services delivered to this population.

In addition to existing quality metrics that are tested and validated, additional measures are needed to evaluate truly person-centered functional outcome measures that are site-neutral, focused on the coordination of services, and based on individual needs and preferences for care. For example, an older adult with severe diabetes complicated by visual problems and neuropathy may identify "the ability to walk safely within the home" as a core preference-based outcome measure. This individual's desired outcome, with these complex health and functional challenges, also has substantial medical and cost implications. The number of providers, sites of care, and services delivered to achieve this outcome may be many. However, the singular fact remains that functional improvement is what the older adult is seeking. The provision of these services and achievement of this outcome could forestall or mitigate negative and costly incidents, such as a fall resulting in a hip fracture and nursing home placement. None of the existing patient satisfaction or quality of care metrics adequately identifies or measures this functional-based, yet medically driven indicator of improvement. Therefore, it is critical that these types of measures be created when evaluating all forms of delivery system improvements, including ACOs, medical/health homes, Special Needs Plans, bundling and other pilot projects, and Innovation Center efforts.

To adequately address the challenges of improving health care quality and reigning in rising costs, providers need to target the right needs with the right intervention, while always considering a person's health and functional status. Solutions include seeing the patient first as a person and focusing on their daily function in light of existing health conditions. These are the keys to a more cost-effective and humane system of care—something that all of us want as we grow older. Moving public policy toward a continuum focus that puts community-based services on par with institutional services, supports choice and self-direction, uses conflict-free care coordination, measures quality outcomes regardless of the site of care, and develops new funding models to allow individuals to prefund these needs are key features of future policy debates.

Association of American Medical Colleges. *What Does Medicare Have to Do with Graduate Medical Education?* Accessed April 25, 2012. Available at: https://www.aamc.org/advocacy/campaigns_and_coalitions/gmefunding/factsheets/253372/medicare-gme.html

Barrett L. *Perceptions of Long-Term Care and the Economic Recession: AARP Bulletin Poll.* 2009. Accessed April 10, 2012. Available at: http://assets.aarp.org/rgcenter/il/bulletin_ltc_09.pdf

Eiken S, Sredl K, Burwell B, Gold L. *Medicaid Expenditures for Long-Term Services and Supports: 2011 Update.* 2011. Accessed April 6, 2012. Available at: http://www.hcbs.org/files/208/10395/2011LTSSExpenditures-final.pdf

Feder J, Komisar H. *Transforming Care for Medicare Beneficiaries with Chronic Conditions and Long-Term Care Needs: Coordinating Care Across All Services.* 2011. Accessed April 25, 2012. Available at: http://www.thescanfoundation.org/sites/default/files/Georgetown_Trnsfrming_Care.pdf

Feder J, Komisar H. *The Importance of Federal Financing to the Nation's Long-Term Care Safety Net.* 2012. Accessed April 6, 2012. Available at: http://www.thescanfoundation.org/sites/thescanfoundation.org/files/Georgetown_Importance_Federal_Financing_LTC_2.pdf

Feinberg L, Reinhard S, Houser A, Choula R. *Valuing the Invaluable: 2011 Update: The Growing Contributions and Costs of Family Caregiving.* 2011. Accessed April 6, 2012. Available at: http://assets.aarp.org/rgcenter/ppi/ltc/i51-caregiving.pdf

Grady A. *CRS Report for Congress: Medicaid Financing: Congressional Research Service.* 2008. Accessed April 25, 2012. Available at: http://aging.senate.gov/crs/medicaid5.pdf

The Henry J. Kaiser Family Foundation. *Projecting Income and Assets: What Might the Future Hold for the Next Generation of Medicare Beneficiaries?* 2011. Accessed April 6, 2012. Available at: http://kaiserfamilyfoundation.files.wordpress.com/2013/01/8172.pdf

Justice D. *Implementing the Affordable Care Act: New Options for Medicaid Home and Community Based Services.* 2010. Accessed April 25, 2012. Available at: http://www.thescanfoundation.org/sites/thescanfoundation.org/files/NASHP_Implementing_ACA_3.pdf

Kaiser Commission on Medicaid and the Uninsured, The Henry J. Kaiser Family Foundation. *Dual Eligibles: Medicaid's Role for Low-Income Medicare Beneficiaries.* 2011. Accessed April 6, 2012. Available at: http://www.kff.org/medicaid/upload/4091-08.pdf

Kemper P, Komisar H, Alecxih L. Long-term care over an uncertain future: what can current retirees expect? *Inquiry.* 2005-2006;42(4):335-350.

Lake Research Partners, American Viewpoint. *California Voters 40 and Older Are Struggling to Make Ends Meet and Financially Unprepared for Growing Older.* 2011. Accessed April 10, 2012. Available at: http://www.thescanfoundation.org/sites/thescanfoundation.org/files/final_poll_report.pdf

National Senior Citizens Law Center. *State Profiles-Dual Eligible Integrated Care Demonstrations: Resources for Advocates.* Accessed April 6, 2012. Available at: http://dualsdemoadvocacy.org/state-profiles

O'Shaughnessy CV. *The Basics: National Spending for Long-Term Services and Supports (LTSS).* 2011. Accessed April 6, 2012. Available at: http://www.nhpf.org/library/the-basics/Basics_LTSS_02-01-13.pdf

Parish S, Grinstein-Weiss M, Yeo Y, Rose R, Rimmerman A, Crossman R. Assets and income: disability-based disparities in the United States. *Soc Work Res.* 2010;31(2):71-82.

RAND. *Assessing Care of Vulnerable Elders (ACOVE).* Accessed April 25, 2012. Available at: http://www.rand.org/health/projects/acove/about.html

Reinhard S, Kassner E, Houser A, Mollica R. *Raising Expectations: A State Scorecard on Long-Term Services and Supports for Older Adults, People with Physical Disabilities, and Family Caregivers.* 2011. Accessed April 6, 2012. Available at: http://www.longtermscorecard.org/~/media/Microsite/Files/AARP_Reinhard_Realizing_Exp_LTSS_Scorecard_REPORT_WEB_v3.pdf

The SCAN Foundation. *Data Brief No. 1: Characteristics of Dual Eligibles.* 2010. Accessed April 6, 2012. Available at: http://www.thescanfoundation.org/sites/default/files/DataBrief_No1.ppt

The SCAN Foundation. *Data Brief No. 3: Dual Eligibles and Medicare Spending.* 2010. Accessed April 6, 2012. Available at: http://www.thescanfoundation.org/sites/thescanfoundation.org/files/1pg_databrief_no3_0.pdf

The SCAN Foundation. *Data Brief No. 10: Dual Eligibles-Health Services Utilization.* 2011. Accessed April 6, 2012. Available at: http://www.thescanfoundation.org/sites/thescanfoundation.org/files/1pg_databrief_no10.pdf

The SCAN Foundation. *Long-Term Care Fundamentals No. 9: Medicaid-Funded Home- and Community-Based Services.* 2011. Accessed April 6, 2012. Available at: http://www.thescanfoundation.org/sites/thescanfoundation.org/files/LTC_Fundamental_9_0.pdf

The SCAN Foundation. *Policy Brief No. 2: A Summary of the Patient Protection and Affordable Care Act (P.L. 111-148) and Modifications by the Health Care and Education Reconciliation Act of 2010 (H.R. 4872).* 2010. Accessed April 25, 2012. Available at: http://www.thescanfoundation.org/sites/default/files/PolicyBrief_2.pdf

Shirk C. *Shaping Medicaid and SCHIP Through Waivers: The Fundamentals.* 2008. Accessed April 6, 2012. Available at: http://www.nhpf.org/library/background-papers/BP64_MedicaidSCHIP.Waivers_07-22-08.pdf

Shugarman L, Whitenhill K. The Affordable Care Act proposes new provisions to build a stronger continuum of care. *Generations.* 2010;35(1):11-18.

Vladeck B. *Testimony on Graduate Medical Education Before the Senate Committee on Finance.* March 12, 1997. Accessed April 25, 2012. Available at: http://www.hhs.gov/asl/testify/t970312a.html

USEFUL WEBSITES

The Henry J. Kaiser Family Foundation. Health Reform Gateway. Accessed April 25, 2012. http://healthreform.kff.org/

The Henry J. Kaiser Family Foundation. *Medicare: A Primer.* 2010. http://www.kff.org/medicare/upload/7615-03.pdf

U.S. Department of Health and Human Services. *Medicare Basics.* http://www.Medicare.gov

Index

Note: Page numbers followed by *b*, *f*, or *t* indicate boxes, figures, or tables, respectively.

INDEX 559

Dextroamphetamine, 331
DI. *See* Diabetes insipidus (DI)
Diabetes, 124
  acute complications, 306
    coma, 306
    diabetic ketoacidosis (DKA), 306
      precipitating factors, 306
    dyspnea symptoms, 306
    hyperglycemia, associated with, 306
    hyperglycemic hyperosmolar state, 306
    insulin deficiency, 306
    lower-extremity soft tissue, 306
    mental status alteration, 306
  chronic complications, 306, 307
    diabetes-related complications, 306
    macrovascular disease, 306, 307
      blood pressure control, 307
      cardiovascular disease
        (CVD), 306
    microvascular disease, 306
      nephropathy, 307
      neuropathy, 307
      retinopathy, 307
  general principles, 305
  geriatric syndromes, 307, 308
    cognitive impairment, 307, 308
    depression, 308
    falls, 308
    fractures, 308
    functional decline, 308
    urinary incontinence, 308
  glycemic treatment, 308, 309
    end-organ complications, 308
    glycemic control targets, 309
      average glucose level, change in, 309*t*
      goals, 309
      hemoglobin A1c targets, guideline
        recommendations for, 309*t*
      hospitalized patients, 309
    hyperglycemia, 308
  insipidus, 263, 264, 267
  mellitus, 41, 61, 207, 305, 306, 308, 341
  nonpharmacologic treatments, 310
    diet, 310
      caloric restriction, 310
      dietary intervention, 310
      recommendations, 310
    exercise, 310
  pathogenesis, 305
  pharmacologic therapy, 310–313
    amylin mimetic, 313
      pramlintide, 313
    biguanides, 310
    α-glucosidase inhibitors, 311, 312
      acarbose (Precose), 311
      miglitol (Glyset), 311
    incretin modulators, 312
      dipeptidyl peptidase-4 (DPP-4)
        inhibitors, 312
      exenatide, 312
      glucagon-like peptide-1 (GLP-1)
        analog, 312
      linagliptin, 312
      liraglutide, 312

saxagliptin, 312
      sitagliptin, 312
    insulin, 312
      commonly uses, 312*t*
      disadvantages, 312
      long-acting, 312
      neutral protamine Hagedorn
        (NPH), 312
      shorter-acting, 312
    meglitinides, 312
      nateglinide, 312
      post-prandial hyperglycemia, 312
      repaglinide, 312
      short-acting insulin
        secretagogues, 312
    noninsulin therapies,
      hyperglycemia, 311*t*
    sulfonylureas, 311
      glipizide, 311
      glyburide, 311
    thiazolidinediones, 312
      insulin sensitizers, 312
      pioglitazone (Actos), 312
      rosiglitazone (Avandia), 312
  prevention, 306
    diabetes prevention program
      (DPP), 306
    metformin, 306
Diabetes insipidus (DI), 263, 264, 267
Diabetes mellitus (DM), 41, 61, 207, 305,
    306, 308, 341
Diabetes neuropathy, 307
Diabetic ketoacidosis (DKA), 306
Diabetic retinopathy, 307, 454, 455
  clincial findings, 455
    asymptomatic, early stages, 455
    blurred vision, 455
    macular edema, subtle signs, 455
    proliferative retinopathy, 455
      visual field scotomas, 455
    signs, 455
      evaluation, 455
  complications, 455
    vision loss caused by, 455
      macular capillary
        nonperfusion, 455
      macular edema, 455
      proliferative retinopathy, 455
  differential diagnosis, 455
  prevention, 455
    annual dilated, funduscopic
      examination, 455
  prognosis, 455
  treatment, 455
    anti-VEGF agents, 455
      intravitreal injections, 455
    clinically significant macular edema
      (CSME), 455
    nonproliferative diabetic
      retinopathy, 455
Diagnostic and statistical manual of
    mental disorders, guidelines,
    119, 120, 328
Dialysis, 273

Diaphoresis, 181
Diarrhea, 249
  clinical findings, 250
  treatment, 250
Diastolic blood pressure (DBP), 202
Diastolic heart failure, 179*t*. *See also* Heart
    failure (HF)
Diastolic hypertension, 202
Diastolic–systolic hypertension, 202.
    See also Hypertension
Diet. *See* Nutrition
Diffuse idiopathic skeletal hyperostosis
    (DISH), 485
  spinal ligaments, ossification, 485
Digital rectal examination (DRE), 284
Digital subtraction angiography
    (DSA), 224
Digoxin, 192, 193
  toxicity, 192
Dihydropyridines, for hypertension, 206*t*
Diltiazem, 184, 210
Diphenhydramine, 387, 388
Disability, 87
Discharge summaries, for older
    adults, 77*t*
Diuretics, 192
  loop, 49, 52
Divalproex sodium, 133*t*
Diverticular disease, 251
  clinical findings, 251
  diverticular bleeding, 251
DM. *See* Diabetes mellitus (DM)
DMARDs. *See* Disease-modifying
    antirheumatic drugs
Docusate, 145
Domiciliary care (assisted-living
    facilities), 108
Do-not-resuscitate (DNR) order, 89
Dorsalis pedis (DP), 224
Dowager's hump, 173
Doxazosin, 210, 286
Doxepin
  anticholinergic properties
    medications, 53*t*
  antidepressants, 330
  sleeping medications, for older
    patients, 387*t*
Doxycycline, 368
  community-acquired pneumonia,
    medication for, 353
  epidermal inclusion cyst, 368
  rosacea, 375
Dressings, 3
  pressure ulcers, 364, 365
Driving
  aging eye, changes in, 451
  cognitive impairment, 124, 133
  conductive hearing loss, 465
  psychoactive medications, 437
  vision impairment, 26
Dronabinol, 499
Dronedarone, 192
Drug–disease interactions, 46, 48,
    404–406, 405*t*